# Clinical Autonomic and Mitochondrial Disorders

Nicholas L. DePace • Joseph Colombo

# Clinical Autonomic and Mitochondrial Disorders

## Diagnosis, Prevention, and Treatment for Mind-Body Wellness

Springer

Nicholas L. DePace, MD, FACC
Franklin Cardiovascular Associates
PA and Autonomic Dysfunction and
POTS Center
Sewell, NJ
USA

Joseph Colombo
TMCAMS, Inc.
Franklin Cardiovascular Associates
PA and Autonomic Dysfunction and
POTS Center
Richboro, PA
USA

ISBN 978-3-030-17015-8 ISBN 978-3-030-17016-5 (eBook)
https://doi.org/10.1007/978-3-030-17016-5



This Springer imprint is published by the registered company Springer Nature Switzerland AG
The registered company address is: Gewerbestrasse 11, 6330 Cham, Switzerland

*To our wives and families, our motivation in all things.*
*Thank you!*

# Foreword

The nervous system comprises the central nervous system (CNS) and the peripheral nervous system (PNS). The peripheral nervous system (PNS) is composed of three parts: the somatic, autonomic, and enteric. The somatic portion functions to control voluntary movement, while the autonomic and enteric function involuntarily to control various bodily functions. The autonomic nervous system (ANS) includes the parasympathetic and sympathetic (P&S) nervous systems. The sympathetics are the "fight or flight system" or the "accelerator of the body," while the parasympathetics act as the "brakes of the body" or the "rest and digest system." Some have coined it the "feed and breed" system. Together, the P&S nervous systems control or coordinate every cell in the body and, thereby, control homeostasis of the entire body, including cardiovascular and respiratory activity, digestion, urination and bowel function, sexual function, sweating, sleep, and ability to maintain upright position. Many physicians, including ourselves, consider the enteric nervous system (ENS) as actually a part of the ANS, specifically the parasympathetic nervous system. It is the most independent functioning component of the ANS and controls gastrointestinal function (secretion and peristalsis).

Anatomically, the ANS is located in both the central and peripheral parts of the nervous system, even though it is considered part of the PNS. Collectively, the P&S are regulated by, and in turn regulate (through feedback), the hypothalamus and the central autonomic network. In the CNS, the P&S are located predominately in the forebrain and brain stem. Therefore, the "mind-to-body" connection by the P&S operates from central (the brain) to peripheral (the body) and back again. The hypothalamus is the highest level of P&S integration under the control of the limbic (emotional influence) and cortical (voluntary influences) structures. By integrating the brain and the body, the P&S controls heart rate regulation, blood pressure regulation (vasomotor), and reflexes such as swallowing, sneezing, vomiting, and coughing.

It is simplistic to state that the sympathetics excite and the parasympathetics inhibit bodily functions since there are exceptions. The "brakes" and "accelerator" concept of the P&S helps the patient better understand the symptoms they are experiencing when a P&S imbalance or dysfunction occurs. P&S imbalances or dysfunctions are known as dysautonomias. They are conditions in which the P&S systems are not functioning properly and are not in balance or not coordinating properly. The P&S can be equated to being a "seesaw" where both ends of the "seesaw" should be level (in balance) or opposing each other when active (one end being high and the other low). There are various abnormalities in which one end of the "see-saw" is too much higher than the other or, at times, the "see-saw" is broken where both ends are up at the same time or are too low at the same time.

Dysautonomia affects the function of the heart, intestine, bladder, pupils, sweat glands, blood vessels, and virtually all organs of the body as the P&S supplies innervation of the smooth muscles and glands throughout the body. Again, the P&S are the regulator of cardiovascular function, arterial baroreceptor reflex, standing response, sweating, gastrointestinal tract motility, and sleep cycle. Imbalance, or malfunction, of the P&S may cause hyperhidrosis and anhydrosis, lightheadedness or dizziness and orthostatic intolerance, and even syncope, high or low heart rates, blood pressure fluctuations, urinary incontinence and retention, insomnia, and swallowing difficulties. Common symptoms of dysautonomia cause exercise intolerance, chronic fatigue, muscle aches and pains, headache or migraine, diffuse sleep, tunnel vision, weakness, blurred vision, constipation, diarrhea, cognitive difficulties, and brain fog. Word-finding difficulties and short-term memory lapses can occur. Gastroparesis is also a common and disabling problem.

Most common symptoms are due to orthostatic intolerance. Standing is a major challenge for a healthy P&S. Gravity causes venous pooling in the lower extremities and lowers central pressures and venous return to the heart. The normal functioning ANS first withdraws the parasympathetics to potentiate and facilitate the sympathetics and then activates the sympathetics. Parasympathetic withdrawal immediately upon standing increases venous return to the heart and also increases heart rate on the initial stand response and avoids venous pooling. In orthostatic-intolerant (OI) individuals, due to dysautonomia, this mechanism is defective. The sympathetics constrict the lower extremity vessels and promote blood flow centrally to the heart. Sympathetic withdrawal inappropriately occurs, blood pools in the legs, and cardiac output and venous return are impaired. The patient may have a drop in blood pressure and orthostatic hypotension or an inappropriate increase in heart rate, overcompensating as in postural orthostatic tachycardia syndrome (POTS), or simply brain fog, fatigue, and exercise intolerance without significant changes in blood pressure or heart rate. The latter is more commonly seen in patients, especially younger patients at presentation. It is estimated that 4 million people in the United States have OI, and this is a major cause of disability and may be responsible for many of the symptoms that we classify as fibromyalgia-type or chronic fatigue. OI and chronic fatigue occur simultaneously.

To treat various forms of dysautonomia, including OI, pharmacology along with lifestyle changes, diet and salt intake, physical maneuvers and compression garments, fluids, stress reduction techniques, and neural feedback may be indicated depending on the patient's symptoms, history, and type of dysautonomia. Experimental pacing and stimulating devices have often been used in various circumstances. Surgical procedures occasionally are indicated, for example, bilateral sympathectomies, for various hyperhidrosis states. Patients with hypermobility syndromes, such as Ehlers-Danlos syndrome (EDS) and other related disorders, are often a significant challenge and occasionally are referred for orthopedic or neurosurgical interventions. Gastroparesis is particularly troublesome, as there may be mixed components of imbalance in the autonomic nervous system affecting the GI tract as compared to other organs, and one pharmacological agent instituted to treat one organ disorder may adversely affect the other. Therefore, pharmacologic treatment of dysautonomia is very complex, and not always successful.

However, one must get at the "root of the problem." Increased oxidative stress is often the real trigger event for causes of mechanism at the cellular level. Deficiency of ATP production and mitochondrial dysfunction leads to significant impairment of neuron function and abnormalities of myelin sheath (neurons are very rich in mitochondrial density). Also, small fibers (the type C fibers, which are sensory and P&S fibers) are susceptible to oxidative stress. Nitric oxide deficiency also contributes to many of the neurological and vascular features of autonomic function and dysfunction. A "cocktail" of antioxidants, anti-inflammatories, and nitric oxide-enhancing agents have been advocated and may be useful empirically, especially at appropriately titrated doses.

When a patient presents to our autonomic center with symptoms consistent with dysautonomia, they have usually seen a minimum of 14 physicians, and a diagnosis has not been made. In fact, most patients arrive at the diagnosis by doing their own independent research on the Internet. Many patients are referred to us via Internet research and not by direct physician referral. One patient, an Indian/Asian young male, stated that he had seen 99 physicians prior to seeing us. These patients with dysautonomia have various presentations. They have oftentimes been labeled with the diagnosis of anxiety and have not had any types of autonomic assessment tests performed, such as sweat testing (sudomotor) or combined heart rate and respiratory variability testing, which are easy noninvasive tests to do in the outpatient center. Most have not had a tilt test performed. There is an obvious problem with identifying these patients due to physicians not being educated in this area sufficiently, both in medical school and within the medical literature. While autonomic dysfunction has in the past been the domain of the neurologist, the cardiologist is also beginning to learn more about it, as many of the diagnostic tests have a cardiac basis and many of the patients present to a cardiologist with shortness of breath, chest pain, and palpitations, which are manifestations of autonomic dysfunction and not intrinsic cardiac disease. In addition, endocrinologists and rheumatologists are beginning to have more awareness of autonomic dysfunction, especially in the diabetic, pain, myalgia, and hypermobility populations.

In fact, the hypermobility populations, which include benign hypermobility and any one of the number of variants of Ehlers-Danlos syndrome, osteogenesis imperfecta, Stickler syndrome, pseudoxanthoma elasticum, and Marfan syndrome, may be the most recent to greatly benefit from the improved autonomic dysfunction/dysautonomia awareness. It has long been known that both Ehlers-Danlos syndrome and dysautonomia are associated with small fiber neuropathy. Recently, testing for both small fiber neuropathy and dysautonomia has become commercially available. It is often difficult to determine which hypermobility disorder the patient suffers from due to the heterogeneity and the expense of gene testing. The Ehlers-Danlos varieties typically have COL1A1 gene abnormalities, while Marfan's has abnormal fibrillin. We have not seen the patient with any of the above disorders that has not suffered from dysautonomia. Some of the more common features, which we recognize, include vascular pooling which mimics Raynaud syndrome, flushing, anxiety, hyperhidrosis, fatigue, and loss of consciousness or POTS.

In this text, we detail the symptoms and diagnoses of dysautonomia and the universal mechanism at the cellular level that causes or contributes to autonomic dysfunction. We propose a six-prong treatment approach that has been useful empirically in clinical practice. This involves not simply pharmacology and physical measures and maneuvers but also diet, an anti-inflammatory approach, an antioxidant approach, and a stress reduction approach. An integrative approach to the treatment of dysautonomia should be holistic. It is our goal to stimulate further research in this area and further education and recognition of this disease entity. Not just physicians and healthcare workers but also the public needs to be educated as to the existence and prevalence of dysautonomia and the related morbidity and mortality risks and the treatment entailed.

Sewell, NJ, USA — Nicholas L. DePace
Richboro, PA, USA — Joseph Colombo
Vineland, NJ, USA — Stephen Soloway

# About the Authors

**Nicholas L. DePace** is board certified in cardiology, echocardiography, internal medicine, lipidology, and nuclear cardiology, with nearly 40 years of clinical practice experience in cardiovascular medicine. He was trained at Mount Sinai Medical School in New York City, and Hahnemann Hospital in Philadelphia. He runs cardiovascular and autonomic practices in south Philadelphia and southern New Jersey. He is a Clinical Professor of medicine at Hahnemann Hospital, with cardiology affiliations and privileges at Jefferson Health Hospitals, NJ, and Pennsylvania Hospital/University Pennsylvania Health System, Philadelphia, PA. In addition to his many hours in clinic and rounding at the hospital, he teaches medical students, interns, and residents and continues to promote research in several fields associated with cardiovascular medicine and autonomic dysfunction. He has published over 100 medical journal articles, abstracts, book chapters, and books in cardiovascular diseases and neurocardiology. He previously served for 10 years on the editorial board of the American Journal of Cardiology. He has many achievements and has received many professional honors and awards throughout his career including being a Fellow of the American College of Cardiology and a Fellow of the American College of Chest Physicians. He has also received honors and awards for his acts of community service. He is a husband of over 35 years and a father of one with one grandchild.

**Joseph Colombo** is trained in neurology with a background in electrical and mechanical engineering. His doctorate from the University of Rochester, NY, is in neuroscience and biomedical engineering. Dr. Colombo currently serves as Chief Technology Officer and Senior Medical Director of TMCAMS, Inc.; and Parasympathetic and Sympathetic Nervous System Consultant, Franklin Cardiovascular Associates, PA. He has been an Adjunct Professor in medicine and lectures worldwide on clinical applications of, and disorders of, the parasympathetic and sympathetic (P&S) nervous systems. His career has included over 17 years developing aircraft crew systems and life support systems for NASA, Military, and FAA, and sensory neural prostheses, including: digital hearing aids, cochlear implants, cochlear nucleus implants, visual prostheses, and vestibular measures. He is a signal processing expert. He has also been involved in developing tele-healthcare and tele-medicine systems. For over 25 years, Dr. Colombo has developed P&S nervous system technologies and has researched and published clinical applications and outcome studies in uses of noninvasive P&S monitoring in critical care (trauma and sepsis), anesthesiology, cardiology, endocrinology, family medicine, internal medicine, pain management, neurology, psychiatry, pulmonology, sleep medicine, and more as positive, patient outcomes data are available. He has (co-)authored over 100 journal articles internationally, book chapters and medical text book on clinical applications of, and outcomes from, noninvasive P&S guided therapy. Dr. Colombo continues to participate in more than 50 clinical research projects worldwide and consults with physicians, clinically, on a global scale. He has a wife of 34 years and two married children, with over 30 years of mentoring hundreds of youths and students.

# Preface

In 1983, I (Dr. DePace) first met, Dr. Jerry Lemole, who was the premier cardiothoracic surgeon in the Philadelphia area at the time. He had previously worked at the Baylor University, Texas Heart Institute, on the team that did the first heart transplant in the United States, and subsequently served as chief of Cardiothoracic Surgery at Temple University Hospital in Philadelphia and Deborah Heart Center in New Jersey. He was renowned for his very quick cross-clamp time and excellent surgical technique.

I noticed that Dr. Lemole's patients had excellent results. Empirically, I compared his results with other cardiothoracic surgeons using stress radionuclide angiography, which we did in our office on our postoperative patients. I noted that his patients had much better left ventricular resting function and reserve compared to other surgeons. This is in an era when cardioplegia[1] was now being perfected and better cardioplegia techniques were making even mediocre surgeons have good results. Therefore, I attempted to understand how Dr. Lemole would get such good results on his patients. Perhaps, he was more fully revascularizing them, and his technique was still far superior to others, which was true at the time, in my opinion. However, I noticed that he put most of his postoperative patients on a coenzyme Q preparation.

I was not familiar with coenzyme Q10 (CoQ10), nor did I know or have any idea about its biological feasibility. There was not really much evidence-based medicine behind its use then. CoQ10 is an essential lipid-soluble antioxidant, which protects cellular membranes and also circulates lipoproteins against free radical-induced oxidative stress, and has significant oxidative stress-reducing properties.

CoQ10 is an essential component of the electron transport chain and is an electron carrier as well as an antioxidant. It made sense that it would be useful in situations where there were deficiencies of mitochondrial energy generation as well as situations in which low cellular antioxidant capacity could be prevalent, such as in the postoperative period.

Significant research has been done since Dr. Lemole first started using CoQ10 (see "coenzyme Q10" section and any of the many references). Of course, Dr. Lemole was not aware of this information or data published as he was using CoQ10 10–20 years before the publication of these data. He was clearly ahead of his time. However, he understood the biological feasibility and advantages of using an antioxidant such as CoQ10 to protect against

[1] Intentional and temporary cessation of cardiac activity, primarily for cardiac surgery.

cardioplegia and postoperative oxidative stress, for these could impair left ventricular function. It is my belief that this is why his patients' postoperative stress radionuclide angiogram studies showed much higher ejection fractions than many of his colleagues' patients at that time.

Heart failure is also due to loss of contractility of the myocardium and is a consequence of a lack of energy in the myocardium. Chronic heart failure patients do show decreased CoQ10 levels on serum studies and endomyocardial biopsies (see "Oxidative Stress in Cardiovascular Diseases"). This research came from Dr. Cooley's lab at Baylor; therefore, Dr. Lemole was probably privy to this research, as he himself had trained at the Texas Heart Institute where Dr. Cooley was operating prior to 1983. Dr. Cooley's data supports that CoQ10 improves the efficiency of energy production, and quantity of energy produced, in human hearts when used as an adjunct to standard medical therapy and heart failure. CoQ10 decreases substances measured that indicate oxidative stress. In heart failure, CoQ10, a neuroprotective against lesions and a significant important antioxidant in both mitochondria and lipid membranes, scavenges free radicals and improves ATP regeneration in cardiac muscles and skeletal muscles in Friedreich's ataxia, another neurodegenerative disease. Data in toto reflects that antioxidant protection with agents, such as CoQ10, is protective in cardiac and neurodegenerative diseases.

In the early 1980s, Dr. Lemole provided me my first introduction to the possibility of using antioxidant therapy in a cardiac setting such as postoperative surgery. I was empirically impressed with the results I saw with my patients postoperatively. Recently, literature has shown that there is increasing interest in introducing CoQ10 for treatment of mitochondrial disorders. Since then, we have had great success in establishing and maintaining wellness in our patients and traditionally carrying lower hospitalizations and pharmaceuticals (and thereby healthcare cost) than most of our colleagues. We believe that this success has everything to do with our cooperative patients, largely adopting and remaining with the Mind-Body Wellness Program described in this book.

Sewell, NJ, USA Nicholas L. DePace

# Contents

# Summary

This book details the science behind the Mind-Body Wellness Program and highlights our clinical successes with the program over the past one and a half decades. This is truly a supplemental approach to standard pharmaceutical, noninvasive, and invasive therapies. An example of its application as a supplemental program is provided in the next paragraph. The program should never be taken as a replacement for standard therapy and may not be for everyone. This program or any portions of this program should be started under close physician supervision.

Someone in the United States dies of a heart disease every 90 seconds. Despite taking statins and lowering cholesterol by 33%, two-thirds (67%) of at-risk patients still have major adverse cardiac events (MACE, e.g., heart attack, sudden death) or stroke, including repeat events. Patients, for example, are not protected from MACE or stroke just because they are on a statin. These patients' disease includes autonomic and mitochondrial dysfunction. A six-pronged approach is used to treat and prevent autonomic and mitochondrial dysfunction and includes the amino acids L-arginine and L-citrulline, as well as inorganic nitrates from beet root and spinach. These amino acids and nitrates may help to protect the two-thirds of the subpopulation, thereby closing that gap. Unfortunately, this will never be heard from the pharmaceutical industry. However, there are peer-reviewed articles in prestigious medical journals that support a lifestyle and supplement (non-pharmaceutical) approach. The pharmaceutical industry will not promote a lifestyle and supplement program because it will detract from their economic profits and require less of their product.

This is just one example of such gaps. Stress, including psychosocial stress, and stress due to anxiety, depression, diabetes, being overweight, excessive consumption of processed and fast foods, sedentary lifestyles, pain, etc., may all lead to chronic diseases, including heart and vascular diseases. While there are pharmaceuticals designed to treat all of these conditions, typically, that is all they do. They only treat these conditions. They do not cure them. In another example, there is a television commercial that says to take another antidepressant if the one prescribed is not (fully) effective. This is another gap, and in this case, the additional antidepressant may only serve to make a bad situation worse. The fish oils, antioxidants (e.g., alpha-lipoic acid), olive oil, and exercise may do more than any (or both) antidepressants, without the myriad of side effects, including suicide risk.

Our point is that despite pharmaceuticals, our patients are still suffering. They suffer from poor quality of life (QoL) due to increased morbidity risk and from reduced longevity due to increased mortality risk. It may be argued that a younger adults' basic definition of QoL is upper GI health, restful sleep, lower GI and bladder health, proper erectile function and vaginal lubrication, and no lightheadedness upon standing. Nowadays, normal blood pressure, cognitive function (including no "brain fog"), and proper energy levels should probably be added. Even when these functions are diminished with time, older adults' QoL would include having the energy and cognitive faculties to spend time with grandchildren, even if the rest of their QoL functions are suffering. By normalizing autonomic and mitochondrial dysfunction, morbidity and mortality risk is minimized, thereby optimizing QoL and possibly longevity. It may also reduce the prescription medication load required to maintain health and establish wellness.

As another example, the vast majority of patients with anxiety, diabetes, heart and kidney diseases, and more have high blood pressure (BP). High BP is arguably the most common condition measured and is not a diagnosis. Consider it more of a warning. High BP is not a problem to be diagnosed until it becomes chronic. Chronic high BP is known as the "silent killer" and is diagnosed as hypertension. High BP must be demonstrated in two or more consecutive doctor visits before a diagnosis of hypertension. Chronic high BP (hypertension) will:

- Damage the organs of the body, like the kidneys (increased morbidity risk), leading to renal failure (increased mortality risk)
- Damage the blood vessels (increased morbidity risk) leading to atherosclerosis, aneurysms, and stroke (increased mortality risk)
- Overwork the heart (increased morbidity risk), leading to heart failure or heart attack (increased mortality risk)
- Damage the nerves and nervous tissue, including the brain (increased morbidity risk) leading to dementia (e.g., Alzheimer's or Parkinson's disease) and autonomic neuropathy (increased mortality risk)

Chronic high BP accelerates the aging process, making one look and feel older before their time.

Over 50% of patients with hypertension are not adequately controlled. They suffer from autonomic and mitochondrial dysfunction causing one or more of headaches or migraines; cognitive difficulties, including "brain fog"; fatigue; lightheadedness or dizziness; anxiety or panic attacks; sleep disorders; and more. A piece of the puzzle is missing. The six prongs of the Mind-Body Wellness Program (Fig. 1) address the autonomic and mitochondrial dysfunction and, thereby, the chasm between well-controlled and current state of most patients. These are (1) a Mediterranean diet, (2) exercise, (3) reduced psychosocial stress, (4) increased nitric oxide to provide better circulation to all cells, (5) decreased oxidative stress to increase energy production and prevent chronic disease or slow its progression, and (6) increased "good" fats to get the energy to all parts of the body.

The six-pronged approach includes three nutraceutical compounds, which are required together for optimal health because all three help support nervous and cardiovascular system health through different mechanisms. One com-

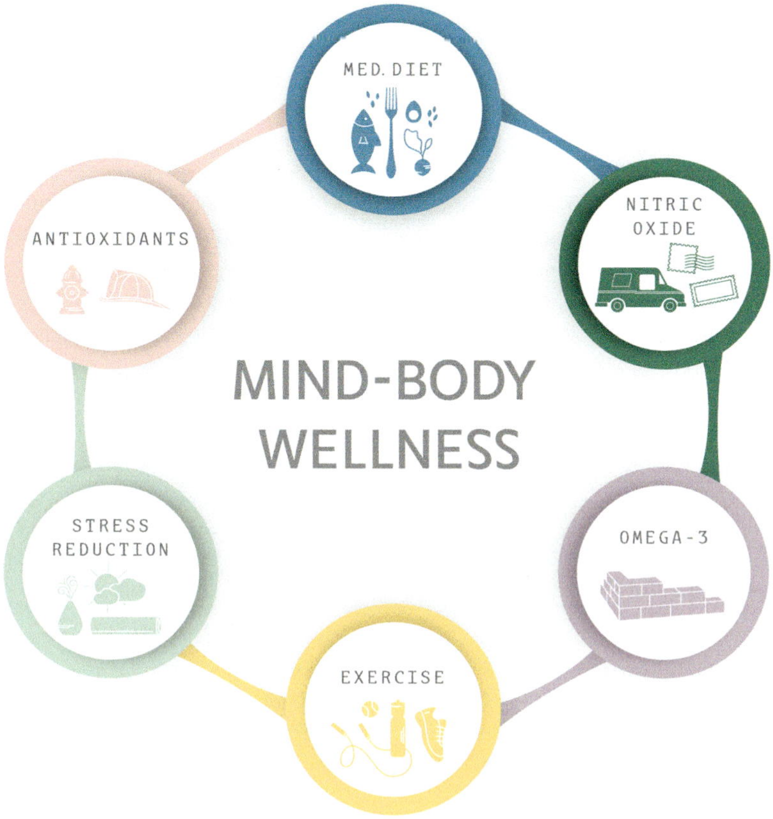


**Fig. 1** The lifestyle and supplement prongs that together comprise a Mind Body-Wellness Program. (Illustrations by Elysian Creative Studio, www.elysiancreativestudio.com, Lizzy Colombo)

pound includes omega-3 fatty acids as obtained from fish oils, for example. These are membrane stabilizers, as well as an anti-inflammatories and antioxidants. Omega-3 or fish oils are provided separately to establish and maintain healthy cell membranes and endothelial function. A nitric oxide compound is included. Nitric oxide, indirectly, supports the heart and vasculature. Both need to be supported at the same time. By providing a nitric oxide compound, nitric oxide production is supported, which promotes endothelial health. The endothelium is the sheet of cells that line all of the blood vessels of the body. Endothelial health promotes proper (smooth) blood flow and flexible and more relaxed blood vessels, both of which may lower blood pressure. Smooth blood flow and lower blood pressure help to protect the heart. Nitric oxide, acting as an antioxidant, together with fish oil, will establish and maintain a healthy lipid balance as supported and perpetuated by the combination of the Mediterranean diet providing more omega-3 fatty acids and exercise inducing additional antioxidant activity. The third compound is an antioxidant compound which supports the brain and the nervous system, especially the autonomic nervous system (ANS), including the parasympathetic and sympathetic (P&S) nervous systems, which are the two components of the ANS. The antioxidant compound includes alpha-lipoic acid (ALA) and coenzyme Q10 (CoQ10), two of the most powerful antioxidants produced in the body. Unfortunately, due to stress, chronic disease, and aging, the body produces less and less of these antioxidants. Fewer antioxidants accelerate the aging process. A high stress lifestyle may reduce the levels of these powerful antioxidants. Levels have been documented as having been reduced to that of a normal 80-year-old individual by the time one is 40 years old. This then reduces QoL and longevity. Diabetes, for example, does the same. It causes a 60-year-old individual with diabetes to have 80-year-old blood vessels. The antioxidant compound, with fish oils and nitric oxide production, provides nutrients and antioxidants to establish and maintain brain and nerve health, thereby reducing psychosocial stress (including anxiety and depression), cognitive difficulties, decreasing oxidative stress, and increasing energy production. It also delays the onset of and reduces the severity of dementia.

> The person who takes medicine must recover twice, once from the disease and once from the medicine. (Sir William Osler, Bt)

The Mind-Body Wellness Program, in part, focuses on the P&S (autonomic) nervous systems. This is the portion of the nervous system that forms the brain-heart (Fig. 2 [1]) and mind-body connection. The P&S nervous sys-

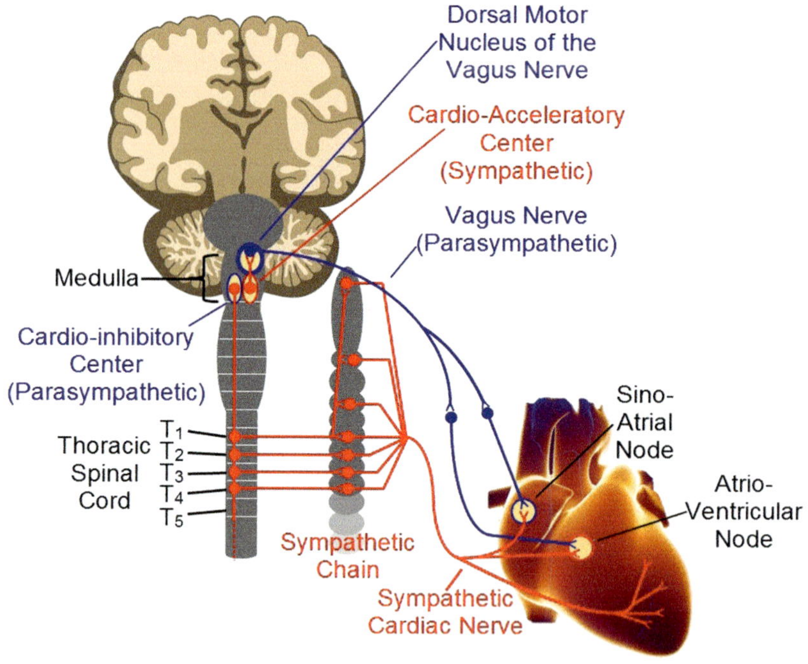


**Fig. 2** Parasympathetic and Sympathetic innervation of the heart: anatomy. Efferent fiber (Vagus) comprises A-beta, A-delta, and unmyelinated C fibers. Coronal Cut illustration modified from Royalty-free stock vector images ID: 1203177505. Coronal and sagittal cut of the human brain. Diagram. Vector illustration, by Olga Bolbot. Heart illustration adapted from Shutterstock Royalty-free stock illustration ID: 82159072 by CLIPAREA l Custom media. (Source: [1]. Reproduced from Martini FH. Fundamentals of Anatomy and Physiology. 8th ed. 2006. Chapter 20, by permission of Pearson Education, Inc Prentice Hall, copyright © 2006. Alternate Source: Agarwal SK, Norby FL, Whitsel EA, Soliman EZ, Chen LY, Loehr LR, Fuster V, Heiss G, Coresh J, Alonso A. Cardiac Autonomic Dysfunction and Incidence of Atrial Fibrillation: Results from 20 years follow-up. JACC. 2017; 69(3): 291–9)

tems regulate blood pressure, heart rate, airway size, airflow to lungs, digestion, bladder and sexual function, depression, anxiety, gland and hormone function, and all of the rest of the body functions. In fact, the P&S nervous systems control or coordinate virtually all cells of the body and all organ and organ systems of the body. The sympathetic nervous system is the reactionary nervous system (known as the "fight or flight" nervous system), responding to stresses and generally expending energy. The parasympathetic nervous system is the protective nervous system (known as the "rest and digest" nervous system) and generally conserves energy. The health of, and balance between, the P&S nervous systems defines QoL, including morbidity and mortality risks.

For example, if the sympathetic nervous system becomes over-reactive, it may damage the parasympathetic nervous system. This may amplify pain reactions and reaction to simple stimuli, causing, in the extreme, anxiety-like, fibromyalgia, or post-traumatic stress disorder symptoms. Prolonged, excess sympathetic activation also leads to chronic inflammation. The P&S systems work together. Excess activity in one branch wears on the other. Most commonly, the overactivation of sympathetic activity, due to the typical stresses of everyday American lifestyles, accelerates the onset of parasympathetic neuropathy leading to early, and persistent, morbidity and mortality risk. The converse has also been noted. Patients that exercise their parasympathetic nervous system too much, through meditation, yoga, and the like, or sympathectomies, have had sympathetic imbalances that also effect morbidity and mortality risk [1]. The main problem is that P&S imbalance increases MACE risk (including stroke). Specifically, low parasympathetic activity levels, especially when compounded by (relatively) high sympathetic activity levels, increase the 5-year mortality rate to over 50% [2]. Clinically speaking, the parasympathetics are not strong enough to prevent a sympathetically mediated ventricular tachy-rhythm from becoming fibrillation or death.

Proper mitochondrial function, including proper amounts of adenosine triphosphate (ATP) produced from the mitochondria, is fundamental to health and wellness. Nerves, including the brain, require lots of energy. Just sitting there, the brain consumes about 70% of the energy produced in the body to control all of the functions of the body. During periods of high activity (whether running or swimming, having an emotional experience like love or rage, or taking a final exam), the brain consumes up to 85% of the energy produced in the body to also control the additional activities. Many cognitive disorders may involve both autonomic and mitochondrial dysfunctions. ATP is needed for all nerve functions and muscle contractions, including cardiovascular muscle contractions.

A lack of ATP causes many mitochondrial and autonomic disorders. Mitochondria produce a significant amount of reactive oxygen species (ROS, a type of free radical). One to three percent (1–3%) of all ROS leak out of the electron transport chain within the mitochondria. ROS damage tissue, including the mitochondria themselves. ROS must be reduced by antioxidants, or they cause damage to proteins, lipids, and cell membranes. In this way, ROS may create atherosclerosis, as well as other damages. Atherosclerosis often blocks blood flow, leading to MACE or stroke. ROS is also associated with various forms of cancer, dementia, and many other diseases and disorders.

ALA and CoQ10 reduce oxidative stress by collecting and neutralizing free radicals, including ROS, that literally burn cell membranes and other structures, including mitochondria. Normally, within the mitochondrial electron transport chains, up to 3% of the time oxygen is incompletely reduced and ROS are produced. Normally, the body's naturally occurring ALA and CoQ10 neutralize these ROS. While there are other antioxidants in the body (i.e., vitamins A, C, and E), these are the most powerful and versatile. They are designed to support P&S and mitochondrial health; they already exist within the nerves and mitochondria, and they recycle vitamins A, C, and E. However, as people age (normally or due to stress, disease, or injury), there are fewer endogenous antioxidants available, and more free radicals leak out of the mitochondria and into the cells, damaging both.

Oxidative stress often causes mitochondrial dysfunction. Mitochondrial dysfunction includes a loss of efficiency, including fewer ATP produced in the electron transport chain and fewer mitochondria to produce ATP. Less ATP means less energy. This is at the core of how chronic stress leads to fatigue and depression. Another result is an increase in free radical production, thereby damaging cells throughout the body. This is a characteristic of aging and is a result of all chronic diseases. Mitochondrial dysfunction can affect all body parts and organs. Oxidative stress can accelerate aging and promote tumor genesis, as well as most chronic diseases, including diabetes, Parkinson's and other neurological diseases, certain types of dementia, and kidney and cardiovascular diseases. Antioxidants react with ROS to prevent or repair damage to tissues.

Because mitochondrial dysfunction relates directly to the aging process, it has been suggested as playing a role in atherosclerotic cardiovascular disease. Mitochondrial DNA copy numbers (mtDNA-CN) are statistics derived from the number of mitochondria per cell and the number of mitochondrial genomes per mitochondria. Analyzing mtDNA-CN in patients at risk for cardiovascular disease could help clinicians predict sudden cardiac death and heart failure in patients up to a decade before anything happens, including symptoms [3, 4]. These findings pave the way for improved outcomes in cardiac patients. The study stated that blood testing for mitochondrial DNA measurements could lead to early detection of cardiovascular disease (CVD) and, therefore, allow at-risk patients to take preventative measures against developing heart problems in the future.

Approximately two out of every three people who experience sudden cardiac death show no symptoms that could have warned their physician of their risk [5]. P&S monitoring already provides a risk indicator for sudden cardiac death, stroke, or other MACE. The P&S indicator is Cardiovascular Autonomic Neuropathy (CAN), which predicts the 5-year risk for MACE [6]. As a risk measure, CAN is more specific when the risk is stratified by Sympathovagal Balance ($SB^2$); predicting the 2-year mortality risk [1]. The

[2] SB is the ratio of resting sympathetic activity (S) to resting parasympathetic activity (P); {SB = S/P: normal adult range: $0.4 < SB < 3.0$}. It is a ratio of averages, rather than an average of ratios. It is a more specific measure of the relative P&S levels as compared to the traditional heart rate variability (HRV) low- to high-frequency ratio (L/H). In P&S

P&S nervous systems rely heavily on mitochondrial function. The lower mitochondrial DNA-CN numbers were, the more at risk a patient was for suffering an adverse CVD event. MTDNA-CN could more accurately predict a 10-year risk for heart failure and augments the P&S findings of CAN with abnormal SB, helping to improve specificity of those who would require early intervention to minimize morbidity and mortality risk, maintain quality of life, reduce hospitalizations and rehospitalizations, reduce healthcare costs, and improve patient outcomes.

The study drew 21,870 participants from the databases of the Cardiovascular Health Study, the Atherosclerosis Risk in Communities Study, and the Multiethnic Study of Atherosclerosis; 92% were CVD-free at baseline. Mitochondrial DNA levels were measured against nuclear DNA levels in these patients, and that number was input into the American College of Cardiology/American Heart Association's Heart Risk Calculator. The calculator includes a patient's cholesterol levels, blood pressure, smoking history, family medical history, weight, and more to predict a 10-year risk for heart attacks and other adverse cardiac events. The study correctly predicted that 6 patients who otherwise wouldn't have been recommended for heart treatment went on to have a life-threatening heart event and 139 patients who would have been recommended for statin treatment under current guidelines actually didn't suffer from CVD.

> One of the first duties of the physician is to educate the masses not to take medicine.
> (Sir William Osler, Bt)

Nutrients included in the Mind-Body Wellness Program are listed below, in no particular order, with a brief description of their function or benefit:

- *Alpha Lipoic Acid (ALA)* – an anti-inflammatory and an antioxidant. At the cellular level, ALA (1) reduces oxidative stress; (2) scavenges (through chelation) and sequesters free radicals, including ROS; (3) brings products to mitochondria; (4) regenerates other antioxidants, including vitamins C and E; (5) increases nitric oxide production; and (6) boosts energy (ATP) production. At the system level, ALA (1) aids in P&S and sensory nervous system function; (2) lowers blood pressure (BP); and (3) slows or relieves the progression of autonomic neuropathy in diabetes and possibly in other chronic diseases [7]. Natural ALA levels in the body decline with age and duration of chronic disease.
- *Coenzyme Q10 (CoQ10)* – an antioxidant. At the cellular level, CoQ10 (1) sequesters active ROS, (2) increases energy (ATP) production, (3) limits electron leak in the electron transport chain (also increasing (ATP) energy production), and (4) reduces mitochondrial dysfunction. At the system level, CoQ10 (1) decreases cholesterol, (2) increases immune function, (3)

terms, "L" is a measure of both P&S activities, but not necessarily all of the P-activity, only that which happens to be in the low-frequency region at the time. "H" is a measure of the rest of the P-activity not in the low-frequency region, plus noise, due to the fact that the high-frequency region is a broad-band, fix measure that may not capture any P-activity. In summary, L/H is approximately (S + P)/(P + noise) and requires assumption and approximation to hypothesize S/P = SB [1].

increases cardiac function by supporting cardiac muscle health, (4) supports skeletal muscle health, (5) reduces inflammation (including reducing inflammatory markers), and (6) lowers BP. A very important note: natural CoQ10 levels in the body decline with age [8].

- *Vitamin B*, vitamins $B_6$ and $B_{12}$, with *magnesium (Mg)* are the potent supporters of parasympathetic nervous system health and thereby help to elevate mood, and protect the heart, among other benefits, such as helping to improve mental health [9].
  - *$B_6$ (Pyridoxine)* – supports nervous system function and boosts energy (ATP) production.
  - *$B_{12}$ (Cobalamin)* – supports nervous system function and boosts energy (ATP) production.
  - *Folic acid ($B_9$)* – cofactor in producing nitric oxide, cofactor in citric acid cycle to trap electrons, and cofactor in reducing the toxin homocysteine. High dose Folic Acids helps to slow or reverse the progression of small fiber disease.
  - *$B_1$ (Thiamine), $B_2$ (Riboflavin), $B_3$ (Niacin), $B_5$ (Pantothenic Acid), and $B_9$ (Folic Acid)* – boosts energy (ATP) production, is a cofactor in citric acid cycle to trap electrons, and attenuates the abnormal effects of asymmetric dimethylarginine (ADMA) by competing with *L-arginine* for nitric oxide synthase (NOS). The arginine part of ADMA, by replacing L-arginine in reactions with NOS, enables ADMA to impair NOS and the synthesis of nitric oxide.
- *Vitamin $D_3$* – helps to strengthen the bones and teeth and helps to decrease diabetes [9].
- *Vitamin E* – a fat-soluble antioxidant that protects cell membranes from ROS, thereby slows the aging process [9].
- *Vitamin K* – supports vascular health, reducing arterial calcification (specifically Vitamin K2), supports healthy blood clotting, and can slow cancer growth [9].
- *Minerals:*
  - *Magnesium (Mg)* – supports parasympathetic nervous system function, boosts energy (ATP) production and reduces anxiety
  - *Zinc (Zn)* – supports immune function and memory, decreases severity of chronic diseases that are age-related, and supports wound healing by contributing to collagen synthesis and epithelialization
  - *Copper (Cu)* – involved in collagen synthesis, supports energy (ATP) production, and increases absorption of iron
  - *Manganese (Mn)* – supports nerve function, involved in fat and carbohydrate metabolism, helps to form connective tissue in bones, and supports blood clotting factors
  - *Selenium (Se)* – an antioxidant that boosts energy (ATP) production
  - *Iron (Fe)* – key to red blood cell function, supports the immune system and involved in energy (ATP) production
- *Amino Acids:*
  - *Glutathione* – an antioxidant that scavenges free radicals and heavy metals and boosts energy (ATP) production.
  - *N-Acetyl Cysteine* – boosts *glutathione* levels.
  - *L-Arginine* – produces nitric oxide naturally through the endogenous nitric oxide synthase (NOS) system. By giving L-arginine exogenously

as well, the L-arginine to ADMA ratio may be increased and tissue damage decreased.
  - *L-Citrulline* – easily absorbed in the liver. L-citrulline is converted to L-arginine and nitric oxide, thereby helping to maintain nitric oxide levels.
  - *L-Carnitine Tartrate* – (1) increases nitric oxide signaling, (2) improves endothelial function, (3) reduces oxidative stress, (4) is important as rate-limiting step in fatty acid oxidation that produces ATP, and (5) supports the metabolism of fat.
  - *L-Lysine* – precursor[3] to *L-carnitine*, boosting *L-carnitine* levels.
- *Beet Root* – a potent, alternate, exogenous source of nitric oxide promoting compounds that does not use the traditional nitric oxide synthesis pathways that involve amino acids.
  - In the body, nitric oxide is generated quickly and dissipates quickly under normal situations. Systemically, it increases endothelial function, thereby enhancing exercise tolerance and lowering blood pressure. It is a natural vasodilator and increases blood flow and circulation. It also inhibits the oxidation of ("bad") LDL cholesterol into "foam cells" that are the precursors to atherosclerosis; as a result, it helps to reduce or lower atherosclerosis. In addition, nitric oxide also (1) kills bacteria, (2) enhances immune function, (3) aids neurotransmission, (4) decreases inflammation, (5) may dilate bronchioles, (6) is an anti-thrombotic, (7) may promote better cerebral circulation, (8) increases Vagal (parasympathetic) tone, (9) slows heart rate, and (10) lowers blood pressure. By increasing parasympathetic tone, including slowing heart rate and lowering blood pressure, nitric oxide is therefore cardio-protective. However, it diminishes with age. By 60 years of age, people have lost, on average, 85% of their nitric oxide production abilities.

## References

1. Colombo J, Arora RR, DePace NL, Vinik AI. Clinical autonomic dysfunction: measurement, indications, therapies, and outcomes. New York: Springer Science + Business Media; 2014.
2. Maser R, Mitchell B, Vinik AI, Freeman R. The association between cardiovascular autonomic neuropathy and mortality in individuals with diabetes, a meta-analysis. Diabetes Care. 2003;26(6):1895–901.
3. Ashar FN, Zhang Y, Longchamps RJ, Lane J, Moes A, Grove ML, Mychaleckyj JC, Taylor KD, Coresh J, Rotter JI, Boerwinkle E, Pankratz N, Guallar E, Arking DE. Association of mitochondrial DNA copy number with cardiovascular disease. JAMA Cardiol. 2017. https://doi.org/10.1001/jamacardio.2017.3683. [Epub ahead of print].
4. Zhang Y, Guallar E, Ashar FN, Longchamps RJ, Castellani CA, Lane J, Grove ML, Coresh J, Sotoodehnia N, Ilkhanoff L, Boerwinkle E, Pankratz N, Arking DE. Association between mitochondrial DNA copy number and sudden cardiac death: findings from the Atherosclerosis Risk in Communities study (ARIC). Eur Heart J. 2017. https://doi.org/10.1093/eurheartj/ehx354. [Epub ahead of print].

[3]...with Methionine...

5. Adabag AS, Luepker RV, Roger VL, Gersh BJ. Sudden cardiac death: epidemiology and risk factors. Nat Rev Cardiol. 2010;7(4):216–25. https://doi.org/10.1038/nrcardio.2010.3.
6. Boulton AJM, Vinik AI, Arrezzo JC, Bril V, Feldman EI, Freeman R, Malik RA, Maser RE, Sosenko JM, Ziegler D. Diabetic neuropathies: a statement by the American Diabetes Association. Diabetes Care. 2005;28(4):956–62.
7. Berkson B. Alpha lipoic acid breakthrough: the superb antioxidant that may slow aging, repair liver damage, and reduce the risk of cancer, heart disease, and diabetes. New York: Three Rivers Press; 1998.
8. Hargreaves IP. Coenzyme Q10: from fact to fiction. New York: Nova Science Publishing, Inc.; 2015.
9. Ferrier DP. Biochemistry. 6th ed. Philadelphia: Lippincott, Williams & Williams, a Wolters Kluwer Business; 2014.

# Disclaimer

Over the years, Drs. DePace and Colombo have worked to avoid, and have even resisted, developing supplements or nutraceuticals. While we recognize that, sometimes, some supplements and nutraceuticals may work for some people, their general reliability in improving patient outcomes, population wide, is less than that for pharmaceuticals. Please understand that the difference between pharmaceuticals and supplements and nutraceuticals is that the FDA ensures that pharmaceuticals work at least 80% of the time (the other 20% may end up in the courts, claiming bad drugs), whereas supplements and nutraceuticals are more a 50-50 proposition. The difference is important to physicians in helping to convince patients that a proposed therapy plan should work. In addition, the lack of scientific rigor and validity and statistical relevance or the poor reputation of many supplements and nutraceuticals turned us off from becoming involved. Do not get us wrong if patients had no other choice or were willing to try supplements and nutraceuticals, then we were were happy to assist. We are not sold out to the pharmaceutical approach either. What we are sold out to is lifestyle modifications: exercise (yes *exercise*, it is not a bad word, especially when we mean an active lifestyle, not necessarily beating one's self up in the gym), the Mediterranean diet, stress reduction (especially reducing psychosocial stress), and building an antioxidant reserve to address what cannot be controlled.

However, recently, many have asked us to create a supplement and nutraceutical program to augment the lifestyle program we have been recommending, including incorporating the antioxidants. So we endeavored to research the literature for those agents that are not only purported to be beneficial but had also the scientific and statistical evidence behind it to validate them. In this way, we have convince ourselves that these agents have a better than 50-50 chance of helping our patients. These are the origins of this book.

While we have packaged the supplements and nutraceuticals with quantities that we recommend for the convenience of our patients, we are not promoting our supplement and nutraceutical package through this book. In fact, we recommend that people choose for themselves and select the ingredients that they wish, after conferring with their physician. For example, a portion of our product includes a nitric oxide supplement, the same benefits of which may be obtained from the product SuperBeets® from human[n] which has been studied by cardiologists and published in the *Journal of the American College of Cardiology*. In fact, as a matter of convenience, we have modeled our product after the published product.

Again, this book is *not* meant to be an advertisement for our product(s). It is meant to be a promotion for the lifelong adoption of the six-pronged Mind-Body Wellness Program, which includes (1) omega-3 fatty acids, (2) nitric oxide, (3) oxidative stress reduction, (4) Mediterranean diet, (5) exercise, and (6) psychosocial stress reduction, that is used to treat and prevent autonomic and mitochondrial dysfunction. Again, the first three prongs may be purchased anywhere. This book is the first of a series of publications designed to help the physician and the patient find reliable and validated forms of omega-3 fatty acid, nitric oxide, and antioxidant products (supplements and nutraceuticals) that have the best chance of helping.

To be clear and for total transparency in this disclaimer, our products include:

- Cardio-Neuro-Mito™, an antioxidant compound
- Vasso-Plus ™, a nitric oxide compound
- Omega-3 Fish Oil

*We wish all a lifetime of health and wellness. Enjoy!*

# Abbreviations

| | |
|---|---|
| AAD | Advanced Autonomic Dysfunction |
| ACE-I | Angiotensin-converting enzyme inhibitor |
| ADD/ADHD | Attention deficit disorder/attention deficit hyperactivity disorder |
| ADMA | Asymmetric dimethylarginine |
| ADP | Adenosine diphosphate |
| AFib | Atrial fibrillation |
| ALA | Alpha-lipoic acid |
| ALLA | Alpha-linoleic acid |
| ANS | Autonomic nervous system |
| ARB | Angiotensin receptor blocker |
| ATP | Adenosine triphosphate |
| BP | Blood pressure |
| btb | Beat-to-beat |
| CABG | Coronary artery bypass grafting |
| CAN | Cardiovascular Autonomic Neuropathy |
| CASS | Composite autonomic scoring scale |
| CBD | Cannabidiol |
| CFS | Chronic fatigue syndrome |
| cGMP | Cyclic guanosine monophosphate |
| CHF | Congestive heart failure |
| CNS | Central nervous system |
| COPD | Chronic obstructive pulmonary disease |
| CoQ10 | Coenzyme Q10 |
| CRP | C-reactive protein |
| CRPS | Chronic regional pain syndrome |
| CVD | Cardiovascular disease |
| DAN | Diabetic Autonomic Neuropathy |
| DB | Deep breathing |
| DHA | Docosahexaenoic acid |
| DNA | Deoxyribonucleic acid |
| ED | Erectile dysfunction |
| EEG | Electroencephalogram |
| EKG | Electrocardiogram |
| EPA | Eicosapentaenoic acid |
| GERD | Gastroesophageal reflux disorder |
| GI | Gastrointestinal |

| | |
|---|---|
| HDL | High-density lipoproteins |
| HPA | Hypothalamic-pituitary-adrenal |
| HR | Heart rate |
| HRV | Heart rate variability |
| HSP | Heat shock proteins |
| LDL | Low-density lipoproteins |
| LOX-1 | Oxidized LDL 1 receptor |
| MACE | Major adverse cardiovascular event |
| MAO | Monoamine oxidase |
| NAC | N-acetylcysteine |
| NMDA | N-methyl-D-aspartate |
| NOS | Nitric oxide synthase (three types: e-, c-, n-, endothelial, constitutive and neural, respectively) |
| OH | Orthostatic hypotension |
| ox-LDL | Oxidize low-density lipoproteins |
| P | Parasympathetic |
| P&S | Parasympathetic and sympathetic nervous systems |
| PAN | Peripheral autonomic neuropathy |
| PC | Postural change |
| PE | Parasympathetic excess |
| PNS | Peripheral nervous system |
| POTS | Postural orthostatic tachycardia syndrome |
| PTSD | Post-traumatic stress disorder |
| PUFA | Polyunsaturated fatty acid |
| QoL | Quality of life |
| QSART | Quantitative Sudomotor Axon Reflex Test |
| RAAS | Renin-angiotensin-aldosterone system |
| RNS | Reactive nitrogen species |
| RONS | Reactive oxygen nitrogen species |
| ROS | Reactive oxygen species |
| RVLM | Rostral ventrolateral medulla |
| S | Sympathetic |
| SB | Sympathovagal balance |
| SE | Sympathetic excess |
| SNRI | Serotonin-norepinephrine reuptake inhibitors |
| SOD | Superoxide dismutase |
| SSRI | Selective serotonin reuptake inhibitors |
| SW | Sympathetic withdrawal |
| THC | Delta-9-tetrahydrocannabinol |
| TMJ | Temporomandibular joint |
| TNF | Tumor necrosis factor |
| VEGF | Vascular endothelial growth factor |
| VNS | Vagal nerve stimulation |

# 1 Introduction

A respected hematologist-oncologist recently stated to the authors that he was "terrified to admit patients to the hospital for comfort care measures and hospice measures, when in fact the gravity of disease may not be as severe as had been prognosticated by the intensivist." This is especially true when a hematologist-oncologist says, or when a patient hears, the word "cancer" or when some cardiologist, or intensivist, hears the diagnosis "congestive heart failure with left ventricular systolic dysfunction." A black cloud is put over the patient, and they are directed toward a palliative-type care route, despite the fact that there may be many medical alternatives which can increase the quality of life and life expectancy in these patients, if they recover from the acute illness.

It is this prevailing attitude that leads individuals and their families into the predicament of facing such harsh alternatives of palliative care and hospice, when indeed these alternatives may not be indicated. Palliative care and hospice have a very important place in medicine, but oftentimes are overdone or are overprescribed. The key is to keep people out of the hospital in the preventive mode, whether it is primary or secondary prevention, by establishing and maintaining wellness.

Franklin Cardiovascular Associates is led by Nicholas L. DePace, M.D., F.A.C.C. He maintains board certification in five areas: cardiology, nuclear cardiology, echocardiography, lipidology (study of cholesterol and related compounds), and internal medicine. He has been practicing clinical cardiology for 34 years, publishing extensively in the fields of cardiovascular disease and autonomic dysfunction. He has authored or coauthored nearly 100 abstracts and journal articles. He has also coauthored two books: *The Heart Repair Manual* [1] and *Clinical Autonomic Dysfunction* – a medical textbook written with Dr. Colombo and others [2]. Dr. DePace treats and diagnoses various diseases that are cardiac or related to cardiology. His major patient population consists of patients with atherosclerosis. In addition, as a certified lipidologist, he treats patients with various disorders due to cholesterol abnormalities. Many cases are very complex and include a genetic basis.

Dr. DePace led the development of a program in the early 1990s, which was dubbed the "Philadelphia Formula for Reversing and Halting Atherosclerosis." Components of this program are in the book, *The Heart Repair Manual* [1]. This program predated risk stratification by the famous Framingham Heart Study [3, 4], which came out several years later. The Framingham Heart Study was an epidemiological study in which a cohort of subjects, residing in Framingham, Massachusetts, USA, was followed prospectively for several decades. Cardiac risk factors were identified as causative agents for coronary heart disease.

Drs. DePace and Colombo first met in 2010. Dr. Colombo introduced Dr. DePace to the ability



N. L. DePace, J. Colombo, *Clinical Autonomic and Mitochondrial Disorders*,
https://doi.org/10.1007/978-3-030-17016-5_1

to noninvasively monitor both the parasympathetic and sympathetic (P&S) systems of the autonomic nervous system, independently and simultaneously, without assumption of approximation. This capability never existed before. We began treating many individuals with autonomic dysfunction and related disorders with good results. Dr. DePace, himself, had had 9 months of autonomic dysfunction with severe orthostatic intolerance.

Drs. DePace and Colombo augmented the Philadelphia Formula for Reversing and Halting Atherosclerosis by adding features that focus on relieving P&S dysfunction, as well. Autonomic dysfunction involves any disorder, disease, or malfunction of the ANS, including one or both of its two branches: the P&S nervous systems (Fig. 1.1). Dr. Colombo is a P&S nervous system consultant. He developed the aforementioned, first, noninvasive technology to independently and simultaneously measure P&S nervous system activity and function, P&S monitoring. Given that the P&S nervous systems control or coordinate all systems of the body, Dr. Colombo continues to research and develop applications for P&S monitoring throughout all of healthcare. P&S monitoring provides physicians more information to improve diagnoses, therapy plans, and outcomes for their patients.

There are six prongs to the treatments developed by Drs. DePace and Colombo, the details of which will be the topic of discussion in this book. The biological feasibility for why these therapies work, or may be helpful, will also be discussed in detail and supported by useful and statistically rigorous basic, applied, and clinical research literature [5].

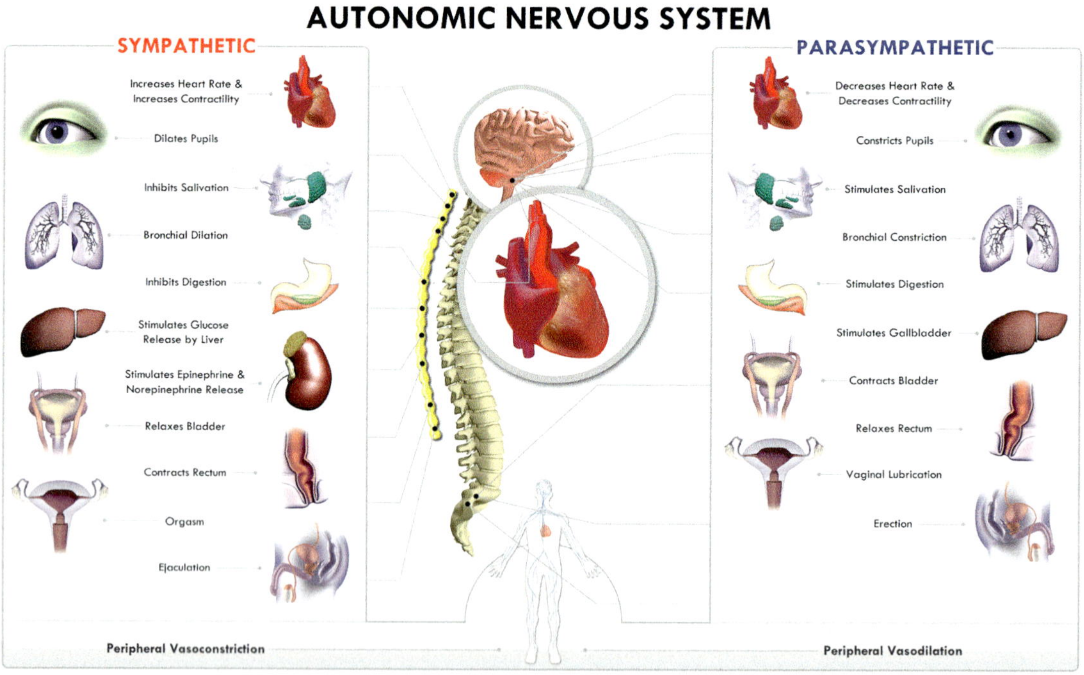


**Fig. 1.1** A schematic of the parasympathetic (right) and sympathetic (left) nervous systems

## References


1. DePace NL, Dowinsky SK, Sherman M. The heart repair manual. New York: WW Norton and Co; 1993.
2. Colombo J, Arora RR, DePace NL, Vinik AI. Clinical autonomic dysfunction: measurement, indications, therapies, and outcomes. New York: Springer Science + Business Media; 2014.
3. Tsuji H, Venditti FJ Jr, Manders ES, Evans JC, Larson MG, Feldman CL, Levy D. Reduced heart rate variability and mortality risk in an elderly cohort. The Framingham Heart Study. Circulation. 1994;90(2):878–83.
4. D'Agostino RB, Vasan RS, Pencina MJ, Wolf PA, Cobain M, Massaro JM, Kannel WB. General cardiovascular risk profile for use in primary care: the Framingham Heart Study. Circulation. 2008;117(6):743–53. https://doi.org/10.1161/CIRCULATIONAHA.107.699579. Epub 2008 Jan 22.
5. DePace NL, Colombo J. Autonomic and mitochondrial dysfunction in clinical diseases: diagnostic, prevention, and therapy. New York: Springer Science + Business Media, Accepted 2019.

# 2 About the Program

The parasympathetic nervous system is commonly referred to as the "rest and digest" nervous system. It is responsible for conserving energy and establishing metabolic baselines. In many situations, it acts like the brakes on a car. It is the "protective" nervous system. The sympathetic nervous system is commonly referred to as the "fight or flight" nervous system. It is responsible for expending energy. In many situations, it acts like the accelerator on a car. It is the "reactionary" nervous system. The ANS is one of the main human systems responsible for our capability and adaptability. The interplay between the P&S branches underlies this ability; they also form the communication network between the mind and the body, including the brain and the heart.

Collectively, the P&S nervous systems are the regulatory branches of the nervous system. Anatomically and physiologically, they exist in both the central and peripheral portions of the nervous system. Together, the P&S nervous systems control bodily functions (Fig. 1.1). To properly affect this control, the two components, P&S, need to be in balance. The specific P&S balance required varies from individual to individual (as it is affected by the individual's genetics) and varies with age, lifestyle, environment, and medical history. It not only includes a resting P&S balance but also a dynamic P&S balance. Autonomic dysfunction results when there is persistent imbalance between the P&S nervous systems, whether it is a resting or static imbalance or a dynamic[1] or response imbalance. This is nicely explained in Dr. Colombo's introductory chapter, specifically page 3, of the textbook, *Clinical Autonomic Dysfunction* [1].

Drs. Colombo and DePace are actively conducting research using P&S monitoring (ANSAR Medical Technologies, Inc., Philadelphia, PA, now TMCAMS, Inc., Atlanta, GA) and vascular endothelial studies to document the benefits of the supplements discussed herein, including on blood vessels (endothelial function) and the P&S nervous systems. There are many disorders involving P&S nervous system dysfunction.

[1] "Dynamic balances" or "dynamic imbalances" are P&S ratios (P&S activity levels relative to each other) under challenging (e.g., non-resting or dynamic) conditions. For example, as measured during the standard clinical autonomic test, during the challenges, the P&S ratio (*aka* sympathovagal balance or SB = S/P) is expected to change as follows: for deep breathing (a parasympathetic challenge), where P is expected to increase and SB is expected to decrease, and for Valsalva and stand or postural change (net sympathetic challenges), where S is expected to increase and SB is expected to increase. There are normal ranges for these SB changes [1]. These normal SB changes define "dynamic balances." Abnormal SB changes define "dynamic imbalances."


N. L. DePace, J. Colombo, *Clinical Autonomic and Mitochondrial Disorders*,
https://doi.org/10.1007/978-3-030-17016-5_2

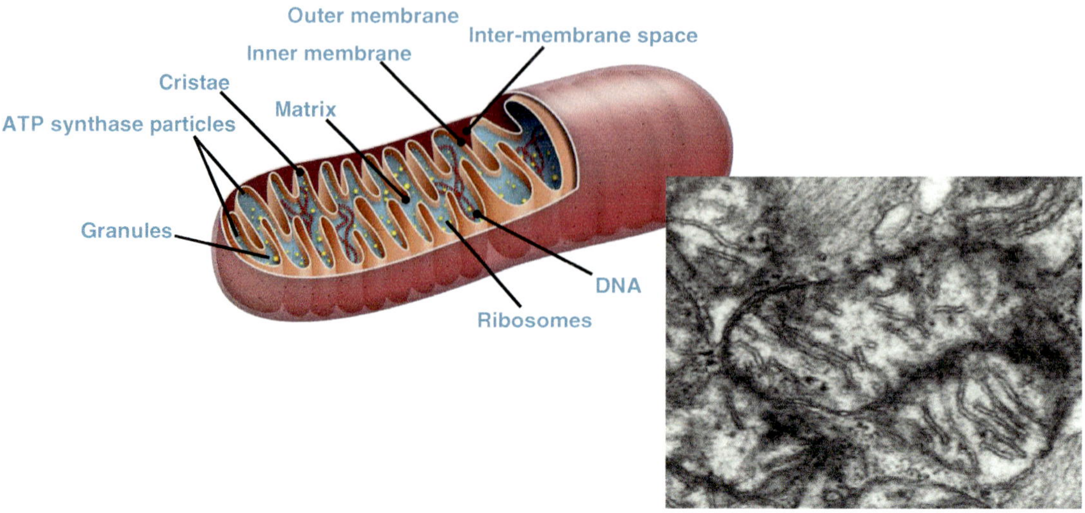


**Fig. 2.1** An illustration of a mitochondrion, including a cutaway diagram of its inner structure, above. To the right is a micrograph of mitochondria in cardiac muscle cells. (Micrograph with permission from Shutterstock Royalty-free stock illustration ID: 1048006219, Mitochondria organelle in cardiac muscle cell tissue electron microscope, by Edgloris Marys. Mitochondrion illustration adapted from Shutterstock Royalty-free stock illustration ID: 1008265135, Section of Mitochondria by Aldona Griskeviciene. Illustration: https://www.umdf.org/what-is-mitochondrial-disease/, Micrograph: https://clinicalgate.com/mitochondria-chloroplasts-peroxisomes/)

These include anxiety, chronic fatigue, fibromyalgia, persistent headache, and various forms of fainting or pre-fainting (involving light-headedness or dizziness), which are, respectively, termed "syncope" and "near syncope." Digestive problems, such as gastroparesis, gastroesophageal reflux disease (GERD), and irritable bowel syndrome, are also affected by P&S nervous system dysfunction. Most importantly, a large percentage of patients in the world have what is termed "orthostatic dysfunction," commonly manifested as "orthostatic intolerance." This form of light-headedness (or dizziness) is arguably the most debilitating symptom of autonomic dysfunction or autonomic neuropathy, as the case may be [2, 3].

Orthostatic dysfunction occurs when people are in the upright position – standing or walking – and develop evidence of lack of cerebral perfusion (blood flow to the head) which can present itself as dizziness, giddiness, brain fog, or cognitive dysfunction. It may also cause visual effects, such as black spots or tunnel vision, headache, or migraine. Up to 97% of the time, this orthostatic intolerance syndrome is associated with chronic fatigue syndrome (CFS) [4], which is defined as 6 months of significant exhaustion associated with, oftentimes, unrefreshing sleep, daytime somnolence, swollen lymph nodes, sore throat, depression, and an inability to function. It is felt that many of these disorders – including migraines; neurodegenerative diseases, such as Parkinson's, Alzheimer's, dementia, and other more complicated neurological syndromes; asthma; and various forms of lung disease, such as COPD – may not only involve the P&S nervous systems but also dysfunction in mitochondria of the cells in the body [5]. These conditions are labeled "mitochondrial dysfunction disorders."

Mitochondria (Fig. 2.1) are small components (organelles) of most cells in the body, the most notable exception being red blood cells [6]. Mitochondria are the power factories of the body. They produce the energy molecule, adenosine triphosphate (ATP). The production of energy (ATP) is somewhat complex and critical to good health, well-being, and life itself. So we will step aside and spend a little time discussing it in detail.

## Energy Production

Cellular energy production from mitochondria via the citric acid cycle and the electron transport chain is well established and is referenced in any biochemistry or cellular physiology texts. Figure 2.2 shows a diagram of a mitochondrion taken from a cell and describes the cell machinery for glucose metabolism, the chemical process for generating ATP. Glucose metabolism is at the core of cellular respiration; it begins with the combination of glucose and oxygen. It is how the cell "breathes." The core chemical equation for cellular respiration is shown in Fig. 2.3. Specifically,

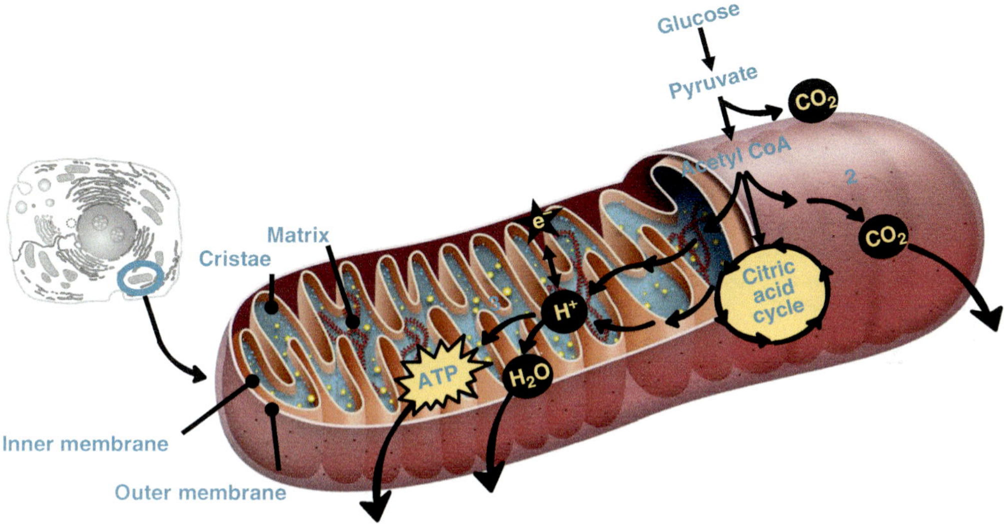


**Fig. 2.2** Cell machinery for glucose metabolism: (1) glycolysis occurs in the cytoplasm, (2) citric acid (or Krebs) cycle takes place mostly in the mitochondrial matrix, and (3) electron transport and oxidative phosphorylation occur on the inner membrane of the mitochondria. (Cell Image from Shutterstock Royalty-free stock vector images ID: 780737359 Animal human cell structure educational science. Microscope 3d eukaryotic nucleus organelle medicine analysis. Glowing white gray biology poster template isolated line art vector illustration by LuckyStep. Mitochondrion illustration adapted from Shutterstock Royalty-free stock illustration ID: 1008265135, Section of Mitochondria by Aldona Griskeviciene. https://basicmedicalkey.com/nutrition-and-metabolism/)

**Fig. 2.3** Cellular respiration – the addition of glucose and oxygen to make energy, chemical energy, in the form of ATP. (Mitochondrion illustration adapted from Shutterstock Royalty-free stock illustration ID: 1008265135, Section of Mitochondria by Aldona Griskeviciene)

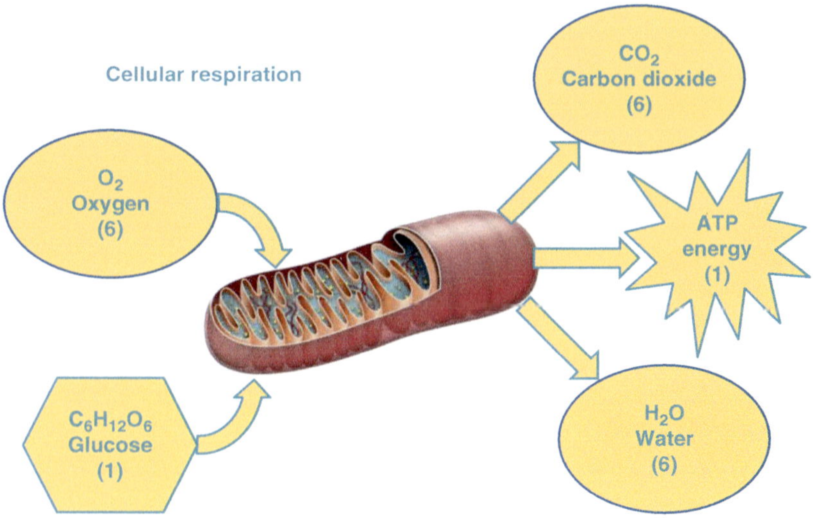

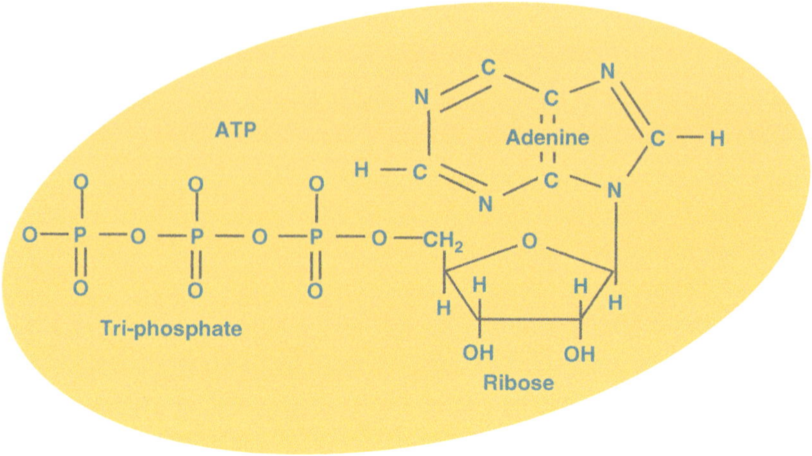


**Fig. 2.4** The chemical structure of ATP. (Illustration by Elysian Creative Studio, www.elysiancreativestudio.com, Lizzy Colombo. https://schoolworkhelper.net/cell-reactions-and-energy/)

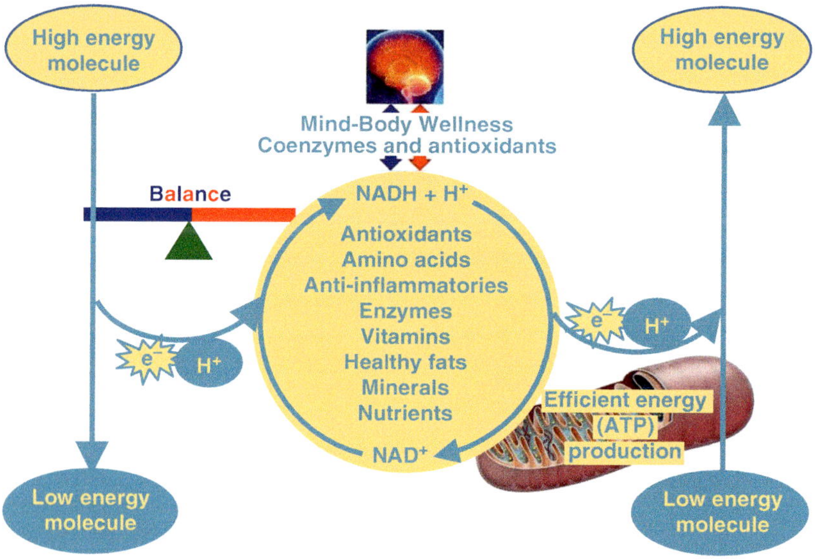


**Fig. 2.5** The coenzymes and antioxidants of the Mind-Body Wellness Program work to enhance the efficiency of transferring chemical energy (ATP). (Mitochondrion illustration adapted from Shutterstock Royalty-free stock illustration ID: 1008265135, Section of Mitochondria by Aldona Griskeviciene. Brain illustration adapted from Shutterstock Royalty-free stock illustration ID: 82159072, Female Brain Xray Anatomy, by CLIPAREA l Custom media. https://basicmedicalkey.com/nutrition-and-metabolism/)

glucose ($C_6H_{12}O_6$) is combined with six oxygens ($6O_2$) to produce ATP (see its molecular structure in Fig. 2.4) and respiratory by-products (water, $H_2O$, and carbon dioxide, $CO_2$).

ATP is derived from food products ingested, which become metabolized and eventually converted to this energy molecule, allowing us to perform our everyday activities. For example, ATP is important for muscle contraction, including heart muscle, and proper nerve function. Because the generation of ATP for energy is so important, the actual chemical process is much more complex, as suggested in Fig. 2.3. The more complex, the greater the number of controls and safeguards there are. Point of fact, there are many cofactors (Fig. 2.5; e.g., enzymes, vitamins, and minerals) required to maintain peak efficiency of this process. With normal aging, or as a result of chronic disease, injury, or pain, efficiency is lost due to the body's loss of natural abilities to pro-

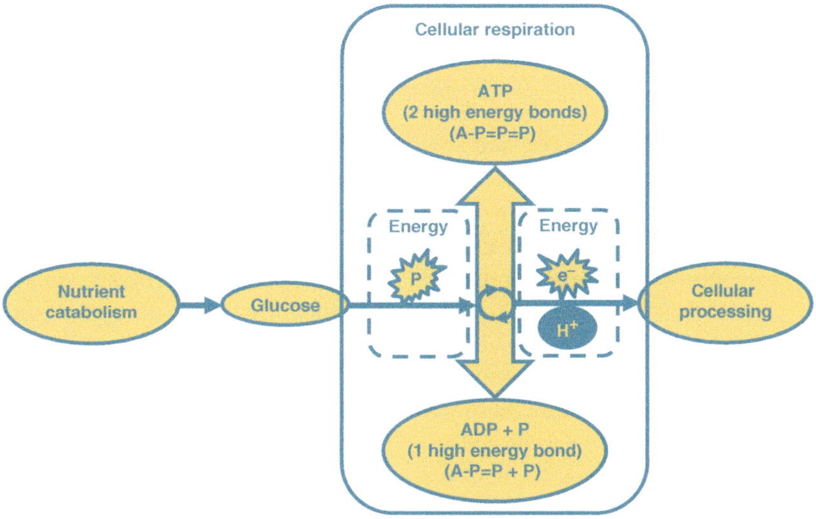


**Fig. 2.6** There is energy stored in the foods we eat. In its base form, energy is stored in the simple sugar molecule sucrose. Several sucrose molecules are stored in the simple carbohydrate glucose. More complex molecules are broken up into glucose molecules through a process called catabolism. Catabolism releases food energy (glucose) into the cellular respiration process to release cellular energy as ATP. ATP temporarily stores energy in its last (third, the "T" in ATP) high-energy phosphate (P, in this diagram) bond. When water is added and the third phosphate breaks free, energy is released to do cellular work. This leaves only two phosphates, and now the molecule is adenosine diphosphate (ADP: "Di" meaning two). ADP can be resynthesized into ATP, capturing additional energy from nutrient catabolism, thereby completing the cycle. (https://basicmedicalkey.com/nutrition-and-metabolism/)

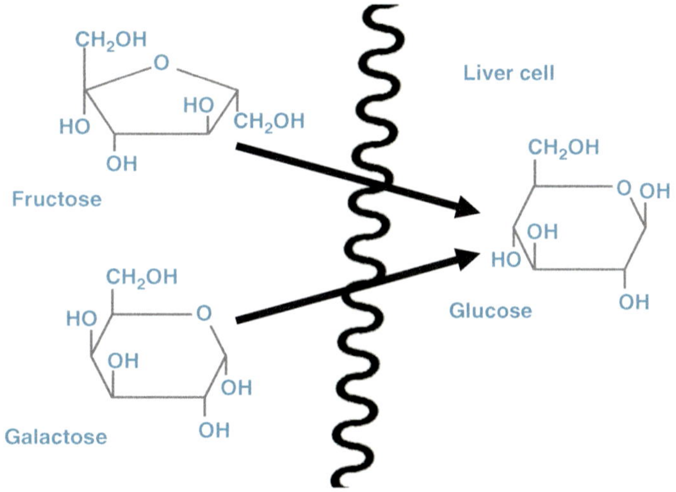


**Fig. 2.7** A simplified example of nutrient catabolism is the conversion of monosaccharides, such as fructose or galactose into the simple sugar, glucose. This process is much more complex and usually occurs in liver cells. Glucose is the carbohydrate used universally by all cells in the body. (https://basicmedicalkey.com/nutrition-and-metabolism/)

duce or retain these factors. It is these factors that are, in part, the subjects of the research and applications discussed in this book.

There is (chemical) energy stored in the foods that are consumed. In its base form, chemical energy is in the simple sugar molecule glucose ($C_6H_{12}O_6$, see Fig. 2.3). Glucose is also the simplest carbohydrate. More complex sugar molecules, carbohydrates, fats, and possibly other molecules under certain conditions (like proteins), are broken into glucose molecules through a process called nutrient catabolism (see Fig. 2.6). Nutrient catabolism releases food energy (glucose, see Fig. 2.7) into the cellular respiration process to combine with oxygen and release cellular energy as ATP. ATP temporarily stores energy in its last (third, the "T" in ATP) high-energy phosphate (P, in Fig. 2.6) bond. When water is added and the third phosphate breaks free, energy is released to do cellular work. This leaves only two phosphates, and now the molecule is adenosine diphosphate (ADP; "Di" meaning two), or ADP. ADP can be resynthesized into ATP, capturing additional energy from nutrient catabolism, thereby completing the cycle.

Nutrient (glucose) catabolism is depicted in Fig. 2.8. Glucose, a simple carbohydrate, is stored in the liver and other tissues as the polymer glycogen, which can then later be hydrolyzed to form individual glucose molecules (see also Fig. 2.7). Glycolysis splits one molecule of glucose, with six carbon atoms, into two pyruvic acid molecules, with three carbon atoms each. The glycolytic pathway is anaerobic, in that it does not require oxygen. A transition reaction removes a carbon dioxide molecule (released as a waste product), converting each pyruvic acid molecule into a two-carbon acetyl group that is escorted by coenzyme A (coA) into the citric acid cycle (aka Krebs cycle). In the citric acid cycle, two more carbon dioxide molecules are released, also as waste products, leaving energy ("$e^-$ "for high-energy electron). This part of glycolysis requires oxygen; therefore, it is aerobic. The "energy particles" ($e^-$) with oxygen then enter the electron transport chain to complete the process of generating energy by converting more ADP into ATP.

The citric acid cycle and the electron transport chain form the core of the energy production process (see Fig. 2.2). Figure 2.9 highlights these two processes. As depicted in Fig. 2.9, glucose from the liver is prepared for cellular respiration through glycolysis. This process also produces ATP and leaves some high-energy electrons, which are collected by the coenzyme, NADH, which is the reduced form of nicotinamide adenine dinucleotide (NAD). This entire process of glycolysis is depicted in schematic form in Fig. 2.10.

Even though glycolysis occurs outside the mitochondria (inside the cytoplasm, see Fig. 2.9), it still generates the energy molecules ATP. As glucose (see Fig. 2.10) is formed into a complex sugar fructose, energy (ATP) is used. Fructose, the sugar first found in fruits, is a common form of sugar found in nature that is made of two sucrose molecules. Even though fructose has two sucrose molecules, it is a healthier sugar because it takes energy to break the chemical bond between the two sucrose molecules. Expending this energy uses more sucrose and causes less excess sucrose.

Excess sucrose in the blood stream turns the blood acidic. If the blood becomes too acidic too often, as in patients with diabetes or who are insulin resistant, then sugar acidosis is possible. Insulin is like the key that unlocks the cell membrane channels that permit sucrose to enter. Insufficient levels of insulin are one way too much sucrose kept in the blood, leading to sugar acidosis. Sugar acidosis can be very damaging, especially (1) to the filtration structures in kidneys (called glomeruli), possibly leading to kidney (renal) disease, and (2) to small nerve fibers, possibly leading to autonomic neuropathy.

Excess sucrose in the blood is often converted to fat. Fat is a highly efficient way to store excess glucose. Fructose is modified by

**Fig. 2.8** Catabolism of glucose. Glucose, a simple carbohydrate, may be stored in the liver and other tissues as the polymer glycogen, which can then later be hydrolyzed to form individual glucose molecules. Glycolysis splits one molecule of glucose, with six carbon atoms, into two pyruvic acid molecules, with three carbon atoms each. The glycolytic pathway is anaerobic, in that it does not require oxygen. A transition reaction removes a carbon dioxide molecule (released as a waste product), converting each pyruvic acid molecule into a two-carbon acetyl group that is escorted by coenzyme A (coA) into the citric acid cycle (Krebs cycle). In the citric acid cycle, two more carbon dioxide molecules are released, also as waste products, leaving energy (indicated by the "e" product). This part of glycolysis requires oxygen and is aerobic. The "energy particles" with oxygen then enter the electron transport chain to complete the process of generating energy by converting more ADP into ATP. (Illustration by Elysian Creative Studio, www.elysiancreativestudio.com, Lizzy Colombo. https://basicmedicalkey.com/nutrition-and-metabolism/)

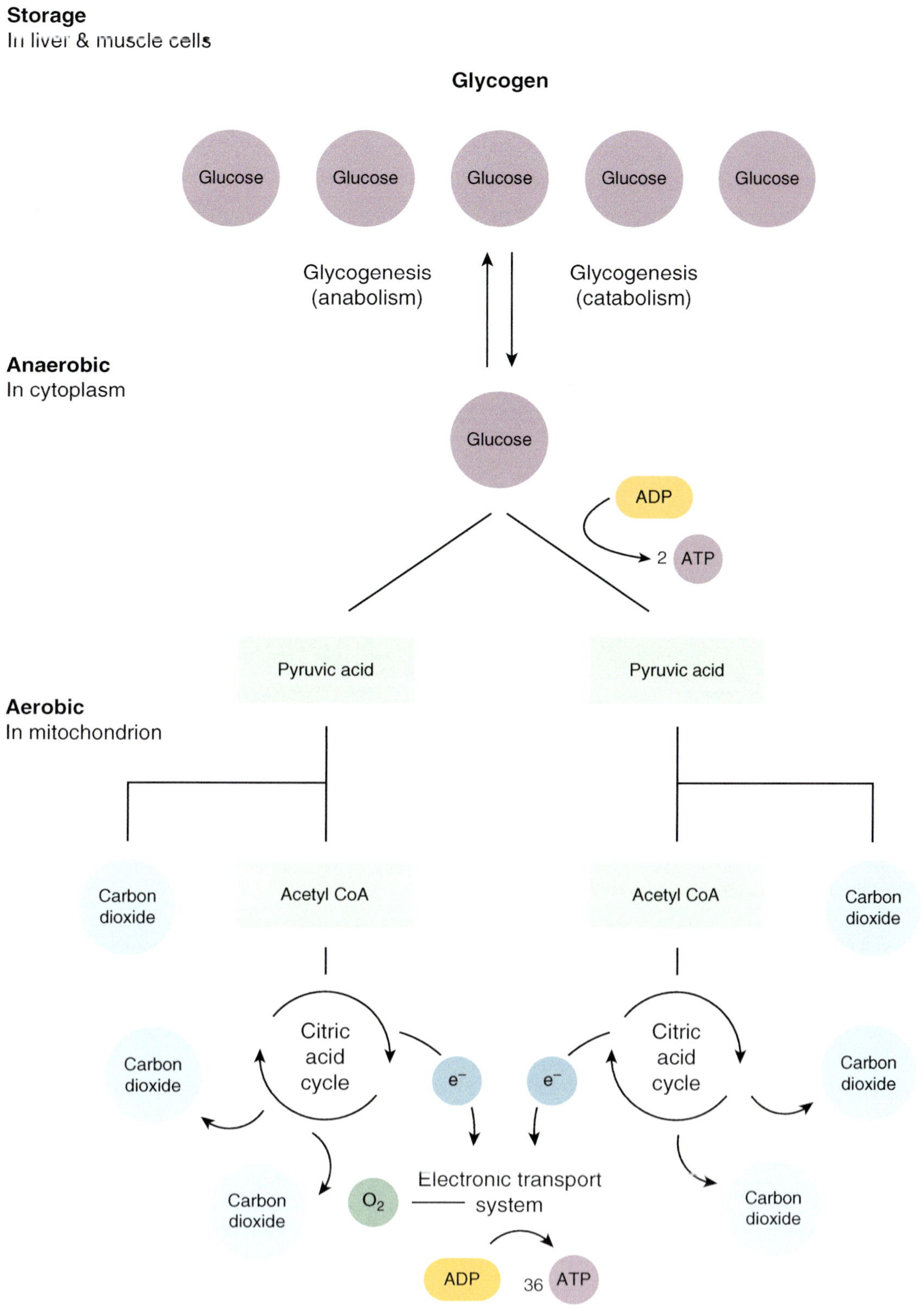
Storage
In liver & muscle cells
Glycogen
Glucose
Glucose
Glucose
Glucose
Glucose
Glycogenesis
(anabolism)
Glycogenesis
(catabolism)
Anaerobic
In cytoplasm
Glucose
ADP
2 ATP
Pyruvic acid
Pyruvic acid
Aerobic
In mitochondrion
Carbon dioxide
Acetyl CoA
Acetyl CoA
Carbon dioxide
Carbon dioxide
Citric acid cycle
e⁻
e⁻
Citric acid cycle
Carbon dioxide
Carbon dioxide
O2
Electronic transport system
Carbon dioxide
ADP
36 ATP

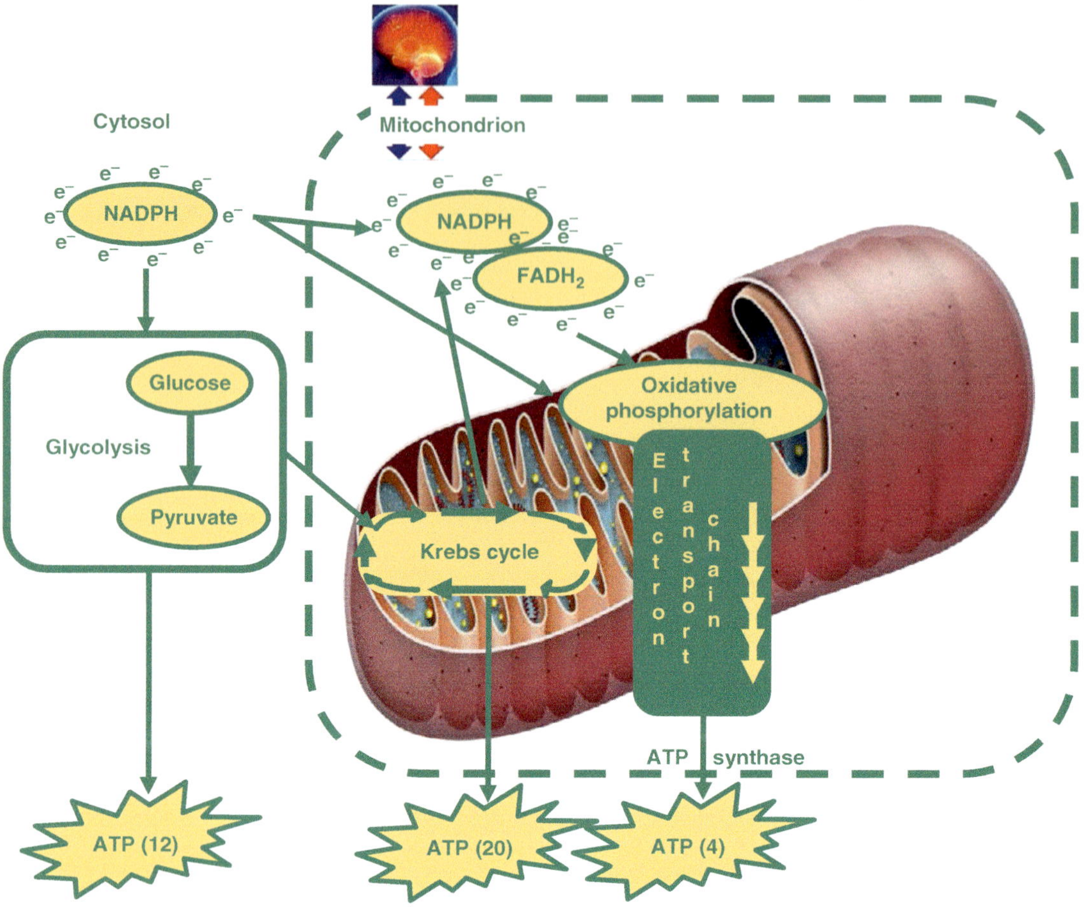


**Fig. 2.9** The heart of energy production in mitochondria: (1) the citric acid cycle (also known as the Krebs cycle) and (2) the electron transport chain. (Mitochondrion illustration adapted from Shutterstock Royalty-free stock illustration ID: 1008265135, Section of Mitochondria by Aldona Griskeviciene. Brain illustration adapted from Shutterstock Royalty-free stock illustration ID: 82159072, Female Brain Xray Anatomy, by CLIPAREA l Custom media. http://sciencewithu.weebly.com/cell-respiration.html)

having a phosphate added, using another energy (ATP) molecule. The modified fructose, with its two phosphates, is spilt into two parts. Each part combines with dihydroxyacetone phosphate and glyceraldehyde 3-phosphate. In this step, each part is also catalyzed by oxidized NAD ($NAD^+$), using yet another phosphate to generate the reduced form of NAD (NADH). The result is diphosphoglycerate which contains two ("Di") phosphates. Then each diphosphoglycerate gives a phosphate to a pair of ADP molecules, and the first two ATP molecules ready for cellular work are released. Left behind are two phosphoglycerates (each containing one phosphate). The phosphoglycerate is restructured, giving off water ($H_2O$) as a waste product and leaving a phosphoenolpyruvate in each spilt. Each phosphoenolpyruvate gives a phosphate to another pair of ADP molecules, and the next two ATP molecules ready for cellular work are released. The net is pyruvic acid which is escorted by coenzyme A (coA) into the citric acid cycle.

Continuing in Fig. 2.10, each pyruvic acid molecule from the glycolysis process is converted in a "transition reaction" (see Fig. 2.11), one each at the top of two separate citric acid cycles (see Fig. 2.8). One of the citric acid cycles is depicted in Fig. 2.12. There is a pyruvate dehydrogenase (PDH) complex (Fig. 2.11) that

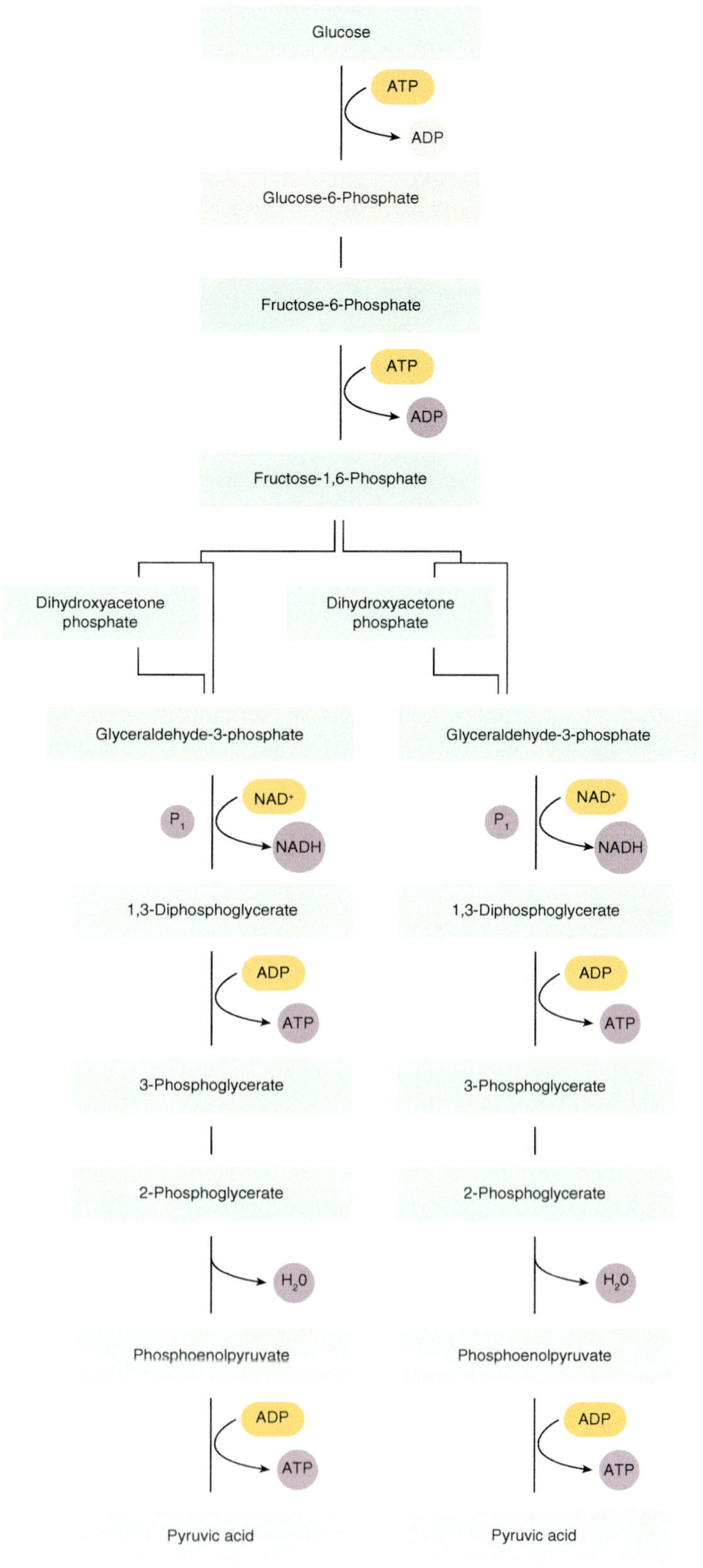


**Fig. 2.10** Glycolysis is a process that prepares the simple carbohydrate glucose, typically from the liver, for use in the citric acid cycle. The citric acid cycle (Krebs cycle) occurs within the mitochondria and is part of cellular respiration. Glycolysis is a series of enzyme-catalyzed reactions that are part of the catabolic pathway. (Illustration by Elysian Creative Studio, www.elysiancreativestudio.com, Lizzy Colombo. https://basicmedicalkey.com/nutrition-and-metabolism/)

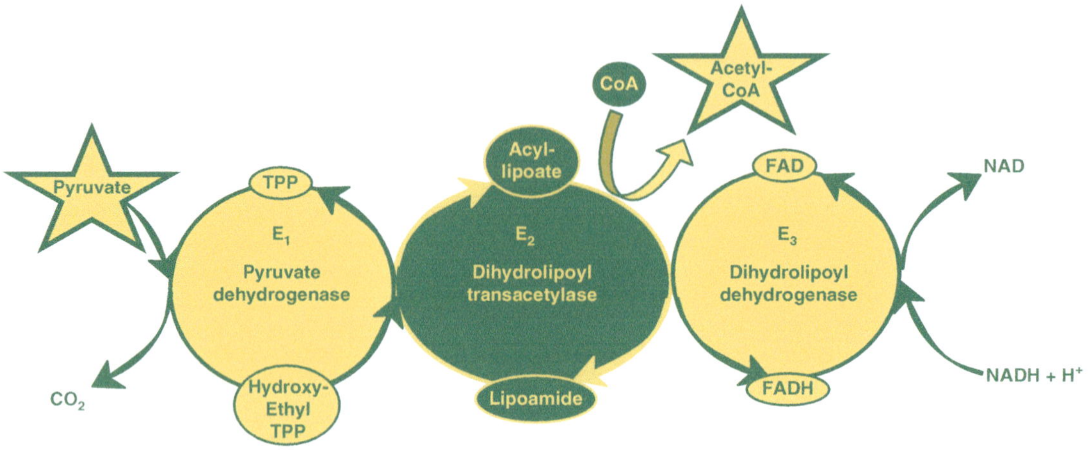


**Fig. 2.11** The pyruvate dehydrogenase (PDH) complex that is the substrate for the transition reaction. See text for more details. (Modified from https://www.youtube.com/watch?v=2HaFHUAwVyQ)

is the substrate for the transition reaction. The PDH complex (PDC) is one of the central enzymes of aerobic metabolism. PDC is a large multienzyme complex comprised of subunits including three enzymes: (E1) pyruvate dehydrogenase, (E2) dihydrolipoyl transacetylase, and (E3) dihydrolipoyl dehydrogenase. It also includes five associated coenzymes. PDC catalyzes the overall oxidation of the end product of glycolysis: pyruvate to acetyl CoA (see Fig. 2.11). PDC breaks down this general reaction into three chemical transformations, requiring all three enzymes in the complex: (1) decarboxylation which results in the loss of $CO_2$, (2) oxidation of keto group (C=O) to a carboxyl group, and (3) activation by linkage to coenzyme A through a thioester bond. Additionally, five coenzymes are utilized by this multienzyme complex: (1) thiamine pyrophosphate (TPP, in the E1 prosthetic group), (2) lipoamide (in the E2 prosthetic group), (3) coenzyme A, (4) flavin adenine dinucleotide (FAD, in the E3 prosthetic group), and (5) the oxidized form of nicotinamide adenine dinucleotide (NAD+).

Just prior to the start of the citric acid cycle, the PDH complex produces acetyl coenzyme A from the pyruvic acid (the glycolysis reaction) and starts the citric acid cycle. Glycolysis also produces carbon dioxide ($CO_2$) and high-energy electrons (denoted as $H^+$ in Fig. 2.12). $CO_2$ is given off as waste. The high-energy electrons are carried off by NADH. The resulting acetyl group is carried by CoA to combine with four-carbon oxaloacetic acid, which is condensed to form citric acid. This is Step 1 of the citric acid cycle (Fig. 2.12). In Step 2, citric acid reacts, in a dehydration-hydration reaction, with a six-carbon substrate, forming isocitric acid. In Step 3, isocitric acid is converted by oxidative decarboxylation to a five-carbon substrate, α-ketoglutaric acid, giving off more $CO_2$. In Step 4, the five-carbon substrate is converted to a four-carbon substrate, succinyl CoA, in another oxidative decarboxylation reaction, giving off another $CO_2$ and more high-energy electrons ($H^+$), which are carried off by more $NAD^+$ as NADH. In Step 5, the four-carbon substrate phosphorylates ADP to create succinic acid and ATP. The ATP is transferred out of the cycle, ready for cellular work. Step 6 dehydrogenates the four-carbon substrate with flavin adenine dinucleotide (FAD) to carry away more high-energy electrons ($H^+$) as the reduced form of FAD and $FADH_2$, leaving fumaric acid (a four-carbon substrate). In Step 7, fumaric acid absorbs water (hydrates) resulting in malic acid (another four-carbon substrate). Step 8 dehydrogenates the four-carbon substrate with $NAD^+$ to carry off more high-energy electrons as NADH (see Fig. 2.12), leaving another four-carbon

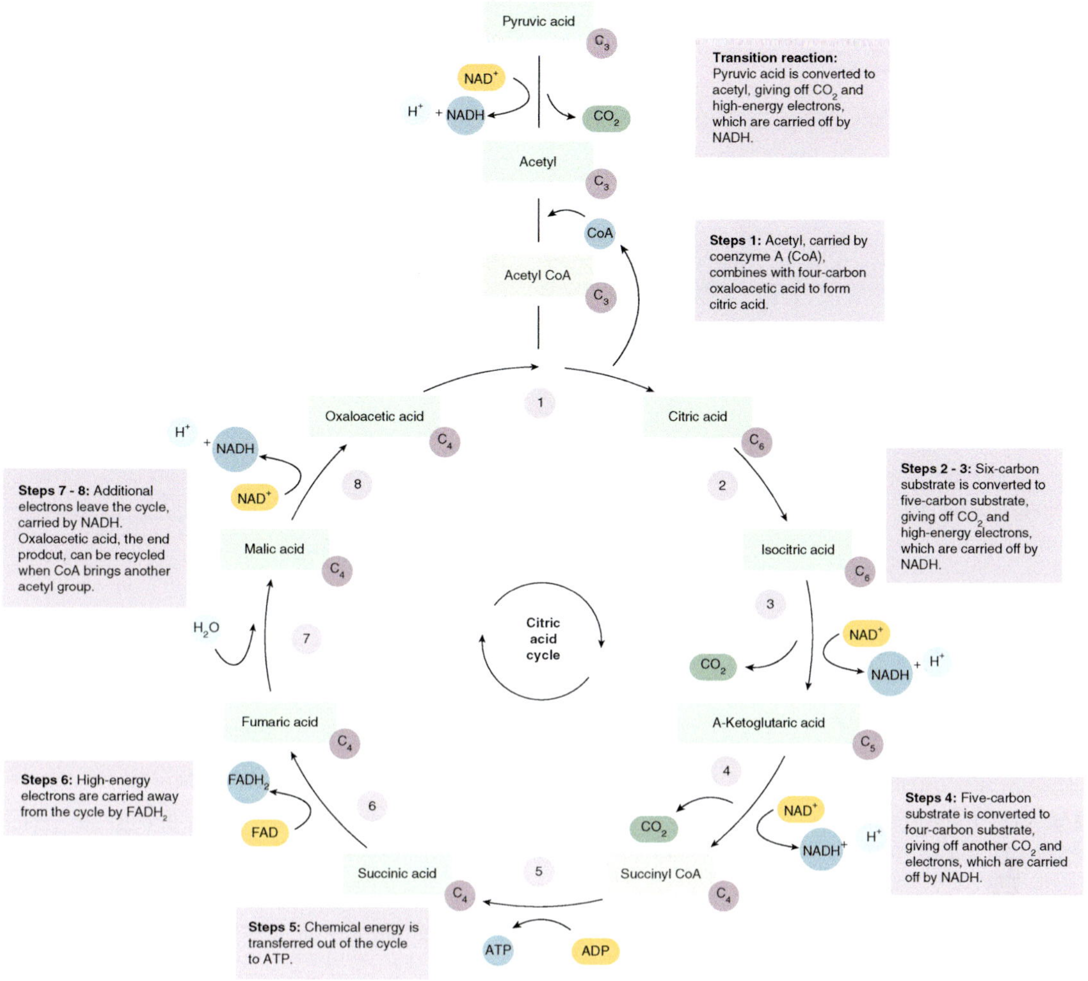


**Fig. 2.12** The citric acid (or Krebs) cycle. Each pyruvic acid molecule from the glycolysis process is prepared to enter the citric acid cycle by the transition reaction, which yields a pair of high-energy electrons and a $CO_2$ molecule. The acetyl group that is formed is picked up by CoA and led into the citric acid cycle itself, which is described herein as a series of eight steps. See text for more detail. High-energy electrons are depicted as $H^+$, or the "H" in NADH or $FADH_2$. (Illustration by Elysian Creative Studio, www.elysiancreativestudio.com, Lizzy Colombo. Source: https://basicmedicalkey.com/nutrition-and-metabolism/)

substrate, oxaloacetic acid. Oxaloacetic acid is recycled when another enzyme CoA brings another acetyl group, taking those two carbons to re-form the initial six-carbon substrate to restart the cycle.

The high-energy electrons carried from the citric acid cycle as NADH or $FADH_2$ are taken to the electron transport chain (Fig. 2.13, which depicts high-energy electrons as "e⁻" and protons as "H⁺"). In Step 1 of the electron transport chain (Fig. 2.13), pairs of high-energy electrons and their accompanying protons are transferred to the components of the electron transport system by NAD and FAD. The entire electron transport chain is wholly contained within the cytoplasm of the mitochondrion. In Step 2, the high-energy particles jump from cytochrome complex to cytochrome complex, transferring energy along the way. In Step 3, the energy being given off is used to pump (transfer) protons into the mitochondrion reservoir (the intermembrane space between the inner and outer membranes of the mitochondrion). In Step 4, the (passive) diffusion of the protons back into the inner compartment

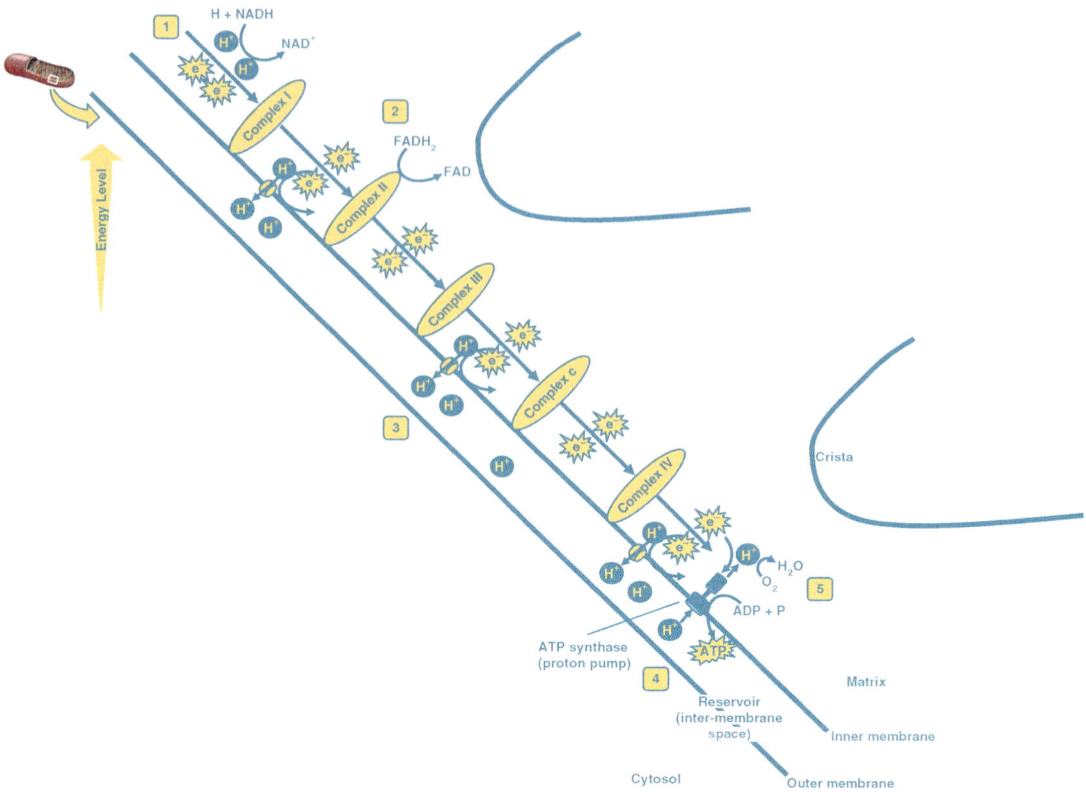


**Fig. 2.13** The electron transport chain. Within a mitochondrion, pairs of high-energy electrons ($e^-$) and their accompanying protons ($H^+$) energize the chain to produce ATP from ADP (an energy-consuming process): (1) The $e^-$ and $H^+$ are transferred to the cytochrome complexes of the electron transport chain by NAD and FAD. (2) The $e^-$'s "jump" from cytochrome complex to complex, losing energy along the way. (3) The energy is used to pump $H^+$ into the intermembrane space, known as the "reservoir." (4) Diffusion of $H^+$ back into the mitochondrial matrix, through the proton pump/ATP synthase complex, drives phosphorylation of ADP to ATP. (5) To minimize ROS formation, at the end of the cytochrome complex chain, $H^+$ are joined with $O_2$, and the now, low-energy $e^-$'s to form water molecules ($H_2O$). (Mitochondrion illustration adapted from Shutterstock Royalty-free stock illustration ID: 1008265135, Section of Mitochondria by Aldona Griskeviciene. https://basicmedicalkey.com/nutrition-and-metabolism/)

provides the energy needed for phosphorylation of ADP to ATP. In Step 5, the protons combine with oxygen ($O_2$) and low-energy electrons at the end of the chain to form water molecules, which is released as waste.

ATP is generated by ATP synthase. Figure 2.14 illustrates how proton wheels, in the inner membrane of the mitochondrion, use the protons from the citric acid cycle. The protons move down their concentration gradient (passively; note: moving charged particles, electrons, or protons are the definition of an electrical current, which in this case provides the energy to drive the cellular machinery). The energy from the rotating proton wheel works to add a phosphate molecule to, or phosphorylate, ADP to become ATP, the energy molecule.

In summary (Fig. 2.15), energy released from the breakdown of glucose is release mostly as heat, but some is transferred to a usable form: the high-energy bonds of ATP. In most human cells, one glucose molecule produces enough useable chemical energy to synthesize 36 energy molecules in the form of ATP molecules. In support of all of this energy production, a number of nutrients are required (see Fig. 2.16), including B vitamins, with zinc, iron, magnesium, copper, manganese, and selenium as cofactors, acting as enzymes making the numerous chemical reactions more efficient, and vitamins A, C, and E,

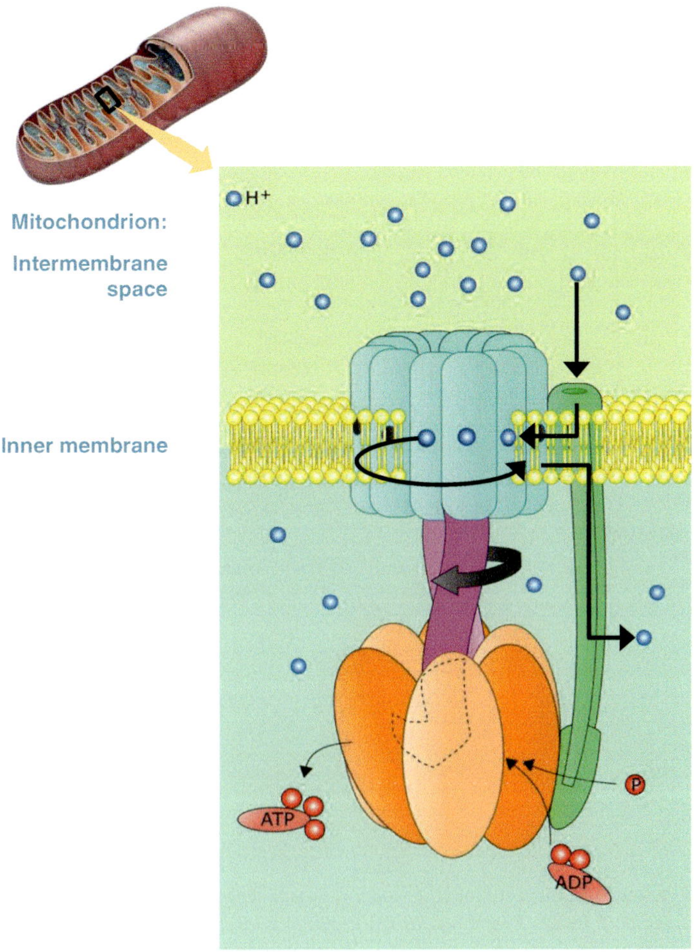


**Fig. 2.14** ATP is generated by ATP synthase. This simple diagram illustrates how the proton wheel in the inner membrane of the mitochondrion uses the protons ($H^+$) from the citric acid cycle to generate ATP from ADP. (Mitochondrion illustration adapted from Shutterstock Royalty-free stock illustration ID: 1008265135, Section of Mitochondria by Aldona Griskeviciene. ATP synthase modified from Shutterstock Royalty-free stock vector images ID: 292748267, Mechanism of action of the ATP synthase, by ellepigrafica [7]. https://basicmedicalkey.com/nutrition-and-metabolism/)

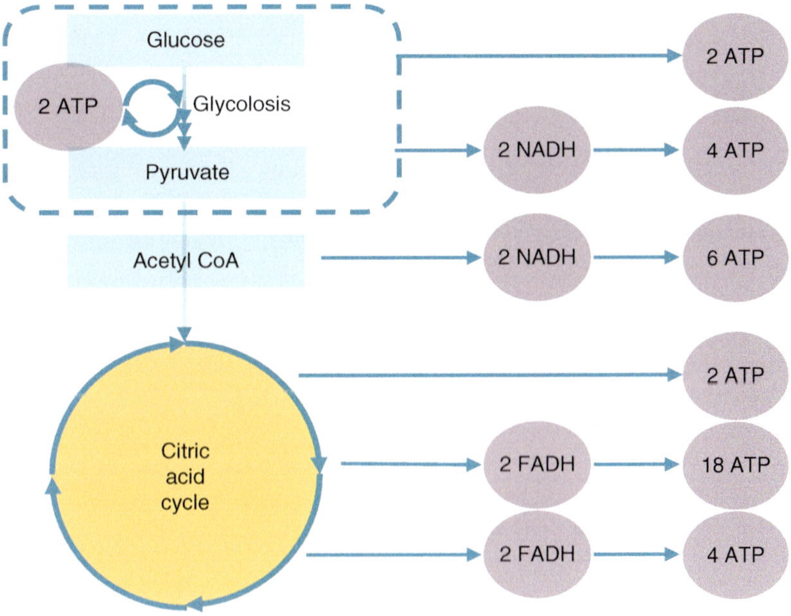


**Fig. 2.15** Energy extracted from glucose. In most human cells, one glucose molecule produces enough useable chemical energy to synthesize 36 energy molecules in the form of ATP molecules (total net ATP yield). (https://basicmedicalkey.com/nutrition-and-metabolism/)

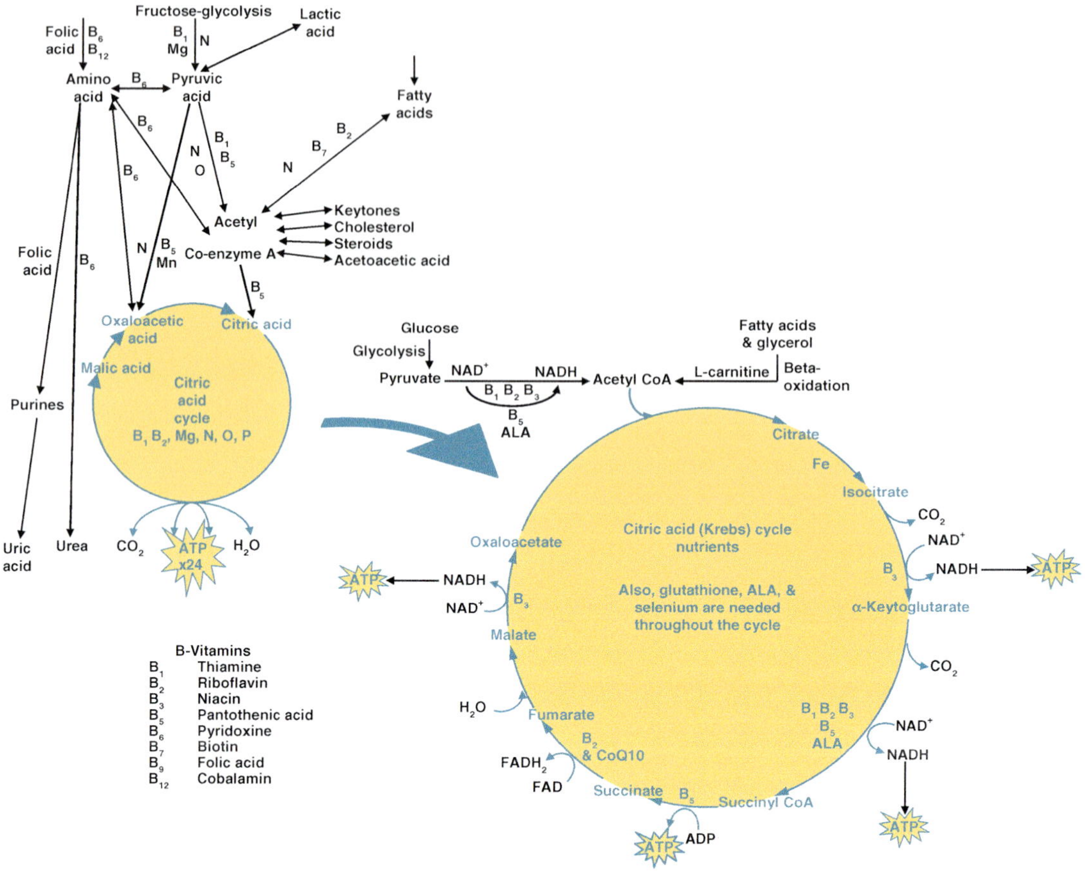


**Fig. 2.16** Nutrients required in support of, and within, the citric acid cycle. The insert to the right provides more detail to the diagram on the left. (Based on [8]. Right panel: http://www.milliesays.com/2015/03/08/nutrient-deficiencies-and-fibromyalgia/)

with ALA and CoQ10 as antioxidants to manage free radicals (including ROS) and other potentially harmful by-products. These nutrients are inherent in, or provided by, the lifestyle or supplements studied herein. While these have many more applications than just for the energy-producing mechanisms,[2] here the focus will only be on energy production. More systemic applications are addressed elsewhere. Nutrients studied include two of the most powerful antioxidants found in the human body. They are alpha-lipoic acid (ALA) and coenzyme Q10 (CoQ10). ALA is required throughout the citric acid cycle, and CoQ10 is required to promote the high-energy electron transfer mediated by FAD. B vitamins and magnesium are also needed throughout, as are amino acids and many other nutrients, as listed in Fig. 2.16.

> Gentlemen, I have a confession to make. Half of what we have taught you is in error, and furthermore we cannot tell you which half it is. (Sir William Osler, Bt)

## Back to the Program

A lack of ATP can cause chronic fatigue syndrome (CFS) and other disorders pertaining to autonomic (P&S) and mitochondrial dysfunction. Even moderate levels of P&S dysfunction are well known to involve many QoL dysfunctions.

[2]These agents help to maintain healthy levels of NADH to boost ATP synthesis. In the brain, NADH increases the production of the neurotransmitters dopamine, norepinephrine, and serotonin, which help elevate mood and improve sleep.

These may include (1) difficult to control BP, blood glucose, or hormone level, (2) difficult to describe pain syndromes (including chronic regional pain syndrome (CRPS) and fibromyalgia), (3) difficult to manage weight loss, (4) unexplained arrhythmia (palpitations) or seizure, (5) symptoms of depression or anxiety, (6) fatigue, (7) exercise intolerance, (8) sex dysfunction, (9) sleep or (10) GI disturbance, (11) occasional to frequent light-headedness or dizziness (orthostatic dysfunction or syncope is arguably the most debilitating symptom of autonomic dysfunction [2, 3]), (12) cognitive dysfunction or "brain fog," (13) attention difficulties, or (14) frequent headache or migraine. Often, none of these symptoms are treated as P&S dysfunctions. They are typically treated in isolation, leading to many medications and often over medication. Often, this is because they occur early in disease processes, when patients are younger. Furthermore, traditional therapies are often not very effective or only mask symptoms. Patients wind up trying many different physicians to no avail and are even recommended for psychiatric evaluation, at which time everyone loses. Everyone loses because the problem is not psychological, but physiological. The problem is that very few know about it. It was not taught in medical school. The stage at which these symptoms present is known as advanced autonomic dysfunction (AAD) or, for patients with diabetes, diabetic autonomic neuropathy (DAN), both of which carry a high morbidity risk (risk of secondary diseases or side effects). Both are defined as low, resting P or S activity. AAD affects QoL [9–11]. This is not reversible; the best that may be done at this time is to preserve what is left. The better option is to start as early as possible to prevent the onset of ADD or DAN. The science behind the lifestyle recommendations and supplements studied herein may delay or prevent the onset of these symptoms and thereby the conditions known as AAD or DAN.

Not long after AAD or DAN, late-stage (end-stage) autonomic dysfunction presents. This is known as cardiovascular autonomic neuropathy (CAN). It is defined as very low, resting parasympathetic activity (e.g., "no brakes"). There are two forms of CAN: functional and structural. Functional CAN patients often find (temporary) relief of CAN once a proper P&S balance is restored for them, the individual patient. Structural CAN is not reversible. Both carry mortality risks. CAN risk is the same as for post-MI and post-CABG patients, as documented in the Framingham Heart Study [12], as well as for other MACE (including stroke) patients. For chronic patients, CAN has been found to carry the same 50% increase in the 5-year mortality rate, as with diabetes [13, 14]. In other words, upon diagnosis, the risk of experiencing a heart attack, stroke, or other MACE within 5 years is 50% or more. CAN is typically normal for post-MI, post-CABG, chronically ill, and geriatric patients. CAN is a normal part of the aging process on the ANS. Again, CAN simply indicates risk of mortality. In other words, it is a sign of age, and people with CAN, who tend to be older, have a greater risk of dying than people without CAN, who tend to be younger and healthier. However, regardless of age, CAN with abnormal P&S balance is not normal. CAN with high P&S balance is high risk [15] and is associated with other risk factors [16, 17], including (1) low ejection fraction [18, 19]; (2) poor cardiac output [20]; (3) arrhythmias [21, 22]; (4) cardiomyopathies [23, 24], including chronic heart failure [25]; (5) poor circulation [26], including poor cardiac circulation (angina or coronary artery disease) [27]; (6) greater mortality [2]; and (7) greater morbidity [3], including silent myocardial infarction and early cardiac death [3, 28]. CAN with high P&S Balance (SB) carries a 50% increase in the 2-year mortality rate [1]. CAN with low P&S balance is associated with "Broken Heart Syndrome" [29] and depression and depression-anxiety syndromes. Often, CAN leads to the need for cardiac intervention or an implanted cardiac device. CAN affects longevity.

Mitochondrial dysfunction is a concern in that it produces a significant amount of harmful compounds in the body, called reactive oxygen species (ROS) and free radicals [30]. Free radicals include nitric oxide (in excess), hydroxyl radicals ($OH^-$), and superoxides (aka ozone, $O_2$ to $O_2^-$). As mentioned above, a source of free radicals is the leakage from the electron transport chain. Free

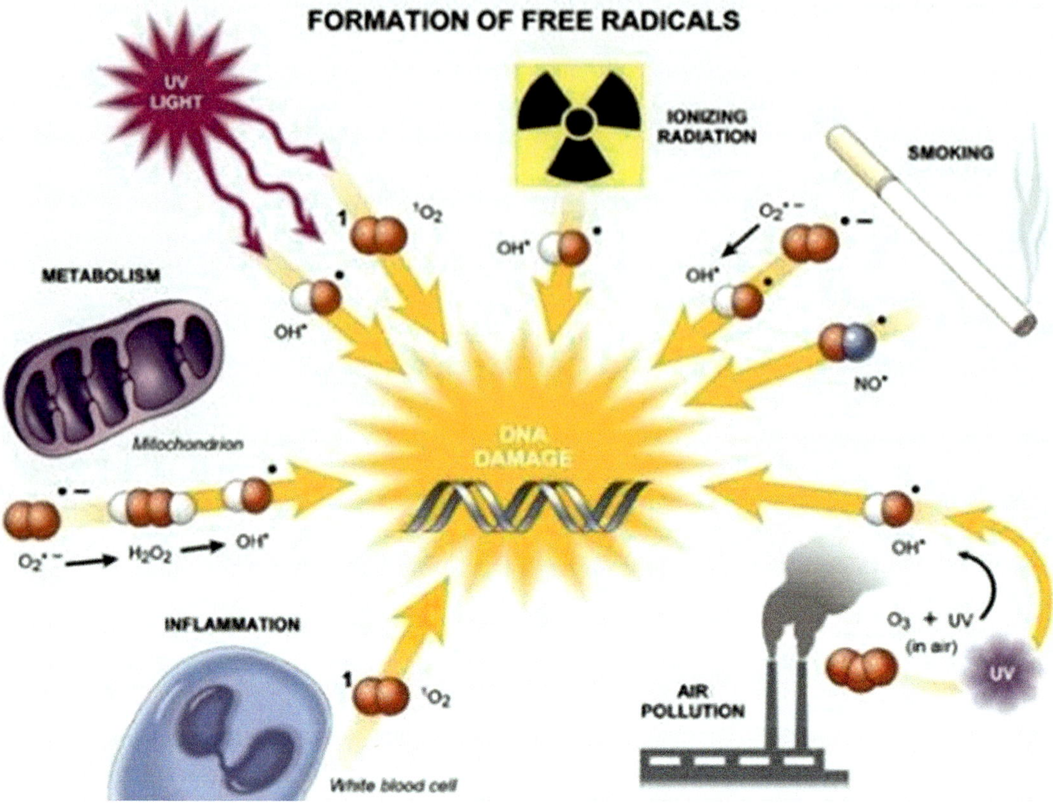


**Fig. 2.17** Free radicals come from many sources: internally (e.g., "leaky" mitochondria and inflammation), externally (e.g., radiation and air pollution), and through lifestyle (e.g., UV from sunbathing and air pollution from living or working in polluted areas and poor nutrition). (Reproduced from Fig. 4 in [31]. Elsevier, Open Access; http://scialert.net/fulltext/?doi=rji.2010.129.145)

radicals are also caused by environmental and lifestyle affects (see Fig. 2.17). They all include an unpaired electron in their outer valence. Antioxidants neutralize free radicals by donating an electron to fill the outer valence pair (see Fig. 2.18). If the electron is not donated by an antioxidant, it will find one elsewhere, thereby damaging the structure from which it takes the electron. On average, the body produces 300 sextillion ($3 \times 10^{23}$) free radicals *per day*! [32]. This number increases with illness or injury. This is the reason exogenous antioxidants are studied herein, especially the more potent antioxidants. Given the harm that is often induced by ROS and free radicals, a brief review is provided to highlight the importance of antioxidants in promoting QoL (reducing morbidity risk) and longevity (reducing mortality risk).

## The Importance of Antioxidants

Reactive oxygen species (ROS) and free radicals are highly reactive and oxygen- and nitrogen-bearing molecules. Sources of ROS are either (1) endogenous (generated within cells or tissues, including mitochondria, peroxisomes, lipoxygenases, NADPH oxidase, and cytochrome P450) or (2) exogenous (generated in the environment, outside the body, including ultraviolet light, ionizing radiation, chemotherapeutics, inflammatory cytokines, and environmental toxins); see Fig. 2.17 [33]. ROS may easily turn into a source of cell and tissue injury, thereby leading to disorders that effect QoL and increase mortality risk. Because humans were made to breath oxygen (molecular oxygen, $O_2$), they have mechanisms and strategies to care-

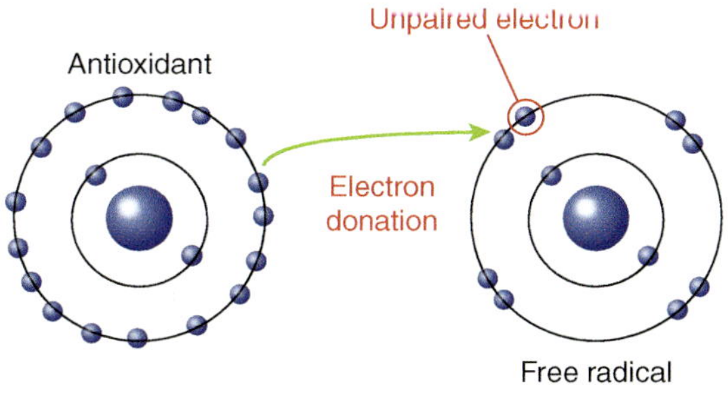


**Fig. 2.18** Free radicals require another electron to complete the electron pairing in their outer valance to be neutral. If the electron is not donated by an antioxidant, it will find one elsewhere, thereby damaging the structure from which it takes the electron. On average, the body produces 300 sextillion ($3 \times 10^{23}$) free radicals *per day*! This number increases with illness or injury. This is the reason for needing antioxidants. (Reproduced from: Presser A. Antioxidants: Our Defense Against Free Radicals. 22 Sep 14 (Free Access). Art Presser is President, Huntington College of Health Sciences. http://blog.primohealthcoach.com/bid/185899/Antioxidants-Our-Defense-Against-Free-Radicals)

fully control the generation of ROS and free other radicals (molecules with an oxygen atom that is missing an electron, $O^+$, or with an extra electron $O^-$); see Fig. 2.18. ROS and free other radicals are highly toxic to cells and tissues [34, 35]. Humans also have mechanisms to "make use" of these molecules under physiological conditions as tools to modulate signal transduction, gene expression, immune support, and cell function [33].

ROS also include molecules that are known as reactive oxygen intermediates (ROI) and reactive nitrogen species (RNS). ROS (collectively) include (1) chemical species formed from incomplete reduction of molecular oxygen, namely, superoxide radical anions ($O_2^-$), hydrogen peroxides ($H_2O_2$), and hydroxyl radicals ($OH^\cdot$); (2) ozone ($O_3$) and singlet oxygen molecules ($^1O_2$), technically known as ROI, as well as compounds such as hypochlorous (HOCl), hypobromous (HOBr), and hypoiodous acids (HOI); (3) molecules such as peroxyl ($ROO^\cdot$), alkoxyl ($RO^\cdot$), semiquinone ($SQ^-$), and carbonate ($CO_3^-$) radicals and organic hydroperoxides (ROOH); and (4) RNS that bear oxygen atoms that include nitric oxide radicals (NO or $NO^\cdot$), nitrogen dioxide radicals ($NO_2^\cdot$), nitrites ($NO_2^-$), and peroxynitrites ($ONOO^-$) [33].

ROS, in particular hydroxyl and peroxyl radicals, hydrogen peroxide, and superoxide radical anion, have long been implicated in oxidative damage inflicted on fatty acids, DNA, and proteins, as well as other cellular components [33, 36]. ROS overproduction is associated with numerous disorders [37]. Oxidative stress caused by the imbalance between excessive formation of ROS and limited antioxidant defenses is connected to many pathologies, including age-related disorders, cancer, cardiovascular and inflammatory diseases, and neurodegenerative diseases, such as Parkinson's and Alzheimer's [38–41].

According to the long-held "free radical theory of aging" [42, 43] advanced by Denham Harman in 1956, the noxious effects of ROS, generated during cellular respiration at the mitochondrial level, are directly involved in aging processes. This hypothesis is, however, currently under revision [36]. Mounting evidence suggests that a little ROS actually may have a beneficial physiological role, acting as messengers in cellular signaling [36, 39, 44–47]. The redox regulation typically involves controlled production of ROSs and RONs (collectively (RONS). They can, in turn, react with specific functional groups of target proteins (e.g., [Fe–S] clusters, cysteines, etc.) that lead to covalent protein modifications. ROS as second messengers are important for the expression of several transcription factors and other signal transduction molecules, such as heat shock-inducing factor and nuclear factor. They also participate in the regulation of cell adhesion, redox-mediated amplification of immune response, and programmed cell death [33].

However, like all things in life, too much of a good thing is no longer good. Too much oxygen burns and destroys. Fire is an oxygen reaction, or oxidative reaction. Excessive oxygen reactions literally burn structures. A derangement in oxygen management results in sustained levels of oxidative stress, which can play a significant role in the development of major human diseases characterized by chronic inflammation, chronic activation of wound healing, and tissue fibrogenesis (essentially, excessive scarring, both inside and out) [33].

Oxidative stress effects pathways by injecting too much energy into the normal oxidative reaction, permitting an incomplete oxygen (or nitrogen, see Fig. 2.18) to be attached to compounds that are used normally. These harmful compounds are very toxic, and, if not neutralized by antioxidants (see Fig. 2.18), they cause damage. This damage promotes disease, especially various forms of cancer, atherosclerosis, and autonomic neuropathy. Antioxidants include those from enzymatic systems (superoxide dismutase, or SOD, catalase, or CAT, and glutathione peroxidase, or GPx) and from nonenzymatic systems (i.e., alpha-lipoic acid, coenzyme Q10, vitamins A, C, or E).

All of these systems (agents) provide an electron to the unpaired oxygen (or nitrogen) outer valence in DNA particles, proteins, lipids, and other components of the body and cell membranes, thereby neutralizing the ROS (see Fig. 2.18). By way of example, the disease atherosclerosis will be considered. To begin with, consider Fig. 2.19. Physiologic stresses, such as

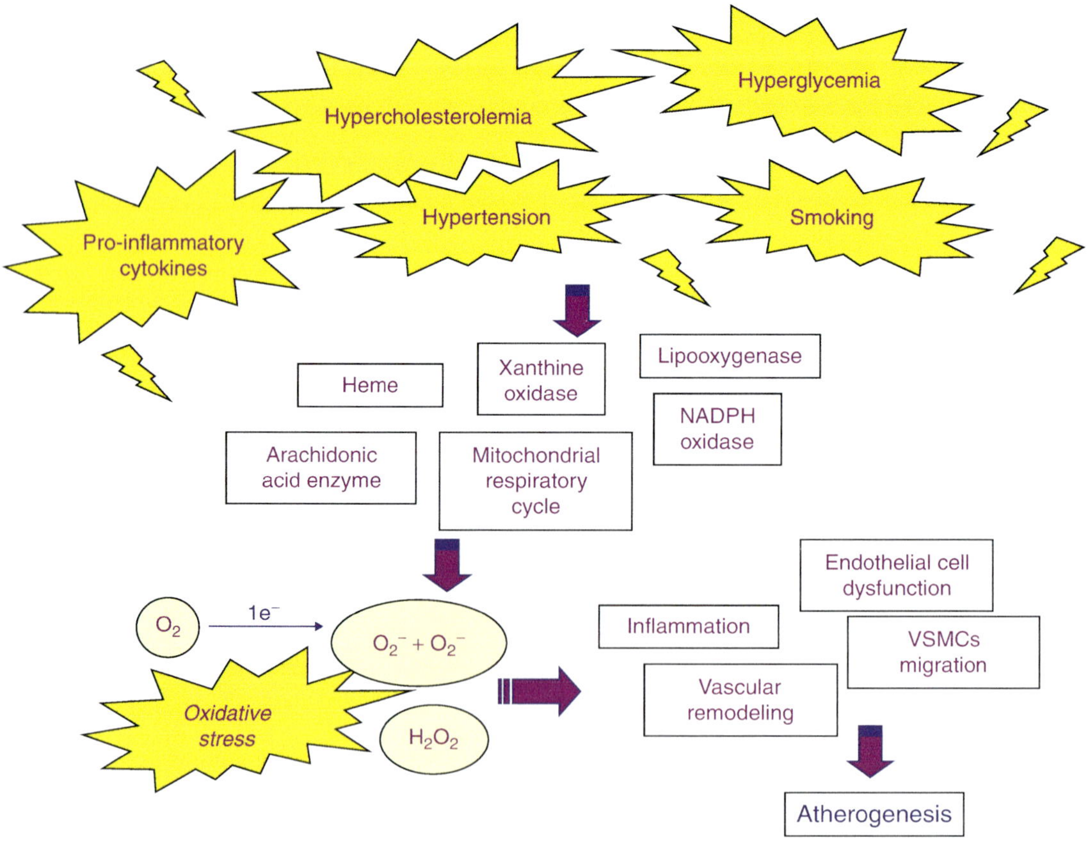


**Fig. 2.19** Role of ROS and oxidative stress in atherosclerosis. $O_2$ oxygen, $O_2^-$ superoxide, $H_2O_2$ hydrogen peroxide, VSMC vascular smooth muscle cell. (Reproduced from Fig. 3 in [48] (InTech, Open Access: https://doi.org/10.5772/53035))

prolonged high BP (hypertension), too much cholesterol (hypercholesterolemia), too much glucose (hyperglycemia), smoking, or excessive inflammation (generating pro-inflammatory cytokines that perpetuate the inflammation), can overstimulate normal functions like mitochondrial respiration (that generates energy, ATP). Persistent overstimulation stresses these normal functions. Note, a little inflammation for a short time is healthy to help with healing and to protect, but prolonged or chronic inflammation is not healthful. This stress may include oxidative stress. Oxidative stress generates ROS or free radicals. At first, ROS and free radicals signal the presence of overstimulation and stress. However, if the ROS signaling persists, the result is persistent inflammation and endothelial cell dysfunction. Endothelial cell dysfunction includes the formation of macrophage foam cells that scavenge ROS, inflammatory cytokines, and other "debris" left by the overstimulation. In excess, foam cells become "sticky," leading to vascular remodeling and the migration of vascular smooth muscle cells, resulting in atherosclerosis.

The result is shown in Fig. 2.20. The whole progression is shown in Figs. 2.21 and 2.22 demonstrating the benefit of antioxidants. Antioxidants limit the number of monocytes that become (differentiate into) macrophages. Antioxidants prevent the oxidation of LDL cholesterol, preventing them from becoming "sticky." Antioxidants also limit the formation of ROS, pro-inflammatory cytokines, and transcription factors, limiting the need for foam cells, not only helping to protect from atherosclerosis but also helping to reduce any pre-existing disease.

The high toxicity attributed to ROS suggests that they are indiscriminate in choosing biological target tissues. The more recent evidence of their signaling role in cells actually suggests the opposite – a well-orchestrated choice of target tissues. The current evidence indicates that individual ROS are selective, based on their precursor's role in normal physiology, and the broad range of target tissues are due to the broad range of reactions for the various species contained within the ROS family [51].

ROS targets include sulfur compounds, both methionine and cysteine [52], also carbon compounds, either in nucleosides or in amino acids such as arginine, lysine, proline, and threonine [53], as well as in polyunsaturated fatty acids

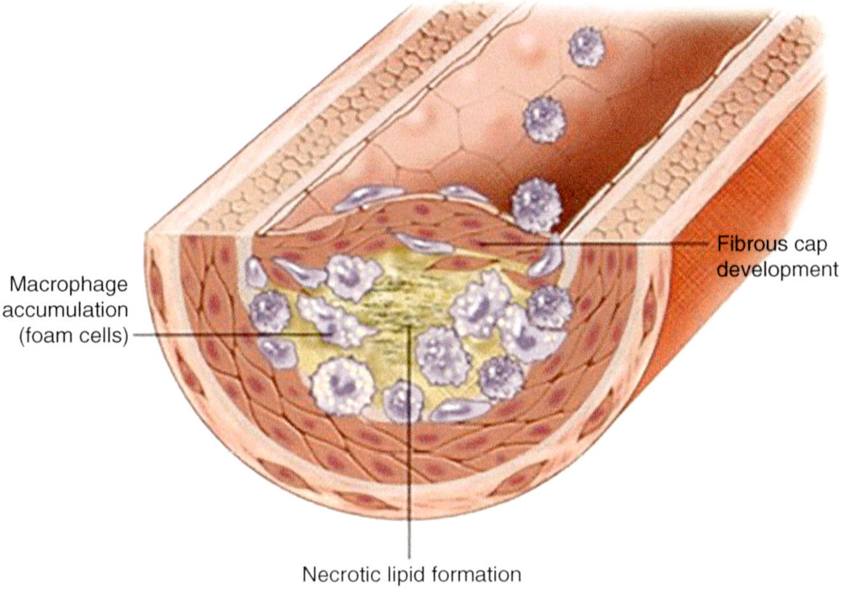


**Fig. 2.20** Atherosclerotic lesion progression. This illustration shows an advanced atherosclerotic plaque with uptake of oxidized LDL by macrophages, which become foam cells. Reactive oxygen species induce necrosis and apoptosis, leading to a necrotic core. Inflammatory cells promote cytokine and growth factor release that stimulates fibrous cap formation. (Modified with permission from [49]. https://radiologykey.com/noninvasive-imaging-of-atherosclerosis/)

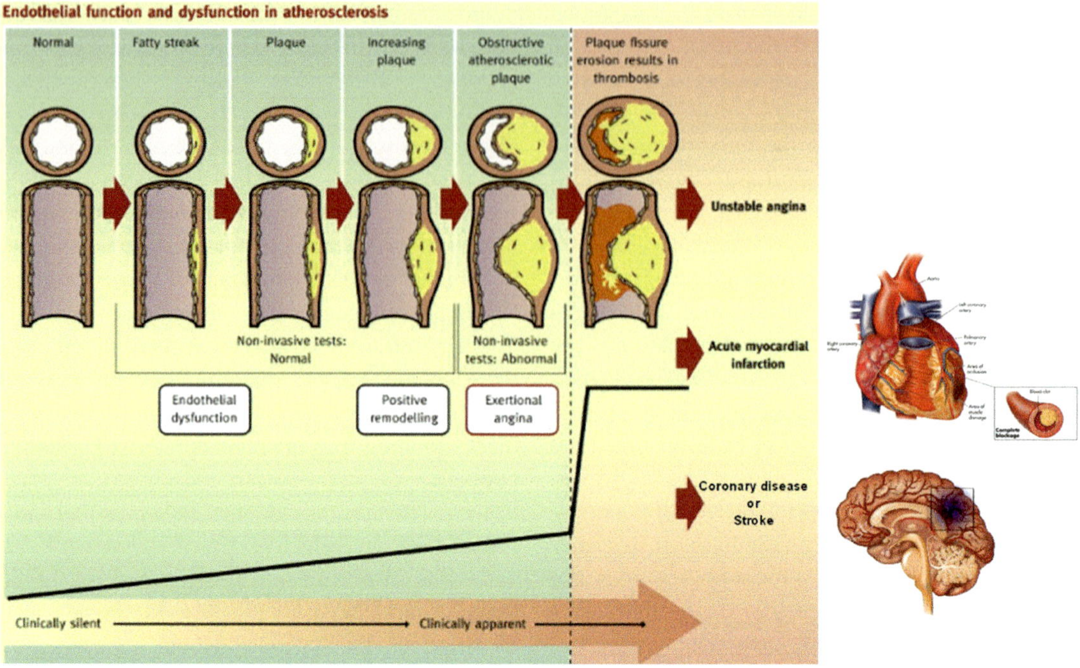


**Fig. 2.21** Progression of atherosclerosis due to endothelial dysfunction, increasing morbidity risk (e.g., unstable angina and other coronary disease) and mortality risk (e.g., including stroke and MI). (Adapted with permission from [50]. Adapted from http://www.cardiachealth.org/heart-information/atherosclerosis)

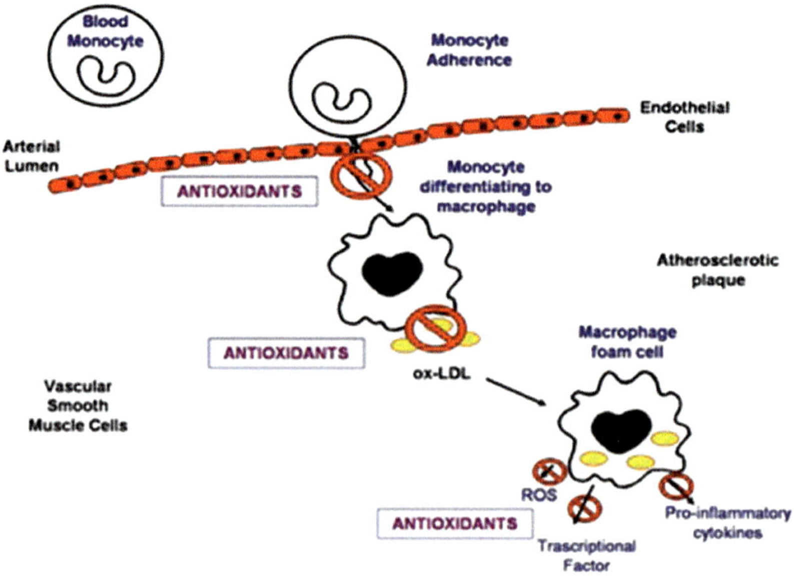


**Fig. 2.22** Potential atheroprotective role of antioxidants in the atherogenic process. ox-LDL oxidized low-density lipoprotein, ROS reactive oxygen species. (Reproduced from Fig. 4 in [48] InTech, Open Access: https://doi.org/10.5772/53035)

[54]. Hydrogen peroxide ($H_2O_2$) typically reacts with thiols in their anionic form [55]. Superoxide radical anion ($O_2^-$) in turn favors reaction with [Fe–S] clusters. A large number of proteins are affected by ROS, where following ROS attack, conformational changes take place that regulate protein activity [56]. Oxidative stress in proteins leads to formation of carbonyl derivatives along their backbone, used as markers of general oxidative stress [57, 58]. Mitochondrial DNA is a major target of ROS. Given that mitochondria are the prevalent source of ROS within cells, this leads to compromised mitochondrial function. ROS reactions with DNA itself, rather than proteins, may serve to promote transcription [52]. Aging cells have an increased level of ROS-damaged nuclear DNA [57]. Lipids, including cell membrane lipids, and organelle membranes, including mitochondria, are common and frequent targets [59].

The lifestyles and supplements (program as depicted in Fig. 1) studied in this book are, collectively, shown to maintain a healthy P&S nervous system and healthy mitochondria. This program also attempts to slow down atherosclerosis production in blood vessels (Fig. 2.21) and suppress oxidative stress. Oxidative stress occurs when there is an imbalance with too much ROS compared to antioxidants (Fig. 2.23). An example at the subcellular (organelle) level is demonstrated in the micrograph shown in Fig. 2.24. The micrograph is of a mitochondrion exposed to high levels of free radicals (ROS). At the cellular level (Fig. 2.25), free radicals ultimately damage cell membranes, causing cells to lyse (thereby be destroyed, accelerating the aging effect, see examples in Fig. 2.26) or grow excessively (possibly leading to cancer).

The aging effect increases morbidity and mortality risk, leading to disease, including life-threatening

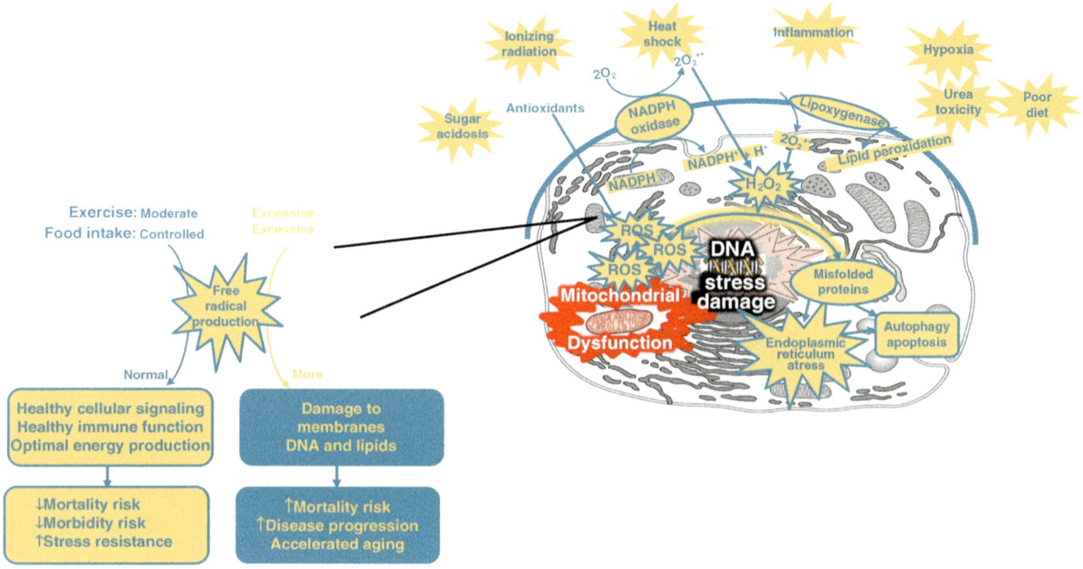


**Fig. 2.23** Oxidative stress affects many pathways, including DNA and protein activity, normal cell development and death (apoptosis), ROS signaling, and mitochondrial function. Proper antioxidant balance relieves oxidative stress. The insert, using mitochondria as the example, illustrates the benefits of a proper balance between ROS (low-level free radicals) and antioxidants. (Cell Image from Shutterstock Royalty-free stock vector images ID: 780737359 Animal human cell structure educational science. Microscope 3d eukaryotic nucleus organelle medicine analysis. Glowing white gray biology poster template isolated line art vector illustration by LuckyStep. Mitochondrion illustration adapted from Shutterstock Royalty-free stock illustration ID: 1008265135, Section of Mitochondria by Aldona Griskeviciene. Adapted from http://www.enzolifesciences.com/platforms/cellular-analysis/oxidative-stress/ (left) and https://fitnessgenes.com/blog/oxidative-stress/ (right))

disease. At the system level, free radicals may affect every system in the body (Fig. 2.27). For example, aging is associated with increased risk of developing cardiovascular diseases (CVDs) in large part through the development of arterial dysfunction due, in part, to vascular endothelial dysfunction and stiffening of arteries (aorta and carotid arteries).

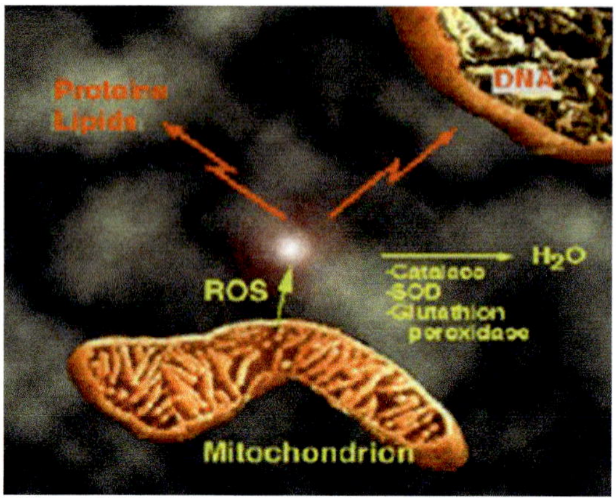


**Fig. 2.24** A micrograph of a mitochondrion damaged by excess free radicals or ROS. (Reproduced from Fig. 13 in [60] (Mary Ann Liebert, Inc., Open Access: https://doi.org/10.5772/53035))

Evidence-based studies of healthy lifestyle, pharmaceutical, and nutraceutical strategies demonstrate that these therapies delay, minimize, or prevent arterial aging or, in late middle-aged or older adults (who already demonstrate features of vascular aging), improve arterial function and reduce the risk of CVD (Fig. 2.28). The body's antioxidant network (Fig. 2.29) is designed to prevent all of these effects: at the organelle, cellular, organ, and system levels. Inflammation exacerbates the aging effect by further damaging mitochondria and blocking the electron transport chain. The imbalance between inflammatory and anti-inflammatory signals contributes to the progression of aging (Fig. 2.30) [63].

The six-pronged lifestyle and supplement approach described herein was developed after many years of empirical and clinical experience with thousands of patients. It is partially based on valuable information obtained from the medical literature, including many significant studies [1]. It also involves incorporating principles of biochemistry and theories of biological feasibility. While this program does not diagnose or treat diseases, it is very useful in promoting wellness.

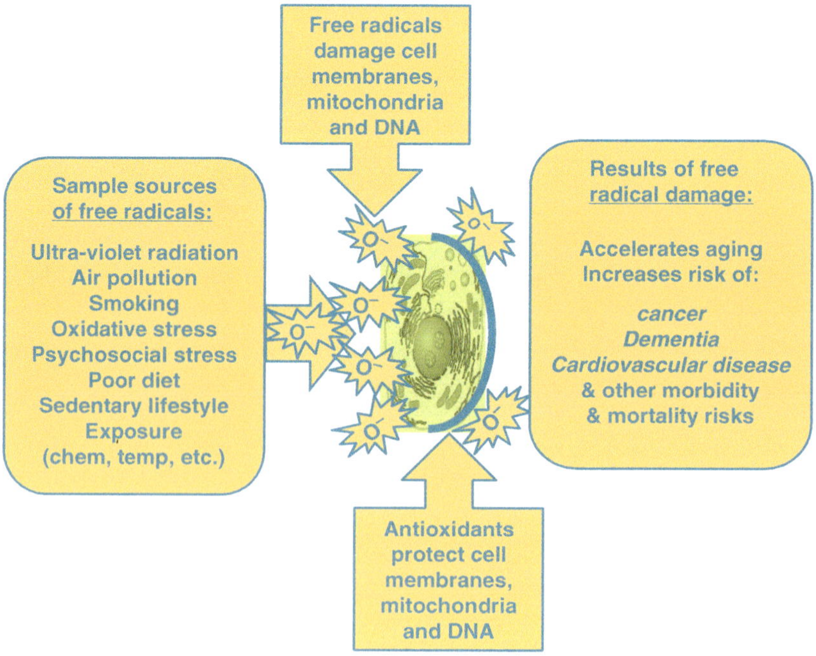


**Fig. 2.25** The effect of free radicals at the cellular level, accelerating aging affects or possibly leading to cancer

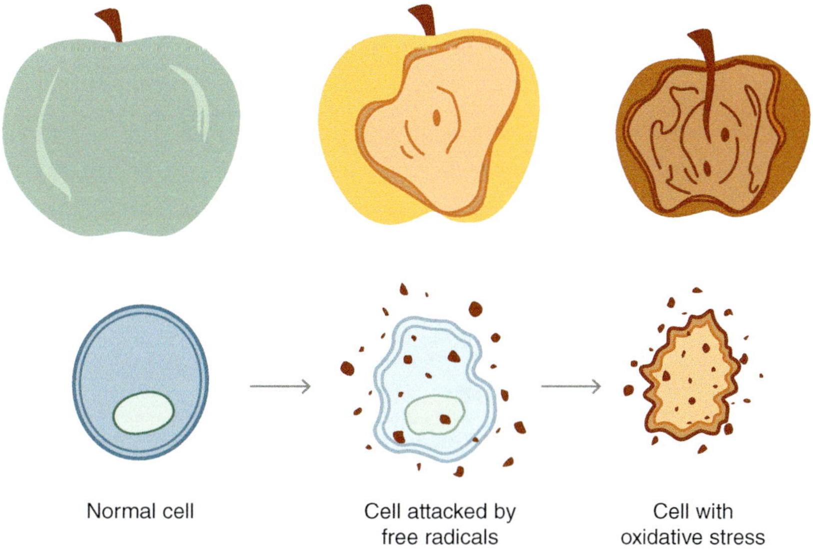


**Fig. 2.26** The oxidation of fruit, like these apples, demonstrates how oxidative stress breaks down cells, causing premature aging and disease. (Illustrations by Elysian Creative Studio, www.elysiancreativestudio.com, Lizzy Colombo)

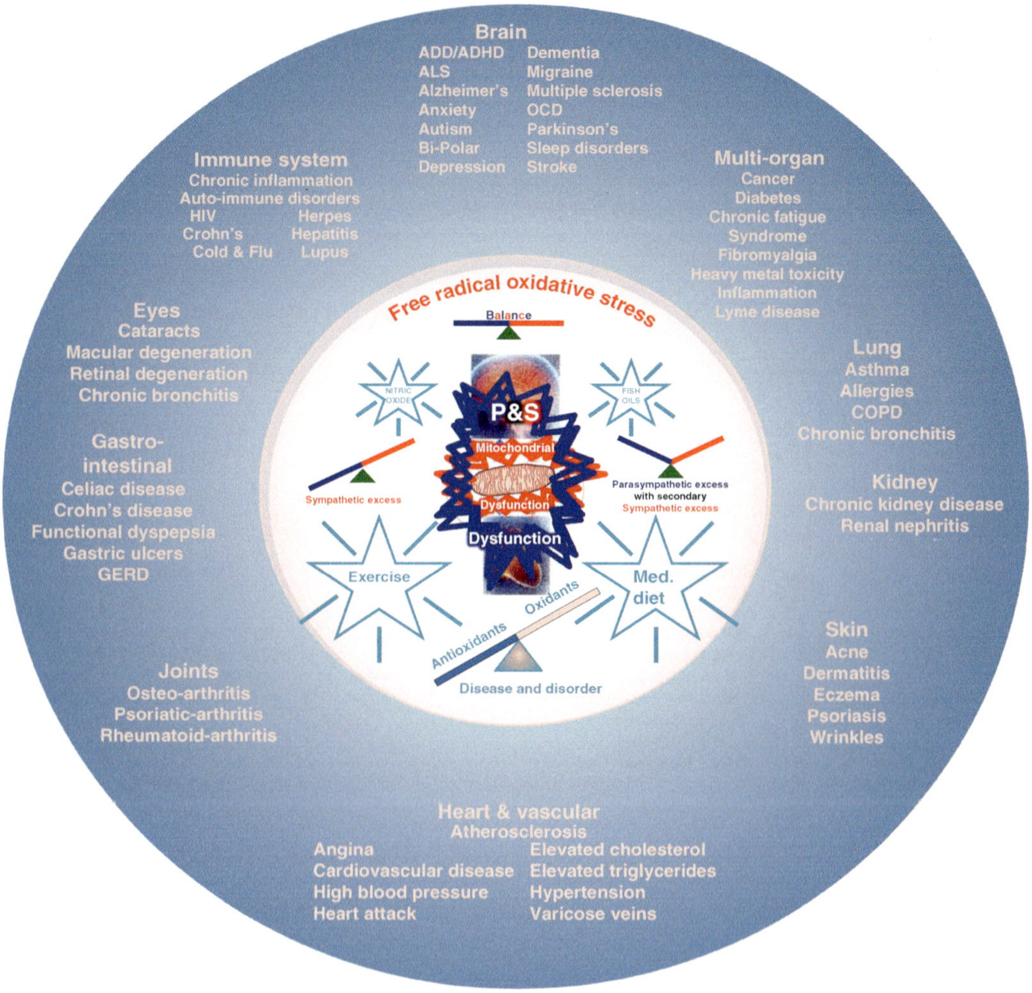


**Fig. 2.27** The effects of oxidative stress at the system level and on the human body. (https://oprocyn.com/oxidative-stress/)

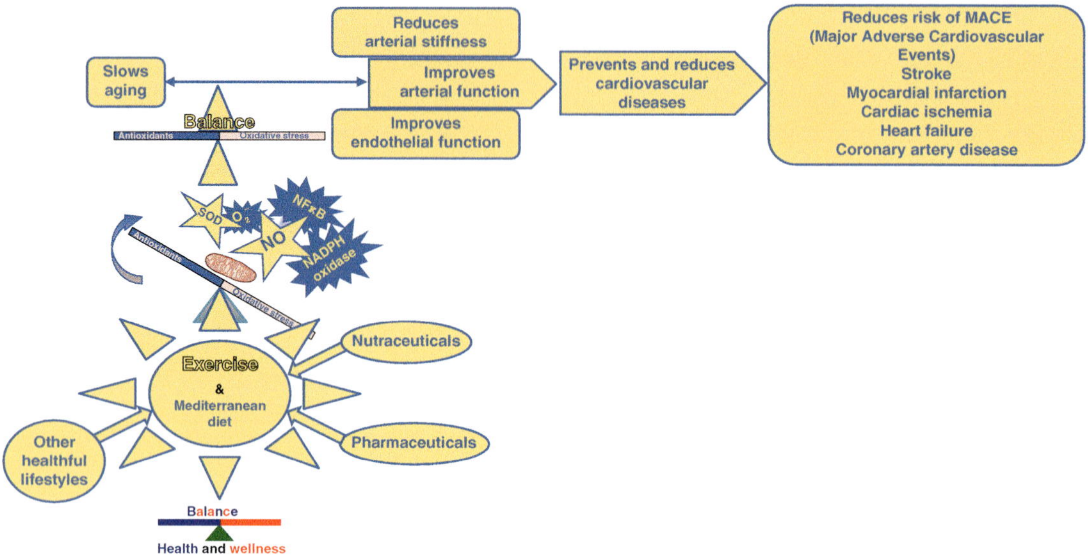


**Fig. 2.28** One of the effects of aging is dysfunction of arteries that leads to cardiovascular disease (CVD). Lifestyle, pharmacology, and nutraceutical strategies slow the aging effects (see Figs. 2.25 and 2.26) and thereby relieve or prevent CVD and other diseases [61]

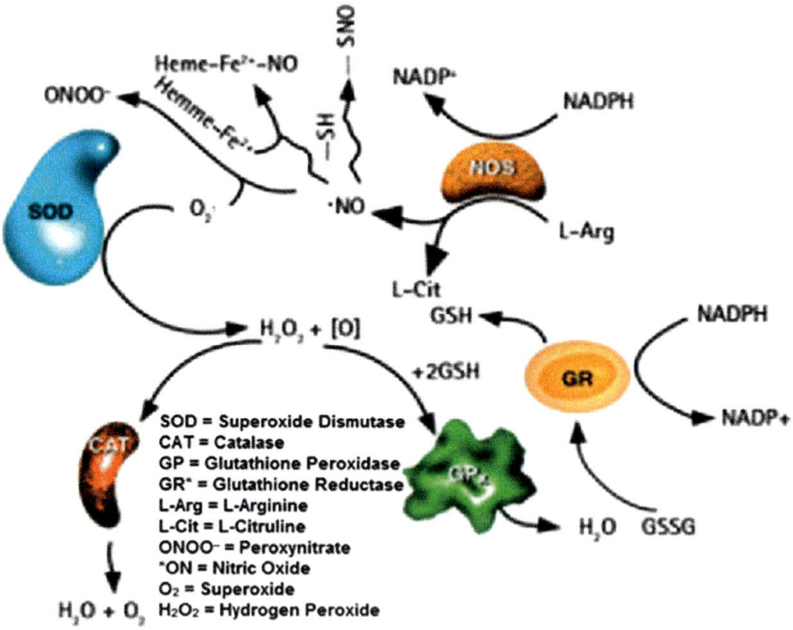


**Fig. 2.29** The antioxidant network. This is the normal system that naturally exists within the body. Notice that some of them are well-known free radicals (e.g., $H_2O_2$). Often, free radicals help to eliminate other free radicals when the balance is right (two negatives can make a positive!). However, as we age and get sick, this network weakens. The Mind-Body Wellness Program is designed to support and strengthen this network. (Reproduced from Fig. 8 in [62] (Open Access, www.nature.com))

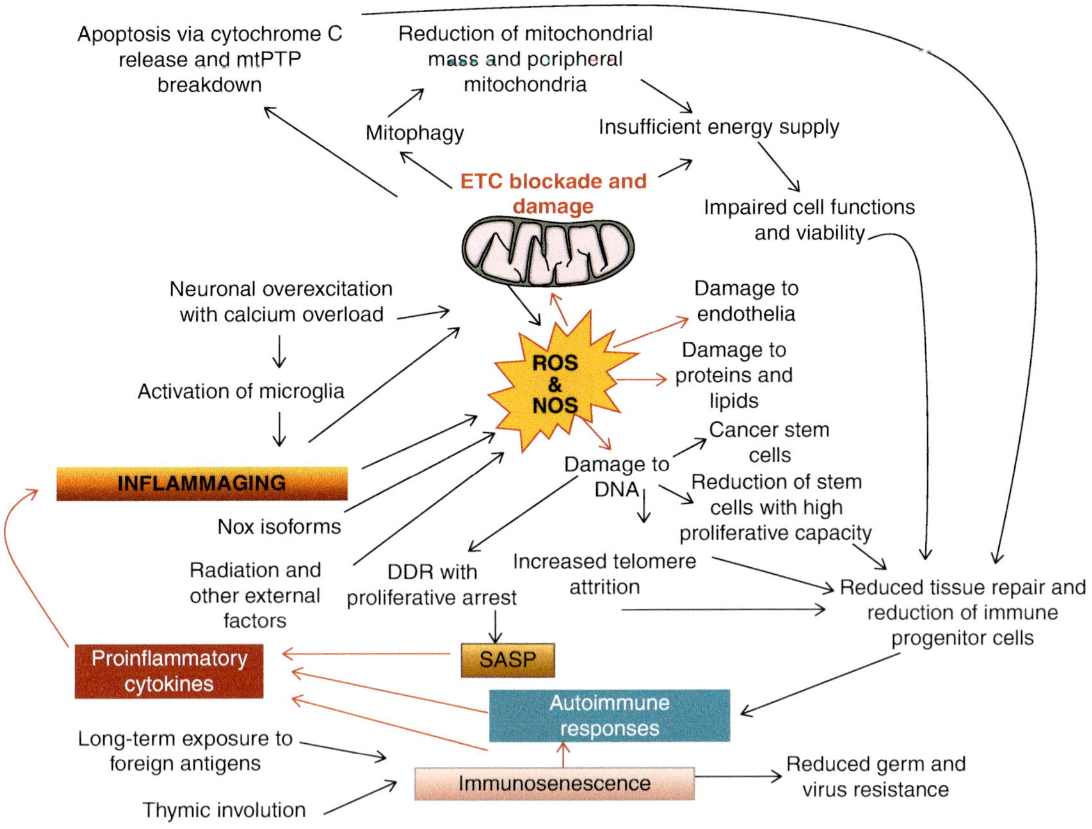


**Fig. 2.30** The imbalance between inflammatory and anti-inflammatory signals is a hallmark of aging and contributes to its progression. An age-related pro-inflammatory tendency ("inflamm-aging" [63]) is mostly unavoidable because of thymic involution and extended germ exposure. Mitochondrial dysfunction ensues with disruption of the electron transport chain and reactive oxygen and nitrogen species generation. (Reproduced with permission from [63] (Springer International Publishing AG). Source: [63, Fig. 8.25])

It does involve a combination of commonly used pharmaceutical agents – for example, statins to lower cholesterol when necessary – along with (1) various nutraceuticals (including vitamins, minerals, and potent antioxidants such as alpha-lipoic acid and coenzyme Q10), (2) beneficial lifestyle behavior (including exercise and stress reduction), and (3) a Mediterranean diet. A general goal should be the creation of an antioxidant milieu so that, in principal, oxidative stress is depressed (Figs. 2.22 and 2.23).

Pharmaceutical agents are developed by research and development companies and pass rigorous protocols before they are accepted by Food and Drug Administration agencies. For the most part, they require prescriptions by licensed physicians. Pharmaceuticals are primarily backed by what are known as randomized, controlled, clinical studies or similar-type well-designed studies, which demonstrate the efficacy of these medicines, especially in treating various ailments. Nutraceuticals are called "functional foods" and are part of functional medicine. A nutraceutical is a food product, such as a fortified food or supplemental dietary product, or vitamin that is believed to provide some health or medical benefit above its nutritional value. They are not used to diagnose or treat diseases.

Hippocrates (Fig. 2.31), the father of ancient medicine, said, "Let food be your medicine." The

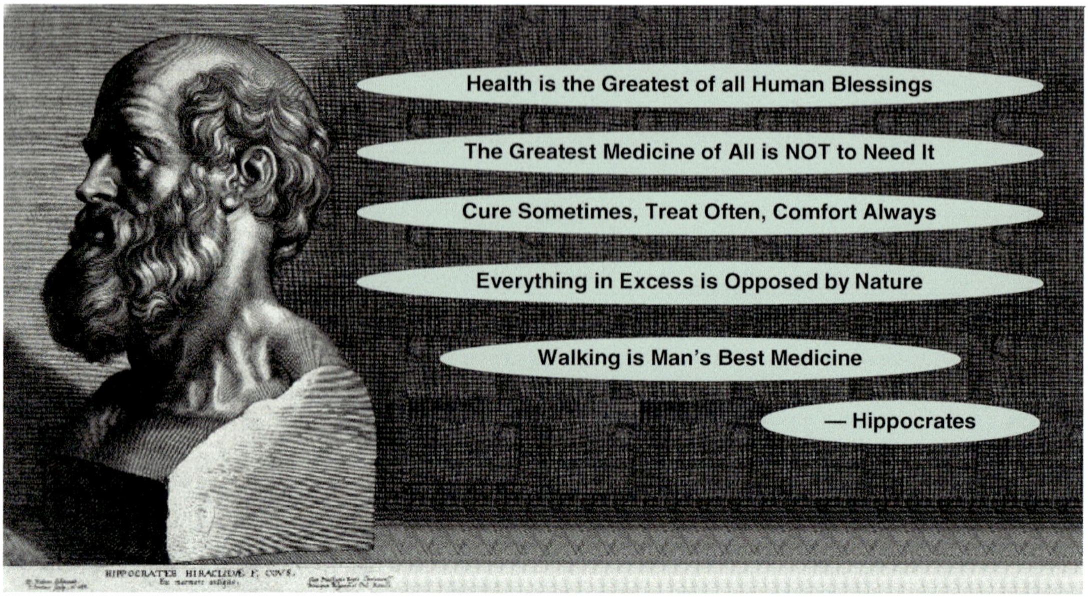


**Fig. 2.31** Hippocrates. (Reproduced from Shutterstock Royalty-free stock illustration ID: 242815789, Hippocrates (460–375 BC). Engraving after an ancient sculpture. By P. Pontius, 17th century French school, by Everett Historical. Source: http://www.skibbereeneagle.ie/latest/hippocrates-of-kos/)

Mediterranean diet (Fig. 2.32) has been shown in numerous studies [see Mediterranean Diet section below] to be efficacious and perhaps the most valuable diet in reducing incidence of heart disease and cancer in large populations of patients. It is very similar to the Japanese diet in many respects. Fish is a component, as are omega-3 fatty acids (Fig. 2.33), which are found in fish. The Mediterranean diet is a plant-based diet consisting of three major components: olives, grapes, and wheat. Small quantities of wine are allowed and known to be beneficial, and organ meats are limited. Healthy dairy products, such as yogurt, are also options. Since the Seven Countries Study [64] was started in the 1970s by Dr. Ancel Keys, numerous studies have validated the importance of this particular diet in maintaining wellness and have demonstrated advantages in (1) weight loss (reduced body mass index) [65], (2) cardioprotective ability [64, 65], (3) cancer-protective ability [66], (4) improvement in diabetes or insulin resistance [66], and (4) providing other major advantages [66]. Initially, Keys pursued the very important question of how dietary fat influenced cholesterol.

Exercise is a key component of wellness as it beneficially affects the antioxidant environment, reduces inflammation in the body, reduces weight and maintains ideal weight, enhances the good cholesterol in the body to work as a vacuum cleaner, reduces blood pressure, reduces stress, improves P&S nervous system dysfunction, and, potentially, improves the function of the millions of mitochondria in the cells of the body ([67], see more in the Exercise section below). There is no better modality, including pharmacological agents, which can do all of these things [68, 69].

Stress in general, and specifically psychosocial stress, is a major risk factor for heart disease. This was highlighted in the INTERHEART Study [70], which involves 52 countries and showed a significant risk of heart attack in individuals experiencing psychosocial stress. Reduction of psychosocial stress is one aim of our six-prong approach to wellness. It may involve meditation, yoga, exercise, biofeedback, relaxation and breathing exercises, or other recreational activities that produce beneficial effects.

Three types of nutraceuticals are utilized in this program. Omega-3 fatty acids are extremely

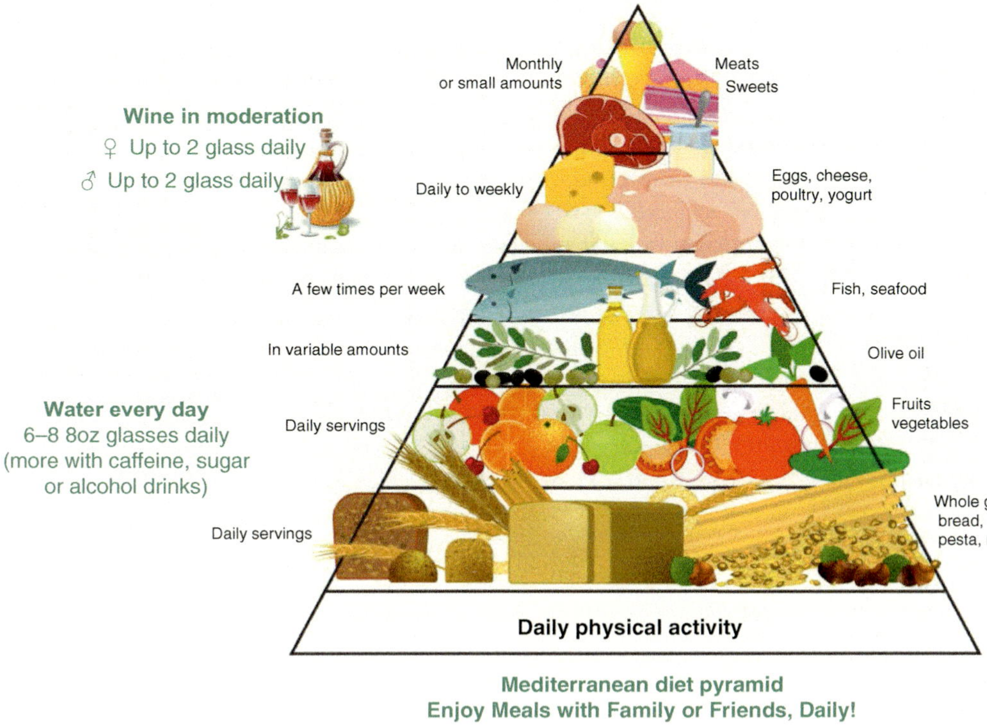


**Fig. 2.32** Mediterranean diet food pyramid. (Adapted from Shutterstock Royalty-free stock vector images ID: 386839267, Mediterranean Diet Image, by Double Brain. Source: https://oldwayspt.org/resources/oldways-mediterranean-diet-pyramid)

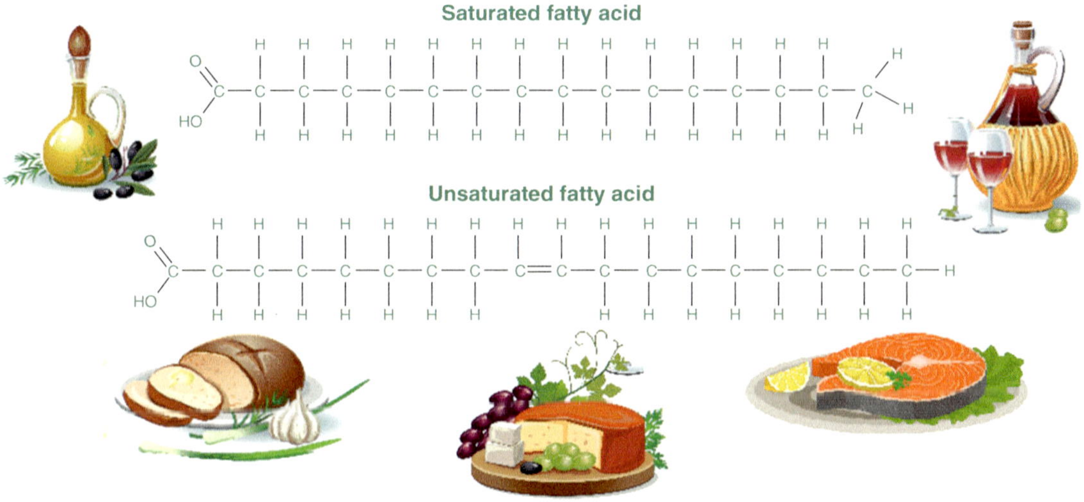


**Fig. 2.33** Fatty-acids molecular structures and food sources. (Adapted from Shutterstock Royalty-free stock vector images ID: 1136773976, Set of Food, by HappyPictures)

important as anti-inflammatory molecules. The others are nitric oxide-promoting compounds or food products, such as L-arginine, L-citrulline, L-carnitine (Fig. 2.34), and beetroot extract (which is a source of inorganic nitrates from the diet). For beneficial antioxidant effects, which is labeled a mitochondrial approach (since most oxidants in the body are produced in the mitochondria), alpha-lipoic acid and coenzyme Q10 specifically are prescribed in concentrations that are deemed optimal (Fig. 2.35). Also, folic acid, B vitamins, vitamin D, and magnesium are very important. As discussed, all of these components have rigorous science and significant statistical data supporting them, individually and in some cases in combination with others.

Dr. Hahnemann, founder of Hahnemann Hospital, Philadelphia, PA, USA, is the father of homeopathic medicine. Homeopathic medicine is a medical philosophy practice using a holistic natural approach to treating illnesses based on the concept that the body can heal itself. It

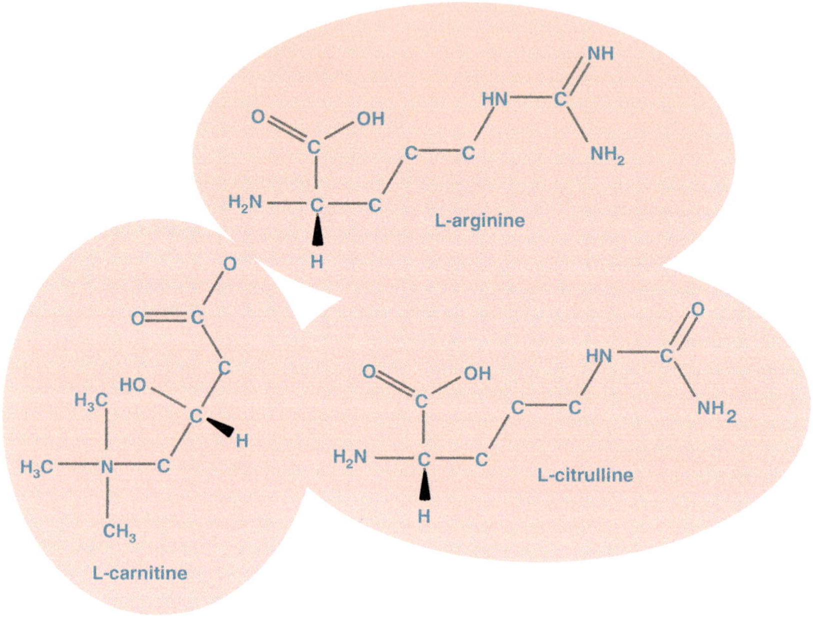


**Fig. 2.34** Amino acid molecular structures. (Source: http://www.chemspider.com/Chemical-Structure.6082.html (L-arginine), http://www.chemspider.com/Chemical-Structure.9367.html (L-citrulline), http://www.chemspider.com/Chemical-Structure.10455.html (L-carnitine))

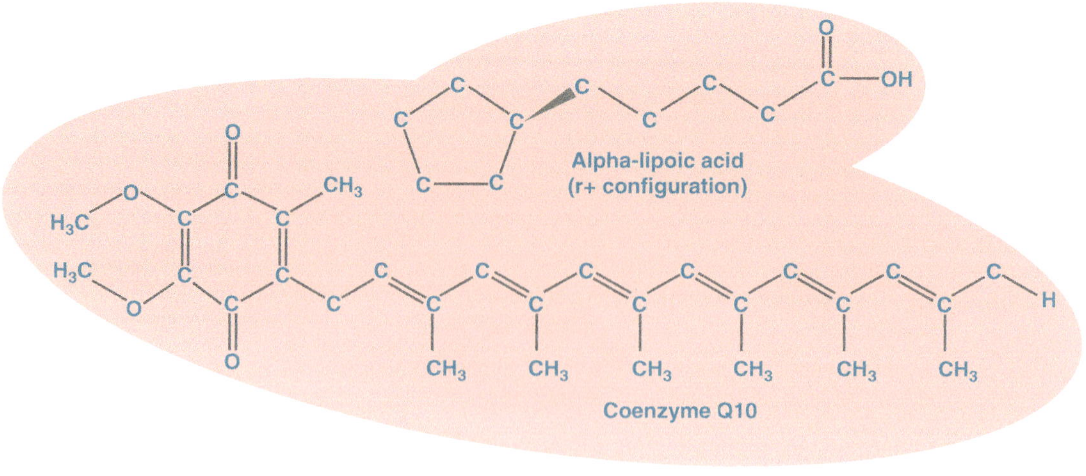


**Fig. 2.35** Antioxidant molecular structures

involves a concept of homeopathic dilution that is "like cures like." In other words, homeopathy uses extremely dilute preparations of natural substances to stimulate the body's own self-healing mechanisms. It is a philosophy of merely providing what may be lacking, rather than attempting to replace or alter what is dysfunctional. Our philosophy modifies this somewhat in that patients are treated holistically with the lowest doses of agents that are necessary to combat a disease.

Sir William Osler (1849–1918), a famous physician, is the father of modern medicine and one of the four founding professors of John Hopkins University. Sir Osler was a physician, pathologist, historian, philosopher, author, teacher, and bibliophile. He created the first residency program for specially trained physicians. He brought students out of lecture halls and into wards. He has had a great impact on modern medicine. Dr. Osler taught, "One of the first duties of physicians is to educate the masses not to take medicine." While he did not believe that no medicines were necessary, it certainly appears that he ascribed to the concept that more is not better; that is, too much medicine may not be beneficial. He also stated, "The person who takes medicine must recover twice, once from the disease and once from the medicine." He went on to state, "The good physician treats the disease. The great physician treats the patient who has the disease." Lastly, he said, "Gentleman, I have a confession to make. Half of what we have taught you is in error, and furthermore, we cannot tell you which half it is." He was a very honest and forthcoming physician whose didactics persist to this day in medical wards.

Dr. Colombo graduated from the University of Rochester School of Medicine with a PhD from the oldest Neuroscience Program, the Center for Brain Research. He studied under Dr. David Felten, the "father" of neuroimmunology. Dr. Felten was the first to discover a nerve synapse on an immune cell. It was an autonomic nerve, a parasympathetic nerve to be exact. Dr. Colombo modeled the interface between the two systems and demonstrated what Dr. Felten hypothesized that the ANS provided the memory for the immune system and that peak immune function occurs when the P&S nervous systems are properly balanced for the individual.

Drs. DePace and Dr. Colombo both have believed in balance. There needs to be balance between work and play (relaxation and the lack of stress), diet and exercise, and secular and spiritual pursuits. There needs to be a proper balance between pharmacological agents that are taken and lifestyle changes. There needs to be a proper balance between the parasympathetic and sympathetic nervous systems. There also needs to be a balance between oxidants and antioxidants. Too many oxidants will favor the process of oxidative stress, which creates a surplus of reactive oxygen species (ROS). ROS damage tissues and proteins and promote many diseases, as mentioned above. All of these are types of "Yin and Yang" balance to help relieve autonomic and mitochondrial dysfunction.

> The good physician treats the disease; the great physician treats the patient who has the disease. (Sir William Osler, Bt)

## References


1. Colombo J, Arora RR, DePace NL, Vinik AI. Clinical autonomic dysfunction: measurement, indications, therapies, and outcomes. New York: Springer Science + Business Media; 2014.
2. Vinik A, Ziegler D. Diabetic cardiovascular autonomic neuropathy. Circulation. 2007;115:387–97.
3. Vinik AI, Maser RE, Nakave AA. Diabetic cardiovascular autonomic nerve dysfunction. US Endocr Dis. 2007;2:2–9.
4. Jay SJ. Orthostatic hypotension and chronic fatigue syndrome. JAMA. 2001;285(11):1441–3. https://doi.org/10.1001/jama.285.11.1441.
5. https://my.clevelandclinic.org/health/articles/what-are-mitochondrial-diseases
6. Zhang ZW, Cheng J, Xu F, Chen YE, Du JB, Yuan M, Zhu F, Xu XC, Yuan S. Red blood cell extrudes nucleus and mitochondria against oxidative stress. IUBMB Life. 2011;63(7):560–5. https://doi.org/10.1002/iub.490.
7. Fillingame RH, Angevine CM, Dmitriev OY. Coupling proton movements to c-ring rotation in F(1)F(o) ATP synthase: aqueous access channels and helix rotations at the a-c interface. Biochim Biophys Acta. 2002;1555(1–3):29–36.
8. Kennedy DO. B vitamins and the brain: mechanisms, dose and efficacy – a review. Nutrients. 2016;8(2):68. https://doi.org/10.3390/nu8020068.

9. Tobias H, Vinitsky A, Bulgarelli RJ, Ghosh-Dastidar S, Colombo J. Autonomic nervous system monitoring of patients with excess parasympathetic responses to sympathetic challenges – clinical observations. US Neurol. 2010;5(2):62–6.
10. Arora RR, Bulgarelli RJ, Ghosh-Dastidar S, Colombo J. Autonomic mechanisms and therapeutic implications of postural diabetic cardiovascular abnormalities. J Diabetes Sci Technol. 2008;2(4):568–71.
11. Nanavati SH, Bulgarelli RJ, Vazquez-Tanus J, Ghosh-Dastidar S, Colombo J, Arora RR. Altered autonomic activity with atrial fibrillation as demonstrated by non-invasive autonomic monitoring. US Cardiol. 2010;7(1):47–50.
12. Tsuji H, Venditti FJ Jr, Manders ES, Evans JC, Larson MG, Feldman CL, Levy D. Reduced heart rate variability and mortality risk in an elderly cohort. The Framingham Heart Study. Circulation. 1994;90(2):878–83.
13. Maser R, Mitchell B, Vinik AI, Freeman R. The association between cardiovascular autonomic neuropathy and mortality in individuals with diabetes, a meta-analysis. Diabetes Care. 2003;26(6):1895–901.
14. Vinik AI, Maser RE, Mitchell BD, Freeman R. Diabetic autonomic neuropathy. Diabetes Care. 2003;26(5):1553–79.
15. Curtis BM, O'Keefe JH. Autonomic tone as a cardiovascular risk factor: the dangers of chronic fight or flight. Mayo Clin Proc. 2002;77:45–54.
16. DePace NL, Mears JP, Yayac M, Colombo J. Cardiac autonomic testing and diagnosing heart disease. "A clinical perspective". Heart Int. 2014;9(2):37–44. https://doi.org/10.5301/heartint.5000218; published online 12/5/2014 12:29:58 PM.
17. DePace NL, Mears JP, Yayac M, Colombo J. Cardiac autonomic testing and treating heart disease. "A clinical perspective". Heart Int. 2014;9(2):45–52. https://doi.org/10.5301/heartint.5000216; published online 11/19/2014 1:16:08 PM.
18. Bullinga JR, Alharethi R, Schram MS, Bristow MR, Gilbert EM. Changes in heart rate variability are correlated to hemodynamic improvement with chronic CARVEDILOL therapy in heart failure. J Card Fail. 2005;11(9):693–9.
19. Fatoni C, Raffa S, Regoli F, Giraldi F, La Rovere MT, Prentice J, Pastori F, Fratini S, Salerno-Uriarte JA, Klein HU, Auricchio A. Cardiac resynchronization therapy improves heart rate profile and heart rate variability of patients with moderate to severe heart failure. J Am Coll Cardiol. 2005;46(10):1875–82.
20. Fathizadeh P, Shoemaker WC, Woo CCJ, Colombo J. Autonomic activity in trauma patients based on variability of heart rate and respiratory rate. Crit Care Med. 2004;32(5):1300–5.
21. Chen JY, Fung JW, Yu CM. The mechanisms of atrial fibrillation. J Cardiovasc Electrophysiol. 2006;17(Suppl 3):S2–7.
22. Copie X, Lamaison D, Salvador M, Sadoul N, DaCosta A, Faucher L, Legal F, Le Heuzey JY, VALID Investigators. Heart rate variability before ventricular arrhythmias in patients with coronary artery disease and an implantable cardioverter defibrillator. Ann Noninvasive Electrocardiol. 2003;8(3):179–84.
23. Alter P, Grimm W, Vollrath A, Czerny F, Maisch B. Heart rate variability in patients with cardiac hypertrophy – relation to left ventricular mass and etiology. Am Heart J. 2006;151(4):829–36.
24. Debono M, Cachia E. The impact of cardiovascular autonomic neuropathy in diabetes: is it associated with left ventricular dysfunction? Auton Neurosci. 2007;132(1–2):1–7.
25. Just H. Peripheral adaptations in congestive heart failure: a review. Am J Med. 1991;90:23S–6S.
26. Nakamura K, Matsumura K, Kobayashi S, Kaneko T. Sympathetic premotor neurons mediating thermoregulatory functions. Neurosci Res. 2005;51(1):1–8.
27. Manfrini O, Morgagni G, Pizzi C, Fontana F, Bugiardini R. Changes in autonomic nervous system activity: spontaneous versus balloon-induced myocardial ischemia. Eur Heart J. 2004;25(17):1502–8.
28. Clarke B, Ewing D, Campbell I. Diabetic autonomic neuropathy. Diabetologia. 1979;17:195–212.
29. Litchman JH, Bigger JT Jr, Blumenthal JA, et al. Depression and coronary heart disease recommendations for screening, referral, and treatment: a science advisory from the American Heart Association Prevention Committee of the Council on Cardiovascular Nursing, Council on Clinical Cardiology, Council on Epidemiology and Prevention, and Interdisciplinary Council on Quality of Care and Outcomes Research: endorsed by the American Psychiatric Association. Circulation. 2008;118:1768–75.
30. Murphy MP. How mitochondria produce reactive oxygen species. Biochem J. 2009;417:1–13 (Printed in Great Britain). https://doi.org/10.1042/BJ20081386.
31. Cadenas E, Davies KJA. Mitochondrial free radical generation, oxidative stress, and aging. Free Radic Biol Med. 2000;29(3–4):222–30.
32. National Institute of Standards and Technology. NIST - https://www.nist.gov/.
33. Novo E, Parola M. Redox mechanisms in hepatic chronic wound healing and fibrogenesis. Fibrogenesis Tissue Repair. 2008;1:5; 1–58. http://www.fibrogenesis.com/content/1/1/5.
34. Gerschman R, Gilbert DL, Nye SW, Dwyer P, Fenn WO. Oxygen poisoning and X-irradiation: a mechanism in common. Science. 1954;119:623–6.
35. Gerschman R, Gilbert DL, Nye SW, Fenn WO. Influence of x-irradiation on oxygen poisoning in mice. Proc Soc Exp Biol Med. 1954;86(1):27–9.
36. Halliwell B, Gutteridge JMC. Free radicals in biology and medicine. 4th ed. Oxford: Oxford University Press; 2007.
37. Finkel T, Holbrook NJ. Oxidants, oxidative stress and the biology of aging. Nature. 2000;408:239–47.
38. Dickinson BC, Chang CJ. Chemistry and biology of reactive oxygen species in signaling or stress responses. Nat Chem Biol. 2011;7(8):504–11.
39. Dröge W. Free radicals in the physiological control of cell function. Physiol Rev. 2002;82(1):47–95.

40. Barnham KJ, Masters CL, Bush AI. Neurodegenerative diseases and oxidative stress. Nat Rev Drug Discov. 2004;3(3):205–14.
41. Finkel T, Serrano M, Blasco MA. The common biology of cancer and aging. Nature. 2007;448(7155):767–74.
42. Harman D. Aging: a theory based on free radical and radiation chemistry. J Gerontol. 1956;11(3):298–300.
43. Harman D. Free radical theory of aging. Mutat Res. 1992;275:257–66.
44. Apel K, Hirt H. Reactive oxygen species: metabolism, oxidative stress, and signal transduction. Annu Rev Plant Biol. 2004;55:373–99.
45. Rhee SG. Cell signaling. H2O2, a necessary evil for cell signaling. Science. 2006;312(5782):1882–3.
46. Kagan VE, Quinn PJ. Toward oxidative lipidomics of cell signaling. Antioxid Redox Signal. 2004;6(2):199–202.
47. West JD, Marnett LJ. Endogenous reactive intermediates as modulators of cell signaling and cell death. Chem Res Toxicol. 2006;19(2):173–94.
48. Rodella LF, Favero G. Atherosclerosis and current anti-oxidant strategies for atheroprotection. Curr Trends Atherogenesis. 2012 (InTech, Open Access). https://doi.org/10.5772/53035.
49. Ross R. Atherosclerosis – an inflammatory disease. N Engl J Med. 1999;340:115.
50. Greenland P, Gidding SS, Tracy RP. Commentary: lifelong prevention of atherosclerosis: the critical importance of major risk factor exposures. Int J Epidemiol. 2002;31:1129–34. https://doi.org/10.1093/ije/31.6.1129.
51. Krumova K, Cosa G. Overview of reactive oxygen species. In: Nonell S, Flors C, editors. Singlet oxygen: applications in biosciences and nanosciences, vol. 1. Cambridge: RSC Publishing; 2016. http://pubs.rsc.org/en/content/chapterhtml/2016/bk9781782620389-00001?isbn=978-1-78262-038-9.
52. Nathan C, Cunningham-Bussel A. Beyond oxidative stress: an immunologist's guide to reactive oxygen species. Nat Rev Immunol. 2013;13(3):349–61.
53. Nathan C, Ding A. SnapShot: reactive oxygen intermediates (ROI). Cell. 2010;140(6):951.
54. Yin H, Xu L, Porter NA. Free radical lipid peroxidation: mechanisms and analysis. Chem Rev. 2011;111(10):5944–72.
55. D'Autreaux B, Toledano MB. ROS as signaling molecules: mechanisms that generate specificity in ROS homeostasis. Nat Rev Mol Cell Biol. 2007;8(10):813–24.
56. Nishii W, Kukimoto-Niino M, Terada T, Shirouzu M, Muramatsu T, Kojima M, Kihara H, Yokoyama S. A redox switch shapes the Lon protease exit pore to facultatively regulate proteolysis. Nat Chem Biol. 2015;11(1):46–51.
57. Finkel T, Holbrook NJ. Oxidants, oxidative stress and the biology of aging. Nature. 2000;408(6809):239–47.
58. Stadtman ER. Protein oxidation and aging. Free Radic Res. 2006;40(12):1250–8.
59. Niki E, Noguchi N. Dynamics of antioxidant action of vitamin E. Acc Chem Res. 2004;37(1):45–51.
60. Caro P, Gomez J, Lopez-Torres M, Sanchez I, Naudiand A, et al. Effect of every other day feeding on mitochondrial free radical production and oxidative stress in mouse liver. Rejuvenation Res. 2008;11:621–9.
61. Seals DR, Edward F. Adolph distinguished lecture: the remarkable anti-aging effects of aerobic exercise on systemic arteries. J Appl Physiol. 2014;117(5):425–39. https://doi.org/10.1152/japplphysiol.00362.2014.
62. Adly AAM. Oxidative stress and disease: an updated review. Res J Immunol. 2010;3:129–45.
63. Cardinali DP. Autonomic nervous system: basic and clinical aspects. Cham: Springer International Publishing AG; 2018.
64. Menotti A, Keys A, Blackburn H, Kromhout D, Karvonen M, Nissinen A, Pekkanen J, Punsar S, Fidanza F, Giampaoli S, Seccareccia F, Buzina R, Mohacek I, Nedeljkovic S, Aravanis C, Dontas A, Toshima H, Lanti M. Comparison of multivariate predictive power of major risk factors for coronary heart diseases in different countries: results from eight nations of the Seven Countries Study, 25-year follow-up. J Cardiovasc Risk. 1996;3(1):69–75.
65. Menotti A, Seccareccia F, Blackburn H, Keys A. Coronary mortality and its prediction in samples of US and Italian railroad employees in 25 years within the Seven Countries Study of cardiovascular diseases. Int J Epidemiol. 1995;24(3):515–21.
66. Toshima H, Koga Y, Menotti A, Keys A, Blackburn H, Jacobs DR, Seccareccia F. The Seven Countries Study in Japan. Twenty-five-year experience in cardiovascular and all-causes deaths. Jpn Heart J. 1995;36(2):179–89.
67. Kostka T, Drai J, Berthouze SE, Lacour JR, Bonnefoy M. Physical activity, aerobic capacity and selected markers of oxidative stress and the anti-oxidant defense system in healthy active elderly men. Clin Physiol. 2000;20(3):185–90.
68. Santos-Parker JR, LaRocca TJ, Seals DR. Aerobic exercise and other healthy lifestyle factors that influence vascular aging. Adv Physiol Educ. 2014;38(4):296–307. https://doi.org/10.1152/advan.00088.2014.
69. Seals DR, Edward F. Adolph Distinguished Lecture: the remarkable anti-aging effects of aerobic exercise on systemic arteries. J Appl Physiol. 2014;117(5):425–39. https://doi.org/10.1152/japplphysiol.00362.2014.
70. Rosengren A, Hawken S, Ounpuu S, Sliwa K, Zubaid M, Almahmeed WA, Blackett KN, Sitthi-amorn C, Sato H, Yusuf S, INTERHEART investigators. Association of psychosocial risk factors with risk of acute myocardial infarction in 11119 cases and 13648 controls from 52 countries (the INTERHEART study): case-control study. Lancet. 2004;364(9438):953–62.

# Omega-3 Fatty Acids (Prong-1)

# 3

All six lifestyle and supplement prongs are equally important. No one is more crucial than any other. They all work together as a team in promoting health and wellness by balancing the parasympathetic and sympathetic (P&S) imbalance that underlies autonomic dysfunction and the antioxidant imbalance that underlies mitochondrial dysfunction. The first prong involves Omega-3 fatty acids (Fig. 3.1). Omega-3 fatty acids are a type of polyunsaturated fatty acid (PUFA; "n-3" is an abbreviation for "Omega-3," the whole abbreviation is n-3 PUFA, or Omega-3). There are also Omega-6 and Omega-9 fatty acids that will be part of the discussion. The "Omega" and the number (3, 6, or 9) designations specify where the fatty acid has sites by which it may bind with other molecules. So it, in part, defines the function of the particular fatty acid (e.g., Omega-3). Why are fatty acids important? You know there are lipoproteins: low-density lipoproteins (LDLs, known as the "bad" cholesterols[1]) and high-density lipoproteins (HDLs, known as the "good" cholesterols). Fatty acids are the "lipo" (fat) part of lipoproteins, regardless of the type. Fatty acids are also the main building blocks of cellular and organelle (i.e., mitochondria and nucleus) membranes (part of the *lipid* bilayer; see Fig. 2.14, ("inner membrane" depicted as the two sheets of yellow balls with yellow "tails" connecting them, the balls represent the lipid parts and the tails represent the protein parts of the lipoproteins). The "Omega" number determines function and flexibility of the membrane. For example, too much Omega-6 makes for stiff membranes that are less permeable. More Omega-3 makes for more supple membranes that are more permeable. The three types of Omega-3 fatty acids that are included in the discussions are alpha-linoleic acid (ALLA[2]), docosahexaenoic acid (DHA), and eicosapentaenoic acid (EPA). It is well known that high LDL levels are a risk factor for atherosclerosis leading to heart attack or stroke, so are low HDL levels. This section will expand on these issues and discuss the fish oil portion of the solution.

As introduced in the previous chapter, oxidized LDLs are a real problem. Granted, reducing the amount of LDL reduces the opportunity for LDLs to be oxidized. Reducing oxidized LDLs reduces the formation of foam cells, which are the start of atherosclerosis. Omega-3 fatty acids help to prevent the oxidation of LDLs and therefore are a key factor in health and wellness. In total, as will be discussed below, fish oil with Omega-3 fatty acids, or Omega-3 fatty acid supplements, causes or promotes (directly and indirectly) antioxidant, anti-inflammatory, and antithrombotic (less clot forming) activities that, among other things, reduces or prevents atherosclerosis.

[1] Note: not all LDLs are "bad." Some LDL is needed in the body to support and promote healthy nervous system function.

[2] Alpha-linolenic acid is abbreviated "ALLA" to differentiate from alpha-lipoic acid (ALA).


N. L. DePace, J. Colombo, *Clinical Autonomic and Mitochondrial Disorders*,
https://doi.org/10.1007/978-3-030-17016-5_3

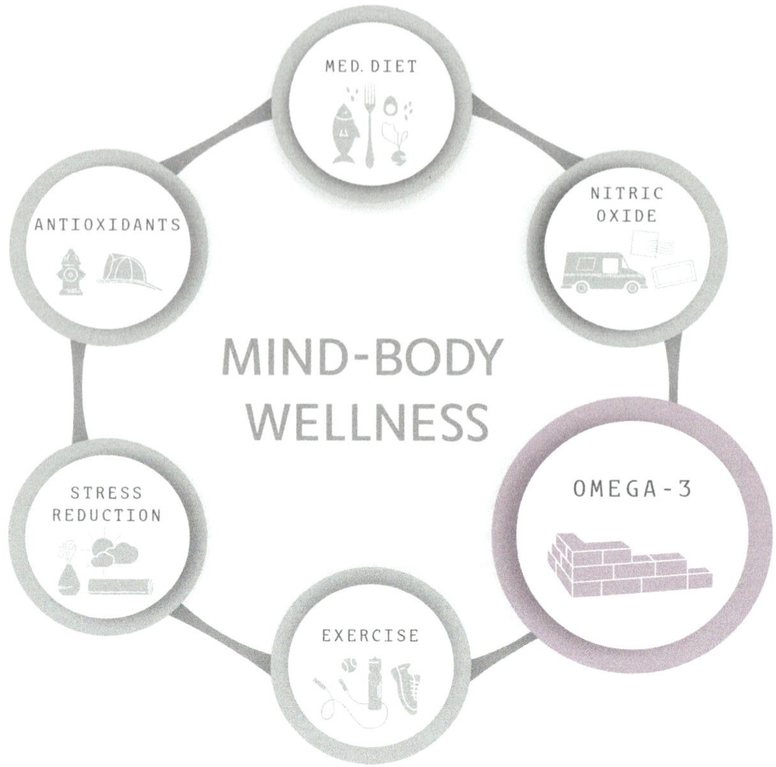


**Fig. 3.1** The Omega-3 fatty acids supplement prong of a Mind-Body Wellness Program. (Illustration by Elysian Creative Studio, www.elysiancreativestudio.com, Lizzy Colombo)

This chapter will discuss the reasons why the Eskimos in Greenland, as an example, do not develop heart disease from atherosclerosis. It is because they take a lot of fish oils through their natural diet. The discussion will include the research behind the reasons and the findings that fish oils help increase the HDL cholesterol, the "good" cholesterol, which may also lower triglycerides in some people. In these people, lower triglycerides also help to prevent atherosclerosis. In fact, while Omega-3 does not lower total LDL cholesterol, it does lower oxidized LDL. This is very important. That this helps with heart health is well known. At the same time, not lowering LDLs may help to preserve healthy nervous system function. In fact, Dr. DePace published an abstract in the late 1980s discussing the effects of Omega-3s on LDLs [1] and cardiovascular health. It was minor research at that time. Then the field of the benefits of fish oils exploded. Fish oils also affect the C fibers in the nerves, including the brain. The autonomic (parasympathetic and sympathetic) nervous system(s) are comprised, primarily, of C fibers. Note, the larger "A" and "B" fibers are in the sensory (hearing, vision, touch, smell, and taste) and motor (muscle control) nervous systems. Fish oil or oily fish products are very important for the brain. Fish is called "brain food."

The two chemicals specifically in fish oils (EPA and DHA) actually go into the membranes of the body, into the phospholipids of the body, and help the membranes and all the cells work better. They keep the blood vessels healthy, the neurons and other tissues healthy, and the axons' myelin sheath healthy. They make the cell membranes flexible. They make the membranes more permeable to the different things that need to go in and out. They improve the workings of receptors. For example, insulin works better with their receptors when the membranes are nice and flexible; whereas, saturated fat makes the membranes rigid, which is not healthful. Fish oils help to relieve inflammatory arthritis. It is thought that they are helpful in reducing plaques in blood vessels; even carotid plaques have been shown to be less involved when fish oils or products containing fish oils are taken.

## Closing the "Statin Gap"

As another example, Omega-3s augment the effect of statins in atherosclerosis. In fact, they help to close the "Statin Gap" (see Fig. 3.2). Despite taking statins and lowering cholesterol by 33%, two-thirds (67%) of at-risk patients still have major adverse cardiac events (MACE, e.g., heart attack, sudden death) or stroke, including repeat events. In other words, statins are not 100% effective. This is the "Statin Gap. Omega-3 fish oils, especially EPA, often help these people and reduce the recurrence of heart attacks and strokes. This is definitively demonstrated by the REDUCE-IT study [2]. REDUCE-IT is a multicenter randomized double-blind placebo-controlled trial involving patients with established cardiovascular disease or diabetes with other risk factors. A total of 8179 patients were enrolled. These patients were all on statin therapy already and had fasting triglyceride levels between 135 and 499 mg/dL. They had LDL cholesterol levels of 41–100 mg/dL. Of these patients, 70.7% were enrolled for secondary prevention of cardiovascular disease (they had already had a heart attack or stroke and were wanting to prevent a second event). The individuals in the fish oil arm received 4 g/day of EPA fish oil, while the placebo group did not receive any. The patients were followed for a median of 14.9 years. The primary endpoint was a five-fold composite of cardiovascular death, nonfatal myocardial infarction, nonfatal stroke, coronary revascularization, or unstable angina. There was also a secondary endpoint, a three-fold composite of cardiovascular death, nonfatal myocardial infarction, or nonfatal stroke (Fig. 3.2).

The study is a landmark study. Given the number and distribution of patients and length of time they were studied, this is a very significant study with good statistical rigor. It is a high-powered study over a prolonged period of time. A previous large study (limited to patients only in Japan), the JELIS study [4, 5], showed benefits of 1.8 grams of EPA. Similar to the REDUCE-IT study, the JELIS study patients were on statin therapy with pure EPA but received a lower dose than in the REDUCE-IT study. They were compared with patients with statin therapy alone and showed an approximate 19% lower risk of ischemic events with statin therapy and EPA compared with statin therapy alone. The REDUCE-IT study showed a 25% reduction in ischemic events despite patients having very low levels of LDL cholesterol and all already on statin therapy. It was noted that the inflammatory marker, C-reactive protein, levels fell in the REDUCE-IT trial for individuals on the EPA arm of the study. It is believed that stabilization and regression of coronary plaque or both may be the operative anti-inflammatory mechanism involved. This anti-inflammatory mechanism has recently been shown in the CANTOS study [6] in which the trial drug included an anti-inflammatory, an IL-6 inhibitor. It is not believed that Omega-3 operates as a lipid-lowering agent to a significant degree in this study. Rather the possible mechanism could be a beneficial antithrombotic affect, in addition to its membrane-stabilizing affects. With pure EPA, LDL and triglyceride levels were not elevated in this study.

The REDUCE-IT study showed both beneficial affects with primary and secondary prevention. Statistically, the number of patients needed to treat to demonstrate a beneficial effect on the endpoints is 28. This study involved over 8000. The fact that so many more patients than statistically necessary were involved speaks to the major impact that this study may have on Western civilizations with high rates of coronary disease and stroke as major causes of morbidity and mortality.

The reason why prior studies with fish oil have been mixed may be explained by the fact that they did not use pure EPA and also did not use high concentrations as were used in the REDUCE-IT trial. In the REDUCE-IT trial, the observed cardiovascular benefits were based on levels of triglycerides: those under 150 mg/dL, those from 150 to 200 mg/dL, and triglycerides greater than 200 mg/dL. There were increased incidents of bleeding in the fish oil arm, but not fatal bleeding or significant cerebral or GI bleeding. Fish oils were shown to be relatively safe in the REDUCE-IT trial. Interestingly, the rate of hospitalization for atrial fibrillation or flutter was actually significantly higher in the fish oil arm in the REDUCE-IT trail compared to the placebo group. There was no explanation for this phenomenon.

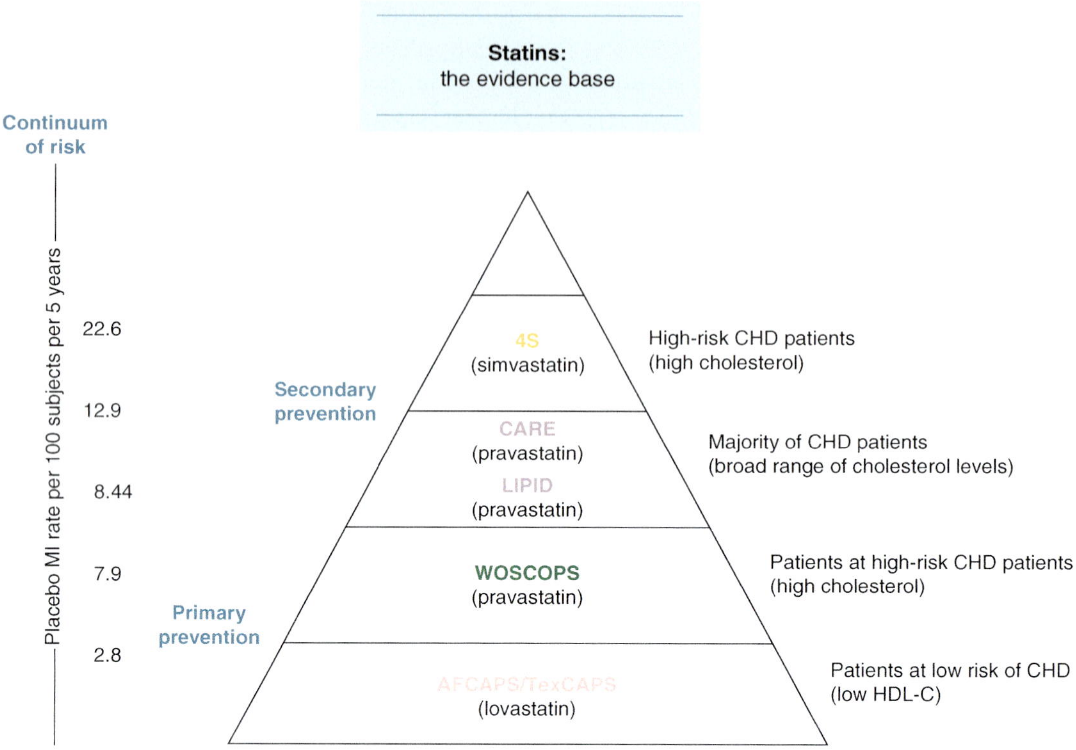


**Fig. 3.2** The Statin Gap. Statins have provided great evidence-based medicine, but they can't work alone. A complete program to combat atherosclerosis is needed [3]. (Illustration by Elysian Creative Studio, www.elysiancreativestudio.com, Lizzy Colombo. Source: https://pace-cme.org/2011/06/16/the-case-for-intensive-lipid-management-the-opportunities-and-issues-for-cardiologists/)

A lot of people do not like to eat fish or do not have time to eat fish, specifically salmon, sardines, albacore tuna, herring, or any of the oily fishes. Yet some of the agencies in this country recommend two fish meals a week. This has become standard in most of the recommendations from the different agricultural and health societies in America, and they are the guidelines. So, how to get around that? It turns out that supplements work, and there is rigorous science to support the fact that EPA fish oil supplements, such as the supplement used in the REDUCE-IT study (Icosapent Ethyl), are healthful. The science will be discussed a little later in this chapter. However, it seems that not everyone benefits from fish oils. No one is harmed by fish oils, but some people do not have a positive effect, only a neutral effect. Those with neutral effects tend to be those who are younger and already eat a healthy diet and exercise regularly (more than 3 days a week).

## Multiple Pathways

There are a number of pathways affected by n-3 PUFAs (see Fig. 3.3). They are used to lower triglycerides (Fig. 3.4, top panel) and make low-density lipoproteins (LDL, the "bad" or "lousy" lipids; Fig. 3.4, bottom panel) more buoyant and less "sticky" so that they do not adhere to artery walls (see Figs. 2.20 and 2.21). Also, the fish oil components prevent the oxygen from combining with the "bad" cholesterol particles in the body to prevent LDLs from oxidizing.

There is a schema of physiologic effects of n-3 PUFA consumption. The relative strength of effect varies by physiologic, and thereby clinic, effect (e.g., triglyceride-lowering). The time course to alter clinical events also varies by duration of consumption for the physiologic effect to alter disease outcomes. For example, the dose-response for anti-arrhythmic effects (the highest

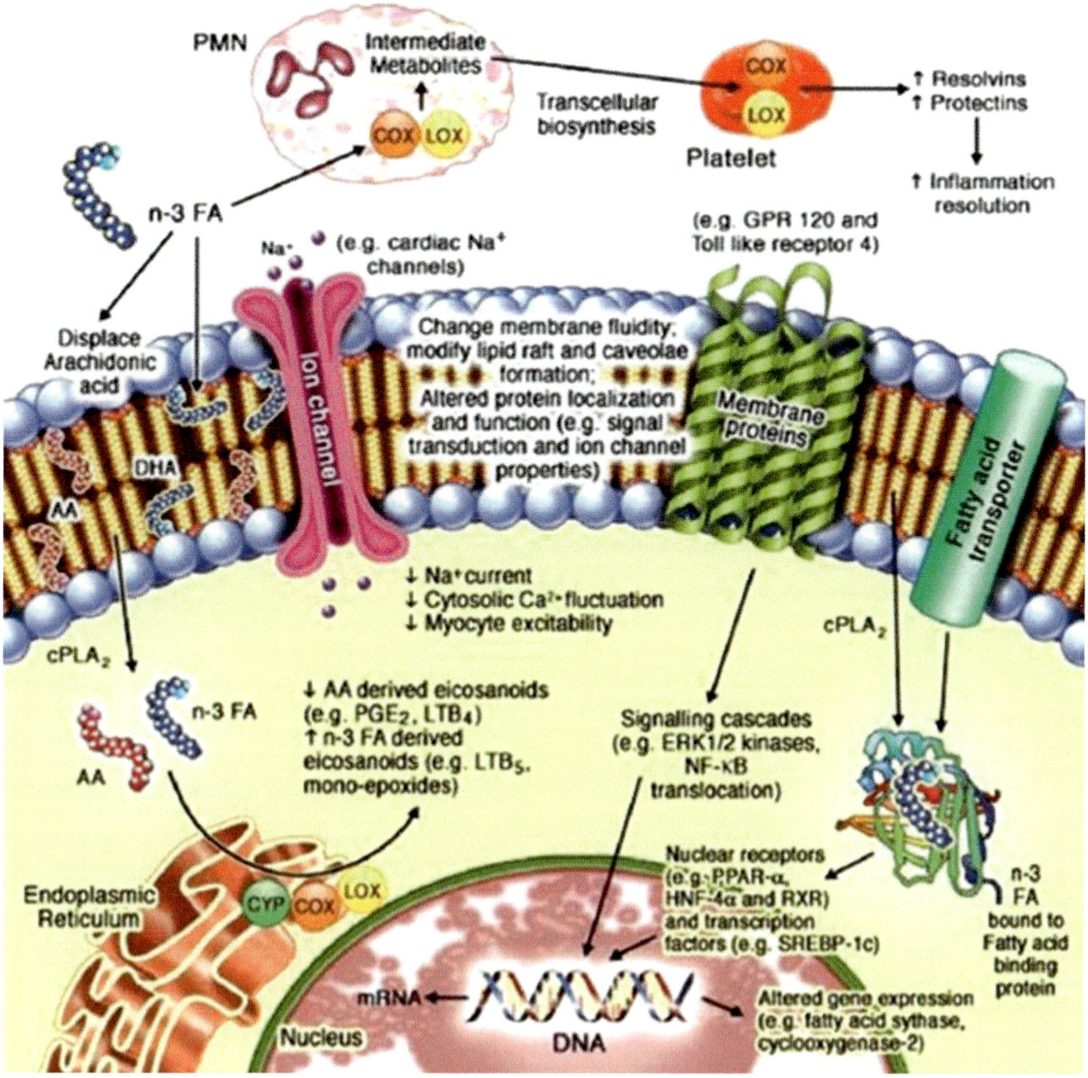


**Fig. 3.3** Pathways affected by n-3 PUFAs. AA arachidonic acid, COX cyclooxygenase, cPLA2 cytosolic phospholipase A2, CYP450 cytochrome P450, DHA docosahexaenoic acid, DNA deoxyribonucleic acid, ERK extracellular signal-regulated kinase, GPR 120 G-protein-coupled receptor 120, HNF hepatic nuclear factor, LOX lipoxygenase, mRNA messenger ribonucleic acid, n-3 FA n-3 fatty acids, NF-κB nuclear factor-kB, PGE2 prostaglandin E2, PMN polymorphonuclear leukocyte, PPAR peroxisome proliferator-activated receptor, RXR retinoid X receptor, SREBP-1c sterol regulatory element binding protein-1c. Cellular and organelle functions are strongly influenced by membrane lipid environments. Lipid micro-domains contribute to the modulation of numerous cellular functions like signal transduction, protein and membrane trafficking, and ion channel kinetics. The incorporation of n-3 PUFA in cell and organelle membrane structures alters their physicochemical properties and influences the localization, function, and signaling of membrane-associated proteins. This might contribute to potential anti-inflammatory and anti-arrhythmic effects [7]. (Open Access, Hindawi Publishing Corp. Source: https://www.researchgate.net/figure/235368999_fig1_Molecular-pathways-affected-by-n-3-PUFA-9-AA-arachidonic acid-COX-cyclooxygenase)

relative strength of effect) appears to be initially steep, reaching a peak around 1000 mg, with a subsequent plateau, and effects on anti-arrhythmic outcomes may occur within weeks. The plateau suggests that further increases in dosage do not further increase the clinic effect or time course to alter clinical effects. For triglyceride-lowering, the dose-response is more

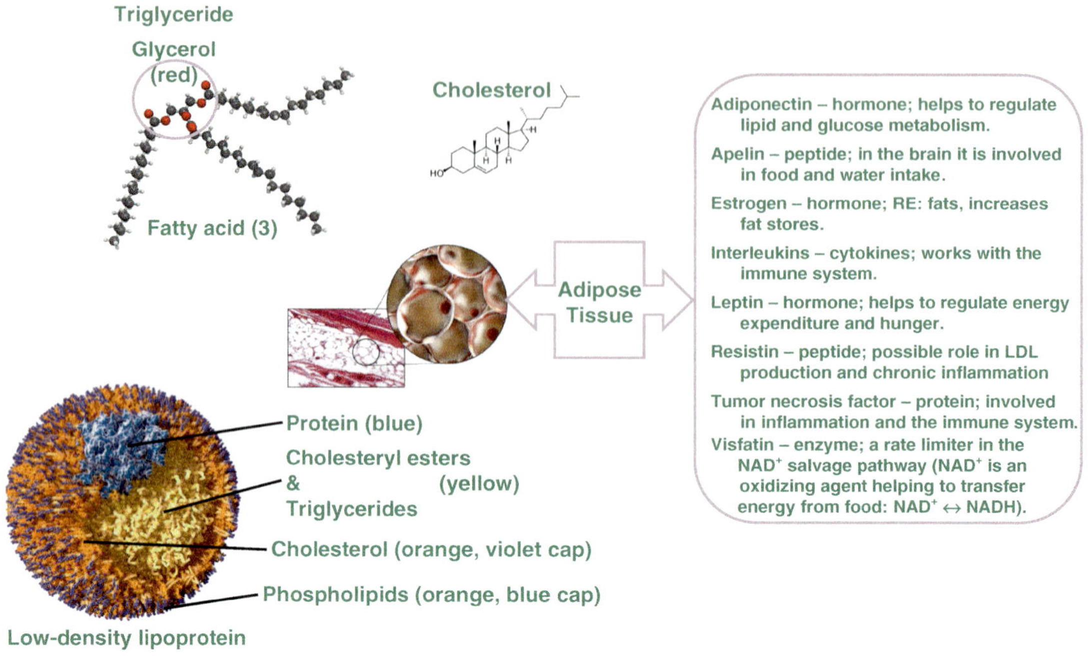


**Fig. 3.4** Triglycerides, cholesterol, and low-density lipoprotein are components of adipose tissue. Triglycerides and cholesterol are also components of low-density lipoproteins (LDLs). Triglycerides are derived from glycerol and three fatty acids. They are the main constituents of body fat. Lipoproteins are derived from cholesterol and triglycerides (both form the lipid part) and proteins. LDLs are composed of (1) a protein (in this case an apolipoprotein, ApoB 100, blue, which binds to lipids), (2) phospholipids (orange with a blue cap, a compound of glycerol, two fatty acids, and choline phosphate, which acts as an emulsifier), (3) cholesterol (orange with a violet cap), (4) triglycerides (yellow), and (5) cholesteryl esters (also yellow, a compound of cholesterol and a fatty acid). All are components of adipose tissue which releases hormones and enzymes involved in food intake and metabolism and immune responses. (Adipose tissue illustration adapted from Shutterstock Royalty-free stock illustration ID: 459227371; white adipose tissue (fat cells), light micrograph, and 3D illustration by Kateryna Kon. LDL illustration adapted from Shutterstock Royalty-free stock illustration ID: 375383317; structure of a low-density lipoprotein (LDL) by Juan Gaertner. Triglyceride illustration adapted from Shutterstock Royalty-free stock illustration ID: 133615109; trans fat containing triglyceride (elaidyl stearyl oleyl triglyceride), molecular model by molekuul_be. Source: triglycerides = http://healthyprotocols.com/3_trigly.htm; lipoprotein = http://www.scientificpsychic.com/health/lipoproteins-LDL-HDL.html)

gradual and monotonic (linear), and effects on disease outcomes may require months or years of intake. HR-lowering and BP-lowering dose-responses are similar to that for the anti-arrhythmic effect, but plateau at levels less than half that for the anti-arrhythmic effect. Unlike the anti-arrhythmic effect, the time course for HR- and BP-lowering is months to years. The dose-response curve for antithrombosis is significantly more gradual than the others, requiring over 2000 mg per day to generate a significant effect; however, the time course is on the order of weeks. Unfortunately, the important effects of n-3 PUFA on endothelial, autonomic, and anti-inflammatory responses are less well known because the dose- and time-responses of these effects are not well-established. Physiologic effects are not necessarily exclusive: e.g., anti-arrhythmic effects may be partly mediated by effects on blood pressure (BP) or heart rate [8].

Oxidized LDL cholesterol becomes incorporated in the blood vessel wall after being engulfed by scavenger cells called macrophages. Oxidized LDL in macrophages form foam cells (Fig. 3.5), and foam cells initiate the development of atherosclerosis [9]. The combination of Omega-3 fish oils and other lifestyle and supplement components is employed to help avoid the formation of

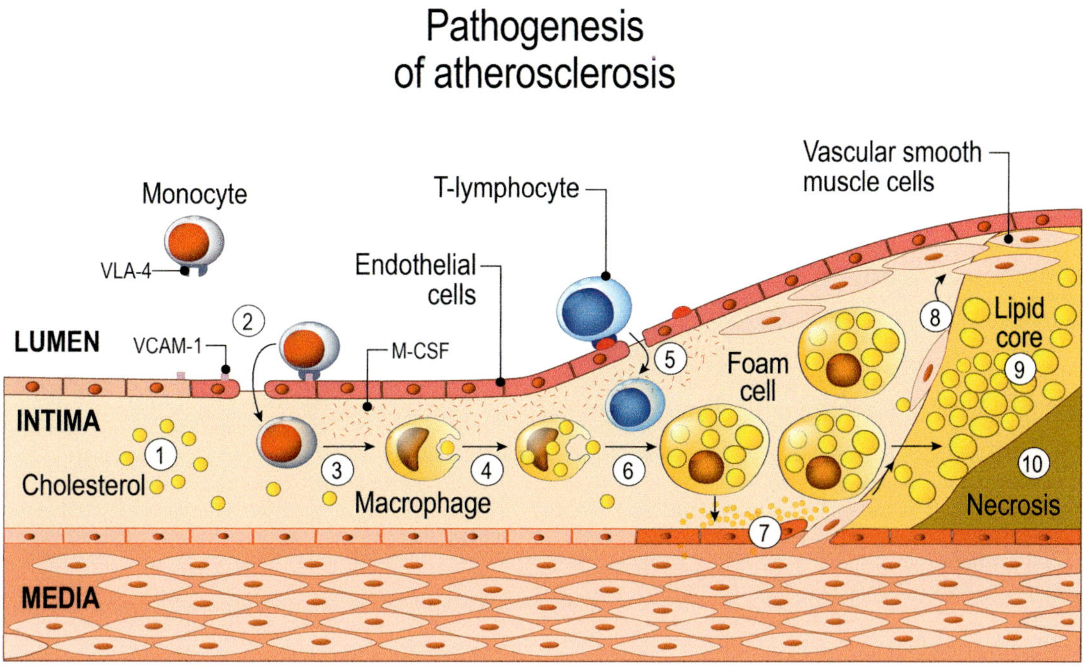


**Fig. 3.5** Pathogenesis of atherosclerosis: formation of foam cells which leads to atherosclerosis. (1) LDL cholesterol enters through intact endothelium and some are oxidized into pro-inflammatory lipids. (2) Monocytes enter. (3) Monocytes are activated (differentiated) as macrophages. (4) Monocyte/macrophage scavenge oxidized LDL. (5) T lymphocytes scavenge inflamed cells. (6) Foam cells are formed from macrophages that are engorged on oxidized LDL. (7) Foam cells release growth factors (cytokines) that initiate atherosclerosis. (8) Foam cells adhere. (9) Atherosclerotic plaque is formed from adhered foam cells forming a lipid pool. (10) Necrosis occurs. (Adapted from Shutterstock Royalty-free stock illustration ID: 1121530022, Pathogenesis of atherosclerosis. Cholesterol plaque, and thrombus formation. Cells structure, by Designua. Source: https://practical-evolutionary-health.com/tag/intestinal-permeability/; Modified from Crawford MH, DiMarco JP, editors. Cardiology. London, 2001, Mosby)

foam cells by lowering serum cholesterol with statins (Fig. 3.6) or other related medicines as necessary. Note, foam cells occur as early as the teenage years and continue throughout the rest of life. Therefore, it is never too soon to start adding fish or Omega-3 supplements to your diet. Once atherosclerosis is suspected, if possible, fish oils are started, with lifestyle and diet changes. If not, two approaches are recommended simultaneously: statins and Omega-3s. Statins inhibit HMG-CoA reductase,[3] which reduces LDL cholesterol production and increases LDL receptors in the liver, preventing LDL release into the bloodstream. By keeping LDL ("bad") cholesterol low, there is less chance of an abundance of these foam cells forming and becoming plaque in the arteries (Fig. 3.5). Statins also help to (1) block macrophages from becoming foam cells in early atherogenesis, (2) prevent platelets from adhering to the endothelium, (3) prevent thrombolysis (clot formation), and (4) block vascular smooth muscle cells from migrating across the endothelium, adding to the atherosclerotic plaque in advanced atherosclerosis. Fish oils help all of this by adding to and keeping a proper antioxidant balance within the body. Together with the

[3]HMG-CoA reductase is a rate-controlling enzyme in the metabolic pathway which produces cholesterol (oxidized LDL) from HMG-CoA (see Fig. 3.6). Statins are HMG-CoA reductase inhibitors that act to block the oxidation of LDL (ox-LDL). Oxidized LDL is a type of ROS. Reducing ox-LDL reduces ROS, thereby reducing the need for more macrophages, thereby limiting their availability to become foam cells. Statins may also cause a small reduction in ubiquinones (CoQ10, see Fig. 3.6).

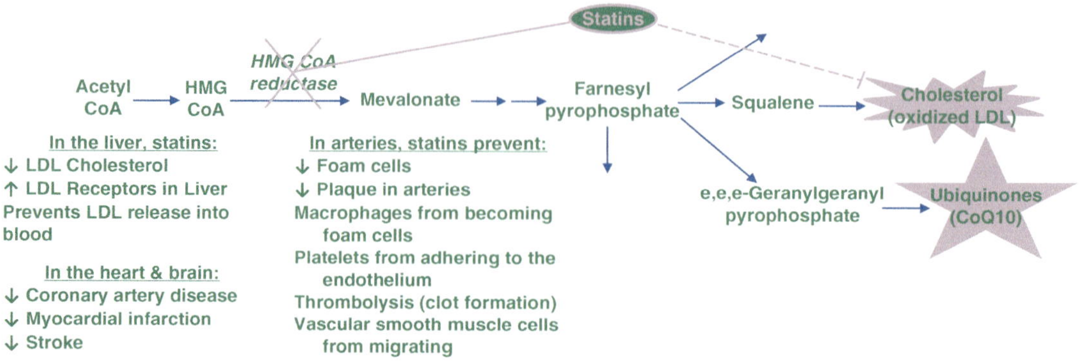


**Fig. 3.6** Statins inhibit HMG-CoA, which reduces LDL cholesterol production and increases LDL receptors in the liver, preventing LDL release into the bloodstream; thereby reducing the amount of excess LDL available for oxidation. Fewer oxidized LDLs results in fewer foam cells, which results in less atherosclerotic plaque. (Sources: https://jleonarddixon.com/2014/05/31/science-unintended-consequences-ancel-keys-cholesterol-and-the-transition-to-an-obese-society-part-xv-discovery-of-the-statin-drugs-rollback-of-ldl-and-protection-from-chd/ (main); http://www.medscape.org/viewarticle/416521_13 (insert); https://www.slideshare.net/drdevb/statins-dr-renuka-joshi-buche (chemical equations in parentheses))

other lifestyle and supplement prongs, the whole Mind-Body Wellness Program helps to prevent excess LDL cholesterol particles from becoming oxidized and more easily incorporated in the blood vessels of the body.

## Details of Oxidized LDL and Atherosclerosis Production

Oxidized LDL (ox-LDL) cholesterol plays a significant role in the development of atherosclerosis (see Figs. 3.3 and 3.5). Reducing ox-LDL cholesterol is always a goal of wellness. A proper antioxidant balance is key in this regard. Simply lowering the LDL particle count may not be enough, and therefore, one needs to prevent even the reduced number of LDL particles from getting oxidized in the first place. One possibility (potential therapeutic target) is the ox-LDL-1 (LOX-1) receptor (aka lecithin-type oxidized LDL-1 receptor, also LOX-1). By blocking the LOX-1 receptor, the receptor's ability to retain ox-LDL is eliminated, preventing it from becoming incorporated into vessel walls and macrophages [10]. This may halt atherosclerosis. As shown in numerous studies, a major complication of LOX-1 is that it promotes myocardial ischemia (a type of heart attack due to blocked arteries preventing the delivery of enough oxygen to the heart) [11]. Atherosclerosis is a chronic inflammatory process that starts collecting ox-LDL in early childhood, causing fatty streaks [12]. LOX-1 is abundantly expressed in atherosclerotic plaques. It is upregulated by conventional risk factors such as diabetes, hypertension, and dyslipidemia.

LOX-1 activates arginase II, which downregulates nitric oxide synthesis in endothelial cells and leads to endothelial dysfunction as less nitric oxide is produced. This is one significant factor in atherosclerosis. Also, ox-LDL, through LOX-1, regulates nitric oxide-mediated vascular reactivity through various pathways, implicating LOX-1 in endothelial dysfunction and endothelial aging. More importantly, recent studies [13] have shown that LOX-1-mediated ROS generation can include mitochondrial DNA damage and enhance expression of inflammatory molecules. This results in the production of inflammatory cytokines, such as interleukins. Inflammatory cytokines sustain the chronic inflammation of atherosclerosis. Antibodies to inhibit LOX-1 have been shown to decrease mitochondrial ROS generation and other free radical processes, which is beneficial.

The normal role of LOX-1 is to participate in the initiation and development of new blood vessels. If a blood vessel is damaged, the damaged section is isolated, and two new vessels are formed to bypass the damaged section. Then the damaged section is sealed off and absorbed. Finally, the two bypass vessels fuse to become a single vessel in place of the original, damaged vessel, with the same size and shape. LOX-1 initiates all of this when a normal amount of ox-LDL is present due to vascular (endothelial) damage or the need for repair. It is only when LOX-1 is over activated due to stress and excess LDL does it turn to making plaque that leads to atherosclerosis.

Specifically, LOX-1 mediates ox-LDL-induced vascular smooth muscle proliferation and neointima formation, as well as blood vessel growth which also occurs in atherosclerotic plaques. Thrombus formation is noted in final stages of atherosclerosis, and LOX-1 has been a mediator in various molecular pathways involved in this. Even platelets have been shown to express LOX-1 and inhibition has been shown to decrease ADP-induced platelet aggregation [14, 15]. Therefore, LOX-1 receptors are extremely important in activating platelets in addition to pro-inflammatory cytokines, such as tumor necrosis factor (TNF), which can be stimulated from fibroblasts. The new vessel formation, angiogenesis, is also regulated by LOX-1. There is, therefore, conclusive evidence that LOX-1 is involved in the development of atherosclerosis. Gene deletions in LOX-1 have shown markedly reduced atherosclerosis and reduced oxidative stress and reduced nitric oxide degradation causing increased NOS and decreased inflammatory effects. Circulating levels of soluble LOX-1 have been proposed as a marker of myocardial ischemia, perhaps even more important than C-reactive protein [16].

LOX-1 also affects HDL. It regulates HDL function. HDL helps to (1) block LDLs from being oxidized; (2) macrophages from becoming foam cells; (3) foam cells from sticking to vessel walls; (4) foam cells from releasing inflammatory products, including cytokines; and (5) platelets from aggregating (see Fig. 3.7). LOX-1 induces endothelial dysfunction by elevating microphage inflammatory proteins. Healthy lev-

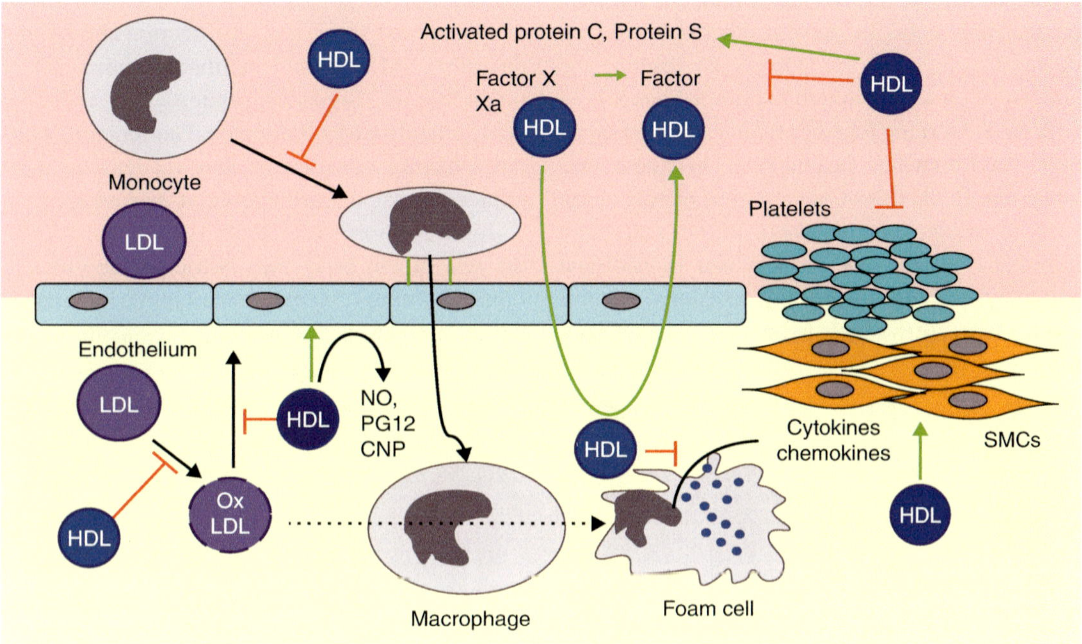


**Fig. 3.7** HDL helps to prevent atherosclerosis by helping to (1) block LDLs from being oxidized; (2) macrophages from becoming foam cells; (3) foam cells from sticking to vessel walls; (4) foam cells from releasing inflammatory products, including cytokines; and (5) platelets from aggregating. (Reproduced from Wikipedia.org, Open Access: https://en.wikipedia.org/wiki/High-density_lipoprotein. Source: Wikipedia)

els of HDL help to promote healthy endothelial cell function. HDL which has been affected by ox-LDL cannot release nitric oxide [17]. It is not surprising that LOX-1 has become a target in prevention of atherosclerosis, especially due to its natural history and related diseases.

In addition to Omega-3s, there are natural LOX-1 modulators. The more important modulators are curcumin (aka., turmeric), flavonoids, and resveratrol, which are provided through the Mediterranean diet, especially by drinking small amounts of red wine (one to two glasses per day); another example of the benefits of the different lifestyle and supplement prongs working together. Other (inducing) therapies to treat heart diseases, including atherosclerosis-induced diseases, that have indirect effects on LOX-1 expression are aspirin, statins, and oral hypoglycemic agents. They may beneficially negate, and therefore, decrease inflammation in atherosclerosis which goes through LOX-1-mediated pathways [18]. In the future, it would not be surprising if LOX-1 becomes a target for reducing atherosclerosis. In summary, the LOX-1 receptor is a novel site to reduce the uptake of oxidized LDL. For the time being, HDL helps to prevent atherosclerosis, as depicted in Fig. 3.7 (see legend). By limiting the amount of ox-LDL through the mutual benefits of Omega-3s working together with a strong antioxidant environment, health and wellness are advanced. In the future, negating the effects of the LOX-1 receptor is expected to be extremely important. While gene models and monoclonal antibodies to LOX-1 are being developed, natural mechanisms are available to be used in the interim.

## Fish Oil Omega-3s as an Anti-inflammatory

Fish oil or Omega-3 compounds are one component of promoting an antioxidant type environment to prevent damage due to oxidation, including the oxidation of LDL. Another of the major components of the brain-heart theory (the brain and heart connection) is anti-inflammatory processes. Inflammation affects all of the organs of the body (Fig. 3.8). As demonstrated with atherosclerosis, chronic inflammation in the body promotes disease; however, there are many other diseases associated with chronic inflammation (Fig. 3.9, 84]. While short-term inflammation contributes to the tissue healing process, chronic inflammation can lead to lifelong debilitation and loss of tissue function and organ failure. Fish oils (rich in Omega-3 fatty acids) help to generate superb anti-inflammatory molecules called resolvins and protectins which are metabolites of Omega-3 fatty acids and may resolve chronic inflammation (Fig. 3.10) [20–22]. Chronic inflammation is important in promoting many diseases including atherosclerosis, various forms of cancer, and autonomic dysfunction and related disorders. Monoclonal antibodies also affect inflammation. Evidence suggests that reducing inflammation using monoclonal antibodies, without affecting lipid levels, may (at least in part) reduce the risk of cardiovascular disease [23].

Inflammation in the brain is different than in the rest of the body (see Nitric Oxide chapter, Figs. 4.50 and 4.51, and related text). In general, the inflammation that accompanies acute injury

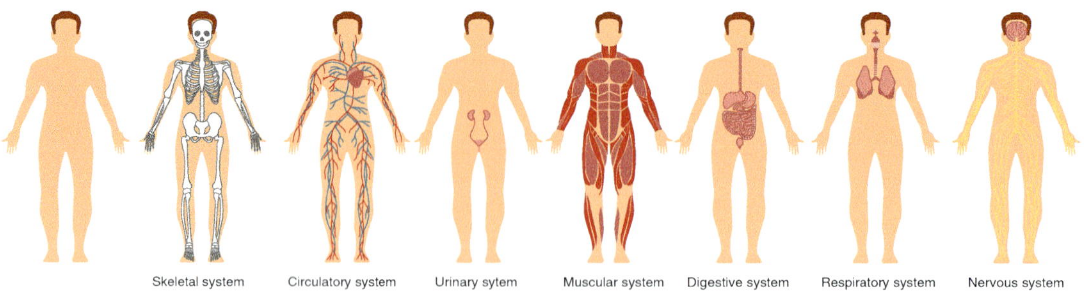


**Fig. 3.8** The P&S nervous systems form the heart-brain connection, and, together with it, the rest of the body's organ systems. Achieving a proper balance between the P&S enables optimal control of the organs, helping to establish and maintain health and wellness. (Illustration by Elysian Creative Studio, www.elysiancreativestudio.com, Lizzy Colombo)

has dual functions: antibacterial action and repair. Antibacterial functions protect damaged tissue from infection. Repair functions are initiated to aid in the recovery of damaged tissue. Brain injury is different in two respects. First, many cases of brain injury are not accompanied by infection: there is no chance of pathogens entering the brain through the skull in ischemia or even in traumatic injury if the skull is intact. Second, neurons are rarely regenerated once damaged. To this end, it seems as if the brain has its own immune system, separate and perhaps unique from the rest of the body (Fig. 3.11). It is separated from the body by the blood-brain barrier. In fact, evidence indicates that immune responses in the brain reduce immune activity in the rest of the body and, if persistent, leads to secondary diseases such as pneumonia which can lead to death [24]. Fish oils or Omega-3 fatty acids, as "brain food," help maintain nerve membrane and myelin health, keeping brain cell membranes and blood-brain vessels flexible, and working with other anti-inflammatories helps maintain brain and nervous system health.

In the cardiovascular system, various epidemiological and observational studies have shown that fish oils (natural or supplements) reduce cardiovascular mortality [25–48]. Greenland Eskimos and Japanese fishing village inhabitants have lower incidents of heart disease than other non-fish consum-

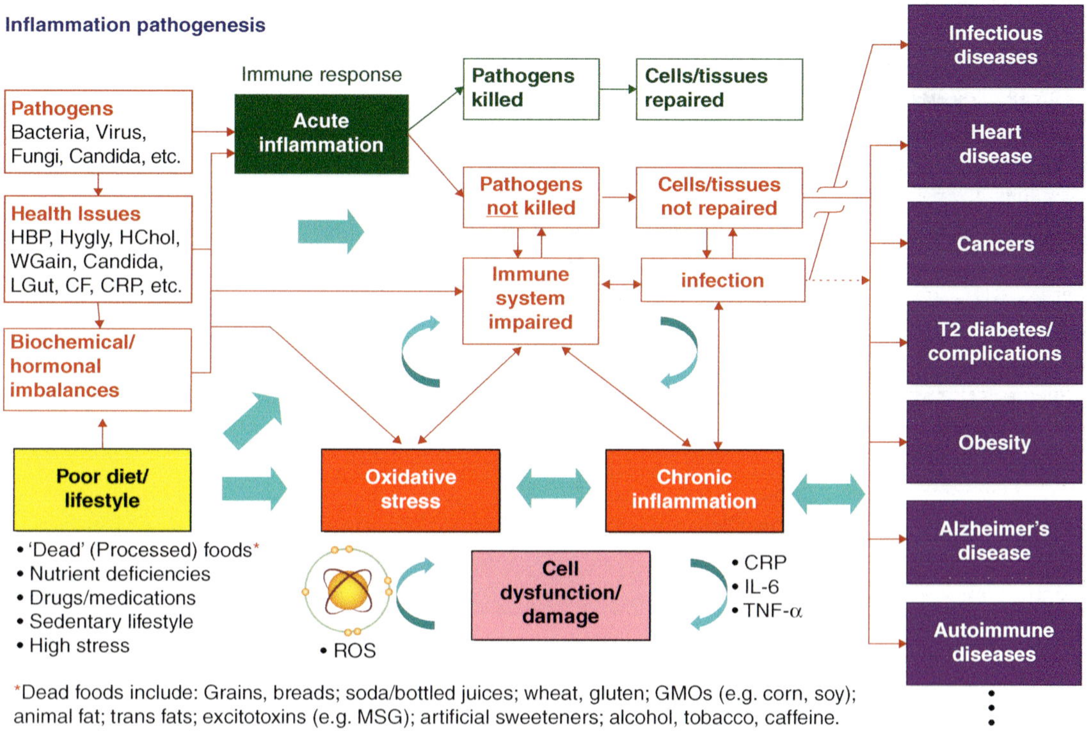


**Fig. 3.9** Inflammation pathogenesis. Inflammation has many sources, including poor diet or lifestyle, which lead to acute inflammation (which is normal and healthy) and oxidative stress (including an overproduction of ROS, which is not normal or healthy). Sources from pathogens and acute (short-term) health issues responded to in a normal, healthy manner (text in green at the top) lead to the pathogens being killed and cells and tissues being repaired. Long-term health issues, including imbalances (which involve P&S imbalances), lead to pathogens not being killed and cells and tissues not being repaired. The abnormal responses (text in red) lead to chronic inflammation and cell damage, which lead to chronic diseases including diabetes, cancers, and heart (cardiovascular) disease, as well as neurological diseases, arthritis, and pulmonary diseases. The Mediterranean diet, exercise, antioxidants, and anti-inflammatories work together to help to prevent the abnormal responses and negative outcomes. (Reproduced with permission from DeWayne McCulley (diabetes engineer and author of "Death to Diabetes") of the Death to Diabetes website https://www.deathtodiabetes.com/root-causes-of-type-2-diabetes.php. Adapted from: http://deathtocancers.blogspot.com/2015/07/cancer-and-inflammation.html)

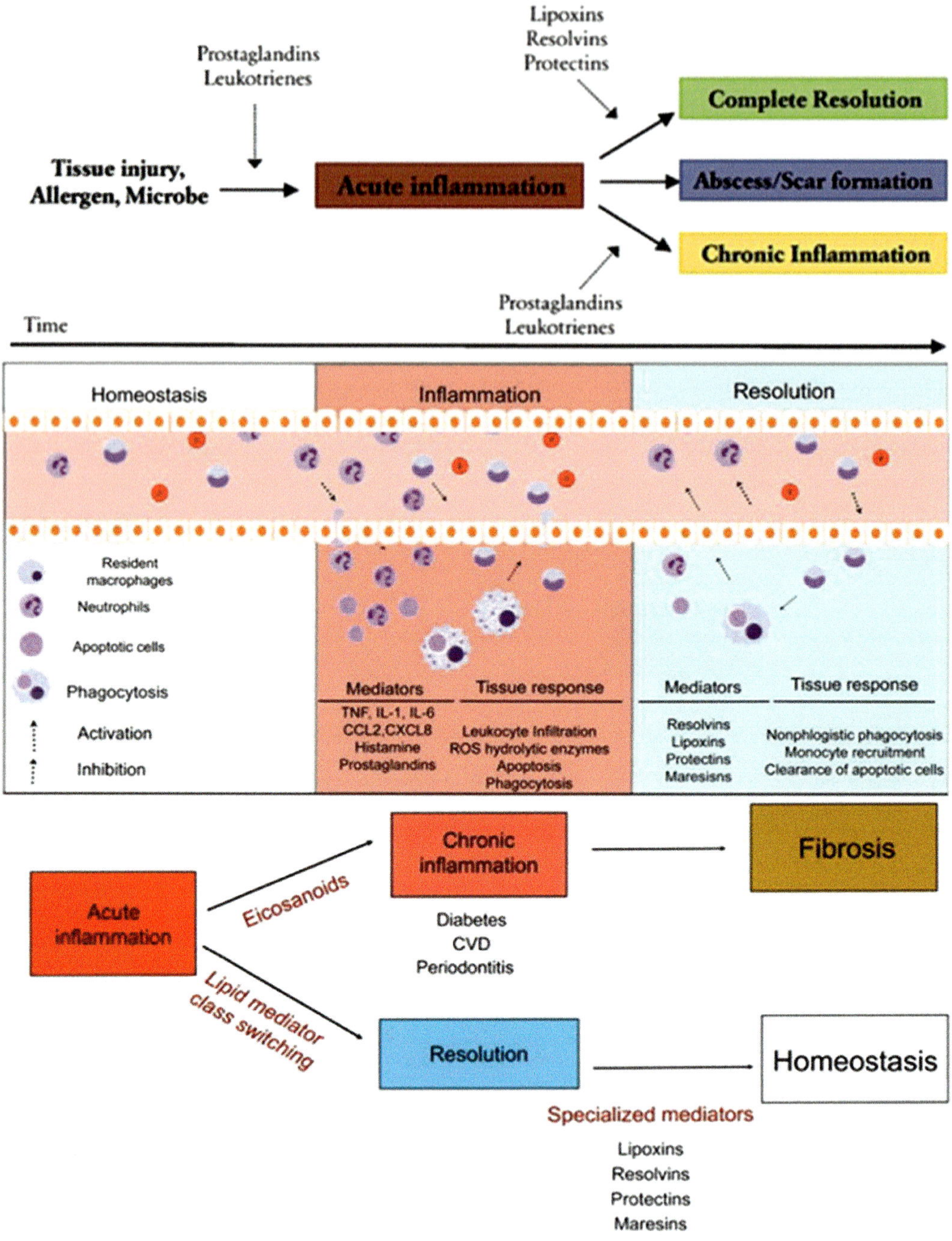


**Fig. 3.10** Role of resolvins and protectins along with lipoxins and maresins (collectively known as "specialized mediators"). Specialized mediators are naturally derived from Omega-3 fatty acids. Increasing Omega-3 fatty acids through supplements increases the numbers of specialized mediators. There are two types of inflammation: acute and chronic. Chronic inflammation is the abnormal resolution of acute inflammation. Specialized mediators prevent chronic inflammation and are influenced by diet, exercise, lifestyle, stress, exposure, etc. Positive influences, including the Mind-Body Wellness Program, proliferate the specialized mediators and prevent chronic inflammation. Negative influences proliferate prostaglandins and leukotrienes (eicosanoids), proliferating macrophages, and lymphocytes which proliferate blood vessels, fibrosis (scar tissue), tissue necrosis, and fewer neutrophils, all leading to chronic inflammation [19]. (Reproduced with permission from John Wiley and Sons. Adapted from http://www.anti-agingfirewalls.com/2016/12/14/inflammation-part-3-resolving-inflammation-resolvins-protectins-maresins-and-lipoxins/)

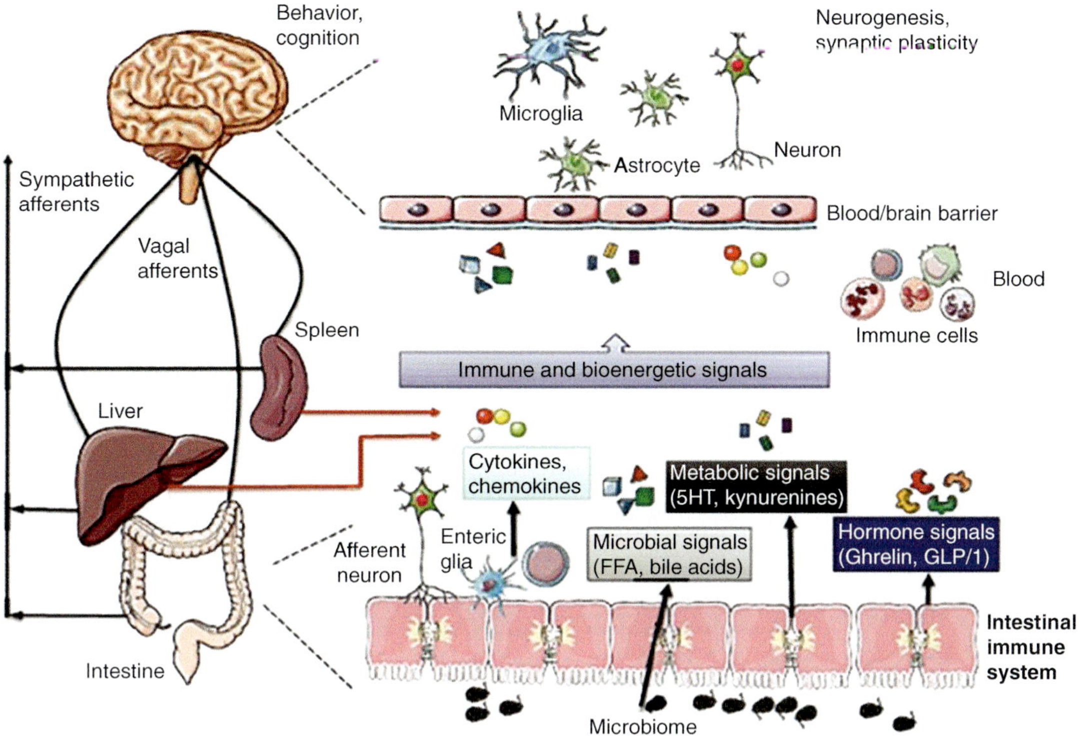


**Fig. 3.11** The basis of the effect of the microbiome on the brain function. The microbiome defines the set of microorganisms that are normally located in different places in the human body, in particular the digestive tract. The microbiome is in a commensal symbiotic relationship with the host. These microbial components aid in the digestion of food, produce vitamins, and protect against colonization of other microorganisms that maybe pathogenic. There are few physiological and immunological parameters that are not significantly affected by the presence and nature of the microbiome, with host resistance to infection being one of the most prominent factors. The gut microbiome is highly dynamic, exhibiting daily cyclic fluctuations that have repercussions for metabolism and circadian rhythm. An essential pathway is neuronal, via innervation of distant organs (e.g., intestine, spleen, and liver) and neuroimmune signals that can be transmitted bidirectionally between the brain and the periphery. Another important route is through the general circulation, where circulating immune signals (e.g., cytokines and chemokines) and bioenergetics signals (e.g., endogenous metabolites of microbial origin) can exert a systemic impact on the brain microenvironment [65, Fig. 3.28]. (Reproduced with permission from Springer International Publishing AG)

ing cultures [49–57]. The Zutphen, Netherlands, study [58–61] was a 20-year study which showed an inverse relationship between fish consumption and mortality from coronary heart disease (Fig. 3.12) [63, 64]. The MRFIT study [65] was another study which showed the benefits of consuming fish. The Chicago Western Electric Study [66–68] was a 30-year study of fish consumption and risk of heart attack. The study showed beneficial effects of fish consumption. Numerous studies have shown that populations that consume fish have a lower incidence of coronary heart disease [69–73]. Omega-3 fatty acids are also promising as a therapy for diseases of other organs (i.e., brain and liver) and cancer, as well [74–103].

The two main types of Omega-3 fatty acids, docosahexaenoic acid (DHA) and eicosapentaenoic acid (EPA), are 22 and 20 carbon chain molecules, respectively (Fig. 3.13). These are known as natural anti-inflammatories or membrane molecules, since they go into the membranes of the body and prevent inflammation (Fig. 3.14). In general, the EPA version of Omega-3 is more functional (gene signaling, cellular processes, energy), and the DHA version of Omega-3 is more structural (acting as the brick in the cell membrane walls). EPA is the precursor parent compound of DHA. Research suggests that 40–60% of DHA in the body is converted from EPA. One way to prevent inflam-

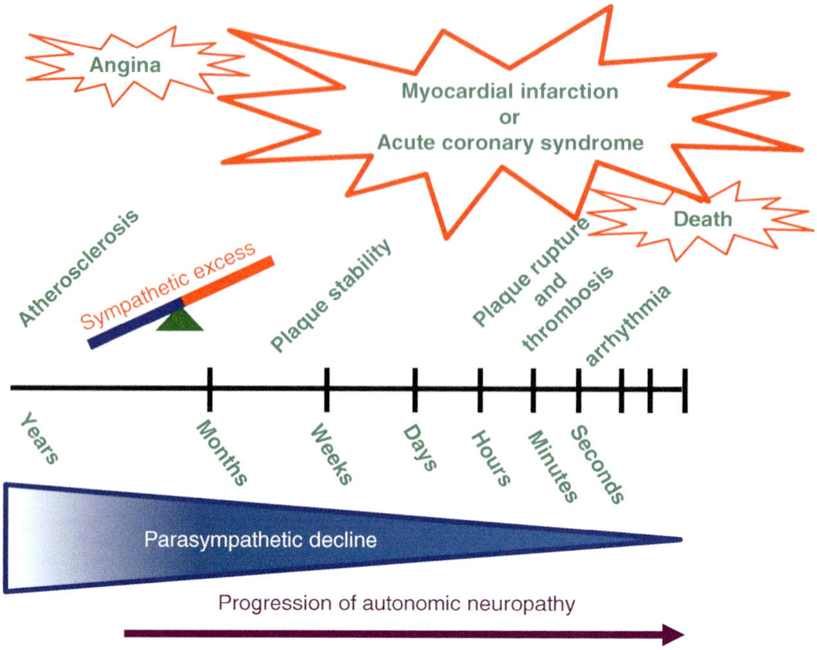


**Fig. 3.12** Mortality risks of coronary heart disease. (Reading from top to bottom:) Events in red are endpoints (MI myocardial infarction, ACS acute coronary syndrome). These are cardiovascular endpoints associated with the time durations indicated below the axis. Atherosclerosis develops slowly over time, and is the result of repeated and chronic offenses (stresses and injuries). Repeated stresses also lead to sympathetic excesses. In both cases short-term (acute) macrophage activity and sympathetic excesses are healthful and protective. However, chronic macrophage activity leads to foam cell development and then progresses to plaque development and atherosclerosis. Similarly, chronic short-term sympathetic excesses, build up and the sympathetics habituate and the sympathetic excess becomes chronic. Once the plaque stabilizes and coronary heart diseases sets in, further insults may cause the plaque to rupture and the final events leading to the endpoints may occur very quickly. In parallel with these cardiovascular events are autonomic events that ultimately facilitate the cardiovascular endpoints. As sympathetic excess (SE) persists, the parasympathetics decline faster (to use the car analogy, persistent "over-acceleration" (SE) wears out the "brakes" (the parasympathetics) faster, and ultimately they cannot stop the car, and it crashes – the heart attack). The decline of the parasympathetics mark the progression of autonomic neuropathy and the increases in, first, morbidity and then mortality risk, facilitating the heart attack (due to no "brakes"). [62]. (Source: http://cursoenarm.net/UPTODATE/contents/mobipreview.htm?2/2/2082)

mation is by impairing the ability of another type of Omega fatty acid, called Omega-6 fatty acid, from entering the membranes and displacing the Omega-3 fatty acids (Fig. 3.15). Again, Omega-3 fatty acids are anti-inflammatory, antithrombotic, and antioxidant [106]. Take, for example, prostaglandins, which are a group of physiologically active lipid compounds having diverse hormone-like effects. They have been found in almost every tissue in humans. In the presence of Omega-3s, the prostaglandins produced are anti-inflammatory, all of which are helpful to the body; whereas, in the presence of Omega-6 fatty acids, the prostaglandins produced are prothrombotic, inflammatory, and promote oxidation [107], all of which are harmful to the body. Omega-6 fatty acids are obtained from various seeds and nuts and vegetable oil such as corn oil or sunflower oil. Replacing Omega-6 fatty acids with Omega-3s in cell membranes can result in decreased cellular response to inflammatory stimuli [108]. The ratio of Omega-3 to Omega-6 fatty acids is important for health. Higher ratios of Omega-3s to Omega-6s promote better health and wellness (Table 3.1) [109]. Another source of Omega-3 is from plants. It is an 18 carbon molecule known as alpha-linolenic acid (ALLA[7], see Fig. 3.16). ALLA, for example, is found in linseed oil. ALLA is converted to EPA and DHA in the body (see Fig. 3.17).

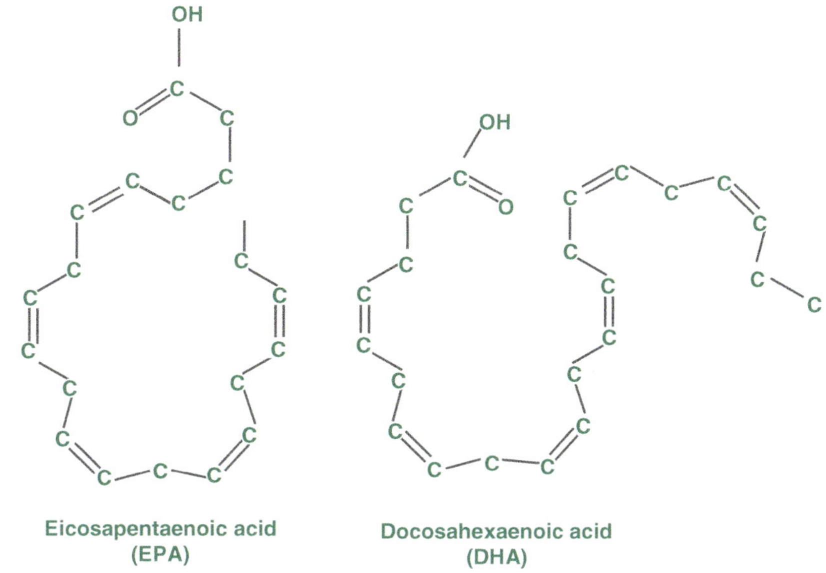


**Fig. 3.13** Molecular structures of EPA and DHA [104]. (Source: http://caloriesproper.com/fish-dark-chocolate-and-red-wine/epa-dpa-dha/)

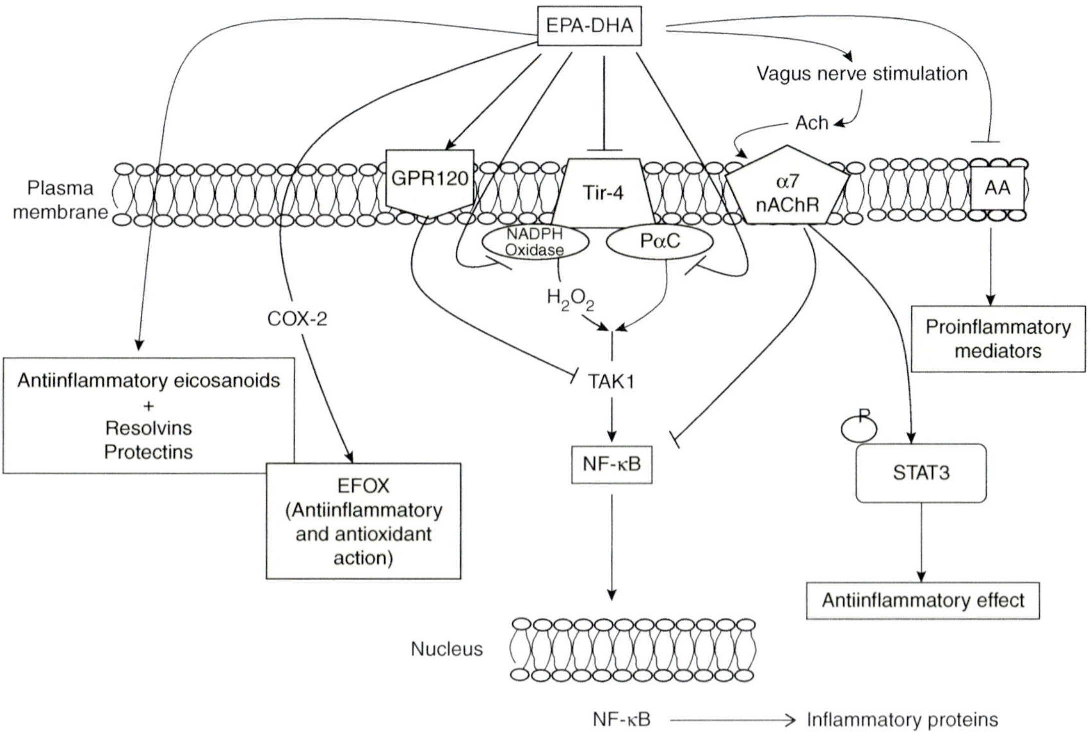


**Fig. 3.14** Omega-3 fatty acid (N-3 PUFA) anti-inflammatory mechanisms. Dietary EPA and DHA supplementation results in an increased incorporation of these fatty acids in cell membranes. EPA and DHA metabolism generates eicosanoids with low inflammatory and pro-resolving effects. Displacing membrane arachidonic acid (AA) reduces the formation of pro-inflammatory mediators. EPA and DHA inhibit cell signaling pathways that result in activation of NF-β, thereby inhibiting toll-like receptor 4 (TLR-4) activation and signaling pathways mediated by G-protein coupled receptor 120 (GPR120) and alpha-7 nicotinic receptor (7 nAChR). EPA and DHA activate the Vagus nerve and acetylcholine (Ach) release, which, in turn, stimulates signal transducer and activator of transcription 3 (STAT3) phosphorylation and thereby anti-inflammatory responses. DHA decreases $H_2O_2$ production and protein kinase C activation, leading to inactivation of the NF-β-mediated response [105]. (Reproduced with permission from Elsevier. Source: https://www.researchgate.net/figure/232246717_fig3_Fig-3-n-3-PUFA-anti-inflammatory-mechanisms-Dietary-EPA-and-DHA-supplementation)

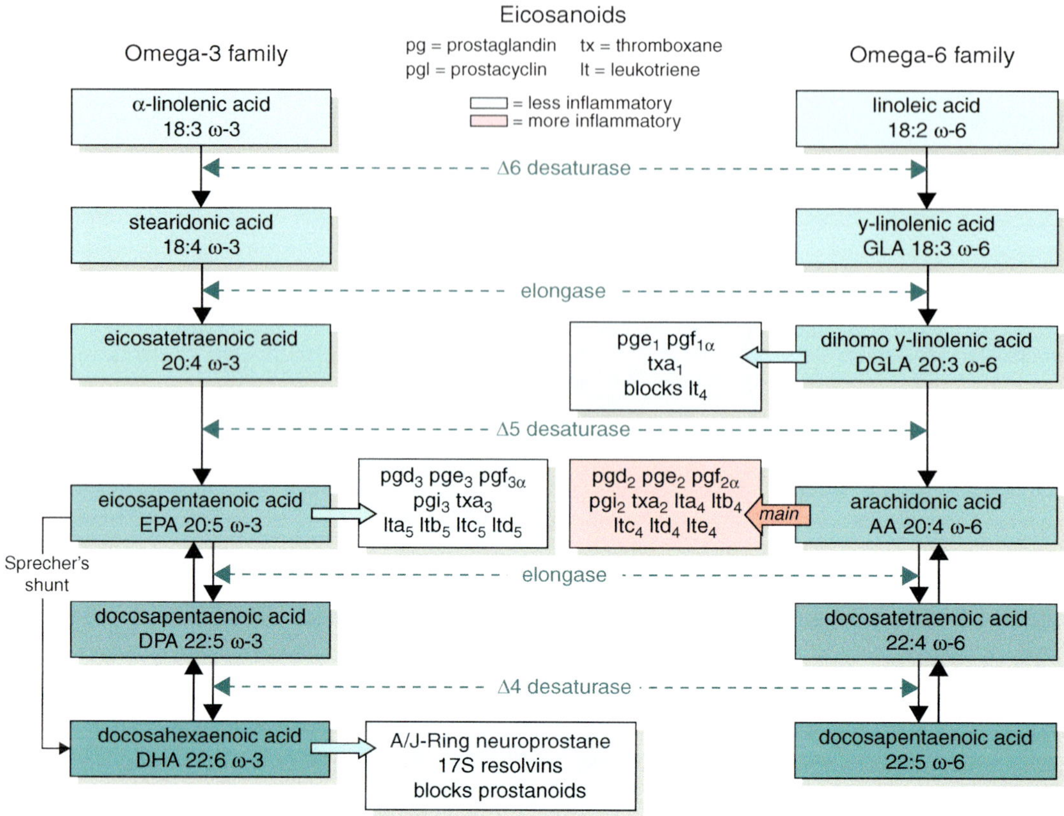


**Fig. 3.15** The eicosanoid pathway is a road map of what happens after consuming Omega-3 or Omega-6. The by-products of these two fats have a big influence on inflammation and immunity. Omega-3s are anti-inflammatory. Omega-6 tends to be pro-inflammatory. (Reproduced with permission from www.Wikipedia.org, David R. Throop, vectorized by Fvasconcellos – w: Image: EFA to Eicosanoid. JPG: https://en.wikipedia.org/wiki/Eicosanoid#/media/File:EFA_to_Eicosanoids.svg. Source: https://omegavia.com/why-omegavia-is-high-in-epa-omega-3-part-1/)

Stress is associated with pro-thrombotic, inflammatory, and oxidative activities. For example, stress from sleep apnea produces inflammation. Stress from being overweight is an inflammation state. Physiologic stress from diabetes is another inflammation state, and so forth. So, anything that reduces inflammation is beneficial. "Natural reduction" of inflammation is possible with exercise, stress reduction, and eating a lot of fish or fish oil and is advantageous to the body. Increasing the Omega-3 to Omega-6 ratio reduces a pro-inflammatory state. It decreases adrenaline and decreases sympathetic nervous system activity, which are both directly associated with inflammation. For example, reducing stress through exercise makes the autonomic nervous system better by increasing parasympathetic (vagal) nerve activity and reducing sympathetic nerve activity. A more vagal physiologic environment is known to be protective for the body. Fish oils appear to have very beneficial effects on autonomic dysfunction, restoring balance and helping the nerves to remain healthy. They also appear to slow heart rate for a more vagally induced (protective) environment [111].

The parasympathetic nervous system is the "breaks" of the body, like the breaks on a car. Typically, it slows things down and protects. The sympathetics are the "accelerator" of the body. The autonomic nervous system, which contains both, has to be in balance with the sympathetics and parasympathetics (adrenaline and vagal activities, respectively), in a (nearly) one to one balance. If there is too much stress at rest, there is too much sympathetic activity, there is too much adrenaline, causing too much inflammation.

**Table 3.1** Omega-6 to Omega-3 fatty acid ratio. Both fatty acids compete for the same enzymes. Omega-6s are pro-thrombotic (pro-clotting), pro-inflammatory, and pro-constrictive (narrows blood vessels, which tends to increase blood pressure). Omega-3s are antithrombotic (impair clotting), anti-inflammatory, dilatory (enlarges blood vessels, which tends to decrease blood pressure), increases healthy nitric oxide production, and improves endothelial function. Ideal ratios of Omega-6 to Omega-3 fatty acids are 4:1 or lower (greater ratios are not healthy, Western diets tend to be 10:1–30:1). Example ratios from different vegetable oils are listed in the table below

| Vegetable oil | Omega-6: Omega-3 |
|---|---|
| Canola | 1:2 |
| Hemp | 2:1 |
| Soybean | 7:1 |
| Corn | 46:1 |
| Olive | 3:1 |
| Cottonseed | * |
| Sunflower | * |
| Peanut | * |
| Flax (preferred) | 1:3 |

*Does not contain Omega-3 fatty acids

What is needed is a little more parasympathetic or vagal activation. Especially for older or chronic disease patients, the recommended autonomic (sympathetic to parasympathetic) ratio, or sympathovagal balance, is a little less than one [112]. It looks like fish oils, in some major studies done by O'Keefe and others, provides that "little extra" vagal activation. In other words, a "little extra" vagal activation at the level of the heart is cardioprotective [113] and protects other organs as well. That is probably the mechanism, like in the heart attack patients of the GISSI International study, by which fish oils reduce the risk of sudden cardiac death. It's probably beneficial in autonomics, not because it lowers triglycerides and not because it increases blood flow, but because it keeps the nerve membranes healthy. The mechanism could be autonomic; however, the anti-inflammatory mechanism of fish oils should not be discounted.

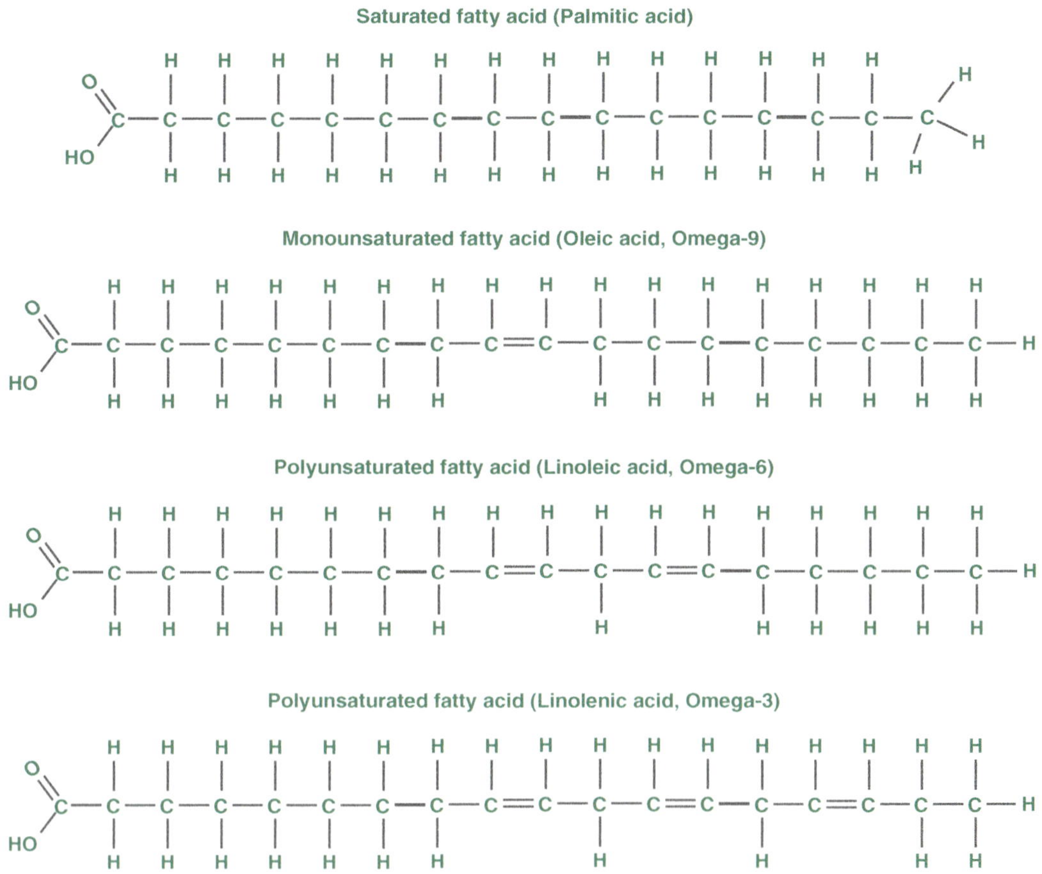


**Fig. 3.16** Molecular structure of Omega-9 fatty acid, with comparison to Omega-3 and Omega-6

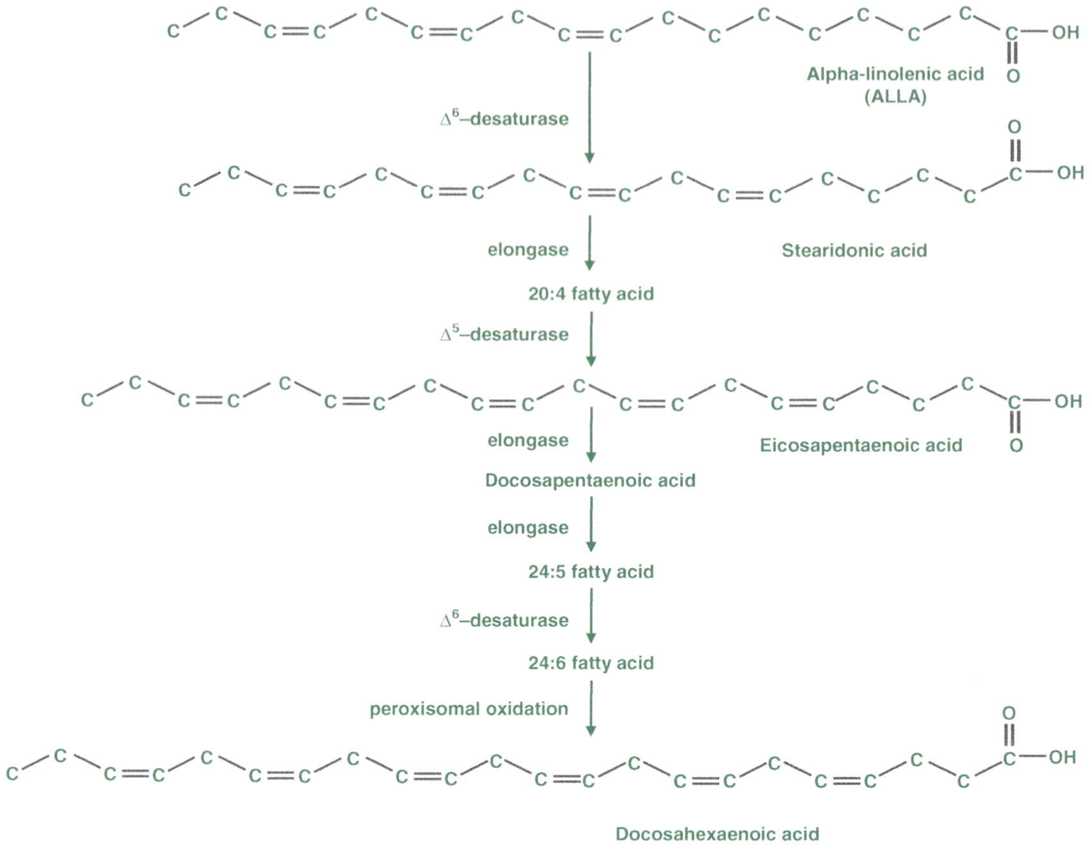


**Fig. 3.17** Pathway for alpha-linolenic acid (ALLA[7]) conversion to eicosapentaenoic acid (EPA) and docosahexaenoic acid (DHA) [110]

These recommendations are not that of any government agency. If there is a family history of coronary heart disease, then 600 mg of EPA plus DHA as a supplement is recommended. If there is a family history of sudden cardiac death or heart disease of significance, at least 1200 mg of EPA plus DHA is recommended. If an individual has a triglyceride level greater than 150, fish oil will be titrated upward to help lower the triglycerides. Up to 3–4 grams of fish oils have been prescribed in many patients, especially those with high triglycerides. These cases are monitored closely for side effects, such as excess bleeding.

These recommendations are based on two major studies: the GISSI study [114–116] and the JELIS study [4–117]. The GISSI study showed that 11,324 patients with recurrent heart attacks prescribed 850 mg of EPA and DHA had, approximately, 50% lower instance of sudden cardiac death. The JELIS study involved 18,645 patients with high cholesterol and a 5-year follow-up (all patients were on statins). The JELIS study showed a major adverse cardiac event (MACE) reduction of 19% with Omega-3 fatty acids. This occurred despite no benefit of Omega-3 lowered LDL counts. These two studies highlight the importance, and potential beneficial effects, of how supplementation with Omega-3 fatty acids can reduce heart disease, including sudden cardiac death. Other studies have not shown such dramatic effect, but have not included such large populations of patients or such large dosages of fish oils as these. In the other studies, patients have been on more modern medications, such as statins, which may have reduced the efficacy of the fish oil supplements. Despite that, the American Heart Association (AHA) has recently recommended (March, 2017) that fish oils are acceptable after heart attack and heart failure and that even a modest 10% reduction of heart disease manifestation would justify treatment with relatively safe therapy [118].

In their recent conclusions, the AHA did not report any new evidence for the use of fish oil in primary prevention of cardiovascular disease. The AHA has previously stated that Omega-3s should be part of a healthy diet and has recommended 1.5–3 g a day of ALLA as also being beneficial, either through plant-based foods or supplement capsule [119]. The AHA dietary guidelines recommend at least two servings of fish per week in a healthy diet [120]. Their diet includes vegetable oils (e.g., soybean, canola, walnut, and flax seed oils) and food such as walnuts and flax seeds, all of which are good sources of ALLA.

Another Omega fatty acid, Omega-9 (see Fig. 3.16), is also an anti-inflammatory. Omega-9 is found in olive oil and will be discussed under the area of Mediterranean diet. One brief note regarding fats, saturated fats have no double bonds. Monounsaturated fats are relatively stable, but not as stable as saturated fat. They only have one double bond. Polyunsaturated fats are the least stable but are the most flexible fats. They have more than one double bond. Omega-3 and fish oils, Omega-6 and vegetable oils, and Omega-9 and extra-virgin or virgin olive oil all have double bonds and are considered polyunsaturated fats. Since the body needs fats for membrane structures, low-fat diets may not be the best option as originally once thought. The body needs some fat. *The key is to pick the right fats!* Omega-3 and Omega-9 are considered most important. Therefore, the liberal consumption of olive oil, Omega-9, and fish oil, Omega-3, fatty acids is recommended.

## More Properties of Fish Oil

Fish oils, in addition to being antithrombotic, in that they impair clotting and inflammation, also dilate blood vessels by increasing nitric oxide production [121]. Nitric oxide is a universal messenger molecule of the body. One of its functions is to improve the health of the endothelial cells lining the insides of arteries. Healthy endothelial cells in the vasculature promote relaxation of the vasculature (i.e., dilation or opening up or relaxing of blood vessels; see Fig. 3.18). These endothelial cells continuously produce an abundance of nitric oxide from the amino acid L-arginine via constitutive nitric oxide synthase (cNOS, see

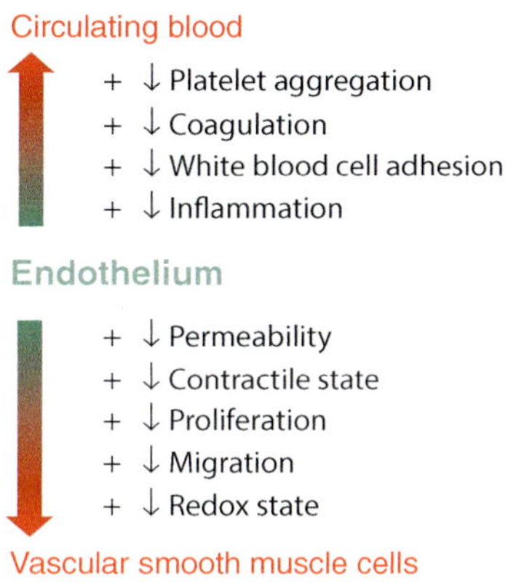


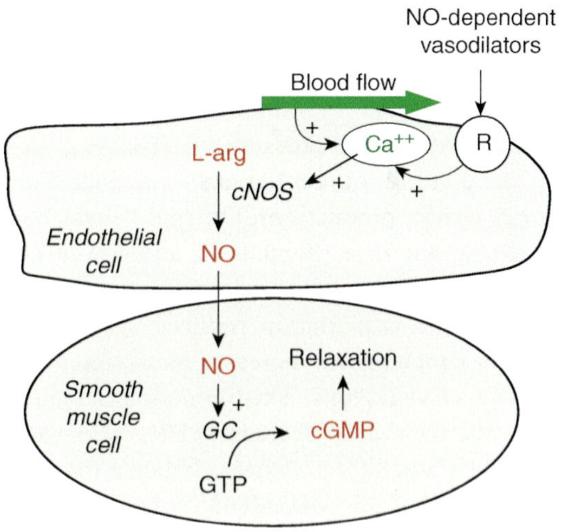


**Fig. 3.18** Nitric oxide improves endothelial cells by reducing free radicals and relaxes vessels. R receptor, L-arg L-arginine, cNOS constitutive nitric oxide synthase, GC guanylyl cyclase, GTP guanosine triphosphate, cGMP cyclic guanosine monophosphate. (Reproduced with permission from Richard E. Klabunde, PhD; in Nitric Oxide Biosynthesis in: Cardiovascular Physiology Concepts. Second Edition, Lippincott Williams & Wilkins, 2012: http://www.cvphysiology.com/Blood%20Flow/BF011. Source: http://www.cvphysiology.com/Blood%20Flow/BF011)

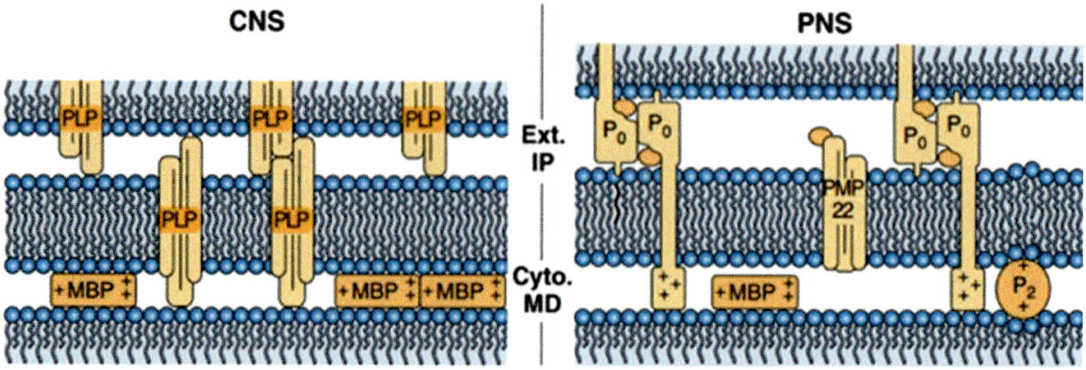


Fig. 3.19 Myelin components, including fatty acid chains (blue), form the lipid bilayers of the myelin cells' plasma membrane. The Omega-3 fatty acids contribute to these fatty acid chains and contribute to the 70–80% fat that insulates nerve fibers to improve the efficiency of nerve conduction. The extracellular surfaces (Ext.) of the myelin cell membranes form the intra-period (IP) lines which are shown in the upperpart of the figure. The cytoplasmic surfaces (Cyto.) of the membranes form the major dense (MD) line. The orange structures are proteins [125]. (Reproduced with permission from Elsevier. Source: https://www.quora.com/What-is-myelin-from-a-structural-perspective-Where-does-the-Schwann-cell-component-end-and-the-fatty-acids-begin)

Fig. 3.18). The vascular endothelium is central to the brain-heart health. Maintaining healthy blood flow to nerves helps to maintain healthy nerves (the brain, and the rest of the nervous system) and the heart. Omega-3s, by keeping endothelial cells and blood vessels healthy, permit them to function continuously and produce nitric oxide. Vasodilation caused by nitric oxide lowers blood pressure [122, 123].

By dilating blood vessels, via increasing nitric oxide production, Omega-3 has been shown to increase vagal tone and lower HR, both of which are cardioprotective [113]. Specifically, vasodilation reduces sympathetic activity which in turn increases parasympathetic activity, or vagal tone. This reduction in sympathetic activity also decreases HR. The vagus (parasympathetic) nerve helps balance the autonomic effects of sympathetic tone. Increased sympathetic tone mediates increases in HR and BP [124]. Fish oils have been shown to counter this by increasing the Vagus nerve activity. The cardioprotective vagal effect may also be the protective mechanism for sudden cardiac death, in that the parasympathetics prevent the sympathetics from driving a ventricular tachycardia (high HR) into ventricular fibrillation which can lead to sudden cardiac death.

Again, fish is also brain food. To maintain a healthy brain and specifically healthy myelin, sufficient amounts of Omega-3 fatty acids are required. Fatty acids are the building blocks of myelin (Fig. 3.19) and other brain tissues (as well as parts of all other tissues, cells, and organelle membranes, throughout the body; Fig. 3.20). Nerve fibers are coated with myelin (Fig. 3.21). *Myelin is 70–80% fat and promotes the efficient transfer of signals through the brain and the nervous system throughout the body.* The brain, on the whole, is about 40% Omega-3 fatty acids. Omega-3 helps myelin sheaths of the nerve cells remain healthy [127]. By doing so, the body's cognitive function stays sharper, mood is stabilized, and muscle coordination is maintained. Fish products, and specifically fish oils, are thought to be extremely protective in maintaining the integrity of these myelin sheaths.

The brain consumes much of the oxygen and nutrients taken in by the body (about 70% at rest and up to 85% when physically or mentally active). Therefore, brain cells are among the cells (liver and cardiac cells) that have the most mitochondria. As mentioned in the introductory chapter, mitochondria are the power plants of cells, producing energy in the form of ATP (Fig. 3.15). By keeping brain cells healthy, mitochondria can

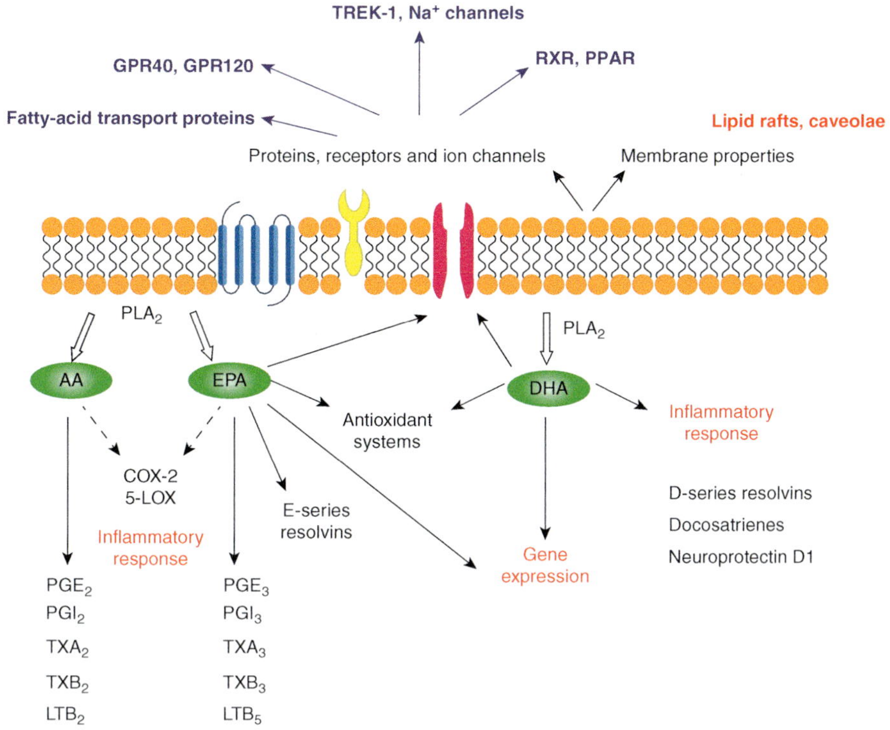


**Fig. 3.20** EPA and DHA are the two main types of Omega-3 fatty acids which play an important role in maintaining normal cell function [126]. (Reproduced with permission from Elsevier. Source: http://www.cell.com/trends/neurosciences/fulltext/S0166-2236(13)00198-7)

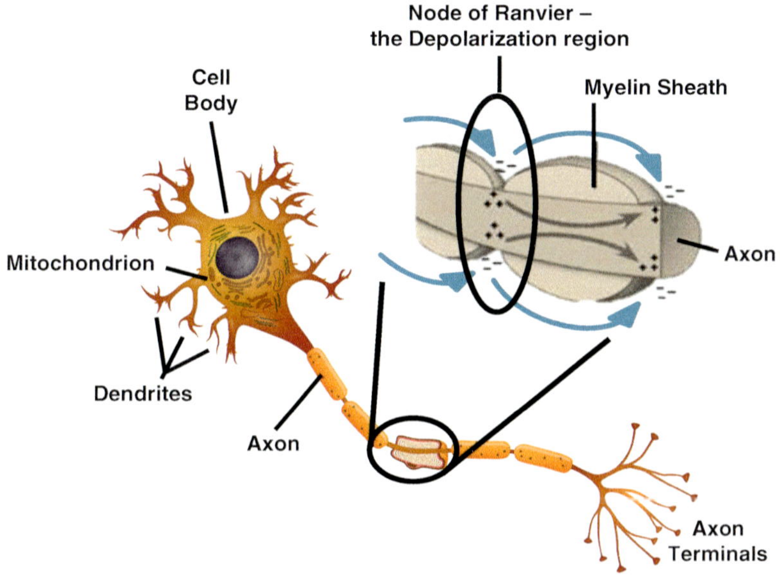


**Fig. 3.21** The function of myelin, forming the myelin sheath, helping to form saltatory conduction. In myelinated axons, the ion current during an action potential at one node of Ranvier spreads along the interior of the axon to the next node (see dark gray arrows), triggering an action potential at the next node. The gated sodium ($Na^+$) and potassium ($K^+$) channels are only at the nodes. Thus, the action potential "jumps" from one node of Ranvier to the next (saltatory conduction, blue arrows). Saltatory conduction greatly increases the speed at which a signal is conducted along an axon. (Adapted from Shutterstock Royalty-free stock vector images ID: 1059570251, Neuron that is the main part of the nervous system, by Netta07)

continue to produce significant amounts of ATP for brain energy. The myelin sheaths are important to protect. When they are damaged (i.e., in multiple sclerosis), they need to be repaired, or else the nerve signal may not make it to its target. Omega-3 is also thought to be helpful in repairing damaged myelin sheaths. To this end, at least 600 mg of Omega-3 supplementation a day is recommended, in addition to eating two to three oily fish meals a week (specifically, fish such as salmon, herring, or mackerel). This is highly encouraged.

If an individual cannot eat fish, they may need to consume more fish oil supplementation. If they have established heart disease, a higher dose is often required [8]. If the triglycerides are significantly above 150, higher doses of fish oil supplements are also used. There are also prescription formulations. Lovaza and Vascepa have been approved by the FDA for very high triglyceride-lowering regiments. As each individual has their own set of different circumstances, and as a result, treatment will vary from individual to individual, starting this program or any of its components should be under close physician supervision.

## Summary of Cumulative Data

In summary (Fig. 3.22), fish oils are anti-inflammatory. They are also vasodilatory. They protect the inner lining of the blood vessels (the endothelium). By enlarging blood vessels, they can lower blood pressure. They are also very important in preserving nerve fibers in the brain and the body. They are very important in pregnancy and the prenatal period with children. So, there are a lot of beneficial effects with fish oil, whether taken naturally, or in supplement form at the appropriate dose for the patient as determined by their physician. While fish oils are, a main component of the six-prong program, they do not work alone. Taking fish oils alone may not help. The whole program is needed, since all six prongs work together: reducing psychosocial stress, exercise, keeping blood vessels healthy with nitric oxide, maintaining a healthy antioxidant reserve, and the Mediterranean diet, including olive oil. Fish oil actually helps nitric oxide levels go up. When the endothelial lining of the vasculature is kept healthy with fish oil, those endothelial cells create nitric oxide. The healthier they are, the more nitric oxide they will make. Indirectly, fish oil helps increase nitric oxide. In addition, nitric oxide will help promote the fish oil anti-inflammatory effect because nitric oxide has anti-inflammatory effects also. The Mind-Body Wellness program all work together as a team. It is a holistic approach that can be tailored to the patient's needs.

**Omega-3 Chapter Science Highlights**

1. *Cardiovascular System* – the best data is with high-dose Omega-3 (1.8 g or more), primarily EPA; this has been shown to reduce cardiovascular (CV) events.
   (a) GISSI (1999) – 11,324 myocardial infarction (MI) patients were given 870 mg Omega-3 (single capsule, 290 mg EPA/580 mg DHA) for 42 months, or vitamin E, or both, or no supplements (the control group). The findings are (1) vitamin E had no effect; (2) Omega-3 lowered CV mortality. Relative risk (RR) was reduced 14% overall, driven primarily by 26% RR reduction in sudden death. At baseline, there was only 4% statin use throughout the cohort. Statin drop-in created 44% statin use by end of the study. The effects of statin use is difficult to determine.
   (b) JELIS (2007) – 18,645 coronary artery disease (CAD) or at-risk patients already prescribed statin and received 1.8 g pre EPA (no DHA) for average 4.7 years. Overall, there was a 19% RR reduction in CV events driven primarily by a reduction in unstable angina. The first study showed a benefit by adding drug to statin therapy. In patients with high triglycerides (>150 mg/dL) and low high-density lipoproteins (<40 mg/dL), there was a 53% RR reduction in CV events.
   (c) At least 16 other CV event reduction studies all used pure or high-dose EPA as

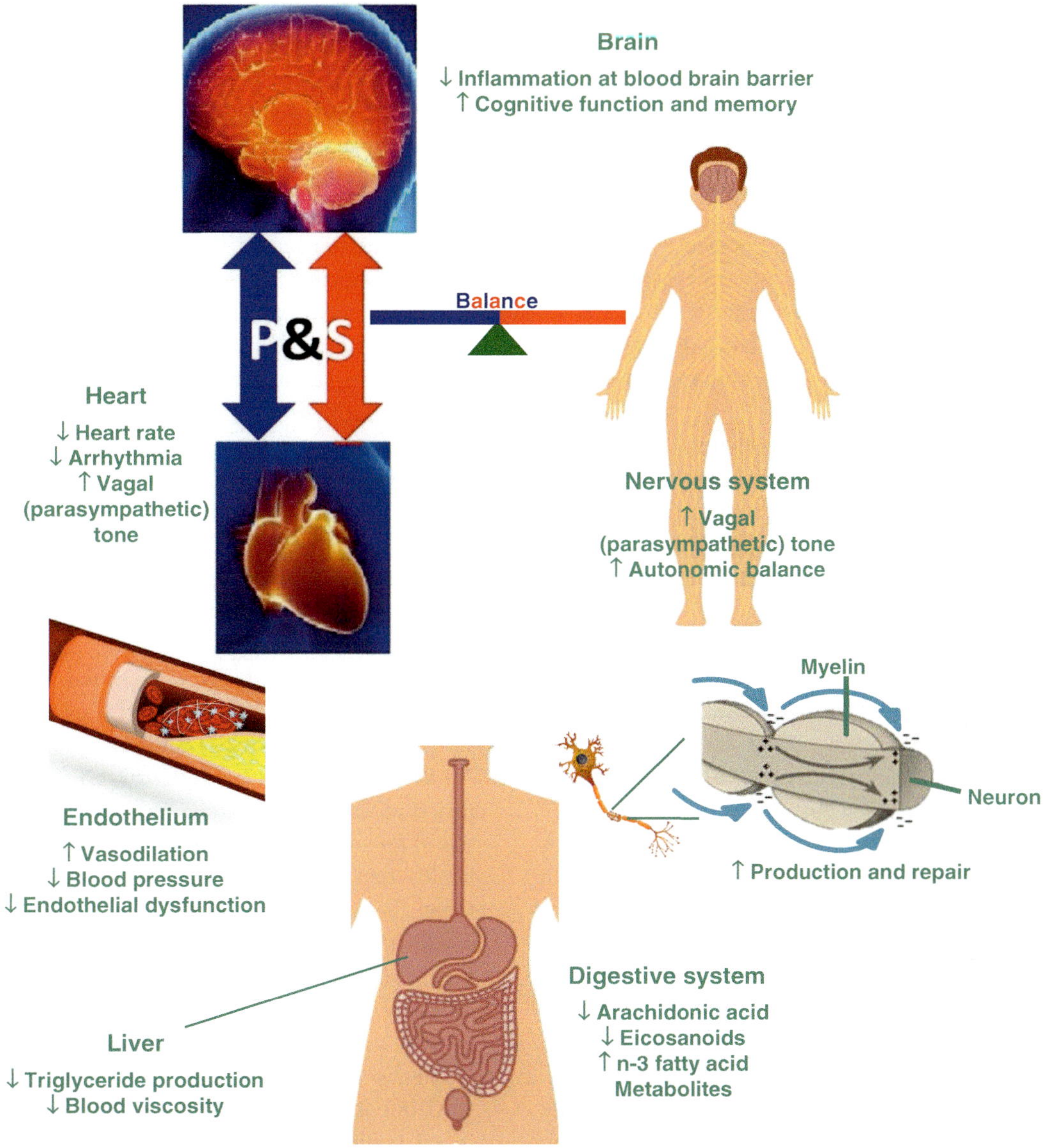


**Fig. 3.22** Physiologic effects of n-3 omega fish oils. See text: "Summary of Cumulative Data"

active treatment versus placebo or no comparator. All 16 were positive for showing a reduction in CV events with pure, or very high, dose EPA. None of these trials (16 other studies and the JELIS study) had elevated triglycerides as an entry criterion (e.g., [117]).

(d) Ocean Trial (2010) – patients receiving Lovaza 1–14 weeks prior to carotidectomy showed that EPA gets into atherosclerotic plaque very rapidly and at a rate eight to ten times greater than DHA.

(e) EPA is shown to thicken and stabilize plaque fibrous cap within days, 150% at 8 weeks, with or without statin.

(f) Low Omega-3 levels in pregnancy leads to subclinical atherosclerosis in the fetus and newborns (as measured by Aortic and Carotid Intima-Media Thickness (AIMT and CIMT, respectively).

(g) Research-supported mechanisms by which EPA reduces CV events include [128]:
   (i) DHA reduces hepatic LDL receptor formation and raises plasma LDL-C; EPA does not.
   (ii) EPA reduces particle number and increases particle size.
   (iii) EPA reduces systemic and vascular-specific inflammation.
   (iv) EPA reduces LDL oxidation.
   (v) EPA reduces remnant cholesterol particles.
   (vi) EPA stabilizes atherosclerotic plaque.
   (vii) EPA reduces thrombus.
   (viii) EPA prevents cellular cholesterol crystallization; DHA does not.
   (ix) EPA demonstrates a slight anticoagulation effect.
   (x) EPA demonstrates a slight antiplatelet effect.
   (xi) EPA demonstrates a normorhythmic or anti-arrhythmic effect.

2. *Anti-inflammatory* – research-supported EPA benefits in [129, 130]:
   (a) Asthma – EPA is more potent than DHA in reducing inflammatory response in human asthmatic alveolar macrophages and decreases reliance on rescue inhalers and medications.
   (b) Attention deficit hyperactivity disorder (ADHD) – EPA benefits pediatric patients, especially at higher doses.
   (c) Brain function – EPA and DHA enter the brain at the same rate and concentration, but EPA is more rapidly burned or beta-oxidized.
   (d) Cancers – EPA improves prognosis in multiple cancers (e.g., colorectal, non-small-cell lung, pancreatic, breast, and others), tumor formation, and tumor advancement reduction, as well as in sarcopenia and cachexia.
   (e) Crohn's disease and inflammatory bowel diseases – EPA reduced Crohn's relapses and improved IBD and joint symptoms.
   (f) Dentition – EPA reduces periodontitis and gingivitis.
   (g) Depression – EPA alone, and with, antidepressant medications show symptom improvement.
   (h) Dermatology – EPA demonstrates benefits in acne vulgaris, dermatitis, psoriasis, and other dermatologic conditions.
   (i) Diabetes, metabolic syndrome, and insulin resistance – EPA improves multiple mechanisms and metrics.
   (j) Lupus –symptomatic relief demonstrated with EPA; studies also showed lower EPA in lupus patients with CVD than without.
   (k) Pregnancy – EPA demonstrated reductions in endometriosis in vitro fertilization (IVF) and miscarriage in patients with antiphospholipid antibodies.
   (l) Rheumatoid arthritis – EPA reduces RA flares, severity of flares, Disease-Modifying Anti-Rheumatic Drugs (DMARD) and Non-Steroidal Anti-Inflammatory Drugs (NSAID) used, and DMARD and NSAID failure.

3. *Health Benefits of Omega-3 Fatty Acids* – proposed in selected research. The following are based on smaller and fewer studies than those health benefits listed above. This does not mean that these benefits are sham. It simply means that more care should be taken when following the referenced recommendations.
   - There is strong evidence that Omega-3 fatty acids have a beneficial effect in bipolar disorder [131, 132].
   - Clinical studies have reported that oral fish oil supplementation has beneficial effects in rheumatoid arthritis and among some asthmatics [133–135].
   - Fish oil improves tubular dysfunction, lipid profiles, and oxidative stress in patients with Immunoglobulin A (IgA) nephropathy [136].
   - Dietary supplementation with flaxseed oil lowers blood pressure in dyslipidemia patients [137].
   - Omega-3 fatty acids improve the cardiovascular risk profile of subjects with metabolic syndrome, including markers of inflammation and autoimmunity [138].

- Omega-3 in modest doses reduces cardiac deaths and in high doses reduces nonfatal cardiovascular events [139].
- Dietary supplementation with Omega-3 fatty acids reduces the incidence of sudden cardiac death in patients with myocardial infarction [140–142].
- Omega-3 fatty acid reduces the total mortality and sudden death in patients with left ventricular systolic dysfunction [143].
- Raising blood levels of Omega-3 fatty acids is up to eight times more effective than automated external defibrillators (AEDs) and up to two times more effective than implanted cardioverter defibrillators (ICDs) in preventing sudden death [144].
- Consuming small quantities of fish is associated with a reduction in coronary heart disease [145].
- Omega-3 fatty acids and vitamin D supplementation results in a substantial reduction in coronary calcium scores and slowed plaque growth [146].
- Omega-3 fatty acid supplementation has a therapeutic effect in children with ADHD [98].
- Omega-3 fatty acids appear to be an effective treatment for children with autism [147].
- Omega-3 fatty acids improve macro- and microvascular function in subjects with type 2 diabetes mellitus [148].
- In patients with stable coronary artery disease, an independent and inverse association exists between n-3 fatty acid levels and inflammatory biomarkers [149].
- Omega-3 fatty acids improve endothelial function in peripheral arterial disease [150].
- Fish oil has a beneficial effect on blood viscosity in peripheral vascular disease [151].
- Fish oil supplementation improves walking distance in peripheral arterial disease [152].
- Omega-3 fish oil reduces the severity of symptoms in patients with systemic lupus erythematosus [153].
- Higher plasma concentrations of EPA and DPA are associated with a lower risk of nonfatal myocardial infarction among women [154–156].
- Fish oil, but not flaxseed oil, decreases inflammation and prevents pressure overload-induced cardiac dysfunction [157].
- The consumption of fish reduces the risk of ischemic stroke in elderly individuals [158, 159].
- A moderate intake of EPA and DHA may postpone cognitive decline in elderly men [160].
- Omega-3 fatty acids may have therapeutic value in the treatment of dry eye syndrome [161, 162].
- Omega-3 fatty acid supplementation exhibits therapeutic value in the treatment of children with attention deficit hyperactivity disorder (ADHD) symptomatology [163].
- Omega-3 fatty acids supplementation prevents and reverses insulin resistance [164].
- Omega-3 fatty acids are beneficial for children with bronchial asthma [165].
- Omega-3 fatty acids alleviate insulin resistance and fatty liver in obese mice [166].
- Intake of EPA and DPA from fish is possibly associated with a reduced prevalence of allergic rhinitis [167].
- Cod liver oil (Omega-3 fatty acids) reduces the need for NSAIDs in patients with rheumatoid arthritis [168].
- Omega-3 fatty acids has significant therapeutic benefits and drug sparing activity in the treatment of rheumatoid arthritis [169].
- Omega-3 fatty acids were shown to be more effective than placebo for depression in both adults and children in small controlled studies and in an open study of bipolar depression [170].
- A diet low in trans-unsaturated fat and rich in Omega-3 fatty acids and olive oil may reduce the risk of age-related macular degeneration [171].

In spite of all of this good news, some of the studies quoted showed only neutral effects. Given these neutral studies, it maybe that the fish oils were only good in certain people and not in others. In a review of this literature, all of the studies that used higher doses of fish oils seemed to do the best in terms of better reductions in only certain diseases, such as heart attacks and deaths. That is also an empiric observation. For example, how can it be that people who live in the middle part of Japan have lower levels of Omega-3 fish oils in their bodies and don't live as long as the people in Japan's fishing villages. It is because those near the ocean are probably eating more fish than those not near the ocean. In another example, how do the Eskimos in Greenland not get heart attacks while eating only the blubber from whales. It is because whale blubber contains fish oils from the algae and plankton they eat. What about supplements, do they actually work? The net of the evidence is positive. It may be that higher doses of fish oils are needed in order to work for people who are sicker. For healthy people, maybe 500–1000 mg of these EPA and DHA compounds from fish oils are needed. However, for patients with high triglycerides or who have heart disease, higher concentrations may be needed. There are a lot of big studies that are ongoing. All of the studies have shown one thing with fish oil capsules. There are no bad or negative effects. The results are either neutral or good. Considering the studies with good results, the populations may have been different. The study dose may have been different. The bioavailability of the compound may have been different. Regardless, there is no question that fish (per say) and probably the fish oils (if taken in the right concentrations and in the right subsets of people) will have beneficial effects. Of course the buyer must beware. The quality of the fish oil is also important. Ultimately, epidemiology cannot be fought. Fish oils do not cause negative results. If the patient is healthy and already eating healthy and living a healthy lifestyle, then the patient is already receiving the benefits that fish oils provide. As soon as the patient becomes sick or if a more typical Western lifestyle (American diet and sedentary) is chosen, then Omega-3 fatty acids from fish oils together with the other five lifestyle and supplement recommendations of the Mind-Body Wellness program are extremely important for relieving autonomic and mitochondrial dysfunction, thereby establishing and maintaining health and wellness.

## References


1. David JKS, DePace N, Noval J, Reichie FA. Cholesterol lowering mechanism of fish oil rich in ω-3 fatty acids in cardiac patients. Arteriosclerosis. 1987;7(5) :512A.
2. Bhatt DL, Steg PG, Miller M, Brinton EA, Jacobson TA, Ketchum SB, Doyle RT Jr, Juliano RA, Jiao L, Granowitz C, Tardif JC, Ballantyne CM; REDUCE-IT Investigators. Cardiovascular risk reduction with icosapent ethyl for hypertriglyceridemia. N Engl J Med. 2018. https://doi.org/10.1056/NEJMoa1812792. [Epub ahead of print].
3. Betteridge DJ. The case for intensive lipid management: The opportunities and issues for cardiologists. PACE-CME Lecture. 2011. https://pace-cme.org/2011/06/16/the-case-for-intensive-lipid-management-the-opportunities-and-issues-for-cardiologists/
4. Yokoyama M, Origasa H, JELIS Investigators. Effects of eicosapentaenoic acid on cardiovascular events in Japanese patients with hypercholesterolemia: rationale, design, and baseline characteristics of the Japan EPA Lipid Intervention Study (JELIS). Am Heart J. 2003;146(4):613–20.
5. Yokoyama M, Origasa H, Matsuzaki M, Matsuzawa Y, Saito Y, Ishikawa Y, Oikawa S, Sasaki J, Hishida H, Itakura H, Kita T, Kitabatake A, Nakaya N, Sakata T, Shimada K, Shirato K, Japan EPA lipid intervention study (JELIS) Investigators. Effects of eicosapentaenoic acid on major coronary events in hypercholesterolemia patients (JELIS): a randomized open-label, blinded endpoint analysis. Lancet. 2007;369(9567):1090–8. Erratum in: Lancet. 2007 Jul 21;370(9583):220.
6. Libby P. Interleukin-1 Beta as a target for atherosclerosis therapy: biological basis of CANTOS and beyond. J Am Coll Cardiol. 2017;70(18):2278–89. https://doi.org/10.1016/j.jacc.2017.09.028.
7. Güttler N, Zheleva K, Parahuleva M, Chasan R, Bilgin M, Neuhof C, Burgazli M, Niemann B, Erdogan A, Böning A. Omega-3 fatty acids and vitamin d in cardiology. Cardiol Res Pract. 2012, Article ID: 729670, 11 pages. https://doi.org/10.1155/2012/729670. Epub 2012 Dec 31.
8. Mozaffarian D, Rimm EB. Fish intake, contaminants, and human health: evaluating the risks and the benefits. JAMA. 2006;296(15):1885–99. Review. Erratum in: JAMA. 2007 Feb 14;297(6):590.
9. Crawford MH, DiMarco JP, editors. Cardiology. London: Mosby; 2001.
10. Chen M, Nagase M, Fujita T, Narumiya S, Masaki T, Sawamura T. Diabetes enhances lectin-like oxidized LDL receptor-1 (LOX-1) expression in the vascular endothelium: possible role of LOX-1 ligand and AGALE. Biophys Res Commun. 2001;287:962–8.
11. Pothineni NVK, Karathanasis SK, Ding Z, Arulandu A, Varughese KI, Mehta JL. LOX-1 in atherosclerosis

and myocardial ischemia: biology, genetics, and modulation. J Am Coll Cardiol. 2017;69(22):2759–68. https://doi.org/10.1016/j.jacc.2017.04.010. Review.
12. Deanfield JE, Halcox JP, Rabelink TJ. Endothelial function and dysfunction: testing and clinical relevance. Circulation. 2007;115(10):1285–95. Review.
13. Ding Z, et al. Mitochondrial DNA damage in NLRP-3 inflammation activation and macrophages implication in atherogenesis. Cardiovasc Res. 2014;103:619–28.
14. Marwali MR, Hu CP, Mohandas B, Dandapat A, Deonikar P, Chen J, Cawich I, Sawamura T, Kavdia M, Mehta JL. Modulation of ADP-induced platelet activation by aspirin and pravastatin: role of lectin-like oxidized low-density lipoprotein receptor-1, nitric oxide, oxidative stress, and inside-out integrin signaling. J Pharmacol Exp Ther. 2007;322(3):1324–32. Epub 2007 May 30.
15. Niwa Y, Iwai N. Nanomaterials induce oxidized low-density lipoprotein cellular uptake in macrophages and platelet aggregation. Circ J. 2007;71(3):437–44.
16. Hayashida K, et al. Serum soluble lectin-like oxidized low-density lipoprotein receptor-1 levels are elevated in acute coronary syndrome, a novel marker for early diagnosis. Circulation. 2005;112:812–8.
17. Besler C, et al. Mechanisms underlying adverse effects of HDL on eNOS-activating pathways in patients with coronary artery disease. J Clin Invest. 2011;121:2693–708.
18. Mehta JL. Aspirin inhibits oxidized LDL-mediated LOX-1 expression and metalloproteinase- 1 in human coronary endothelial cells. Cardiovasc Res. 2004;64(2):243–9.
19. Freire MO, Van Dyke TE. Natural resolution of inflammation. Periodontol 2000. 2013;63(1):149–64. https://doi.org/10.1111/prd.12034.
20. Kohli P, Levy BD. Resolvins and protectins: mediating solutions to inflammation. Br J Pharmacol. 2009;158(4):960–71. https://doi.org/10.1111/j.1476-5381.2009.00290.x.
21. Chandrasekharan JA, Sharma-Walia N. Lipoxins: nature's way to resolve inflammation. J Inflamm Res. 2015;8:181–92. Published online 2015 Sep 30. https://doi.org/10.2147/JIR.S90380.
22. Serhan CN, Yang R, Martinod K, Kasuga K, Pillai PS, Porter TF, Oh SF, Spite M. Maresins: novel macrophage mediators with potent anti-inflammatory and pro-resolving actions. J Exp Med. 2009;206(1):15–23. https://doi.org/10.1084/jem.20081880.
23. Ridker PM, Everett BM, Thuren T, MacFadyen JG, Chang WH, Ballantyne C, Fonseca F, Nicolau J, Koenig W, Anker SD, Kastelein JJP, Cornel JH, Pais P, Pella D, Genest J, Cifkova R, Lorenzatti A, Forster T, Kobalava Z, Vida-Simiti L, Flather M, Shimokawa H, Ogawa H, Dellborg M, Rossi PRF, Troquay RPT, Libby P, Glynn RJ, CANTOS Trial Group. Anti-inflammatory therapy with canakinumab for atherosclerotic disease. N Engl J Med. 2017;377(12):1119–31. https://doi.org/10.1056/NEJMoa1707914. Epub 2017 Aug 27.
24. Hu PJ, Pittet JF, Kerby JD, Bosarge PL, Wagener BM. Acute brain trauma, lung injury and pneumonia: more than just altered mental status and decreased airway protection. Am J Physiol Lung Cell Mol Physiol. 2017. https://doi.org/10.1152/ajplung.00485.2016. [Epub ahead of print].
25. Kromhout D, Bosschieter EB, de Lezenne Coulander C. The inverse relation between fish consumption and 20-year mortality from coronary heart disease. N Engl J Med. 1985;312(19):1205–9.
26. Kenny D, Warltier DC, Pleuss JA, Hoffmann RG, Goodfriend TL, Egan BM. Effect of omega-3 fatty acids on the vascular response to angiotensin in normotensive men. Am J Cardiol. 1992;70(15):1347–52.
27. Chin JP, Gust AP, Nestel PJ, Dart AM. Marine oils dose-dependently inhibit vasoconstriction of forearm resistance vessels in humans. Hypertension. 1993;21(1):22–8.
28. Bjerregaard P, Mulvad G, Pedersen HS. Cardiovascular risk factors in Inuit of Greenland. Int J Epidemiol. 1997;26(6):1182–90.
29. Nordøy A. Fish consumption and cardiovascular diseases. Eur Heart J Suppl. 2001;3(Suppl D):D4–7.
30. Leaf A, Kang JX, Xiao YF, Billman GE. Clinical prevention of sudden death by n-3 polyunsaturated fatty acids and mechanism of prevention of arrhythmias by n-3 fish oils. Circulation. 2003;107(21):2646–52. Review.
31. Kris-Etherton PM, Harris WS, Appel LJ, American Heart Association. Nutrition Committee. Fish consumption, fish oil, omega-3 fatty acids, and cardiovascular disease. Circulation. 2002;106(21):2747–57. No abstract available. Erratum in: Circulation. 2003 Jan 28;107(3):512.
32. Wang C, Harris WS, Chung M, Lichtenstein AH, Balk EM, Kupelnick B, Jordan HS, Lau J. n-3 Fatty acids from fish or fish-oil supplements, but not alpha-linolenic acid, benefit cardiovascular disease outcomes in primary- and secondary-prevention studies: a systematic review. Am J Clin Nutr. 2006;84(1):5–17. Review.
33. Chrysohoou C, Panagiotakos DB, Pitsavos C, Skoumas J, Krinos X, Chloptsios Y, Nikolaou V, Stefanadis C. Long-term fish consumption is associated with protection against arrhythmia in healthy persons in a Mediterranean region – the ATTICA study. Am J Clin Nutr. 2007;85(5):1385–91.
34. O'Keefe JH Jr, Abuissa H, Sastre A, Steinhaus DM, Harris WS. Effects of omega-3 fatty acids on resting heart rate, heart rate recovery after exercise, and heart rate variability in men with healed myocardial infarctions and depressed ejection fractions. Am J Cardiol. 2006;97(8):1127–30. Epub 2006 Mar 3.
35. von Schacky C, Harris WS. Cardiovascular benefits of omega-3 fatty acids. Cardiovasc Res. 2007;73(2):310–5. Epub 2006 Sept 1. Review.
36. Artham SM, Lavie CJ, Milani RV, Anand RG, O'Keefe JH, Ventura HO. Fish oil in primary and secondary cardiovascular prevention. Ochsner J. 2008;8(2):49–60.

37. Weitz D, Weintraub H, Fisher E, Schwartzbard AZ. Fish oil for the treatment of cardiovascular disease. Cardiol Rev. 2010;18(5):258–63. https://doi.org/10.1097/CRD.0b013e3181ea0de0. Review.
38. Kromhout D, Yasuda S, Geleijnse JM, Shimokawa H. Fish oil and omega-3 fatty acids in cardiovascular disease: do they really work? Eur Heart J. 2012;33(4):436–43. https://doi.org/10.1093/eurheartj/ehr362. Epub 2011 Sept 19. Review.
39. Moertl D, Hammer A, Steiner S, Hutuleac R, Vonbank K, Berger R. Dose-dependent effects of omega-3-polyunsaturated fatty acids on systolic left ventricular function, endothelial function, and markers of inflammation in chronic heart failure of nonischemic origin: a double-blind, placebo-controlled, 3-arm study. Am Heart J. 2011;161(5):915.e1–9. https://doi.org/10.1016/j.ahj.2011.02.011.
40. Albert CM. Omega-3 fatty acids, ventricular arrhythmias, and sudden cardiac death: antiarrhythmic, proarrhythmic, or neither. Circ Arrhythm Electrophysiol. 2012;5(3):456–9. https://doi.org/10.1161/CIRCEP.112.971416.
41. Kotwal S1, Jun M, Sullivan D, Perkovic V, Neal B. Omega 3 fatty acids and cardiovascular outcomes: systematic review and meta-analysis. Circ Cardiovasc Qual Outcomes. 2012;5(6):808–18. https://doi.org/10.1161/CIRCOUTCOMES.112.966168. Epub 2012 Oct 30.
42. Kwak SM, Myung SK, Lee YJ, Seo HG, Korean Meta-analysis Study Group. Efficacy of omega-3 fatty acid supplements (eicosapentaenoic acid and docosahexaenoic acid) in the secondary prevention of cardiovascular disease: a meta-analysis of randomized, double-blind, placebo-controlled trials. Arch Intern Med. 2012;172(9):686–94. https://doi.org/10.1001/archinternmed.2012.262. Review.
43. Rizos EC, Ntzani EE, Bika E, Kostapanos MS, Elisaf MS. Association between omega-3 fatty acid supplementation and risk of major cardiovascular disease events: a systematic review and meta-analysis. JAMA. 2012;308(10):1024–33. https://doi.org/10.1001/2012.jama.11374. Review.
44. Ohnishi H, Saito Y. Eicosapentaenoic acid (EPA) reduces cardiovascular events: relationship with the EPA/arachidonic acid ratio. J Atheroscler Thromb. 2013;20(12):861–77. Epub 2013 Sept 18. Review.
45. Casula M, Soranna D, Catapano AL, Corrao G. Long-term effect of high dose omega-3 fatty acid supplementation for secondary prevention of cardiovascular outcomes: a meta-analysis of randomized, placebo controlled trials [corrected]. Atheroscler Suppl. 2013;14(2):243–51. https://doi.org/10.1016/S1567-5688(13)70005-9. Review. Erratum in: Atheroscler Suppl. 2014 Mar;233(1):122.
46. Nosaka K, Miyoshi T, Iwamoto M, Kajiya M, Okawa K, Tsukuda S, Yokohama F, Sogo M, Nishibe T, Matsuo N, Hirohata S, Ito H, Doi M. Early initiation of eicosapentaenoic acid and statin treatment is associated with better clinical outcomes than statin alone in patients with acute coronary syndromes: 1-year outcomes of a randomized controlled study. Int J Cardiol. 2017;228:173–9. https://doi.org/10.1016/j.ijcard.2016.11.105. Epub 2016 Nov 9.
47. Watanabe Y, Tatsuno I. Omega-3 polyunsaturated fatty acids for cardiovascular diseases: present, past and future. Expert Rev Clin Pharmacol. 2017;29:1–9. https://doi.org/10.1080/17512433.2017.1333902. [Epub ahead of print].
48. Siscovick DS, Barringer TA, Fretts AM, Wu JH, Lichtenstein AH, Costello RB, Kris-Etherton PM, Jacobson TA, Engler MB, Alger HM, Appel LJ, Mozaffarian D, American Heart Association Nutrition Committee of the Council on Lifestyle and Cardiometabolic Health; Council on Epidemiology and Prevention; Council on Cardiovascular Disease in the Young; Council on Cardiovascular and Stroke Nursing; and Council on Clinical Cardiology. Omega-3 polyunsaturated fatty acid (fish oil) supplementation and the prevention of clinical cardiovascular disease: a science advisory from the American Heart Association. Circulation. 2017;135(15):e867–84. https://doi.org/10.1161/CIR.0000000000000482. Epub 2017 Mar 13. Review.
49. Bjerregaard P, Pedersen HS, Mulvad G. The associations of a marine diet with plasma lipids, blood glucose, blood pressure and obesity among the inuit in Greenland. Eur J Clin Nutr. 2000;54(9):732–7.
50. Yamagishi K, Iso H, Date C, Fukui M, Wakai K, Kikuchi S, Inaba Y, Tanabe N, Tamakoshi A, Japan Collaborative Cohort Study for Evaluation of Cancer Risk Study Group. Fish, omega-3 polyunsaturated fatty acids, and mortality from cardiovascular diseases in a nationwide community-based cohort of Japanese men and women the JACC (Japan Collaborative Cohort Study for evaluation of cancer risk) study. J Am Coll Cardiol. 2008;52(12):988–96. https://doi.org/10.1016/j.jacc.2008.06.018.
51. Nakamura Y, Hozawa A, Turin TC, Takashima N, Okamura T, Hayakawa T, Kita Y, Okayama A, Miura K, Ueshima H, NIPPON DATA80 Research Group. Dietary habits in middle age and future changes in activities of daily living – NIPPON DATA80. Gerontology. 2009;55(6):707–13. https://doi.org/10.1159/000235906. Epub 2009 Aug 28.
52. Hirai Y, Geleijnse JM, Adachi H, Imaizumi T, Kromhout D. Systolic blood pressure predicts cardiovascular mortality in farming but not in a fishing community. -A 40-year follow up of the Japanese cohorts of the Seven Countries Study. Circ J. 2011;75(8):1890–6. Epub 2011 Jun 15.
53. Eguchi E, Iso H, Tanabe N, Wada Y, Yatsuya H, Kikuchi S, Inaba Y, Tamakoshi A, Japan Collaborative Cohort Study Group. Healthy lifestyle behaviors and cardiovascular mortality among Japanese men and women: the Japan Collaborative Cohort Study. Eur Heart J. 2012;33(4):467–77. https://doi.org/10.1093/eurheartj/ehr429.
54. Tsugane S, Sawada N. The JPHC study: design and some findings on the typical Japanese diet. Jpn J Clin

Oncol. 2014;44(9):777–82. https://doi.org/10.1093/jjco/hyu096. Epub 2014 Aug 7.
55. Nakamura Y, Okuda N, Okamura T, Kadota A, Miyagawa N, Hayakawa T, Kita Y, Fujiyoshi A, Nagai M, Takashima N, Ohkubo T, Miura K, Okayama A, Ueshima H, NIPPON DATA Research Group. Low-carbohydrate diets and cardiovascular and total mortality in Japanese: a 29-year follow-up of NIPPON DATA80. Br J Nutr. 2014;112(6):916–24. https://doi.org/10.1017/S0007114514001627.
56. Menotti A, Puddu PE. How the Seven Countries Study contributed to the definition and development of the Mediterranean diet concept: a 50-year journey. Nutr Metab Cardiovasc Dis. 2015;25(3):245–52. https://doi.org/10.1016/j.numecd.2014.12.001. Epub 2014 Dec 12.
57. Nanri A, Mizoue T, Shimazu T, Ishihara J, Takachi R, Noda M, Iso H, Sasazuki S, Sawada N, Tsugane S, Japan Public Health Center-Based Prospective Study Group. Dietary patterns and all-cause, cancer, and cardiovascular disease mortality in Japanese men and women: the Japan public health center-based prospective study. PLoS One. 2017;12(4):e0174848. https://doi.org/10.1371/journal.pone.0174848. eCollection 2017.
58. Oomen CM, Feskens EJ, Räsänen L, Fidanza F, Nissinen AM, Menotti A, Kok FJ, Kromhout D. Fish consumption and coronary heart disease mortality in Finland, Italy, and The Netherlands. Am J Epidemiol. 2000;151(10):999–1006.
59. Oomen CM, Ocké MC, Feskens EJ, van Erp-Baart MA, Kok FJ, Kromhout D. Association between trans fatty acid intake and 10-year risk of coronary heart disease in the Zutphen Elderly Study: a prospective population-based study. Lancet. 2001;357(9258):746–51.
60. Streppel MT, Ocké MC, Boshuizen HC, Kok FJ, Kromhout D. Long-term fish consumption and n-3 fatty acid intake in relation to (sudden) coronary heart disease death: the Zutphen study. Eur Heart J. 2008;29(16):2024–30. https://doi.org/10.1093/eurheartj/ehn294. Epub 2008 Jul 18.
61. Keli SO, Feskens EJ, Kromhout D. Fish consumption and risk of stroke. The Zutphen Study. Stroke. 1994;25(2):328–32.
62. Mozaffarian D, Wu JHY. Omega-3 fatty acids and cardiovascular disease: effects on risk factors, molecular pathways, and clinical events. J Am Coll Cardiol. 2011;58(20):2047–67. https://doi.org/10.1016/j.jacc.2011.06.063.
63. Woodside JV, Kromhout D. Fatty acids and CHD. Proc Nutr Soc. 2005;64(4):554–64.
64. Alexander DD, Miller PE, Van Elswyk ME, Kuratko CN, Bylsma LC. A meta-analysis of randomized controlled trials and prospective cohort studies of eicosapentaenoic and docosahexaenoic long-chain omega-3 fatty acids and coronary heart disease risk. Mayo Clin Proc. 2017;92(1):15–29. https://doi.org/10.1016/j.mayocp.2016.10.018. Review.
65. Gorder DD, Dolecek TA, Coleman GG, Tillotson JL, Brown HB, Lenz-Litzow K, Bartsch GE, Grandits G. Dietary intake in the Multiple Risk Factor Intervention Trial (MRFIT): nutrient and food group changes over 6 years. J Am Diet Assoc. 1986;86(6):744–51.
66. Miura K, Greenland P, Stamler J, Liu K, Daviglus ML, Nakagawa H. Relation of vegetable, fruit, and meat intake to 7-year blood pressure change in middle-aged men: the Chicago Western Electric Study. Am J Epidemiol. 2004;159(6):572–80.
67. Daviglus ML, Stamler J, Orencia AJ, Dyer AR, Liu K, Greenland P, Walsh MK, Morris D, Shekelle RB. Fish consumption and the 30-year risk of fatal myocardial infarction. N Engl J Med. 1997;336(15):1046–53.
68. Orencia AJ, Daviglus ML, Dyer AR, Shekelle RB, Stamler J. Fish consumption and stroke in men. 30-year findings of the Chicago Western Electric Study. Stroke. 1996;27(2):204–9.
69. Liu XQ, Li YH. Epidemiological and nutritional research on prevention of cardiovascular disease in China. Br J Nutr. 2000;84(Suppl 2):S199–203.
70. Hunter DJ, Kazda I, Chockalingam A, Fodor JG. Fish consumption and cardiovascular mortality in Canada: an inter-regional comparison. Am J Prev Med. 1988;4(1):5–10.
71. McLaughlin J, Middaugh J, Boudreau D, Malcom G, Parry S, Tracy R, Newman W. Adipose tissue triglyceride fatty acids and atherosclerosis in Alaska Natives and non-Natives. Atherosclerosis. 2005;181(2):353–62.
72. Shay CM, Stamler J, Dyer AR, Brown IJ, Chan Q, Elliott P, Zhao L, Okuda N, Miura K, Daviglus ML, Van Horn L. Nutrient and food intakes of middle-aged adults at low risk of cardiovascular disease: the international study of macro−/micronutrients and blood pressure (INTERMAP). Eur J Nutr. 2012;51(8):917–26. https://doi.org/10.1007/s00394-011-0268-2. Epub 2011 Nov 6.
73. Menotti A, Puddu PE. How the Seven Countries Study contributed to the definition and development of the Mediterranean diet concept: a 50-year journey. Nutr Metab Cardiovasc Dis. 2015;25(3):245–52. https://doi.org/10.1016/j.numecd.2014.12.001. Epub 2014 Dec 12.
74. McVeigh GE, Brennan GM, Johnston GD, McDermott BJ, McGrath LT, Henry WR, Andrews JW, Hayes JR. Dietary fish oil augments nitric oxide production or release in patients with type 2 (non-insulin-dependent) diabetes mellitus. Diabetologia. 1993;36(1):33–8.
75. Rossi E, Costa M. Fish oil derivatives as a prophylaxis of recurrent miscarriage associated with antiphospholipid antibodies (APL): a pilot study. Lupus. 1993;2(5):319–23.
76. Belluzzi A, Brignola C, Campieri M, Pera A, Boschi S, Miglioli M. Effect of an enteric-coated fish-oil preparation on relapses in Crohn's disease. N Engl J Med. 1996;334(24):1557–60.
77. Teitelbaum JE, Allan Walker W. Review: the role of omega 3 fatty acids in intestinal inflammation. J Nutr Biochem. 2001;12(1):21–32.

78. Nemets B, Stahl Z, Belmaker RH. Addition of omega-3 fatty acid to maintenance medication treatment for recurrent unipolar depressive disorder. Am J Psychiatry. 2002;159(3):477–9.
79. MacLean CH, Newberry SJ, Mojica WA, Khanna P, Issa AM, Suttorp MJ, Lim YW, Traina SB, Hilton L, Garland R, Morton SC. Effects of omega-3 fatty acids on cancer risk: a systematic review. JAMA. 2006;295(4):403–15. Review. Erratum in: JAMA. 2006 Apr 26;295(16):1900.
80. Reisman J, Schachter HM, Dales RE, Tran K, Kourad K, Barnes D, Sampson M, Morrison A, Gaboury I, Blackman J. Treating asthma with omega-3 fatty acids: where is the evidence? A systematic review. BMC Complement Altern Med. 2006;6:26. Review.
81. Mita T, Watada H, Ogihara T, Nomiyama T, Ogawa O, Kinoshita J, Shimizu T, Hirose T, Tanaka Y, Kawamori R. Eicosapentaenoic acid reduces the progression of carotid intima-media thickness in patients with type 2 diabetes. Atherosclerosis. 2007;191(1):162–7. Epub 2006 Apr 17.
82. Brunborg LA, Madland TM, Lind RA, Arslan G, Berstad A, Frøyland L. Effects of short-term oral administration of dietary marine oils in patients with inflammatory bowel disease and joint pain: a pilot study comparing seal oil and cod liver oil. Clin Nutr. 2008;27(4):614–22. https://doi.org/10.1016/j.clnu.2008.01.017. Epub 2008 Apr 18.
83. Caughey GE, James MJ, Proudman SM, Cleland LG. Fish oil supplementation increases the cyclooxygenase inhibitory activity of paracetamol in rheumatoid arthritis patients. Complement Ther Med. 2010;18(3–4):171–4. https://doi.org/10.1016/j.ctim.2010.05.032.
84. Gogus U, Smith C. n-3 Omega fatty acids: a review of current knowledge. Int J Food Sci Technol. 2010;45:417–36. Review.
85. Huang TL. Omega-3 fatty acids, cognitive decline, and Alzheimer's disease: a critical review and evaluation of the literature. J Alzheimers Dis. 2010;21(3):673–90. https://doi.org/10.3233/JAD-2010-090934. Review.
86. Masterton GS, Plevris JN, Hayes PC. Review article: omega-3 fatty acids – a promising novel therapy for non-alcoholic fatty liver disease. Aliment Pharmacol Ther. 2010;31(7):679–92. https://doi.org/10.1111/j.1365-2036.2010.04230.x. Review.
87. Naqvi AZ, Buettner C, Phillips RS, Davis RB, Mukamal KJ. n-3 fatty acids and periodontitis in US adults. J Am Diet Assoc. 2010;110(11):1669–75. https://doi.org/10.1016/j.jada.2010.08.009.
88. Aghdassi E, Ma DW, Morrison S, Hillyer LM, Clarke S, Gladman DD, Urowitz MB, Fortin PR. Alterations in circulating fatty acid composition in patients with systemic lupus erythematosus: a pilot study. JPEN J Parenter Enteral Nutr. 2011;35(2):198–208. https://doi.org/10.1177/0148607110386378.
89. Bloch MH, Qawasmi A. Omega-3 fatty acid supplementation for the treatment of children with attention-deficit/hyperactivity disorder symptomatology: systematic review and meta-analysis. J Am Acad Child Adolesc Psychiatry. 2011;50(10):991–1000. https://doi.org/10.1016/j.jaac.2011.06.008. Epub 2011 Aug 12. Review.
90. Kiecolt-Glaser JK, Belury MA, Andridge R, Malarkey WB, Glaser R. Omega-3 supplementation lowers inflammation and anxiety in medical students: a randomized controlled trial. Brain Behav Immun. 2011;25(8):1725–34. https://doi.org/10.1016/j.bbi.2011.07.229. Epub 2011 Jul 19.
91. Sublette ME, Ellis SP, Geant AL, Mann JJ. Meta-analysis of the effects of eicosapentaenoic acid (EPA) in clinical trials in depression. J Clin Psychiatry. 2011;72(12):1577–84. https://doi.org/10.4088/JCP.10m06634. Epub 2011 Sept 6.
92. Swanson D, Block R, Mousa SA. Omega-3 fatty acids EPA and DHA: health benefits throughout life. Adv Nutr. 2012;3(1):1–7. https://doi.org/10.3945/an.111.000893. Epub 2012 Jan 5.
93. Wu JH, Micha R, Imamura F, Pan A, Biggs ML, Ajaz O, Djousse L, Hu FB, Mozaffarian D. Omega-3 fatty acids and incident type 2 diabetes: a systematic review and meta-analysis. Br J Nutr. 2012;107(Suppl 2):S214–27. https://doi.org/10.1017/S0007114512001602. Review.
94. Desbois AP, Lawlor KC. Antibacterial activity of long-chain polyunsaturated fatty acids against Propionibacterium acnes and Staphylococcus aureus. Mar Drugs. 2013;11(11):4544–57. https://doi.org/10.3390/md11114544.
95. Robinson LE, Mazurak VC. N-3 polyunsaturated fatty acids: relationship to inflammation in healthy adults and adults exhibiting features of metabolic syndrome. Lipids. 2013;48(4):319–32. https://doi.org/10.1007/s11745-013-3774-6. Epub 2013 Mar 1. Review.
96. Skilton MR, Mikkilä V, Würtz P, Ala-Korpela M, Sim KA, Soininen P, Kangas AJ, Viikari JS, Juonala M, Laitinen T, Lehtimäki T, Taittonen L, Kähönen M, Celermajer DS, Raitakari OT. Fetal growth, omega-3 (n-3) fatty acids, and progression of subclinical atherosclerosis: preventing fetal origins of disease? The Cardiovascular Risk in Young Finns Study. Am J Clin Nutr. 2013;97(1):58–65. https://doi.org/10.3945/ajcn.112.044198. Epub 2012 Nov 14.
97. Bauer I, Hughes M, Rowsell R, Cockerell R, Pipingas A, Crewther S, Crewther D. Omega-3 supplementation improves cognition and modifies brain activation in young adults. Hum Psychopharmacol. 2014;29(2):133–44.
98. Hawkey E, Nigg JT. Omega-3 fatty acid and ADHD: blood level analysis and meta-analytic extension of supplementation trials. Clin Psychol Rev. 2014;34(6):496–505. https://doi.org/10.1016/j.cpr.2014.05.005. Epub 2014 Jun 2.
99. Pappalardo G, Almeida A, Ravasco P. Eicosapentaenoic acid in cancer improves body composition and modulates metabolism. Nutrition. 2015;31(4):549–55. https://doi.org/10.1016/j.nut.2014.12.002. Epub 2014 Dec 12. Review.

100. Yang P, Jiang Y, Fischer SM. Prostaglandin E3 metabolism and cancer. Cancer Lett. 2014;348(1–2):1–11. https://doi.org/10.1016/j.canlet.2014.03.010. Epub 2014 Mar 18. Review.
101. Brinton EA, Ballantyne CM, Bays HE, Kastelein JJ, Braeckman RA, Soni PN. Effects of icosapent ethyl on lipid and inflammatory parameters in patients with diabetes mellitus-2, residual elevated triglycerides (200–500 mg/dL), and on statin therapy at LDL-C goal: the ANCHOR study. Cardiovasc Diabetol. 2013;12:100. https://doi.org/10.1186/1475-2840-12-100. Erratum in: Cardiovasc Diabetol. 2015 Jul–Aug;9(4):618.
102. Proudman SM, Cleland LG, Metcalf RG, Sullivan TR, Spargo LD, James MJ. Plasma n-3 fatty acids and clinical outcomes in recent-onset rheumatoid arthritis. Br J Nutr. 2015;114(6):885–90. https://doi.org/10.1017/S0007114515002718. Epub 2015 Aug 18.
103. Wani AL, Bhat SA, Ara A. Omega-3 fatty acids and the treatment of depression: a review of scientific evidence. Integr Med Res. 2015;4(3):132–41.
104. Harris WS, Mozaffarian D, Lefevre M, et al. Towards establishing dietary reference intakes for eicosapentaenoic and docosahexaenoic acids. J Nutr. 2009;139(4):804S–19S. https://doi.org/10.3945/jn.108.101329.
105. Giudetti AM, Cagnazzo R. Beneficial effects of n-3 PUFA on chronic airway inflammatory diseases. Prostaglandins Other Lipid Mediat. 2012;99(3–4):57–67. https://doi.org/10.1016/j.prostaglandins.2012.09.006.
106. Bradberry JC, Hilleman DE. Overview of omega-3 fatty acid therapies. P T. 2013;38(11):681–91.
107. Patterson E, Wall R, Fitzgerald GF, Ross RP, Stanton C. Health implications of high dietary omega-6 polyunsaturated fatty acids. Published online 2012 Apr 5. https://doi.org/10.1155/2012/539426.
108. Bagga D, Wang L, Farias-Eisner R, Glaspy JA, Reddy ST. Differential effects of prostaglandin derived from omega-6 and omega-3 polyunsaturated fatty acids on COX-2 expression and IL-6 secretion. Proc Natl Acad Sci U S A. 2003;100(4):1751–6. Epub 2003 Feb 10.
109. Simopoulos AP. An increase in the omega-6/omega-3 fatty acid ratio increases the risk for obesity. Nutrients. 2016;8(3):128. Published online 2016 Mar 2. https://doi.org/10.3390/nu8030128.
110. Calder PC. Fatty acids and inflammation: The cutting edge between food and pharma. Eur J Pharmacol. 2011;668(Supplement 1):S50–8.
111. Macartney MJ, Hingley L, Brown MA, Peoples GE, McLennan PL. Intrinsic heart rate recovery after dynamic exercise is improved with an increased omega-3 index in healthy males. Br J Nutr. 2014;112(12):1984–92. https://doi.org/10.1017/S0007114514003146. Epub 2014 Oct 30.
112. Ali MA, Waheed A, Jurivich DA, Colombo J, Singer DH. Short-term time domain HRV measures: comparisons with 24-hr Holter monitoring. Chicago: Geriatric Medicine Society Meeting; 2006.
113. Umetani K, Singer DH, McCraty R, Atkinson M. Twenty-four hour time domain heart rate variability and heart rate: relations to age and gender over nine decades. J Am Coll Cardiol. 1998;31(3):593–601.
114. Rovelli F, De Vita C, Feruglio GA, Lotto A, Selvini A, Tognoni G. GISSI trial: early results and late follow-up. Gruppo Italiano per la Sperimentazione della Streptochinasi nell'Infarto Miocardico. J Am Coll Cardiol. 1987;10(5 Suppl B):33B–9B.
115. Fresco C, Franzosi MG, Maggioni AP, Tognoni G. The GISSI-2 trial: premises, results, epidemiological (and other) implications. Gruppo Italiano per lo Studio delia Sopravvivenza nell'Infarto Miocardico. Clin Cardiol. 1990;13(8 Suppl 8):VIII32–6.
116. Marchioli R, Barzi F, Bomba E, Chieffo C, Di Gregorio D, Di Mascio R, Franzosi MG, Geraci E, Levantesi G, Maggioni AP, Mantini L, Marfisi RM, Mastrogiuseppe G, Mininni N, Nicolosi GL, Santini M, Schweiger C, Tavazzi L, Tognoni G, Tucci C, Valagussa F, GISSI-Prevenzione Investigators. Early protection against sudden death by n-3 polyunsaturated fatty acids after myocardial infarction: time-course analysis of the results of the Gruppo Italiano per lo Studio della Sopravvivenza nell'Infarto Miocardico (GISSI)-Prevenzione. Circulation. 2002;105(16):1897–903.
117. Cleland JG, Freemantle N, Coletta AP, Clark AL. Clinical trials update from the American Heart Association: REPAIR-AMI, ASTAMI, JELIS, MEGA, REVIVE-II, SURVIVE, and PROACTIVE. Eur J Heart Fail. 2006;8(1):105–10. Review.
118. http://news.heart.org/fish-oil-supplements-provide-some-benefit-after-heart-attack-heart-failure/
119. Tong X, Christian P, Zhao M, Wang H, Moreau R, Su Q. Activation of hepatic CREBH and Insig signaling in the anti-hypertriglyceridemic mechanism of R-α-lipoic acid. J Nutr Biochem. 2015;26(9):921–8. https://doi.org/10.1016/j.jnutbio.2015.03.011. Epub 2015 May 7.
120. http://www.heart.org/HEARTORG/HealthyLiving/HealthyEating/HealthyDietGoals/Fish-and-Omega-3-Fatty-Acids_UCM_303248_Article.jsp#.WUKmyMq7qpo
121. McVeigh GE, Brennan GM, Johnston GD, McDermott BJ, McGrath LT, Henry WR, Andrews JW, Hayes JR. Dietary fish oil augments nitric oxide production or release in patients with type 2 (non-insulin dependent) diabetes mellitus. Diabetologia. 1993;36(1):33–8.
122. Omura M, Kobayashi S, Mizukami Y, Mogami K, Todoroki-Ikeda N, Miyake T, Matsuzaki M. Eicosapentaenoic acid (EPA) induces Ca(2+)-independent activation and translocation of endothelial nitric oxide synthase and endothelium-dependent vasorelaxation. FEBS Lett. 2001;487(3):361–6.

123. De Caterina R, Liao JK, Libby P. Fatty acid modulation of endothelial activation. Am J Clin Nutr. 2000;71(1 Suppl):213S–23S. Review.
124. Curtis BM, O'Keefe JH. Autonomic tone as a cardiovascular risk factor: the dangers of chronic fight or flight. Mayo Clin Proc. 2002;77:45–54.
125. Quarles RH, Macklin WB, Morell P. Myelin formation, structure and biochemistry. In: Basic neurochemistry: molecular, cellular, and medical aspects. Siegel: Elsevier, Inc; 2006.
126. Michael-Titus AT, et al. Omega-3 fatty acids and traumatic neurological injury: from neuroprotection to neuroplasticity? Trends Neurosci. 2014;37(1):30–8. https://doi.org/10.1016/j.tins.2013.10.005. Epub 2013 Nov 22.
127. Pu H, Guo Y, Zhang W, Huang L, Wang G, Liou AK, Zhang J, Zhang P, Leak RK, Wang Y, Chen J, Gao Y. Omega-3 polyunsaturated fatty acid supplementation improves neurologic recovery and attenuates white matter injury after experimental traumatic brain injury. J Cereb Blood Flow Metab. 2013;33(9):1474–84. https://doi.org/10.1038/jcbfm.2013.108. Epub 2013 Jun 26.
128. Ohnishi H, Saito Y. Eicosapentaenoic acid (EPA) reduces cardiovascular events: relationship with the EPA/arachidonic acid ratio. J Atheroscler Thromb. 2013;20(12):861–77. Epub 2013 Sept 18.
129. Calder PC. Omega-3 fatty acids and inflammatory processes. Nutrients. 2010;2(3):355–74. https://doi.org/10.3390/nu2030355. Epub 2010 Mar 18.
130. Calder PC. Omega-3 fatty acids and inflammatory processes: from molecules to man. Biochem Soc Trans. 2017;45(5):1105–15. https://doi.org/10.1042/BST20160474. Epub 2017 Sept 12.
131. Arnold LE, Young AS, Belury MA, Cole RM, Gracious B, Seidenfeld AM, Wolfson H, Fristad MA. Omega-3 fatty acid plasma levels before and after supplementation: correlations with mood and clinical outcomes in the omega-3 and therapy studies. J Child Adolesc Psychopharmacol. 2017;27(3):223–33. https://doi.org/10.1089/cap.2016.0123. Epub 2017 Feb 3.
132. Pompili M, Longo L, Dominici G, Serafini G, Lamis DA, Sarris J, Amore M, Girardi P. Polyunsaturated fatty acids and suicide risk in mood disorders: a systematic review. Prog Neuro-Psychopharmacol Biol Psychiatry. 2017;74:43–56. https://doi.org/10.1016/j.pnpbp.2016.11.007. Epub 2016 Dec 8. Review.
133. Abdulrazaq M, Innes JK, Calder PC. Effect of ω-3 polyunsaturated fatty acids on arthritic pain: asystematic review. Nutrition. 2017;39–40:57–66. https://doi.org/10.1016/j.nut.2016.12.003. Epub 2016 Dec 21. Review.
134. Senftleber NK, Nielsen SM, Andersen JR, Bliddal H, Tarp S, Lauritzen L, Furst DE, Suarez-Almazor ME, Lyddiatt A, Christensen R. Marine oil supplements for arthritis pain: a systematic review and meta-analysis of randomized trials. Nutrients. 2017;9(1). pii: E42. https://doi.org/10.3390/nu9010042. Review.
135. Beermann C, Neumann S, Fußbroich D, Zielen S, Schubert R. Combinations of distinct long-chain polyunsaturated fatty acid species for improved dietary treatment against allergic bronchial asthma. Nutrition. 2016;32(11–12):1165–70. https://doi.org/10.1016/j.nut.2016.04.004. Epub 2016 May 6. Review.
136. Barnadas MA, Díaz Encarnación MM. Refractory cutaneous IgA vasculitis treated with omega-3 fatty acids. Case Rep Dermatol. 2016;8(3):333–40. https://doi.org/10.1159/000452320. eCollection 2016 Sept–Dec.
137. Chauhan S, Kodali H, Noor J, Ramteke K, Gawai V. Role of omega-3 fatty acids on lipid profile in diabetic dyslipidemia: single blind, randomized clinical trial. J Clin Diagn Res. 2017;11(3):OC13–6. https://doi.org/10.7860/JCDR/2017/20628.9449. Epub 2017 Mar 1.
138. Ebrahimi M, Ghayour-Mobarhan M, Rezaiean S, Hoseini M, Parizade SM, Farhoudi F, Hosseininezhad SJ, Tavallaei S, Vejdani A, Azimi-Nezhad M, Shakeri MT, Rad MA, Mobarra N, Kazemi-Bajestani SM, Ferns GA. Omega-3 fatty acid supplements improve the cardiovascular risk profile of subjects with metabolic syndrome, including markers of inflammation and auto-immunity. Acta Cardiol. 2009;64(3):321–7.
139. Ong HT, Cheah JS. Statin alternatives or just placebo: an objective review of omega-3, red yeast rice and garlic in cardiovascular therapeutics. Chin Med J. 2008;121(16):1588–94. Review.
140. Zhao YT, Chen Q, Sun YX, Li XB, Zhang P, Xu Y, Guo JH. Prevention of sudden cardiac death with omega-3 fatty acids in patients with coronary heart disease: a meta-analysis of randomized controlled trials. Ann Med. 2009;41(4):301–10. https://doi.org/10.1080/07853890802698834.
141. Artham SM, Lavie CJ, Milani RV, Anand RG, O'Keefe JH, Ventura HO. Fish oil in primary and secondary cardiovascular prevention. Ochsner J. 2008;8(2):49–60.
142. Christensen JH. n-3 fatty acids and the risk of sudden cardiac death. Emphasis on heart rate variability. Dan Med Bull. 2003;50(4):347–67. Review.
143. Katsi V, Georgiopoulos G, Laina A, Koutli E, Parissis J, Tsioufis C, Nihoyannopoulos P, Tousoulis D. Left ventricular ejection fraction as therapeutic target: is it the ideal marker? Heart Fail Rev. 2017. https://doi.org/10.1007/s10741-017-9624-5. [Epub ahead of print] Review.
144. Khoueiry G, Abi Rafeh N, Sullivan E, Saiful F, Jaffery Z, Kenigsberg DN, Krishnan SC, Khanal S, Bekheit S, Kowalski M. Do omega-3 polyunsaturated fatty acids reduce risk of sudden cardiac death and ventricular arrhythmias? A meta-analysis of randomized trials. Heart Lung. 2013;42(4):251–6. https://doi.org/10.1016/j.hrtlng.2013.03.006. Epub 2013 May 25.

145. Harris WS, Del Gobbo L, Tintle NL. The omega-3 index and relative risk for coronary heart disease mortality: estimation from 10 cohort studies. Atherosclerosis. 2017;262:51–4. https://doi.org/10.1016/j.atherosclerosis.2017.05.007. Epub 2017 May 6.
146. Davis W, Rockway S, Kwasny M. Effect of a combined therapeutic approach of intensive lipid management, omega-3 fatty acid supplementation, and increased serum 25 (OH) vitamin D on coronary calcium scores in asymptomatic adults. Am J Ther. 2009;16(4):326–32. https://doi.org/10.1097/MJT.0b013e31817a8f3c.
147. Mazahery H, Stonehouse W, Delshad M, Kruger MC, Conlon CA, Beck KL, von Hurst PR. Relationship between long chain n-3 polyunsaturated fatty acids and autism spectrum disorder: systematic review and meta-analysis of case-control and randomised controlled trials. Nutrients. 2017;9(2). pii: E155. https://doi.org/10.3390/nu9020155. Review.
148. Stirban A, Nandrean S, Götting C, Tamler R, Pop A, Negrean M, Gawlowski T, Stratmann B, Tschoepe D. Effects of n-3 fatty acids on macro- and microvascular function in subjects with type 2 diabetes mellitus. Am J Clin Nutr. 2010;91(3):808–13. https://doi.org/10.3945/ajcn.2009.28374. Epub 2010 Jan 13
149. Nishizaki Y, Shimada K, Daida H. The balance of omega-3 polyunsaturated fatty acids for -reducing residual risks in patients with coronary artery disease. Acta Cardiol. 2017;21:1–9. https://doi.org/10.1080/00015385.2017.1305174. [Epub ahead of print].
150. Drudi LM, Schaller MS, Hiramoto J, Gasper W, Harris WS, Hills NK, Grenon SM. Predictors of change in omega-3 index with fish oil supplementation in peripheral artery disease. J Surg Res. 2017;210:124–31. https://doi.org/10.1016/j.jss.2016.11.011. Epub 2016 Nov 11.
151. Woodcock BE, Smith E, Lambert WH, Jones WM, Galloway JH, Greaves M, Preston FE. Beneficial effect of fish oil on blood viscosity in peripheral vascular disease. Br Med J (Clin Res Ed). 1984;288(6417):592–4.
152. Enns JE, Yeganeh A, Zarychanski R, Abou-Setta AM, Friesen C, Zahradka P, Taylor CG. The impact of omega-3 polyunsaturated fatty acid supplementation on the incidence of cardiovascular events and complications in peripheral arterial disease: a systematic review and meta-analysis. BMC Cardiovasc Disord. 2014;14:70. https://doi.org/10.1186/1471-2261-14-70. Review.
153. Arriens C, Hynan LS, Lerman RH, Karp DR, Mohan C. Placebo-controlled randomized clinical trial of fish oil's impact on fatigue, quality of life, and disease activity in systemic lupus erythematosus. Nutr J. 2015;14:82. https://doi.org/10.1186/s12937-015-0068-2.
154. Sun Q, Ma J, Campos H, Rexrode KM, Albert CM, Mozaffarian D, Hu FB. Blood concentrations of individual long-chain n-3 fatty acids and risk of nonfatal myocardial infarction. Am J Clin Nutr. 2008;88(1):216–23.
155. Hu FB, Bronner L, Willett WC, Stampfer MJ, Rexrode KM, Albert CM, Hunter D, Manson JE. Fish and omega-3 fatty acid intake and risk of coronary heart disease in women. JAMA. 2002;287(14):1815–21.
156. Hu FB, Stampfer MJ, Manson JE, Rimm EB, Wolk A, Colditz GA, Hennekens CH, Willett WC. Dietary intake of alpha-linolenic acid and risk of fatal ischemic heart disease among women. Am J Clin Nutr. 1999;69(5):890–7.
157. Ghule AE, Kandhare AD, Jadhav SS, Zanwar AA, Bodhankar SL. Omega-3-fatty acid adds to the protective effect of flax lignan concentrate in pressure overload-induced myocardial hypertrophy in rats via modulation of oxidative stress and apoptosis. Int Immunopharmacol. 2015;28(1):751–63. https://doi.org/10.1016/j.intimp.2015.08.005. Epub 2015 Aug 14.
158. Song TJ, Chang Y, Shin MJ, Heo JH, Kim YJ. Low levels of plasma omega 3-polyunsaturated fatty acids are associated with cerebral small vessel diseases in acute ischemic stroke patients. Nutr Res. 2015;35(5):368–74. https://doi.org/10.1016/j.nutres.2015.04.008. Epub 2015 Apr 16.
159. Virtanen JK, Siscovick DS, Lemaitre RN, Longstreth WT, Spiegelman D, Rimm EB, King IB, Mozaffarian D. Circulating omega-3 polyunsaturated fatty acids and subclinical brain abnormalities on MRI in older adults: the cardiovascular health study. J Am Heart Assoc. 2013;2(5):e000305. https://doi.org/10.1161/JAHA.113.000305.
160. Bo Y, Zhang X, Wang Y, You J, Cui H, Zhu Y, Pang W, Liu W, Jiang Y, Lu Q. The n-3 polyunsaturated fatty acids supplementation improved the cognitive function in the Chinese elderly with mild cognitive impairment: a double-blind randomized controlled trial. Nutrients. 2017;9(1). pii: E54. https://doi.org/10.3390/nu9010054.
161. Molina-Leyva I, Molina-Leyva A, Bueno-Cavanillas A. Efficacy of nutritional supplementation with omega-3 and omega-6 fatty acids in dry eye syndrome: a systematic review of randomized clinical trials. Acta Ophthalmol. 2017; https://doi.org/10.1111/aos.13428. [Epub ahead of print].
162. Mohammadpour M, Mehrabi S, Hassanpoor N, Mirshahi R. Effects of adjuvant omega-3 fatty acid supplementation on dry eye syndrome following cataract surgery: a randomized clinical trial. J Curr Ophthalmol. 2016;29(1):33–8. https://doi.org/10.1016/j.joco.2016.05.006. eCollection 2017 Mar.
163. Königs A, Kiliaan AJ. Critical appraisal of omega-3 fatty acids in attention-deficit/hyperactivity disorder treatment. Neuropsychiatr Dis Treat. 2016;12:1869–82. https://doi.org/10.2147/NDT.S68652. eCollection 2016. Review.
164. Kalupahana NS, Claycombe K, Newman SJ, Stewart T, Siriwardhana N, Matthan N, Lichtenstein AH,

Moustaid-Moussa N. Eicosapentaenoic acid prevents and reverses insulin resistance in high-fat diet-induced obese mice via modulation of adipose tissue inflammation. J Nutr. 2010;140(11):1915–22. https://doi.org/10.3945/jn.110.125732. Epub 2010 Sept 22.

165. Best K, Makrides M. Possible protective effect of prenatal omega-3 long-chain polyunsaturated fatty acids supplementation on persistent wheeze and asthma in early childhood. Evid Based Med. 2017;22(3):104. https://doi.org/10.1136/ebmed-2017-110696. Epub 2017 May 12.
166. Oliveira V, Marinho R, Vitorino D, Santos GA, Moraes JC, Dragano N, Sartori-Cintra A, Pereira L, Catharino RR, da Silva AS, Ropelle ER, Pauli JR, De Souza CT, Velloso LA, Cintra DE. Diets containing α-linolenic (ω3) or oleic (ω9) fatty acids rescues obese mice from insulin resistance. Endocrinology. 2015;156(11):4033–46. https://doi.org/10.1210/en.2014-1880. Epub 2015 Aug 17.
167. Best KP, Sullivan T, Palmer D, Gold M, Kennedy DJ, Martin J, Makrides M. Prenatal fish oil supplementation and allergy: 6-year follow-up of a randomized controlled trial. Pediatrics. 2016;137(6). pii: e20154443. https://doi.org/10.1542/peds.2015-4443.
168. Galarraga B, Ho M, Youssef HM, Hill A, McMahon H, Hall C, Ogston S, Nuki G, Belch JJ. Cod liver oil (n-3 fatty acids) as an non-steroidal anti-inflammatory drug sparing agent in rheumatoid arthritis. Rheumatology (Oxford). 2008;47(5):665–9. https://doi.org/10.1093/rheumatology/ken024. Epub 2008 Mar 24.
169. Proudman SM, Cleland LG, James MJ. Dietary omega-3 fats for treatment of inflammatory joint disease: efficacy and utility. Rheum Dis Clin N Am. 2008;34(2):469–79. https://doi.org/10.1016/j.rdc.2008.03.003.
170. Chhetry BT, Hezghia A, Miller JM, Lee S, Rubin-Falcone H, Cooper TB, Oquendo MA, Mann JJ, Sublette ME. Omega-3 polyunsaturated fatty acid supplementation and white matter changes in major depression. J Psychiatr Res. 2016;75:65–74. https://doi.org/10.1016/j.jpsychires.2015.12.007. Epub 2016 Jan 11.
171. Souied EH, Delcourt C, Querques G, Bassols A, Merle B, Zourdani A, Smith T, Benlian P, Nutritional AMD Treatment 2 Study Group. Oral docosahexaenoic acid in the prevention of exudative age-related macular degeneration: the Nutritional AMD Treatment 2 study. Ophthalmology. 2013;120(8):1619–31. https://doi.org/10.1016/j.ophtha.2013.01.005. Epub 2013 Feb 8.

# 4 Nitric Oxide (Prong-2)

The second prong to treating autonomic and mitochondrial dysfunction to be discussed is the nitric oxide prong (Fig. 4.1). Again all prongs are integral to the whole, and all work together in concert to establish and maintain health and wellness. Omitting even one prong significantly reduces the opportunity to establish and maintain long-term wellness. The objective of the nitric oxide prong is to increase nitric oxide levels in the body.

Nitric oxide (Fig. 4.2) is a gas that lasts only a few seconds. It is produced when L-arginine is

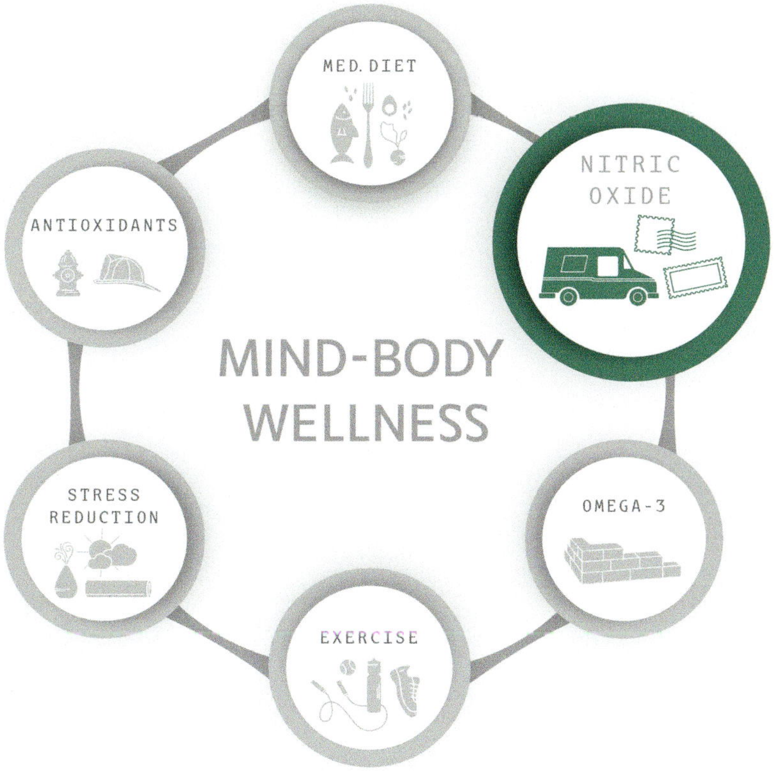


**Fig. 4.1** The Mind-Body Wellness Program – nitric oxide prong. (Illustration by Elysian Creative Studio, www.elysiancreativestudio.com, Lizzy Colombo)


N. L. DePace, J. Colombo, *Clinical Autonomic and Mitochondrial Disorders*,
https://doi.org/10.1007/978-3-030-17016-5_4

converted by nitric oxide synthase (NOS) to L-citrulline. Nitric oxide and water are the other products (see Fig. 4.3). The doctors recognized for the discoveries of nitric oxide as a universal signaling molecule won the Nobel Prize in Physiology or Medicine in 1998 (see Fig. 4.3). They found it throughout the body (see Fig. 4.4).

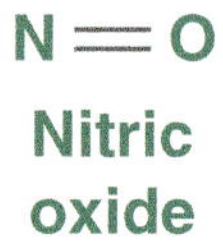


**Fig. 4.2** Molecular structure of nitric oxide (aka, nitrogen monoxide). (Source: http://www.mensanswer.com/articles/fitness/best-nitric-oxide-supplements-available/)

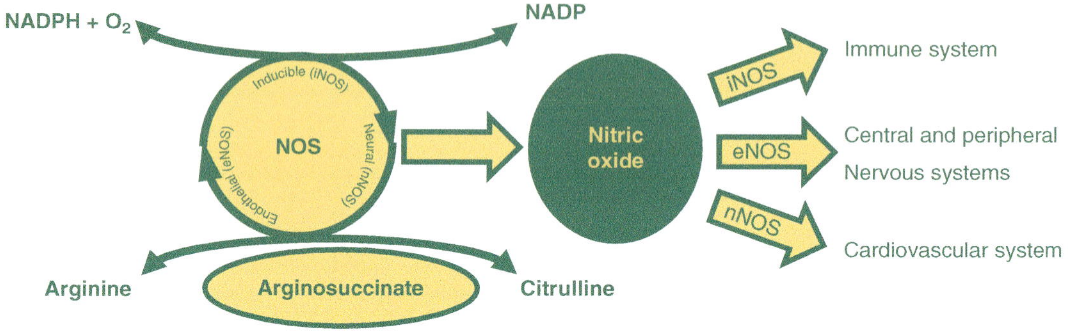


**Fig. 4.3** Different types of NOS in different tissues to create nitric oxide throughout the body. nNOS production of nitric oxide in the (1) central nervous system (CNS) supports (**a**) synaptic plasticity and (**b**) blood pressure regulation, and (2) peripheral nervous system supports (**c**) atypical neurotransmission (acts as a type of neurotransmitter) and (**d**) penile erection. iNOS production of nitric oxide in the immune system (**e**) supports nonspecific immune defense (e.g., against pollen and throughout the body, including the lungs), (**f**) mediates inflammation (i.e., in joints as well as arteries and elsewhere), and (**g**) mediates the response to septic shock. eNOS production of nitric oxide in the cardiovascular system endothelium mediates (**h**) vasodilation, (**i**) vasoprotection, and (**j**) prevention of atherosclerosis

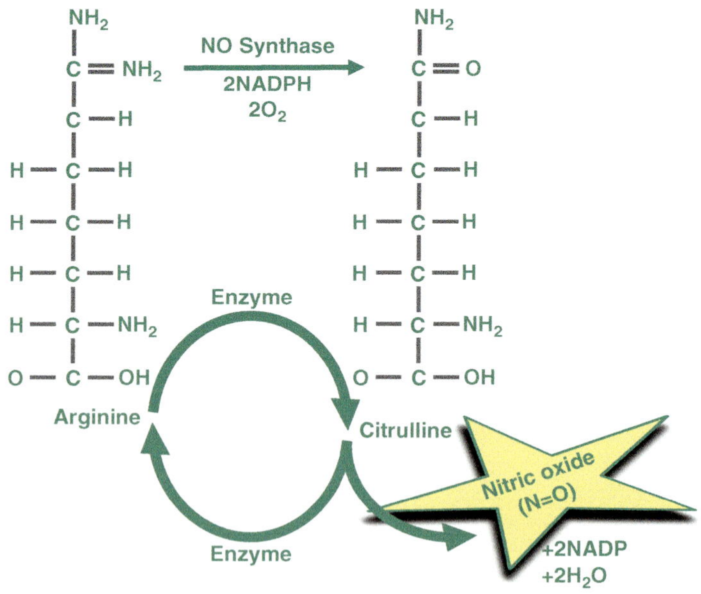


**Fig. 4.4** Nitric oxide synthase (NOS) converts L-arginine to L-citrulline, plus nitric oxide and water. (Insert: Adapted from Shutterstock Royalty-free stock illustration ID: 108941690, by Alila Medical Media)

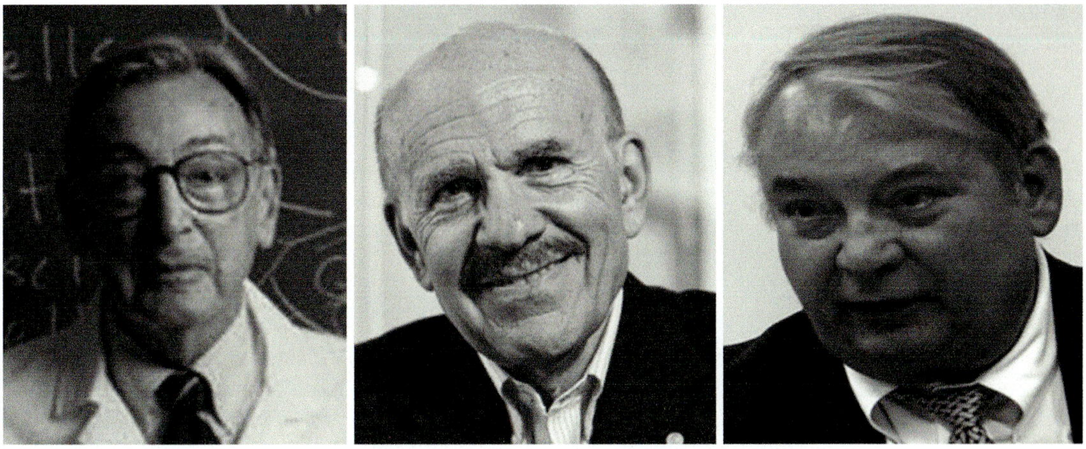


**Fig. 4.5** The doctors that shared the 1998 Nobel Prize for discoveries of nitric oxide as a signaling molecule: Drs. Robert F. Furchgott, Louis J. Ignarro, and Ferid Murad. (Photos from Wikipedia, by: (Furchgott) J.A. Zubrovich, (Ignarro) C. Barretta, and (Murad) J. Dahl)

For example, in the cardiovascular system (see Figs. 4.6 and 4.7), nitric oxide signals endothelial cells to cause vasodilation. In this way, it is a natural dilator of blood vessels. It increases blood flow and circulation. In the brain this improves cognitive function. Endothelial cells, in part, make up the blood-brain barrier (BBB). A healthy BBB optimizes brain function, including memory, cognition, and control and coordination throughout the body. It is interesting that all six lifestyle and supplement prongs increase nitric oxide either directly or indirectly. By keeping endothelial cells healthy throughout the body, nitric oxide is more readily produced. When endothelial cells become damaged, diseased, or defaced, nitric oxide deficiency occurs. For example, endothelial dysfunction is a cardiovascular risk factor [1]. When endothelial dysfunction is treated by increasing nitric oxide levels in the body, cardiovascular risk factors are improved. Also, when cardiovascular risk factors are treated, the endothelial dysfunction is reversed [2, 3]. Endothelial dysfunction is an independent predictor of cardiac events. Nitric oxide mediates distinct signaling profiles depending on its concentration and the antioxidant buffer balance in the body.

NOS is the enzyme involved, and there are several types of these depending on what tissues are generating the gas. The three known forms of NOS are endothelial NOS (eNOS), inducible NOS (iNOS), and neural NOS (nNOS) (Fig. 4.3). eNOS and nNOS are dependent on high concentrations of calcium ($Ca^{++}$), whereas, iNOS is calcium-independent because of its high affinity for $Ca^{++}$/calmodulin (Calm), which activates the enzyme even at basal levels of intracellular $Ca^{++}$. When coupled to a cofactor (such as nicotinamide adenine dinucleotide phosphate, NADPH, or flavin adenine dinucleotide, FAD) and in the presence of oxygen ($O_2$), NOS converts L-arginine to nitric oxide and L-citrulline (Fig. 4.4). Nitric oxide has a low solubility in water with a very short half-life. It therefore needs to be made constantly and locally, which is part of why it is ubiquitous. Nitric oxide is the only gas that is known to act as a messenger molecule in the body.

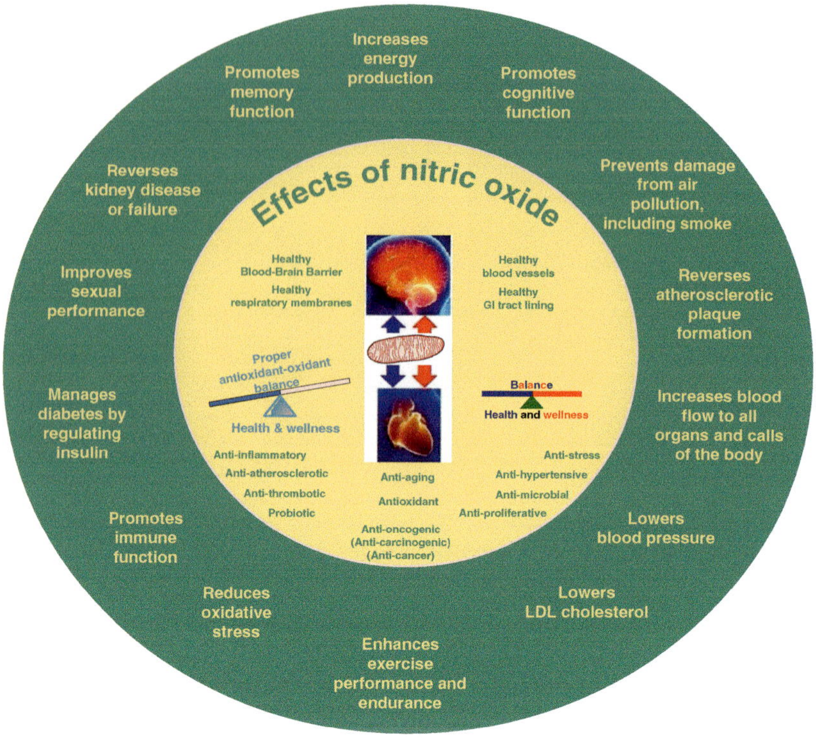


**Fig. 4.6** Nitric oxide is a ubiquitous messenger, also known as the "universal messenger"

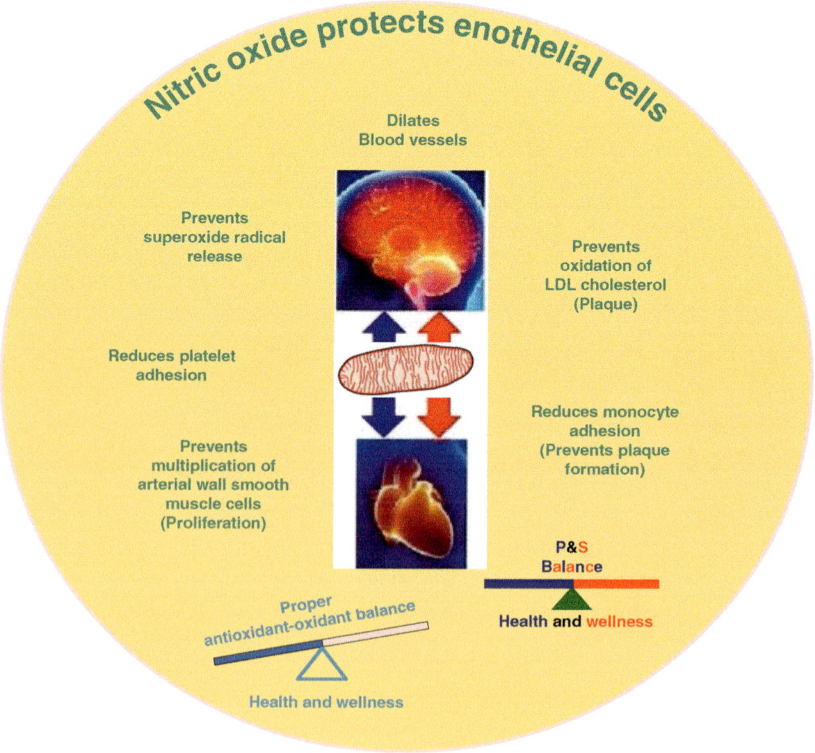


**Fig. 4.7** Nitric oxide protects endothelial cells

## The "Universal Messenger"

As mentioned before, under healthy conditions, nitric oxide is a ubiquitous messenger (see Fig. 4.6), considered by some to be the "universal messenger" within the human body [4] (see Table 4.1). Nitric oxide works as a neurotransmitter and vasodilator [5, 6]. It dilates blood vessels by acting like a hormone, diffusing out of the endothelial cell and into the blood vessel smooth muscle cell, working against sympathetic nerve input to the vessel (see insert, below). In the smooth muscle cell, nitric oxide activates guanylyl cyclase, a second messenger, to convert guanosine triphosphate (GTP) to guanosine monophosphate (GMP), reducing $Ca^{++}$ levels in the smooth muscle cells, relaxing the smooth muscle cell, and thereby helping to dilate the vessel. Nitric oxide is bactericidal and can fight infections and bacteria [7–9]. It is also anti-inflammatory, not only reducing but also preventing inflammation [10]. Very importantly, it is an antioxidant and performs many antioxidant activities, including neutralizing ROS as well as free radicals, superoxides, and peroxides (Figs. 4.6 and 4.7) [11].

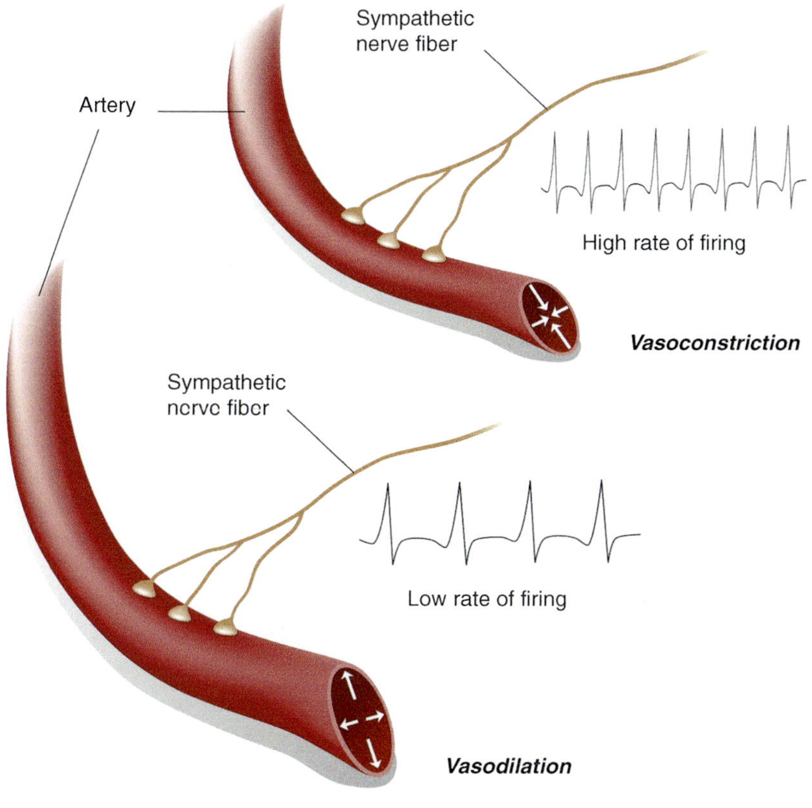


It can promote cerebral circulation [12], so that people who have "brain fog" actually feel better and have fewer cognitive difficulties. Endothelium, neurons, and glia can all produce nitric oxide which is a potent vasodilator. Nitric oxide is a mediator of endothelium-dependent relaxation (endothelium-derived relaxing factor, EDRF). These cells produce nitric oxide under basal conditions and in response to a variety of vasoactive stimuli in large cerebral arteries and the cerebral microcirculation. Endothelium-dependent relaxation is impaired in the presence of several pathophysiological conditions. Increases in cerebral blood flow during hypercapnia also appear to be dependent on impaired nitric oxide production. This impairment may contribute to cerebral ischemia or stroke, which of course increases brain fog and cognitive

**Table 4.1** Nitric oxide, the universal messenger

| | |
|---|---|
| Vasodilates blood vessels | Improves erectile dysfunction |
| | Increases blood flow to organs and organ systems |
| | Lowers blood pressure |
| | Improves intermittent claudication in subjects with peripheral vascular disease |
| Bactericidal | Combats infections (both bacterial and viral) |
| Anti-inflammatory | Reduces and prevents inflammation causing atherosclerosis and arthritis and impairs leukocyte adhesion |
| Antioxidant | Neutralizes ROS/RNS and free radicals |
| Regulates cell proliferation | Angiogenesis, neurogenesis |
| Inhibits platelet aggregation | Prevents pathological clotting |
| Prevents oxidation of lipoproteins (LDL) | Inhibits foam cell proliferation and propagation of atherosclerosis (acts as anti-atherosclerotic molecule) |
| Enhances the immune system | Tumor suppression properties |
| Regulates mitochondrial respiration and gene expression | Promotes production of new mitochondria after insult (e.g., stroke or heart attack) |
| Promotes bone remodeling and healing | Prevents osteoporosis |
| Increases parasympathetic (vagal) tone | Reduces stress through balancing sympathetic overactivity |
| Detoxifies ammonia | As nitric oxide is produced, citrulline is recycled to arginine which works to detoxify ammonia |

issues. Activation of glutamate receptors in brain endothelial cells, neurons, and glia appears to be a major stimulus for production of nitric oxide by neurons. Neuronally derived nitric oxide may mediate local increases in cerebral blood flow during increases in cerebral metabolism. Nitric oxide synthase-containing neurons also innervate large cerebral arteries and cerebral arterioles on the brain surface. Activation of parasympathetic fibers that innervate cerebral vessels produces nitric oxide-dependent increases in cerebral blood flow. Astrocytes and microglia can release relatively large quantities of nitric oxide after induction of NOS in response to endotoxin or some cytokines. Thus there are several pathways by which nitric oxide helps to reduce cognitive difficulties and "brain fog" [13].

Nitric oxide promotes sexual health. How it affects erectile dysfunction (ED) [14] and possibly vaginal lubrication [15] and other reproductive functions will be discussed (see "Erectile Dysfunction" section). By decreasing the tone of the blood vessel and causing them to dilate, nitric oxide can lower blood pressure (vasodilation). Nitric oxide is an inhibitory messenger in other endothelial systems [16], for example, endothelin-1, which is a substance that acts as a constrictor of blood vessels. So, nitric oxide naturally opens up the arteries (vasodilation) and inhibits those agents (e.g., endothelin-1) that constrict the vasculature when vasoconstriction is an adverse event, such as when vasoconstriction significantly increases blood pressure.

Nitric oxide regulates the local cell growth in the walls of blood vessels, helping to regulate cell proliferation. Too much proliferation begins to occlude the lumen of the artery and constricts blood flow. Nitric oxide protects the arteries from the adverse effects of "sticky" or too many platelets and products of platelets aggregating to cause blood clots, further occluding the vessel. As a result, it is antithrombotic (Fig. 4.8) [17]. Another very important function is that nitric oxide keeps leukocytes, white blood cells (Fig. 4.9), from traveling to, and adhering to, the surface of the endothelial cells [18]. Leukocyte adhesion (Fig. 4.10) causes inflammation and damages endothelial cells, promoting plaque buildup. This is another mechanism by which nitric oxide acts an anti-inflammatory [19]. Another very important activity of nitric oxide is that it helps to prevent the oxidation of lipoproteins which carry LDL ("bad") cholesterol in the body (Fig. 4.11). As discussed previously (see "The Importance of

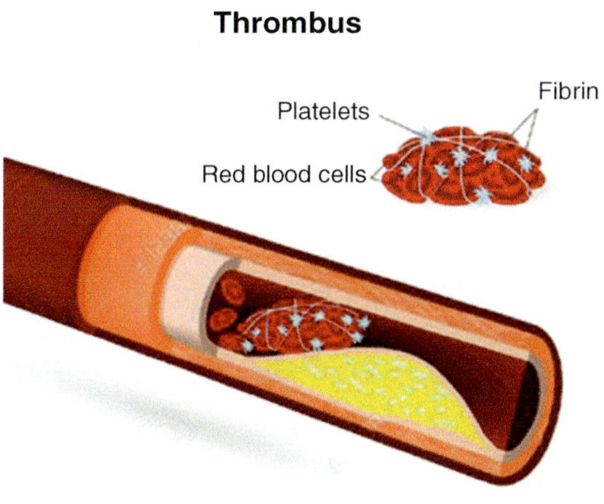


**Fig. 4.8** Thrombus formation with plaque. (Adapted from Shutterstock Royalty-free stock illustration ID: 196102103, Thrombus. Blood clot. Diagram. Illustration depicting thrombus formation over arterial plaque, by Designua)

Antioxidants"), oxidized LDL collect in the blood vessels as foam cells, when taken up by macrophages that are stimulated by nitric oxide from endothelial cells. This process occurs very easily. Unfortunately, foam cells are the beginning of atherosclerosis, more on this later in "The Anti-atherosclerotic Molecule" section of this chapter.

Nitric oxide benefits the immune system. It is antimicrobial with probiotic activities [21, 22], and it upregulates the immune system, including facilitating T cells [23–25]. Nitric oxide regulates processes involved in sepsis defense [26]. It strengthens the body's defense against infection and retards tumor growth by enhancing immune function, and through an ample production of nitric oxide in white blood cells (Fig. 4.12) [28], it kills invading bacteria and parasites. Every day

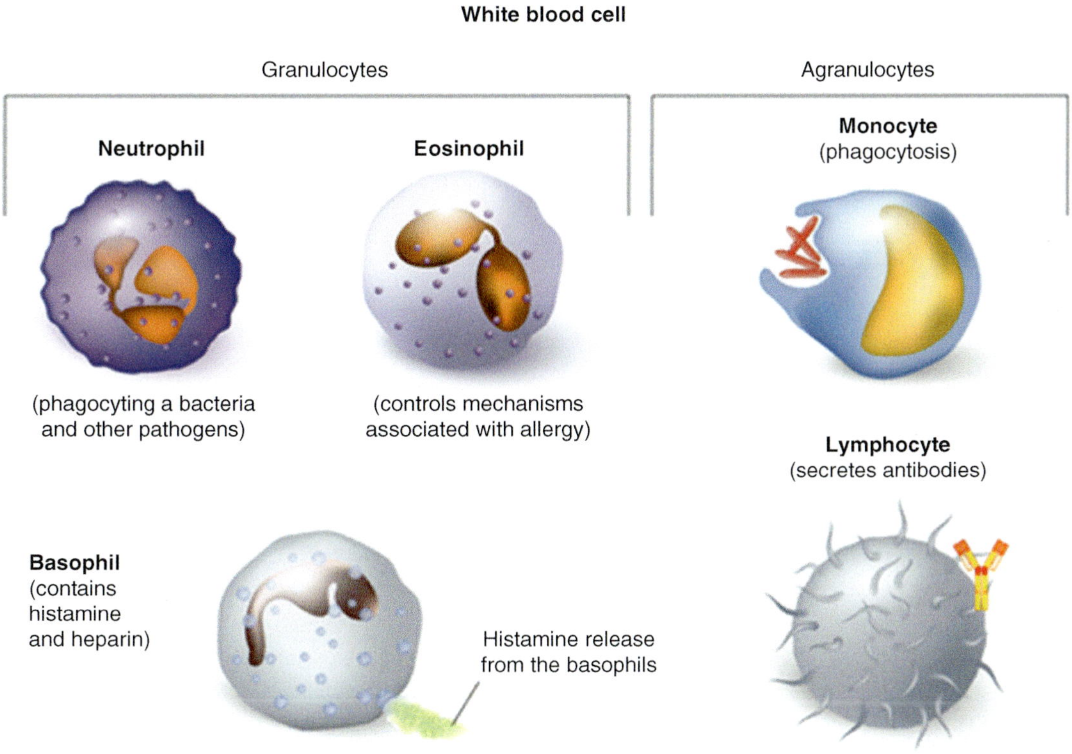


**Fig. 4.9** The types of white blood cells ("leukocytes"). (Adapted from Shutterstock Royalty-free stock illustration ID: 387954859, types of white blood cells. Infographics. leukocytes or leucocytes, by Designua)

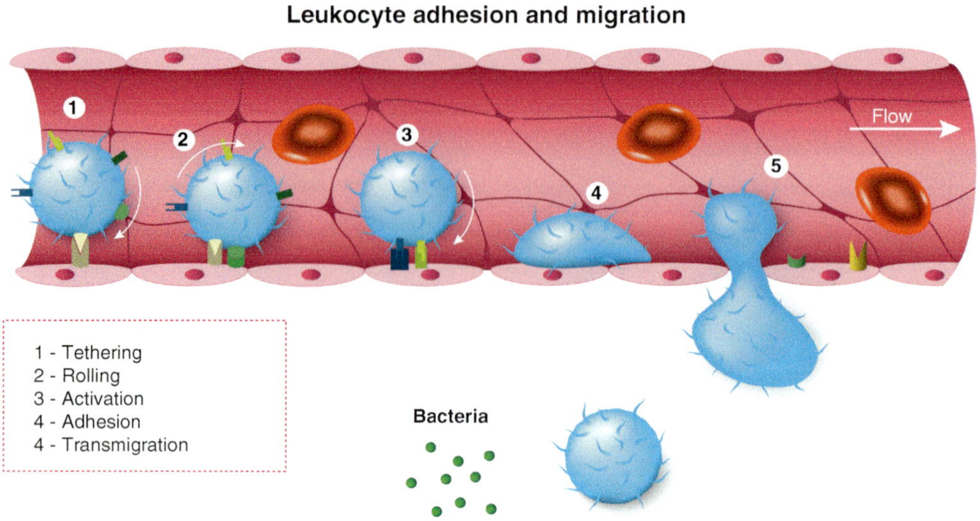


**Fig. 4.10** Leukocyte adhesion and formation. (Adapted from Shutterstock Royalty-free stock vector images ID: 358701779, Leukocyte adhesion and migration, by Designua)

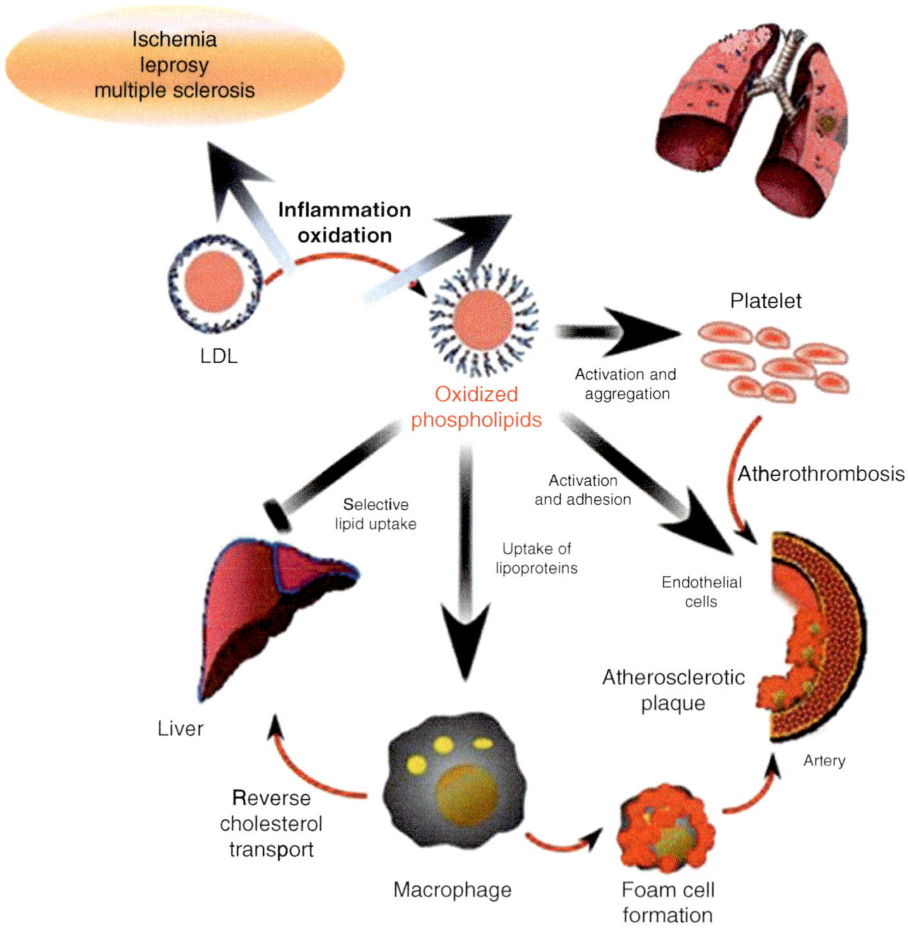


**Fig. 4.11** Effects of oxidized LDL cholesterol [20, Fig. 4.3]. (Open Access, IntechOpen: http://www.intechopen.com/books/lipoproteins-role-in-health-and-diseases/oxidized-phospholipids-introduction-and-biological-significance)

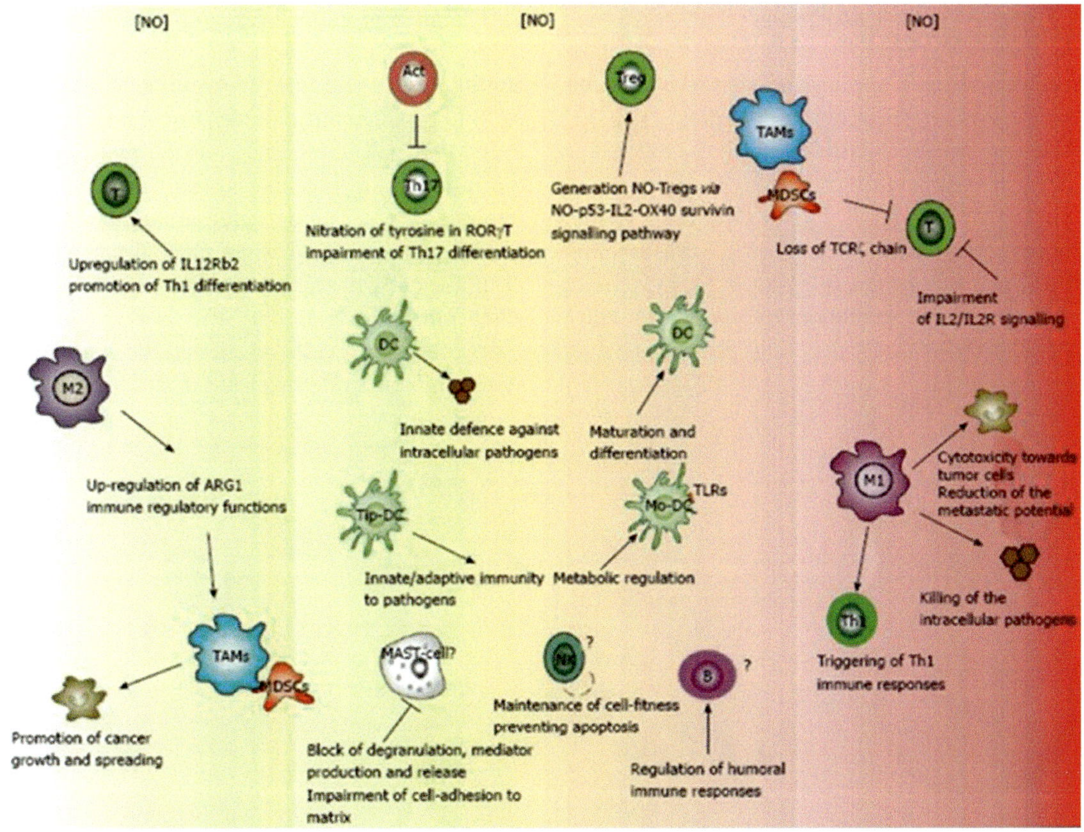


**Fig. 4.12** Distinctive effects of nitric oxide in immune cell subsets. Nitric oxide (NO) represents one of the key players involved in immunity and inflammation. The figure depicts the distinctive effects of NO within immune system, including controversial behavior. Low levels of nitric oxide (left) could either favor Th1 (helper T-cell) response or immune-regulatory environment, while high levels of nitric oxide (right) are either necessary for macrophage effector function or could impair T-cell activation. This opposite behavior is more evident where nitric oxide concentration is poorly defined (middle), where nitric oxide sources and effects are more debated. Question marks tag open issues in the field. → or ⊣ point out the effects of nitric oxide directly produced by the indicated cell on different targets. ← or ⊢ point out the effects of nitric oxide originated by different (not specifically indicated) sources on different targets. TAM tumor-associated macrophage, MDSCs myeloid-derived suppressor cells, IL interleukin, DC dendritic cell, NK natural killer cell [27]. (Open Access, WJEM)

from birth, the body produces millions of cancer cells. Finding them and eliminating them is one of the functions of the immune system. Studies show conflicting results on how nitric oxide affects cancer cells. However, recent research is discovering the specific conditions which can trigger nitric oxide-related and nitric oxide-mediated tumor suppression, making it potentially one of the strongest, yet little-known, cancer fighters.

Since nitric oxide is also a promoter of cell growth, it can be both a cancer tumor promoter under certain circumstances and a cancer suppressor. One of the most powerful ways it can help heal cancer is by encouraging the growth of healthy cells. It has been suggested that nitric oxide modulates different cancer-related events, including angiogenesis, apoptosis, cell cycle, invasion, and metastasis. On the other hand, it is also emerging as a potential anti-oncogenic agent [29, 30]. It appears that high levels of NOS expression (e.g., generated by activated macrophages) are either cytostatic or cytotoxic for tumor cells, whereas low-level activity can have the opposite effect and promote tumor growth. Paradoxically therefore, nitric oxide (and related reactive nitrogen species) may have both genotoxic and angiogenic properties [31–33]. Although the jury is still out as to the exact "low point" at which nitric oxide may increase cancer tumor growth, what is crystal clear (and verified by countless studies) is that nitric oxide at a high level is a tumor suppressor (Fig. 4.13) [35]. Being proactive with prevention by increasing nitric oxide levels naturally may help prevent and even heal cancer.

The most promising research regarding nitric oxide levels and cancer has been around the amino acid L-arginine. L-Arginine works with NOS to produce nitric oxide (Fig. 4.14). A study found that with the highest nitric oxide activity, the nitric oxide present caused cancer cells to implode [36]. Tumor cells are destroyed by "active macrophages" when nitric oxide activity in tumor cells is stimulated. On the other hand, when nitric oxide activity was lowered significantly, the tumor cells developed the capacity to avoid immune system-related destruction. Nitric

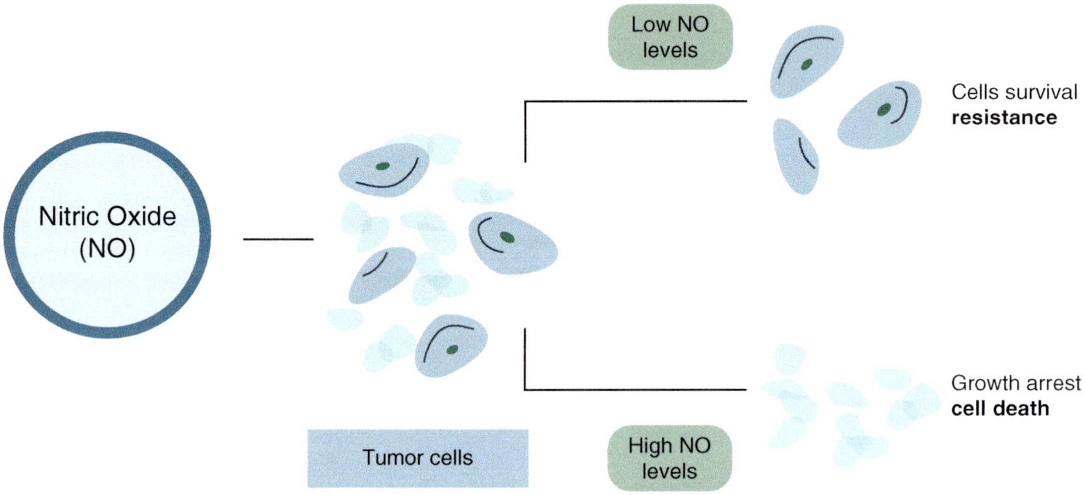


**Fig. 4.13** Nitric Oxide (NO) level determines activity in cancer cells [34]. (Illustration by Elysian Creative Studio, www.elysiancreativestudio.com, Lizzy Colombo)

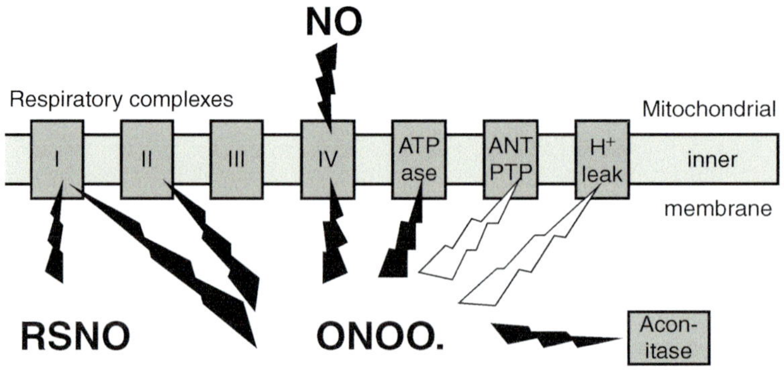


**Fig. 4.14** Main actions of nitric oxide (NO), peroxynitrite ($ONOO^-$), and nitrosothiols (RSNO) on mitochondria. Nitric oxide specifically and reversibly inhibits cytochrome oxidase (complex IV; see Fig. 2.12); nitrosothiols inactivate complex I, whereas peroxynitrite inhibits multiple respiratory complexes and aconitase and activates the proton leak and permeability transition pore (ANT-PTP), which may contribute to nitric oxide-induced cell death. Inhibitions are indicated by dark arrows/bolts, while light ones indicate activations [16]. (Republished with permission from Elsevier)

oxide appears to inhibit the enzymes responsible for growth of cancer cells, and high levels of nitric oxide lead to anticancer effects [30, 37].

Nitric oxide helps to regulate other functions [4, 38] (Fig. 4.14 [39]), including mitochondrial respiration and gene expression (as a pleiotropic regulator [40]). How nitric oxide regulates (inhibits) mitochondrial respiration is a little bit complicated and very specific (see Fig. 4.15). However, like anything, too much is also not good. For example, after an injury, such as a stroke or a heart attack, new mitochondria are rapidly proliferated to power the healing process. Nitric oxide initiates this proliferation, but also helps to prevent too much proliferation, all to counterbalance the effects of the injury. By limiting the regeneration and proliferation of mitochondria, nitric oxide helps prevent too much damage. Nitric oxide can also prevent cells from dying too soon, or the nitric oxide can make cells die that are no longer healthy, helping to remove damaged, dead, or alien cells [41]. Therefore, it regulates cell death (Fig. 4.16) [42], especially blood vessel cells. This wasn't appreciated until recent years. Interestingly, nitric oxide also enhances a process called angiogenesis which is the process of forming new blood vessels from pre-existing blood vessels. The mechanism helps stimulate a substance called vascular endothelial growth factor (VEGF) [43–47]. VEGF is important in stem cell transplants and making heart muscle cells with transplants. VEGF makes new blood vessels come out of old blood vessels and works

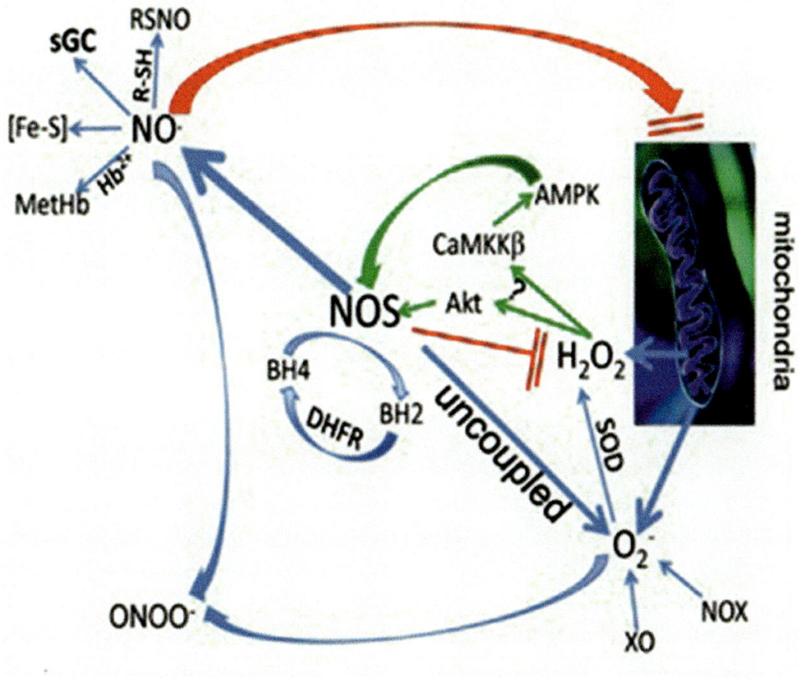


**Fig. 4.15** NOS-derived NO can inhibit mitochondrial respiration, as shown by the red arrow. Superoxide not only is formed by uncoupled NOS but also may arise from oxidative metabolism in mitochondria. Nicotinamide adenine dinucleotide phosphate (NADPH) oxidases (NOX), xanthine oxidoreductases (XO), and other oxidases also lead to the formation of reactive oxygen species (ROS). Superoxide can undergo rapid dismutation to form hydrogen peroxide ($H_2O_2$), a stable ROS that plays key roles in cellular signaling. $H_2O_2$ promotes activation of eNOS through protein kinase-, and Akt-, dependent phosphorylation, as noted by the green arrows. $H_2O_2$ leads to activation of the adenosine monophosphate (AMP)-activated protein kinase (AMPK), a process that depends on specific AMPK kinases, including the calcium-/calmodulin-dependent protein kinase-β (calmodulin KKβ). eNOS tonically inhibits endogenous $H_2O_2$ formation in endothelial cells [4]. (Republished with permission from SpringerLink)

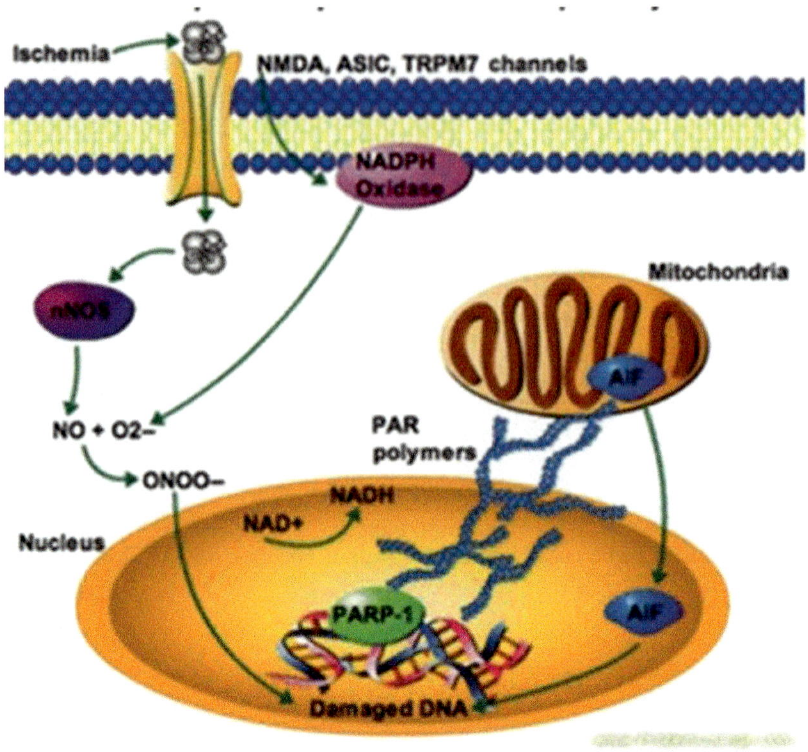


**Fig. 4.16** An example of nitric oxide-mediated cell death. Ischemia causes calcium influx through multiple channels including N-methyl-D-aspartate (NMDA) receptor, acid-sensing ion channel (ASIC), and TRPM7, which leads to increased neuronal nitric oxide synthase (nNOS) and generation of peroxynitrite ($ONOO^-$) from nitric oxide (NO) and superoxide ($O2^-$), damaging DNA. $O2^-$ is generated from NMDA receptor activation of nicotinamide adenine dinucleotide phosphate oxidase. The DNA repair enzyme poly(ADP-ribose) polymerase-1 (PARP-1) is activated utilizing cellular nicotinamide adenine dinucleotide ($NAD^+$), forming poly-ADP-ribose (PAR) polymers, which cause nuclear translocation of apoptosis-inducing factor (AIF) further damaging DNA. Cell death occurs from AIF-mediated DNA degradation and $NAD^+$ depletion, causing energy failure [41]. (Republished with permission from John Wiley and Sons)

with nitric oxide to repair other tissues, including nerve cells and brain cells. Damage releases nitric oxide, and the released nitric oxide stimulates the repair or new tissue generation process (Fig. 4.17) [48]. Another function of nitric oxide is to help form the endothelial progenitor cells in bone marrow to also support the formation of new blood vessels (Fig. 4.17). These progenitor cells make new endothelial cells to replenish them. Taken all together, nitric oxide is significantly involved in the repair of injury, including injury to blood vessels and brain cells.

Nitric oxide promotes bone remodeling and healing and may improve bone density [49]. It has a role in stimulating the hypothalamic-pituitary axis (Figs. 4.18, [50] and 4.19). Nitric oxide can release growth hormone, and there are now standard tests in endocrinology where L-arginine is used to show this stimulation. Nitric oxide affects the autonomic (P&S) nervous system(s). It increases vagal (parasympathetic) tone, helping to decrease sympathetic activity, thereby helping to reduce stress throughout the body. Nitric oxide, therefore, has a good balancing effect on the P&S nervous systems, helping to protect the heart and the other systems of the body; that is a whole lecture in and of itself and is for another time. Nitric oxide regulates inflammatory mechanisms. It is a reparative molecule, a reparative gas. Nitric oxide repairs tissues any-

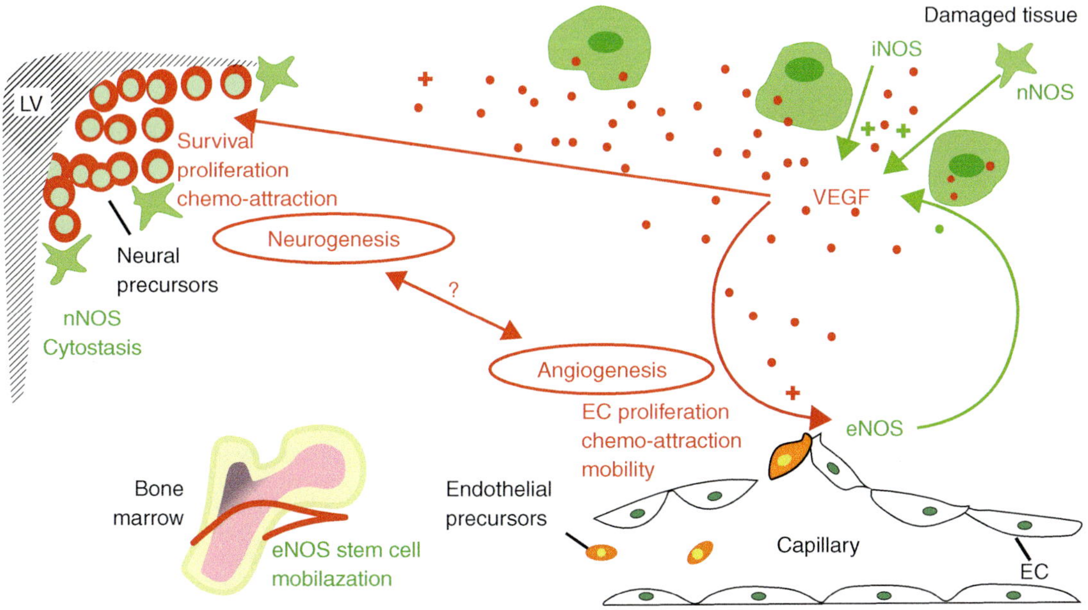


**Fig. 4.17** A model of nitric oxide-VEGF action in the brain. This model includes both angiogenesis (repair of blood vessels, capillaries in this illustration) and neurogenesis (repair of brain cells). In damaged areas, VEGF and nitric oxide synthase (specifically, the neural type, nNOS, and the inducible type, iNOS) are upregulated, generating nitric oxide. A positive feedback is created in which nitric oxide enhances VEGF expression and VEGF increases endothelial nitric oxide synthase (eNOS) expression in capillary damaged endothelial cells, thereby increasing the quantity of nitric oxide. Together nitric oxide and VEGF cause migration and proliferation of new capillary endothelial cells, which form the foundation for the new capillaries. The foundation of new endothelial cells causes chemoattraction and homing of hematopoietic stem cell-derived endothelial precursors, generating more endothelial cells, leading to angiogenesis. Meanwhile, VEGF increases nNOS expression, generating more nitric oxide on the brain side of the blood-brain barrier, enhancing proliferation of neural precursors, neuroblasts, and the migration of neuroblasts to the lesion area. nNOS-generated nitric oxide also promotes the survival of the remaining and repairable neurons in the lesion area. VEGF also acts as a chemoattractor for material needed to repair surviving brain (nerve) cells. In addition, nitric oxide produced by eNOS in the bone marrow promotes hematopoietic stem cell mobilization and, therefore, contributes to angiogenesis and revascularization of the damaged area. Meanwhile, continued expression of nitric oxide attracts scavenger cells to isolate, remove, and recycle unrepairable and necrotic tissue [48]. (Republished with permission from SAGE Publications)

where there is local injury, not just in vessels but in other tissue, including the brain and nervous system. Nitric oxide is released to stimulate and regulate repair and "cleanup." Having as much of it around as healthy is very helpful for the body to keep maintaining these important properties and functions, but still (like oxygen and water) not too much.

## Detoxification and the Urea Cycle

Nitric oxide helps as a detoxifying agent. The body makes ammonia ($NH_3$), especially in the muscles during exercise, for example. Ammonia is highly toxic. It needs to be detoxified before it may be eliminated. The urea cycle (see Fig. 4.20) is the process that rids the body of ammonia. The urea cycle occurs in the liver (Fig. 4.21). As discussed, L-arginine may become nitric oxide and L-citrulline via NOS (see Fig. 4.22). Ammonia is taken into the urea cycle, for example, by carbonyl phosphate (see Fig. 4.20). In the urea cycle, L-citrulline couples with the ammonia (indicated as $NH_2$ in Fig. 4.20) to start detoxification. The modified ammonia is then coupled with L-arginine, using water, to complete the detoxification process and produce urea. Here is another reason to maintain healthy levels of these amino acids to maintain wellness. This processing occurs partially in the

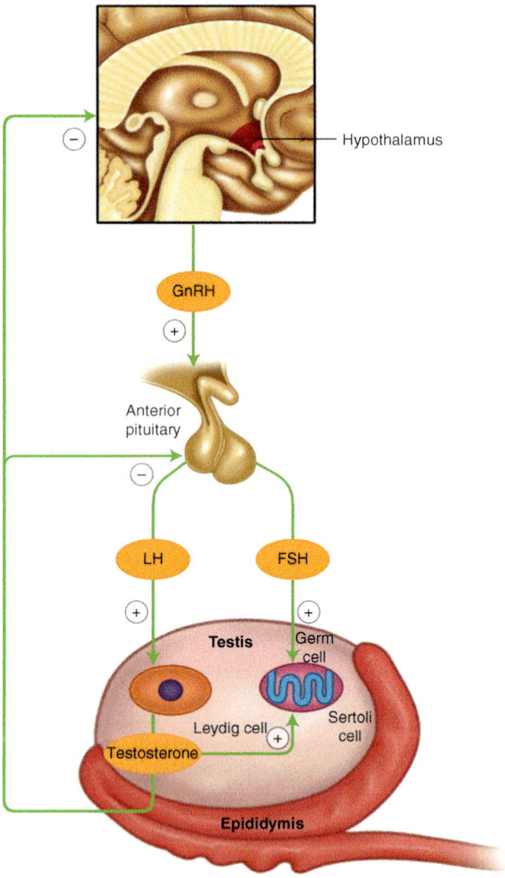


**Fig. 4.18** Male regulation of hypothalamic-pituitary axis. (1) NO stimulates LHRH secretion from the hypothalamus. (2) LHRH affects release of LH from the pituitary gland. (3) LH effects testosterone secretion in the testis. (4) Testosterone affects germ cell apoptosis and survival. (5) Germ cell survival leads to secretion or absorption of epididymal fluids and spermatozoa maturation. (6) Nitric oxide also regulates testicular microcirculation. Abbreviations: LHRH, luteinizing hormone-releasing hormone; GnRH, gonadotropin-releasing hormone; LH, luteinizing hormone; FSH, follicle-stimulating hormone [50]. (Open Access, IntechOpen)

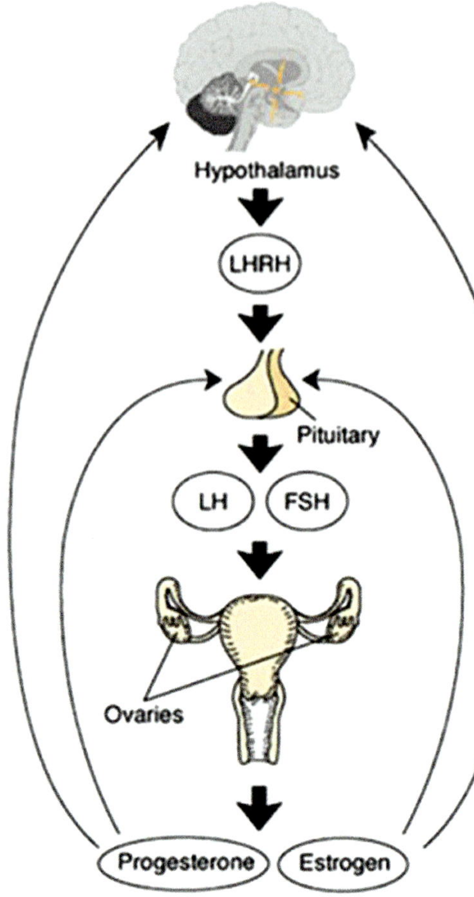


**Fig. 4.19** Female regulation of hypothalamic-pituitary axis. (1) NO stimulates LHRH secretion from the hypothalamus. (2) LHRH affects release of LH from the pituitary gland. (3) LH effects progesterone and estrogen secretion in the ovaries. (4) Progesterone and estrogen affect ovulation. (5) Nitric oxide also regulates uterine microcirculation. Abbreviations: LHRH, luteinizing hormone-releasing hormone; LH, luteinizing hormone; FSH, follicle-stimulating hormone [51]. (Republished with permission from NIAAA)

cytoplasm of liver cells and partially in those cells' mitochondria (see Fig. 4.20). The urea is then passed into the bloodstream and filtered by the kidneys to be excreted as urine (see Fig. 4.21). Nitric oxide is a product of the urea cycle and helps to regulate ammonia detoxification.

The urea cycle and the nitric oxide cycle (Fig. 4.22) are interconnected by L-arginine (arginine as indicated in the Fig. 4.22) as follows: L-citrulline (citrulline as indicated in the Fig. 4.22), made from ammonia and ornithine, is recycled to L-arginine in the urea cycle. L-Arginine then enters the nitric oxide cycle where it is converted to L-citrulline and nitric oxide by NOS. As discussed, L-citrulline takes part in two important processes: (1) L-citrulline is active in the production of nitric oxide, and (2) L-citrulline is important for the removal of ammonia from the blood in the form of urea. In the net, both processes are equal in the body. As a supplement, L-arginine is readily broken down into ornithine and urea before most of it reaches

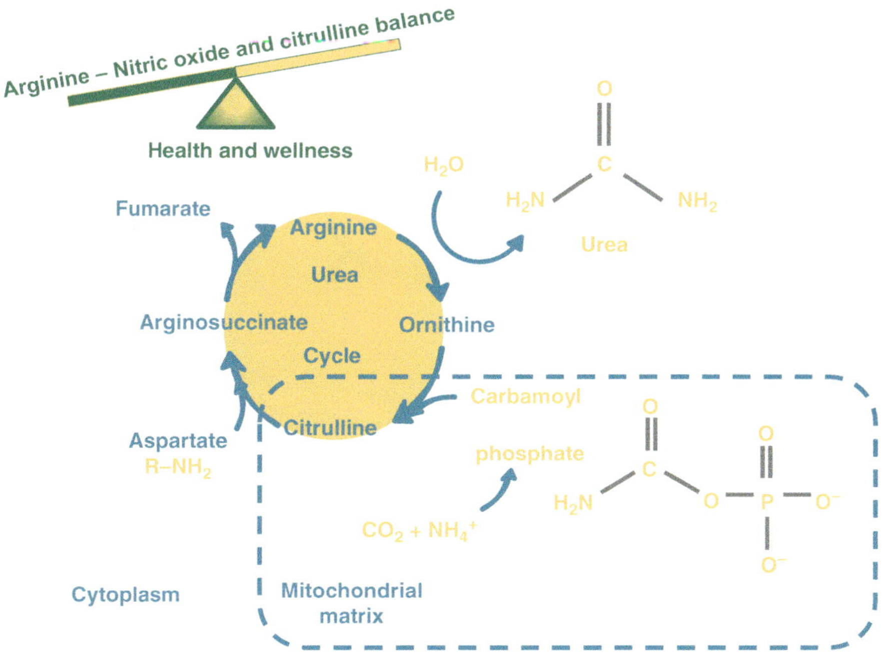


**Fig. 4.20** Simplified urea cycle

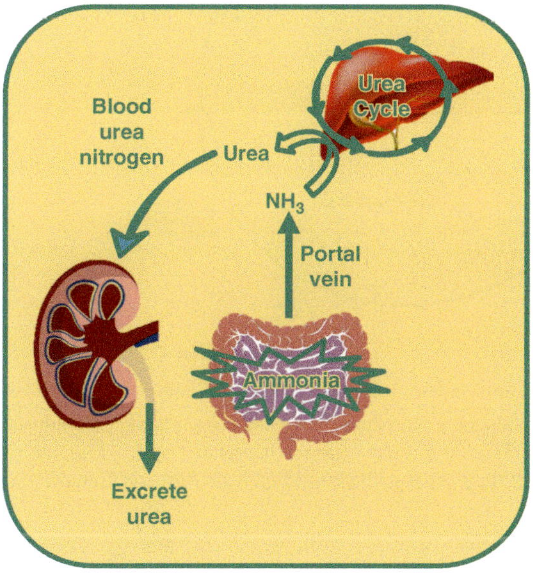


**Fig. 4.21** Ammonia detoxification occurs in the liver. (Adapted from Shutterstock Royalty-free stock vector images ID: (Intestines) 789,679,084 by Christos Georghiou, (Kidney) 1,039,345,291 by gst)

the blood. L-Citrulline, on the other hand, is not susceptible to arginase in the stomach and, therefore, makes it into the body where it eventually produces L-arginine which supports both pathways: the urea cycle and the nitric oxide cycle.

The urea cycle is also interconnected with the arginine-citrulline cycle (see Fig. 4.23) through argininosuccinate lyase (ASL). Although ASL is involved in the urea cycle with no net synthesis of L-arginine in the liver (all that is synthesized is used in the urea cycle), many tissues depend on it for the regeneration of L-arginine to ensure sufficient levels to purge ammonia, for example. In most tissues, the arginine-citrulline cycle couples L-arginine recycling to L-citrulline by NOS, with the generation of nitric oxide as a by-product.

Figure 4.24 depicts a summary of the various detoxification or neutralization processes that involve nitric oxide. The lungs deactivate nitric oxide by adding oxygen to make nitrogen dioxide ($NO_2$). Saliva reduces nitrogen dioxide to nitro-

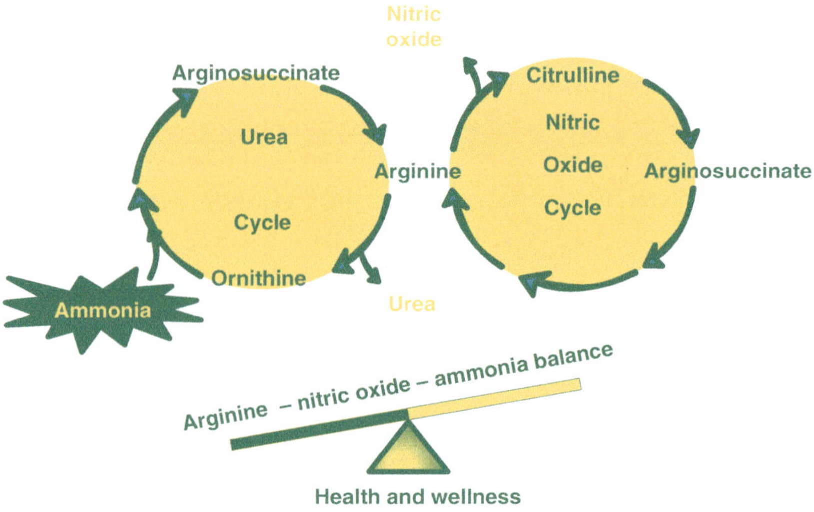


**Fig. 4.22** Urea cycle and nitric oxide cycle coupled through L-arginine. Enzymes: (1) arginase, (2) ornithine carbamoyltransferase, (3) argininosuccinate synthase, (4) argininosuccinate lyase, (5) nitric oxide synthase (NOS) [52]

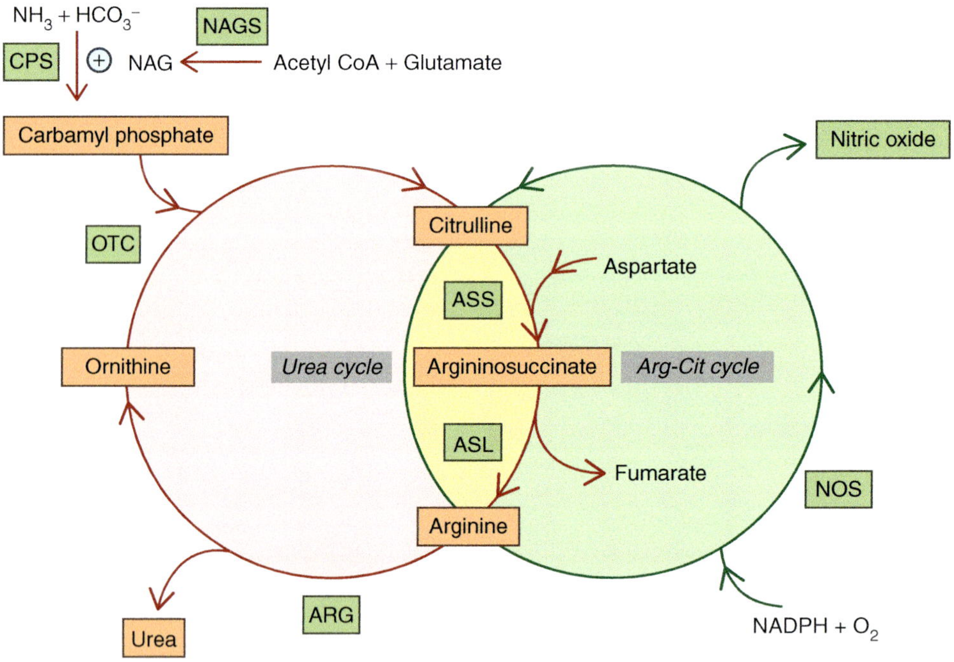


**Fig. 4.23** Urea cycle interconnected with the arginine-citrulline cycle. ARG arginase, ASL argininosuccinate lyase, ASS argininosuccinate synthase, CPS carbamoyl phosphate synthetase, NAGS N-acetylglutamate synthase, OTC, ornithine transcarbamylase [53, Fig. 4.3]. (Republished with permission from Springer Nature)

gen gas, an inert product which composes over 75% of the air. In the blood, nitric oxide is involved in other functional nitrate groups such as $NO_2$ and $NO_3$, with RSNO (nitric oxide, "NO," attached to a sulfur atom, "S," and an organic functional group, "R") serving to transmit nitric oxide bioactivity and to regulate protein function. In the bowels, functional nitrate groups are reclaimed, leaving behind ammonia, which is collected and transferred to the liver for detoxification. Excess superoxide variants of nitrate groups are also filtered by the kidneys and are passed in urine or feces. Nitric oxide equilibrium is maintained throughout the body, mostly in the

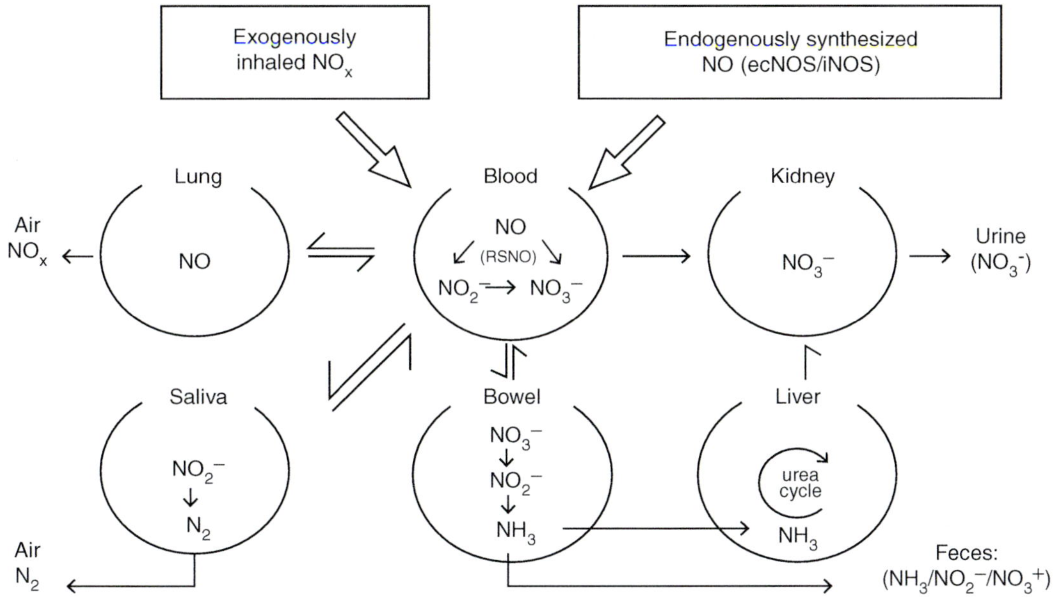


**Fig. 4.24** Biotransformation of nitric oxide and its related N-oxides [54]. (Republished with permission from Elsevier)

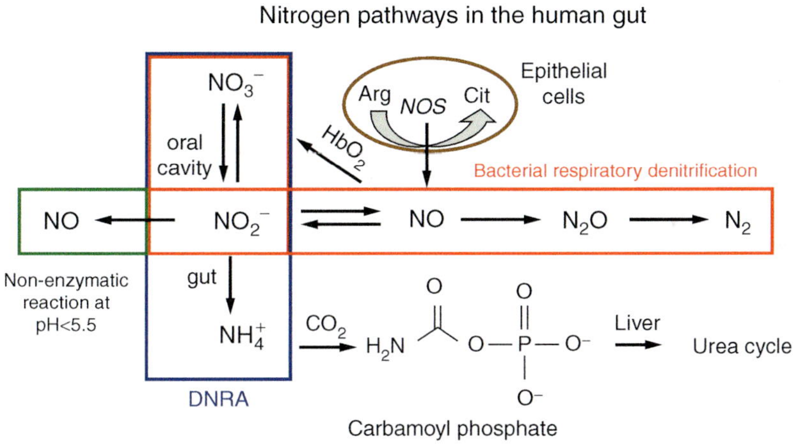


**Fig. 4.25** Schematic representation of the link between different pathways of nitrogen oxide reduction in the human gut and the fate of ammonia. Each colored box represents a distinct pathway: bacterial respiratory denitrification to dinitrogen in red box, the dissimilatory nitrate reduction to ammonia (DNRA) in blue box, and the non-enzymatic conversion of nitrite to NO in green box (this route becomes significant only at pH < 5.5). The endogenous L-arginine/NO synthase pathway from epithelial cells of the intestinal mucosa lining is also noted [55, Fig. 4.5]. (Open Access, PloS ONE)

gut, as depicted in Fig. 4.25. Nitric oxide is involved with L-arginine in slowing the aging effect of oxidization. Note the urea cycle (outlined in yellow in Fig. 4.33) is at the center of the antiaging process [56].

## Nitric Oxide Production

Again, a major producer of nitric oxide is the endothelium. The endothelial cell system is the largest organ system in the body, and if it were stretched out, it would cover the area of several football fields. As discussed, the endothelial cell system functions as barriers throughout the body and prevents harmful substances from reaching organs and tissues. It is a monolayer of cells and regulates blood pressure, blood flow, nutrient flow, and immune access (i.e., protecting gametes because they carry only half the genetic information of a normal cell). In the cardiovascular system, it controls growth of new blood vessels and controls clotting and inflammation. In the brain, it forms the blood-brain barrier. When there is damage to these endothelial cells, nitric oxide is not produced in abundance, and, for example, clotting and inflammation are facilitated. This can cause vascular disease and stoppage of circulation and cause heart attacks and strokes. The heart has small blood vessels, which when afflicted by endothelial dysfunction cause microvascular disease. More nitric oxide (e.g., from L-arginine supplement) also improves blood flow through those small blood vessels. Often, people with chest pains have small vessel disease. They have a normal coronary catheterization, but their stress test is abnormal due to endothelial dysfunction.

The quantification, or measurement, of endothelial health has commonly been divided into peripheral endothelial function (a systemic measure of endothelial function) versus coronary endothelial function (which must be assessed with invasive angiography) [1]. Testing involves pharmacological or physiological stimulation of the endothelial release of nitric oxide and other vasoactive substances. All these techniques have in common a measure of the response of the vessels to endothelial-dependent stimuli, mainly reactive hyperemia (shear stress) or vasoactive substances. Indeed, both macrovascular endothelial dysfunction, as measured by flow-mediated dilation [57, 58], and microvascular endothelial dysfunction [59, 60] have been found to be independent predictors of future cardiovascular events (MACE) in large cohort studies in healthy individuals over and above traditional risk factor assessment.

As introduced above, L-arginine is crucial for nitric oxide production. While L-arginine has many functions throughout the body (see below, “L-Arginine Requirements in Humans”), for the purposes herein it is followed into endothelial cells. eNOS is activated by $Ca^{++}$ levels in the endothelial cell. $Ca^{++}$ level is mediated by shear stress level due to blood flow outside the endothelial cell. eNOS converts L-arginine to nitric oxide using a cofactor, BH4 [61–63] (Fig. 4.26 [64]). Folic acid (vitamin $B_9$) accelerates the effect of BH4 (Fig. 4.26) [65]. Folic acid is also important in reducing homocysteine levels. Homocysteine is a substance which is toxic to blood vessel and endothelial cells if it is allowed to become elevated (see “Homocysteine” section in Chap. 5). Homocysteine also allows for another harmful substance, asymmetric dimethylarginine (ADMA), which is an L-arginine derivative produced and causes damage to tissues. L-Citrulline is a by-product of this. L-Citrulline can then be recycled through the nitric oxide cycle (see Fig. 4.22). Increasing the intake of L-arginine is very beneficial in increasing nitric oxide production, especially in people with heart disease, vascular disease, or the beginnings of endothelial dysfunction.

L-Arginine is a precursor of nitric oxide [66], and L-arginine’s effects can be measured by what is called brachial flow-mediated dilatation. After taking L-arginine for a prolonged period of time, a blood pressure cuff is placed on the arm, and blood flow through the brachial artery is measured with ultrasound and with other devices. Certain subsets of people who take more L-arginine over a period of time will have more blood flow through the brachial artery. That’s because the endothelium has a healthier supply of L-arginine. As a precursor of nitric oxide, it is a good vasodilator. In some people, more L-arginine, including when taken exogenously, removes more ammonia from the body; in the process more nitric oxide is produced, helping to maintain wellness.

ADMA (Fig. 4.27) is produced in cytoplasm of cells from a methylation process. It is either elevated by oxidized LDL cholesterol or derived from homocysteine. It impairs medicines, like statins, from lowering cholesterol and raising nitric oxide levels, by competing with L-arginine

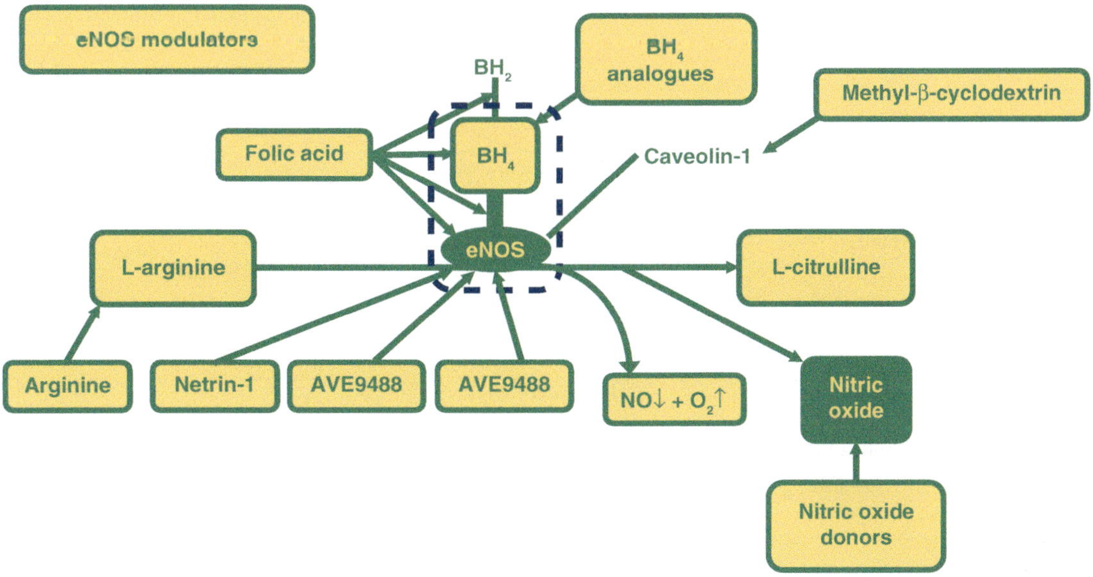


**Fig. 4.26** Schematic overview of the different endothelial nitric oxide synthase (eNOS) modulators, including BH4 (tetrahydrobiopterin). BH4 has been recognized as an essential cofactor of eNOS since it was first described in 1989. In its coupled state, BH4 is tightly bound to eNOS, and the amount of binding is correlated with eNOS activity. In the presence of its substrates (L-arginine and oxygen), eNOS catalyzes the formation of L-citrulline and nitric oxide. In the presence of subsaturating levels of BH4, the electron transfer in eNOS becomes uncoupled from L-arginine oxidation and nitric oxide formation. This uncoupling results in superoxide production by eNOS. Netrin-1, AVE9488, and AVE3085 are transcription enhancers of eNOS [64]. See text for details

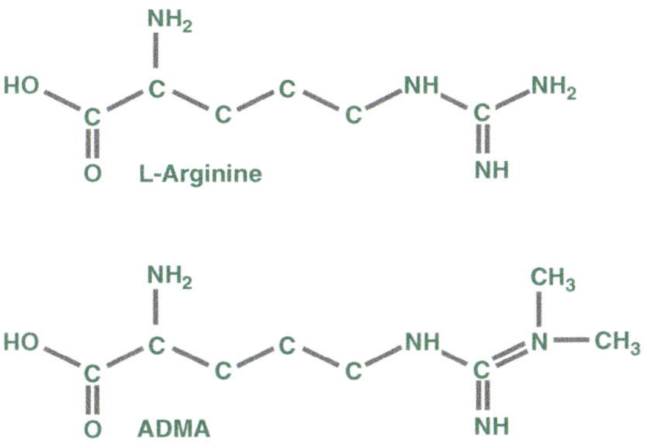


**Fig. 4.27** Asymmetric dimethylarginine (ADMA) is an L-arginine derivative that chemically resembles and opposes L-arginine and causes damage to tissues [67, Fig. 4.3]

for NOS enzyme. ADMA may also be generated when there is an excess of nitric oxide in the presence of excess $Ca^{++}$, as when there is too much shear stress from high, turbulent blood flow (see "The Anti-atherosclerotic Molecule" section for more information). B vitamins and folic acid attenuate the abnormal effects of ADMA competing with L-arginine for the enzyme NOS by accelerating the effects of BH4 in coupling NOS (see Fig. 4.28). There is a ratio of L-arginine to ADMA which is important, and if it becomes reduced, *it is a significant risk factor for cardiovascular and other diseases* (Fig. 4.29). Increasing this ratio reduces the risk, especially in patients with underlying heart disease or endothelial dysfunction.

There are many processes in the body which elevate ADMA. These include high cholesterol, smoking, diabetes, and high homocysteine levels. Elevated ADMA is associated with congestive heart failure, liver failure, preeclampsia, hypertension, chronic renal disease, erectile dysfunction, as well as atherosclerosis. Again, ADMA is the endogenous competitive inhibitor of NOS and regarded as a novel cardiovascular risk factor. While these processes are treatable or preventable, there is one process that is neither: aging. Aging is well known as a major risk factor for development of cardiovascular disease. One

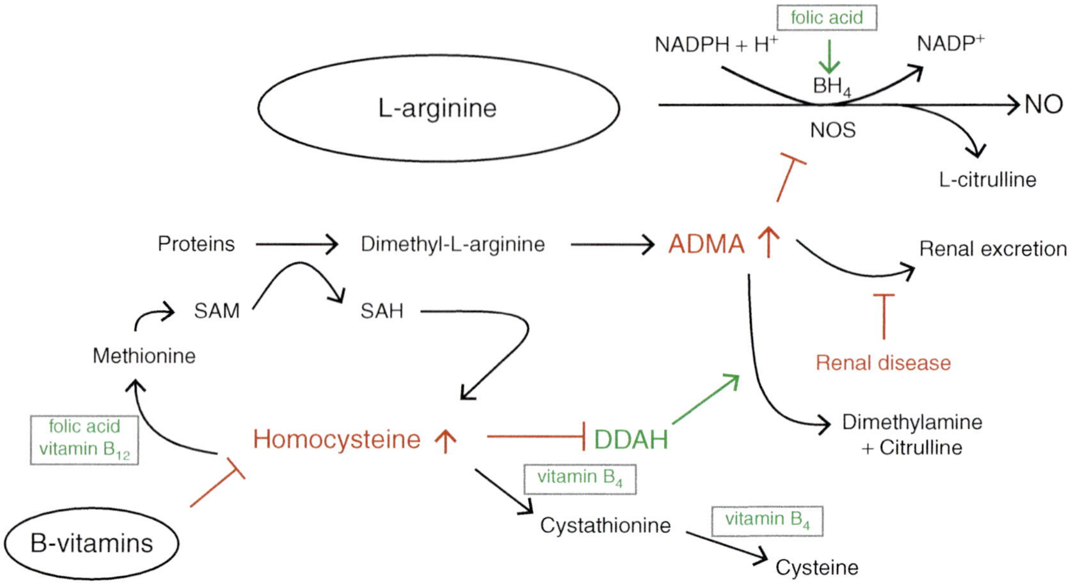


**Fig. 4.28** ADMA competes for L-arginine-binding sites on NOS. Folic acid helps to accelerate BH4 coupling to reduce the competition [65, Fig. 4.6]. (Open Access, SpringerLink)

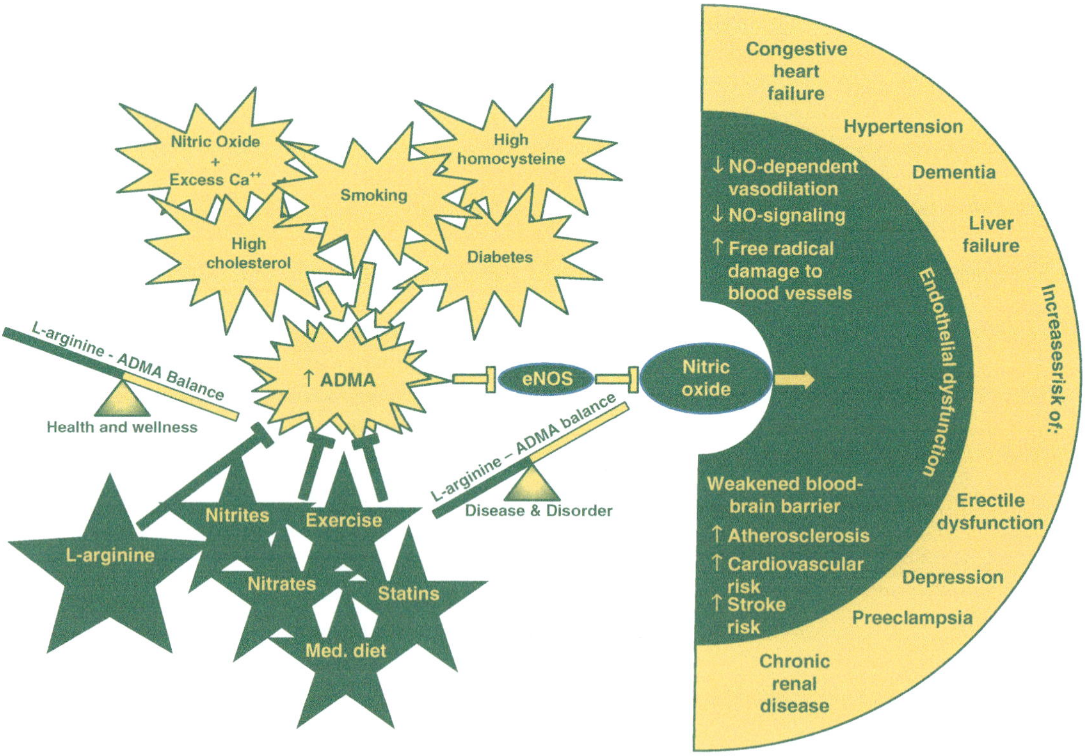


**Fig. 4.29** High ADMA to L-arginine ratios is a significant morbidity risk factor [68]

pathophysiological mechanism through which increasing age may lead to cardiovascular damage is the promotion of endothelial dysfunction via the nitric oxide-ADMA (NO-ADMA) imbalance. Biologically aging (senescent) endothelial cells produce less nitric oxide, thereby reducing the availability of cGMP signaling cascade, enabling more ADMA to be produced. This process could account for endothelial dysfunction and the development of cardiovascular diseases [68]. Senescence of endothelial cells can be altered by several different factors that influence the NO-ADMA system, contributing to delay or acceleration of the senescent process. The close interaction between the NO-ADMA system and biomarkers of endothelial cell senescence suggests that modulation of the NO-ADMA system could influence the process of human endothelial senescence. Biomarkers of endothelial cell senescence include telomere length[1] [69–72] (see also "Telomere Length, Longevity, Fish Oils and Antioxidants" in Chap. 9).

Therapeutic intervention aimed at preserving bioavailable nitric oxide or reducing ADMA levels (increasing the NO-ADMA ratio) helps to attenuate aging-related cardiovascular diseases [68]. This is another reason for older or chronic disease patients to supplement their diet with L-arginine, L-citrulline, or nitrates (e.g., beetroot). As a bonus, aspirin increases the NO-ADMA ratio by positively effecting both (increased) nitric oxide and (decreased) ADMA [73]. Note exogenous agents such as angiotensin II [74], and ibuprofen and acetaminophen [73], are known to decrease the NO-ADMA ratio. Statins are mixed and depend on the specific agent, some increase the ratio, some have no apparent effect, and some decrease the ratio [68]; take care in prescribing and include follow-up testing. Patients needing to take agents that reduce the ratio are recommended to supplement their diet with L-arginine or L-citrulline or nitrates (e.g., beetroot) to compensate and maintain a high NO-ADMA ratio.

Exogenous L-arginine beneficially affects the NO-ADMA ratio. The enzyme NOS can be induced in endothelial cells to produce more nitric oxide. This will prevent ADMA from competing with this enzyme and producing harmful oxidants instead of nitric oxide. L-Arginine is more beneficial in people with established illness and older subjects than in healthy young subjects in this regard. The L-arginine-ADMA competition is known as the L-arginine paradox.[2] While there is typically plenty of L-arginine (the rate limiter in the production of nitric oxide) in the cell, ADMA is promoted under conditions of too much nitric oxide (during prolonged illness or prolonged inflammation). Again, overwhelming the ADMA with L-arginine prevents the ADMA from binding and reduces health risks (i.e., morbidity and mortality risks).

L-Arginine and L-citrulline are both important substrates which help sustain nitric oxide levels. While they can be obtained through diet, one would have to take significant quantities of dietary substances to achieve what can be achieved in supplements. For example, watermelon is an excellent source of L-citrulline. However, over 2 lbs. of watermelon yields only 1 g of L-citrulline. L-Citrulline is easily absorbed and goes to the liver where it is converted to L-arginine, which becomes nitric oxide. It appears that half the dose of L-citrulline is required to produce the same amount of nitric oxide as a full dose of L-arginine. As mentioned, L-arginine and L-citrulline can interconvert with each other.

Nitric oxide production from endothelial cells is stimulated by a variety of mechanical forces such as shear stress (from blood flowing through the vessel), cyclic strain (from constriction and dilation), and humoral factors (ranging from

[1]Telomeres are nucleoprotein complexes located at both ends of eukaryotic chromosomes. These complexes consist of a six-base-pair DNA repeat (TTAGGG) and a growing list of associated proteins [69,70]. Telomeres are important structures involved in cell cycle control and essential for maintaining genome stability and integrity and for an extended proliferative life span in both cultured cells and the whole organism [71,72].

[2]L-Arginine is the substrate for the endothelial nitric oxide synthase (eNOS) to generate nitric oxide. The L-arginine paradox refers to the phenomenon that exogenous L-arginine causes nitric oxide-mediated biological effects despite the fact that NOS are saturated with the substrate L-arginine.

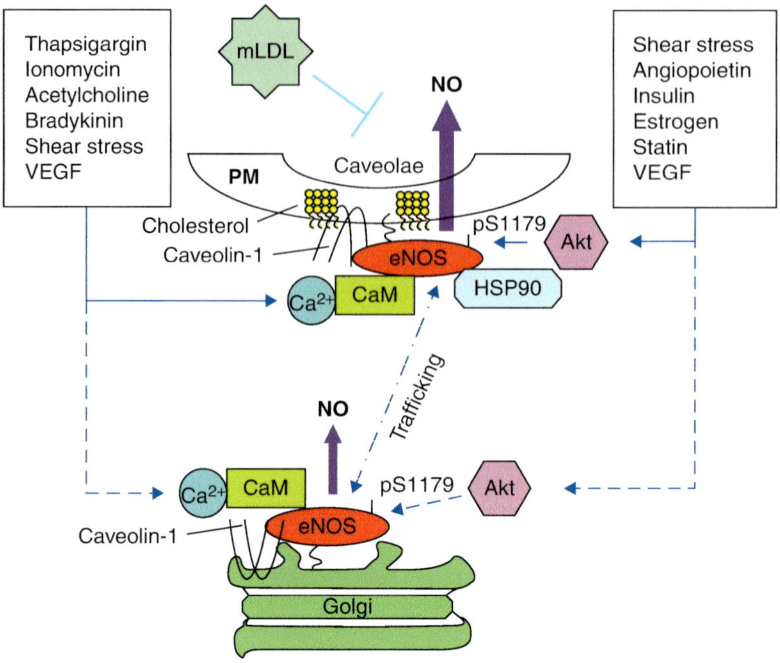


**Fig. 4.30** Putative mechanisms for the functional difference of the plasma membrane (PM)- and the Golgi-eNOS. In endothelial cells, eNOS is mainly localized in caveolae, cholesterol-enriched PM micro-domains, and the Golgi complex, in which eNOS is associated with caveolin-1. $Ca^{++}$-mobilizing agents such as thapsigargin increase intracellular $Ca^{++}$ levels and result in $Ca^{++}$/calmodulin binding to eNOS that stimulates eNOS activation and subsequently nitric oxide (NO) production. Other stimuli such as angiopoietin mediate Akt and other protein kinase activation, leading to eNOS phosphorylation that increases eNOS activation even in low levels of intracellular $Ca^{++}$. The PM-localized eNOS is more efficient in producing nitric oxide in response to various agonists compared with Golgi-eNOS, which may be attributable to higher phosphorylation and calmodulin affinity of the PM-eNOS relative to the Golgi-eNOS. HSP90 binding to eNOS may facilitate Akt-induced eNOS phosphorylation at S1179. However, the PM-eNOS is much more sensitive to the modification of cholesterol levels in cells such as by the treatment of mLDL. In addition, subcellular localization of eNOS is dynamic, and eNOS can traffic between the PM and the Golgi complex. Of note, the availability of eNOS substrate L-arginine and its cofactors such as BH4 in particular subcellular localization (not shown) may affect the ability of eNOS to produce nitric oxide as well [75]. (Republished with permission from Wolters Kluwer Health, Inc.)

growth factors to peptide hormones, including acetylcholine (Ach), vascular endothelial growth factor (VEGF), bradykinin, estrogen, sphingosine-1-phosphate, hydrogen peroxide ($H_2O_2$), and angiotensin II). Specifically, eNOS is a dually acylated peripheral membrane protein that is targeted to endothelial plasmalemmal caveolae[3] (see Fig. 4.30) through an interaction with the caveolae structural protein, Cav1 (caveolin-1). Cav1 inhibition of eNOS is relieved by calmodulin, which causes dissociation of eNOS from caveolin. This regulatory mechanism is further modified by heat shock protein 90 (HSP90), which binds to eNOS and facilitates displacement of Cav1 by calmodulin (see Fig. 4.30), [75]. In addition to these protein interactions that modulate calmodulin binding, other cellular signaling cascades also regulate eNOS activity. [76].

Physiologically, endothelial cells are exposed to the hemodynamic forces of blood, including laminar shear stress. The circulation of cerebrospinal fluid may also create a shear force to stimulate nitric oxide production from the endothelial cells of the blood-brain barrier. Shear stress, via G-proteins, activates several signal transduction pathways, including the phosphatidylinositol

[3] Small (50–100 nanometer) flask-shaped invaginations of the plasma membrane in many vertebrate cell types, especially in endothelial cells

3-kinase, phosphoinositide-dependent kinase, and adenylate cyclase via cyclic adenosine monophosphate (cAMP), leading to eNOS activation by phosphorylation of serine residues (S617 and S1179 for the protein kinase B (Akt) and S635 and S1179 for PKA), which promote eNOS activation. Additional stimuli, such as VEGF, estrogen, S-1P, and bradykinin (Bdk), bind to their cognate receptors (RTKs, VEGFR, ESR, EDG, and BdkR) and stimulate PI3K/Akt. However, they also activate phospholipase C-gamma and phosphatidylinositol 4,5-bisphosphate to increase cytoplasmic $Ca^{++}$ and diacylglycerol levels. The increase in cytoplasmic $Ca^{++}$ levels activates calmodulin, which binds to the canonical calmodulin-binding domain in eNOS to promote the alignment of the oxygenase and reductase domains of eNOS, leading to efficient nitric oxide synthesis. In addition, calmodulin activates calmodulin kinase-II, which phosphorylates eNOS on S1179. Increases in diacylglycerol (DAG) levels activate protein kinase-C pathway, which may negatively regulate eNOS or influence its coupling [77].

Finally, metabolic stress triggering the breakdown of ATP stimulates AMP kinase to phosphorylate eNOS on S1179. Phosphorylation of this residue by protein kinase-A is also associated with increased enzyme activity. Other proteins which are associated with increased eNOS activity or nitric oxide release are dynamin-2 (a GTP-binding protein) and porin, which colocalize and directly interact with eNOS. Their interactions with eNOS are stimulated by intracellular $Ca^{++}$ and lead to eNOS activation. Efficient supply with substrate during all this is ensured by localization of the L-arginine transporter cationic amino acid transporter-1 in caveolae and its direct interaction with eNOS [78].

eNOS can interact with various proteins in its "less active" and "more active" states. Myristoylation of eNOS occurs co-translationally and targets eNOS to cellular membranes, where eNOS is then palmitoylated. These lipidations promote eNOS association with cell membranes and are essential for linking upstream signal transduction pathways to eNOS activity in cells. N-Myristoylated and N-palmitoylated membrane-bound eNOS associates with the caveolae coat protein Cav1 and with HSP90. C-Terminal HSP70-interacting protein (CHIP) interacts with both HSP70 and HSP90 and negatively regulates eNOS trafficking into the Golgi complex. By contrast, nitric oxide synthase-interacting protein (NOSIP), a 34 kDa protein, and nitric oxide synthase traffic inducer (NOSTRIN) negatively regulate eNOS localization in the plasma membrane. Acute activation of eNOS in blood vessels in response to agonist such as acetylcholine (Ach) or Bdk results in the activation of the soluble guanylyl cyclase (sGC) in smooth muscle cells, production of cyclic guanosine monophosphate (cGMP), and degradation of cyclin A. An increase in intracellular cGMP levels affects vascular tone by decreasing the intracellular concentration of free $[Ca^{++}]$I by channel cyclic nucleotide-gated (cNG) ion channel complex modulation, as well as by activating protein kinase G (PKG) and phosphorylating HSP20, which regulate force by binding to thin filaments and inhibiting cross-bridge cycling [79]. Nitrosylation of caspase3 and caspase8 deactivates the proteins, thus leading to inhibition of apoptosis.

eNOS is an important regulator of cardiovascular homeostasis because it is the major source of nitric oxide production in vascular endothelial cells. eNOS plays a crucial role in the state of blood vessel vasodilatation and hence blood pressure regulation. In addition, nitric oxide released from the endothelium modulates other processes including platelet aggregation, platelet and leukocyte adhesion to the endothelium, endothelin-1 generation, vascular smooth muscle cell proliferation, and angiogenesis. Because of the important role of nitric oxide in each of these processes, abnormalities in vascular nitric oxide production are thought to contribute to the pathogenesis of certain vascular disorders, such as those of atherosclerosis and hypertension [80, 81]. The above description of the complexity of endothelial cell nitric oxide regulation and activity is summarized in Fig. 4.31.

Nitric oxide production diminishes with age [82]. When one is in their 20s, 100% of nitric oxide is available. By age 60, as little as only 15% of nitric oxide may be available. With aging,

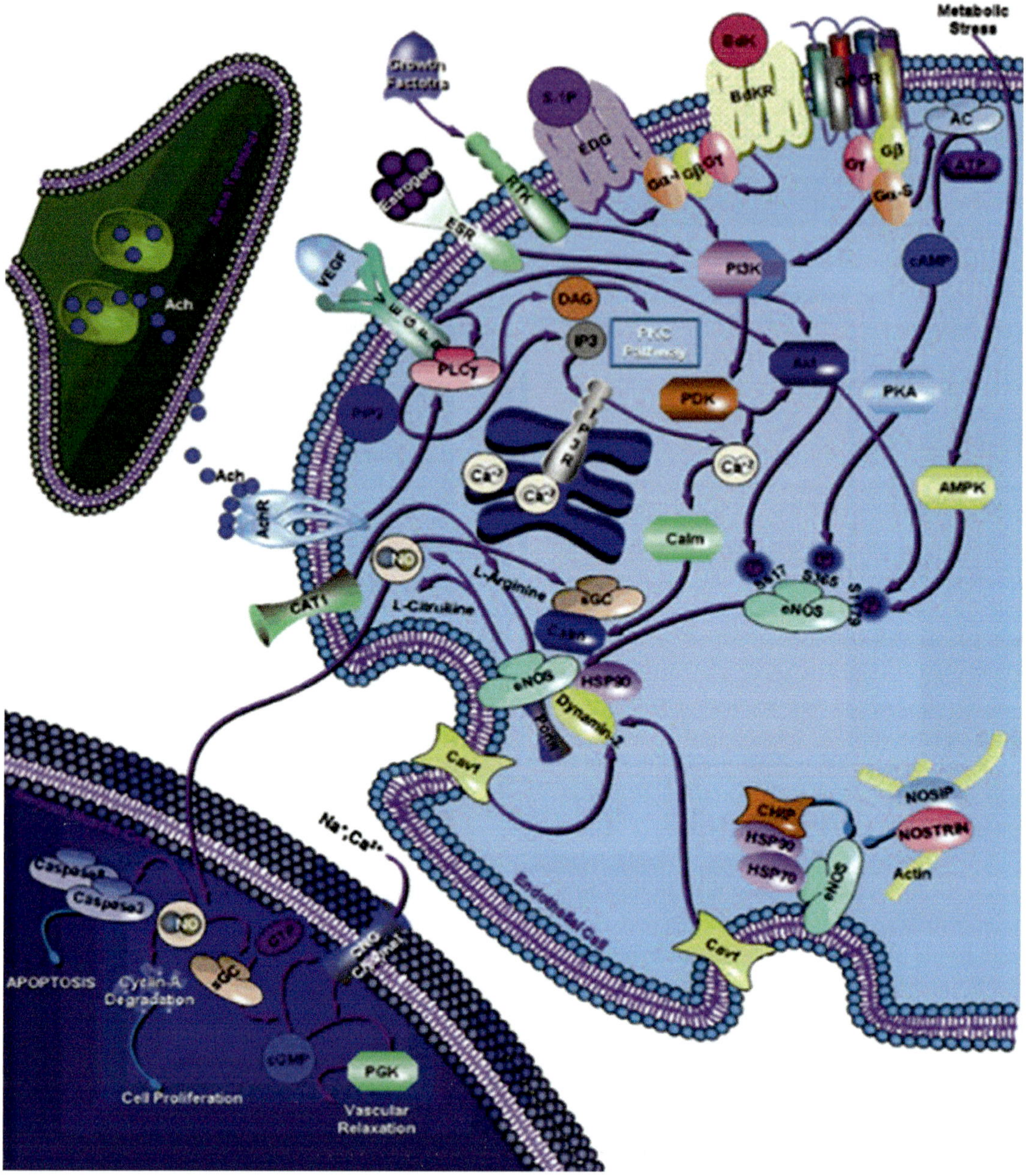


Fig. 4.31 Summary of endothelial cell nitric oxide activity in blood vessels. (© 2009 QIAGEN, all rights reserved)

80% of the ability to make nitric oxide will be lost. Taking nitrates in a diet, such as with beetroot, is an excellent way to increase nitric oxide [83–87]. Studies have shown that beetroot consumption does improve endothelial function as measured by brachial flow dilatation with various testing techniques (see section on "Beetroot Powder"). Generally, nitrate ingestion from any dietary rich source helps to increase nitric oxide [88]. However, it is important to emphasize that supplements cannot take the place of medications that are prescribed (e.g., antihypertensive or cholesterol-lowering pharmacological agents). Close physician supervision is required when working with supplements in conjunction with pharmacological agents. Also, supplements may cause adverse interactions with other pharmacological agents, and one's personal physician input is important in this regard.

## Beetroot Powder

The NOS system is the primary endogenous system that causes continuous production of nitric oxide in the body. The exogenous system is known as the alternate non-enzymatic pathway. It is an alternate way of producing nitric oxide, through an alternate pathway that does not involve NOS or L-arginine. Through the exogenous system, nitric oxide is produced in the body from dietary nitrates such as from beetroot and green leafy vegetables (Fig. 4.32). These are sources of inorganic nitrates which are converted to nitrates by mouth bacteria then eventually to nitric oxide. Both routes of production of nitric oxide vasodilate blood vessels and are important for killing invading bacteria by enhancing immune function, cause neurotransmission between nerve cells which is important for avoidance learning, and may also dilate the bronchioles in the lung and decrease inflammation.

Beetroot powder, made into a drink, is an excellent way to exogenously increase nitric oxide levels in the body. Beetroot, arguably, has the highest concentration of nitrates of any natural exogenous source. Beetroot is converted by the saliva and bacteria in the body to nitrites and nitric oxide. A meta-analysis that looked at 16 trials of over 250 people that took beetroot compounds up to 15 days [89] showed that beetroot decreased systolic blood pressure by 4.4 mmHg. It has been shown that it does lower blood pressure in other studies [90–97].

It is well known that hypertension is a very important mortality and morbidity risk factor. It has a high attributable risk for heart attacks, myocardial infarctions, and stroke, perhaps more significant than the other risk factors. Lowering blood pressure, even a little bit, is very important in reducing heart attack and stroke risk. Blood pressure is only controlled in approximately 50% of patients with pharmaceutical treatment alone. Therefore, based on meta-analysis data, ingesting beetroot juice will provide the added benefit of lowering blood pressure through the production of additional nitric oxide, which causes increased vasodilation, reduced atherosclerotic plaque and blockages, and more compliant blood vessels. However, there is evidence that additional nitrate ingestion, as from beetroot, does not further

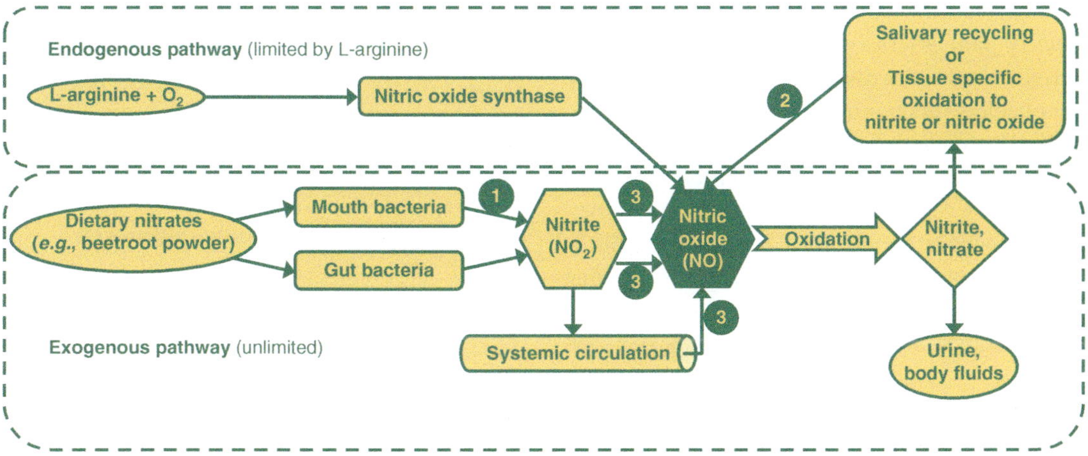


**Fig. 4.32** A schematic of the physiologic disposition of nitrate, nitrite, and nitric oxide from exogenous (dietary) and endogenous sources. Key: (1) the action of bacterial nitrate reductases on the tongue and enzymes that have nitrate reductase activity in tissues, (2) bacterial nitrate reductases, (3) enzymes with nitrite reductase activity [88]

reduce blood pressure once a hypertensive patient is well managed or well controlled [98]. This seems to be due to the fact that well-managed hypertensive patients have also modified their lifestyles to include proper exercise, diet, and stress reduction to naturally produce and consume more nitric oxide and permit the nitric oxide that is present to focus on maintenance rather than repair.

In fact, beetroot has been shown to be an excellent blood pressure-lowering agent in many studies [99–109]. Beetroot also improves submaximal exercise tolerance in older patients with heart failure and preserved ejection fractions. It has been shown to speed recovery from exercise [110]. It is important to note that the benefits from beetroot are long term. Short-term, or acute, doses of beetroot have not demonstrated any additional nitric oxide benefits [111–113]. It is so rich in vegetable nitrates that it may be the main mechanism for the "Dietary Approaches to Stop Hypertension" (DASH) diet being effective in lowering blood pressure, not the low sodium in the DASH diet but the high nitrates, which can convert to nitric oxide and lower blood pressure. Beetroot also lowers the oxygen costs of exercise from the cardiovascular system [114]. Recent studies in 2016 in the *American Journal of Cardiology* showed that patients with congestive heart failure had benefits of using beetroot, because of its ability to vasodilate arteries [115, 116].

Beetroot may also increase patients' walking time if their arteries are blocked or they have peripheral vascular disease [117]. It helps to keep the platelets functioning well and prevents endothelial dysfunction, as do other products that beneficially affect nitric oxide; maximal doses of beetroot are recommended. It seems to work better in younger people than L-arginine. This is because the L-arginine already saturates that enzyme pathway. So people that want better exercise tolerance are recommended with beetroot. Beetroot in combination with L-arginine and L-citrulline lowers blood pressure in patients with hypertensive disorders and in many instances reduces their pre-existing blood pressure medicines or even discontinues them all together. Beetroot is recommended as a multifaceted, natural approach to raising nitric oxide in the body. In addition to L-arginine supplementation with L-citrulline supplementation, exercise with reduced stress, fish oil supplementation, and antioxidant supplementation (alpha-lipoic acid and CoQ10), beetroot is recommended. All will directly or indirectly increase nitric oxide in the body and will be beneficial, and beetroot also has the additional benefit of taking advantage of a different pathway to produce nitric oxide than do the others.

## L-Arginine

L-Arginine is one of the most metabolically versatile amino acids (Table 4.2) [56]. It is classified as a semi-essential or conditionally essential amino acid. It is essential in children and nonessential in adults [118]. Proper plasma concentrations are maintained by dietary intake, protein turnover, arginine synthesis, and metabolism. The highest concentration of L-arginine is found in turkey and then pork loin, chicken, pumpkin seeds, soybeans, peanuts, and dairy products, in descending order. The main tissue in which endogenous L-arginine synthesis occurs is the

**Table 4.2** Properties of L-arginine. These properties are in addition to helping to produce nitric oxide (see Table 4.1)

| Properties | Methods |
|---|---|
| Promotes wound healing | Helps to build collagen |
| Aids in waste removal | Detoxifies urea in the urea cycle |
| Aids in releasing hormones | Especially growth hormone |
| Aids in healing gastric ulcers | Inhibits gastric hyperacidity |
| Aids in reducing atherosclerosis | Improves the function of statins and helps to close the "Statin Gap" |
| Improves insulin sensitivity | Increases insulin release and recovery of beta cells |
| Important for immune function | Has anticarcinogenic effect |
| Beneficial in weight loss | Improves exercise tolerance, due to improved blood flow to the lower extremities |

kidney, where L-arginine is formed from L-citrulline, which is released mainly by the small intestine [119]. The liver is also capable of synthesizing considerable amounts of L-arginine; however, this is completely recycled in the urea cycle so that the liver contributes little or no net L-arginine to the body [120]. Note the urea cycle (outlined in yellow in Fig. 4.33 [56]) is at the center of the antiaging process. In addition to nitric oxide production, L-arginine is involved in tissue repair, protein synthesis, and immune cell maintenance.

L-Arginine may also make different metabolites which may interfere with other processes in the body. It may make other products, which seem to help build collagen. So, L-arginine has a lot of functions, not just making nitric oxide (see Table 4.1) or waste removal in the form of urea detoxifying the body through the urea cycle (see above). Again, the urea cycle through L-arginine and arginine succinate is linked into the Krebs cycle, or the citric acid cycle, where ATP is made. It is interesting how nature has an interconnection between different cycles: the nitric oxide cycle (Fig. 4.22), the urea cycle (Fig. 4.22), the citric acid cycle (Krebs cycle, Fig. 2.11), and the arginine-citrulline cycle (Fig. 4.23). L-Arginine is right in the middle of all of that. It is a product of arginine succinate.

L-Arginine is important in cell division and therefore wound healing. When L-arginine converts to L-ornithine and L-citrulline, collagen is formed. L-Arginine, as a precursor for L-ornithine through the urea cycle, promotes the involvement of L-ornithine in collagen buildup for healthy tissues and wound healing. L-Arginine is important for immune function. It is important in hormone release, especially growth hormone. It helps to release growth hormone by binding an inhibitor of growth hormone release. Growth hormone

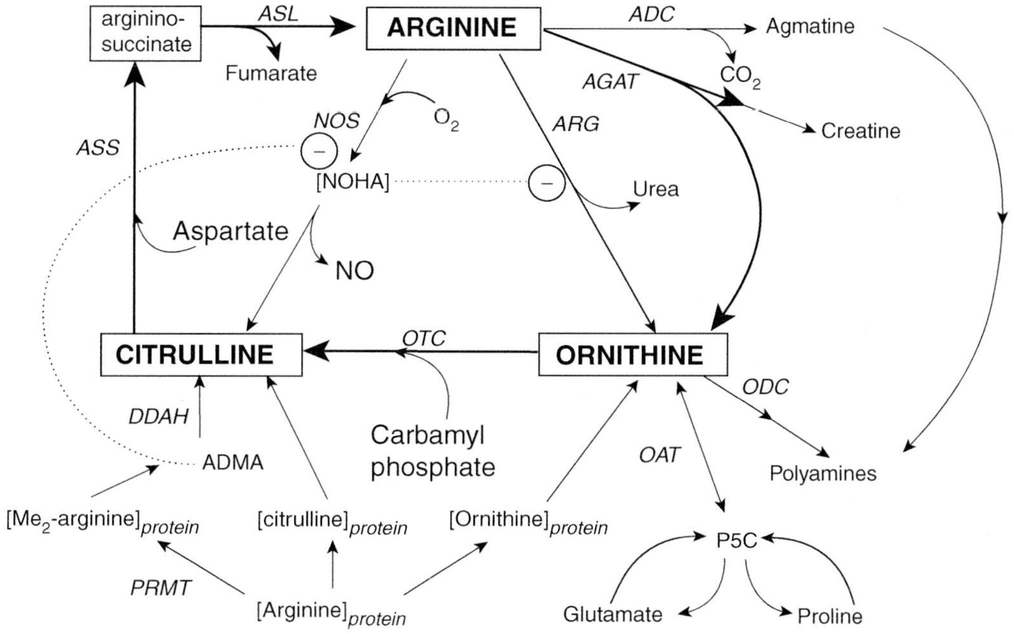


**Fig. 4.33** Overview of L-arginine metabolism (not all reactants and products are shown). Inhibition of specific enzymes is indicated by dashed lines and the dash within a circle. Amino acid residues within proteins are identified by brackets. Abbreviations: ADC, arginine decarboxylase; AGAT arginine:glycine amidinotransferase, ARG arginase; ASL argininosuccinate lyase, ASS argininosuccinate synthase, DDAH dimethylarginine dimethylaminohydrolase, Me2 dimethyl, OAT ornithine aminotransferase, ODC ornithine decarboxylase, OTC ornithine transcarbamylase, P5C l-D1-pyrroline-5-carboxylate, PRMT protein-arginine methyltransferase. (Republished with permission from Elsevier [56, Fig. 4.1])

causes muscle buildup, including from exercise, and so forth. L-Arginine may improve cognitive behavior. It inhibits gastric hyperacidity.

As shown in some studies, L-Arginine is very effective when patients do not respond to statins as expected. L-Arginine seems to improve statin efficacy. These studies indicate that when nitric oxide formation is blocked or impaired, L-arginine given with simvastatin is helpful. L-Arginine can lower blood pressure. It has an antihypertensive effect which has been shown in studies via a nitric oxide mechanism (see Table 4.1). In another endocrine (hormone) effect, L-arginine improves insulin sensitivity. It seems to increase insulin release and recovery of beta cells in the pancreas and improves control of blood sugar. There have been some studies that suggest that it has anticarcinogenic effect and it is an essential nutrient for rapidly growing intestines in the regulation of the "gut barrier" immune function [121].

L-Arginine is beneficial in weight loss and, also, people with claudication. Of course, people should ask their physicians first. Years ago, doctors used to prescribe wafers with L-arginine in them, a couple of milligrams of L-arginine in each wafer. People would actually walk further when they took it because it made for better blood flow to the lower extremities by reducing claudication. It also increases blood flow in type 1 and type 2 diabetics by improving factors of vasodilatation and nitric oxide. Some studies suggest that people who are prediabetic, or glucose intolerant, are beneficially affected by L-arginine. A bonus with L-arginine is that it doesn't have to go through the nitric oxide pathway. It can reduce copper and induced lipid oxidation and can decrease hormones like angiotensin II to prevent it from raising blood pressure. L-Arginine is considered an essential amino acid during pregnancy. Insufficient amounts may lead to retarded intrauterine growth rate and low birth weight. L-Arginine has a lot of beneficial effects that are important to realize, and it is just starting to be used due to its many advantages in health and wellness. But, the main mechanism of L-arginine in a lot of these processes is not endocrine but nitric oxide [122].

L-Arginine as a supplement is effective [123]. As discussed above, brachial flow dilatation improves with increases in nitric oxide. L-Arginine increases nitric oxide bioavailability, thereby improving brachial flow and reducing associated MACE risk factors. These studies demonstrate that blood pressure and blood flow are also improved. Meta-analyses demonstrate that L-arginine certainly helps people who have endothelial dysfunction. They already have problems with risk factors or with atherosclerosis. L-Arginine augments nitric oxide production and helps to relieve the risk factors and atherosclerosis. In healthy, young people, it might not be so effective [124–126]. Athletes have taken arginine for three main reasons: (1) its role in the secretion of endogenous growth hormone, (2) its involvement in the synthesis of creatine, and (3) its role in augmenting nitric oxide. However, because they are young and healthy, often they are already rate limited (NOS saturated) on the manufacture of nitric oxide (there is already enough L-arginine in the body to make nitric oxide) [124, 127, 128]. Therefore, it might be a waste of money looking to enhance exercise performance by taking L-arginine. To really increase exercise tolerance, there are data that involve L-arginine and beetroot. As discussed above, this pathway uses saliva and is absorbed through the mouth, making nitric oxide there and augmenting nitric oxide availability. So, for the young who are healthy and want to try and increase nitric oxide, L-arginine is not recommended. It really only helps people who are starting to age or have atherosclerotic problems or other risk factors. Beetroot or other forms of nitrates such as natural green leafy vegetables and walnuts are the preferred methods for healthier, younger people.

For the most part, people who are young and healthy, if they follow the Mediterranean diet and exercise and reduce stress, will experience the better part of this program. With age the body becomes more vulnerable, and more supplemental help may be needed. As soon as someone does not "feel 20 anymore" is when this program becomes effective. It is primarily designed for the person over 30. If one under 30 has symptoms and signs, then this program will also help. Examples of those under 20 who may benefit include those with symptoms of autonomic dysfunction or premature vascular disease or the like or premature cholesterol disorders like familial hypercholesterolemia where cholesterol levels are very high.

Only about 40% of the L-arginine ingested survives to enter the bloodstream [129]. Most dietary proteins have a relatively balanced mixture of amino acids; therefore, the only way to selectively deliver more L-arginine is to supplement it. There is little evidence to support an absolute dietary deficiency as a cause of vascular dysfunction in humans. However, there is evidence that supports the importance of an exogenous supply of L-arginine for a healthy vascular system [130]. In this study, vascular endothelial function was examined in the cardiovascular system. Exogenous L-arginine caused a rapid reduction in systolic and diastolic pressures when infused into healthy humans and patients with various forms of hypertension. Furthermore, oral L-arginine supplementation attenuates platelet reactivity and improves endothelial function in animal models of hypercholesterolemia and atherosclerosis [56].

Clinical studies of L-arginine have also been highly positive in improving endothelial dysfunction and even preventing restenosis after balloon angioplasty. Most reports ascribe the clinical benefits of L-arginine in CVD to the provision of nitric oxide. L-Arginine is the only precursor for NOS reaction. Nitric oxide is produced by all tissues of the body and plays particularly important roles in cardiovascular homoeostasis. Several studies have shown that L-arginine improves vascular function by overcoming the deleterious effects of ADMA (a novel cardiovascular risk factor). ADMA, as a competitive inhibitor of NOS, has been found to be elevated in serum in many diseases [131]. L-Arginine is required for normal spermatogenesis [132, 133]. Wound healing involves platelets, inflammatory cells, fibroblasts, and epithelial cells. All of these cell types are capable of producing nitric oxide either constitutively or in response to inflammatory cytokines. Nitric oxide produced by both iNOS and eNOS plays many important roles in wound healing, from the inflammatory phase through to scar remodeling. Nitric oxide has cytostatic, chemotactic, and vasodilatory effects during early wound repair and regulates proliferation and differentiation of several cell types, modulates collagen deposition and angiogenesis, and affects wound contraction (Fig. 4.34) [135].

L-Arginine was first noted to enhance wound healing in 1978 [136]. Since then, dietary L-arginine has been shown to improve collagen deposition and wound strength [137, 138]. This effect may be due in part to the subsequent increase in production of ornithine by the action of arginase enzyme, a precursor of L-proline during collagen synthesis [139]. The direct role of nitric oxide as a cofactor in the promotion of wound healing by L-arginine has also been reported [140]. L-arginine might improve wound immune cell function by decreasing the inflammatory response at the wound site [141]. The healing effect of L-arginine is also extended to cover burn injuries. Oral dietary L-arginine supplementation of 100–400 mg/kg/day shortened re-epithelialization times, increased amounts of

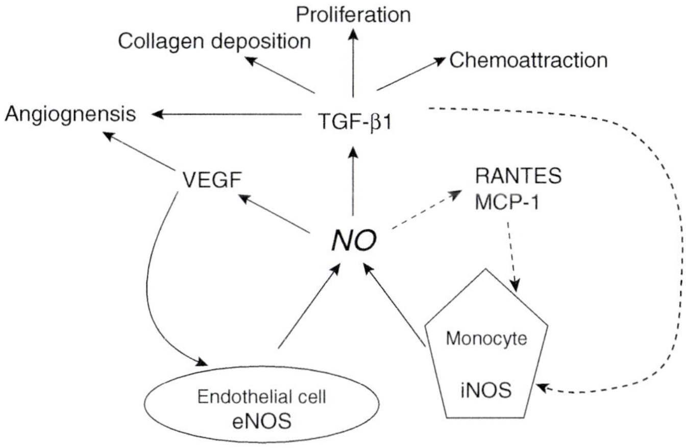


**Fig. 4.34** Schematic of the hypothesized roles of nitric oxide (NO) in wound healing. Production of nitric oxide from eNOS or iNOS leads to modulation of cytokines (e.g., MCP-1, RANTES, VEGF, and TGF-β1), which in turn modulates the various facets of wound healing (e.g., chemoattraction, proliferation, collagen deposition, and angiogenesis) [134]. (Republished with permission from Elsevier [56, Fig. 4.4])

hydroxyproline, and accelerated the synthesis of reparative collagen in burned rats [142]. Burn injuries significantly increase arginine oxidation and fluctuations in L-arginine reserves. Total parenteral nutrition (TPN) increases conversion of L-arginine to L-ornithine and proportionally increases irreversible L-arginine oxidation. These make L-arginine conditionally essential in severely burned patients receiving TPN [143]. Diabetes is also associated with reduced plasma levels of L-arginine [144] and elevated levels of the NOS inhibitor ADMA [145].

Evidence suggests that L-arginine supplementation is an effective way to improve endothelial function in individuals with diabetes mellitus (DM) [146–149]. Accumulating evidence is beginning to indicate that nitric oxide from L-arginine via NOS plays a part in the formation of memory [150]. Nitric oxide generated from L-arginine is released from a postsynaptic source to act presynaptically on one or more neurons. This leads to a further increase in the release of glutamate and, as a result, to a stable increase in synaptic transmission, a phenomenon known as long-term potentiation. This is thought to be linked to memory function (Fig. 4.35) [151].

In summary, L-arginine directly, or indirectly through nitric oxide, is involved or promotes many functions throughout the body. It is purported to have ergogenic potential [152]. L-Arginine has been demonstrated to improve peripheral circulation [153], renal function [154], and immune function [155]. It also possesses anti-stress and adaptogenic capabilities [156]. L-Arginine stimulates the release of growth hormone [157], pancreatic insulin and glucagon, and pituitary prolactin [158]. The antioxidant property of L-arginine has been well documented in several reports [148, 159]. L-Arginine has demonstrated an acute and transient improvement of pulmonary function in cystic fibrosis patients [160]. Nebulized L-arginine significantly increased exhaled nitric oxide concentrations. Manufacturers have tried to enrich apples, which already contain L-Arginine, with additional L-arginine to further increase apples' antioxidant levels. L-Arginine and apples appear to be a good combination. This supports the old saying that an apple a day keeps the doctor away. Perhaps this should be modified to say take L-arginine with an apple a day, and you may not only keep the doctor away, but you may keep the hospital away. In other words, they augment each other.

## L-Citrulline

L-Citrulline is the other compound created in the creation of nitric oxide from L-arginine (see Fig. 4.4). L-Citrulline is a nonessential amino acid, since it can be produced from L-arginine. In the diet, L-citrulline can be found in watermelon (where it was discovered) and in very low levels in cucumbers, cantaloupe, and milk. L-Citrulline operates primarily in the liver and in the urea cycle (see Fig. 4.20) to help to detoxify the body of ammonia. In the nitric oxide cycle, L-citrulline is recycled to L-arginine by argininosuccinate (see Fig. 4.22) to produce more nitric oxide. Because L-citrulline can be converted into L-arginine again and vice versa, it can promote and do the things L-arginine can do (see "L-Arginine" section). In fact, a significant synergism between the two taken together has been documented in studies, especially with blood flow (including blood flow to the brain to reduce fatigue) and erectile dysfunction (see section below). This is because together they help to produce more nitric oxide to help maintain optimal levels of that messenger throughout the body. L-Citrulline is well absorbed by the GI tract. It is more well absorbed than L-arginine. As stated above, only about 40% of the L-arginine ingested is absorbed through the GI tract. Virtually all of the L-citrulline ingested is absorbed. Therefore, L-Citrulline makes for a more efficient supplement. To that end, only about half the amount of L-citrulline is required to make as much L-arginine in the body as compared to the amount of L-arginine needed to be consumed to achieve the same levels. Therefore, the two are recommended together.

L-Citrulline is an alternative to think about. If a patient is reluctant to take statins or they only want to take in low dose, they should think about taking the antioxidant benefit of L-arginine and L-citrulline to keep oxidization of LDL from happening and utilize the nitric oxide mechanism to restore and promote healthy blood vessels. This is one example of the need to close the "Statin Gap"

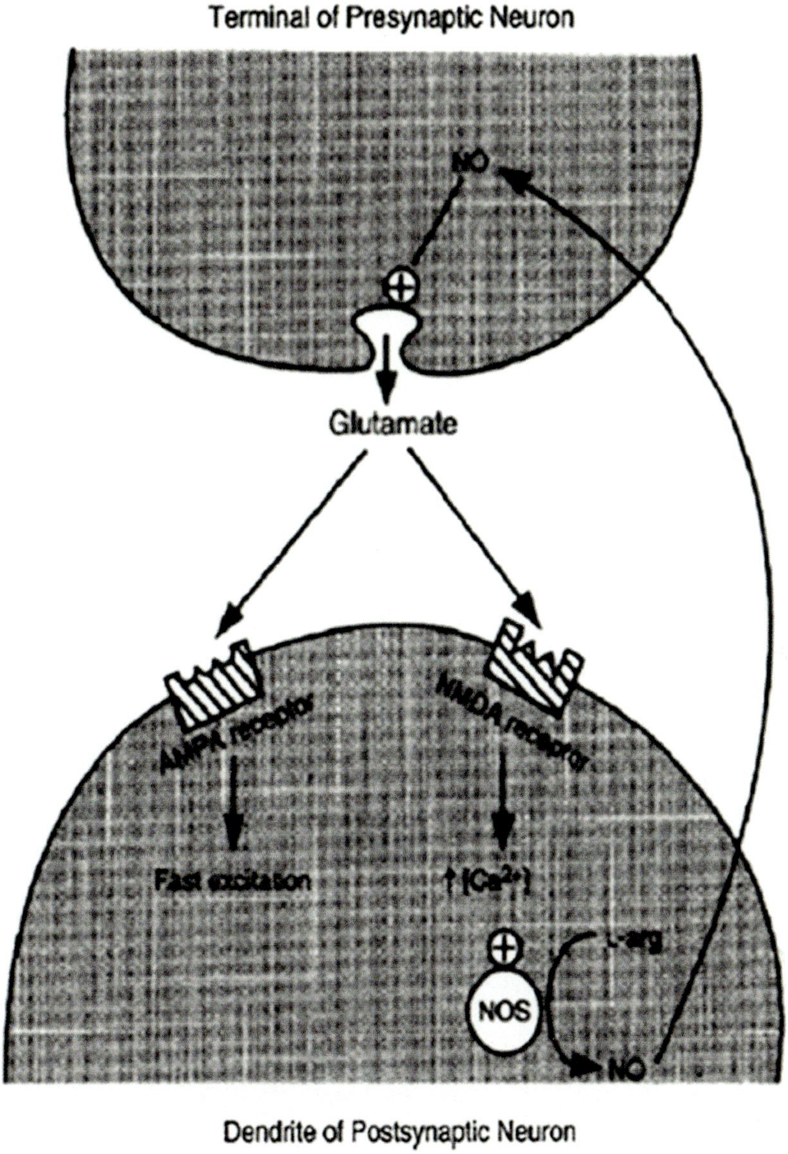


**Fig. 4.35** The role of nitric oxide (NO) in the long-term potentiation of neuronal activity. Glutamate released from the presynaptic nerve terminal activates different types of receptors on the dendrites of the postsynaptic neuron. Under normal conditions, the alpha-amino-3-hydroxy-5-methyl-4-isoxazole propionate (AMPA) receptors mediate most of the effects of glutamate. During high-frequency synaptic transmission, however, the activation of N-methyl-d-aspartate (NMDA) receptors results in an increase in intracellular calcium, which stimulates the constitutive nitric oxide synthase (NOS). The nitric oxide that is produced diffuses back to the presynaptic neuron, where it enhances the release of glutamate. The increased glutamate release leads to greater activation of postsynaptic glutamate receptors, thereby increasing the effectiveness of that synapse. Plus signs indicate stimulation. L-Arginine (l-Arg) [134]. (Republished with permission from Elsevier [56, Fig. 4.5])

(see Chap. 3 "Closing the Statin Gap"). Closing the Statin Gap is important since statins are not 100% protective. Patients are still having cardiac events, including heart attacks, and strokes while they are taking the statins. Statins may also damage the myelin sheath of nerves, causing patients to complain of muscle weakness and reduced coordination. This is due to the fact that statins not only reduce the LDLs in the bloodstream to prevent oxidation and the process leading to athero-

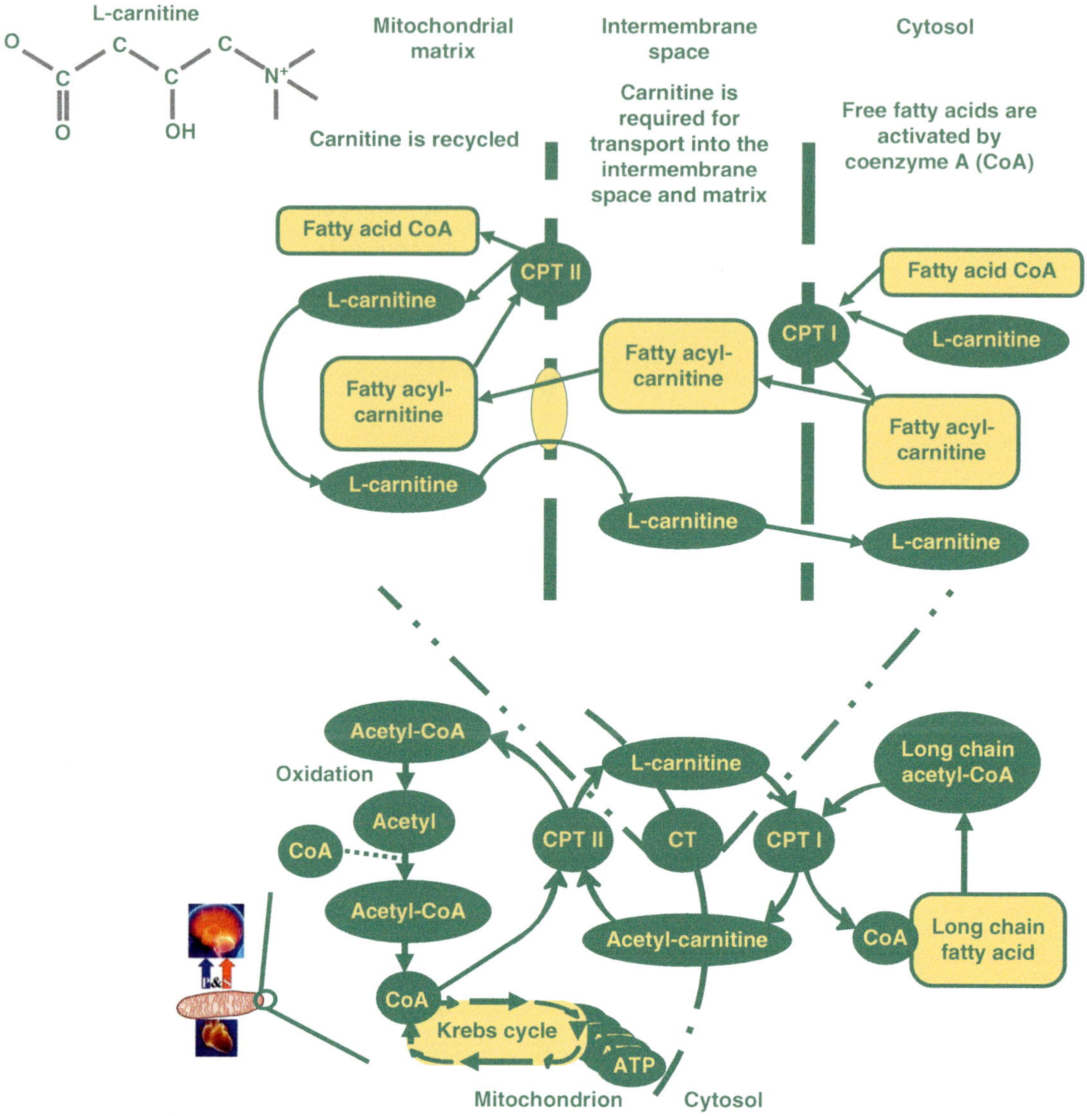


**Fig. 4.36** The L-carnitine fatty acid shuttle. The insert, top, left, depicts the chemical structure of L-carnitine. L-carnitine transports ("shuttles") fatty acids through the intermembrane spaces of mitochondria, into their matrices (details depicted top, right). Fatty acids are required in the production of ATP, which occurs in the matrices of the cell's mitochondria (below, right) [52]

sclerosis, but they also reduce the LDLs needed to repair and refurbish the myelin required for healthy, functioning nerves. The protective measures for this will be discussed below.

## L-Carnitine

L-Carnitine is antioxidant as well as anti-inflammatory (see Fig. 2.34). It is important for (1) fatty acid oxidation which generates ATP and energy in the mitochondria,[4] (Fig. 4.36) (2) keeping the blood vessels open, and (3) helping nitric oxide signal and improving endothelial function. It has been labeled as a fat burner

[4]When fatty acids undergo beta oxidation in mitochondria, L-carnitine facilitates transports of fatty acids into the matrix of the mitochondria, and this is called the "L-carnitine fatty acid shuttle," see Fig. 4.37.

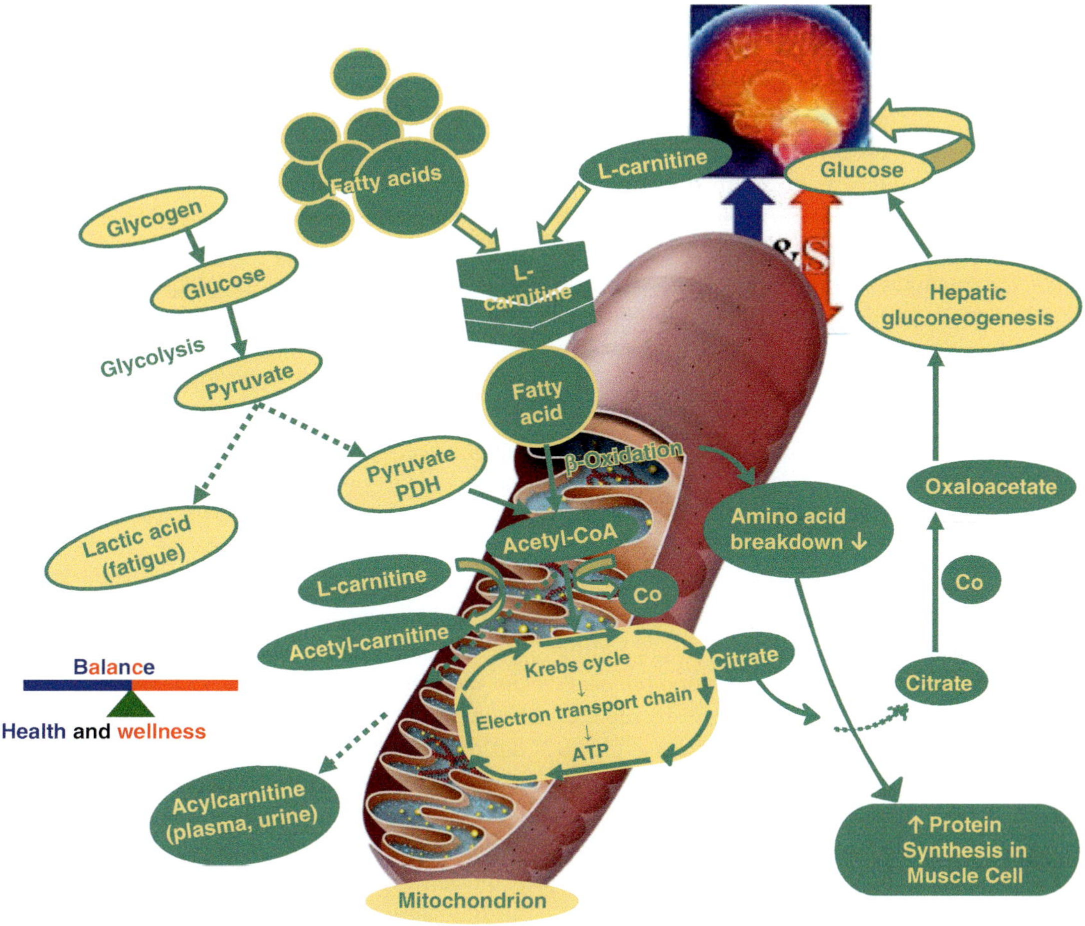


**Fig. 4.37** Details of the role of L-carnitine in weight management. Although carnitine is well known for its fat-burning properties, it can also improve performance and recovery after intense exercise. In fact, carnitine plays a key role in muscle glycogen metabolism, ATP production, muscle tissue repair, and even free radical scavenging. Supplementation with carnitine before exercise can increase muscle glycogen storage and improve ATP production, which improves strength and delays fatigue. When an abundance of fatty acids has been mobilized in cells, carnitine gets to work and shuttles them over to the mitochondria so they can be burned off as fuel. From a recovery standpoint, carnitine decreases production of free radicals and reduces muscle tissue damage and soreness from exercise via improvements in muscle cell biomechanics. When it comes to fat loss, it's best to take carnitine before workouts or in the earlier part of the day. It also works best when it's stacked with other fat-burning ingredients that help mobilize fatty acids, such as caffeine and raspberry ketone. Carnitine works to support fat loss by transporting long-chain fatty acids into the mitochondria, which are the energy powerhouses (or fat-burning furnaces) found in cells [52]

(Fig. 4.37). L-Carnitine is made in the body by glycine and methionine and helps to oxidize fats and fatty acids and bring them into the mitochondria to produce ATP (see Fig. 2.16). However, in reality, it is not a great fat burner unless the patient is L-carnitine deficient. If normal, there is no additional fat-burning effect by taking supplemental L-carnitine. It is not recommend as a fat burner or for weight loss in the majority of people if they don't have a deficiency. It is recommended for mitochondrial wellness if a mitochondrial disorder is suspected. It is healthy for the endothelial system because it promotes the nitric oxide signaling; therefore, it has multiple advantages as an antioxidant and an anti-inflammatory. In this regard, L-carnitine is an important component in wellness; 1000 mg a day is recommended.

There are several forms of L-carnitine. It is also found naturally in the body as acetyl-L-carnitine (ALCAR) and easily crosses the blood-brain barrier and may provide mental focus and better memory. L-Carnitine/L-tartrate (LCLT) provides antioxidants, is found in fruits, is usually a preferred form, and is the most stable. Another form, glycine propionyl-L-carnitine (GPLC), promotes strong blood flow to muscles, compensates oxygen loss during workout, enhances fat metabolism, and has been shown in many studies to be excellent in enhancing exercise. GPLC increases nitric oxide and blood flow. Increases in nitrite and nitrate plasma levels are seen after 4 weeks of supplementation with GPLC. Remember, nitric oxide has many health benefits. It may have antiaging and cognitive ability benefits, limit cigarette damage, promote increased libido, prevent kidney disease, and promote better cholesterol profile by preventing LDL oxidation, thereby lowering blood pressure. L-Carnitine may also prevent diabetes by regulating insulin, as well as helping to increase physical endurance, blood flow, and energy production in patients diagnosed with diabetes.

## The Anti-atherosclerotic Molecule

Atherosclerosis comes from the Greek word *athero* which means arteries and *sclerosis* which means hardening. It is the number one killer in America. One-third of deaths in America are cardiovascular including heart disease, stroke, and other vascular diseases. Any advantage in combating atherosclerosis would be welcomed. Increasing nitric oxide levels are very useful tools in the armamentarium to fight atherosclerosis. The heart attacks and strokes are mostly due to atherosclerotic arteries in the heart or brain, respectively.

Nitric oxide is known as the "anti-atherosclerotic molecule." It helps to prevent the process leading to atherosclerosis. As discussed before, when there is excess amount of LDL cholesterol, the LDLs may become oxidized. Oxidized LDLs are damaging and are consumed by macrophages to protect the system. However, when the system is overwhelmed by oxidized LDLs, the macrophages become engorged on oxidized LDLs and become "sticky," and they stick to the walls of blood vessels (see Fig. 4.38). The system often becomes overwhelmed when there are insufficient amounts of nitric oxide caused by too many injured endothelial cells. A sticky macrophage is a foam cell. Foam cells are the beginning of atherosclerosis. The foam cells stick and build up, forming plaque, and so forth (see Figs. 2.20 and 4.8). However, if there is enough nitric oxide, the oxidized LDLs, or better yet the LDLs themselves (before being oxidized), are neutralized by an electron from nitric oxide, and the need for the macrophages is reduced, and the process toward foam cells and atherosclerosis is prevented (see Fig. 2.22). This way nitric oxide is also a natural antioxidant.

The process leading to atherosclerosis can start in the teenage years. This is why it is important to eat healthy from a young age. This does not mean not eating any fat (LDL). There is still brain and nerve development occurring throughout the childhood years and continuing into the teenage years which requires LDL for proper nervous system development, health, and wellness. Even adults continue to need a low level of LDL cholesterol to maintain (repair and replace) healthy nerves and membranes. Cholesterol is needed for all of the membranes in the body. Cholesterol is good, *in appropriate amounts*. Too much cholesterol is not good. Like everything else, moderation is best. A serum cholesterol level of 150 mg/dL is a target for keeping membranes intact. Cholesterol levels above 150 mg/dL, for the most part, and LDLs start sticking to the arteries. Eating healthy means limiting fat, such as with the Mediterranean diet, as discussed below. Starting this healthy lifestyle while young will (hopefully) perpetuate it into the adult years. For as people slow down (due to age or disease), the beginning stages of atherosclerosis take hold, and the disease and associated risk factors catch up with us, causing the earlier heart disease observed in many practices.

Again, the sequence of events is: foam-cell induced plaque builds up when the endothelial cells in the body become injured. Fewer, healthy, endothelial cells mean less nitric oxide synthases

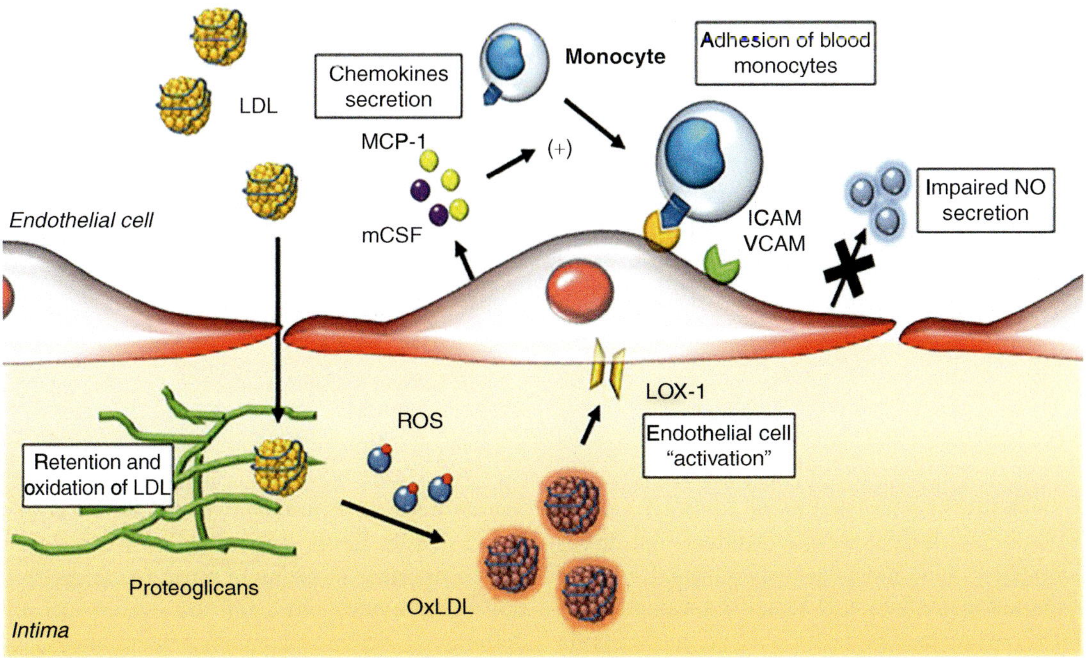


**Fig. 4.38** Role of OxLDL in endothelial dysfunction [161–174]. OxLDL formed and retained in the subendothelial space and activates endothelial cells (ECs) through the induction of the cell surface adhesion molecules which, in turn, induce the rolling and adhesion of blood monocytes and T cells. OxLDL induces the expression of intercellular adhesion molecule-1 (ICAM-1) and vascular cell adhesion molecule-1 (VCAM-1), increasing the adhesive properties of endothelium. The blood leukocytes recruited migrate into the tunica intima, guided by chemokines. OxLDL stimulates endothelial cells to secrete monocyte chemotactic protein-1 (MCP-1) and monocyte colony-stimulating factor (mCSF) that induce the recruitment of monocytes. OxLDL is also chemotactic for monocytes, T lymphocytes, and macrophages. These adhesions cause oxidative stress in endothelial cells, (1) producing significant amounts of superoxide, which chemically inactivates nitric oxide, forming peroxynitrite, and (2) inhibiting eNOS activity by dislocating eNOS from plasmalemmal caveolae [175, Fig. 4.3]. (Open Access, IntechOpen)

to produce nitric oxide, which means more LDLs become oxidized, which causes more foam cells. It becomes a downward spiral. Several factors and events injure endothelial cells. The oxidative hypothesis of lipids states that when LDL cholesterol gets oxidized (now the "lousy" or "bad" LDL), it becomes incorporated into the vessel walls as foam cells and plaques. The goal is to keep the LDL particles under 100 mg/dL in people who are at high risk for heart disease. In diabetics, who are at very high risk, the goal is to keep it under 70 mg/dL. However, this may not be enough. In the Statin Gap, lower LDL cholesterol is still only 33% protective, on average. With a rich, antioxidative environment, LDL is less susceptible to becoming oxidized, thereby reducing the Statin Gap. Two-thirds of patients still may have cardiac events. This is because the remaining LDL particles, even though they become reduced, still become oxidized, especially if there are insufficient antioxidant defenses. The sixfold approach of the Mind-Body Wellness program discussed herein, including increasing nitric oxide, attempts to create a more beneficial antioxidant milieu, thereby creating a more beneficial antioxidant defense, preventing atherosclerosis.

The flow of blood through blood vessels causes a shear stress on the walls of the vessels. This shear stress is the primary mechanism to stimulate endothelial cell production of nitric oxide (see the section on "Nitric Oxide

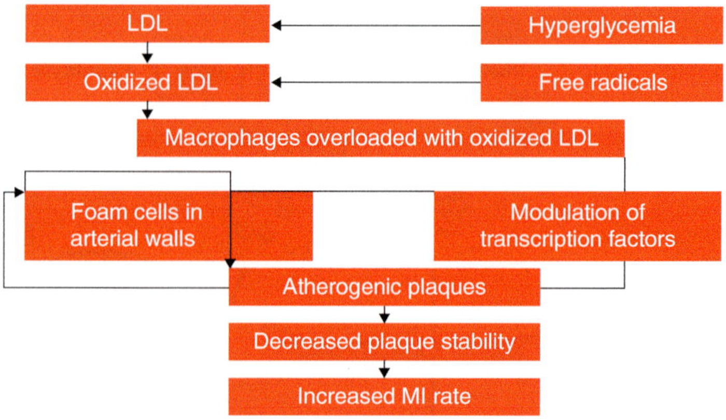


**Fig. 4.39** Diabetes- and atherosclerosis-induced cardiovascular disease [176, Fig. 4.6]. (Republished with permission from John Wiley and Sons)

Production"). Shear stress is minimal during smooth, or what is known as laminar (not turbulent), flow. Laminar flow is the optimal level of stimulation for endothelial cells' production of nitric oxide and is facilitated by nitric oxide "greasing the skids" and "widening" the way. Turbulence in the blood flow across the endothelial cells will injure them. High blood pressure and hardened vessels cause turbulence. In the atherosclerosis process, turbulence caused by the plaque that is deposited on the vessel walls ("fatty streaks") is the first cause of turbulence. As plaques grow, more turbulence is created, causing higher stress on the endothelial cells. Ultimately with blood clots, the blockage (partially occluding the vessel) causes very high flow rates, as the blood is forced through, causing very high shear stress, virtually stripping the endothelial cells from the walls of the vessels.

Even without plaque, high blood pressure causes high shear stresses that injure endothelial cells. Hardened arteries, due to calcification and other disorders, increase shear stress because it reduces the flexibility of the vessel walls injuring endothelial cells. With less flexibility, there is less give and take with each heartbeat, potentially causing damage with the systolic blood pressure. Cigarettes and diabetes and other poor lifestyle choices and diseases (see Fig. 4.39) lead to high blood pressure, LDL oxidation, hardened arteries, etc.; each results in compounding the other, multiplying the turbulence effect on endothelial cells. Even male gender is a risk factor, as the higher testosterone levels in men potentiate the factors that cause turbulent blood flow through blood vessels. Given these risk factors, it is even more important to promote nitric oxide production to provide sufficient anti-atherosclerotic defenses as well as maintain a proper antioxidant milieu.

People can have a complex genetic susceptibility with family history of plaque formation in their arteries. There are also nontraditional risk factors which can cause injury to endothelial cells like stress (e.g., psychosocial stress; see related chapter below). A sedentary lifestyle and not exercising is a big risk factor. Exercise is arguably the best way to keep arteries healthy. Reducing obesity helps to prevent or reduce atherosclerosis. These risk factors injure the endothelial cells, in one way or another, ultimately causing too much stress against the endothelial cell lining of the artery walls. In a sense, nitric oxide helps to keep the artery walls slippery ("greasing the skids") to minimize stress and make it more difficult for things to stick to it, thereby preventing plaque. Actually, in this process, nitric oxide is both anti-atherosclerotic (slippery walls) and antioxidant (preventing LDLs from becoming oxidized).

After foam cells start forming (see Fig. 4.40), little cells inside the vessel wall start dying (a process known as apoptosis). The smooth muscle cells then begin proliferating and thicken. Thickening progresses as more foam cells are formed. During this process, inflammation begins. Micro-blood vessels start coming in to support the additional smooth muscle cells,

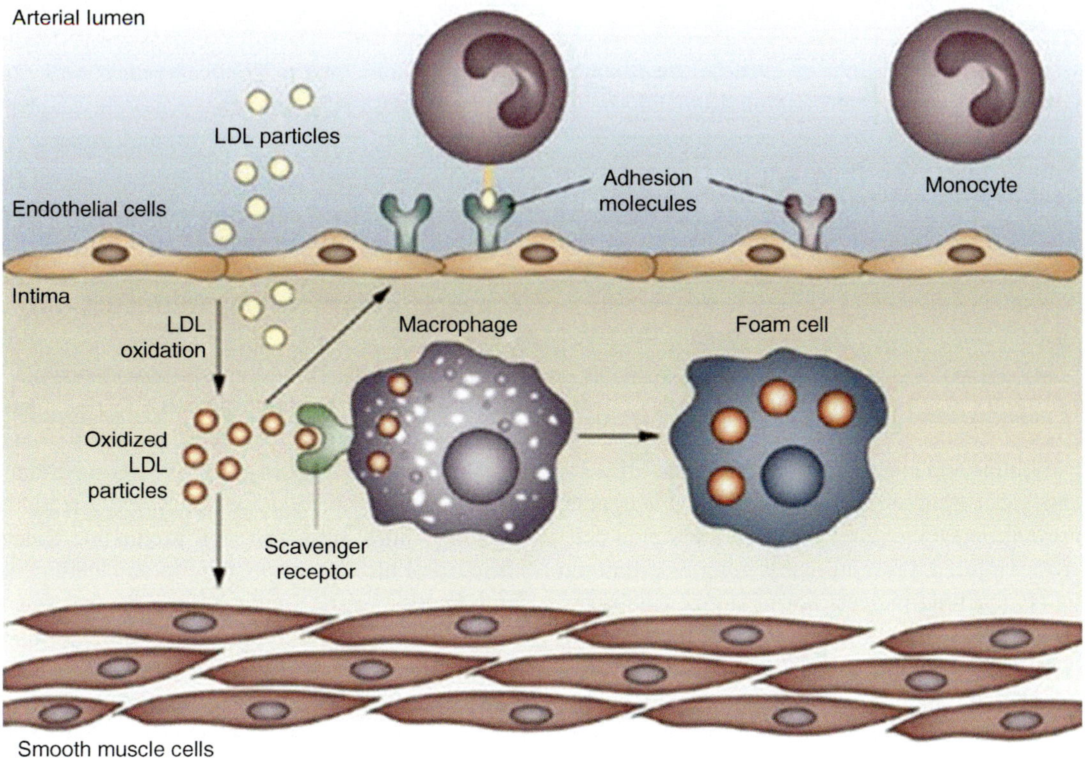


**Fig. 4.40** Foam cell formation [177, Fig. 4.6]. (Republished with permission from Springer Nature)

bringing more inflammatory products, adding to plaque formation. Plaque eventually becomes vascularized, and a cap forms over it as the plaque gets bigger and bigger. Not only is this a danger because it blocks the vessel and reduces blood flow to the area of the body the vessel supplies (an ischemic event[5]), but a cap may rupture, and if the blockage is near the heart, it may cause a heart attack (an infarct[1]). If the blockage is near the brain, it is known as a stroke. As with the brain or the heart, ischemia anywhere in the body may cause the death of cells being supplied by the blocked blood vessel, and this can cause disease (e.g., kidney disease leading to renal failure), including sepsis. Even though there is reduced flow downstream of the blockage, blood is still being forced through the narrowed lumen at very high rates, causing very high shear rates in the area, further damaging the endothelial cells and reducing nitric oxide production in that area, exacerbating the pro-atherosclerotic process. Often blood clots form on top of plaque (see Fig. 4.8). Nitric oxide is the body's own way of keeping the platelets from clumping together, making nitric oxide antithrombotic as well as anti-atherosclerotic and antioxidant. The result of nitric oxide on the platelets is replicated in other therapies typically recommended to patients that have atherosclerosis problems, often due to endothelial dysfunction. The other therapies include baby aspirin, fish oil, and blood thinners like Plavix.

[5]Ischemia is an inadequate blood supply to an area of the body. Infarct is an obstruction of a blood vessel, which can cause ischemia. If the blockage is near the heart, it may cause a heart attack. If the heart attack is due to ischemia, it is usually not as severe. If the heart attack is due to an infarct (called a myocardial infarct), it can lead to sudden (cardiac) death. If the ischemia or infarct is near the brain, it is known as a stroke. As with the brain or the heart, ischemia anywhere in the body may cause the death of cells being supplied by the blocked blood vessel, and this can cause disease, including sepsis.

However, prevention and maintaining wellness are preferred. The goal is to attack the plaque when it is first starting, or even before it starts, when the artery is healthy. This way, endothelial cells are preserved so that corrective therapy or mere maintenance is avoided. Again, to keep these cells healthy, high levels of nitric oxide are needed in the bloodstream; much like it is when people are young and active. Teach patients the benefits of exercise, because it is a great way to produce nitric oxide. Teaching patients the benefits of proper levels of L-arginine, whether it is from leafy greens or beetroot, or walnuts or pistachios, furthers health and wellness. Keeping the L-arginine and nitric oxide pathway (see Figs. 4.4 and 4.22) optimal is recommended. Of course, prevention also requires that the endothelial cells are not injured. Preventing this injury is promoted by (1) teaching patients not to smoke (including quitting if the patient is a smoker); (2) preventing type 2 diabetes or, if the patient has diabetes, treating it (more) aggressively; (3) reducing weight or correcting obesity or, better yet, teaching patients lifestyles to avoid obesity; (4) minimizing saturated fats in the diet; (5) reducing and avoiding stress, especially psychosocial stress, which is highly pro-inflammatory and significantly inhibits nitric oxide production; (6) reducing, and maintaining healthy levels of, cholesterol; and (7) exercising. Exercise is probably better than any medicine in increasing nitric oxide production and decreasing inflammation and stress. Anyone of these seven actions goes a long way to inhibit the atherosclerotic process.

From the previous chapter, fish oil is also a powerful anti-atherosclerotic. Fish oil also increases nitric oxide levels. By maintaining healthy endothelial cells with fish oil, the endothelial cells will, again, produce more nitric oxide. Therefore, indirectly, fish oil helps with nitric oxide production. In addition, nitric oxide will help the fish oil anti-inflammatory effect because nitric oxide has anti-inflammatory effects also. They all tie together. Add to fish oil the seven prevention actions from the last paragraph, and all of them together virtually guarantee the inhibition of the atherosclerotic process. The six-pronged Mind-Body Program, which is holistic, should be tailored to the patient's needs based on history, lifestyle, and genetic makeup. Having said that, it is still not possible to "fight genetics," and pharmaceuticals may still be required. If risk is a significant possibility, a physician will order tests to confirm and, if needed, augment the Mind-Body Program with prescription medication.

## The Anti-inflammatory Molecule

As mentioned above and in addition to being an anti-atherosclerotic agent, nitric oxide also interrupts inflammatory processes caused by foam cells (apoptosis, smooth muscle cells proliferation, and micro-blood vessel vascularization, bringing more inflammatory products). Since nitric oxide also interrupts the process leading to inflammation, nitric oxide is also known as an anti-inflammatory. Inflammation will, among other things, raise C-reactive protein (CRP) levels in the blood. CRP can be measured. CRP is produced in the liver. It is a chemical that is accepted as a marker of inflammation and even may cause inflammatory reactions. CRP is triggered by interleukins which can restrict the production of NOS. By restricting (binding to) NOS, inflammation (from CRP and other inflammatory substances) causes less NOS to be available to convert L-arginine to nitric oxide. An example of another inflammatory substance is the metabolite asymmetric dimethylarginine (ADMA; see Figs. 4.27 and 4.28), which has oxygen-like properties and therefore is itself inflammatory. ADMA can also bind NOS, exacerbating its inflammatory effects (see above).

Free radicals are also inflammatory substances. Free radicals have a free electron floating around in the outer ring of the molecule. This free electron is looking to steal another electron from nearby tissue so the free radical molecule becomes stable (see Fig. 2.18 and Chap. 2: "The Importance of Antioxidants"). In stealing an electron from tissue, it damages that tissue. Then that tissue becomes a free radical. As a new free radical, the damaged tissue looks to steal an electron from something else, and the cascade continues. As the cascade continues, all of the tissues involved are damaged, becoming free radicals, working as oxidants. This is not healthy. Nitric oxide neutralizes free radicals[6], not only for free radicals but also for many other pro-inflammatory processes and substances, including infection, tobacco, and diabetes.

Another amino acid, L-carnitine, is also an anti-inflammatory. L-Carnitine decreases nuclear factor-kB (NF-kB) production from scavenger cells, thereby decreasing inflammation. There are other anti-inflammatory substances and processes, many of them are included in the Mind-Body Wellness Program. Fish oils are anti-inflammatory. The cofactors, including coenzyme Q10 and alpha-lipoic acid, have anti-inflammatory (as well as antioxidant) effects. Again (it cannot be stressed enough), probably the best anti-inflammatory is exercise, recommended every day. Weight loss is a great way to combat inflammation. Keeping blood sugar and stress levels low, and an ideal weight, combats inflammation. Red wine, in moderation,[7] is a great anti-inflammatory agent, and it also relaxes. All of these substances and processes attack inflammation in different ways and associate with, or augment, the antioxidant effects of nitric oxide. This is why the Program should be taken as a whole and not in parts.

Not only in blood vessels, but throughout the body, a nitric oxide equilibrium, or balance, maintains a proper antioxidant milieu required to maintain health. As discussed, too much nitric oxide can cause the very problems nitric oxide is meant to prevent. Nitric oxide deficiency, or insufficiency, can be just as bad. For example, in blood vessels, nitric oxide balance reduces inflammation. Healthy endothelial cells produce appropriate amounts of nitric oxide which keep the vessel walls smooth. Smooth vessel walls keep blood flow smooth (known as laminar flow). Laminar flow minimizes friction between the blood and the endothelial cells, thereby preventing or reducing inflammation. Excess nitric oxide may cause too much vasodilation and blood pressure will be too low. Insufficient nitric oxide, resulting in turbulent flow and friction with the blood vessel walls, initiates inflammation intended to protect the vessels. If this condition is prolonged and the inflammation persists, the vessel lumen narrows, causing blood flow to become more turbulent; damaging endothelial cells, reducing the (local) production of nitric oxide, leading to vasoconstriction, which promotes more inflammation attracting more oxidants; causing more turbulence; and so on. Low nitric oxide promotes inflammation. Again, with more of nitric oxide's diverse properties (anti-inflammatory, antioxidant, and anti-atherosclerotic), an increase in nitric oxide levels aborts and possibly reverses this adverse cascade.

Nitric oxide insufficiency may result from L-arginine insufficiency and the other injurious substances as discussed above. Another process that leads to nitric oxide insufficiency results from uncoupled NOS. The enzyme, endothelial NOS (eNOS; see Fig. 4.34) or the other NOS enzymes (see Fig. 4.33) which are key to producing nitric oxide, may become uncoupled by substances like ADMA or other inflammatory products, including ROS and oxidized nitrogen compounds, causing more free radicals. Uncoupled NOS enzymes cannot produce nitric oxide. Uncoupled NOS enables L-arginine to be processed down other pathways, further reducing the production of nitric oxide. A nitric oxide deficient patient has a lot of vasoconstriction. The arteries are no longer big and healthy, and blood flow is restricted (at least due to vasoconstriction) and more turbulent. Again, the inflammation leads to plaque buildup and eventually atherosclerosis.

With plaque buildup, platelets are activated, and they accumulate in inflammatory sites, causing damage to the endothelial cells and reducing nitric oxide production. A pro-thrombotic environment is created by low nitric oxide and thromboses are formed and so forth. As atherosclerosis formation progresses and blood clots begin to form, morbidity and mortality (stroke and heart attack) risk increases significantly. Meanwhile, with low nitric oxide levels, local mitochondria go unchecked, adding to the inflammation through the production of more oxides (ROS). The additional ROS are not neutralized due to the lack of nitric oxide and lead to more oxidized

[6]True, once Nitric oxide give up an electron, it then becomes a free radical. However, Nitric Oxide has a very short half-life and breaks down quickly, so it little time if any to oxidize anything else.

[7]One to two 4 oz. glasses a day for men and one 4 oz. glass a day for women is recommended.

LDLs, and the downward spiral of inflammation leading to atherosclerosis continues. Insufficient nitric oxide levels also enable the endothelin-1 compound which is a really strong vasoconstrictor. Without proper amounts of nitric oxide, endothelin-1 goes unopposed and causes the arteries to constrict. Similar inflammatory processes occur elsewhere throughout the body, leading to more inflammation, promoting all of the risk factors that lead to reduced quality of life and reduced continuation of life (longevity).

Nitric oxide insufficiency and the resulting inflammation stimulate the sympathetic nervous system, leading to too much cortisol and adrenaline throughout the body, which exacerbates inflammation. Excessive sympathetic activity pulls the autonomic nervous system out of balance, promoting the risk factors (e.g., diabetes-induced heart disease, high cholesterol, high blood pressure, persistent obesity). As sympathetic activity, relative to parasympathetic activity, becomes excessive, it further suppresses the protective parasympathetics, and there are even more adrenaline-type compounds around. In the extreme, suppressed parasympathetic activity cannot prevent heart attack, stroke, aneurysms, sepsis, and other potentially life-ending events. Nitric oxide has a strong influence within the parasympathetic nervous system as the neurotransmitter of the family of parasympathetic neurons known as nitrergic neurons, adding to the well-known cholinergic family. Through its mediation of parasympathetic activity by nitrergic neurons, nitric oxide indirectly reduces sympathetic activity (balancing the ANS), reducing cortisol and adrenaline and helping to reduce inflammation and symptoms associated with sympathetic excess.

## Erectile Dysfunction

An example of nitric oxide insufficiency is erectile dysfunction (ED). ED also stands for endothelial dysfunction. They are synonymous. With this type of erectile dysfunction, endothelial cells are not working well, causing vessels to constrict and restricting blood flow to vital organs. As discussed, nitric oxide causes vasodilatation which brings more blood, in this case, promoting erection. Prescription phosphodiesterase inhibitors like Viagra, Levitra, and Cialis inhibit an enzyme known as phosphodiesterase type 5 (PDE5), which

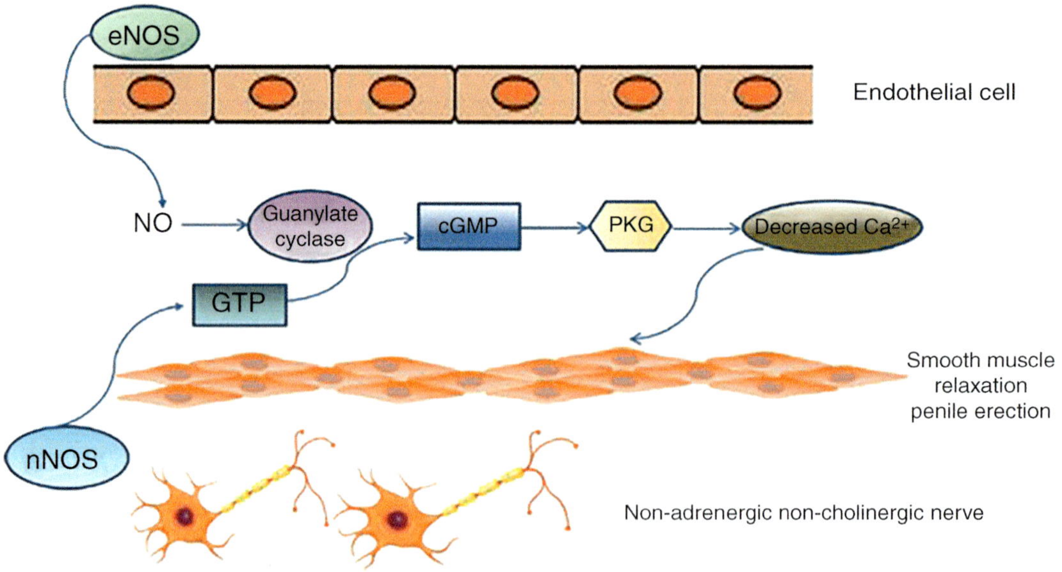


**Fig. 4.41** Role of NOS and nitric oxide in penile erection. The nNOS and iNOS regulate penile erection through nitric oxide/cGMP/PKG pathway. Abbreviations: eNOS endothelial nitric oxide synthase, nNOS neuronal nitric oxide synthase, NO nitric oxide, GTP guanosine triphosphate, cGMP cyclic guanosine monophosphate, PKG protein kinase G [50]. (Open Access, IntechOpen)

prevents phosphodiesterase from binding GMP, a secondary messenger that nitric oxide activates (see Fig. 4.41). This leads to vasodilation. L-Citrulline and L-arginine reduce ED by increasing nitric oxide through the NOS pathway, which is a different mechanism and is complimentary to PDE5 inhibition as well as to Viagra, Cialis, and other similar medicines. Some data has shown that L-citrulline, L-arginine, and PDE5 inhibitors work synergistically to reverse this type of ED [178].

In an indirect way, they turn on the same protein kinase through the nitric oxide mechanism and vasodilate along a different pathway than L-arginine. The two of them together are working by different mechanisms. L-Arginine is not as potent as the impotence drugs. However, there have been studies that show that when the two are used together, they seem to be better for ED. Some studies show that just using L-arginine in someone who has mild ED is all that is needed. Vaginal lubrication is the female corollary to male erection [179], and dysfunction due to endothelial dysfunction might be similarly affected by nitric oxide.

## An Antioxidant Molecule

As an anti-atherosclerotic agent, nitric oxide also interrupts oxidative processes by neutralizing ROS, other free radicals, superoxides, and peroxides (see Fig. 4.7). This interruption occurs regardless of how nitric oxide is produced. Whether through L-arginine and L-citrulline with NOS, or through nitrates such as beetroot, nitric oxide is extremely important as an antioxidant. As discussed, nitric oxide prevents the oxidation of LDLs, which is why it is also an anti-atherosclerotic (see Fig. 2.20). In a dose-dependent manner, it helps in limiting the oxidative processes involved in cancer (see Figs. 4.12 and 4.13). Figure 2.21 depicts nitric oxide's role in the antioxidant network within the body.

Nitric oxide, like oxygen, could potentially be damaging as well. Excess nitric oxide becomes an oxidant under the right circumstances ("right" as in "perfect storm"; see "The Dark Side of Nitric Oxide" section). Maintaining a proper antioxidant milieu prevents nitric oxide from becoming an oxidant, restoring proper levels of nitric oxide to act as its own antioxidant.

## Heart Failure

Heart failure (HF) with preserved ejection fraction accounts for at least half of the HF hospitalizations in North America. The symptoms of HF generally center around two main features: (1) dyspnea, likely reflective of pulmonary congestion, and (2) exertional intolerance, consistent with inefficient oxygen delivery or utilization. After an HF hospitalization, survival is poor. Despite the scope and seriousness of this problem, no targeted therapeutic intervention has been clearly identified to decrease the morbidity or mortality from this syndrome [180]. Nitric oxide plays a pivotal role in the maintenance of cardiovascular homeostasis. A reduction in the bioavailability of endogenous nitric oxide, manifested as a decrease in production or impaired signaling, is associated with many cardiovascular diseases including hypertension, atherosclerosis, stroke, as well as HF. Figure 4.42 is an example of nitric oxide insufficiency in HF. The role of ROS and decreased nitric oxide in HF with preserved ejection fraction is depicted in Fig. 4.42. ROS generated from comorbidity-induced systematic inflammation stimulate additional ROS production in the coronary endothelium, leading to a cascade involving depletion of nitric oxide and subsequent cardiac alterations that are manifested in HF with preserved ejection fraction [115, 116, 180–190].

As indicated in Fig. 4.42, there is substantial evidence that ROS, generated predominantly from NADPH oxidases (NOX), are responsible for the reduced nitric oxide bioavailability in vascular and cardiac pathologies. ROS can compromise nitric oxide function via a direct inactivation of nitric oxide, together with a reduction in nitric oxide synthesis and oxidation of its receptor, soluble guanylyl cyclase. Unfortunately, even with administration of nitrogen-based vasodilators to compensate for the ROS-mediated loss in nitric oxide bioactivity, their clinical utility is limited due to the development of tolerance and resistance and systemic hypotension. Efforts to directly scavenge ROS with antioxidants also has had limited clinical efficacy [186], primarily due to the broad spectrum of antioxidants and the general use of the less efficacious agents. This is why the antioxidants alpha-lipoic acid and CoQ10 are specifically recommended. These antioxidants are

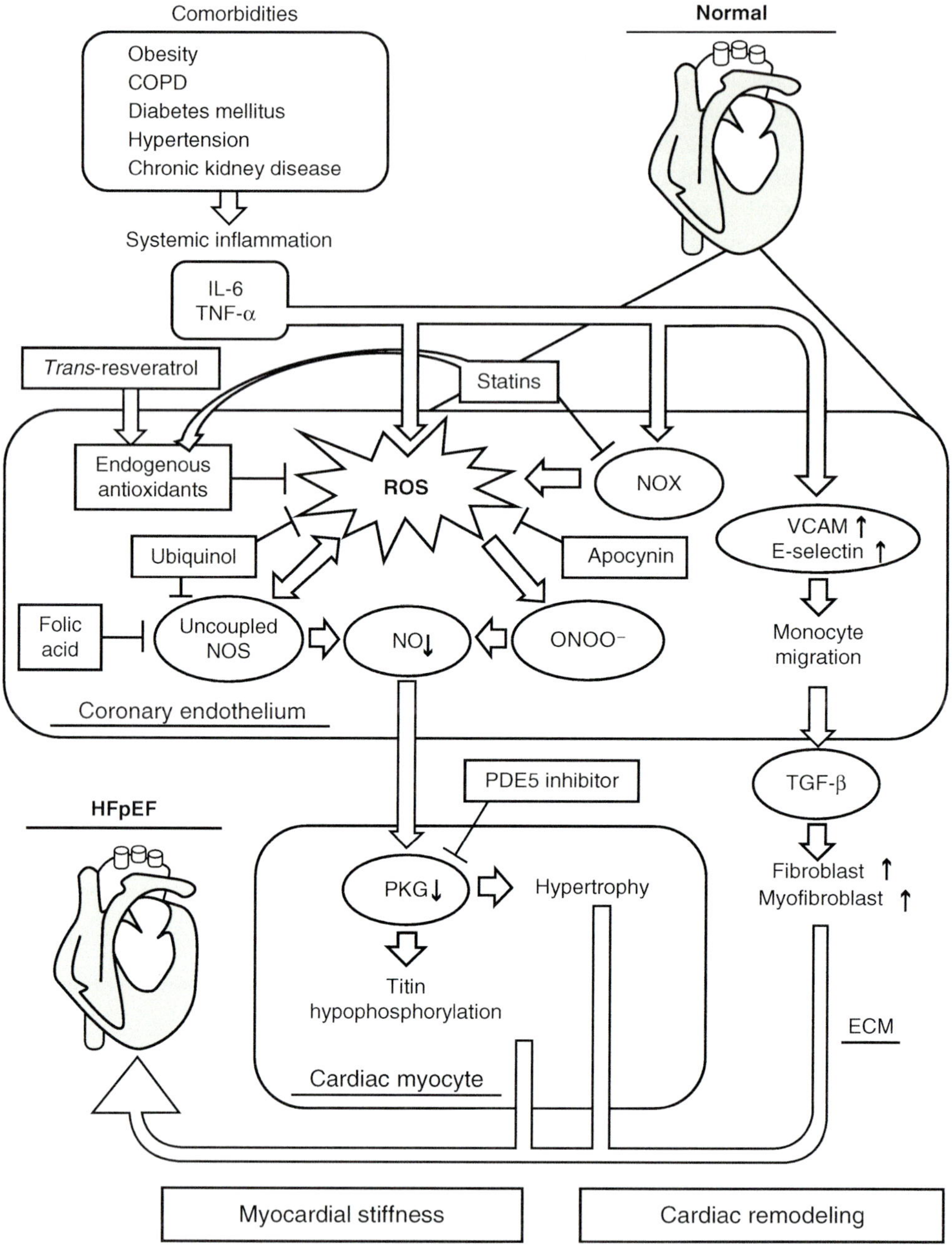


**Fig. 4.42** The role of reactive oxygen species (ROS) and nitric oxide (NO) in heart failure with preserved ejection fraction. ROS generated from comorbidity-induced systematic inflammation stimulate additional ROS production in the coronary endothelium, leading to a cascade involving depletion of NO and subsequent cardiac alterations that are manifested in heart failure with preserved ejection fraction. COPD chronic obstructive pulmonary disease, ECM extracellular matrix, HFpEF heart failure with preserved ejection fraction, IL-6 interleukin 6, NOS nitric oxide synthase, NOX NADPH oxidase, $ONOO^-$ peroxynitrite, PDE5 phosphodiesterase type 5, PKG cGMP-dependent protein kinase, TGF-β transforming growth factor-β, TNF-α tumor necrosis factor-α, VCAM vascular cell adhesion molecule [181]. (Republished with permission from the American Physiological Society)

not only known to directly scavenge ROS but also recycle the less efficacious agents (e.g., vitamins C and E), increasing the antioxidant milieu.

In the cardiovascular system, nitric oxide acts as the policeman of the circulation, or the blood vessel system of the body, by regulating hemostatic mechanisms of blood flow. It also acts as the firemen of the body by preventing white blood cells from adhering to blood vessel walls and causing inflammation (in essence, it is the fireman that prevents fires from occurring by preventing inflammation). As an antioxidant, it acts as a recycler, turning free radicals and reactive oxygen and nitrogen species into useable and safe elements. Nitric oxide can also be represented by the Red Cross ambulance and first aid crew, because it is a reparative gas. Lastly, by stopping clots from forming and causing traffic jams, it acts as the engineer and architect in the building of new roads and throughways (blood vessels) in the circulatory system.

## Nitric Oxide in the Nervous System

Heart failure and hypertension, diabetes mellitus, chronic renal failure, etc. are impacted by the health of the autonomic nervous system and its control of circulation and the associated organs or organ systems. Nitric oxide synthesized via neuronal NOS (nNOS) plays a significant role in regulation and modulation of autonomic (parasympathetic and sympathetic) control of circulation [187]. Sympathetic activation increases nitric oxide release [191]. As a result of autonomic neuropathy, excessive sympathetic activation may be secondary to abnormal parasympathetic activation, which may cause excessive nitric oxide levels. Heart failure and other pathological states are associated with diminished nNOS expression and blunted autonomic effects of nitric oxide in the central nervous system. From P&S monitoring, heart failure is associated with excessive sympathetic activation with depleted parasympathetic

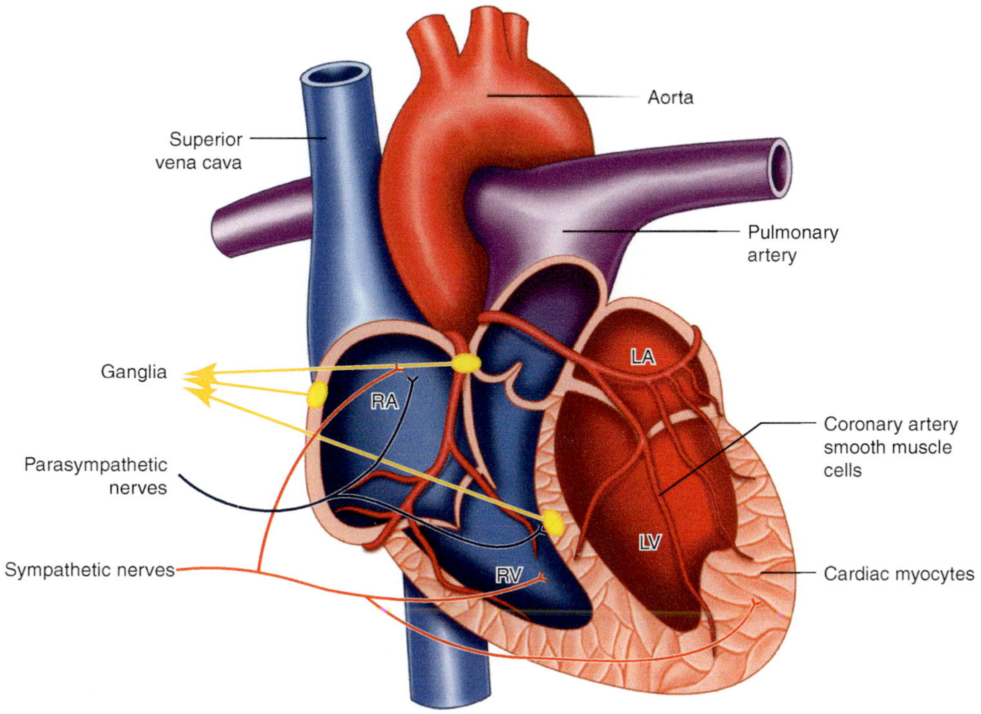


**Fig. 4.43** Distribution and structure of neuronal nitric oxide synthase (nNOS) protein in the heart. nNOS is expressed in cardiac myocytes, coronary artery smooth muscle cells, cardiac ganglia, and sympathetic and parasympathetic nerves [193]. (Republished with permission from John Wiley and Sons)

activation, the latter associated with cardiovascular autonomic neuropathy (CAN) [192].

nNOS is the major endogenous source of myocardial nitric oxide. Myocardial nitric oxide facilitates cardiac relaxation and modulates contraction (Fig. 4.43) [193]. In the healthy heart, it regulates intracellular $Ca^{++}$ signaling pathways and oxidative homeostasis and is upregulated in the early phases of pathology. nNOS plays pivotal roles in protecting the myocardium from increased oxidative stress, systolic and diastolic dysfunction, adverse structural remodeling, and arrhythmias in the failing heart. nNOS-derived nitric oxide is involved in early hypertension in the failing myocardium. The spatial compartmentation of nNOS, its diverse binding partners in the diseased heart, and regulation in response to pathological stress are possible explanations for the varied underlying mechanisms and functions. The dynamic localization and various mediating mechanisms of nNOS ensure that it is able to regulate functions effectively in the heart under stress [193]. nNOS is also the only NOS isoform that is expressed in intrinsic cardiac neurons from autonomic nerves and ganglions [194–196] and controls parasympathetic and sympathetic regulation of cardiac rhythm and contractility. nNOS is also expressed in human coronary artery smooth muscle cells [197] and maintains the basal blood flow [198].

Nitric oxide, derived from NOS, plays an important role in regulating sympathetic nerve activity [199]. It is well known that stress is mediated by sympathetic activity and excess sympathetic activity is associated with amplified stress responses and its corresponding symptoms, including hypertension and heart disease (e.g., heart failure) and cerebrovascular disease. Any reduction in stress [200], including an increase in parasympathetic activity [192], relieves excessive sympathetic activation and corresponding symptoms. nNOS is expressed throughout the central and peripheral nervous system. nNOS has a sympatho-inhibitory effect under physiological conditions by acting on different sites of the nervous system, including the paraventricular nucleus, the nucleus of the solitary tract, the rostral ventrolateral medulla, the carotid body, and the nerves in the kidney. The nucleus of the solitary tract, the rostral ventrolateral medulla, and the carotid body are all parasympathetic nuclei. nNOS is sympatho-inhibitory in a range of diseases, including chronic heart failure, chronic renal failure, hypertension, and diabetes. nNOS is believed to mediate sympatho-inhibitory effects induced by a range of signaling pathways, including those promoted by angiotensin-converting enzyme 2 overexpression, statin therapy, angiotensin II type 1 receptor blockers, exercise training, tumor necrosis factor-α blockade, superoxide dismutase mimetics, and estrogen replacement therapy [199]. Increases in nNOS can increase sympatho-inhibitory (gamma-aminobutyric acid) activity and decrease sympatho-excitatory (angiotensin II signaling and glutamate) activity. nNOS may have sympatho-excitatory effects in some circumstances, such as chronic heart failure induced by prolonged high salt treatment [199].

To maintain cardiovascular homeostasis in non-pathological conditions, discrete neural networks using specified signaling mechanisms at both cellular and molecular levels are required. In heart failure, the cell signaling protein partners CAPON[8] and PIN[9] decrease the bioavailability of nitric oxide by inhibiting nNOS activity, leading to the removal of tonic neuronal inhibition [201]. Following a myocardial infarction, proinflammatory cytokines in the paraventricular nucleus, and the subsequent generation of ROS via angiotensin II activation of the angiotensin II type 1 receptor, increase sympathetic excitation (Fig. 4.44). A pathological feature of heart failure is abnormal (excessive) control of the sympathetic nervous system. The paraventricular nucleus (PVN) of the hypothalamus is one of the most important central sites involved in regulating sympathetic tone and is, in part, responsible for the dysregulation of the sympathetic nervous system evident in heart failure.

[8]CAPON is an nNOS-associated protein which is highly enriched in the brain and has numerous co-localizations with nNOS. CAPON interacts with the nNOS PDZ domain through its C-terminus. CAPON competes with PSD95 for interaction with nNOS, and overexpression of CAPON results in a loss of PSD95/nNOS complexes in transfected cells. CAPON may influence nNOS by regulating its ability to associate with PSD95/NMDA receptor complexes.

[9]PIN is a protein inhibitor of nNOS known to dissociate nNOS dimers into monomers.

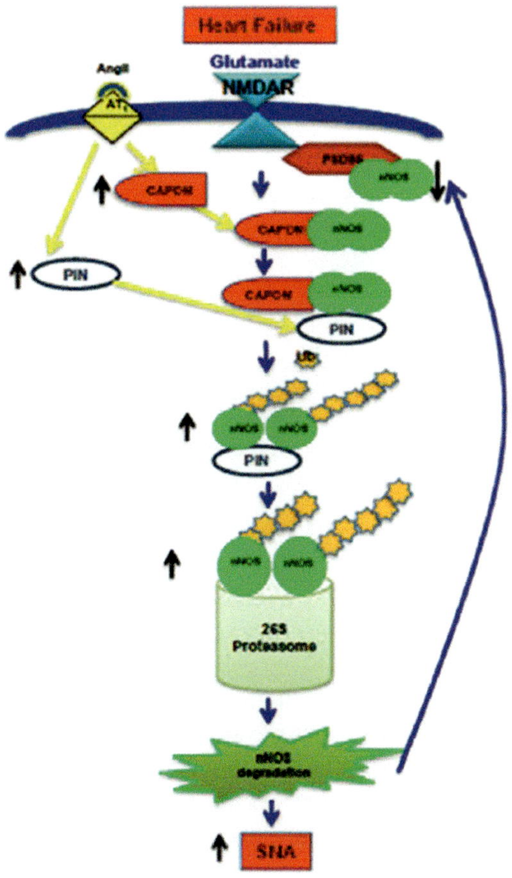


**Fig. 4.44** Posttranslational modification of neuronal nitric oxide synthase (nNOS) alters the regulation of the paraventricular nucleus (PVN) in heart failure. Overactivation of the angiotensin II type 1 receptor (AT1R) leads to overexpression of CAPON and PIN. CAPON and PIN interfere with nNOS activation, reducing nitric oxide (NO) production in the PVN and causing an increase in sympathetic nerve activity (SNA) [201, Fig. 2A]. (Republished with permission from John Wiley and Sons)

Generation of sympathetic tone in response to fluctuations in cardiovascular regulation uses discrete anatomical pathways and neurochemical modulators (Fig. 4.45). Direct and indirect projections from the PVN pre-autonomic neurons innervate the sympathetic preganglionic neurons in the spinal cord, which in turn innervate sympathetic ganglia that give rise to the sympathetic nerves. Pre-autonomic neurons of the PVN themselves receive an afferent input arising from the nucleus tractus solitarius (NTS, parasympathetic inputs), and visceral sensory receptors convey cardiovascular fluctuations to the NTS. The PVN contains excitatory and inhibitory neurons, whose balance determines the sympathetic tone.

In non-pathological conditions, the tonic inhibition of the PVN pre-autonomic neurons is mediated by GABA- and nitric oxide-releasing neurons. In heart failure, the pre-autonomic neurons are disinhibited by the actions of the excitatory neurotransmitters glutamate and angiotensin II, leading to increased sympathetic activity. A key feature of the disinhibition is a reduction in the bioavailability of nitric oxide as a consequence of disrupted CAPON and PIN signaling mechanisms within the neuron. Another critical feature that contributes to increased neuronal excitation within the PVN is the production of pro-inflammatory cytokines immediately following a myocardial infarction, the activation of the angiotensin II type 1 receptor, and the production of ROS [201].

Hypertension is a prevalent condition worldwide and is the key risk factor for fatal cardiovascular complications, including heart failure as well as stroke and sudden cardiac death. Reduced bioavailability of nitric oxide in the endothelium is an important precursor for impaired vasodilation and hypertension. In the heart, nitric oxide deficiency deteriorates the adverse consequences of pressure overload and causes cardiac hypertrophy, fibrosis, and myocardial infarction which lead to fatal heart failure and sudden cardiac death (Fig. 4.46). Recent consensus is that both eNOS and nNOS are the constitutive sources of nitric oxide in the myocardium. Between the two, nNOS is the predominant isoform of NOS that controls intracellular $Ca^{++}$ homeostasis, myocyte contraction, relaxation, and signaling pathways, including nitrous-redox balance [187]. Notably, recent research indicates that cardiac eNOS protein is reduced, but nNOS protein expression and activity are increased in hypertension. Furthermore, nNOS is induced by the interplay between angiotensin II type 1 receptors and angiotensin II type 2 receptors, as mediated by NADPH oxidase and ROS-dependent eNOS activity in cardiac myocytes. nNOS, in turn, protects the heart from abnormal myocardial relaxation in hypertension [188].

Inhaled nitrite, as a source of nitric oxide, is safe in pulmonary hypertension patients and has

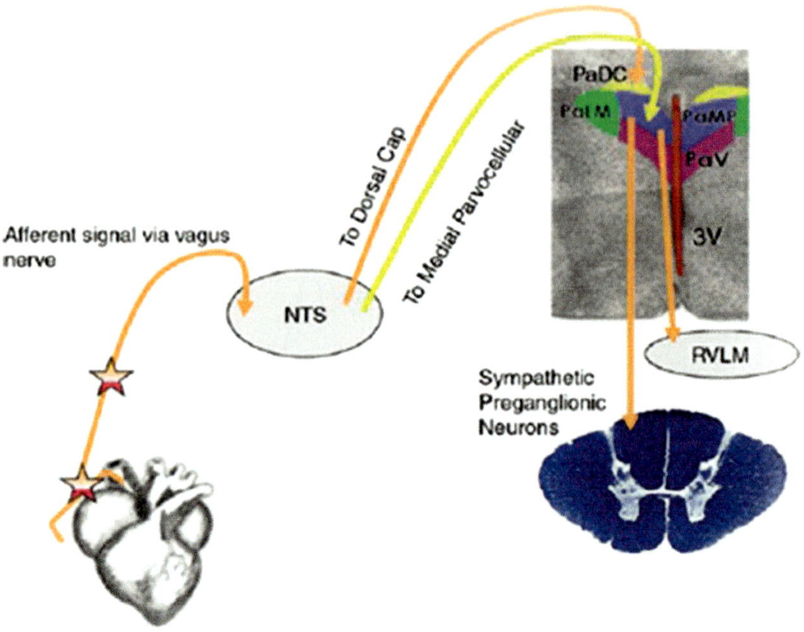


**Fig. 4.45** Schematic diagrams to show the components of the volume reflex arc. Volume receptors in the heart provide the vagal (parasympathetic) afferent signals to the nucleus tractus solitarius (NTS), which are then conducted to the paraventricular nucleus (PVN). Direct and indirect efferent projections influence sympathetic outflow at the level of the sympathetic preganglionic neurons [405, Fig. 1A]. (Republished with permission from John Wiley and Sons)

been shown to be efficacious in pulmonary hypertensive heart failure patients with preserved ejection fraction primarily via improvements in left and right ventricular filling pressures and pulmonary artery compliance due to increased nitric oxide production [189]. In general, increased nitric oxide may relieve symptoms of heart failure and may help to slow its progression.

Again, heart failure is highlighted by symptom-limited exercise capacity and recurrent hospitalizations. Despite substantial advances in pharmacopeia, heart failure with reduced ejection fraction still requires additional therapeutic strategies to improve quality of life. Currently, iron deficiency is overwhelmingly recognized in over 30–50% of patients with stable chronic heart failure, which worsens prognosis. The established pathophysiological mechanisms of progressive heart failure may be intertwined with increasingly reduced myocardial iron, wherein one begets the other. Most importantly, iron deficiency constitutes a novel target for symptom relief in carefully selected patients. In this regard, intravenous iron may be a safe and efficacious intervention, potentially reducing heart failure hospitalizations (see Fig. 4.47) [202].

It may be hypothesized that lower citric acid cycle activity impairs the normal bioenergetics in the cardiomyocytes in heart failure. This is similar to the phenomenon observed in myocytes of exercising skeletal muscles. Abnormal bioenergetics could lead to impaired maximal exercise capacity in iron-deficient heart failure patients with reduced ejection fraction due to limited left ventricular contractile reserve (i.e., an inability to increase cardiac output with exercise). For instance, in these patients, decreasing ROS scavenging enzymes may intensify local oxidative stress in myocardial iron deficiency) with ensuing myocardial damage (see Fig. 4.47) [202].

Nitric oxide plays multiple roles in the entire nervous system (not just the P&S nervous systems), as well as in glial regulated pathways. Nitric oxide roles are both physiologic and pathologic. Pathologic roles, including neuroinflammation and neurodegenerative diseases, will be discussed in the "Dark Side of Nitric Oxide" section later. Under physiological conditions, nitric oxide (1) contributes to regulating proliferation, survival, and differentiation of neurons; (2) is involved in synaptic activity, neural plasticity, and cognitive function (i.e., memory); (3) exerts long-lasting effects through regulation of transcription factors and modulation of gene expression; and (4) promotes better cerebral circulation, thereby improving "brain fog" symp-

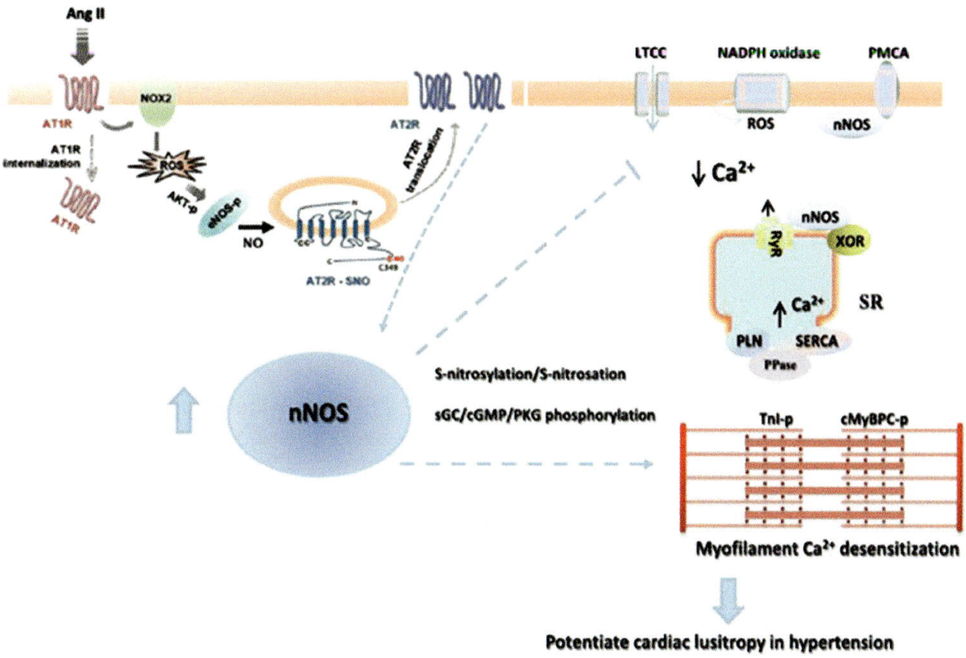


**Fig. 4.46** Schematic diagram of nNOS upregulation by angiotensin II (Ang II) in cardiac myocytes and the potential target proteins. Mechanism of regulation in cardiac myocytes from hypertension (left). Ang II stimulates AT1R and NADPH oxidase in cardiac myocytes. AT1R and intracellular ROS activate Akt and phosphorylate endogenous eNOS to produce nitric oxide (NO). Endothelial nitric oxide synthase (eNOS) and NO-dependent S-nitrosylation of AT2R lead to the translocation of AT2R to the plasma membrane and induces neural NOS (nNOS) protein and increases NO production. In hypertension, cardiac nNOS is upregulated and facilitates myocyte relaxation. nNOS reduces $Ca^{++}$ influx via LTCC and promotes $Ca^{++}$ reuptake via SERCA through PLN phosphorylation (secondary to PPase-dependent PKA phosphorylation) in healthy hearts. In hypertension, nNOS inhibits LTCC and phosphorylates cMBP-C Ser273 and cTnI Ser23/Ser24 via cGMP-/PKG-dependent mechanism. As a result, myofilament $Ca^{++}$ sensitivity is reduced which accounts for nNOS-dependent positive lusitropy (myocardial relaxation or systolic function) in hypertension [193]. (Republished with permission from John Wiley and Sons)

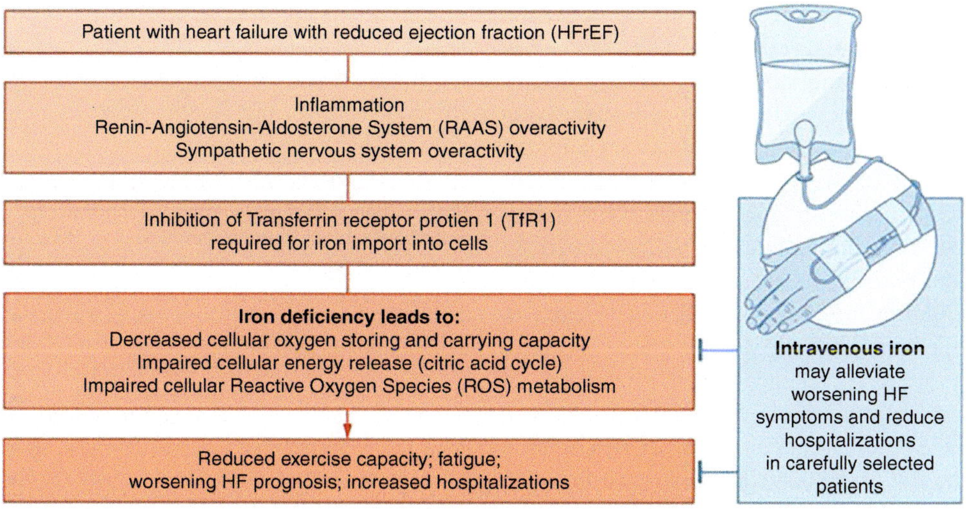


**Fig. 4.47** Involvement of iron deficiency in heart failure patients with reduced ejection fraction due to limited left ventricular contractile reserve [202]. (Republished with permission from Elsevier)

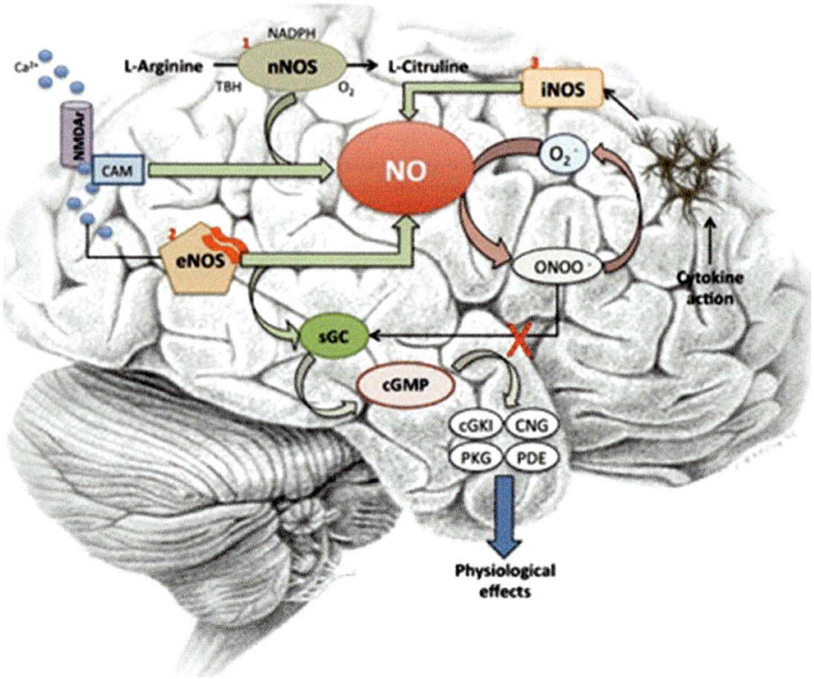


**Fig. 4.48** Nitric oxide is a primary messenger in the brain's inflammation and immune responses [1983, Fig. 24.2]. (Open Access, Frontiers in Cellular Neuroscience)

toms in individuals with autonomic dysfunction. Interestingly, nitric oxide may help balance the parasympathetic and sympathetic branches of the autonomic nervous system. It increases vagal tone, which slows heart rate, and decreases sympathetic tone, which decreases blood pressure. This is another way (in addition to the vascular effects) that nitric oxide is cardioprotective.

Inflammation in the brain is different than in the rest of the body. Throughout the body, the inflammation that accompanies acute injury has dual functions: antibacterial action and repair. Antibacterial functions protect damaged tissue from infection, and repair functions are initiated to aid in the recovery of damaged tissue. Brain injury is different in two respects. First, many cases of brain injury are not accompanied by infection: there is no chance of pathogens (infection) entering the brain in ischemia or even in traumatic injury, if the skull is intact. Second, neurons are rarely regenerated once damaged. To this end, it seems as if the brain has its own immune system, separate, and perhaps unique from the rest of the body. It is separated from the body by the blood-brain barrier. In fact, evidence indicates that immune responses in the brain reduce immune activity in the rest of the body and, if persistent, lead to secondary diseases such as pneumonia, which can lead to death [203].

A primary messenger in the brain's inflammation and immune response is nitric oxide (Fig. 4.48). There are parasympathetic nerves that respond to nitric oxide, called "nitrergic," that are now known to accompany the well-known cholinergic class of nerves. Throughout the body, the nitrergic class of nerves effect cerebral vasodilation[10] (Fig. 4.49),

[10]Cerebral vasodilation is the vasodilation of the vessels in the meninges and in the circle of Willis. In the brain itself, there are no blood vessels, and, normally, there is no blood. Blood carries different salts, also known as electrolytes. The introduction of blood into the brain will change the electrical environment of that area of the brain and cause a change in brain patterns and damage cells (which will change brain patterns permanently). The meninges are the protective tissues surrounding the brain. They help to maintain proper pressures within the brain and contain the cerebral spinal fluid which bathes the brain in the nutrients it needs to function. The circle of Willis is the blood vessels supplying "blood to the brain." In actuality, they bring blood close to the brain so that the nutrients needed may diffuse into the cerebral spinal fluid. Also, the brain has "sensors" that monitor the blood so that the brain "knows" what is needed by the rest of the body, as it works to help maintain homeostasis. Cerebral vasodilation helps to facilitate the delivery of nutrients to the brain and allows the meninges to be more flexible, thereby relieving pressure in the brain.

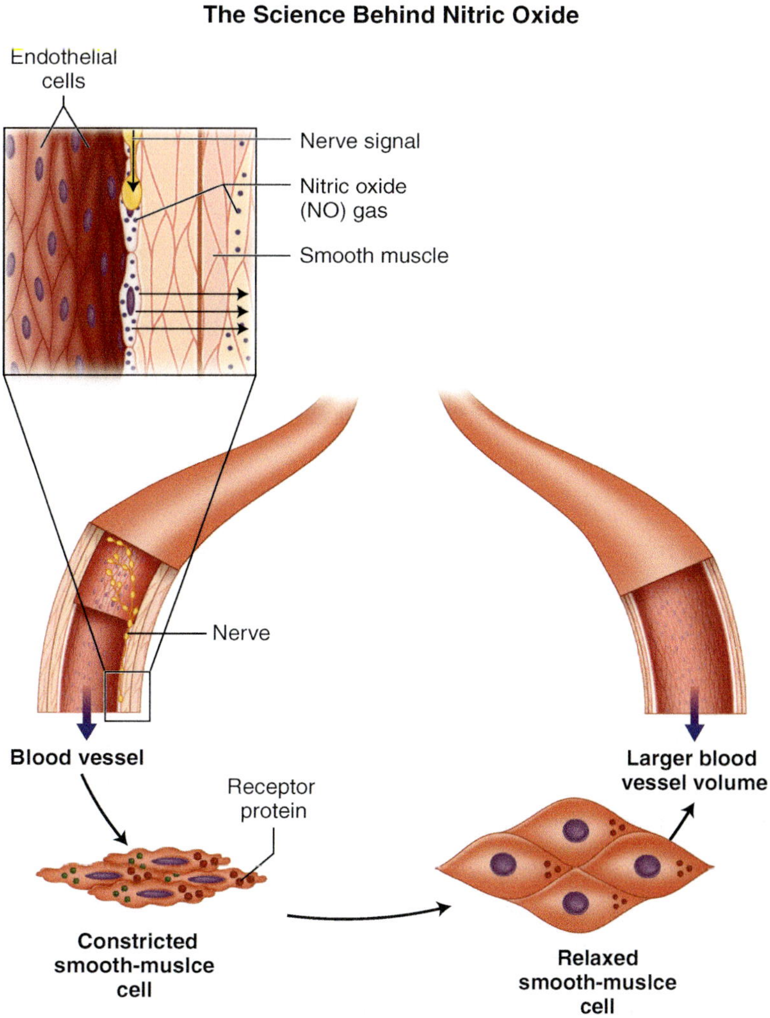


**Fig. 4.49** Nitrergic parasympathetic nerves mediate cerebral vasoconstriction. (Springer Nature, Garth Haller, 2018)

penile erection, and relaxation of sphincters. Normally, nitric oxide via parasympathetic activation causes vasodilation of cerebral vasculature. Normally, nitric oxide from (1) eNOS or (2) oxidative stress in the rostral ventrolateral medulla (RVLM) in the brain stem helps regulate sympathetic activity. The RVLM is an autonomic vasomotor center. Normally, eNOS in the RVLM inhibits sympathetic activity via an increase in γ-aminobutyric acid (GABA). Angiotensin II type 1 receptor (AT1R)-induced oxidative stress in the RVLM affects sympathetic excitation. Normally, increases in AT1R-induced oxidative stress or decreases in nitric oxide in the RVLM cause sympathetic excitation.

In the brain, nitric oxide can stimulate both pro- and anti-inflammatory cytokines, depending on the conditions under which the nitric oxide is produced (see Fig. 4.50) [204]. Anti-inflammatory nitric oxide activity increases collateral blood flow and decreases neuronal apoptosis and platelet aggregation, all leading to neuroprotection. Pro-inflammatory nitric oxide activity will be discussed in the "Dark Side of Nitric Oxide" section later.

Interleukins are proteins that regulate immune and inflammatory responses. Anti-inflammatory cytokines are IL-10 and transforming growth factor-β (TGF-β). Interleukins are produced by leukocytes (white blood cells) for regulating immune responses. Lymphokines are cytokines that are produced by lymphocytes (a type of small white blood cell). Lymphokines send signals out to other cells, such as macrophages (a type of large white blood cell) and other lympho-

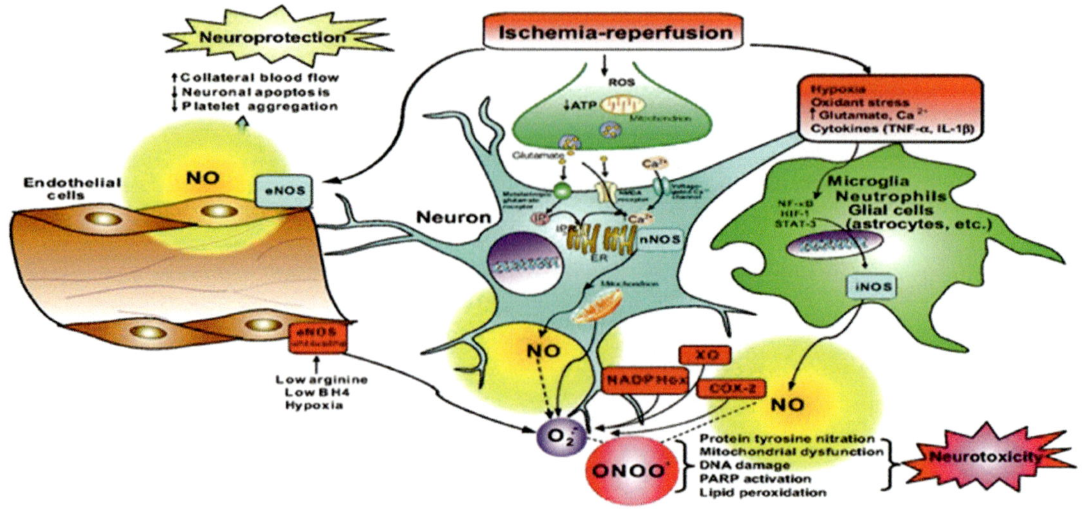


**Fig. 4.50** Pro- and anti-inflammatory roles of nitric oxide. Brain ischemia and reperfusion lead to transient stimulation of the activity of eNOS, resulting in brief increases in endothelial nitric oxide generation, associated with neuroprotective actions in stroke. In parallel, ischemic energy depletion and oxidant (ROS) production trigger the release of glutamate, which results in neuronal calcium overload from extracellular (activation of calcium channels) and intracellular (phosphoinositol-3-kinase-endoplasmic reticulum signaling) sources. Calcium overload results in prolonged synthesis of nitric oxide, due to stimulated activity of the neuronal isoform of NOS (nNOS). Enhanced nitric oxide generation also depends on the induced expression of inducible NOS (iNOS) in various types of reactive inflammatory cells, upon the activation of several cell signaling pathways (HIF-1, STAT3, and NF-κB) in response to hypoxia, cytokines, oxidants, and glutamate. During the same period of time, superoxide production is enhanced due to the uncoupling of eNOS, mitochondrial dysfunction, and the stimulated activity of NADPH oxidase, xanthine oxidase, and cyclooxygnease-2 (COX-2). Formation of peroxynitrite ($ONOO^-$) is then markedly favored, damaging lipids, proteins, and DNA and triggering the activation of poly(ADP-ribose) polymerase (PARP), which all contribute significantly to neurotoxicity [408, Fig. 15]. (Republished with permission from the American Physiological Society)

cytes, recruiting them to help fight the infection. Cytokines are a large group of proteins, peptides, or glycoproteins that are secreted by specific cells of the immune system. They are a category of signaling molecules that mediate and regulate immunity, inflammation, and hematopoiesis (the production of blood cells and platelets, which occurs in the bone marrow). They are produced by a broad range of cells, including immune cells like macrophages, B lymphocytes, T lymphocytes, and mast cells, as well as endothelial cells, fibroblasts, and various stromal cells. A given cytokine is produced by more than one type of cell. Nitric oxide from the endothelial cells and others helps regulate immune responses.

The N-methyl-D-aspartate (NMDA) receptor, a specific type of glutamate receptor, is very important for controlling synaptic plasticity and learning and memory function. As a result, it is located throughout the brain in almost every brain cell. In neurons with NMDA receptors that mediate pain, pleasure, and emotional responses and behaviors, nitric oxide acts as a retrograde messenger. The activation of the guanylyl cyclase and the resulting elevation of cGMP is a major downstream signal of nitric oxide in neurons (see Fig. 4.51) [205]. For the pain, pleasure, and emotional responses, such as those that lead to alcoholism (ETOH, in the Fig. 4.51), nNOS is blocked, and insufficient levels of nitric oxide are produced, causing disinhibition of learned responses that avoid harmful excesses, such as excess consumption of alcohol, which would reinforce addictive behaviors.

Nitrergic parasympathetic neurons work to regulate the vascular tone of the large cerebral arteries (Fig. 4.52). Nicotine activates presynaptic receptors on sympathetic nerves, causing release of norepinephrine, which then activates the presynaptic β2-adrenoceptors located on neighboring nitrergic, parasympathetic nerves, causing nitric oxide release from the nitrergic nerve terminals. Nitric oxide activates guanylate

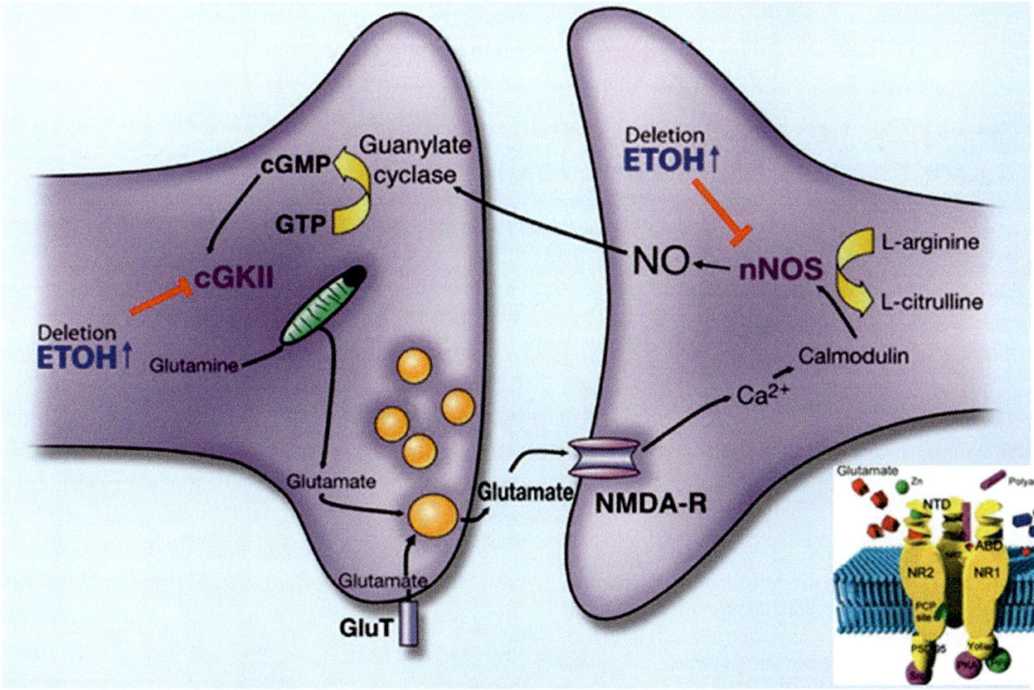


**Fig. 4.51** nNOS/nitric oxide (NO)/cGMP/cGMP-dependent protein kinase II (cGKII) signaling is involved in mediating alcohol reinforcement. The stimulation of NMDA receptors (insert) leads to $Ca^{++}$ influx, and binding of $Ca^{++}$ to calmodulin activates nNOS, which produces nitric oxide from arginine. Nitric oxide acts as a retrograde messenger. The activation of the guanylyl cyclase and the resulting elevation of cGMP are major downstream signals of nitric oxide in neurons. In neurons, the target of cGMP is cGKII. Genetic deletion or blockade of nNOS and cGKII, respectively, leads to enhanced alcohol (ETOH) self-administration or disinhibition of learned responses or behaviors (Main: [409], Fig. 7. Insert: [1984], Fig. 3; Adapted from Shutterstock Royalty-free stock illustration ID: 390561898, by Juan Gaertner. Main and insert illustrations republished with permission from the American Physiological Society)

cyclase in the smooth muscle cell to increase the synthesis of cGMP from GTP and relaxes the smooth muscle. Nitric oxide is synthesized from L-arginine in the presence of NOS. The by-product of nitric oxide synthesis, L-citrulline, is actively recycled to L-arginine [206]. The net result is depicted in Fig. 4.49.

Resting parasympathetic activation is known to stimulate microglia (see insert). Microglia are a type of glial cell located throughout the brain and spinal cord and account for 10–15% of all cells found within the brain. As the resident macrophage cells, they act as the first and main form of active immune defense in the central nervous system (CNS) [207]. Microglia are known to be mobilized with brain injury. The parasympathetics are activated when organs require protection and upregulate the immune system. For example, by the third concussion, a persistent dynamic parasympathetic excess (PE) is typically demonstrated.

Microglia
(stained blue)

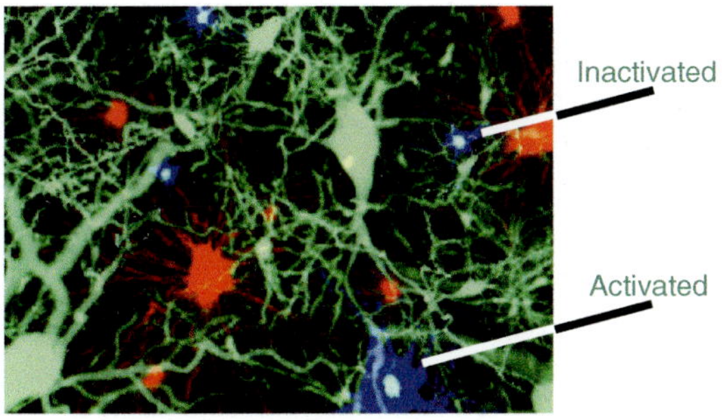


Neurons – green, Astrocytes - red

PE is only measured by P&S monitoring technology. Evidence indicates that with brain injury, the parasympathetics shift immune priority to the brain, leaving other organs, i.e., the lungs, susceptible to infections, leading to (for example) pneumonia and high risk of death.

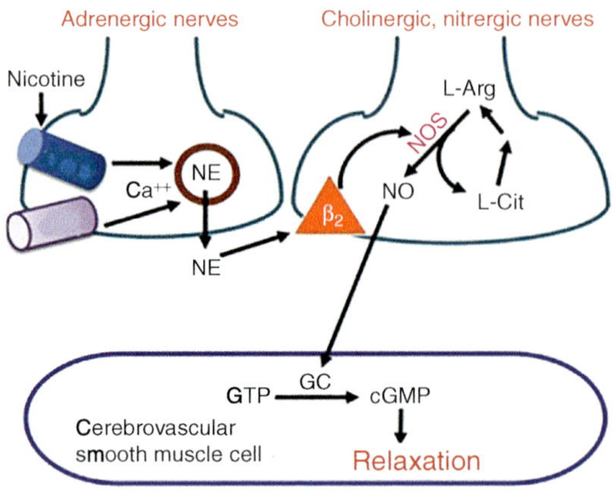


**Fig. 4.52** An axo-axonal interaction between adrenergic and nitrergic nerves in the regulation of the tone of the large cerebral arteries. Nicotine activates presynaptic receptors on sympathetic nerves, causing release of norepinephrine (NE), which then activates the presynaptic β2-adrenoceptors located on neighboring nitrergic nerves, causing nitric oxide release from the nitrergic nerve terminals. Nitric oxide activates guanylate cyclase (GC) in the smooth muscle cell to increase the synthesis of cGMP from GTP and relaxes the smooth muscle. Nitric oxide is synthesized from L-arginine (L-Arg) in the presence of NOS. The by-product of nitric oxide synthesis, L-citrulline (L-Cit), is actively recycled to L-Arg [206, Fig. 6]. (Open Access, PLoS One)

Sympathetic activation promotes inflammation. In the acute stage (short term), this helps to protect and heal. Excessive sympathetic activation (SE) leads to disorder and disease. Chronic (resting) sympathetic activation due to stressful lifestyles is well known to lead to disorder and disease. Dynamic PE[11] promotes SE. The parasympathetics set the threshold around which the sympathetics react. Dynamic PE is an abnormal autonomic response to stress, causing an excessive stress reaction (secondary SE). It is possible that nitric oxide is the parasympathetic agent mediating microglial proliferation. Therefore, the possible proliferative pathway is PE leads to SE, which leads to chronic inflammation and then to excess microglia proliferation. This causes continued brain injury and diseases of the brain, including ADHD, Alzheimer's, Parkinson's, and MS.

## The Dark Side of Nitric Oxide

Earlier in this chapter, the nitric oxide paradox[12] was introduced. This paradox is an example of the possible effects of an overproduction of nitric oxide (e.g., during prolonged illness or prolonged inflammation; see Fig. 4.53), the "dark side of nitric oxide." The dark side of nitric oxide is caused by its immediate environment. However, there are global differences inside and outside the blood-brain barrier, as well. Either place, nitric oxide, itself, is a free radical. As discussed above, outside the blood-brain barrier, nitric oxide normally facilitates the relaxation of vascular smooth muscles, promoting proper blood flow and blood pressure throughout the body. Inside the blood-brain barrier, nitric oxide normally facilitates synaptic activity, neural plasticity, memory, and more (see above). However, sometimes it does not.

Sometimes, outside the blood-brain barrier, excess nitric oxide is produced. If it is produced in an environment with excess $Ca^{++}$, nitric oxide remains a free radical. If there is an excess of free radicals or an excess of oxygen in an environment, nitric oxide can combine with them as a super oxide radical. In the presence of excess oxygen, nitric oxide can go down an alternate pathway and form a peroxide nitrate compound which can damage cells. As a free radical, it contributes to the production of ROS and promotes the opposite of its normal physiologic activity, leading to inflammation, cell death, and oxidized LDL (which, as discussed above, can become atherosclerosis). Another "dark side" example of

[11]Dynamic PE is an abnormal, "hidden" parasympathetic excess. It is hidden in a sympathetic challenge. Normally with a sympathetic challenge, the parasympathetics first decrease then the sympathetics react, increase. With a dynamic PE, the parasympathetics instead increase abnormally. This forces a (secondary) sympathetic excess (SE), causing abnormal increases in heart rate, blood pressure, and cardiac output, as well as anxiety and exaggerated pain and stress responses. The secondary SE also often masks the (primary) PE. If the SE responses are treated, often the PE is exacerbated. Rather treat the PE [192], then the SE is relieved, and then the results of SE are eventually relieved.

[12]The L-arginine-ADMA competition: while there is typically plenty of L-arginine (the rate limiter in the production of nitric oxide) in the cell, ADMA is promoted under conditions of too much nitric oxide (during prolonged illness or prolonged inflammation).

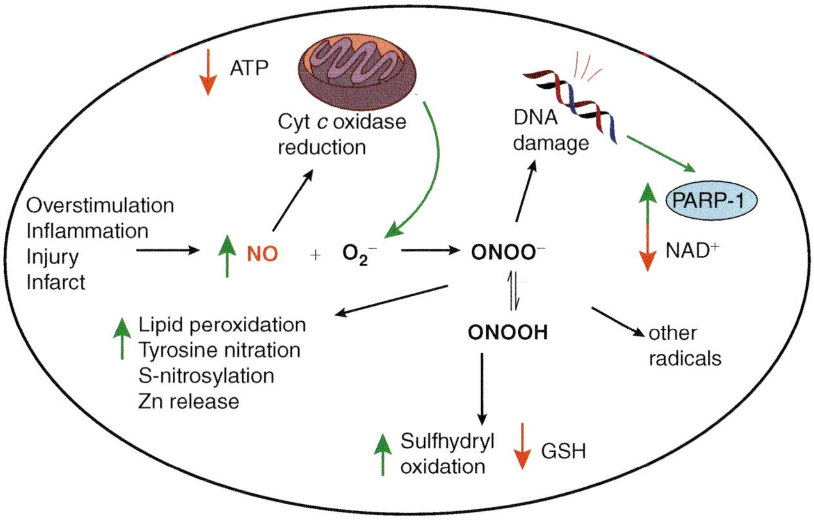


**Fig. 4.53** Nitric oxide overproduction. There are two dysfunctional nitric oxide signaling and damage mechanisms following inflammation, infarct, or NMDA receptor overstimulation: decreased ATP (energy) production due to mitochondrial dysfunction and increased inflammation due to oxidative stress [208]. (Republished with permission from Royal Society of Chemistry)

nitric oxide outside the brain is when excess nitric oxide combines with oxygen to produce pernitrate. Pernitrate is also a potent-free radical that causes tissue and cell damage.

In the brain, pathologic roles of nitric oxide include neuro-inflammation and neurodegenerative diseases. A pro-inflammatory nitric oxide activity example is depicted in Fig. 4.50 (above) which demonstrates two conditions: (1) low L-arginine or low BH4 and (2) excess $Ca^{++}$. Low L-arginine or BH4 enables eNOS (in the endothelial cell) to produce free radicals, rather than stable nitric oxide. Excess $Ca^{++}$ causes excessive nitric oxide production by both (1) nNOS (in the neuron), which may add to the free radical population, and (2) iNOS in microglial cells, which both add to the free radical population and the release of pro-inflammatory cytokines (interleukin-1, interleukin-6, tumor necrosis factor). The latter may cause autoimmune reactions or induce mitochondrial dysfunction [209] in the brain, which can lead to depression, autism, poor memory, Alzheimer's disease, and multiple sclerosis. While maintaining normal $Ca^{++}$ is the direct method for preventing these poor outcomes, lower $Ca^{++}$ to do so may not be safe, especially with aging and chronic disease and the associated difficulty of knowing the correct balance for $Ca^{++}$. It may be safer in these patients to promote, establish, and maintain as high an antioxidant-oxidant ratio as possible.

Under normal conditions, nitric oxide in the brain stimulates microglial activation for regular "housekeeping" activities (overall brain maintenance). The CNS is not usually accessed directly by pathogenic factors in the body's circulation due to a series of endothelial cells known as the blood-brain barrier, which prevents most infections from reaching the vulnerable nervous tissue. In the case where infectious agents are directly introduced to the brain, microglial cells must react quickly to decrease inflammation and destroy the infectious agents before they damage the sensitive neural tissue. Due to the unavailability of antibodies from the rest of the body, microglia must be able to recognize foreign bodies, swallow them, and activate T cells. They are constantly scavenging the CNS for plaques, damaged or unnecessary neurons and synapses, and infectious agents [210]. Since these processes must be efficient to prevent potentially fatal damage, microglia are extremely sensitive to even small pathological changes in the CNS, including excess nitric oxide production. Again, excess nitric oxide may turn the microglia against the host and destroy healthy tissue (see Fig. 4.50). Pathologically, an intimate relationship exists between microglial activation, nitric oxide, and neuro-inflammation in the human brain (Fig. 4.54) [208].

Microglial cells physically survey their domains on a regular basis. This action is car-

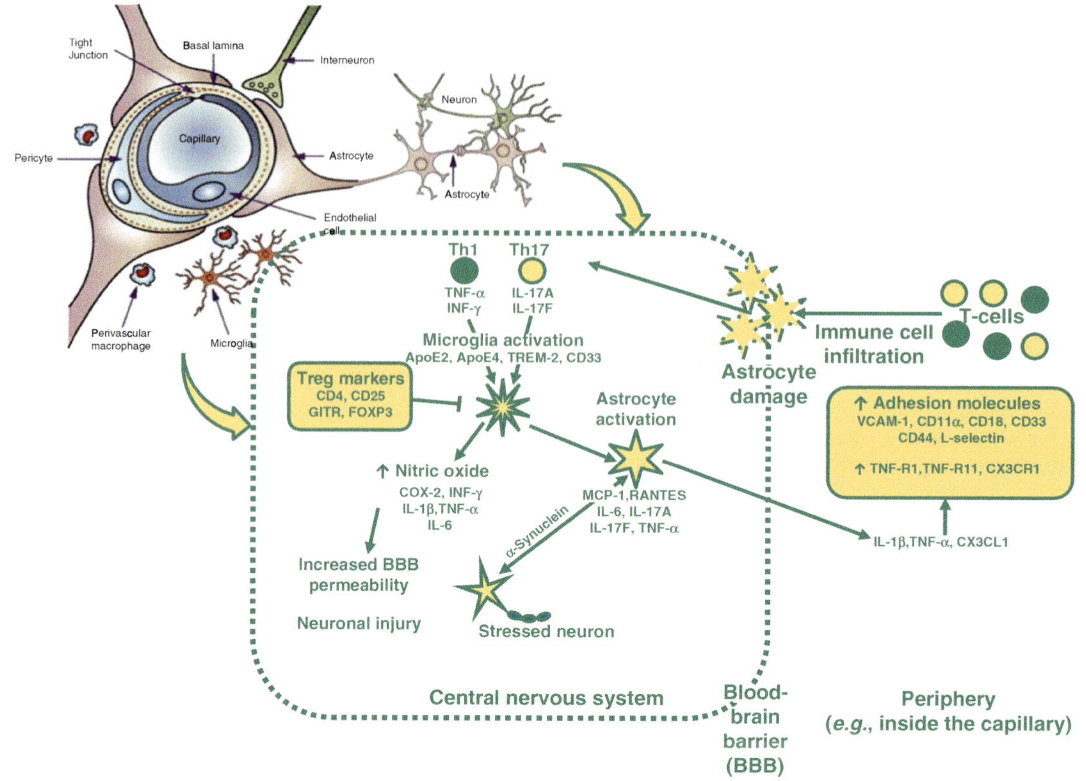


**Fig. 4.54** After compromise of the blood-brain barrier (BBB; either by skull fracture or cerebrovascular event, where blood enters the brain), T cells can infiltrate the central nervous system, releasing cytokines that contribute to neuronal inflammation by activating microglia, astrocytes, T cells, and other immune cells. Chronic neuronal inflammation can lead to neuronal death and the release of toxic protein aggregates (Tau, β-amyloid, and α-synuclein), accessory molecules (ApoE), and other cellular components leading to neurodegeneration and disease [211]. (Republished with permission from Elsevier)

ried out in the amoeboid and resting states. When the microglial cell finds foreign material, damaged cells, apoptotic cells, neurofibrillary tangles, DNA fragments, or plaques, it will activate and phagocytose the material or cell. Chronic activation of CNS microglia (neuro-inflammation) may produce neurodegenerative symptoms such as plaque formation and dystrophic neurite growth. It is important to distinguish between acute and chronic neuro-inflammation. Acute neuro-inflammation is generally caused by some neuronal injury, after which microglia migrate to the injured site, engulfing dead cells and debris [212]. The term neuro-inflammation generally refers to more chronic, sustained injury when the responses of microglial cells (due to persistent and excessive nitric oxide production) contribute to and expand the destructive effects of the inflammation, worsening the disease process.

When microglia are activated, they take on an amoeboid shape and they alter their gene expression. Increased parasympathetic activity associated with healing helps to activate microglia. Decreased parasympathetic activity following healing deactivates microglia. Prolonged, chronic, or abnormal parasympathetic activation (Parasympathetic Excess or PE) prolongs the activation of microglia, possibly preventing healing. Altered gene expression leads to the production of numerous potentially neurotoxic mediators. These mediators are important in the normal functions of microglia, and their production is usually decreased once their task is complete. In chronic neuro-inflammation, microglia remain activated for an extended period during

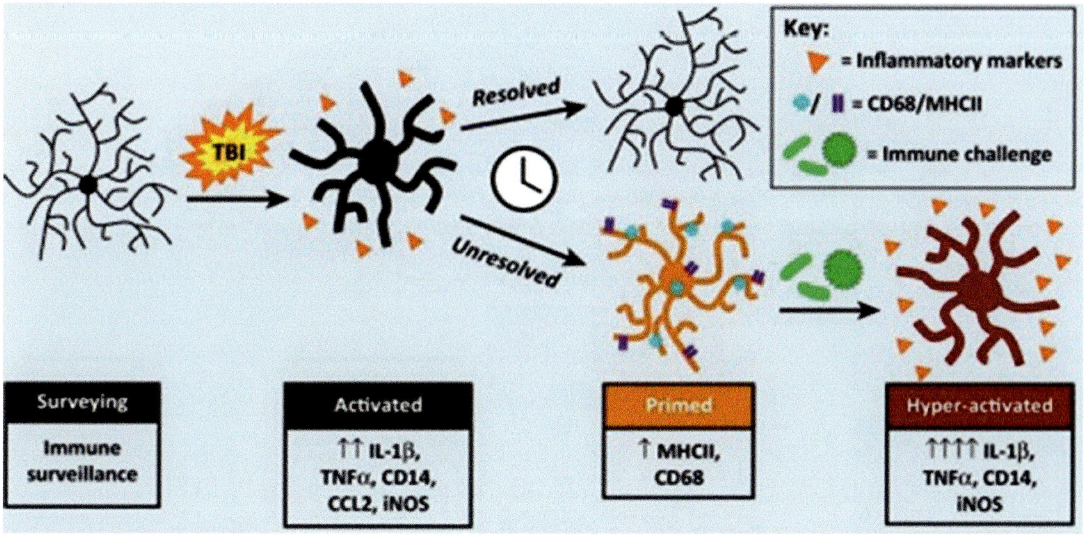


**Fig. 4.55** Nitric oxide production is increased by activated microglia via the iNOS gene [217, Fig. 4]. (Republished with permission from Elsevier)

which the production of neurotoxic mediators is sustained longer than usual and they contribute to neuronal death [213]. In brain injury, microglia have been implicated in neuropathic pain. They become activated in response to nerve injury, which includes the release and production of nitric oxide. Once activated, microglia release substances that excite pain-sensitive neurons, including prostaglandins and ROS. Overproduction of nitric oxide by nNOS is one of the fundamental causes underlying neurodegenerative disorders and neuropathic pain. Overproduction promotes microglia release of pro-inflammatory molecules, including IL-1β [214], IL-6 [215], and TNF-α [216]. The release of these pro-inflammatory molecules creates a positive feedback loop, exacerbating the pain response.

After compromise of the blood-brain barrier (either by skull fracture or cerebrovascular event, where blood enters the brain), excess nitric oxide in the presence of inflammatory cytokine may help to increase blood-brain barrier permeability, thereby increasing neuronal injury and further increasing microglial activation (Fig. 4.54). Nitric oxide production is increased by activated microglia via the iNOS gene. Prolonged, hyper-activation of microglia causes prolonged, overproduction of nitric oxide (including from the microglia themselves), reversing the benefits of nitric oxide (Fig. 4.55). This is treatable. Under the Mind-Body Wellness Program, antioxidants, including from the Mediterranean diet, and exercise help to maintain normal $Ca^{++}$ levels, normal nitric oxide levels, and relieve prolonged PE, which deactivates prolonged microglial activation, which permits the brain to (finally) finish healing. Very low-dose anticholinergics may replace, help to augment, or help to accelerate the relief of PE.

## Nitric Oxide Summary

Nitric oxide is an important signaling molecule in the human body. It has crucial roles in the support of the brain-heart, or mind-body, system health and wellness, including cellular communication, especially endothelial cell communication, neuronal communication, blood flow and blood pressure regulation, and immune system activation including central nervous system microglial activation. Underlying mind-body health and wellness is parasympathetic and sympathetic health and wellness and vascular and mitochondrial health and wellness. In all of this, nitric oxide is the ubiquitous messenger, with the following (Fig. 4.56):

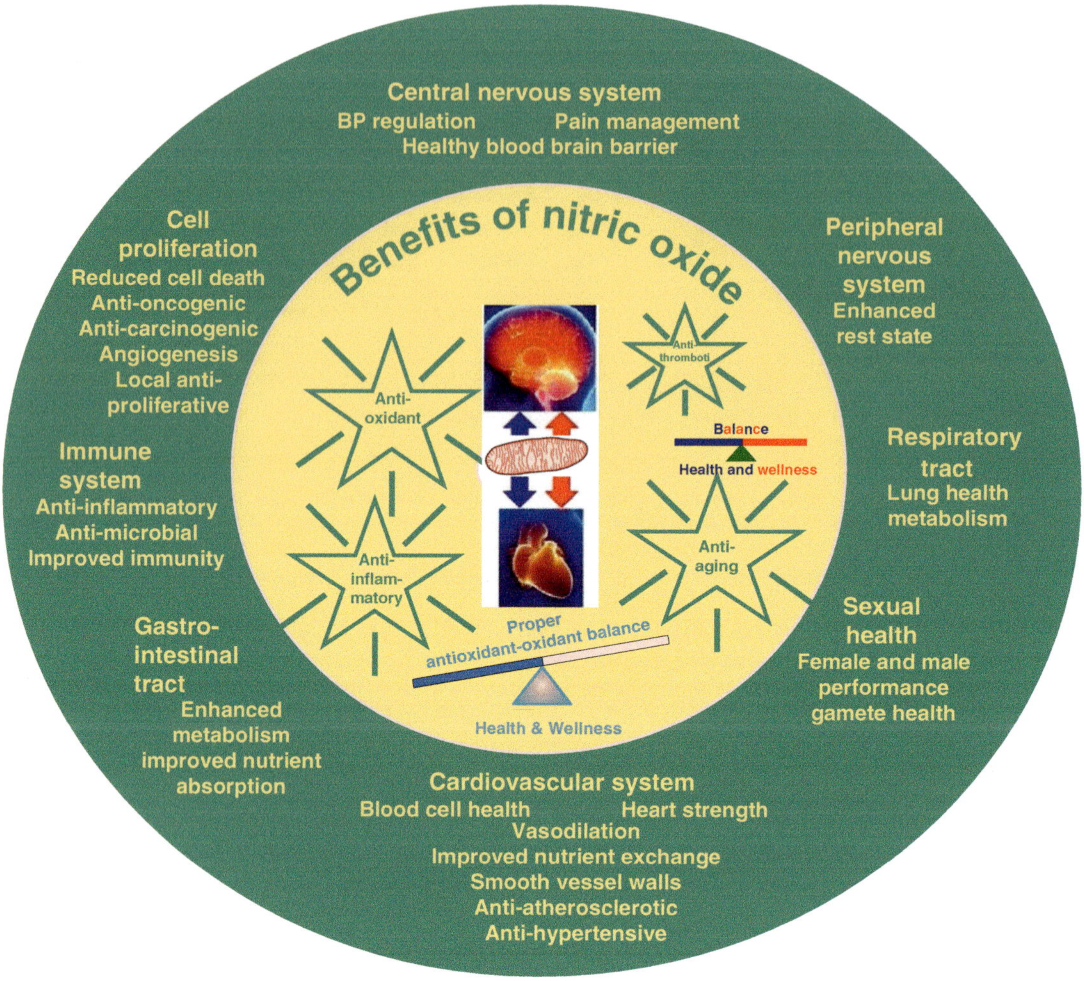


**Fig. 4.56** Nitric oxide functions, summary

- It functions as a neurotransmitter.
- It functions as a bactericide (antimicrobial: nitric oxide produced in phagocytes is cytotoxic to microbes).
- It regulates hemostatic mechanisms of blood vessels and vasodilates and lowers blood pressure (acts like a policeman of traffic flow).
- It functions as an anti-inflammatory and inhibits white blood cell from adhering to blood vessel (acts like a fireman that extinguishes fires and prevents them from occurring).
- It functions as a reparative gas (represents the Red Cross ambulance).
- It functions as an antithrombotic – by preventing platelets from clumping together to clot off blood vessels (acts like a policeman preventing "traffic jams," stopping clots from causing slowing or stopping blood flow).
- It functions in angiogenesis – by stimulating VEGF for growth of new blood vessels on top of old blood vessel (the engineers and architects that build new highways).
- It functions as an antioxidant (inhibits LDL cholesterol from becoming oxidized, preventing "foam cells" from forming).
- It upregulates the immune system by enhancing T-cell function.
- It promotes sexual health (both penile erection and vaginal lubrication).
- It promotes better cerebral circulation, possibly preventing "brain fog" or cognitive difficulties.

- It regulates local cell growth (antiproliferative).
- It inhibits mitochondrial respiration in times of stress.
- It prevents more damage when heart attacks or strokes occur.
- It regulates cell death.
- It helps form endothelial progenitor cells in the bone marrow (replenishes endothelial cells).
- It increases vagal tone and thereby protects the autonomic nervous system.
- It decreases sympathetic tone.
- It helps repair damaged tissues.
- It is cardioprotective (balances vagal and sympathetic tone).
- It promotes bone remodeling and healing and may improve bone density
- It reduces joint pain and may minimize further cartilage damage by increasing blood flow to joints.

While there is a good side, just like too much oxygen or water, under extreme circumstances, too much nitric oxide may also not be good. Excess nitric oxide by itself is not harmful as the gas dissipates in a few seconds. However, excess nitric oxide becomes very harmful as it becomes unstable. Unstable nitric oxide is an oxidant and may reverse the good that it does. This is why the complete Mind-Body Wellness program is needed to prevent the processes that leads to unstable nitric oxide (e.g., NOS uncoupling, excess $Ca^{++}$, excess oxygen, persistent microglial activation in the brain, low L-arginine to ADMA ratio, or low BH4). The program establishes and maintains a healthy milieu, a healthy environment, for the nitric oxide to remain beneficial and prevent disease.

The opposite is also not good. Nitric oxide insufficiency is caused by injury to endothelial cells or uncoupling of NOS in any form: eNOS, nNOS, or iNOS. Risk factors that cause endothelial cell injury include:

- High blood pressure (increases blood vessel wall shear force and injuring endothelial cells)
- Cigarette smoking
- Diabetes
- High lipid values
- Male gender
- Stress, especially psychosocial stress
- Familial traits, genetic susceptibility
- Sedentary lifestyle
- Obesity

Nitric oxide insufficiency leads to vasoconstriction, high blood pressure, atherosclerosis, cognitive dysfunction, autonomic dysfunction, immune dysfunction, and mitochondrial dysfunction. All dysfunctions may lead to a constellation of negative symptoms.

Again, the L-arginine-nitric oxide pathway is controlled by eNOS which converts L-arginine into nitric oxide. Young, healthy people naturally have low ADMA levels (high L-arginine to ADMA ratios). Therefore, L-arginine level supplementation doesn't really affect the ratio. Young, healthy individuals also do not benefit from L-arginine supplementation in terms of atherosclerosis because the ratio is high. L-Arginine supplementation is often more beneficial for individuals over age 40 or those with established chronic disease with underlying vascular, endothelial, or mitochondrial disease. In these patients, increased L-arginine/ADMA ratio is more beneficial. In individuals with cardiovascular or cerebral risk factors (heart attack, stroke, or sudden death), exogenous L-arginine supplementation may beneficially increase the L-arginine/ADMA ratio. This is often the reason that eNOS works better with L-arginine supplementation despite therapeutic levels of L-arginine in cells at baseline. This is known as the L-arginine paradox. Intracellular L-arginine is the rate-limiting step in nitric oxide production.

Even in people not taking any L-arginine supplements, blood levels of L-arginine may already be high enough to saturate eNOS. When an enzyme (in this case eNOS) is saturated with substrate (in this case L-arginine), more substrate won't have an effect on a reaction. Therefore, supplementing L-arginine (even in large doses) in healthy people won't lead to more nitric oxide from the L-arginine-nitric oxide pathway, simply because L-arginine is not rate limiting for eNOS. However, it is a different story in clinical conditions such as high blood pressure [218], elevated or abnormal cholesterol levels [219, 220], heart disease [221], insulin resistance [222], diabetes [223, 224], and in the elderly [218, 225, 226]. Under clinical conditions, L-arginine supplementation may exert beneficial effects, at least in part, due to increased nitric oxide production [218]. Again, this is the "L-arginine paradox," and it refers specifically to these situations in which L-arginine supplementation stimulates eNOS activity and nitric oxide production, even when blood L-arginine levels are within the normal range [227]. One explanation for the L-arginine paradox is the presence of high levels of ADMA (asymmetric dimethylarginine). ADMA inhibits eNOS [228–231]. ADMA is produced as part of the body's normal metabolism [232–234], but in clinical conditions, ADMA levels are elevated severalfold [231]. In the presence of elevated ADMA blood levels, eNOS activity is impaired, causing reduced nitric oxide production.

The six prongs of the Mind-Body Wellness Program work together to enhance endothelial wellness, as well as mitochondrial wellness and nervous system wellness. The last, specifically, targets the small, C nerve fibers, which include the autonomic nervous systems. Antioxidants promote nitric oxide by helping to establish the "proper milieu" for the individual. This then directs nitric oxide production down the pathways that promote vasodilation and healthy brain function and away from forming free radicals. A proper antioxidant balance for the individual provides a good buffer system from free radicals and damaging oxidative substances, keeping nitric oxide around to maintain blood vessel, nerve, and mitochondrial health. Nitric oxide as an anti-atherosclerotic supports fish oil (omega-3 fatty acids), statins (e.g., Zetia or Welchol), the Mediterranean diet, exercise, the right weight, stress reduction, and antioxidants in preventing atherosclerosis, through maintaining low LDL particle count and minimizing the amount of LDL becoming oxidized. In this sense, nitric oxide is a double bonus. In fact, it is a triple bonus when its action as an anti-inflammatory (as discussed above) is added to its anti-atherosclerotic and antioxidant activities.

Nitric oxide is produced by NOS from L-arginine which also produces L-citrulline. The L-citrulline may then be recycled and made into L-arginine. Both are available and may increase nitric oxide production, exogenously. Dietary sources of L-arginine include:

- Animal proteins, which is the richest source
- Nuts, specifically walnuts, pistachios, and peanuts
- Dairy products
- Soybeans
- Pumpkin seeds
- Chicken and turkey
- Pork loin
- Spirulina
- Chick peas
- Lentils
- Legumes and grains
- Tuna, salmon, shrimp, and crab
- Eggs (whole or raw)

Dietary sources of L-citrulline, which can sustain nitric oxide levels longer than L-arginine, include:

- Watermelon, which is the richest source, and where it was first discovered (over 2 lbs. of watermelon are required for 1 g of L-citrulline)
- Dark chocolate
- Nuts
- Fish and meat
- Fruits
- Legumes
- Vegetables

From these sources, however, it is difficult to get therapeutic quantities of L-arginine and L-citrulline by diet alone. There is the L-citrulline example, above. Another example is milk. Almost 2 gallons of milk is required to get 5 g of L-arginine. Folic acid is also helpful as it promotes nitric oxide production. Folic acid may also be obtained from diet, including:

- Eggs
- Peas
- Bananas
- Spinach

The other main amino acid in the Mind-Body Wellness Program is L-carnitine. Its dietary sources are:

- Red meat is one of the highest sources of L-carnitine, at about 56–162 mg per serving.
- Pork, seafood, and chicken have much lower levels, between 3 and 7 mg per serving.
- Dairy, like ice cream, milk, and cheese, has between 3 and 8 mg per serving.

As always, close physician supervision is recommended before prescribing any of the Mind-Body Wellness Program changes or any of these supplements.

## References


1. Widmer RJ, Lerman A. Endothelial dysfunction and cardiovascular disease. Glob Cardiol Sci Pract. 2014;2014(3):291–308. https://doi.org/10.5339/gcsp.2014.43. eCollection 2014. Review.
2. Endemann DH, Schiffrin EL. Endothelial dysfunction. J Am Soc Nephrol. 2004;15(8):1983–92. Review.
3. Hadi HA, Carr CS, Al SJ. Endothelial dysfunction: cardiovascular risk factors, therapy, and outcome. Vasc Health Risk Manag. 2005;1(3):183–98. Review.
4. Michel T, Vanhoutte PM. Cellular signaling and NO production. Pflugers Arch. 2010;459(6):807–16. https://doi.org/10.1007/s00424-009-0765-9. Epub 2010 Jan 16. Review.
5. Snyder SH. Nitric oxide: first in a new class of neurotransmitters. Science. 1992;257(5069):494–6.
6. Groneberg D, Voussen B, Friebe A. Integrative control of gastrointestinal motility by nitric oxide. Curr Med Chem. 2016;23(24):2715–35. Review.
7. Hibbs JB Jr, Taintor RR, Vavrin Z, Rachlin EM. Nitric oxide: a cytotoxic activated macrophage effector molecule. Biochem Biophys Res Commun. 1988;157(1):87–94. Erratum in: Biochem Biophys Res Commun 1989 Jan 31;158(2):624.
8. Hibbs JB Jr. Synthesis of nitric oxide from L-arginine: a recently discovered pathway induced by cytokines with antitumour and antimicrobial activity. Res Immunol. 1991;142(7):565–9; discussion 596–8. Review.
9. Nathan CF, Hibbs JB Jr. Role of nitric oxide synthesis in macrophage antimicrobial activity. Curr Opin Immunol. 1991;3(1):65–70. Review.
10. Margel D, Mizrahi M, Regev-Shoshani G, Ko M, Moshe M, Ozalvo R, Shavit-Grievink L, Baniel J, Kedar D, Yossepowitch O, Lifshitz D, Nadu A, Greenberg D, Av-Gay Y. Nitric oxide charged catheters as a potential strategy for prevention of hospital acquired infections. PLoS One. 2017;12(4):e0174443. https://doi.org/10.1371/journal.pone.0174443. eCollection 2017.
11. Tsukiyama Y, Ito T, Nagaoka K, Eguchi E, Ogino K. Effects of exercise training on nitric oxide, blood pressure and antioxidant enzymes. J Clin Biochem Nutr. 2017;60(3):180–6. https://doi.org/10.3164/jcbn.16-108. Epub 2017 Apr 7.
12. Faraci FM. Reactive oxygen species: influence on cerebral vascular tone. J Appl Physiol (1985). 2006;100(2):739–43. Review.
13. Faraci FM, Brian JE Jr. Nitric oxide and the cerebral circulation. Stroke. 1994;25(3):692–703.
14. Musicki B, Lagoda G, Goetz T, La Favor JD, Burnett AL. Transnitrosylation: a factor in nitric oxide-mediated penile erection. J Sex Med. 2016;13(5):808–14. https://doi.org/10.1016/j.jsxm.2016.03.003.
15. Elder JA, Braver Y. Female sexual dysfunction. http://www.clevelandclinicmeded.com/medicalpubs/diseasemanagement/womens-health/female-sexual-dysfunction/
16. Brown GC. Regulation of mitochondrial respiration by nitric oxide inhibition of cytochrome c oxidase. Biochim Biophys Acta. 2001;1504(1):46–57. Review.
17. Damodaran VB, Leszczak V, Wold KA, Lantvit SM, Popat KC, Reynolds MM. Anti-thrombogenic properties of a nitric oxide-releasing dextran derivative: evaluation of platelet activation and whole blood clotting kinetics. RSC Adv. 2013;3(46). https://doi.org/10.1039/C3RA45521A.
18. Lefer AM. Nitric oxide: nature's naturally occurring leukocyte inhibitor. Circulation. 1997;95(3):553–4. Review.
19. Lefer AM, Lefer DJ. Nitric oxide. II. Nitric oxide protects in intestinal inflammation. Am J Phys. 1999;276(3 Pt 1):G572–5. Review.
20. Ashraf MZ, Srivastava S. Oxidized phospholipids: introduction and biological significance. In: Lipoproteins. Gerhard Kostner; 2012. https://doi.org/10.5772/50461.
21. Predonzani A, Calì B, Agnellini AH, Molon B. Spotlights on immunological effects of reactive nitrogen species: when inflammation says nitric oxide. World J Exp Med. 2015;5(2):64–76.
22. Korhonen R, Korpela R, Saxelin M, Mäki M, Kankaanranta H, Moilanen E. Induction of nitric oxide synthesis by probiotic lactobacillus rhamnosus GG in J774 macrophages and human T84 intestinal epithelial cells. Inflammation. 2001;25(4):223–32.
23. Geiger R, Rieckmann JC, Wolf T, Basso C, Feng Y, Fuhrer T, Kogadeeva M, Picotti P, Meissner F, Mann M, Zamboni N, Sallusto F, Lanzavecchia A. L-arginine modulates T cell metabolism and enhances survival and anti-tumor activity. Cell. 2016;167(3):829–842.e13. https://doi.org/10.1016/j.cell.2016.09.031. Epub 2016 Oct 13.
24. Niedbala W, Cai B, Liew FY. Role of nitric oxide in the regulation of T cell functions. Ann Rheum Dis. 2006;65(Suppl 3):iii37–40. Review.

25. Niedbala W, Besnard AG, Jiang HR, Alves-Filho JC, Fukada SY, Nascimento D, Mitani A, Pushparaj P, Alqahtani MH, Liew FY. Nitric oxide-induced regulatory T cells inhibit Th17 but not Th1 cell differentiation and function. J Immunol. 2013;191(1):164–70. https://doi.org/10.4049/jimmunol.1202580. Epub 2013 May 29.
26. Winkler MS, Kluge S, Holzmann M, Moritz E, Robbe L, Bauer A, Zahrte C, Priefler M, Schwedhelm E, Böger RH, Goetz AE, Nierhaus A, Zoellner C. Markers of nitric oxide are associated with sepsis severity: an observational study. Crit Care. 2017;21(1):189. https://doi.org/10.1186/s13054-017-1782-2.
27. Predonzani A, Calì B, Agnellini AH, Molon B. Spotlights on immunological effects of reactive nitrogen species: when inflammation says nitric oxide. World J Exp Med. 2015;5(2):64–76. https://doi.org/10.5493/wjem.v5.i2.64. eCollection 2015 May 20.
28. Predonzani A, Calì B, Agnellini AH, Molon B. Spotlights on immunological effects of reactive nitrogen species: when inflammation says nitric oxide. World J Exp Med. 2015;5(2):64–76.
29. Ying L, Hofseth LJ. An emerging role for endothelial nitric oxide synthase in chronic inflammation and cancer. Cancer Res. 2007;67:1407–10.
30. Choudhari SK, Chaudhary M, Bagde S, Gadbail AR, Joshi V. Nitric oxide and cancer: a review. World J Surg Oncol. 2013;11:118. https://doi.org/10.1186/1477-7819-11-118. Review.
31. Li LM, Kibourn RG, Adams J, Filder IJ. Role of NO in lysis of tumor cells by cytokine activated endothelial cells. Cancer Res. 1991;51:2531–5.
32. Shang ZJ, Li JR. Expression of endothelial nitric oxide synthase and vascular endothelial growth factor in oral squamous cell carcinoma: its correlation with angiogenesis and disease progression. J Oral Pathol Med. 2005;4:134–9.
33. Lechner M, Lirk P, Rieder J. Inducible nitric oxide synthase (iNOS) in tumor biology: the two sides of the same coin. Semin Cancer Biol. 2005;15:277–89.
34. Rapozzi V, Della Pietra E, Bonavida B. Dual roles of nitric oxide in the regulation of tumor cell response and resistance to photodynamic therapy. Redox Biol. 2015;6:311–7. https://doi.org/10.1016/j.redox.2015.07.015. Epub 2015 Jul 31. Review.
35. Rapozzi V, Della Pietra E, Bonavida B. Dual roles of nitric oxide in the regulation of tumor cell response and resistance to photodynamic therapy. Redox Biol. 2015;6:311–7. https://doi.org/10.1016/j.redox.2015.07.015. Epub 2015 Jul 31. Review.
36. Reveneau S, Arnould L, Jolimoy G, Hilpert S, Lejeune P, Saint-Giorgio V, Belichard C, Jeannin JF. Nitric oxide synthase in human breast cancer is associated with tumor grade, proliferation rate, and expression of progesterone receptor. Lab Investig. 1999;79:1215–25.
37. Seabra AB, de Lima R, Calderón M. Nitric oxide releasing nanomaterials for cancer treatment: current status and perspectives. Curr Top Med Chem. 2015;15(4):298–308. Review.
38. Brown GC. Regulation of mitochondrial respiration by nitric oxide inhibition of cytochrome c oxidase. Review. Biochim Biophys Acta Bioenerg. 2001;1504(1):46–57.
39. Brown GC. Regulation of mitochondrial respiration by nitric oxide inhibition of cytochrome c oxidase. Review. Biochim Biophys Acta Bioenerg. 2001;1504(1):46–57.
40. Chakraborty S, Ain R. Nitric-oxide synthase trafficking inducer is a pleiotropic regulator of endothelial cell function and signaling. J Biol Chem. 2017;292(16):6600–20. https://doi.org/10.1074/jbc.M116.742627. Epub 2017 Feb 24.
41. Siegel C, McCullough LD. NAD+ depletion or PAR polymer formation: which plays the role of executioner in ischemic cell death? Acta Physiol (Oxf). 2011;203(1):225–34. https://doi.org/10.1111/j.1748-1716.2010.02229.x.
42. Siegel C, McCullough LD. NAD+ depletion or PAR polymer formation: which plays the role of executioner in ischemic cell death? Acta Physiol (Oxf). 2011;203(1):225–34. https://doi.org/10.1111/j.1748-1716.2010.02229.x.
43. Morbidelli L, Chang CH, Douglas JG, Granger HJ, Ledda F, Ziche M. Nitric oxide mediates mitogenic effect of VEGF on coronary venular endothelium. Am J Phys. 1996;270(1 Pt 2):H411–5.
44. Ziche M, Morbidelli L, Choudhuri R, Zhang HT, Donnini S, Granger HJ, Bicknell R. Nitric oxide synthase lies downstream from vascular endothelial growth factor-induced but not basic fibroblast growth factor-induced angiogenesis. J Clin Invest. 1997;99(11):2625–34.
45. Uhlmann S, Friedrichs U, Eichler W, Hoffmann S, Wiedemann P. Direct measurement of VEGF-induced nitric oxide production by choroidal endothelial cells. Microvasc Res. 2001;62(2):179–89.
46. Kimura H, Esumi H. Reciprocal regulation between nitric oxide and vascular endothelial growth factor in angiogenesis. Acta Biochim Pol. 2003;50(1):49–59. Review.
47. Zhang HH, Chen JC, Sheibani L, Lechuga TJ, Chen DB. Pregnancy augments VEGF-stimulated in vitro angiogenesis and vasodilator (NO and H2S) production in human uterine artery endothelial cells. J Clin Endocrinol Metab. 2017. https://doi.org/10.1210/jc.2017-00437.
48. Estrada C, Murillo-Carretero M. Nitric oxide and adult neurogenesis in health and disease. Neuroscientist. 2005;11(4):294.
49. Wimalawansa SJ. Nitric oxide and bone. Ann N Y Acad Sci. 2010;1192:391–403. https://doi.org/10.1111/j.1749-6632.2009.05230.x. Review.
50. Yu Q, Li T, Li J, Zhong L, Mao X. Nitricoxidesynthase in male urological and andrologic functions. Nitric oxide synthase – simple enzyme-complex roles. 113–36. http://www.intechopen.com/books/nitric-oxide-synthase-simpleenzyme-complex-roles

51. Emanuele MA, Wezeman F, Emanuele NV. Alcohol's effect on female reproductive function. Alcohol Res Health. 2002;26(4):274–81. National Institute on Alcohol Abuse and Alcoholism (NIAAA). June, 2003. https://pubs.niaaa.nih.gov/publications/arh26-4/274-281.htm
52. Ferrier DP. Biochemistry. 6th ed. Philadelphia: Lippincott, Williams & Williams, a Wolters Kluwer Business; 2014.
53. Erez A. Arginosuccinate acidura: from monogenic to a complex disorder. Genet Med. 2013;15:251–7. https://doi.org/10.1038/gim.2012.166. Epub 2013 Jan 10.
54. Kelm M. Nitric oxide metabolism and breakdown. BBA. 1999;1411:273–89. https://doi.org/10.1016/S0005-2728(99)00020-1.
55. Tiso M, Schechter AN. Nitrate reduction to nitrite, nitric oxide and ammonia by gut bacteria under physiological conditions. PLoS One. 2015;10(3):e0119712. https://doi.org/10.1371/journal.one.0119712.
56. Gad MZ. Anti-aging effects of L-arginine. J Adv Res. 2010;1:169–77. Review.
57. Yeboah J, Folsom AR, Burke GL, Johnson C, Polak JF, Post W, Lima JA, Crouse JR, Herrington DM. Predictive value of brachial flow-mediated dilation for incident cardiovascular events in a population-based study: the multi-ethnic study of atherosclerosis. Circulation. 2009;120(6):502–9.
58. Huang A, Silver AE, Shvenke E, Schopfer DW, Jahangir E, Titas MA, Shpilman A, Menzoian JO, Watkins MT, Raffetto JD, Gibbons G, Woodson J, Shaw PM, Dhadly M, Eberhardt RT, Keaney JF Jr, Gokce N, Vita JA. Predictive value of reactive hyperemia for cardiovascular events in patients with peripheral arterial disease undergoing vascular surgery. Arterioscler Thromb Vasc Biol. 2007;27(10):2113–9.
59. Anderson T, Charbonneau F, Title LM, Buithieu J, Rose MS, Conradson H, Hildebrand K, Fung M, Verma S, Lonn EM. Microvascular function predicts cardiovascular events in primary prevention: long-term results from the firefighters and their endothelium (FATE) study. Circulation. 2011;123(2):163–9.
60. Lind L, Berglund L, Larsson A, Sundström J. Endothelial function in resistance and conduit arteries and 5-year risk of cardiovascular disease. Circulation. 2011;123(14):1545–51.
61. Gorren AC, Mayer B. Tetrahydrobiopterin in nitric oxide synthesis: a novel biological role for pteridines. Curr Drug Metab. 2002;3(2):133–57. Review.
62. Michel T. NO way to relax: the complexities of coupling nitric oxide synthase pathways in the heart. Circulation. 2010;121(4):484–6. https://doi.org/10.1161/CIR.0b013e3181d1e24e. Epub 2010 Jan 18.
63. Channon KM. Tetrahydrobiopterin: a vascular redox target to improve endothelial function. Curr Vasc Pharmacol. 2012;10(6):705–8. Review.
64. Zhang Y, Janssens SP, Wingler K, Schmidt HH, Moens AL. Modulating endothelial nitric oxide synthase: a new cardiovascular therapeutic strategy. Am J Physiol Heart Circ Physiol. 2011;301(3):H634–46. https://doi.org/10.1152/ajpheart.01315.2010. Epub 2011 May 27. Review. Erratum in: Am J Physiol Heart Circ Physiol. 2012 Jul 15;303(2):H241.
65. Menzel D, Haller H, Wilhelm M, et al. L-arginine and B vitamins improve endothelial function in subjects with mild to moderate blood pressure elevation. Eur J Nutr. 2018;57(2):557–68. https://doi.org/10.1007/s00394-016-1342-6 (Springer Berlin Heidelberg).
66. Stuehr DJ. Enzymes of the L-arginine to nitric oxide pathway. J Nutr. 2004;134(10 Suppl):2748S–51S; discussion 2765S–2767S. Review
67. Lai WK, Kan MY. Homocysteine-induced endothelial dysfunction. Ann Nutr Metab. 2015;67:1–12. https://doi.org/10.1159/000437098.
68. Scalera F, Bode-Böger SM. Nitric oxide–asymmetric dimethylarginine system in endothelial cell senescence. In: Ignarro LJ, editor. Nitric oxide biology and pathobiology. 2nd ed. San Diego: Elsevier; 2010.
69. Moyzis RK, Buckingham JM, Cram LS, Dani M, Deaven LL, Jones MD, Meyne J, Ratliff RL, Wu JR. A highly conserved repetitive DNA sequence, (TTAGGG)n, present at the telomeres of human chromosomes. Proc Natl Acad Sci U S A. 1988;85(18):6622–6.
70. Blackburn EH. Telomere states and cell fates. Nature. 2000;408:53–6.
71. Blackburn EH. Switching and signaling at the telomere. Cell. 2001;106:661–73.
72. Blasco MA. Mammalian telomeres and telomerase: why they matter for cancer and aging. Eur J Cell Biol. 2003;82:441–6.
73. Bode-Böger SM, Martens-Lobenhoffer J, Täger M, Schröder H, Scalera F. Aspirin reduces endothelial cell senescence. Biochem Biophys Res Commun. 2005;334:1226–32.
74. Scalera F, Martens-Lobenhoffer J, Bukowska A, Lendeckel U, Täger M, Bode-Böger SM. Effect of telmisartan on nitric oxide-asymmetrical dimethylarginine system. Role of angiotensin II type 1 receptor and peroxisome proliferator activated receptor γ signaling during endothelial aging. Hypertension. 2008;51:696–703.
75. Jin ZG. Where is endothelial nitric oxide synthase more critical: plasma membrane or Golgi? Arterioscler Thromb Vasc Biol. 2006;26(5):959–61.
76. Petruson K, Stalfors J, Jacobsson KE, Ny L, Petruson B. Nitric oxide production in the sphenoidal sinus by the inducible and constitutive isozymes of nitric oxide synthase. Rhinology. 2005;43(1):18–23.
77. Fleming I, Busse R. Molecular mechanisms involved in the regulation of the endothelial nitric oxide synthase. Am J Physiol Regul Integr Comp Physiol. 2003;284(1):R1–12.
78. Ostrom RS, Bundey RA, Insel PA. Nitric oxide inhibition of adenylyl cyclase type 6 activity is dependent upon lipid rafts and caveolin signaling complexes. J Biol Chem. 2004;279(19):19846–53.
79. Minshall RD, Sessa WC, Stan RV, Anderson RG, Malik AB. Caveolin regulation of endothelial

function. Am J Physiol Lung Cell Mol Physiol. 2003;285(6):L1179–83.
80. Ho FM, Lin WW, Chen BC, Chao CM, Yang CR, Lin LY, Lai CC, Liu SH, Liau CS. High glucose-induced apoptosis in human vascular endothelial cells is mediated through NF-kappaB and c-Jun NH(2)-terminal kinase pathway and prevented by PI3K/Akt/eNOS pathway. Cell Signal. 2006;18(3):391–9. Epub 2005 Jun 20.
81. Boo YC, Jo H. Flow-dependent regulation of endothelial nitric oxide synthase: role of protein kinases. Am J Physiol Cell Physiol. 2003;285(3):C499–508.
82. Goubareva I, Gkaliagkousi E, Shah A, Queen L, Ritter J, Ferro A. Age decreases nitric oxide synthesis and responsiveness in human platelets and increases formation of monocyte-platelet aggregates. Cardiovasc Res. 2007;75(4):793–802. Epub 2007 May 24.
83. Eggebeen J, Kim-Shapiro DB, Haykowsky M, Morgan TM, Basu S, Brubaker P, Rejeski J, Kitzman DW. One week of daily dosing with beetroot juice improves submaximal endurance and blood pressure in older patients with heart failure and preserved ejection fraction. JACC Heart Fail. 2016;4(6):428–37. https://doi.org/10.1016/j.jchf.2015.12.013. Epub 2016 Feb 10.
84. Shaltout HA, Eggebeen J, Marsh AP, Brubaker PH, Laurienti PJ, Burdette JH, Basu S, Morgan A, Dos Santos PC, Norris JL, Morgan TM, Miller GD, Rejeski WJ, Hawfield AT, Diz DI, Becton JT, Kim-Shapiro DB, Kitzman DW. Effects of supervised exercise and dietary nitrate in older adults with controlled hypertension and/or heart failure with preserved ejection fraction. Nitric Oxide. 2017;69:78–90. https://doi.org/10.1016/j.niox.2017.05.005. Epub 2017 May 23.
85. Woessner MN, McIlvenna LC, Ortiz de Zevallos J, Neil C, Allen JD. Dietary nitrate supplementation in cardiovascular health: an ergogenic aid or exercise therapeutic? Am J Physiol Heart Circ Physiol. 2017:ajpheart004142017. https://doi.org/10.1152/ajpheart.00414.2017.
86. Notay K, Incognito AV, Millar PJ. Acute beetroot juice supplementation on sympathetic nerve activity: a randomized, double-blind, placebo-controlled proof-of-concept study. Am J Physiol Heart Circ Physiol. 2017;313(1):H59–65. https://doi.org/10.1152/ajpheart.00163.2017. Epub 2017 May 5.
87. Ashor AW, Lara J, Siervo M. Medium-term effects of dietary nitrate supplementation on systolic and diastolic blood pressure in adults: a systematic review and meta-analysis. J Hypertens. 2017;35(7):1353–9. https://doi.org/10.1097/HJH.0000000000001305.
88. Clements WT, Lee SR, Bloomer RJ. Nitrate ingestion: a review of the health and physical performance effects. Nutrients. 2014;6(11):5224–64. https://doi.org/10.3390/nu6115224. Review.
89. Siervo M, Lara J, Ogbonmwan I, Mathers JC. Inorganic nitrate and beetroot juice supplementation reduces blood pressure in adults: a systematic review and meta-analysis. J Nutr. 2013;143(6):818–26. https://doi.org/10.3945/jn.112.170233. Epub 2013 Apr 17. Review.
90. Coles LT, Clifton PM. Effect of beetroot juice on lowering blood pressure in free-living, disease-free adults: a randomized, placebo-controlled trial. Nutr J. 2012;11:106. https://doi.org/10.1186/1475-2891-11-106.
91. Hobbs DA, Goulding MG, Nguyen A, Malaver T, Walker CF, George TW, Methven L, Lovegrove JA. Acute ingestion of beetroot bread increases endothelium-independent vasodilation and lowers diastolic blood pressure in healthy men: a randomized controlled trial. J Nutr. 2013;143(9):1399–405. https://doi.org/10.3945/jn.113.175778. Epub 2013 Jul 24.
92. Jajja A, Sutyarjoko A, Lara J, Rennie K, Brandt K, Qadir O, Siervo M. Beetroot supplementation lowers daily systolic blood pressure in older, overweight subjects. Nutr Res. 2014;34(10):868–75. https://doi.org/10.1016/j.nutres.2014.09.007. Epub 2014 Sep 28.
93. Wong RH, Garg ML, Wood LG, Howe PR. Antihypertensive potential of combined extracts of olive leaf, green coffee bean and beetroot: a randomized, double-blind, placebo-controlled crossover trial. Nutrients. 2014;6(11):4881–94. https://doi.org/10.3390/nu6114881.
94. Clements WT, Lee SR, Bloomer RJ. Nitrate ingestion: a review of the health and physical performance effects. Nutrients. 2014;6(11):5224–64. https://doi.org/10.3390/nu6115224. Review.
95. Lara J, Ashor AW, Oggioni C, Ahluwalia A, Mathers JC, Siervo M. Effects of inorganic nitrate and beetroot supplementation on endothelial function: a systematic review and meta-analysis. Eur J Nutr. 2016;55(2):451–9. https://doi.org/10.1007/s00394-015-0872-7. Epub 2015 Mar 13. Review.
96. Lee JS, Stebbins CL, Jung E, Nho H, Kim JK, Chang MJ, Choi HM. Effects of chronic dietary nitrate supplementation on the hemodynamic response to dynamic exercise. Am J Physiol Regul Integr Comp Physiol. 2015;309(5):R459–66. https://doi.org/10.1152/ajpregu.00099.2015. Epub 2015 Jun 17.
97. Clifford T, Howatson G, West DJ, Stevenson EJ. The potential benefits of red beetroot supplementation in health and disease. Nutrients. 2015;7(4):2801–22. https://doi.org/10.3390/nu7042801. Review.
98. Bondonno CP, Liu AH, Croft KD, Ward NC, Shinde S, Moodley Y, Lundberg JO, Puddey IB, Woodman RJ, Hodgson JM. Absence of an effect of high nitrate intake from beetroot juice on blood pressure in treated hypertensive individuals: a randomized controlled trial. Am J Clin Nutr. 2015;102(2):368–75. https://doi.org/10.3945/ajcn.114.101188. Epub 2015 Jul 1.
99. Kelly J, Vanhatalo A, Wilkerson DP, Wylie LJ, Jones AM. Effects of nitrate on the power-duration relationship for severe-intensity exercise. Med Sci Sports Exerc. 2013;45(9):1798–806. https://doi.org/10.1249/MSS.0b013e31828e885c.

100. Muggeridge DJ, Howe CC, Spendiff O, Pedlar C, James PE, Easton C. The effects of a single dose of concentrated beetroot juice on performance in trained flatwater kayakers. Int J Sport Nutr Exerc Metab. 2013;23(5):498–506. Epub 2013 Apr 9. Erratum in: Int J Sport Nutr Exerc Metab. 2013 Dec;23 (6):642.
101. Hoon MW, Jones AM, Johnson NA, Blackwell JR, Broad EM, Lundy B, Rice AJ, Burke LM. The effect of variable doses of inorganic nitrate-rich beetroot juice on simulated 2,000-m rowing performance in trained athletes. Int J Sports Physiol Perform. 2014;9(4):615–20. https://doi.org/10.1123/ijspp.2013-0207. Epub 2013 Sep 30.
102. Breese BC, McNarry MA, Marwood S, Blackwell JR, Bailey SJ, Jones AM. Beetroot juice supplementation speeds O2 uptake kinetics and improves exercise tolerance during severe-intensity exercise initiated from an elevated metabolic rate. Am J Physiol Regul Integr Comp Physiol. 2013;305(12):R1441–50. https://doi.org/10.1152/ajpregu.00295.2013. Epub 2013 Oct 2.
103. Lowery RP, Joy JM, Dudeck JE, Oliveira de Souza E, McCleary SA, Wells S, Wildman R, Wilson JM. Effects of 8 weeks of Xpand® 2X pre workout supplementation on skeletal muscle hypertrophy, lean body mass, and strength in resistance trained males. J Int Soc Sports Nutr. 2013;10(1):44. https://doi.org/10.1186/1550-2783-10-44.
104. Thompson KG, Turner L, Prichard J, Dodd F, Kennedy DO, Haskell C, Blackwell JR, Jones AM. Influence of dietary nitrate supplementation on physiological and cognitive responses to incremental cycle exercise. Respir Physiol Neurobiol. 2014;193:11–20. https://doi.org/10.1016/j.resp.2013.12.015. Epub 2013 Dec 31.
105. Pinna M, Roberto S, Milia R, Marongiu E, Olla S, Loi A, Migliaccio GM, Padulo J, Orlandi C, Tocco F, Concu A, Crisafulli A. Effect of beetroot juice supplementation on aerobic response during swimming. Nutrients. 2014;6(2):605–15. https://doi.org/10.3390/nu6020605.
106. Flanagan SD, Looney DP, Miller MJ, DuPont WH, Pryor L, Creighton BC, Sterczala AJ, Szivak TK, Hooper DR, Maresh CM, Volek JS, Ellis LA, Kraemer WJ. The effects of nitrate-rich supplementation on neuromuscular efficiency during heavy resistance exercise. J Am Coll Nutr. 2016;35(2):100–7. https://doi.org/10.1080/07315724.2015.1081572. Epub 2016 Feb 17.
107. Petrie M, Rejeski WJ, Basu S, Laurienti PJ, Marsh AP, Norris JL, Kim-Shapiro DB, Burdette JH. Beet root juice: an ergogenic aid for exercise and the aging brain. J Gerontol A Biol Sci Med Sci. 2016. https://doi.org/10.1093/gerona/glw219. [Epub ahead of print].
108. Domínguez R, Cuenca E, Maté-Muñoz JL, García-Fernández P, Serra-Paya N, Estevan MC, Herreros PV, Garnacho-Castaño MV. Effects of beetroot juice supplementation on cardiorespiratory endurance in athletes. A systematic review. Nutrients. 2017;9(1). pii: E43. https://doi.org/10.3390/nu9010043. Review.
109. Montenegro CF, Kwong DA, Minow ZA, Davis BA, Lozada CF, Casazza GA. Betalain-rich concentrate supplementation improves exercise performance and recovery in competitive triathletes. Appl Physiol Nutr Metab. 2017;42(2):166–72. https://doi.org/10.1139/apnm-2016-0452. Epub 2016 Oct 14.
110. Vanhatalo A, Jones AM, Blackwell JR, Winyard PG, Fulford J. Dietary nitrate accelerates postexercise muscle metabolic recovery and O2 delivery in hypoxia. J Appl Physiol (1985). 2014;117(12):1460–70. https://doi.org/10.1152/japplphysiol.00096.2014. Epub 2014 Oct 9.
111. Kim JK, Moore DJ, Maurer DG, Kim-Shapiro DB, Basu S, Flanagan MP, Skulas-Ray AC, Kris-Etherton P, Proctor DN. Acute dietary nitrate supplementation does not augment submaximal forearm exercise hyperemia in healthy young men. Appl Physiol Nutr Metab. 2015;40(2):122–8. https://doi.org/10.1139/apnm-2014-0228. Epub 2014 Oct 15.
112. MacLeod KE, Nugent SF, Barr SI, Koehle MS, Sporer BC, MacInnis MJ. Acute beetroot juice supplementation does not improve cycling performance in normoxia or moderate hypoxia. Int J Sport Nutr Exerc Metab. 2015;25(4):359–66. https://doi.org/10.1123/ijsnem.2014-0129. Epub 2015 Mar 26.
113. Arnold JT, Oliver SJ, Lewis-Jones TM, Wylie LJ, Macdonald JH. Beetroot juice does not enhance altitude running performance in well-trained athletes. Appl Physiol Nutr Metab. 2015;40(6):590–5. https://doi.org/10.1139/apnm-2014-0470. Epub 2015 Feb 4.
114. Flueck JL, Bogdanova A, Mettler S, Perret C. Is beetroot juice more effective than sodium nitrate? The effects of equimolar nitrate dosages of nitrate-rich beetroot juice and sodium nitrate on oxygen consumption during exercise. Appl Physiol Nutr Metab. 2016;41(4):421–9. https://doi.org/10.1139/apnm-2015-0458. Epub 2015 Dec 23.
115. Chirinos JA, Akers SR, Trieu L, Ischiropoulos H, Doulias PT, Tariq A, Vassim I, Koppula MR, Syed AA, Soto-Calderon H, Townsend RR, Cappola TP, Margulies KB, Zamani P. Heart failure, left ventricular remodeling, and circulating nitric oxide metabolites. J Am Heart Assoc. 2016;5(10). pii: e004133. Erratum in: J Am Heart Assoc. 2017 Feb 14;6(2).
116. Zamani P, Tan V, Soto-Calderon H, Beraun M, Brandimarto JA, Trieu L, Varakantam S, Doulias PT, Townsend RR, Chittams J, Margulies KB, Cappola TP, Poole DC, Ischiropoulos H, Chirinos JA. Pharmacokinetics and pharmacodynamics of inorganic nitrate in heart failure with preserved ejection fraction. Circ Res. 2017;120(7):1151–61. https://doi.org/10.1161/CIRCRESAHA.116.309832. Epub 2016 Dec 7.
117. Jacob T, Ascher E, Vorsanger M, Hingorani A, Kallakuri S, Yorkovich W, Schuzter R. Decreased production of nitric oxide by peripheral blood mono-

nuclear cells of patients with peripheral vascular disease. Vasc Endovasc Surg. 2005;39(2):175–81.
118. Tapiero H, Mathé G, Couvreur P, Tew KD. L-Arginine. Biomed Pharmacother. 2002;56(9):439–45.
119. Dhanakoti SN, Brosnan JT, Herzberg GR, Brosnan ME. Renal arginine synthesis: studies in vitro and in vivo. Am J Phys. 1990;259(3 Pt1):E437–42.
120. Watford M. The urea cycle: a two-compartment system. Essays Biochem. 1991;26:49–58.
121. Fritz JH. Arginine cools the inflamed gut. Infect Immun. 2013;81(10):3500–2. https://doi.org/10.1128/IAI.00789-13. Epub 2013 Jul 29.
122. Patel VB, Preedy VR, Rajendram R, editors. L-arginine in clinical nutrition. Cham: Humana Press, Springer International Publishing; 2017.
123. Pahlavani N, Jafari M, Sadeghi O, Rezaei M, Rasad H, Rahdar HA, Entezari MH. L-arginine supplementation and risk factors of cardiovascular diseases in healthy men: a double-blind randomized clinical trial. Version 2. F1000Res. 2014 [revised 2017 Jun 1];3:306. https://doi.org/10.12688/f1000research.5877.2. eCollection 2014.
124. Clifford T, Howatson G, West DJ, Stevenson EJ. The potential benefits of red beetroot supplementation in health and disease. Nutrients. 2015;7(4):2801–22. https://doi.org/10.3390/nu7042801. Review.
125. Flanagan SD, Looney DP, Miller MJ, DuPont WH, Pryor L, Creighton BC, Sterczala AJ, Szivak TK, Hooper DR, Maresh CM, Volek JS, Ellis LA, Kraemer WJ. The effects of nitrate-rich supplementation on neuromuscular efficiency during heavy resistance exercise. J Am Coll Nutr. 2016;35(2):100–7. https://doi.org/10.1080/07315724.2015.1081572. Epub 2016 Feb 17.
126. Domínguez R, Cuenca E, Maté-Muñoz JL, García-Fernández P, Serra-Paya N, Estevan MC, Herreros PV, Garnacho-Castaño MV. Effects of beetroot juice supplementation on cardiorespiratory endurance in athletes. A systematic review. Nutrients. 2017;9(1). pii: E43. https://doi.org/10.3390/nu9010043. Review.
127. Bondonno CP, Liu AH, Croft KD, Ward NC, Shinde S, Moodley Y, Lundberg JO, Puddey IB, Woodman RJ, Hodgson JM. Absence of an effect of high nitrate intake from beetroot juice on blood pressure in treated hypertensive individuals: a randomized controlled trial. Am J Clin Nutr. 2015;102(2):368–75. https://doi.org/10.3945/ajcn.114.101188. Epub 2015 Jul 1.
128. Arnold JT, Oliver SJ, Lewis-Jones TM, Wylie LJ, Macdonald JH. Beetroot juice does not enhance altitude running performance in well-trained athletes. Appl Physiol Nutr Metab. 2015;40(6):590–5. https://doi.org/10.1139/apnm-2014-0470. Epub 2015 Feb 4.
129. Boger RH, Bode Boger SM. The clinical pharmacology of L-arginine. Annu Rev Pharmacol Toxicol. 2001;41:79–99.
130. Kamada Y, Nagaretani H, Tamura S, Ohama T, Maruyama T, Hiraoka H, et al. Vascular endothelial dysfunction resulting from L-arginine deficiency in a patient with lysinuric protein intolerance. J Clin Invest. 2001;108(5):717–24.
131. Boger RH, Ron ES. L-arginine improves vascular function by overcoming deleterious effects of ADMA, a novel cardiovascular risk factor. Altern Med Rev. 2005;10(1):14–23.
132. Holt LE Jr, Albanese AA. Observations on amino acid deficiencies in man. Trans Assoc Am Phys. 1944;58:143–56.
133. Tanimura J. Studies on arginine in human semen. II. The effects of medication with L-arginine-HCL on male infertility. Bull Osaka Med Sch. 1967;13(2):84–9.
134. Finkel T, Holbrook NJ. Oxidants, oxidative stress and the biology of aging. Nature. 2000;408(6809):239–47.
135. Schwentker A, Vodovotz Y, Weller R, Billiar TR. Nitric oxide and wound repair: role of cytokines? Nitric Oxide. 2002;7(1):1–10.
136. Seifter E, Rettura G, Barbul A, Levenson SM. Arginine: an essential amino acid for injured rats. Surgery. 1978;84(2):224–30.
137. Kirk SJ, Hurson M, Regan MC, Holt DR, Wasserkrug HL, Barbul A. Arginine stimulates wound healing and immune function in elderly human beings. Surgery. 1993;114(2):155–9.
138. Arbss MA, Ferrando JM, Vidal J, Quiles MT, Huguet P, Castells J, et al. Early effects of exogenous arginine after the implantation of prosthetic material into the rat abdominal wall. Life Sci. 2000;67(20):2493–512.
139. Albina JE, Mills CD, Henry WL Jr, Caldwell MD. Temporal expression of different pathways of L-arginine metabolism in healing wounds. J Immunol. 1990;144(10):3877–80.
140. Shi HP, Efron DT, Most D, Tantry US, Barbul A. Supplemental dietary arginine enhances wound healing in normal but not inducible nitric oxide synthase knockout mice. Surgery. 2000;128(2):374–8.
141. Angele MK, Nitsch SM, Hatz RA, Angele P, Hernandez Richter T, Wichmann MW, et al. L-arginine: a unique amino acid for improving depressed wound immune function following hemorrhage. Eur Surg Res. 2002;34(1–2):53–60.
142. Chen X, Li Y, Cai X, Xu W, Lu S, Shi J. Dose–effect of dietary L-arginine supplementation on burn wound healing in rats. Chin Med J. 1999;112(9):828–31.
143. Yu YM, Ryan CM, Castillo L, Lu XM, Beaumier L, Tompkins RG, et al. Arginine and ornithine kinetics in severely burned patients: increased rate of arginine disposal. Am J Physiol Endocrinol Metab. 2001;280(3):E509–17.
144. Pieper GM, Siebeneich W, Dondlinger LA. Short-term oral administration of L-arginine reverses defective endothelium-dependent relaxation and cGMP generation in diabetes. Eur J Pharmacol. 1996;317(2–3):317–20.
145. Abbasi F, Asagmi T, Cooke JP, Lamendola C, McLaughlin T, Reaven GM, et al. Plasma concentrations of asymmetric dimethylarginine are increased

in patients with type 2 diabetes mellitus. Am J Cardiol. 2001;88(10):1201–3

146. Giugliano D, Marfella R, Verrazzo G, Acampora R, Nappo F, Ziccardi P, et al. L-arginine for testing endothelium-dependent vascular functions in health and disease. Am J Phys. 1997;273(3 Pt 1):E606–12.
147. Wascher TC, Graier WF, Dittrich P, Hussain MA, Bahadori B, Wallner S, et al. Effects of low-dose L-arginine on insulin-mediated vasodilatation and insulin sensitivity. Eur J Clin Investig. 1997;27(8):690–5.
148. Lubec B, Hayn M, Kitzmuller E, Vierhapper H, Lubec G. L-arginine reduces lipid peroxidation in patients with diabetes mellitus. Free Radic Biol Med. 1997;22(1–2):355–7.
149. Piatti PM, Monti LD, Valsecchi G, Magni F, Setola E, Marchesi F, et al. Long-term oral L-arginine administration improves peripheral and hepatic insulin sensitivity in type 2 diabetic patients. Diabetes Care. 2001;24(5):875–80.
150. Bohme GA, Bon C, Stutzmann JM, Doble A, Blanchard JC. Possible involvement of nitric oxide in long-term potentiation. Eur J Pharmacol. 1991;199(3):379–81.
151. Moncada S, Higgs A. The L-arginine–nitric oxide pathway. N Engl J Med. 1993;329(27):2002–12. [73] Campbell BI, La Bounty PM, Roberts M. The ergogenic potential of arginine. J Int Soc Sports Nutr 2004;1(2):35–8.
152. Campbell BI, La Bounty PM, Roberts M. The ergogenic potential of arginine. J Int Soc Sports Nutr. 2004;1(2):35–8.
153. Fossel ET. Improvement of temperature and flow in feet of subjects with diabetes with use of a transdermal preparation of L-arginine: a pilot study. Diabetes Care. 2004;27(1):284–5.
154. Klahr S. Can L-arginine manipulation reduce renal disease? Semin Nephrol. 1999;19(3):304–9.
155. Park KG, Hayes PD, Garlick PJ, Sewell H, Eremin O. Stimulation of lymphocyte natural cytotoxicity by L-arginine. Lancet. 1991;337(8742):645–6.
156. Gupta V, Gupta A, Saggu S, Divekar HM, Grover SK, Kumar R. Antistress and adaptogenic activity of L-arginine supplementation. Evid Based Complement Alternat Med. 2005;2(1):93–7.
157. Collier SR, Casey DP, Kanaley JA. Growth hormone responses to varying doses of oral arginine. Growth Hormon IGF Res. 2005;15(2):136–9.
158. Boger RH, Bode Boger SM. The clinical pharmacology of L-arginine. Annu Rev Pharmacol Toxicol. 2001;41:79–99.
159. Boger RH, Bode Boger SM, Mugge A, Kienke S, Brandes R, Dwenger A, et al. Supplementation of hypercholesterolaemic rabbits with L-arginine reduces the vascular release of superoxide anions and restores NO production. Atherosclerosis. 1995;117(2):273–84.
160. Grasemann H, Kurtz F, Ratjen F. Inhaled L-arginine improves exhaled nitric oxide and pulmonary function in patients with cystic fibrosis. Am J Respir Crit Care Med. 2006;174(2):208–12.
161. Frostegard J, Haegerstrand A, Gidlund M, Nilsson J. Biologically modified LDL increases the adhesive properties of endothelial cells. Atherosclerosis. 1991;90:119–26.
162. Rajavashisth TB, Andalibi A, Territo MC, Berliner JA, Navab M, Fogelman AM, Lusis AJ. Induction of endothelial cell expression of granulocyte and macrophage colony-stimulating factors by modified low-density lipoproteins. Nature. 1990;344:254–7.
163. Yla-Herttuala S, Lipton BA, Rosenfeld ME, Sarkioja T, Yoshimura T, Leonard EJ, Witztum JL, Steinberg D. Expression of monocyte chemoattractant protein 1 in macrophage-rich areas of human and rabbit atherosclerotic lesions. Proc Natl Acad Sci U S A. 1991;88:5252–6.
164. Catapano AL, Maggi FM, Tragni E. Low density lipoprotein oxidation, antioxidants, and atherosclerosis. Curr Opin Cardiol. 2000;15:355–63.
165. Quinn MT, Parthasarathy S, Fong LG, Steinberg D. Oxidatively modified low density lipoproteins: a potential role in recruitment and retention of monocyte/macrophages during atherogenesis. Proc Natl Acad Sci U S A. 1987;84:2995–8.
166. Forstermann U, Sessa WC. Nitric oxide synthases: regulation and function. Eur Heart J. 2012;33:829–37, 837a–837d.
167. Blair A, Shaul PW, Yuhanna IS, Conrad PA, Smart EJ. Oxidized low density lipoprotein displaces endothelial nitric-oxide synthase (eNOS) from plasmalemmal caveolae and impairs eNOS activation. J Biol Chem. 1999;274:32512–9.
168. Cominacini L, Rigoni A, Pasini AF, Garbin U, Davoli A, Campagnola M, Pastorino AM, Lo Cascio V, Sawamura T. The binding of oxidized low density lipoprotein (ox-LDL) to ox-LDL receptor-1 reduces the intracellular concentration of nitric oxide in endothelial cells through an increased production of superoxide. J Biol Chem. 2001;276:13750–5.
169. Chen M, Masaki T, Sawamura T. LOX-1, the receptor for oxidized low-density lipoprotein identified from endothelial cells: implications in endothelial dysfunction and atherosclerosis. Pharmacol Ther. 2002;95:89–100.
170. Kataoka H, Kume N, Miyamoto S, Minami M, Moriwaki H, Murase T, Sawamura T, Masaki T, Hashimoto N, Kita T. Expression of lectinlike oxidized lowdensity lipoprotein receptor-1 in human atherosclerotic lesions. Circulation. 1999;99:3110–3117. Role of Oxidized LDL in Atherosclerosis. https://doi.org/10.5772/5937573.
171. Li D, Mehta JL. Antisense to LOX-1 inhibits oxidized LDL-mediated upregulation of monocyte chemoattractant protein-1 and monocyte adhesion to human coronary artery endothelial cells. Circulation. 2000;101:2889–95.
172. Li D, Chen H, Romeo F, Sawamura T, Saldeen T, Mehta JL. Statins modulate oxidized low-density

lipoprotein-mediated adhesion molecule expression in human coronary artery endothelial cells: role of LOX-1. J Pharmacol Exp Ther. 2002;302:601–5.
173. Cominacini L, Fratta Pasini A, Garbin U, Pastorino A, Rigoni A, Nava C, Davoli A, Lo Cascio V, Sawamura T. The platelet-endothelium interaction mediated by lectin-like oxidized low-density lipoprotein receptor-1 reduces the intracellular concentration of nitric oxide in endothelial cells. J Am Coll Cardiol. 2003;41:499–507.
174. Valente AJ, Irimpen AM, Siebenlist U, Chandrasekar B. OxLDL induces endothelial dysfunction and death via TRAF3IP2: inhibition by HDL3 and AMPK activators. Free Radic Biol Med. 2014;70C:117–28.
175. Leiva E, Wehinger S, Guzmán L, Orrego R. Role of oxidized LDL in atherosclerosis. In: Kumar SA, editor. Hypercholesterolemia; 2015. https://doi.org/10.5772/59375.
176. Rosen P, Nawroth PP, King G, Möller W, Tritschler H-J, Packer L. The role of oxidative stress in the onset and progression of diabetes and its complications: a summary of a Congress Series sponsored by UNESCO-MCBN, the American Diabetes Association and the German Diabetes Society. Diabetes Metab Res Rev. 2001;17(3):189–209. https://doi.org/10.1002/dmrr.196.
177. Rocha VZ, Libby P. Obesity, inflammation, and atherosclerosis. Nat Rev Cardiol. 2009;6(6):399–409. https://doi.org/10.1038/nrcardio.2009.55. Epub 2009 Apr 28. Review.
178. Shindel AW, Kishore S, Lue TF. Drugs designed to improve endothelial function: effects on erectile dysfunction. Curr Pharm Des. 2008;14(35):3758–67. Review.
179. Enzlin P, Mathieu C, Vanderschueren D, Demyttenaere K. Diabetes mellitus and female sexuality: a review of 25 years' research. Diabet Med. 1998;15(10):809–15.
180. Ryan JJ, Fang JC. Taking NO for an answer: exploring the therapeutic potential of nitrite in HFpEF. Circ Res. 2016;119(7):782–4. https://doi.org/10.1161/CIRCRESAHA.116.309623.
181. Zuo L, Chuang CC, Hemmelgarn BT, Best TM. Heart failure with preserved ejection fraction: defining the function of ROS and NO. J Appl Physiol. 2015;119(8):944–51. https://doi.org/10.1152/japplphysiol.01149.2014.
182. Gevaert AB, Shakeri H, Leloup AJ, Van Hove CE, De Meyer GRY, Vrints CJ, Lemmens K, Van Craenenbroeck EM. Endothelial senescence contributes to heart failure with preserved ejection fraction in an aging mouse model. Circ Heart Fail. 2017;10(6). pii: e003806. https://doi.org/10.1161/CIRCHEARTFAILURE.116.003806.
183. Octavia Y, Kararigas G, de Boer M, Chrifi I, Kietadisorn R, Swinnen M, Duimel H, Verheyen FK, Brandt MM, Fliegner D, Cheng C, Janssens S, Duncker DJ, Moens AL. Folic acid reduces doxorubicin-induced cardiomyopathy by modulating endothelial nitric oxide synthase. J Cell Mol Med. 2017. https://doi.org/10.1111/jcmm.13231. [Epub ahead of print].
184. Lahera V. Nitric oxide: a possible new biomarker in heart failure? Relationship with pulmonary hypertension secondary to left heart failure. Clin Investig Arterioscler. 2017;29(3):127–8. https://doi.org/10.1016/j.arteri.2017.04.001.
185. Kraehling JR, Sessa WC. Contemporary approaches to modulating the nitric oxide-cGMP pathway in cardiovascular disease. Circ Res. 2017;120(7):1174–82. https://doi.org/10.1161/CIRCRESAHA.117.303776. Review.
186. Ritchie RH, Drummond GR, Sobey CG, De Silva TM, Kemp-Harper BK. The opposing roles of NO and oxidative stress in cardiovascular disease. Pharmacol Res. 2017;116:57–69. https://doi.org/10.1016/j.phrs.2016.12.017. Epub 2016 Dec 15.
187. Sharma NM, Patel KP. Post-translational regulation of neuronal nitric oxide synthase: implications for sympathoexcitatory states. Expert Opin Ther Targets. 2017;21(1):11–22. Epub 2016 Dec 2. Review.
188. Zhang YH. Neuronal nitric oxide synthase in hypertension – an update. Clin Hypertens. 2016;22:20. eCollection 2016. Review.
189. Simon MA, Vanderpool RR, Nouraie M, Bachman TN, White PM, Sugahara M, Gorcsan J 3rd, Parsley EL, Gladwin MT. Acute hemodynamic effects of inhaled sodium nitrite in pulmonary hypertension associated with heart failure with preserved ejection fraction. JCI Insight. 2016;1(18):e89620.
190. Forte M, Conti V, Damato A, Ambrosio M, Puca AA, Sciarretta S, Frati G, Vecchione C, Carrizzo A. Targeting nitric oxide with natural derived compounds as a therapeutic strategy in vascular diseases. Oxidative Med Cell Longev. 2016;2016:7364138. https://doi.org/10.1155/2016/7364138. Epub 2016 Aug 29. Review.
191. Shabeeh H, Seddon M, Brett S, Melikian N, Casadei B, Shah AM, Chowienczyk P. Sympathetic activation increases NO release from eNOS but neither eNOS nor nNOS play an essential role in exercise hyperemia in the human forearm. Am J Physiol Heart Circ Physiol. 2013;304(9):H1225–30. https://doi.org/10.1152/ajpheart.00783.2012. Epub 2013 Feb 22.
192. Colombo J, Arora RR, DePace NL, Vinik AI. Clinical autonomic dysfunction: measurement, indications, therapies, and outcomes. New York: Springer Science + Business Media; 2014.
193. Zhang YH, Jin CZ, Jang JH, Wang Y. Molecular mechanisms of neuronal nitric oxide synthase in cardiac function and pathophysiology. J Physiol. 2014;592(15):3189–200. https://doi.org/10.1113/jphysiol.2013.270306. Epub 2014 Apr 22. Review.
194. Mohan RM, Choate JK, Golding S, Herring N, Casadei B, Paterson DJ. Peripheral pre-synaptic pathway reduces the heart rate response to sympathetic activation following exercise training: role of NO. Cardiovasc Res. 2000;47:90–8.

195. Choate JK, Danson EJ, Morris JF, Paterson DJ. Peripheral vagal control of heart rate is impaired in neuronal NOS knockout mice. Am J Physiol Heart Circ Physiol. 2001;281:H2310–7.
196. Danson EJ, Choate JK, Paterson DJ. Cardiac nitric oxide: emerging role for nNOS in regulating physiological function. Pharmacol Ther. 2005;106:57–74.
197. Han G, Ma H, Chintala R, Miyake K, Fulton DJ, Barman SA, White RE. Nongenomic, endothelium-independent effects of estrogen on human coronary smooth muscle are mediated by type I (neuronal) NOS and PI3-kinase-Akt signalling. Am J Physiol Heart Circ Physiol. 2007;293:H314–21.
198. Seddon M, Melikian N, Dworakowski R, Shabeeh H, Jiang B, Byrne J, Casadei B, Chowienczyk P, Shah AM. Effects of neuronal nitric oxide synthase on human coronary artery diameter and blood flow in vivo. Circulation. 2009;119:2656–62.
199. Wang Y, Golledge J. Neuronal nitric oxide synthase and sympathetic nerve activity in neurovascular and metabolic systems. Curr Neurovasc Res. 2013;10(1):81–9. Review.
200. Curtis BM, O'Keefe JH. Autonomic tone as a cardiovascular risk factor: the dangers of chronic fight or flight. Mayo Clin Proc. 2002;77:45–54.
201. Pyner S. The paraventricular nucleus and heart failure. Exp Physiol. 2014;99(2):332–9. https://doi.org/10.1113/expphysiol.2013.072678. Epub 2013 Dec 6. Review.
202. Rocha BML, Cunha GJL, Menezes Falcão LF. The burden of iron deficiency in heart failure: therapeutic approach. J Am Coll Cardiol. 2018;71(7):782–93.
203. Hu PJ, Pittet JF, Kerby JD, Bosarge PL, Wagener BM. Acute brain trauma, lung injury and pneumonia: more than just altered mental status and decreased airway protection. Am J Physiol Lung Cell Mol Physiol. 2017:ajplung.00485.2016. https://doi.org/10.1152/ajplung.00485.2016. [Epub ahead of print].
204. Pacher P, Beckman JS, Liaudet L. Nitric oxide and peroxynitrite in health and disease. Physiol Rev. 2007;87(1):315–424. Review.
205. Spanagel R. Alcoholism: a systems approach from molecular physiology to addictive behavior. Physiol Rev. 2009;89(2):649–705. https://doi.org/10.1152/physrev.00013.2008. Review.
206. Lee RH, Tseng TY, Wu CY, Chen PY, Chen MF, Kuo JS, Lee TJ. Memantine inhibits α3β2-nAChRs-mediated nitrergic neurogenic vasodilation in porcine basilar arteries. PLoS One. 2012;7(7):e40326. https://doi.org/10.1371/journal.pone.0040326. Epub 2012 Jul 5.
207. Filiano AJ, Gadani SP, Kipnis J. Interactions of innate and adaptive immunity in brain development and function. Brain Res. 2015;1617:18–27. PMC 4320678. PMID 25110235. https://doi.org/10.1016/j.brainres.2014.07.050.
208. Mukherjee P, Cinelli MA, Kang S, Silverman RB. Development of nitric oxide synthase inhibitors for neurodegeneration and neuropathic pain. Chem Soc Rev. 2014;43(19):6814–38. https://doi.org/10.1039/c3cs60467e. Review.
209. Bowerman M, Vincent T, Scamps F, Perrin FE, Camu W, Raoul C. Neuroimmunity dynamics and the development of therapeutic strategies for amyotrophic lateral sclerosis. Front Cell Neurosci. 2013;7:214. https://doi.org/10.3389/fncel.2013.00214. Review.
210. Gehrmann J, Matsumoto Y, Kreutzberg GW. Microglia: intrinsic immuneffector cell of the brain. Brain Res Rev. 1995;20(3):269–87.
211. Chen Y, Liu L. Modern methods for delivery of drugs across the blood-brain barrier. Adv Drug Deliv Rev. 2012;64(7):640–65. https://doi.org/10.1016/j.addr.2011.11.010. Epub 2011 Nov 28.
212. Streit WJ. Microglial senescence: does the brain's immune system have an expiration date? Trends Neurosci. 2006;29(9):506–10.
213. Wood P. Neuroinflammation: mechanisms and management. Totowa: Humana Press; 2003.
214. Clark AK, Staniland AA, Marchand F, Kaan TKY, McMahon SB, Malcangio M. P2X7-dependent release of interleukin-1 and nociception in the spinal cord following lipopolysaccharide. J Neurosci. 2010;30(2):573–82.
215. Shigemoto-Mogami Y, Koizumi S, Tsuda M, Ohsawa K, Kohsaka S, Inoue K. Mechanisms underlying extracellular ATP-evoked interleukin-6 release in mouse microglial cell line, MG-5. J Neurochem. 2001;78(6):1339–49.
216. Hide I, Tanaka M, Inoue A, Nakajima K, Kohsaka S, Inoue K, Nakata Y. Extracellular ATP triggers tumor necrosis factor-α release from rat microglia. J Neurochem. 2002;75(3):965–72.
217. Witcher KG, Eiferman DS, Godbout JP. Priming the inflammatory pump of the CNS after traumatic brain injury. Trends Neurosci. 2015;38(10):609–20. https://doi.org/10.1016/j.tins.2015.08.002. Review.
218. Gokce N. L-arginine and hypertension. J Nutr. 2004;134(10 Suppl):2807S–11S; discussion 2818S–2819S.
219. Higashi Y, Oshima T, Ozono R, et al. Aging and severity of hypertension attenuate endothelium-dependent renal vascular relaxation in humans. Hypertension. 1997;30(2 Pt 1):252–8.
220. Clarkson P, Adams MR, Powe AJ, et al. Oral L-arginine improves endothelium-dependent dilation in hypercholesterolemic young adults. J Clin Invest. 1996;97(8):1989–94.
221. Kawano H, Motoyama T, Hirai N, et al. Endothelial dysfunction in hypercholesterolemia is improved by L-arginine administration: possible role of oxidative stress. Atherosclerosis. 2002;161(2):375–80.
222. Adams MR, McCredie R, Jessup W, et al. Oral L-arginine improves endothelium-dependent dilatation and reduces monocyte adhesion to endothelial cells in young men with coronary artery disease. Atherosclerosis. 1997;129(2):261–9.
223. Sydow K, Mondon CE, Cooke JP. Insulin resistance: potential role of the endogenous nitric oxide syn-

thase inhibitor ADMA. Vasc Med. 2005;10(Suppl 1):S35–43.
224. Piatti PM, Monti LD, Valsecchi G, et al. Long-term oral L-arginine administration improves peripheral and hepatic insulin sensitivity in type 2 diabetic patients. Diabetes Care. 2001;24(5):875–80.
225. Pieper GM, Siebeneich W, Dondlinger LA. Short-term oral administration of L-arginine reverses defective endothelium-dependent relaxation and cGMP generation in diabetes. Eur J Pharmacol. 1996;317(2–3):317–20.
226. Bode-Boger SM, Muke J, Surdacki A, et al. Oral L-arginine improves endothelial function in healthy individuals older than 70 years. Vasc Med. 2003;8(2):77–81.
227. Alvares TS, Meirelles CM, Bhambhani YN, et al. L-arginine as a potential ergogenic aid in healthy subjects. Sports Med. 2011;41(3):233–48.
228. Vallance P, Chan N. Endothelial function and nitric oxide: clinical relevance. Heart. 2001;85(3):342–50.
229. Boger RH, Cooke JP, Vallance P. ADMA: an emerging cardiovascular risk factor. Vasc Med. 2005;10(Suppl 1):S1–2.
230. Cooke JP. ADMA: its role in vascular disease. Vasc Med. 2005;10(Suppl 1):S11–7.
231. Boger RH. Asymmetric dimethylarginine, an endogenous inhibitor of nitric oxide synthase, explains the "L-arginine paradox" and acts as a novel cardiovascular risk factor. J Nutr. 2004;134(10 Suppl):2842S–7S; discussion 2853S.
232. Sibal L, Agarwal SC, Home PD, et al. The role of asymmetric dimethylarginine (ADMA) in endothelial dysfunction and cardiovascular disease. Curr Cardiol Rev. 2010;6(2):82–90.
233. Cooke JP. Asymmetrical dimethylarginine: the Uber marker? Circulation. 2004;109(15):1813–8.
234. Tran CT, Leiper JM, Vallance P. The DDAH/ADMA/NOS pathway. Atheroscler Suppl. 2003;4(4):33–40.

# 5 Oxidative Stress Reduction (Prong-3)

The third prong of the Mind-Body Wellness Program (Fig. 5.1) focuses on reducing oxidative stress. The purpose is to (1) decrease reactive oxygen species (ROS; see Fig. 2.26) and free radicals (see Figs. 2.24 and 2.25) when they are harmful to the body and (2) increase antioxidant defenses (Fig. 5.60) to establish and maintain an appropriate antioxidant-oxidant balance that promotes health and wellness. In essence, the goal of this approach is to increase antioxidant buffer capacity. The preceding sections of this book already introduce a number of issues regarding oxidation

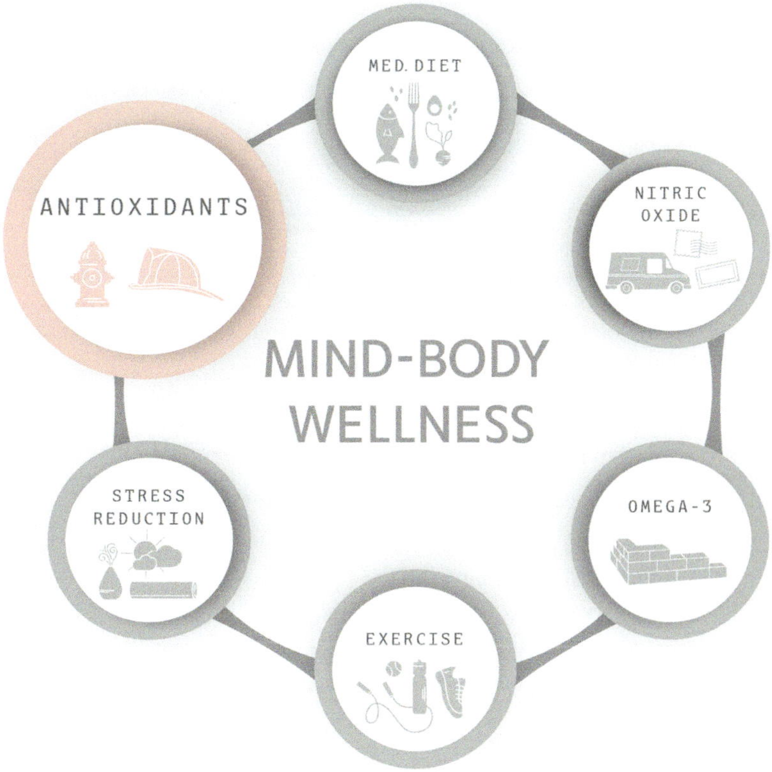


**Fig. 5.1** The Mind Body-Wellness Program – Oxidative stress reduction prong. (Illustration by Elysian Creative Studio, www.elysiancreativestudio.com, Lizzy Colombo)


N. L. DePace, J. Colombo, *Clinical Autonomic and Mitochondrial Disorders*,
https://doi.org/10.1007/978-3-030-17016-5_5

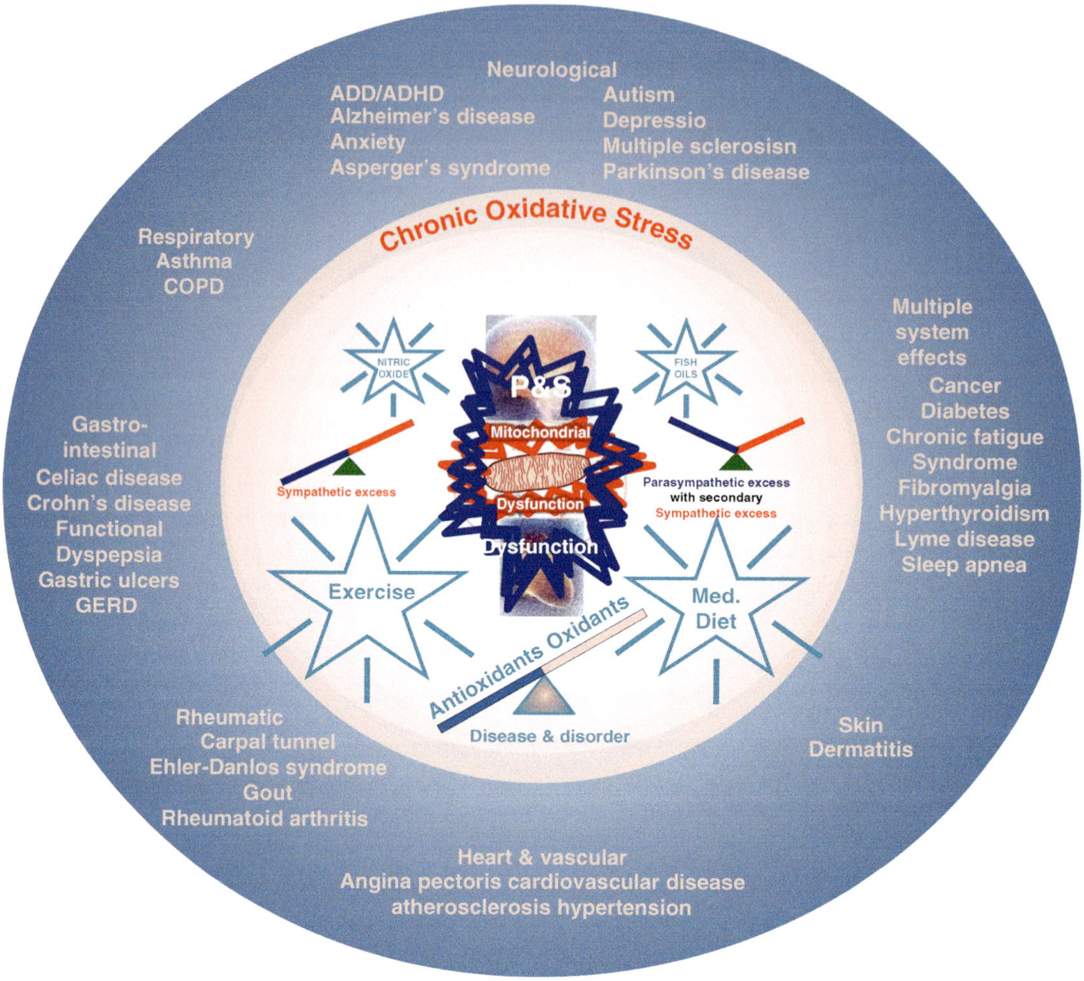


**Fig. 5.2** Clinical examples of the effects of chronic oxidative stress. Chronic oxidative stress may lead to P&S disorders (S-excess and P-excess with secondary S-excess. Chronic oxidative stress may be relieved by exercise, diet, nitric oxide supplements, and fish oil supplements. (Adapted from: http://bestincorporatehealth.com/oxidative-stress-stress)

(see Fig. 2.25) and its causes: oxidative stress and its contributors (including the "dark side" of very necessary processes: mitochondrial function and nitric oxide function) and the antioxidant natures of omega-3 fatty acids and nitric oxide [1]. The last three chapters will also involve oxidants, oxidative stress, and antioxidants in natural, non-pharmaceutical, and non-nutraceutical forms. The Mediterranean diet (see Fig. 2.32) provides a number of exogenous sources of antioxidants, which will be discussed in that chapter. As mentioned earlier, exercise is arguably the best and most efficient of all antioxidants and will be discussed in that chapter. Psychosocial stress is arguably the most pervasive of all oxidative stresses, and how reducing it is an antioxidant in itself will be discussed it that chapter. Antioxidants repair, remove, and prevent radical oxygen and nitrogen species and other free radical damage by adding electrons to all types of free radicals. The clinical manifestations of oxidative stress are numerous (see Fig. 5.2) and, under chronic conditions, often present in multiples.

As stated above, sources of oxidative stress are ubiquitous (e.g., Fig. 2.16). They are internal as well as external. Antioxidants themselves,

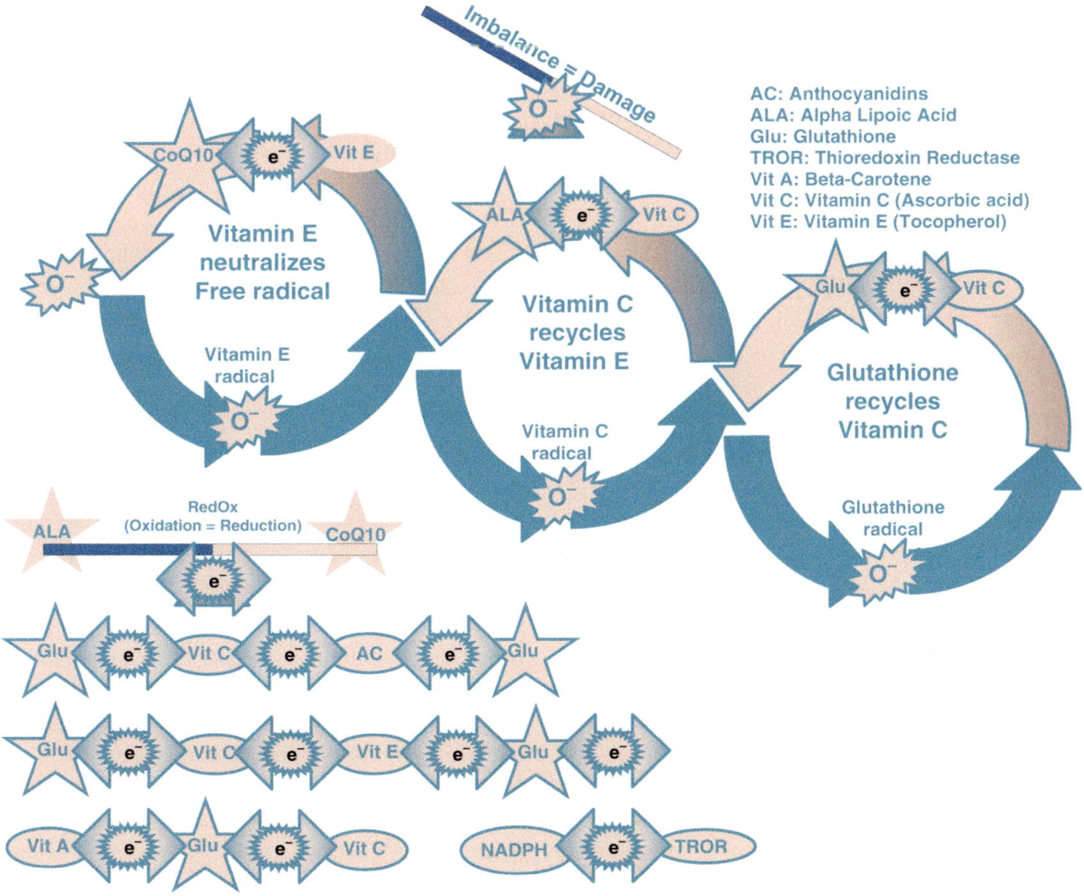


**Fig. 5.3** Antioxidant buffer requires several antioxidants, in surplus, working together to share electrons between themselves to remain antioxidants and provide electrons to neutralize ROS, RNS, and free radicals before they damage healthy tissue. (Source: http://www.happyliving.com/2016/09/02/use-the-power-of-antioxidants-to-take-down-free-radicals/) An example of antioxidant recycling. The antioxidants work together to maintain a healthy antioxidant buffer and to prevent themselves from becoming oxidants. In this example, a free radical is eliminated by vitamin E, which will be recovered by vitamin C. Vitamin C then will be recycled by glutathione, which will be restored by anthocyanidins. Coenzyme Q10, beta-carotene, and alpha-lipoic acid help each other. (Source: http://www.buyvitaminsonline.com.au/blog/tag/usana-healthpak/)

once they have given up their electron, become oxidants and need an electron from somewhere else. If this electron comes from atoms or molecules in healthy positions or situations, the oxidative process is perpetuated. Fortunately, there is an antioxidant network (Fig. 2.28) where many antioxidants work together to keep the giving and receiving of electrons "within the family." The network helps to prevent other molecules from having to get involved. This is known as the antioxidant buffer (see Fig. 5.3). Even critical processes generate oxidants. As discussed, mitochondria generate oxidants as a normal course of function (Fig. 2.17). Not all oxidants are bad. Nitric oxide is a natural oxidant. The immune system recruits oxidants of all sorts, and even generates oxidants, to combat invading pathogens. Oxidative stress affects many pathways (Fig. 2.23).

Again, not all are bad. Like nitric oxide, a little (in time and space) is healthful; in addition to helping the immune system, they are used in signaling, among other physiologic activities. As with everything else in life, moderation; a little is actually good. This moderation is the antioxidant-oxidant balance. The way red blood cells carry oxygen from the lungs to the rest of the body is an oxidation reaction. The iron atoms in the red blood cells literally rust (oxidize) as they collect oxygen to enable the red blood cell to carry the oxygen (that is why they are red, from the rust). Remember oxidation is a type of burning, and the body uses oxidation to literally help to "recycle the trash." Definitely, though, too much oxidation is never good. Small fires are helpful (cooking, staying warm, burning trash, and making things). Large fires destroy.

To reduce oxidative stress, first a balance between oxidants and antioxidants must be achieved (see Fig. 5.4). Then, to maintain the balance and promote wellness, an antioxidant buffer must be established and maintained. A healthy diet and exercise are important but may not be enough; supplements may add the antioxidants that may be in deficit or missing, especially as systems age (physiologic age may be years ahead of chronological age due to injury, disease, lifestyle, or genetics). At the subcellular level, this will maintain healthy mitochondrial and nitric oxide function to help maintain (1) supple, well integrated, and properly functioning membranes; and (2) healthy DNA. At the cellular level, antioxidants combat oxidative stress and help to maintain proper endothelial function, provide (virtually) all cells with sufficient energy supplies, and maintain proper communications, growth, replication, repair, and recycling.

At the organ and system level, antioxidants combat oxidative stress and help to maintain (1) a healthy cardiovascular system to ensure proper blood supply; (2) a healthy immune system to (a) keep the body free of debris, (b) attack pathogens (bacterial, viral, and parasite infections) before they are able to establish themselves, (c) scavenge pre-cancer cells as they form, (d) decrease the incidence of autoimmune disease, (e) decrease the level of incidence and prevalence of various malignancies, (f) decrease allergies, and (g) slow the progression of aging to all parts of the body [2]; and (3) maintain a healthy nervous system to (a) coordinate and control both the cardiovascular and immune systems and all other systems of the body to promote proper bodily functions and to (b) maintain proper brain (including the central autonomic nervous system) and cognitive functions. Oxidative stress is associated with

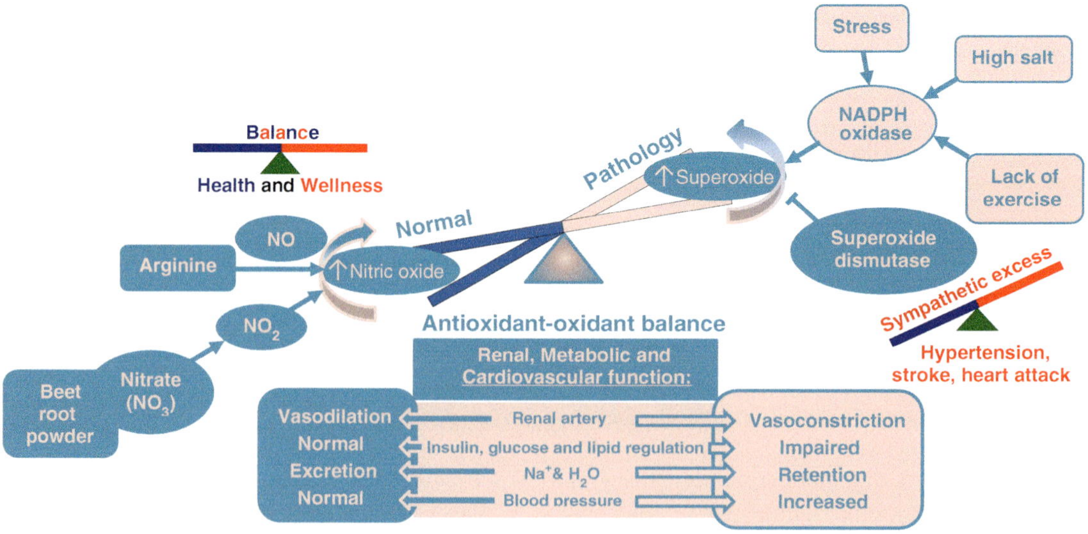


**Fig. 5.4** An example of the effects of balance and imbalance between antioxidants and oxidants. Imbalance between nitric oxide (NO) and reactive oxygen species (ROS) signaling has been linked to renal dysfunction, metabolic syndrome, cardiovascular disease, and type 2 diabetes. (Source: http://ki.se/en/fyfa/reactive-oxygen-species-and-nitric-oxide-signaling-in-renal-and-cardiovascular-function)

depression-anxiety syndromes, chronic fatigue, fibromyalgia, migraines, neurodegenerative diseases, ADD/ADHD, autonomic dysfunction, atherosclerosis, and COPD, to name a few. Supplements to help reduce oxidative stress and to minimize the risk of, or help to relieve, these disorders and diseases include alpha-lipoic acid; coenzyme Q10, vitamins A, C, and E; beta-carotene; cysteine; and zinc. Note, alpha-lipoic acid and coenzyme Q10 provide bonus antioxidant action, in that they also recycle the vitamins and more, including glutathione (Fig. 5.5).

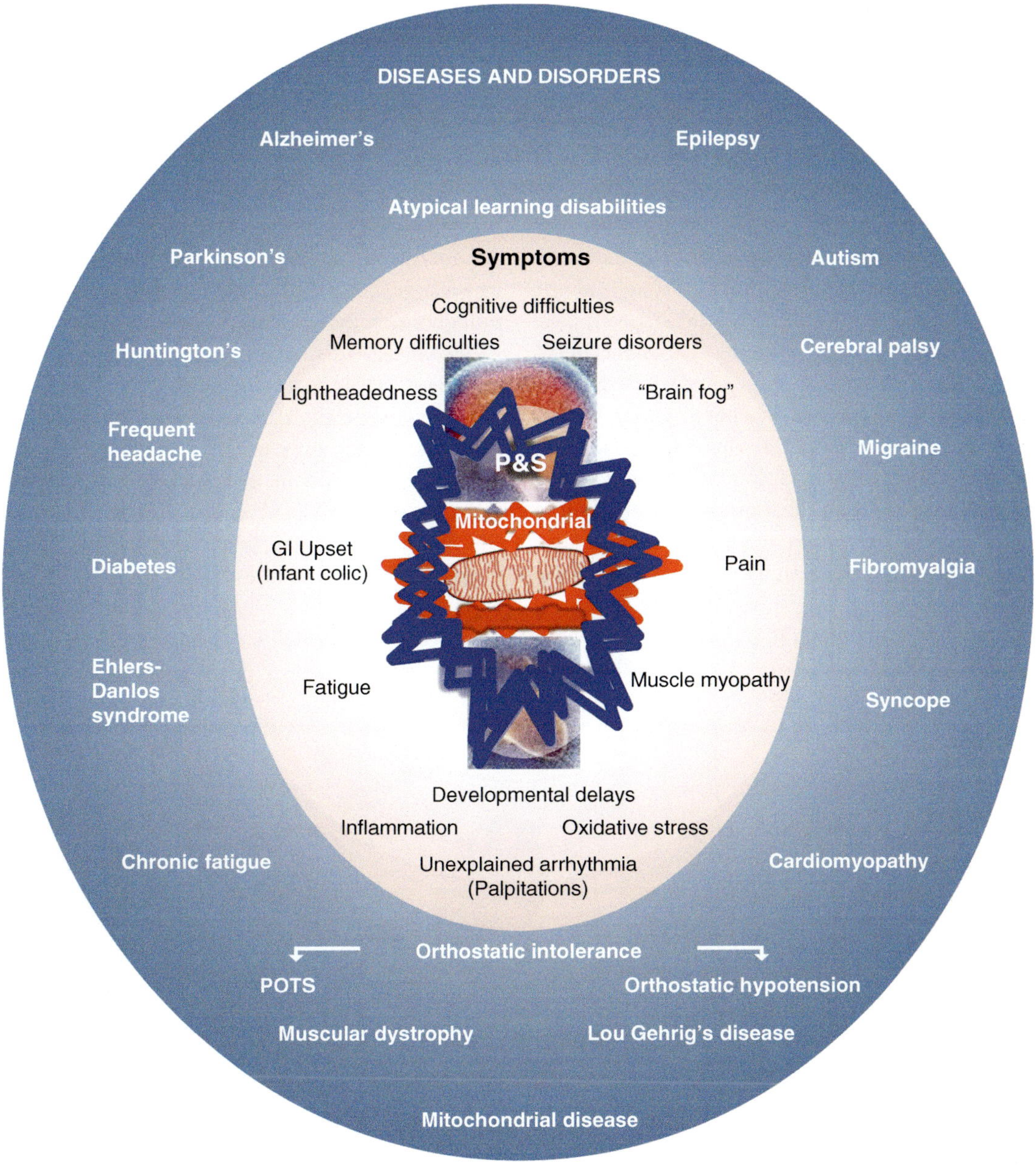


**Fig. 5.5** Mitochondrial dysfunction underlies autonomic (P&S) dysfunction which is associated with many diseases and disorders throughout the body and morbidity and mortality risks. Mitochondrial and autonomic dysfunction go together like Laurel and Hardy, Bud and Lou, Sears and Roebuck, or Funk and Wagnall. (Sources: Adapted from https://adultonsetmitochondrialdisease.wordpress.com/ and http://www.myquinstory.info/fluoroquinolones-mitochondrial-dysfunction/)

## Reduce Mitochondrial Dysfunction

As a reminder, mitochondria are organelles in cells. There are up to 2000 mitochondria in virtually every cell in the human body, with the most notable exception being red blood cells. Mitochondria require oxygen for cellular respiration. They make the ATP which is the energy molecule in the body (Fig. 2.14). As introduced in the Summary chapter at the beginning of the book, oxidative stress often causes mitochondrial dysfunction, not that mitochondria are perfect to begin with. As also introduced at the beginning of the book, mitochondria, themselves, contribute to oxidative stress (see Fig. 2.15), perhaps only very little per mitochondrion (1–3%), but there are thousands of trillions of them throughout the body. Doing the math, mitochondria are the greatest producers of oxidants within the body. Antioxidants help keep the oxidants (ROS) produced by mitochondria in check. Other factors that lead to mitochondrial dysfunction include decrease in (cellular) respiratory complex activity, increase in free radical production (including reactive nitrogen species, RNS), increase in mitochondrial synthase activity, increase in nitric oxide production, impaired electron transport system, and mitochondrial permeability.

Mitochondria are the factories, or powerhouses, of the cells and are the key organelles in the process of cellular respiration. As a reminder, mitochondria house (Fig. 2.8) the citric acid cycle (or Krebs cycle, Fig. 2.12) and the electron transport chain (Fig. 2.13) which produces ATP, the energy molecule of the body. Mitochondrial dysfunction includes a loss of efficiency in the production of ATP and a decrease in the number of ATP produced [3]. It also includes a reduction in the numbers of mitochondria to produce ATP, resulting in fewer ATP. This results in less energy for the systems of the body to function properly, especially the nervous system (including the brain), which is the greatest energy consumer. Another result of the loss of efficiency is an increase in free radical (ROS) production by the mitochondria themselves.

Given their distribution throughout the body, mitochondrial leakage damages cells throughout the body, especially if there are not enough antioxidants already present. This is a characteristic of aging and results in, and is a result of, chronic diseases (Fig. 5.5). Mitochondrial dysfunction can affect all body parts and organs (Fig. 5.6). Persistent oxidative stress also destroys mitochondria (see Fig. 2.24). Cumulatively, oxidative stress accelerates the aging (see Fig. 2.25,

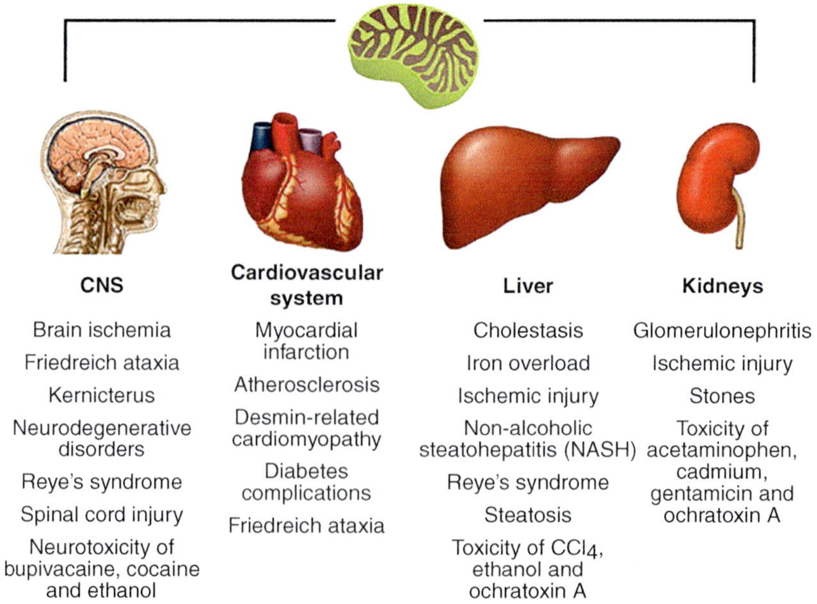


**Fig. 5.6** Mitochondrial dysfunction affects many organ systems throughout the body and may also cause chronic fatigue, fibromyalgia, and migraine. (Republished with permission from the American Physiological Society. Source: [4, Fig. 12])

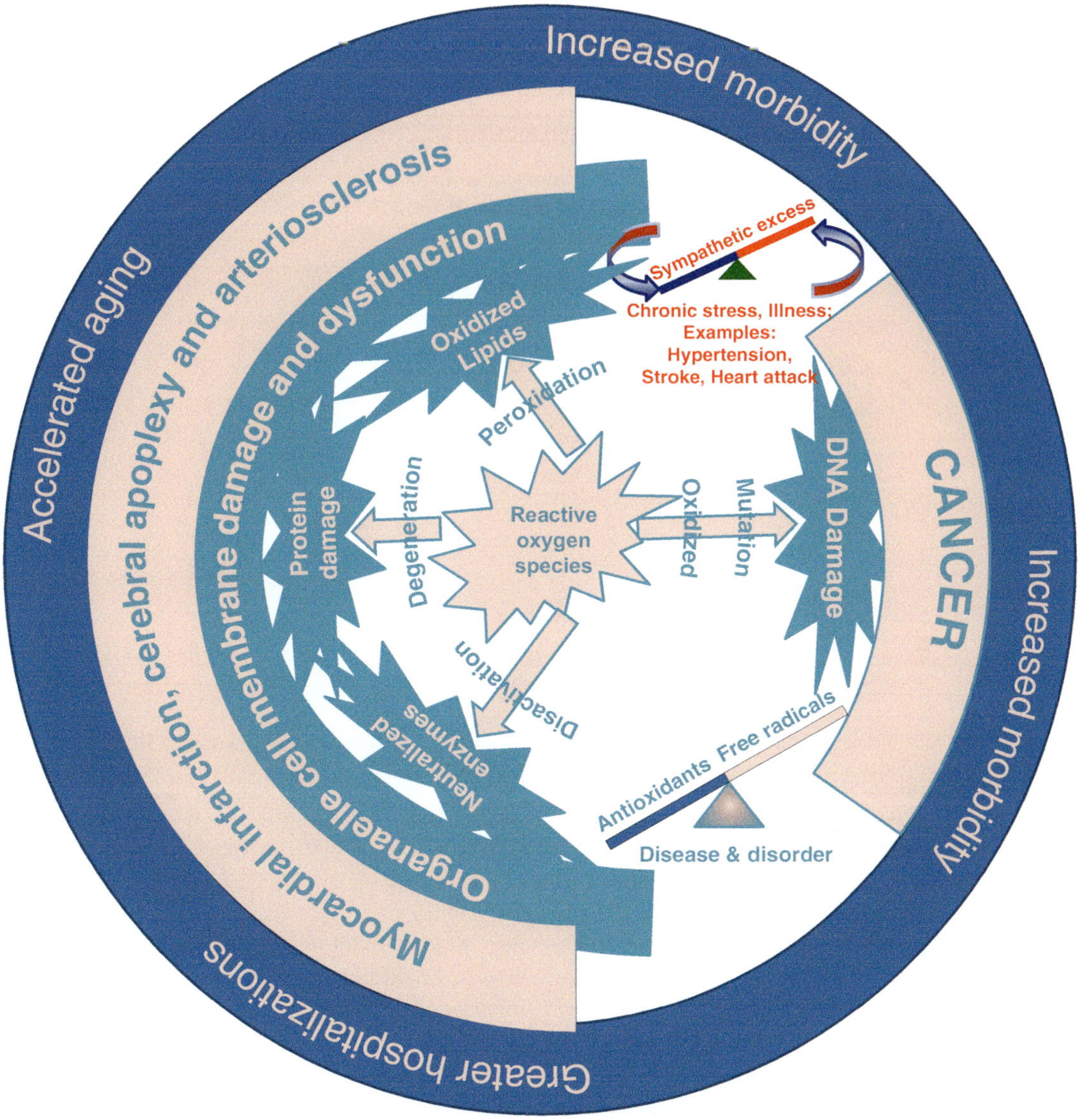


**Fig. 5.7** Cell and tissue damage by reactive oxygen species (ROS). (Source: https://www.cosmobio.com/contents/products_nns_20060421.html)

Fig. 2.26) and chronic diseases processes (see Figs. 2.27 and 2.28), including by slowing the immune system. Slowing the immune system enables and promotes tumor genesis[1] (Fig. 5.7).

Mitochondrial dysfunction may cause mitochondrial disease. Mitochondrial disease may be genetic, thereby inherited, presenting from infancy when they are primary mitochondrial diseases [5]. In primary mitochondrial disorders, stroke like

[1]The day you are born, your body creates pre-cancer cells. Cancer is simply a mass of your own cells that did not divide properly so that they begin to grow outside the checks and balances of your own body. It is a purpose of your immune system, beginning the day you are born, to find all of these cells and destroy them. As immune systems age and slow, some cells may be missed, and a tumor is permitted to start because the tumor cells are not "tagged" for destruction and therefore are assumed to be a normal part of the body.

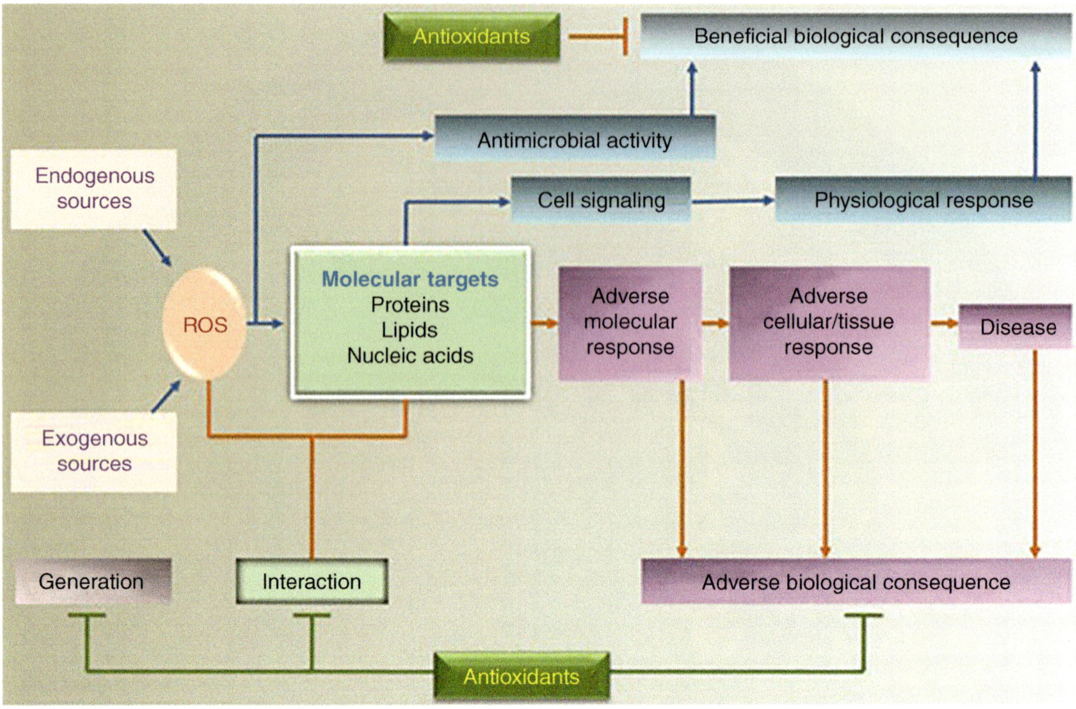


**Fig. 5.8** The ROS paradigm defines the scope of ROS activity which includes generation of ROS and related reactive species (RNS), the interactions of these reactive species with target biomolecules, and the resulting biological consequences (adverse or beneficial: *the paradigm*). This paradigm also depicts the antioxidant-based intervention of diseases associated with ROS, emphasizing the importance of selectively controlling ROS-mediated adverse effects without compromising the physiological functions of these species. (Open Access, Cell Med Press, AIMSCI Scientific Publishing. Source: [8, Fig. 5])

syndromes, migraines, cortical blindness, developmental delays, seizures, muscle weakness, peripheral neuropathies, and many other abnormalities are associated. In these mitochondrial disorders, increased ROS, abnormal calcium regulation, and reduced synaptic plasticity are seen [6]. However, the more common types of mitochondrial dysfunction occur with aging [7].

Key ROS products produced in the body include the superoxide radical ($O_2$), hydroperoxyl radical (HOO-), hydroxyl radical (OH), lipid peroxyl radical (ROO), nitric oxide, and peroxynitrate (OONO-). The singlet oxygen[2] and hydrogen peroxide ($H_2O_2$) are also included (Figs. 2.29). Antioxidants react with ROS to prevent or repair damage to tissues (see Figs. 2.18). However, ROS (as well as RNS and free radicals) may, themselves, be healthful in addition to harmful. This is the "ROS paradigm" (Fig. 5.8). The deleterious effects of ROS, when turned against invading microbes, turn positive as they demonstrate, beneficially, antimicrobial activity (Fig. 5.9). They are still damaging, but in these cases they damage cells that are themselves damaging. (This demonstrates the adaptability of the body, and two negatives can make a positive.) ROS can attack a diverse range of targets to exert antimicrobial activity, which accounts for their versatility in mediating host defense against a broad range of pathogens [10]. Antibiotics kill bacteria in part by inducing ROS [9, 11]. The ROS paradigm underlies important mechanisms for the integrity and fitness of life and aging. The pathways that regulate ROS homeostasis are crucial for neutralizing the toxicity of ROS and demonstrate ROS cellular signaling activity (Fig. 5.10) [12–16]. This is another example of how the body can use all things for good, as long as the "things" are kept in moderate amounts. Note: antioxidants also block the

[2] The singlet oxygen which is not a free radical per se, yet it is still unstable. $O_2$ is preferred, not O.

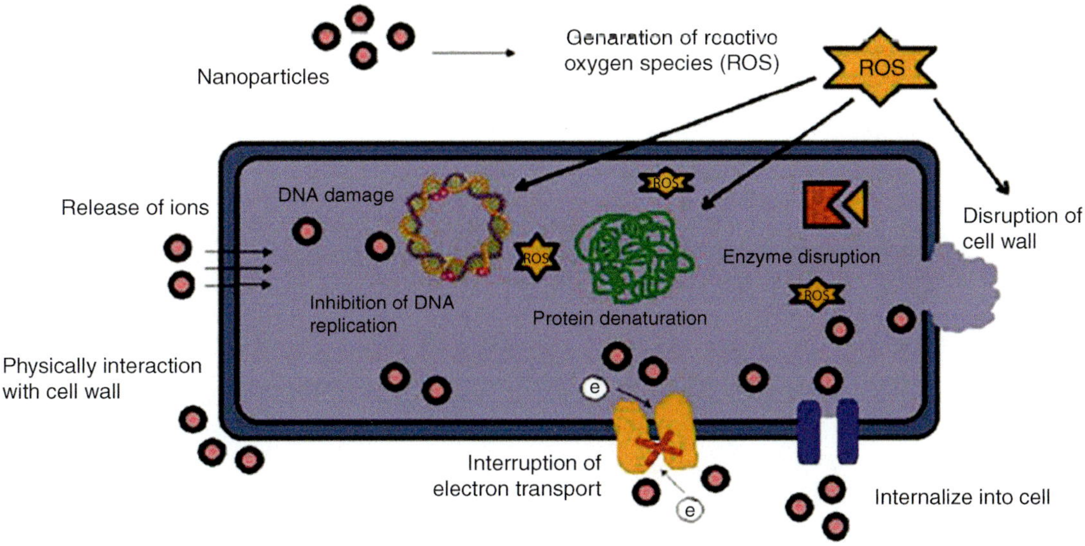


**Fig. 5.9** Various mechanisms of antimicrobial activity of ROS (from metal nanoparticles, e.g., zinc, copper, and magnesium). (Republished with permission from Elsevier. Source: [9])

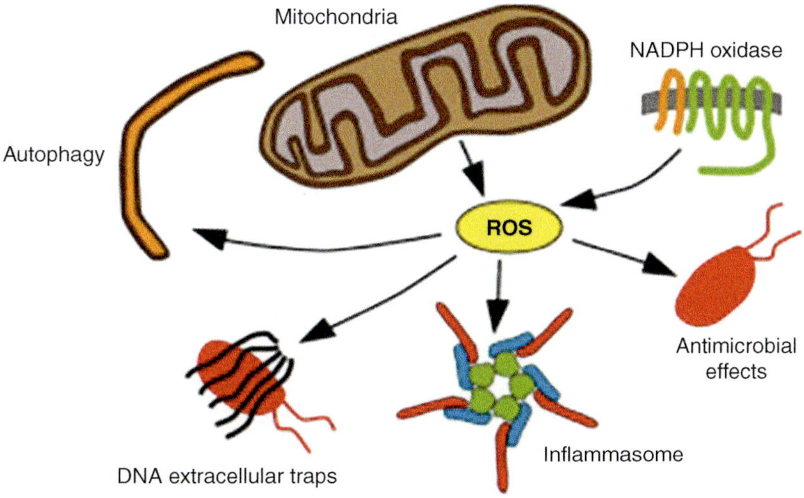


**Fig. 5.10** ROS signaling. Reactive oxygen species (ROS) are integral components of multiple cellular pathways, even though excessive or inappropriately localized ROS damage cells. ROS function as antimicrobial effector molecules and as signaling molecules that regulate such processes as autophagy (an intracellular degradation system that delivers cytoplasmic constituents to the lysosome), inflammasomes (a multiprotein molecule of the immune system), and the production of DNA-based neutrophil extracellular traps (used to control microbial infections). (Republished with permission from Elsevier. Source: [12])

"good" results of ROS functions (see Fig. 5.10), but this should not prevent the establishment and maintenance of a proper antioxidant milieu within the body, including a sufficient antioxidant buffer. The buffer will keep the ROS local to where they are produced for a beneficial purpose and keep them from migrating, or spreading, to where they are harmful (Fig. 5.11).

Decreasing ATP, the energy source, can produce chronic fatigue [19]. Other disorders associated with mitochondrial dysfunction are also associated with autonomic dysfunction, most likely the result

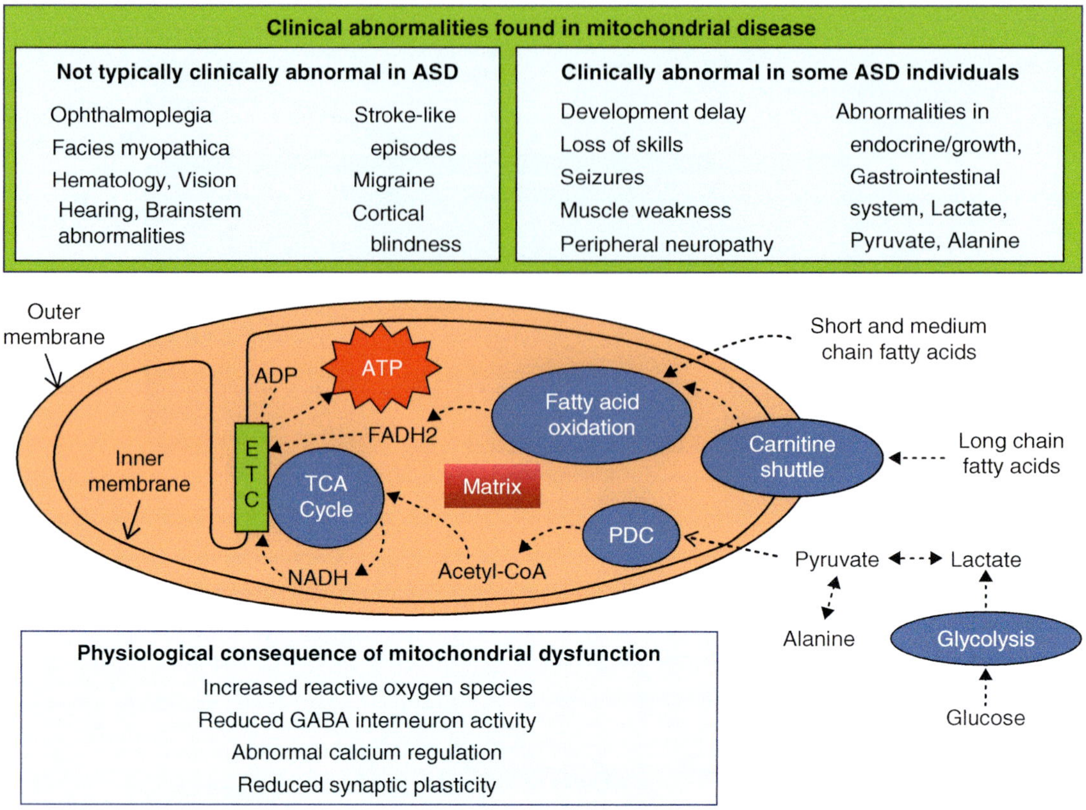


**Fig. 5.11** Consequences of mitochondrial disease in the brain. This example is based on autism spectrum disorders (ASD). The top panel outlines some of the features and metabolic markers used to diagnose mitochondrial disease. The features are divided up into those that are not typically clinically abnormal in ASD and those found to be clinically abnormal in some individuals with ASD. These features are found in many diagnoses associated with mitochondrial disease. The mitochondrion is represented diagrammatically in the middle of the figure. Glucose and fatty acids are processed through separate but overlapping pathways to create ATP. The fatty acid oxidation pathway, tricarboxylic acid (TCA) cycle, and pyruvate dehydrogenase complex (PDC) are located within the mitochondrion matrix, which is located inside the inner mitochondrial membrane. Long-chain fatty acids require the carnitine shuttle to enter the mitochondrial matrix, whereas medium- and short-chain fatty acids do not require the carnitine shuttle. One of the enzymes for the TCA cycle, succinate dehydrogenase, is complex II of the electron transport chain (ETC). Electron carriers, NADH and FADH2, transfer energy from the TCA cycle, and fatty acid oxidation pathway to the ETC. The ETC is the final common pathway for the generation of ATP from ADP. The bottom panel lists some of the physiological consequences of mitochondrial dysfunction [17]. (Open Access, Springer Nature Publishing Group. Source: [18])

of damage to mitochondria in neurons and decreased production of energy to those neurons. Therefore, autonomic dysfunction is often associated with chronic fatigue in mitochondrial dysfunction entities [20, 21]. Mitochondrial dysfunction has been established as associated with cardiomyopathies [22], various developmental delays (e.g., Fig. 5.11), genetic dysfunctions (Fig. 5.11), mitochondrial diseases at birth, and acquired mitochondrial dysfunctions such as muscular dystrophies. More recently, evidence is building that associates mitochondrial dysfunction with brain ischemia, neurotoxicity, autism, Parkinson's, epilepsy, learning disability, ALS, fibromyalgia, diabetes and its complications, developmental disease, Alzheimer's disease, Huntington's disease, cerebral palsy, and other neurodegenerative diseases, myocardial infarction, atherosclerosis, ischemia/reperfusion, aging process, and septic shock (see Fig. 5.12) [18, 24]. Alpha-lipoic acid is one of the most powerful antioxidants naturally occurring in the body and is known to be selective for nerves. This may the basis for the benefit of alpha-lipoic acid as a preventative and therapy for slowing the progression

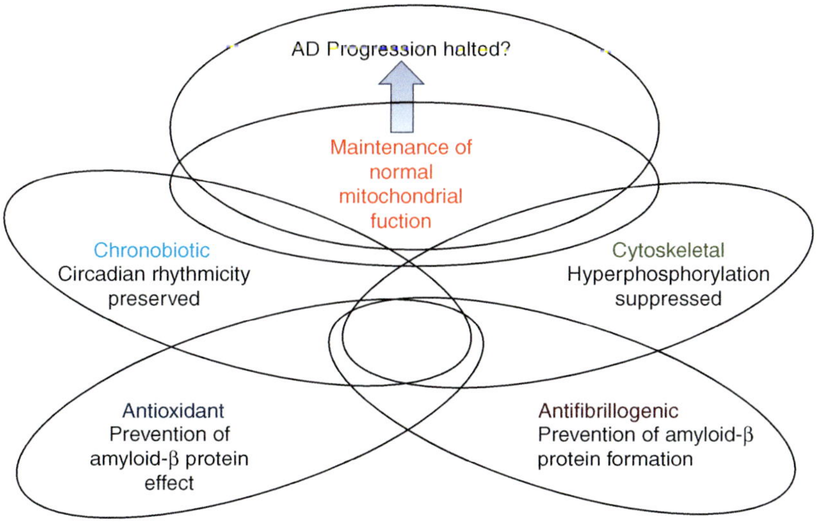


**Fig. 5.12** Maintenance of normal mitochondrial function with normal melatonin function may help halt the progression of Alzheimer's disease and other neurodegenerative diseases. The multiple effects and the different degrees of overlap (interrelations and mutual influences) are indicated by their respective intersections. (Republished with permission from Springer International Publishing AG. Source: [23, Fig. 8.23])

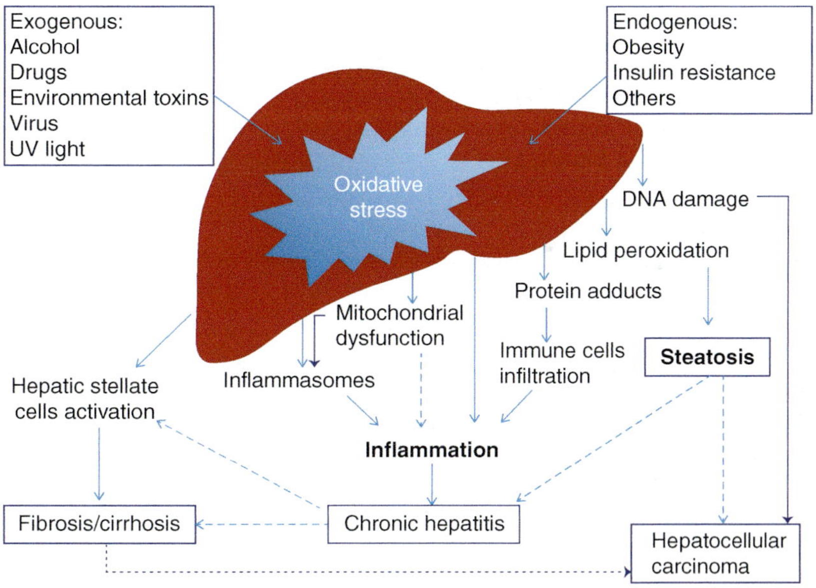


**Fig. 5.13** Consequences of mitochondrial disease outside the brain. This example depicts the general mechanistic scheme of oxidative stress induced by various factors of liver disease. (Open Access, MDPI. Source: [25])

of autonomic neuropathy. Maintenance of normal mitochondrial function with normal melatonin function may help halt the progression of Alzheimer's disease (see Fig. 5.12) and other neurodegenerative diseases (Fig. 5.13).

Again, dysfunction of the mitochondria can affect all organ systems, including the GI tract, the liver (ischemic injury, fatty liver, iron over-load, see Fig. 5.13), and the kidney (ischemic injury, various forms of nephritis). It may cause chronic pain, muscle myopathies, fibromyalgia-like syndromes, seizure disorders, neurodegenerative disorders, cancer, and many cognitive dysfunction states [26, 27]. These are often acquired and are not genetic. Although there is a genetic susceptibility in some individuals who develop mitochondrial, and perhaps thereby autonomic, dysfunction during their lifetime, there are those who do not. Many demonstrate familial connections with mitochondrial dysfunction and several familial diseases.

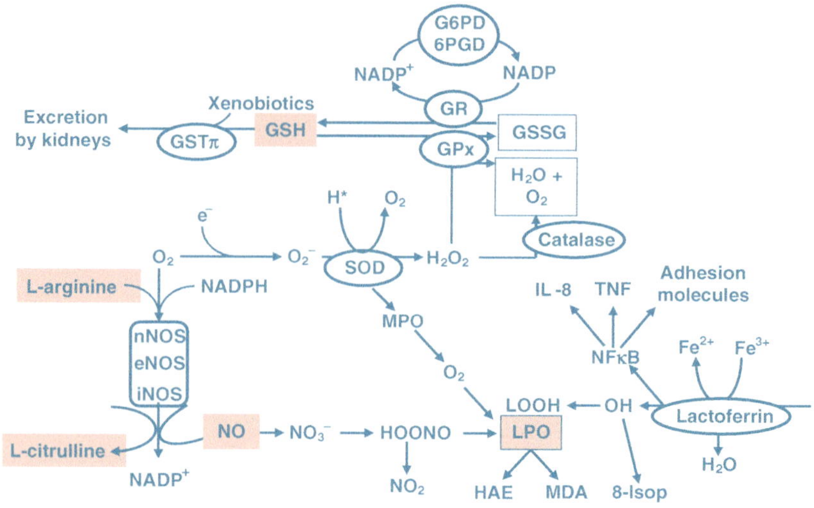


**Fig. 5.14** Oxidative stress pathways. See text for details. (Source: http://www.deltaclon.com/secciones/catalogo-assay/)

Free radicals (ROS, RNS, and other free radicals, generally known as activated oxygen species, or AOS) and increased oxidative stress have been associated with disease entities similar to what has been seen with mitochondrial dysfunction [28]. The basis for this association is that both mitochondrial dysfunction and formation of free radicals (ROS) and oxidative stress are interconnected, as discussed earlier in the book.

As an example, excessive ROS in the liver disturbs homeostasis, resulting in oxidative stress and often mitochondrial disease (Fig. 5.14). Oxidative stress plays a critical role in liver diseases and other chronic and degenerative disorders [29]. Oxidative stress not only triggers hepatic damage by inducing irretrievable alteration of lipids, proteins, and DNA but more importantly modulating pathways they support that control normal biological functions. Since these pathways regulate gene transcription, protein expression, cell apoptosis, and hepatic stellate cell activation, validating oxidative stress as one of the pathological mechanisms is important in establishing and maintaining health and wellness. Oxidative stress may result in the initiation and progression of various liver diseases, such as chronic viral hepatitis, alcoholic liver diseases, and nonalcoholic steatohepatitis [30, 31]. The cross talk among pathological factors (inflammation and free radicals) and immune responses [25–31] may be complicated, but again, understanding it is important for wellness.

## Oxidative Stress

The shift in antioxidant-oxidant balance in favor of oxidants is termed "oxidative stress" and leads to oxidative damage (see Insert[3] below [33]). Oxidative stress contributes to many pathological conditions, including cancer, neurological disorders, atherosclerosis,

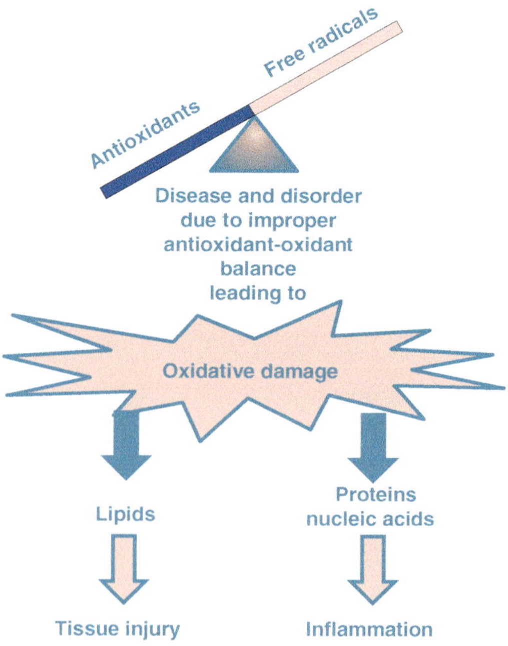


[3]Open Access, Springer Nature.

hypertension, ischemia-reperfusion, diabetes, acute respiratory distress syndrome, idiopathic pulmonary fibrosis, COPD, and asthma [34]. As previously introduced, ROS are a type of oxygen-derived free radical. There are also nitrogen-derived free radicals (RNS) and others (generally termed "free radicals") that are produced by, or introduced into, the body that are considered contributors to oxidative stress, even though they are not oxygen-based. RNS and other free radicals still need another electron to stabilize, and antioxidants are still suitable donors; therefore, they are included in oxidative stress. Focusing on ROS, they are chemically reactive substances containing oxygen, such as oxygen ions and peroxide ions. ROS are produced in moderate amounts naturally during normal oxygen metabolism, such as during mitochondrial respiration and energy generation, but they are quickly removed by cellular defense mechanisms or natural antioxidants (natural electron donors) [35]. Thus, cells can in fact maintain a transient state of low concentrations of ROS without damaging the cell. As mentioned, ROS actually have functional roles, some more of which were not mentioned including cellular signaling, modulation of gene expression, activation of mitogen-activated protein (MAP) kinases (involved in insulin signaling), and reversible gene modulations. However, an increase in ROS production or a decrease in ROS scavenging leads to an excess of these oxygen-derived free radicals, resulting in oxidative stress. This is usually resisted by cellular defense mechanisms so long as they are active, including antioxidants [36].

As shown in Fig. 5.14, release of ROS, such as superoxide ($O_2^-$) or peroxide (e.g., hydrogen peroxide, $H_2O_2$), can be triggered by exogenous or endogenous oxidizing agents, such as therapeutics or their metabolites. $O_2^-$ can be converted to $H_2O_2$ by superoxide dismutase (SOD). Glutathione reductase (GSR) utilizes NADPH to convert oxidized glutathione (GSSG) to reduced glutathione (GSH). GSH is then oxidized back to GSSG by glutathione peroxidase (GPX) in a cyclical reaction to neutralize $2H_2O_2$ into $2H_2O$ and $O_2$. When oxidative stress occurs, G6PD enzyme activity enables cells to cope with low NADPH levels. Myeloperoxidase (MPO) is a source of oxidative stress in the human artery wall. Macrophages use ROS to kill invading pathogens [37]. One oxidative pathway involves MPO, a secreted heme-protein expressed at high levels in atherosclerotic lesions, where it co-localizes in part with macrophages [38]. The enzyme uses hydrogen peroxide ($H_2O_2$) to execute oxidative reactions in the macrophage and extracellular milieu. This process also leads to lipid peroxidation (LPO), the oxidative degradation of lipids. In cell membranes, without a proper antioxidant-oxidant balance [39], LPO is the process in which free radicals "steal" electrons from the lipids in cell membranes, resulting in cell damage. In macrophages, LPO reduces LDL, resulting in ox-LDL, which can turn macrophages into foam cells and contribute to the progression of atherosclerosis (see "Details of Oxidized LDL and Atherosclerosis Production"). 8-Isoprostaglandin F2α (8-Isop) is a biomarker of lipid oxidation and, therefore, inflammation and oxidative stress. S-Glutathionylation of hemoglobin (HAE) is a marker of oxidative stress [40] and is increased in patients with diabetes, hyperlipidemia, and renal failure. Glutathionylation uncouples eNOS, causing nitric oxide insufficiency, promoting endothelial disease.

Conceptually similar to the blood-brain barrier, the testis and ovaries (gametes) are also isolated from the blood by an endothelial barrier. However, instead of working to maintain an electrically neutral environment in the brain, the endothelium around the gametes works to isolate, and preserve, the gametes[4] from the immune system. Malondialdehyde (MDA, Fig. 5.14) is a pro-inflammatory and oxidative stress biomarker of spermatogenesis in the testis and therefore the health of this endothelial barrier.

The catalase enzyme (Fig. 5.14) neutralizes $H_2O_2$, producing water and (stable) oxygen

[4]The sperm and ovaries do not have a full complement of chromosomes, only half. If the immune system had access to them, as it does most of the rest of the body, they would be considered foreign and would constantly be attacked.

($O_2$). NADPH prevents catalase from its inactive state [41]. As an example that promotes oxidative stress, lactoferrin (a catalase) and $H_2O_2$ from $H_2O$ and hydroxide (OH). OH, when combined with NF-κB, results in inflammatory cytokines and adhesion molecules (see insert below [42]).

In the brain, oxidative stress may result in metabolic disorders related to overnutrition [43–45]. Overnutrition activates NF-κB (specifically IKKβ/NF-κB) and associated pro-inflammatory pathways (Fig. 5.15). The effects of NF-κB-mediated metabolic inflammation are deleterious and can give rise to impairments of normal intracellular signaling and disruptions of metabolic physiology [47]. These impairments and disruptions, particularly in the hypothalamus, could account for the development of overnutrition-induced metabolic syndrome and related disorders such as obesity, insulin resistance, type 2 diabetes, and obesity-related hypertension [48–51]. Oxidative stress and mitochondrial dysfunction seem to mediate hypothalamic NF-κB activation and overnutrition. The resulting inflammation is reciprocally related to the induction of various stresses, such as mitochondrial oxidative stress and endoplasmic reticulum stress [47].

In addition to metabolic syndrome and diabetes, oxidative stress contributes to neurodegenerative diseases [52, 53]. When ROS homeostasis is disrupted, excessive ROS are accumulated in the mitochondria and cytoplasm and can cause oxidative damage to nerve cells (Fig. 5.15) [54]. Since it can also activate cellular inflammatory pathways, it is associated with impaired neuronal functions that also lead to metabolic disorders [55] and neurodegenerative diseases [56, 57]. Unresolved endoplasmic reticulum stress can induce mitochondrial changes leading to cell apoptosis [58]. Intraventricular infusion of an endoplasmic reticulum stress inhibitor suppresses the activation of IKKβ/NF-κB pathway activity, and neither high-fat diet nor central administration of chemical endoplasmic reticulum stress inducer is able to induce hypothalamic endoplasmic reticulum stress with central inhibition of the IKKβ/NF-κB pathway [48, 59]. Finally, endoplasmic reticulum stress also causes cellular accumulation of ROS associated with oxidative stress [60], which in turn reciprocally can promote endoplasmic reticulum stress [46].

In summary, oxidative stress outside the brain (Fig. 5.16), regardless of its source (failure of regulation or excessive free radicals), leads to (1) impairment of intracellular signaling, (2) mitochondrial dysfunction, (3) accelerated cellular aging and apoptosis, (4) disruption of membrane integrity, and (5) lipid, protein, and nucleic acid (DNA) damage. Inside the brain (Fig. 5.17), oxidative stress leads to (1) neuro-inflammation, (2) acceleration of aging and apoptosis, (3) dysfunctional neuronal integrity, (4) impaired neurotransmission, and (5) impaired neuroplasticity. The systemic effects of oxidative stress are listed in Fig. 5.18.

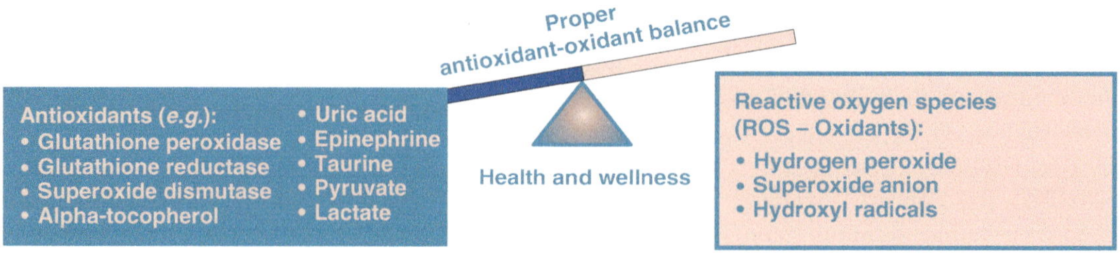

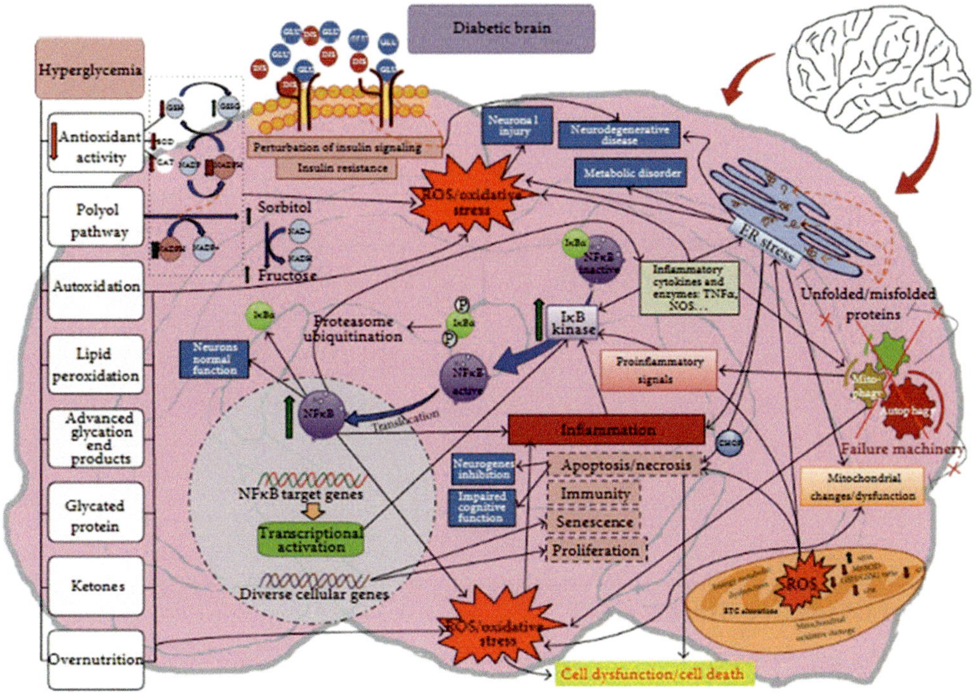


**Fig. 5.15** Brain oxidative stress, including endoplasmic reticulum (ER) stress, using diabetes as the model. Scheme summarizing the involvement of oxidative stress (mitochondrial dysfunction and ER stress), inflammation, and autophagy in the diabetic brain. GSH reduced glutathione, GSSG glutathione disulfide, SOD superoxide dismutase, NAD+ nicotinamide adenine dinucleotide (NAD) oxidized, NADP+ NAD phosphate (NADP) oxidized, NADPH NADP reduced, NADH NAD reduced, CAT catalase, IκBa nuclear factor of kappa light polypeptide gene enhancer in B cell inhibitor, $\alpha$ alpha, NFκB nuclear factor kappa-light-chain-enhancer of activated B cells, ER endoplasmic reticulum, GLU glucose, INS insulin, P phosphate, MDA malondialdehyde, ATP adenosine triphosphate, ETC electron transport chain, ROS reactive oxygen species, MnSOD manganese superoxide dismutase, GSR glutathione reductase CHOP C/EBP homology protein, TNF$\alpha$ tumor necrosis factor alpha, NOS nitric oxide synthases. (Open Access, Hindawi. Source: [46])

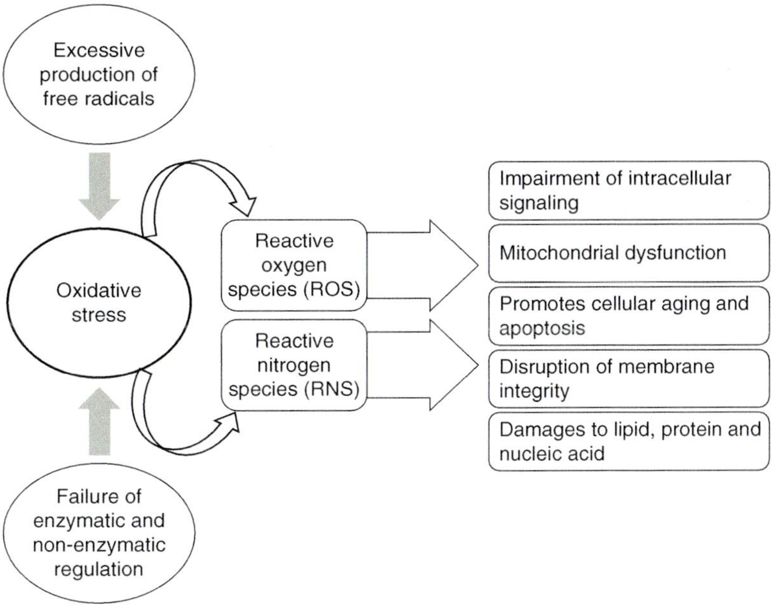


**Fig. 5.16** Effects of oxidative stress outside the brain. (Republished with permission from Wolters Kluwer Medknow Publications. Source: [61, Fig. 3])

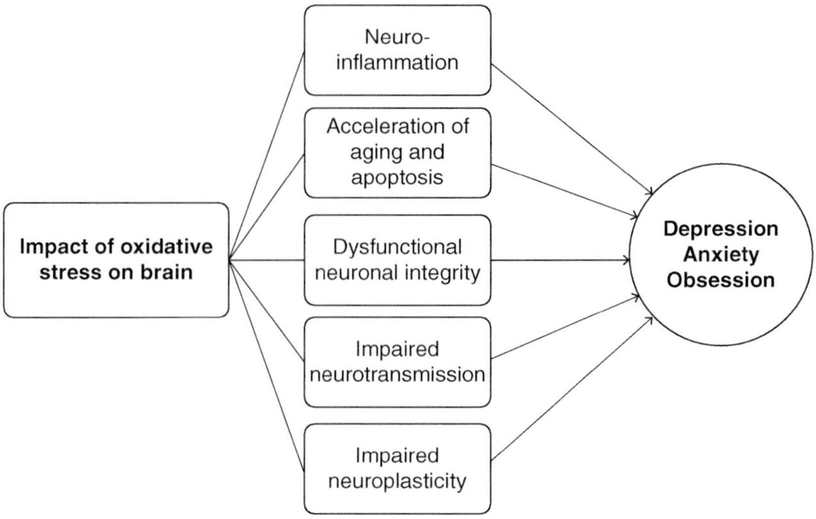


**Fig. 5.17** Effects of oxidative stress inside the brain. (Republished with permission from Wolters Kluwer Medknow Publications. Source: [61, Fig. 4])

## Markers of Oxidative Stress

A persistent prooxidant environment in cells can modify redox-sensitive molecules. A common approach to assess oxidative stress involves the measurement of the increase or decrease in a redox-sensitive molecule that responds to oxidative stress. In general, reliable markers of oxidative stress possess the following qualities: (1) chemically unique and detectable, (2) increased or decreased during periods of oxidative stress, (3) relatively long half-lives, and (4) not impacted by other cellular processes (e.g., cell cycle, energy metabolism, etc.) [63, 64]. Many molecules that fit one or more of these criteria have been identified, and techniques to measure these biomarkers have been reported [65–73].

During periods of oxidative stress, prooxidants overwhelm the antioxidant defenses in cells and damage cellular components. Oxidative stress is often characterized by a(n): (1) increase in the formation of radicals and other oxidants, (2) decrease in small-molecular-weight or lipid-soluble antioxidants, (3) disturbance in cellular redox balance, and (4) oxidative damage to cellular components (i.e., lipids, proteins, and/or DNA). As a result, biomarkers of oxidative stress typically fall into one of the four categories [64]. The first category of biomarkers involves the detection of oxidants (e.g., superoxide anions, hydroxyl radicals, hydrogen peroxide, peroxynitrate, and other radicals) [64]. Unfortunately, direct measurement of radical production in living cells is difficult because radicals are highly reactive and have a short half-life. Exogenous molecules such as fluorescent probes or spin traps are commonly used to measure oxidant production in cells. When employed, the probe, or spin trap, is converted into a uniquely modified radical product with a relatively long half-life that can be quantified as a measurement of oxidant production [68, 69]. Nonetheless, because an increase in oxidant production does not necessarily define a prooxidant condition, measures of increased oxidant production alone are not definitive markers of oxidative stress. A disadvantage of using probes or spin traps is that these molecules may perturb the biological system being investigated [63]. Another drawback is that many spin traps and fluorescent probes are toxic to cells [63].

A second group of oxidative stress biomarkers incorporates the measurement of antioxidants in tissues (e.g., glutathione, ascorbate (vitamin C), α-tocopherol (vitamin E), etc.) and total antioxidant capacity. In theory, decreases in antioxidants commonly occur during oxidative insults. Measurement of a decline in tissue antioxidant levels is a biomarker of oxidative stress. While a decline is used as a biomarker of oxidative stress, the approach is not without weaknesses. For

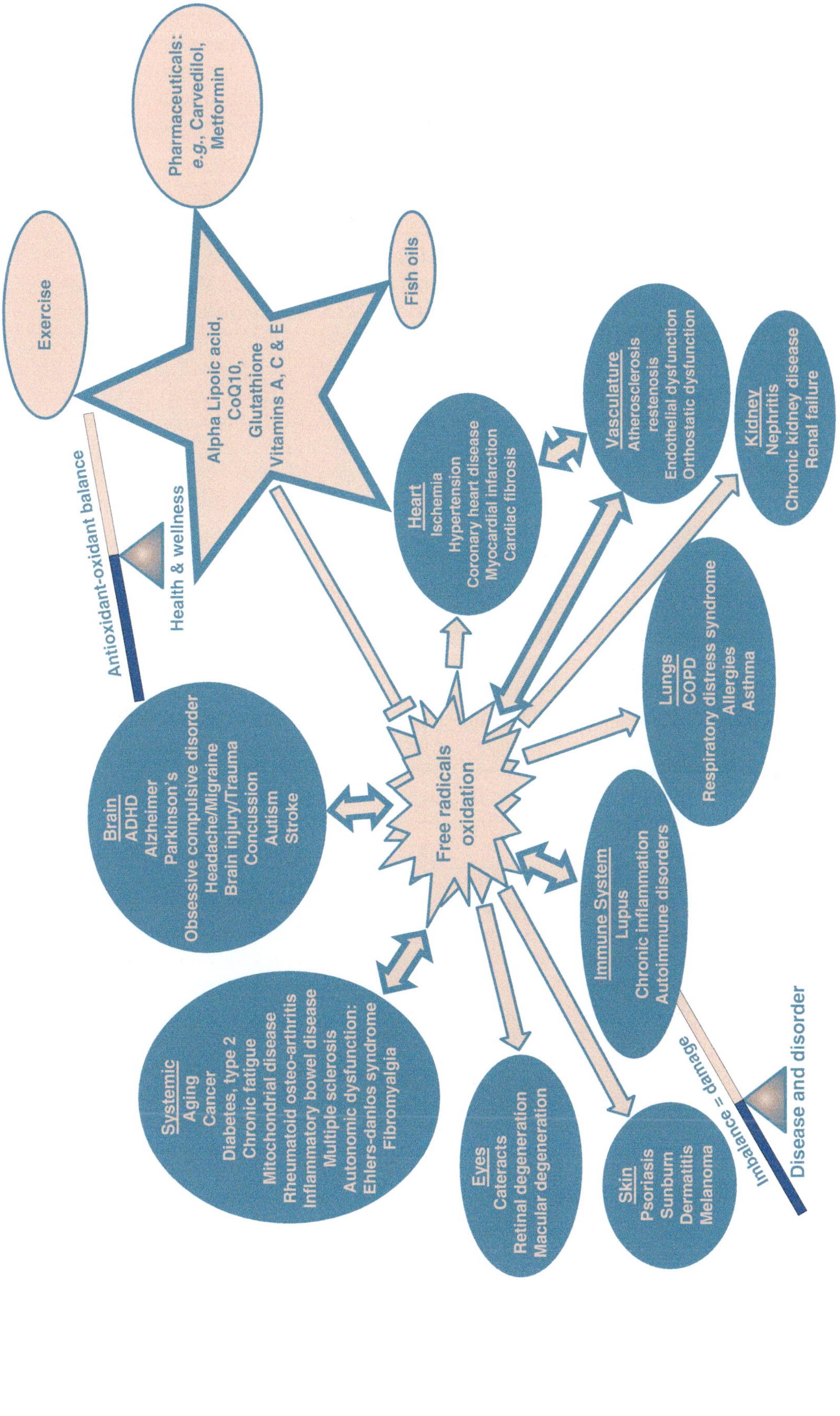


**Fig. 5.18** Systemic effects of oxidative stress. Double-headed arrows indicate that small amounts of oxidative stress are healthy, such as when the immune system uses oxidants as part of the passive defense. Single-headed arrows indicate oxidative stress only [62]. (Source: https://www.pinterest.com/explore/oxidative-stress/)

example, factors such as changes in cellular metabolism and diet can influence antioxidant levels in cells. Another weakness is the potential for auto-oxidation during sample handling, resulting in measurement of associated antioxidant depletion, artificially increasing the measurement of the oxidant [63].

A third class of biomarkers for oxidative stress involves the evaluation of oxidatively modified molecules (e.g., protein carbonyls, isoprostanes, nitrotyrosine, 8-OH-dG, 4-hydroxy-nonenal, and malondialdehyde). Reactions of ROS with lipids, proteins, or DNA generate uniquely oxidized biomolecules that can be used as "fingerprints" to detect oxidative stress in cells. Common measures of oxidation include the measurement of protein carbonyls as an indicator of protein oxidation; assessment of isoprostanes, malondialdehyde, and 4-hydroxy-2-nonenal as signs of lipid peroxidation; and evaluation of DNA oxidation by assaying the levels of the oxidized base, 8-hydroxy-2′-deoxyguanosine (8-OH-dG) [65, 69, 71, 74]. Although it can be argued that oxidized molecules are the most important biomarker of oxidative stress, their measurement in biological systems is often difficult because oxidized molecules exist in limited amounts in cells even during periods of oxidative stress. Moreover, identical to other biomarker methodologies, measurement of oxidation products is subject to assay artifacts if tissue samples are handled improperly [63].

The fourth category of oxidative stress biomarkers involves the measurement of cellular redox balance (antioxidant-prooxidant balance, e.g., GSH/GSSH ratio, cysteine redox state, and thiol/disulfide state). One of the most commonly measured markers of cellular redox balance is the ratio of GSH to GSSH. This assay is useful because increased oxidant production results in a decrease in the GSH/GSSH ratio. The decrease indicates lower levels of reduced GSH in favor of increased oxidized GSH (i.e., GSSG). Although this assay is conceptually simple, experimental artifacts are common and can occur during tissue removal and sample processing due to improper tissue handling permitting auto-oxidation [63].

Although there are many parameters to quantify oxidative stress, the development of a single and ideal biomarker has proven difficult. It appears that no one biomarker best assesses oxidative stress and that, in most cases, the measurement of multiple biomarkers is required to confirm the presence of oxidative stress in tissues [63].

## Aldehydes: Oxidative Stress and ROS Production Versus Alpha-Lipoic Acid, as Modeled in Diabetes

Aldehydes have a carbonyl group (a carbon double-bonded to an oxygen) with a single hydrogen and a defining carbon chain bonded with the carbon (see insert). The carbonyl group

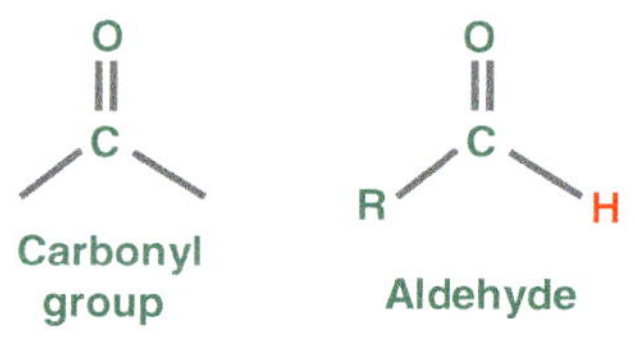


is the functional group. Carbonyl groups are highly reactive. The classical sequence of events is that oxidative stress triggers lipid peroxidation which in turn produces aldehyde by-products. Lipid aldehydes are able to also induce the production of ROS (Fig. 5.19) [76–82]. This is thought to be of importance in their deleterious effects [63]. This concept is reinforced by the fact (1) that an increase in local glutathione can prevent the deleterious effects of aldehyde (i.e., 4-hydroxy-2-nonenal, or HNE, a well-studied and notably toxic aldehyde) on ROS production [81] (2) and that dysfunction of glutathione S-transferase, a major enzyme for aldehyde detoxification, leads to oxidative stress [83, 84]. These examples demonstrates how lipid by-products are parts of a vicious circle in which increased ROS production generates aldehydes which further amplify the generation of oxidative species and so on (Fig. 5.19). Aldehydes regulate gene expression, including the expression of several antioxidant enzymes [63]. Aldehydes induce cellular growth, apoptosis and inflammatory responses, and they have been implicated in insu-

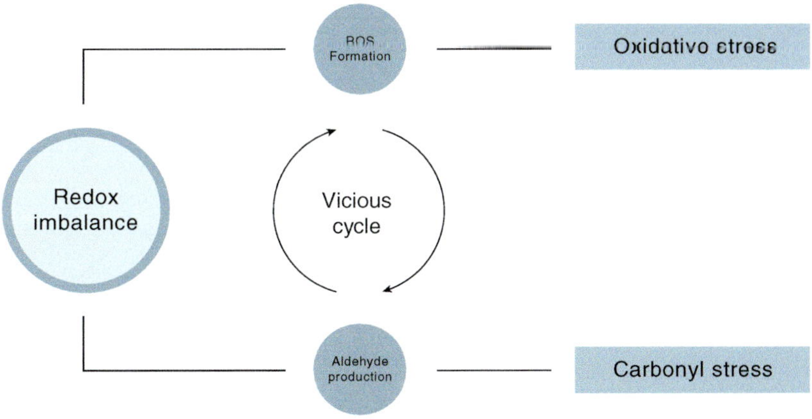


**Fig. 5.19** The vicious circle linking ROS and lipid aldehyde production promotes stress [63, 75]. (Illustration by Elysian Creative Studio, www.elysiancreativestudio.com, Lizzy Colombo. Source: [63])

lin production. As a result, aldehydes seem to have both a beneficial and deleterious effect. The local concentration of aldehydes seems to determine the effect; low concentrations are beneficial and high concentrations are deleterious [63].

Considering metabolic syndrome as a precursor to type 2 diabetes, significant aldehyde production through lipid peroxidation is tightly linked to high-fat diet and obesity. Increased oxidative stress in accumulated fat is an important pathogenic mechanism of obesity-associated metabolic syndrome [85]. Chronic, low-grade inflammation of white adipose tissue is a hallmark of obesity and a major contributor to oxidative stress and lipid peroxidation [86]. In the expanding adipose tissue, hypertrophied adipocytes contribute to the inflammation by upregulating the expression and release of pro-inflammatory cytokines. Aldehydes also decrease the expression of the anti-inflammatory, insulin-sensitizing hormone, adiponectin [87, 88], therefore linking lipid peroxidation by-products and chronic inflammation.

Epidemiological studies demonstrate that fasting glycemia is positively correlated with oxidative stress markers and negatively correlated with plasma glutathione [89, 90]. Diabetes is associated with decreased vitamin C and glutathione [91, 92], enabling oxidative stress. Insulin sensitivity can be improved through antioxidant or carbonyl scavenging treatment [93, 94], demonstrating the tight link existing between oxidative stress, oxidation by-products, and insulin resistance. Pancreatic islet cells are known to be affected by aldehydes [63].

With diabetes, aldehyde concentration is increased in several tissues including in the pancreas, liver, brain, and heart. Oxidative stress, through ROS, can positively and negatively regulate insulin signaling, depending on time, dose, model, and free radical used [95]. However, prolonged oxidative stress impairs insulin signaling and glucose uptake. While aldehyde inhibition of mitochondrial aconitase (a hydroxyl radical) enables the generation of precursors of fatty acid synthesis (see Fig. 5.20) [97], data suggest that accumulation of lipid aldehydes and fat deposition could be mutually inductive leading to a vicious circle promoting fat accretion (see Fig. 5.20).

## Alpha-Lipoic Acid

Preventing the deleterious effects of aldehydes with alpha-lipoic acid (ALA), as demonstrated by type 2 diabetes, has been known for decades. ALA has many applications throughout the body, including the fact that it improves immune responses and glucose tolerance and insulin sensitivity [98]. ALA may lower resting blood pressure and slows or even reverses (temporarily) the progression of autonomic neuropathy [99–104]. Similarly in obese and insulin-resistant patients, increased intake of vitamin E (an antioxidant recycled by ALA) reduces fasting glycemia and insulin

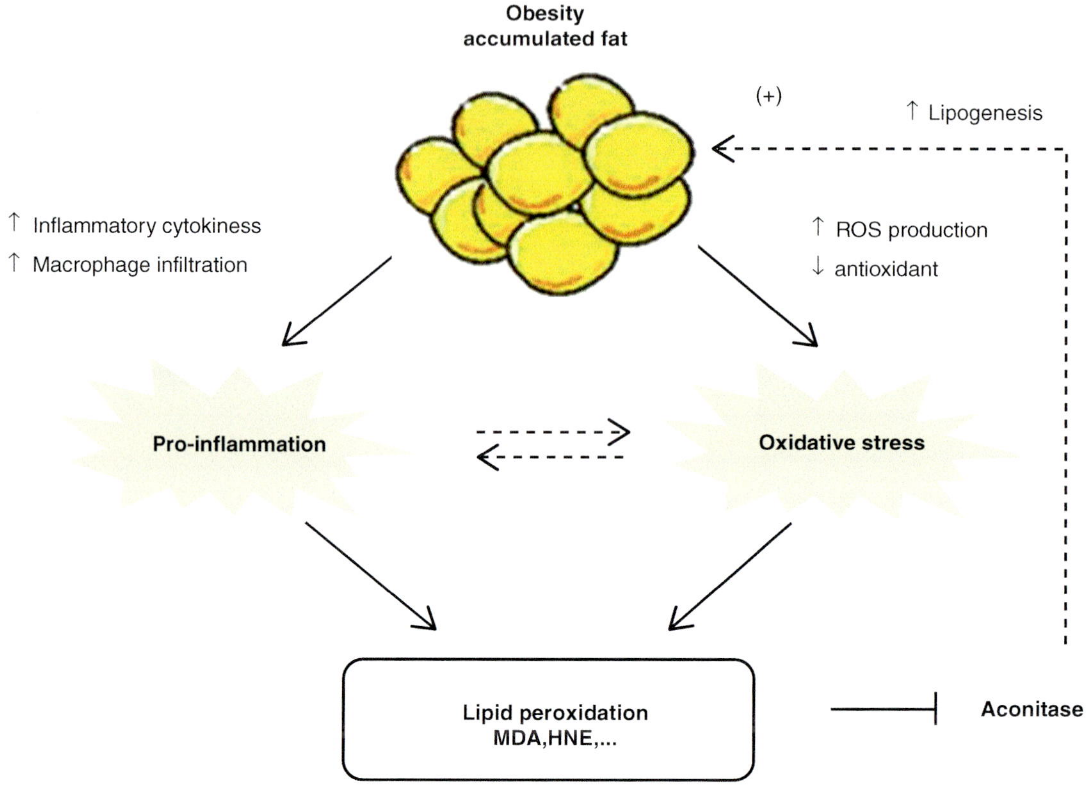


**Fig. 5.20** The obesity-lipid peroxidation vicious circle [63, 75, 96]. (Open Access, Intech Open)

resistance. This is correlated with a decrease in the concentration of peroxides in plasma [105]. This adds further evidence for a causative role of oxidative stress in the metabolic syndrome and opens new therapeutic perspectives using antioxidant or scavenging of toxic aldehydes.

ALA prevents the development of glucose-induced insulin resistance by decreasing oxidative stress in both adipocytes and muscle cells [106, 107] and also decreases lipid peroxidation markers. Glutathione (GSH) is present in high concentration in the cytoplasm [108, 109]. GSH is an important coenzyme of several enzymatic reactions and exerts its antioxidant activity mainly through regeneration of vitamin E and also through direct interaction with free radical and aldehydes. GSH is necessary for the activity of glutathione-S-transferases (GSTs), a family of enzymes responsible for detoxifying electrophile by-products, such as those derived from lipid peroxidation. On insulin-sensitive tissues (muscle, adipose tissue), aldehydes lead to insulin resistance. In the pancreas, aldehydes impair insulin secretion. Together with the carbonylation of the insulin peptide itself, aldehydes could contribute to the defects in insulin action, leading to the metabolic syndrome. The role of aldehydes is mitigated by the mild effect obtained with antioxidants or aldehyde scavengers in the treatment of diabetic complications. Oxidative stress and its derivatives are nevertheless important in the metabolic syndrome. Prevention or treatment of some of the associated complications of oxidative stress, such as with ALA, seems to be accessed through the reduction of both ROS and toxic aldehyde by-products [63].

As mentioned above, the carbonyl group is highly reactive. Carbonyl groups are attached to other types of molecules, such as ketones (see insert). Carbonyl radicals cause carbonyl stress. Similar to oxygen radicals in oxidative stress, carbonyl radicals in carbonyl stress generally

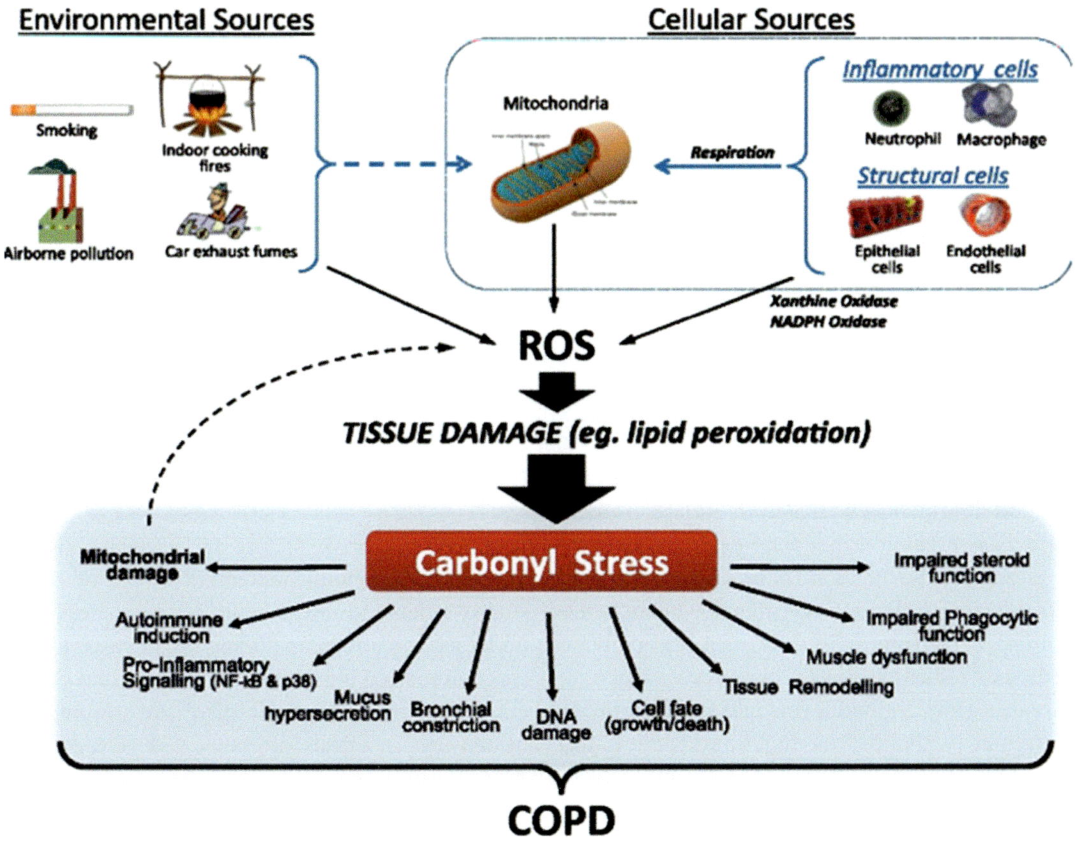


**Fig. 5.21** Carbonyl stress leads to many pathological processes which, cumulatively, lead to diseases such as COPD [111]. (Republished with permission from Elsevier)

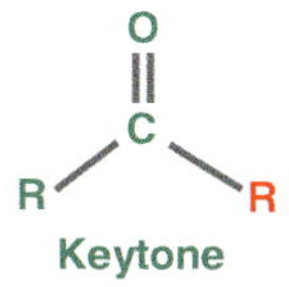


cause similar types of damage. Carbonyl stress is increased carbonyl modification of tissue and cellular proteins, primarily in uremia. Carbonyl stress has been implicated in the pathogenesis of long-term uremic complications such as dialysis-related amyloidosis [110]. As shown in Fig. 5.21, carbonyl stress leads to many pathological processes which, cumulatively, lead to diseases such as COPD [111].

ALA [112–115] is a key antioxidant. It is a sulfur coenzyme and was isolated in 1951. It is also known as thioctic acid. It is not a vitamin. ALA is a natural cofactor in the body and is seen both in the enzyme pyruvate dehydrogenase and in an enzyme in the Krebs cycle. Arsenic is lethal and kills because it complexes with lipoic acid in the pyruvate dehydrogenase complex.[5] ALA lowers blood pressure because it enhances nitric oxide production. Good sources of ALA in foods include broccoli, spinach, carrots, red meats and organ meats, brussels sprouts, brewer's yeast, tomatoes, beets, and peas. Again, it helps to regenerate other antioxidants, such as glutathione, in addition to vitamins A, C, and E (see Figs. 5.3). It modulates inflammation. It sequesters free radicals in ROS. It aids in cardiac func-

[5]Arsenic is found in trace amounts in apple seeds, among others, and, perhaps due to its affinity to ALA, helps to kill pre-cancer cells, another example where "bad things" are not all bad. However, any more than trace amounts and arsenic becomes bad. This gives more meaning to "an apple a day keeps the doctor away."

tion and helps restore autonomic and sensory nerves [116, 117, 118]. ALA has been shown to help burn carbohydrates and bring glucose metabolic products into mitochondria. It acts as both antioxidant and anti-inflammatory. ALA has been called the universal antioxidant. It is unique because it is both lipid and water soluble. It protects both the interior and exterior parts of cells from cell-damaging free radicals. Not only is it involved in free radical scavenging but also protein repair and chelation of metals.

ALA may be useful in migraine and vision problems [119], helping reduce the risk of type 2 diabetes by increasing insulin sensitivity [117, 118] and metabolic syndrome by improving brain function. It is evidenced that 200–600 mg of ALA twice a day is beneficial depending on the severity of autonomic dysfunction (neuropathy). Because ALA can lower glucose, care must be taken to not promote hypoglycemia if one is on oral diabetic medicines. ALA decreases insulin resistance. It increases acetylcholine levels and has benefits in this regard with P&S dysfunction [120]. It has been shown to lower lipids in the liver and may be effective in treating fatty liver [544 and empirical evidence]. ALA can lower blood pressure, and as with glucose, care must be taken to not promote hypotension. Most importantly, ALA appears to increase energy and ATP [121], and it has been used in chronic fatigue syndromes. Lipoic acid reduces lipid peroxidation and may be important in treating atherosclerosis [122].

Some data suggests that ALA protects against memory loss and aging [120] and may be beneficial in treating patients with Alzheimer's disease [123, 124], Parkinson's disease [125, 126], and stroke victims [127]. It increases blood flow to nerve endings, which is also helpful in neuropathy. Therefore, it has many vascular and neurological potential benefits. In addition, because of its wellness-promoting effects on mitochondrial function, it appears to be very versatile. ALA and Co-Q10 are currently being tested in patients with autonomic dysfunction with P&S Monitoring. ALA can be part of an anti-obesity therapy and can be used for its lipid-lowering properties [128]. It has also been noted that excess amounts of heavy metals in the body increase oxidative stress. ALA has been shown to be an excellent chelating agent, helping to remove excess amounts of heavy metals.

In summary, ALA enhances nitric oxide production, lowers blood pressure, makes insulin work better, increases ATP, is a potent antioxidant and anti-inflammatory compound, both lipid and water soluble, and may have potential uses in weight loss, fatty liver disease, and autonomic and peripheral neuropathies, especially diabetic neuropathy. It is a healthy supplementation to the Mediterranean diet.

## Oxidative Stress in Cardiovascular Diseases

Cardiovascular risk factors and vascular disease are associated with increased levels of ROS. Improvement in circulation is very important under all conditions, including cardiovascular diseases. Impaired blood flow to muscles and organs causes dysfunction, morbidity, and chronic illnesses and increases mortality risk. Excess free radicals (ROS and RNS, referred to in combination as RONS, and other free radicals) decrease endothelial nitric oxide production by uncoupling eNOS. Traditional risk factors for circulatory diseases have been identified, and excellent pharmacological and lifestyle measures to improve these risk factors have been developed. Traditional risk factors include diabetes, high LDL cholesterol, low HDL cholesterol, family history of premature cardiovascular disease,[6] male gender[6], hypertension, being sedentary, aging, obesity, and tobacco [129, 130]. Nontraditional risk factors include psychosocial stress, inflammation, endothelial dysfunction, kidney disease, and poor brachial index measurements [129, 130]. Oxidative stress has typically not been considered a nontraditional risk factor since it is difficult to measure and measurements are usually done in experimental situations in a laboratory (see "Markers of Oxidative Stress," above).

Atherosclerosis is a common circulatory disease and is highly associated with endothelial dysfunction. A vicious cycle between oxidative stress and oxidative stress-induced atheroscleropathy

[6]This is considered a non-modifiable risk factor.

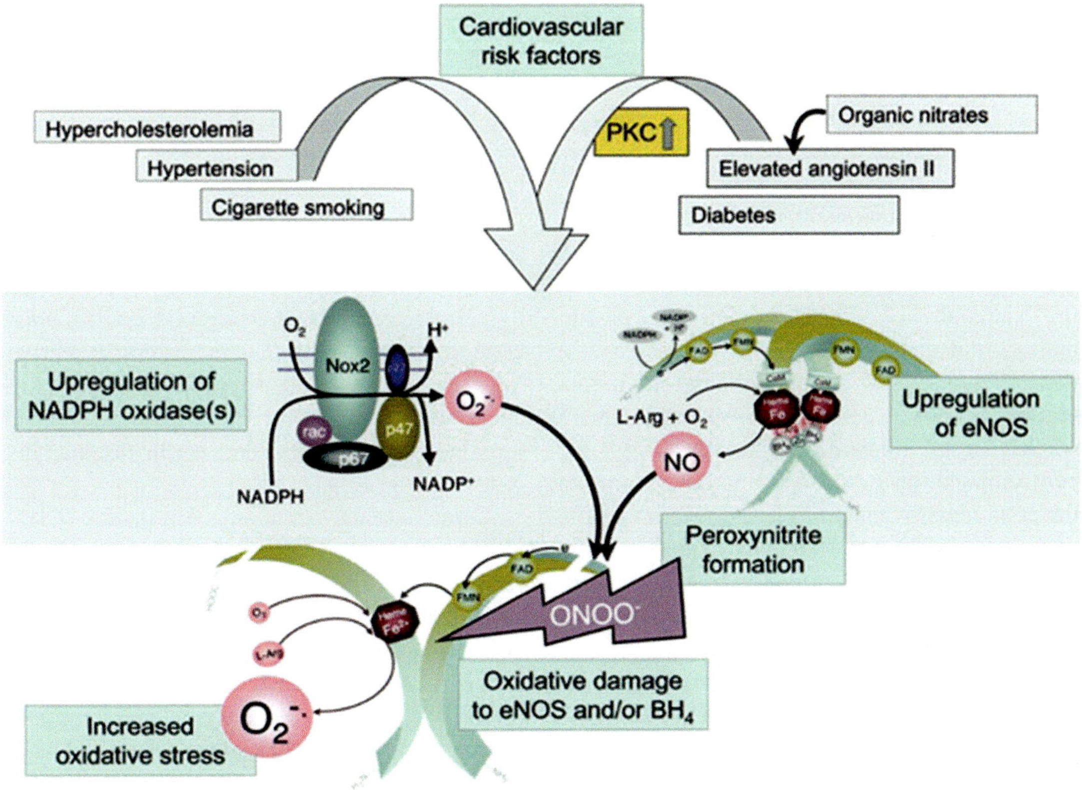


**Fig. 5.22** Potential mechanisms by which cardiovascular risk factors lead to endothelial dysfunction. In many types of vascular disease, NADPH oxidases and eNOS are upregulated in parallel. Their respective products rapidly recombine to form the ROS, $ONOO^-$. This oxidizes BH4, the essential cofactor of eNOS, or produces oxidative damage to the zinc-thiolate cluster of eNOS. Thus, $O_2$ reduction by eNOS is uncoupled from nitric oxide formation, and a functional NOS is converted into a dysfunctional $O_2^-$-generating enzyme that contributes to vascular oxidative stress. (Republished with permission from Wolters Kluwer Health, Inc. Source: [132, 133])

sis leads to the development and progression of atherosclerosis (see Figs. 2.19). Cardiovascular risk factors increase the expression or activity of NADPH oxidases (NOX) in atherosclerotic arteries, including increased expression of NOX2 and NOX4 (which has been observed in the vascular wall [131]; see Fig. 5.22), thereby enhancing the production of RONS (e.g., $O_2^-$ and peroxynitrate). Endothelial dysfunction could be due to decreased eNOS expression. However, several studies have shown that cardiovascular risk factors are associated with an increase, rather than a decrease, in eNOS expression [134]. Increased expression of eNOS in vascular disease seems to be a consequence of an excess production of $H_2O_2$. $H_2O_2$, the dismutation[7] product of $O_2^-$, can increase eNOS expression through transcriptional and posttranscriptional mechanisms [135]. An accelerated degradation of nitric oxide by its reaction with $O_2^-$ is another pathway to increase eNOS expression. Nitric oxide and $O_2^-$ react rapidly to form the ROS, $ONOO^-$, which in turn leads to eNOS uncoupling, enzyme dysfunction, and vascular disease (see Fig. 5.22) [133].

In addition to atherosclerosis being a cause of heart attacks, oxidative stress is another cause of heart attacks. This relationship is based on cyclic guanosine monophosphate (cGMP) and cyclic adenosine monophosphate (cAMP). cGMP transmits the messages of the parasympathetic nervous system in the cells of the heart muscles, as it does in other cells in the body.

[7]Dismutation is the simultaneous oxidation and reduction chemical reaction.

cAMP transmits the messages of the sympathetic nervous system. Sympathetic activity increases the content of cAMP. Parasympathetic activity increases cGMP in cells. An increase in cAMP activates numerous reactions in the cell; likewise, a cGMP increase sets off other processes that often counteract one another. These messengers transmit the commands of the P&S control centers in the brain. The commands of the sympathetics stimulate activity, performance, and energy consumption, whereas the parasympathetics command relaxation, regeneration, economy, cell protection, and "homeostasis." In its concern for "homeostasis," the parasympathetics ensure that the functioning of the cells remains balanced and does not get out of control (Fig. 5.23). However, oxidative stress stimulates sympathetic activity. Excessive sympathetic activity, associated with heart attack, is associated with high levels of oxidative stress. In other words, oxidative stress due to an imbalance in the oxidant-antioxidant ratio leads to a P&S imbalance as described above. If the P&S imbalance presents while the patient demonstrates CAN (cardiovascular autonomic neuropathy), a condition of very weak parasympathetic activity at rest, then there may not be sufficient parasympathetic activity to prevent a sympathetically mediated ventricular tachy-rhythm from becoming ventricular fibrillation and perhaps resulting in an infarction or sudden death.

Sleep apnea is well known to cause sympathetic excess which leads to hypertension and cardiovascular disease. The pathophysiology of cardiovascular morbidity in obstructive sleep apnea is complex and involves neural, humoral, mechanical, and hemodynamic components that are modified either by genetic makeup, nutrition, or lifestyle-related variables [136, 137]. Sleep apnea is associated with elevated sympathetic discharge during sleep and waking that has been linked with increased systemic blood pressure and could be, partially, ameliorated by CPAP treatment [138–141]. It is important to note, however, that CPAP is not sympatholytic. It only has an indirect effect on the sympathetics. It relieves the stress of not sleeping well but does not actively, and directly, reduce sympathetic excess. If there are other reasons for sympathetic excess (e.g., hypertension, obesity, or diabetes), CPAP alone is typically not sufficient to relieve sympathetic excess.

Oxidative stress with obesity can initiate cardiovascular consequences in sleep apnea. Sleep apnea, itself, is a cause of oxidative stress, compounding the stress, leading to associated conditions and comorbidities, such as sympathetic over-activation, persistent obesity, hypertension, hyperlipidemia, and diabetes. Of course, these conditions also cause oxidative stress, exacerbating the condition and perpetuating this vicious cycle, eventually involving inflammatory and immune cell activation and cardiovascular disease (see Fig. 5.24) [142].

Cardiovascular autonomic neuropathy (CAN) is a risk factor for major adverse cardiac events (MACE, e.g., heart attack, stroke, heart failure, cardiomyopathy, aneurysm, etc.). Again, CAN is defined as very low resting parasympathetic activity [116]. CAN carries a 5-year, 50% mortality rate [143–145]. CAN is associated with other risk factors [146, 147], including (1) low ejection fraction [148, 149]; (2) poor cardiac output [150]; (3) arrhythmias [151, 152]; (4) cardiomyopathies [153, 154], including chronic heart failure [155]; (5) poor circulation [156], including poor cardiac circulation (angina or coronary artery disease) [157]; (6) greater mortality [117]; and (7) greater morbidity [118], including silent myocardial infarction and early cardiac death [118, 158]. Very low parasympathetic activity (measured as high Sympathovagal Balance, or SB, by P&S Monitoring) may lead to the need for cardiac intervention or an implanted cardiac device [116]. CAN with high SB carries a 2-year, 50% mortality risk.

Whether it is hypertension, sleep apnea, diabetes, or most types of cardiovascular disease, all involve excessive sympathetic over-activation,[8]

[8]This sympathetic over-activation, as referenced three times in this section, is a relative term. It is not an absolute term. In other words, it is a sympathetic level that is excessive when compared to the corresponding parasympathetic level. There should be a balance. In the resting state, sympathetic to parasympathetic balance (aka sympathovagal balance or SB, as measured by P&S Monitoring) should be near 1.0. Sympathetic excess is defined as resting SB > 3.0, regardless of the absolute levels of sympathetic or parasympathetic activity.

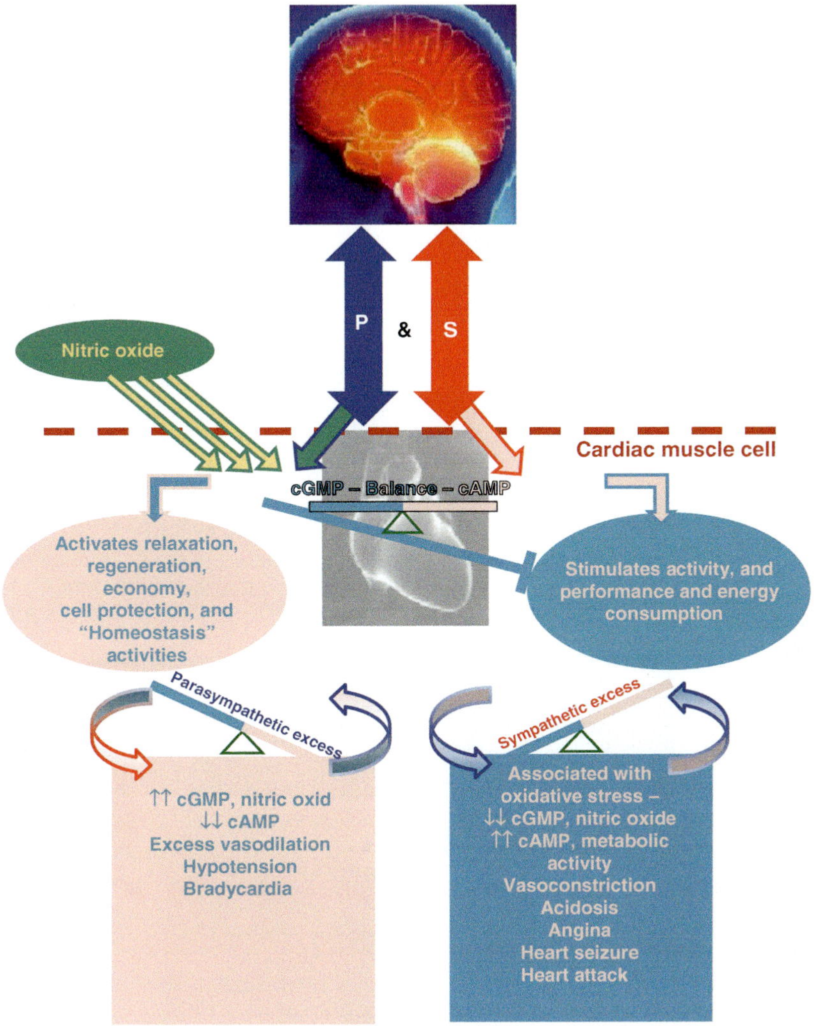


**Fig. 5.23** Balance between cAMP and cGMP. These rapid messengers are central to the relationship between oxidative stress and heart attacks. As in the rest of the body, cGMP transmits the messages of the parasympathetic nervous system, and cAMP transmits the messages of the sympathetic nervous system into cells, in this case cardiac muscle cells. P-activity increases cGMP concentrations in cells and S-activity increases cAMP concentrations. An increase in cGMP activates relaxation, regeneration, economy, cell protection, and "homeostasis" activities within cells. An increase in cAMP stimulates activity, performance, and energy consumption. The actions of the two often counteract one another. The parasympathetics, via cGMP, ensures that the functioning of the cells remains balanced and does not get out of control. A large increase in cAMP causes an automatic rise in the level of cGMP. Due to this protective action, even if stress levels are critical, the heart muscle is not damaged. Nitric oxide also increases cGMP levels in cells. With aging, disease, or stress, P-activity declines, reducing cGMP levels in cells. This is not critical as long as there are sufficient levels of nitric oxide. When both P-activity and nitric oxide levels are low, the "metabolic brake" fails, permitting significant increases in cellular metabolic activity leading to acidosis and then heart seizure and heart attack. This is compounded by the damaging vascular effects of low nitric oxide throughout the body (e.g., a lack of vasoconstriction, a lack of vascular compliance, increase in blood coagulation) [133]. Abbreviations: cAMP, cyclic adenosine monophosphate; cGMP, cyclic guanosine monophosphate. (Source: Sroka K. http://heartattacknew.com/faq/what-is-the-connection-between-oxidative-stress-and-heart-attacks/)

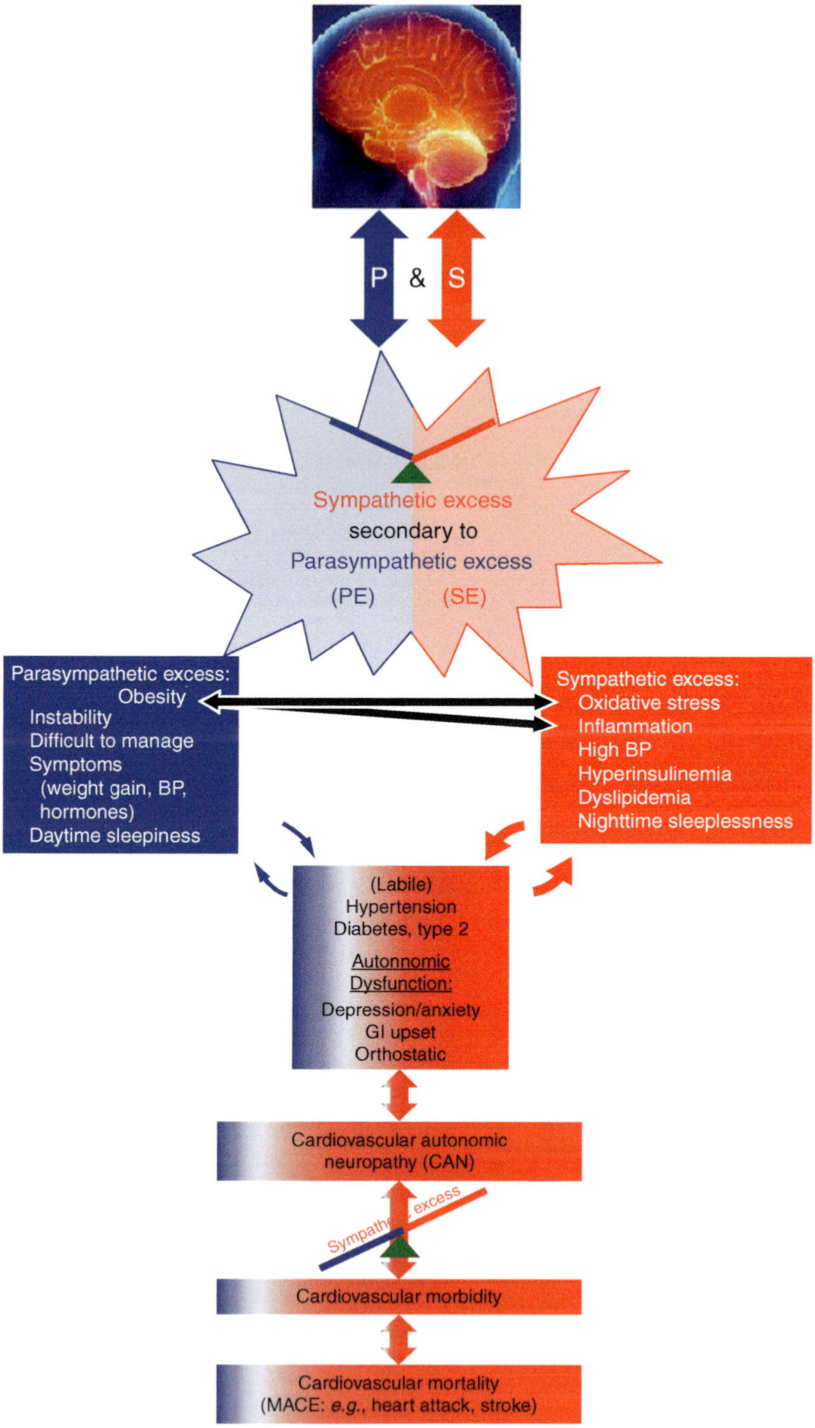


**Fig. 5.24** A schematic illustration of the possible role of oxidative stress and inflammation in obstructive sleep apnea and the development of associated conditions and comorbidities. Associated conditions and comorbidities can be induced by oxidative stress or developed independently. Once these conditions and comorbidities develop, regardless of the initiating factors, they elicit a series of intricate interactions with various transduction pathways, promoting oxidative stress and inflammation. The enhanced oxidative stress exacerbates inflammation, which in turn further exacerbates oxidative stress, generating a vicious cycle, eventually leading to cardiovascular morbidity. Abbreviations: SA sympathetic activation, HTN hypertension, DM type 2 diabetes. (Source: [134])

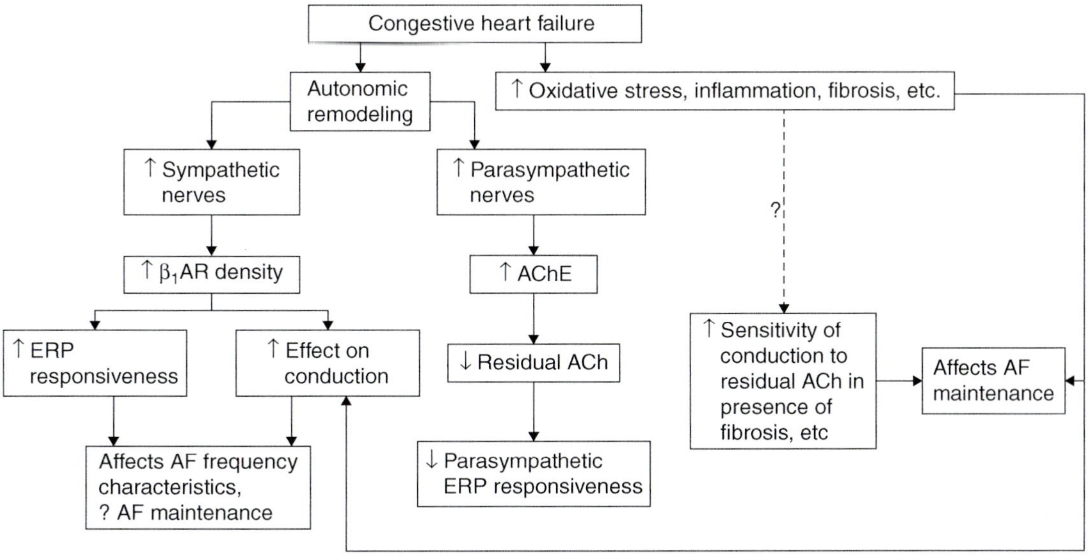


**Fig. 5.25** Proposed model of the creation of an autonomic substrate for atrial fibrillation (AF) in congestive heart failure. The model suggests the likely presence of synergistic interactions between structural changes (fibrosis) and autonomic remodeling in the creation of AF substrate in heart failure. Ach, acetylcholine; AChE, acetylcholinesterase; $\beta_1$AR, $\beta_1$1 adrenergic receptor; ERP, effective refractory period. (Republished with permission from Wolters Kluwer Health, Inc. Source: [159], modified from [160].)

which eventually, and more rapidly than normal aging, reduces (further) parasympathetic activity (Fig. 5.25), thereby more rapidly progressing to CAN. This progression is typically slowed by normalizing (for the individual) the P&S balance, known as sympathovagal balance [116]. For example, CPAP in sleep apnea may reduce sympathetic activity. If the patient also has hypertension, CPAP is often not enough. Antihypertensives (which are either direct or indirect sympatholytics, e.g., angiotensin; see Fig. 5.26), supplements, or lifestyle changes are needed to both reduce blood pressure and, in the process, also further reduce sympathetic activation. If the patient also has diabetes, again, CPAP may not be enough. More aggressive blood glucose and diabetes management, including pharmaceuticals, supplements, or lifestyle changes, may be needed to further reduce sympathetic activity directly. Again, this may not be enough. If the patient is also obese with atherosclerosis, then weight loss and statins, and supplements (*i.e.*, Omega-3 fish oils with statins) or lifestyle changes, are needed to further reduce sympathetic activity and weight loss by reducing stress and statins by improving blood flow and endothelial function. Once the sympathetics are balanced with the parasympathetics, then CAN risk is normal.

As indicated above, CAN risk is associated with multiple risk factors. For example, with congestive heart failure (CHF) and oxidative stress, atrial fibrillation is a common comorbidity, perhaps due in large part to the underlying P&S imbalance caused by CHF (see Fig. 5.26) [159, 160]. The nervous system is highly sensitive to oxidative stress, especially the autonomic nervous system, with its thinner myelin sheath and smaller fiber diameter (C fibers). This is especially true for the parasympathetic nervous system, of which approximately 70% (outside the brain) is the vagus nerve. The vagus nerve is one of the longest nerves in the body and highly exposed and therefore highly susceptible to oxidative stress, as well as to many other toxic processes in the body.

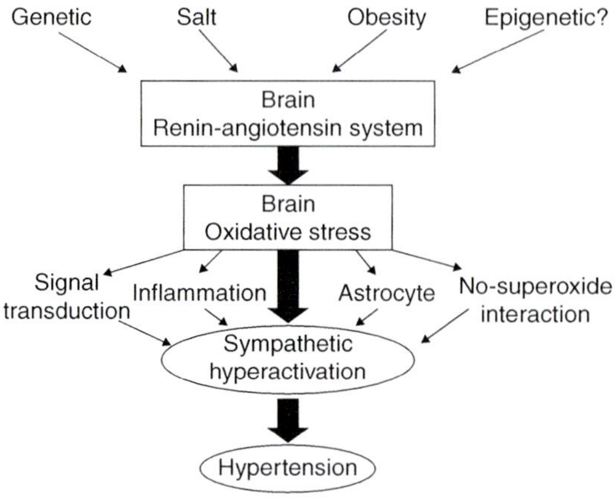


**Fig. 5.26** A conceptual schema showing the regulation of sympathetic nerve activity via brain renin-angiotensin system and oxidative stress. (Open Access, Frontiers in Physiology. Source: [161])

Inside the brain, there is an interaction between superoxide and nitric oxide [161]. In the brain, nitric oxide inhibits the activation of the sympathetic nervous system [162, 163]. The rostral ventrolateral medulla (RVLM; Fig. 5.27) is known as the pressor area of the medulla. It is a brain region that is responsible for basal and reflex control of sympathetic activity associated with cardiovascular function. Abnormally elevated sympathetic activity in the RVLM is associated with various cardiovascular diseases, such as heart failure and hypertension. The RVLM is notably involved in the baroreflex. It receives inhibitory GABAergic (GABA is an amino acid) input from the caudal ventrolateral medulla (Fig. 5.27). The RVLM is a primary regulator of the sympathetic nervous system. Oxidative stress modulates the balance between excitatory amino acid glutamate and the inhibitory amino acid GABA in the RVLM. The balance between excitatory and inhibitory amino acids determines the neural activity in this region [165, 166]. An increase in nitric oxide in the RVLM reduces sympathetic activity which reduces baroreceptor reflex, which reduces blood pressure. It also reduces heart rate. The same responses are produced with a decrease in the inhibitory GABA input to RVLM sympathetic neurons [162] (Fig. 5.27). Nitric oxide in the RVLM increases GABA release. The reduced availability of nitric

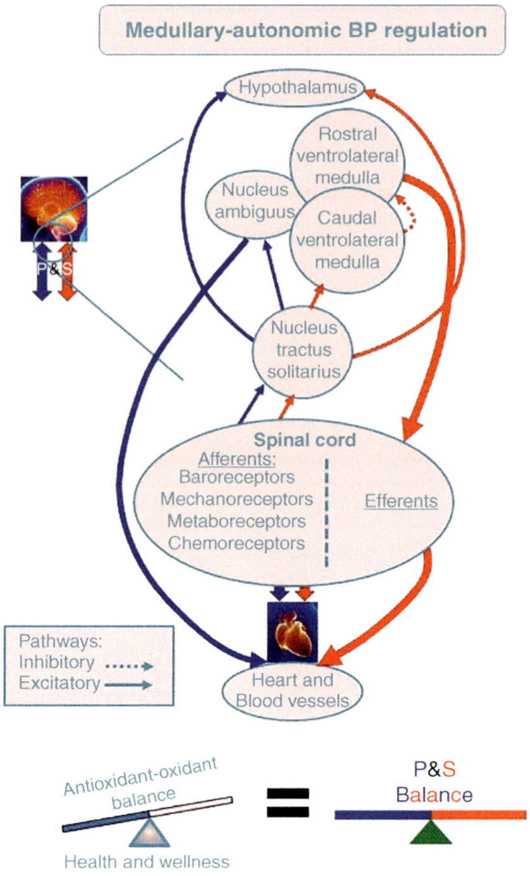


**Fig. 5.27** Blood pressure regulation by medulla. Major pathways in medulla are concerned with blood pressure regulation [164]. Chronic increased sympathetic outflow suppresses nitric oxide activity (red arrows) leading to increased oxidative stress and reduced GABA release, sustaining or further increasing blood pressure. The opposite is also true (blue arrows). See also Fig. 7.5, in Chap. 7. CVLM caudal ventrolateral medulla, NA nucleus ambiguus, NTS nucleus tractus solitarius, RVLM rostral ventrolateral medulla. (Source: https://clinicalgate.com/arterial-blood-pressure/)

oxide is associated with increased oxidative stress which reduces GABA release, thereby increasing sympathetic excitation, which increases baroreceptor reflex and blood pressure and leads to hypertension. This pathway to hypertension starts with oxidative stress which reduces nitric oxide levels by causing an overexpression of iNOS in the RVLM [167]. iNOS overexpression seems to be caused by NOS uncoupling due to reduced levels of L-arginine or BH4. Upregulation of angiotensin II, type 1 receptor,

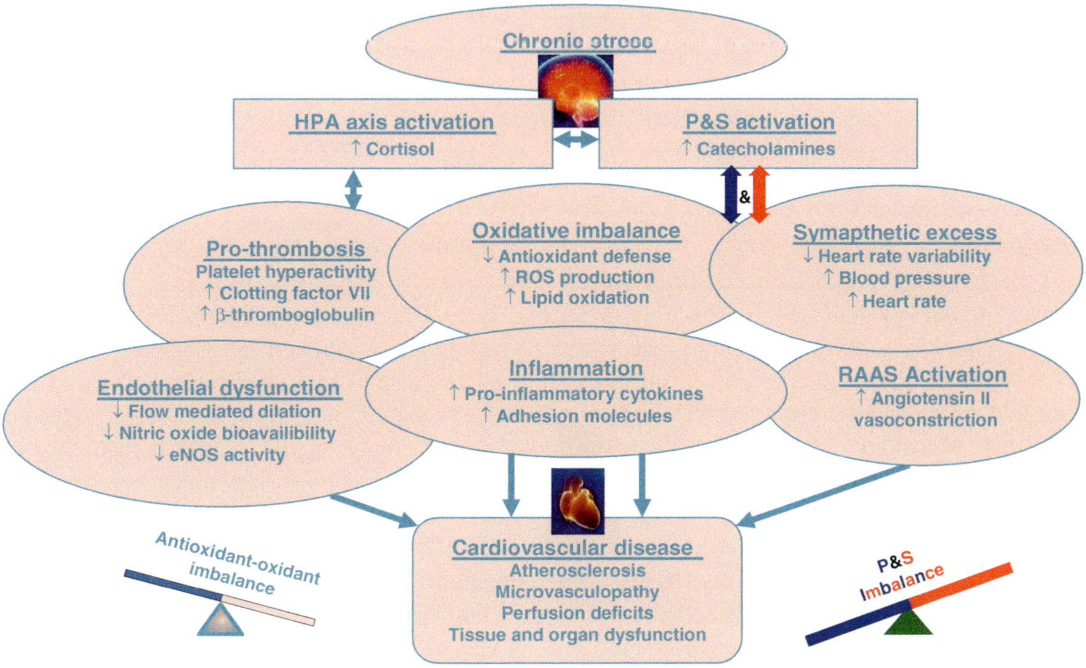


**Fig. 5.28** Some of the mechanisms involved in stress-induced cardiovascular adverse effects. Abbreviations: HPA hypothalamic-pituitary-adrenal, RAAS renin-angiotensin-aldosterone system, ROS reactive oxygen species, eNOS endothelial nitric oxide (NO) synthase. (Source: [169])

and iNOS in the RVLM is also associated with the maintenance of high blood pressure and renal sympathetic activation [168] and is another possible pathway to iNOS overexpression.

Pharmacology and "functional medicine" are complimentary. Prescription medicines are needed to ensure the disease or disorder is stabilized and at least partially relieved, and then functional medicine (i.e., supplements and lifestyle modifications, including diet and exercise) completes the therapy and helps to establish and maintain wellness. Examples (as discussed above) include: type 2 Diabetes medications (i.e., Metformin) and Alpha-Lipoic Acid, or Statins and Omega-3 fish oils. Traditional approaches should not be discounted but should incorporate complimentary (nontraditional) approaches as well.

Another mind-body effect of chronic stress involves the P&S branches of the autonomic nervous system and the complimentary hormonal centers, the hypothalamic-pituitary-adrenal (HPA) axis (Fig. 5.28) [169]. Consider the relationship between the P&S and HPA axis and the cardiovascular system. Under stress, the sympathetic nervous system activates and increases communication with the heart and vasculature by increasing catecholaminergic communications, specifically the β-sympathetic nerves that communicate with the heart to increase heart rate (chronotropic) or blood pressure (ionotropic) activity. The α-sympathetic nerves communicate with the vasculature and cause vasoconstriction, peripherally also raising blood pressure. The HPA axis increases cortisol release into the body, effecting increased fat retention (especially abdominal), mood (including increasing anxiety), poor sleep causing fatigue, menstrual and fertility issues for women, changes in libido in both genders, depressed immune activity, high blood pressure, increased osteoporosis, dehydration, and more. Increased cortisol increases systemic inflammation, further increasing sympathetic (catecholamine) activity. This leads to chronic inflammation and renin-angiotensin-aldosterone system activation increasing or supporting chronically elevated blood pressure.

Chronically elevated sympathetic output causes P&S (autonomic) and oxidative imbalance, high blood pressure (including hypertension), high heart rate (including arrhythmia), and endothelial dysfunction. These abnormalities promote micro- and macrovascular diseases (e.g., arteriosclerotic coronary disease or ASCD) and abnormal perfusion of organs and tissues.

For short durations, these activities are protective and perhaps even lifesaving. However, under chronic conditions, all three activities accelerate the onset and increase the severity of heart disease and stroke and thereby morbidity and mortality risk. Morbidity risk readily involves renal disorder, cognitive function, and "quality of life" disorders, including upper and lower GI upset, bladder dysfunction, sleep disorders, and sex dysfunction. Mortality risk involves CAN with high risk of MACE and typically reduces possible life span. Again, stress reduction through exercise, diet, relaxation (meditation, breathing exercises, yoga, etc.), and antioxidant supplements help to stay, and potentially reverse, the effects of chronic stress.

## Coenzyme Q10

Like ALA, CoQ10 is the other powerful antioxidant made by the body. It also has many applications throughout the body, especially in the mitochondria which is critical for proper cardiac and nerve function. As mentioned in the Preface, arguably the first serious application of CoQ10 in cardiology was by Dr. Lemole. Dr. Lemole's cardiac bypass patients had excellent results on CoQ10, as compared with other cardiothoracic patients empirically with stress radionuclide angiography. His patients had much better left ventricular resting function and reserve compared to other surgeons. This was in an era when cardioplegia[9] was then being more perfected, and better cardioplegia techniques were making even mediocre surgeons to have good results. Dr. Lemole's patients' good results were perhaps likely because they were more fully revascularized and because his technique was still far superior to others, which arguably was true at the time. However, he also put most of his postoperative patients on a CoQ preparation, even before many were familiar with CoQ10 or had knowledge about its biological feasibility. There was very little evidence-based medicine behind its use when he first started using it.

CoQ10 is an essential, lipid-soluble antioxidant which protects cellular membranes and also circulates lipoproteins against free radical-induced oxidative stress. CoQ10 has significant oxidative stress-reducing properties. CoQ10 is an essential component of the electron transport chain and functions as an electron carrier as well as an antioxidant. It made sense that it would be useful in situations where there were deficiencies of mitochondrial energy generation as well as situations in which cellular antioxidant capacity, such as in the postoperative period, could be prevalent.

Reactive oxygen species (ROS) and reactive nitrogen species (RNS, collectively abbreviated as RONS) play a significant role in pathophysiology of cardiovascular disease, and this was beginning to be appreciated at that time. Subsequently, it has been shown that CoQ10 has a protective effect on the endothelia or the cells that line the inner layer of the blood vessels [170]. It also improves the preservation of mitochondrial ATP production, especially after ischemia and reperfusion injury. CoQ10 has been used in the cardiothoracic surgical setting to compensate reperfusion-related increases in ROS and generation of oxidative damage because of its ability to scavenge hydroxyl free radicals directly. It had been postulated that the action of CoQ10 could reduce myocardial injury from cardioplegia and decrease troponin I[10] release and therefore protect against post-stress contractile dysfunction [171, 172]. The formation of hydroxyl peroxide arising from ischemia perfusion injury can trigger myoglobin oxidation to ferrimyoglobin, which can be detrimental to the myocardium. Mordente and coworkers in 1993 showed that

[9]Intentional and temporary cessation of cardiac activity, primarily for cardiac surgery

[10]Troponin I is involved in muscle contraction and is a marker of heart attack in the bloodstream.

UQ10-H2[11] was capable of reducing both ferrimyoglobin and metmyoglobin to oxymyoglobin[12] and thus displayed a process by which antioxidant mechanisms can occur with CoQ10 in ischemia-reperfusion-induced damage [173].

The biological feasibility and advantages of using an antioxidant such as CoQ10 are to protect against cardioplegia and postoperative oxidative stress which could impair left ventricular function. Arguably, the addition of CoQ10 improves stress radionuclide angiogram studies done postoperatively and shows much higher ejection fraction than without.

Heart failure is also due to loss of contractility of the myocardium. This is a consequence of insufficient energy in the myocardium. Chronic heart failure patients do show decreased CoQ10 levels on serum studies and endomyocardial biopsies [174, 175]. Data supports findings that CoQ10 improves the efficiency of, and quantity of, energy production in human hearts as an adjunct to standard medical therapy in heart failure [176–178]. Further studies showed that CoQ10 decreased thiobarbituric acid-reactive substances (TBARS) and malondialdehyde (MDA), which are substances measured which indicate oxidative stress. This is supported in heart failure; CoQ10 scavenges free radicals [179].

However, trials with CoQ10 have been small and in some cases incomplete. Some have shown improvement in the New York Heart Association Heart Failure rating. Overall biochemical data [180] support a favorable effect of CoQ10 in outcomes and trials in heart failure, but these are limited and none of the small trials have shown a difference in mortality. Some reported studies have shown reduced hospital stay and reduced ionotropic requirements to improve patients' cardiac output postoperatively.

There are many randomized studies of CoQ10 supplementation in chronic stable heart failure. There are many differences in the methodologies and some of the outcomes. A long-term multicenter and randomized study [181] reports clinical outcomes of hospitalization and mortality. This was the largest randomized placebo-controlled trial in the treatment of heart failure reported in peer review literature to date and had 641 patients and long follow-up duration of 1 year. The data showed impressive reduction in hospitalizations for heart failure of 23% for placebo and 37% for CoQ10, but no difference in mortality. However, only 30% of patients were taking ACE inhibitors and none were taking beta-blockers. Today, patients are taking beta-blockers and ACE inhibitors, some of both of which do now have antioxidant effects. Given that CoQ10 is known to recycle other antioxidants (e.g., vitamins A, C, and E), without these other antioxidants, the effects of CoQ10 are reduced. Therefore, to do a study would be difficult based on the fact that patients are already taking significant pharmacology. It is unlikely that further trials or even meta-analysis will provide more information. The data, however, says that by itself CoQ10 has (1) a biological feasibility of a protective mechanism in patients to preserve left ventricular function or treat patients with left ventricular dysfunction and (2) offers a rationale to use it in postoperative cardiothoracic patients. Given that CoQ10 recycles other antioxidants, thereby increasing its own potency as an antioxidant, theoretically amplifies these findings in heart failure.

Literature has shown that there is increasing interest in introducing CoQ10 for treatment of mitochondrial disorders. CoQ10, as noted, has been reported to improve ATP regeneration in vitro and is a significant important antioxidant in both mitochondria and lipid membranes. CoQ10 is neuroprotective against lesions produced by the mitochondrial toxin malonate [182].

CoQ10 improves ATP regeneration in cardiac muscles and skeletal muscles in Friedreich's ataxia, another neurodegenerative disease [183–185]. Another study in Huntington's disease and other neurodegenerative diseases showed that

[11] UQ10-H2 is the molecular name for CoQ10. UQ is the abbreviation for ubiquinone, the oxidized form, or ubiquinol, the reduced form. The latter is the useable form. The former is immediately transformed to the latter in the body. Either way, it is essential in the function and health of mitochondrial electron transport and the production of ATP.

[12] Myoglobins provide muscle cells reserve stores of oxygen for periods of intense activity. Ferri and Met forms of myoglobin provide more efficient means of storing oxygen.

CoQ10 produced a 14% slowing in disease progression over 30 months [186]. This study did not quite lead to statistical significance; however, their data in toto do reflect that antioxidant protection with agents such as CoQ10 is protective in cardiac and neurodegenerative diseases.

## Oxidative Stress I: Biology and Cardiovascular Disease

Oxidative stress and inflammation contribute to most human diseases. ROS play a major role in cellular and mitochondrial signaling and functioning. However, if ROS reach an excessive amount, they can cause tissue damage, including to mitochondria [187]. Mitochondria contribute approximately one-quarter the volume of cardiomyocytes or myocardial cells. This is because the heart requires high ATP production for energy on a continuous basis [188]. Mitochondria serve to generate ATP through a sequence of oxidizing and reducing reactions, which donate electrons down the electron transfer chain, utilizing oxygen to generate ATP. This is termed oxidative phosphorylation.

When electron transfer in the electron transport chain is not complete, the partial reduction of oxygen creates a superoxide ($O_2^-$) and can subsequently cause other ROS, such as hydrogen peroxide ($H_2O_2$) and hydroxyl radicals. The partial reduction is due to a small "leak," in which oxygen that was supposed to be consumed by the process of ATP production was lost and becomes a free radical. Less than 0.1% of electrons from the electron transport chain "leak." If not neutralized by antioxidants, these leaked electrons, or oxygen atoms, may damage and eventually destroy the mitochondria or nearby organelles or tissues. This requires mitochondria to contain antioxidant mechanisms to extinguish ROS, primarily the "leaked" oxygen. One system is the superoxide dismutase enzymes that dismutase $O_2$-$2H_2O_2$. Mitochondria $H_2O_2$ then undergoes catabolism by other enzymes, including glutathione peroxidase, and is ultimately reduced to water. Experimental studies have shown that excess mitochondrial ROS formation exacerbates ischemia reproduced in injury, heart failure, and diabetic cardiomyopathy [189–191]. Interestingly, at low or physiologic levels, ROS are signaling molecules within the mitochondria to modulate mitochondrial and cardiomyocyte function in a beneficial way. Apoptosis is tightly regulated cell death. Breakdown of organelles and cells can cause necrosis. Mitochondrial roles in cell death pathways are not completely distinguished during necrosis and apoptosis.

Evidence suggests that mitochondrial damage can directly give rise to immune activation in numerous organs including the heart [192]. Following myocardial infarction, necrosis in myocardial DNA can be released into circulation, which activates neutrophils and initiates systemic inflammation [193]. Oxidative stress can damage cells as noted due to mitochondrial dysfunction. Strategies including lifestyle changes, such as caloric restriction, exercise training, and therapeutic agents [194, 195], help to control mitochondrial ROS production, supporting mitochondrial function and preventing apoptosis, necrosis, and inflammation.

There is a complex association between oxidative stress, telomere biology, and cell senescence. Cell division and aging are the most important causes of telomere shortening [187]. Oxidative stress can promote telomere shortening and dysfunction [196]. This drives cell aging or senescence and apoptosis. Factors which cause telomere attrition are age, cell division, genetic factors, oxidative stress, inflammation, and renin-angiotensin system activation. Factors which counteract telomere shortening include telomerase enzymes, genetic factors, estrogen, and antioxidants [187]. Environmental factors inhibiting shortening of telomere length include a healthy lifestyle [197–201]. Circulating leukocyte, telomere length, and oxidative stress may be targets for statin therapy and metformin [202]. High-level physical activity in leisure time is associated with longer leukocyte telomere length [203]. Weight loss and bariatric surgery also increase leukocyte telomere length in obese patients [204]. Environmental factors negatively affecting telomere length include smoking, alcohol abuse, and air pollution [187].

Mental stress also negatively effects telomere length. In addition to a healthy lifestyle and estrogen treatment, vitamins C, D, and E, omega-3 fatty acids, statin, metformin, and bariatric surgery counteract telomere shortening.

ROS accelerates telomere shortening and causes DNA damage. ROS induces a DNA damage response and senescence [205]. Telomere shortening and cellular senescence are involved in aging and the development of age-related disease, but to what extent this is causal or secondary has not been fully developed. Many of the factors which cause telomere shortening and dysfunction are modifiable. Some are non-modifiable. Healthy lifestyle is modifiable. A healthy lifestyle remains a cornerstone of preventing age-related cardiovascular disease. The question is can antioxidants or certain drugs (e.g., metformin or renin-angiotensin blockers) be clinically beneficial at protecting telomeres and preventing premature cardiovascular aging? Research is being done to develop new antioxidants to prevent age-related diseases and promote healthy aging [206].

## Oxidative Stress II: Impact on the Heart and Vasculature

ROS regulate multiple vascular cell functions including endothelial cell and smooth muscle cell growth proliferation, angiogenesis, vascular, tone, etc. [207]. Heart failure is categorized by activation of sympathetic nervous system and renin-angiotensin system. These neuroendocrine activations are associated with oxidative stress in the myocardium and vasculature. Oxidative stress is an imbalance between a generation of ROS and its detoxification. In heart failure, oxidative stress occurs in the myocardium [208, 209] and plasma and correlates with left ventricular dysfunction [210]. ROS adversely affect the disposition of myocardial calcium, causing arrhythmia and abnormal cardiac remodeling and left ventricular hypertrophy, apoptosis, and necrosis. Enzymatic sources for ROS include nicotinamide adenine dinucleotide phosphate (NADPH) and oxidases. Also, they include uncoupled nitric oxide synthase (NOS), and lastly, mitochondria are considered relevant sources of ROS in heart failure.

In the mitochondria, the Krebs cycle generates NADH which donates electrons to the electron transport chain to produce ATP. The Krebs cycle also produces substrates that regenerate NADPH, which in turn regenerates antioxidative enzymes. Mitochondrial calcium is responsible for regeneration of NADH and NADPH which compromises ATP production and produces ROS from mitochondria. Uncoupled endothelial NOS is also seen in heart failure. This is seen both in blood vessels and in myocardial cells.

Antioxidants such as vitamins E and C have not been beneficial in heart failure. This is because these vitamins are not specifically targeted to the site of ROS generation in the mitochondrion. These vitamins react more slowly with ROS, and ROS can interact with nitric oxide to induce damage quicker. In fact, high doses of vitamin E worsen rather than improve vascular function, which may be related to the pro-oxidative vitamin E radical that is produced. This may be why long-term vitamin E does not prevent but rather induces heart failure with acute left heart decompensation, as shown in the HOPE trial [211]. This was also found in the HOPE-TOO study [212].

Angiotensin-converting enzymes and angiotensin receptor blockers exert their beneficial effects in part through antioxidative mechanisms. They are a primary therapy of blocking ROS production at the enzymatic source, whereas vitamin E therapy can be considered only a secondary therapy that scavenges already formed ROS. Hydralazine is also an important drug and affects the balance between $O_2^-$ and NO, the so-called nitrous-redox balance, which is impaired in heart failure. In fact, nitrate tolerance is prevented when combined with hydralazine because hydralazine inhibits nitroglycerin-induced vascular $O_2^-$ and $ONOO^-$ formation in vitro and in vivo. Again, it is emphasized that low concentrations of ROS are physiological and protective. High concentrations of ROS cause oxidative stress and play a casual role in the initiation and progression of heart failure.

Under conditions of oxidative stress, ROS mediate vascular changes such as endothelial dysfunction by disrupting the vaso-protective nitric oxide signaling cascade [213]. Nitric oxide is a key anti-atherosclerotic component and has been called the anti-atherosclerotic molecule. Nitric oxide (1) inhibits platelet adhesion, (2) inhibits platelet aggregation, (3) powerfully augments vasodilation or stimulation of CGMP production by smooth muscle cells, (4) decreases leukocyte-endothelial interaction, and (5) reduces smooth muscle cell proliferation [214]. Nitric oxide is generated from L-arginine by endothelial nitric oxide synthetization in the presence of its essential cofactor BH4. Superoxides ($O_2^-$) rapidly scavenge nitric oxide to produce $ONOO^-$ [215]. Rapid reaction between $O_2^-$ and nitric oxide yields $ONOO^-$ approximately three to four times faster than dismutation of $O_2^-$ by the superoxide dismutase (SOD). ROS plays a role in the inflammatory component of atherosclerosis by secreting pro-inflammatory cytokines, interleukins IL-1β and IL-8 [216].

Inflammatory pathways drive atherogenesis and link conventional risk factors to atherosclerosis and its complications. One inflammatory mediator has come to the fore as a therapeutic target in cardiovascular disease. The experimental and clinical evidence reviewed here support interleukin-1 beta (IL-1β) as both a local vascular and systemic contributor in this regard (Fig. 5.29). Intrinsic vascular wall cells and lesional leukocytes alike can produce this cytokine. Local stimuli in the plaque favor the generation of active IL-1β through the action of a molecular assembly known as the inflammasome. Clinically applicable interventions that interfere with IL-1 action can improve cardiovascular outcomes, ushering in a new era of anti-inflammatory therapies for atherosclerosis. The translational path described in Fig. 5.30 illustrates how advances in basic vascular biology may transform therapy. Biomarker-directed application of anti-inflammatory interventions may help achieve a more precise and individualized therapy for cardiovascular patients.

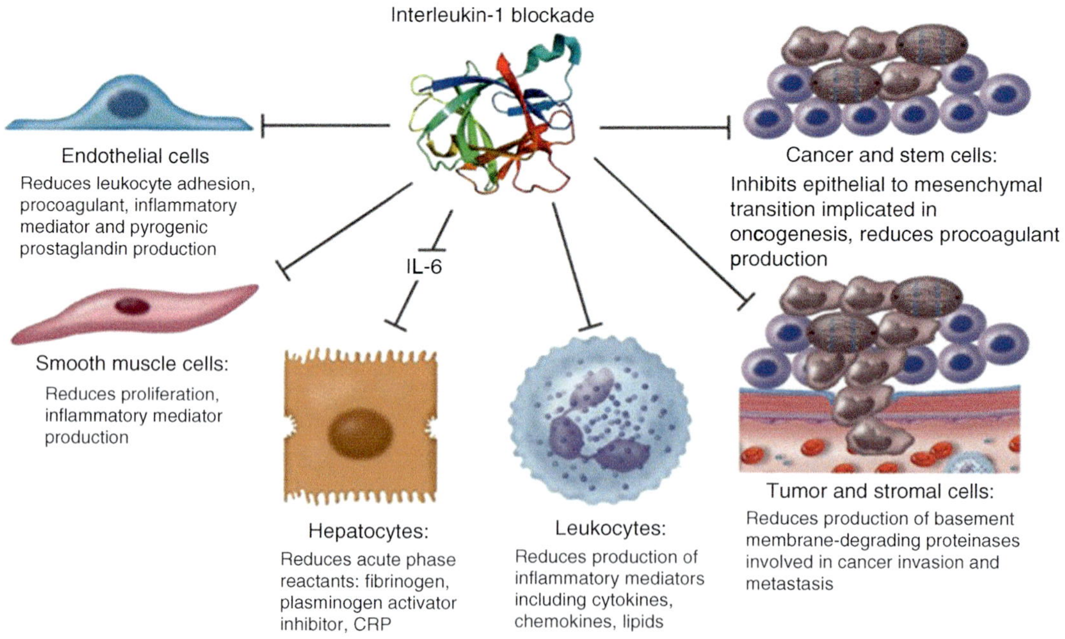


**Fig. 5.29** Interleukin (IL)-1 exerts many actions on cells that can contribute to pathogenesis of diseases, including atherosclerosis, thrombosis, oncogenesis, and invasion and metastasis of tumors. Many of the effects of IL-1 on hepatocytes, including the induction of the acute phase response, depend on the intermediary IL-6, a cytokine potently induced by IL-1. Strong human genetic evidence implicates IL-6 as a causal factor for atherothrombosis. CRP C-reactive protein [217]

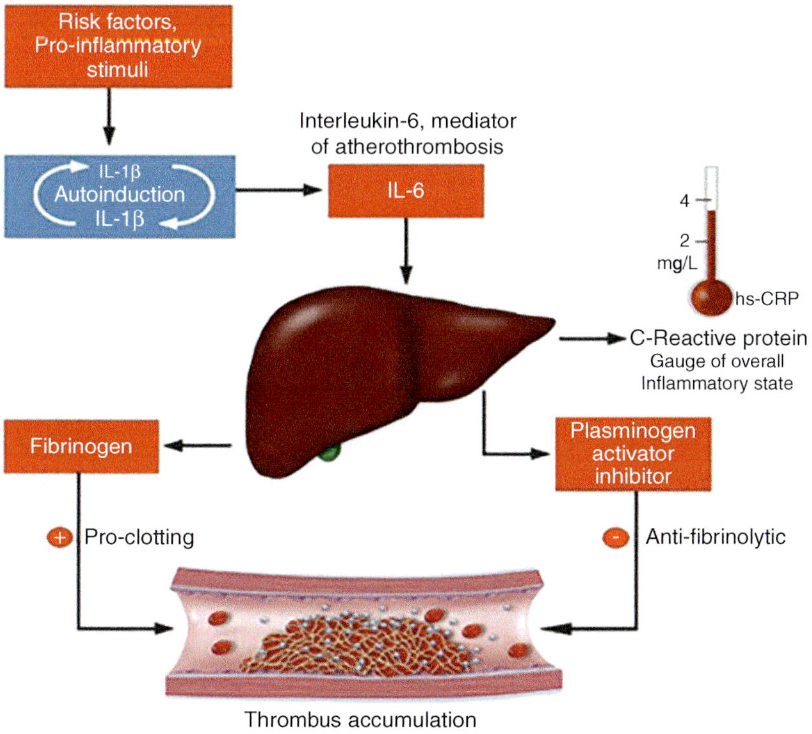


**Fig. 5.30** Interleukin-1 can induce its own gene expression in many cell types, including those implicated in atherosclerosis. This property provides a positive feedback amplification loop for boosting IL-1 levels at sites of inflammation. IL-1 also strongly augments the production of IL-6 by various cell types. IL-6 mediates the acute phase response through which the liver produces proteins that participate in host defenses but that also augments thrombosis and inhibits fibrinolysis as explained in the text. hs-CRP = high-sensitivity C-reactive protein [217]. (Republished with permission from Elsevier)

Experimental and clinical data suggest that reducing inflammation without affecting lipid levels, with human monoclonal antibodies, may reduce the risk of cardiovascular disease. Yet, the inflammatory hypothesis of atherothrombosis has remained unproved. Anti-inflammatory therapy targeting the interleukin-1β innate immunity pathway may significantly lower the rate of recurrent cardiovascular events, independent of lipid level lowering (CANTOS Clinical Trials). Trial evidence suggests a 15% reduction in death from myocardial infarction, cardiovascular disease, and combined cardiovascular diseases [218]. These results suggest that abnormal antibodies associated with inflammation play at least a partial role in atherogenesis leading to cardiovascular disease and that reducing inflammation, by reducing abnormal antibodies, may ultimately reduce cardiovascular disease.

Multiple bodies of experimental and clinical evidence correlate inflammation with atherogenesis and its complications [219–226]. Inflammatory status, monitored by C-reactive protein (CRP) concentrations measured with a high-sensitivity CRP (hsCRP) assay, improves the prediction of first occurrence and recurrent cardiovascular events, improved beyond the predictions of conventional risk algorithms [227, 228]. Targeting therapies with anti-inflammatory actions based on inflammatory status can reduce cardiovascular events [229]. Reductions of events by statin therapy may result in part from muting inflammation both by reduction in LDL and by direct effects [230–232]. However, this is often not enough (see "Statin Gap," Fig. 3.2). There are strong correlations between inflammation and atherosclerosis, and anti-inflammatory therapies (e.g., agents such as statins which alter both the causal risk factor (LDL) and inflammatory pathways) and reduced risk of atherosclerosis. However, high-dose statin treatment and other current standard measures only prevent a fraction of recurrent events in survivors of myocardial infarction (MI) [233–235] and may involve other disorders or dysfunctions that involve neuromuscular and cognitive processes. This residual burden of events presents a pressing unmet medical need [217], which may be filled with the Mind-Body Program, as discussed throughout this book.

Oxidative stress causes endothelial dysfunction through $O_2$-scavenging of nitric oxide to produce ONOO-, followed by uncoupling of oxygen regeneration from nitric oxide synthase (NOS) by endothelial nitric oxide, causing it to produce atherosclerotic lesions [236]. ROS favor pro-inflammation, vascular cell adhesion molecules, and NF-kB activation. These are transcription factors that play a role in the proliferative singling associated with smooth muscle cell growth in vascular remodeling. Oxidative stress is a critical component of hypertension where NATPH oxidase represents the primary source of ROS. In vascular aging, two characteristics of ROS-related features have been defined in the endothelial dysfunction in essential artery stiffness [237].

Unfortunately, there is confusion within the industry. Some large meta-analyses have shown that antioxidant supplements show no beneficial effects. Further, some even suggest that they may potentially raise overall mortality. This is unfortunate because these studies are not consistent nor are their results assessed against consistent, let alone common measures. For example, someone who is already consuming recommended daily allowances of vitamin C, through eating and drinking fruits, vegetables, and juices that contain the vitamin, is permitted to enter a study where 1000 mg of supplemental vitamin C is administered. These patients may show no advantage, because they are already consuming what the body needs and is able to use. In fact, these patients may complain of additional symptoms (like their urine burning them when they void). This is then taken as a negative without any explanation, and now there is "evidence" that vitamin C is potentially harmful. Well the urine burns because there was too much vitamin C taken, and the body is trying to eliminate it, causing the urine to become too acidic (as you know, vitamin C is an acid). Now people are worried about renal damage, due to the high acid content in the blood, and many other possibilities, no matter how remote.

This is how bad research, or research reported with a bias, is harmful. As in this example, the report that "vitamin C is harmful" does not inform anyone that the people for whom there was some discomfort did not report that they were already consuming significant quantities of vitamin C. It does not state that the researchers did not screen for baseline levels of vitamin C to begin with or that healthy people who did not need more vitamin C were not excluded from the study. The study also does not state that the subjects were or were not taking alpha-lipoic acid (ALA). As discussed earlier in this book, ALA recycles and, therefore, potentiates vitamin C. So if the study does not control for ALA, the results will be more varied. The subjects taking ALA will have much more significant vitamin C benefit than those who do not; and this has nothing to do with vitamin C itself. This confusion is a main reason for the writing of this book. This book is an attempt to bring some order to the confusion and chaos in the supplement and nutraceutical world.

To that end, care is still needed, for there are many mechanisms that are still poorly understood or not, yet, known. With regard to the failure of antioxidants and vitamins, there are many mechanisms that have been hypothesized. Antioxidants and vitamins, for example, do not scavenge hydrogen peroxide ($H_2O_2$) creating water ($H_2O$) and hypochlorous acid (HClO). Hydrogen peroxide is strongly implicated in vascular damage. Another possibility is that many antioxidants are likely oxidized rapidly to an inactive form. Dosage inconsistencies have been noted, as has disease state inconsistencies (e.g., clinical trials were performed in high-risk patients in which vascular disease was advanced and who needed much more help that just supplements).

Fortunately, certain areas of research have been standardized. For example, considerable advancements have been made in the delivery of antioxidants to the individual mitochondrion. There is a new compound, MitoQ, that follows this principle of diminishing radical production in mitochondrial damage without interfering with respiratory function. It has been shown to blunt myocardial ischemia-reperfusion injury, nitrate-related endothelial damage, blood pressure, and doxorubicin-induced heart damage and sepsis-associated heart and liver damage [195].

In summary, vascular aging causes endothelial dysfunction and arterial stiffness. ROS negatively affect calcium handling and regulate multiple vascular functions. At low levels, they are beneficial. At high levels, they promote vascular disease through direct and irreversible oxidative damage to macromolecules as well as disruption of redox-dependent vascular wall signaling processes [207].

## Oxidative Stress III: Cardiovascular Risk of Obesity, Diabetes, Smoking, and Pollution

Diabetes and obesity have similarities in that fatty acid uptake and fatty acid oxidation are increased as levels of intra-myocardial circulating triglycerides, circulating free fatty acids, glucose uptake, and glucose oxidation are reduced [238, 239]. The ability of obese or diabetic hearts to use glucose results in reliance on fatty acid oxidation and reduces metabolic flexibility. Free fatty acids increase ROS production in mitochondria, which increases mitochondrial dysfunction leading to (among other dysfunctions) increased myocardial ROS emission [240]. Mitochondria are not the only source for ROS. ROS from any source damages mitochondrial DNA. Since mitochondria have no repair capacity because they lack histones, and because they are in close proximity to the electron transport chain, many mitochondrial proteins in livers are damaged. These are the mechanism by which high-fat diets have detrimental effects.

Hyperglycemia induces the mitochondria to produce excess superoxide ($O_{2^-}$, a type of ROS) from increased flux in the electron transport chain. This is a major cause of the clinical consequences associated with diabetes and obesity [241]. In this way, hyperglycemia activates four major pathways in the pathogenesis of cardiovascular complications of diabetes and obesity including (1) a path that increases production of advanced glycation end products (AGEs), (2) the polyol pathway, (3) the hexosamine pathway, and (4) the protein kinase C-dependent signal transduction [241]. In addition to increasing ROS production by mitochondria and other sources, cardiac expression or the activity of many antioxidant enzymes is reduced in obese or diabetic hearts along with reductions in circulating antioxidant enzymes [242, 243]. This may involve a phenomenon called metabolic memory resulting from prolonged hyperglycemia inclusive of metabolic changes that alter inflammatory and oxidative stress pathways [244].

Non-myocardial sources of ROS include NOX, xanthine oxidase (XO), uncoupled endothelial nitric oxide synthase (eNOS), mitochondrial monoamine oxidase A (MAO-A), lipoxygenase, cyclooxygenase, and other hemoproteins [245]. NOX2 prevents oxidative stress in mitochondrial abnormalities caused by saturated fat and cardiomyocytes. The ability of cardiomyocytes to respond to increased fatty acid load is significantly reduced with age and obesity, resulting in accumulation of lipids and ceramides, mitochondrial dysfunction, increased ROS production, and possibly reduced cell viability [246–248].

In addition, telomere length is a sensitive indicator of cumulative oxidative stress in post-mitotic cells, such as cardiomyocytes, and is significantly reduced in cardiomyocytes from young subjects with obesity [249]. Ectopic lipid accumulation in the heart is associated with cardiac hypertrophy, cardiac dysfunction, and apoptosis [248].

Increased oxidative stress in the heart and heart muscle cells is induced by multiple mechanisms, including mitochondrial dysfunction and uncoupling, increased fatty acid oxidation, enhanced NOX activity, and reduced antioxidant capacity. Recent data suggests metabolic memory is an important contributor to cardiovascular disease, as cells remember exposure to hyperglycemia and oxidative stress. Large-scale clinical trials using antioxidant therapy to treat cardiovascular disease have failed, especially vitamin E, as mentioned before [250]. Remember without alpha-lipoic acid (ALA), vitamin E is less potent. In large-scale studies, ALA has indeed been shown to significantly reduce heart disease in diabetes. It appears a more comprehensive approach may be required that prevents ROS generation while also promoting ROS scavenging, in particular, of damaged or aged cellular components and invaders of the body such as bacteria and viruses.

Cigarettes and pollution have also been shown to increase oxidative stress. Cigarette-related products and combustion-derived environmental air pollution (C-DEAP), which are principally found in urban pollution, have similarities. Tobacco smoke is comprised of a mixture of gases, aerosolized liquids, and small particles. The gas vapor phase of cigarette-related products contains nitrogen, carbon dioxide, and carbon monoxide with smaller but significant amounts of hydrogen, cyanide, nitric acid, methane, benzene, hydrogen sulfide, and a wide selection of hydrocarbons, aldehydes, carbonyls, and nitrosamines [251]. Air pollution derives from a large number of man-made (including industry, power plants, household, traffic, cooking, construction, mechanical, agriculture) and environment (forest fires, volcanic eruptions, pollen, molds, dust) sources. Epidemiology studies have shown a clear association between various cardiovascular diseases from smoking and from air pollution, including coronary artery disease, peripheral artery disease, heart failure, cerebrovascular disease, cardiac arrhythmia, and venous thromboembolism [252–265]. A substantial body of work demonstrates that these pollutants impair cardiovascular function [266, 267].

Air pollution is associated with elevated blood pressure and abnormal vascular function. This promotes vasoconstriction and decreased vasodilatory responses [268–270]. Exposure to pollution is accompanied by increases in inflammatory markers [271–273]. There is increased adherence of leukocytes to vessel wall in early events in atherosclerosis [274]. In addition to its effects on the pulmonary and peripheral vasculature, C-DEAP has also shown to have detrimental effects on coronary circulation [275–278]. Exposure to high levels of air pollution is associated with numerous biomarkers of oxidative stress [279–285]. Acute exposure to C-DEAP suggests a role for oxidative stress which attenuates vasodilatation in response to nitric oxide donor drugs. Reducing exposure to air pollution will undoubtedly remain a principal means of preventing the associated adverse health effects [286].

There is now overwhelming evidence that air pollution is associated with cardiovascular disease. There are striking similarities between composition of cigarette smoke and combustion-derived air pollution, both associated with multiple detrimental effects on the cardiovascular system. Certain individuals are more susceptible to cigarette smoke and air pollution. Particle size is important. Oxidative stress is a key mediator in air pollution and smoking in causing both lung and vascular injury. There is a question of whether pharmacological agents or supplements can limit the harmful effects of air pollution. It is possible. Antioxidant agents could represent a useful preventative strategy due to the clear involvement of oxidative stress in cardiovascular actions of air pollution. Research is ongoing.

## Oxidative Stress and Aging

Aging is a multidimensional irreversible accumulation of physiological, physical, environmental, and social changes [287]. Oxidative stress breaks down cells (damages cell membranes; alters gene (DNA) expression, which causes loss of genetic information; and interrupts signal transduction), leading to uncontrolled (not physiologically beneficial) cell death, causing premature aging and disease (see Fig. 2.25 and Fig. 5.31). Antioxidants (1) slow cell membrane damage, (2) slow gene alteration, (3) and promote normal signal transduction, thereby facilitating gene and tissue repair, which slows and perhaps (temporarily) reverses the aging process and degenerative disorders.

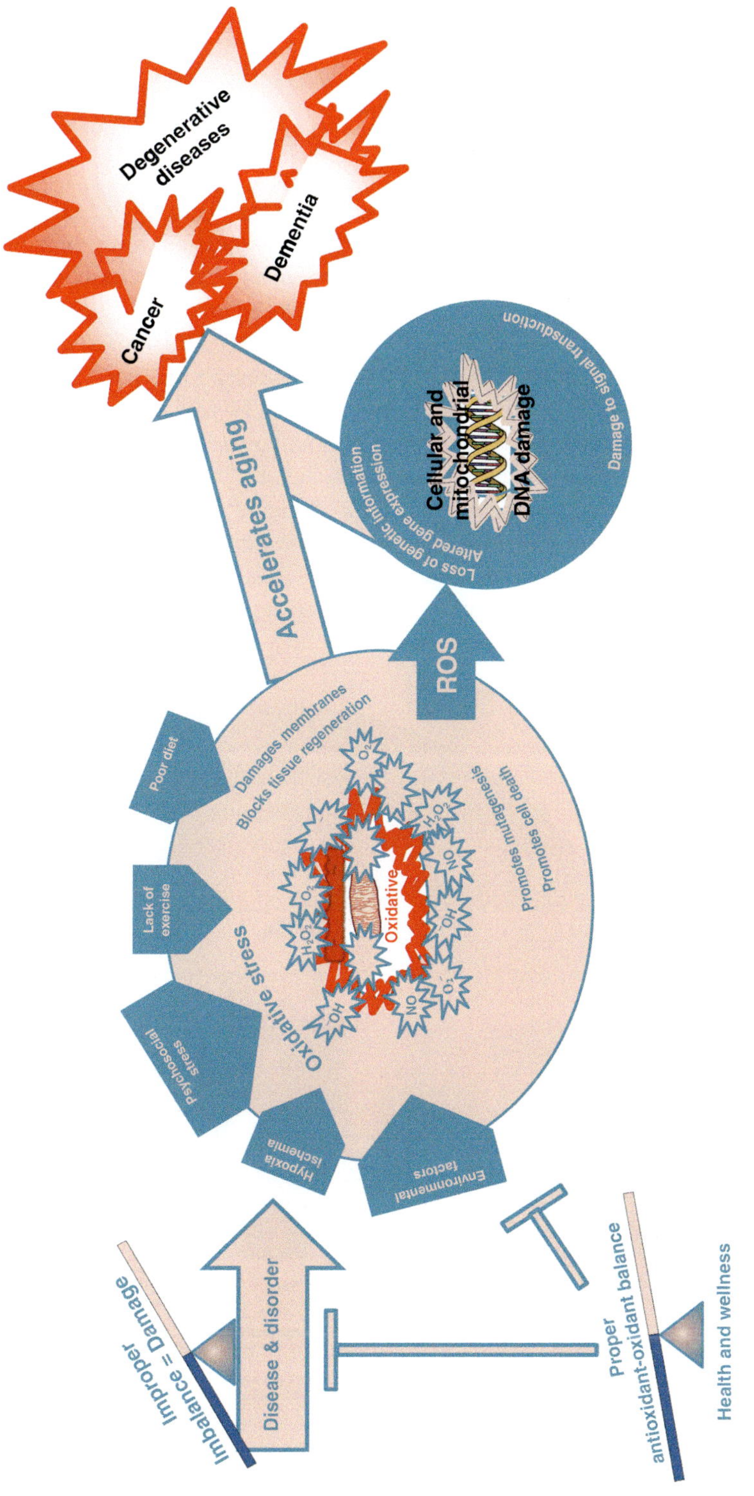


**Fig. 5.31** Oxidative stress and cellular damage during aging [217]. (Republished with permission from Elsevier. Source: http://realhealthcareclinic.com/2016/11/mitochondrial-dysfunction-and-chronic-disease/)

The "normal" aging process involves slowing of processes and reduction of process efficiencies (Fig. 5.32). A hallmark of aging is the decline in the autonomic nervous system. This decline seems to precede the decline in all other systems, including the immune system. This is logical, given that the P&S branches control and coordinate all other systems of the body. Figure 5.33 [288] displays the average declines in P&S activity (blue and red curves, respectively), with age, in a cohort of 239 normal subjects. Figure 5.34 displays the curves from Fig. 5.33 and from patient cohorts diagnosed with diabetes, hypertension, coronary artery disease (CAD), and HIV/AIDS. Notice that regardless of the disease and the system(s) affected (cardiovascular or not), disease accelerates the aging process. From the normal data, the P&S curves present with the parasympathetics higher than the sympathetics earlier in life. They overlie themselves, indicating P&S balance through the middle years, and again resume the trend of the parasympathetics higher than the sympathetics later in life. Parasympathetics higher than the sympathetics indicates a low-normal P&S balance, which is known to be cardioprotective.

From the four inserts of Fig. 5.34, disease processes cause the sympathetics to be higher than the parasympathetics, including later in life, which is associated with higher numbers of comorbidities and associated secondary symptoms and increase in medication load. Using type 2 diabetes as a model of chronic disease, Fig. 5.35 presents the normal subject P&S data from Fig. 5.33 with the average P&S data from over 500 type 2 diabetic patients. These data are age-matched. On average, P&S levels are up to 50% depleted upon first diagnosis, *and it is asymptomatic*. This seems to reflect the American Diabetes Association's indication that by the time of diagnosis, a type 2 diabetic has had the disease for up to 5 years [289, 290]. This confirms the

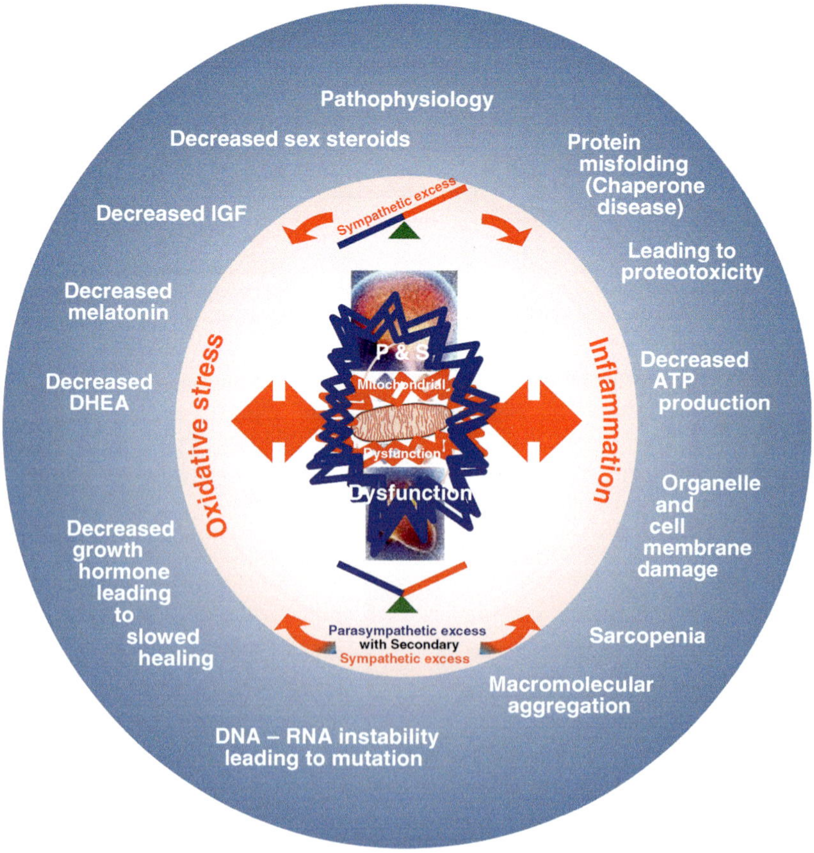


**Fig. 5.32** The consequences of aging. (Source: [23])

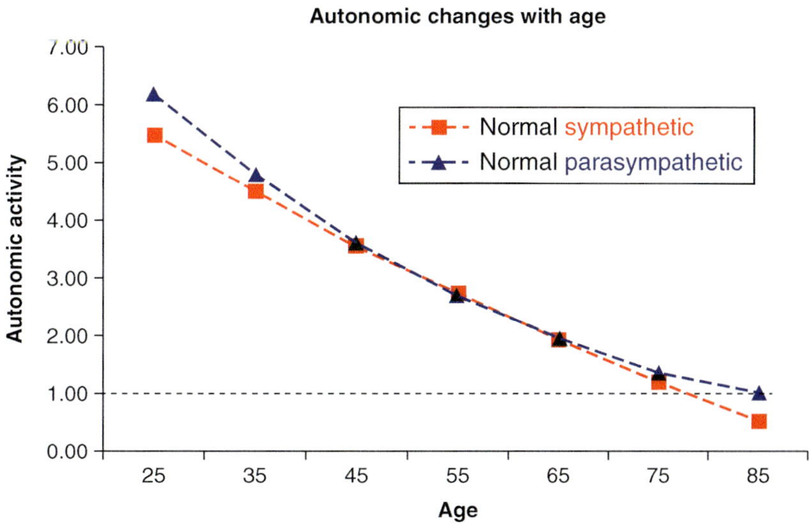


**Fig. 5.33** The effect of normal aging on the P (blue) and S (red) nervous systems (autonomic activity, bpm²). The horizontal broken line is the threshold of autonomic neuropathy. (Adapted from [288], with a population of 239 normal subjects (74 female). See text for details. Republished with permission from Springer Science + Business Media [116, Fig. 12.1])

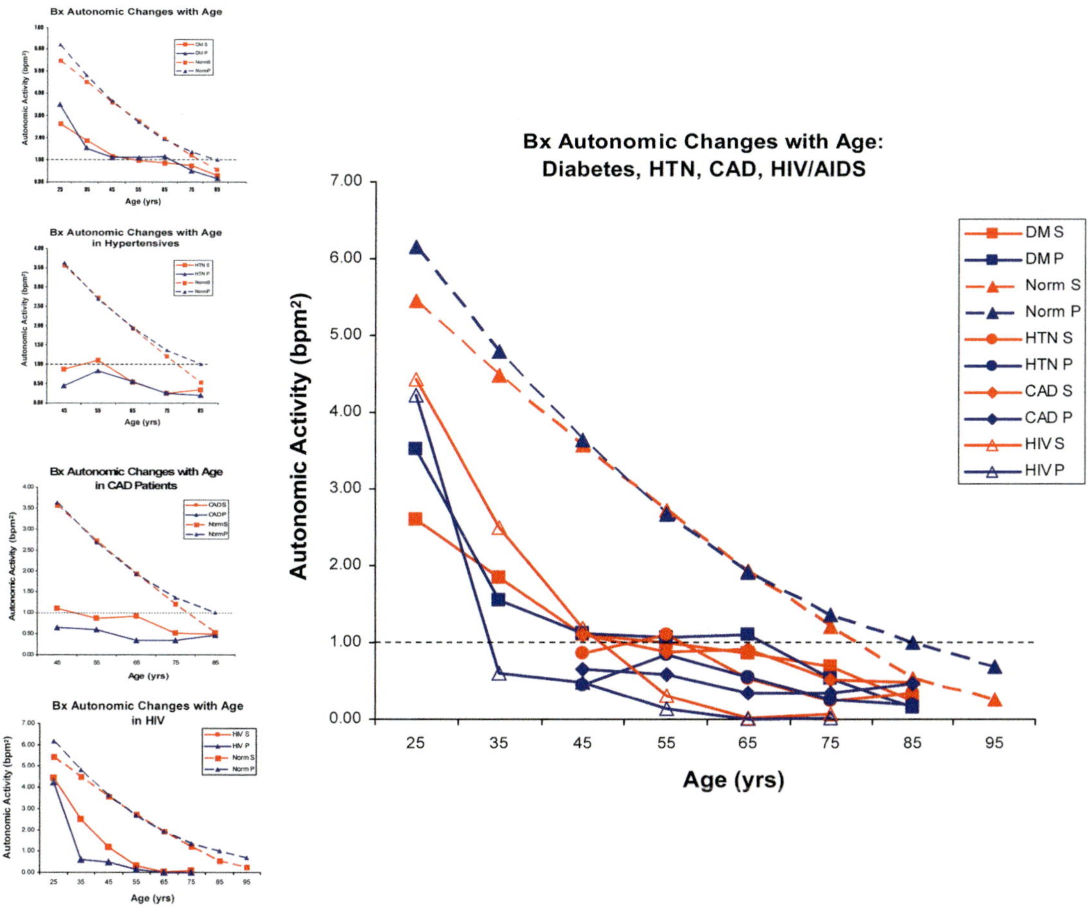


**Fig. 5.34** Age-matched comparisons between normal subjects and patients with diabetes, hypertension, CAD, and HIV/AIDS. P (blue) and S (red) nervous system activity (autonomic activity, bpm²) [116, Fig. 12.10]. See text for details. (Republished with permission from Springer Science + Business Media)

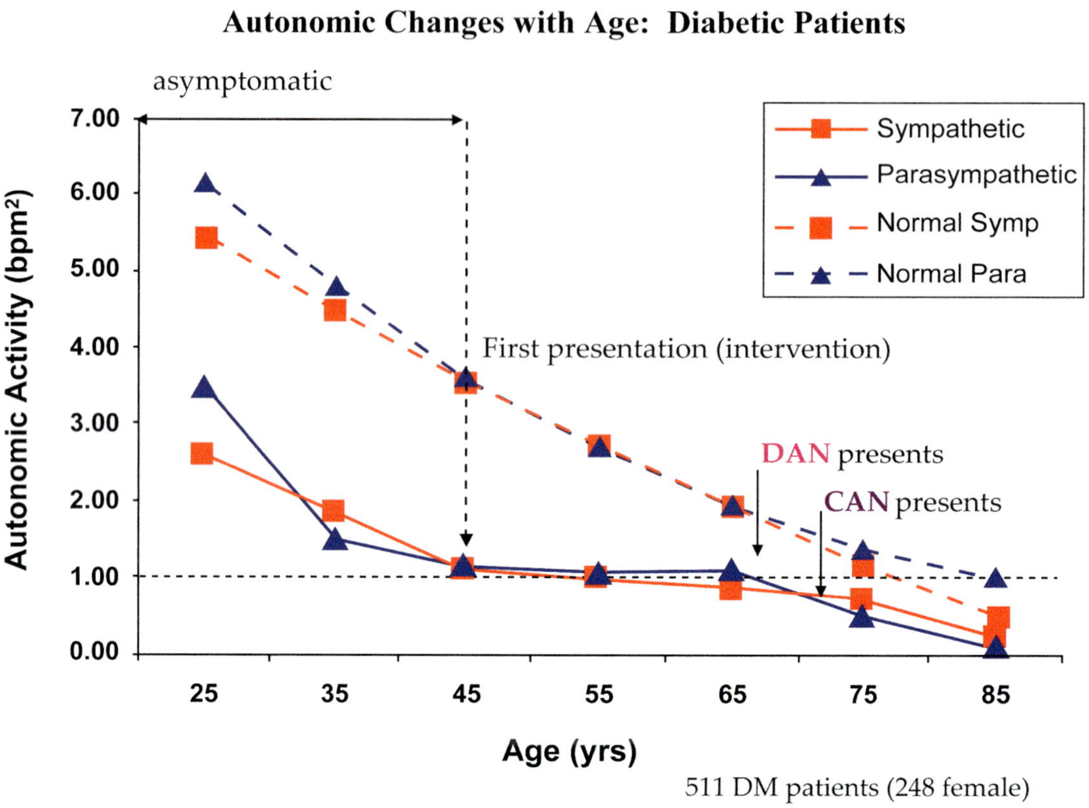


**Fig. 5.35** An age-matched comparison between normal subjects and patients with diabetes. P (blue) and S (red) nervous systems (autonomic activity, bpm$^2$) [116] See text for details. (Republished with permission from Springer Science + Business Media)

ADA recommendation for P&S monitoring within 2 years of a diagnosis of type 2 diabetes [289, 290]. The 7 years (five plus two) of the disease and the prediabetic conditions have already significantly depleted the P&S nervous systems, before the disease is even detected. By time symptoms present, P&S levels are up to 80% depleted, *and the decline was asymptomatic.*

Chronic disease seems to cause late-stage (relative) sympathetic dominance (SB > 1.0), which is known to increase morbidity and mortality, whereas the normal subjects demonstrate low-normal SB (0.4 < SB < 1.0). Low-normal SB is known to reduce morbidity and mortality [291]. Low-normal SB is titrated either with pharmaceuticals, nutraceuticals, or lifestyle changes, usually a combination of the three. Intervention slows P and S decline. Note how flat the patients' curves (solid lines) are after the "first presentation" and intervention around age 45 until decline continues (in parallel with normals) around age 65. Therapy to establish and restore normal SB, especially early, is known to slow autonomic decline. Figure 5.36 suggests that if the intervention that "flattens" (slows) the decline in P&S response is adopted earlier, the therapy could translate the patient's P&S response curves to the more normal autonomic decline curves of the normal subjects, minimizing morbidity and mortality and improving outcomes.

In the last decade (Fig. 5.36), even now that (on average) CAN is demonstrated by both cohorts, the normal subjects' parasympathetic levels are higher than their sympathetic levels.

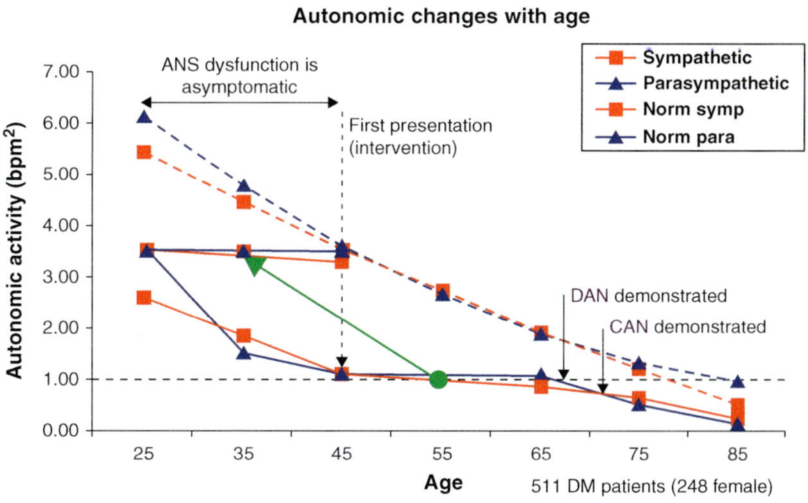


**Fig. 5.36** The effects of restoring and maintain autonomic (sympathovagal) balance [116]. See text for details. (Republished with permission from Springer Science + Business Media)

Again, this is known to be cardioprotective and is associated with fewer comorbidities and a reduced mediation load. Even though the chronic disease patients demonstrate (on average) a normal balance, their sympathetics are still higher than their parasympathetics. This is the main reason why the chronic disease patients also carry a greater comorbidity burden and higher medication load. Injury, lifestyle, genetics, and oxidative stress cause, or are caused by, P&S imbalance. P&S imbalance accelerates the progression of autonomic neuropathy and accelerates aging.

Higher parasympathetic levels than sympathetic levels at rest (low-normal sympathovagal balance) are also neuroprotective. One mechanism involves afferent vagus nerve (parasympathetic) stimulation of the nucleus tractus solitarius via the dorsal vagal complex. Stimulation of nucleus tractus solitarius stimulates the locus coeruleus, which causes the release of norepinephrine. Finally, norepinephrine stimulates neurogenesis, as well as excitation of cholinergic neurons, which leads to acetylcholine release and inhibition of inflammation. This pathway leads to a second mechanism in which norepinephrine also stimulates the release of serotonin from the dorsal raphe nucleus. Serotonin stimulates neurogenesis as well as suppresses the toxicity of excess sympathetic excitation. In the third pathway, the central cholinergic system releases acetylcholine, which inhibits inflammation in the brain by activating a nicotinic acetylcholine receptor (nAChR a 7), leading to suppression of cytokine (pro-inflammatory) release. The central cholinergic system also drives the cholinergic anti-inflammatory pathway systemically via the efferent vagus nerve. In the fourth pathway, nitrergic parasympathetic cerebrovascular innervation releases nitric oxide, which stimulates the sphenopalatine ganglion which causes vasodilation and increased perfusion, also leading to neuroprotection (see Fig. 5.37) [293]. Mechanisms promoting normal and pathological central nervous system aging are depicted in Fig. 5.38.

The decline with age in the P&S nervous systems seems to correlate with the decrease in the body's defense against oxidative stress and free radicals. The nerves are quite sensitive to oxidative stress and therefore are quite vulnerable to its effects, which contribute to their decline and premature aging. Oxidative stress is the key in the aging process triggering premature cell death. As the P&S nerves become dysfunctional and undergo premature cell death, organs eventually become dysfunctional, and morbidity and mortality risk increases sooner than in age-matched normal subjects.

In fact, not just the P&S nervous systems and the immune system but all systems of the body normally decline. From puberty throughout the rest of life, the efficiency of all physiological processes progressively declines [294, 295]. The

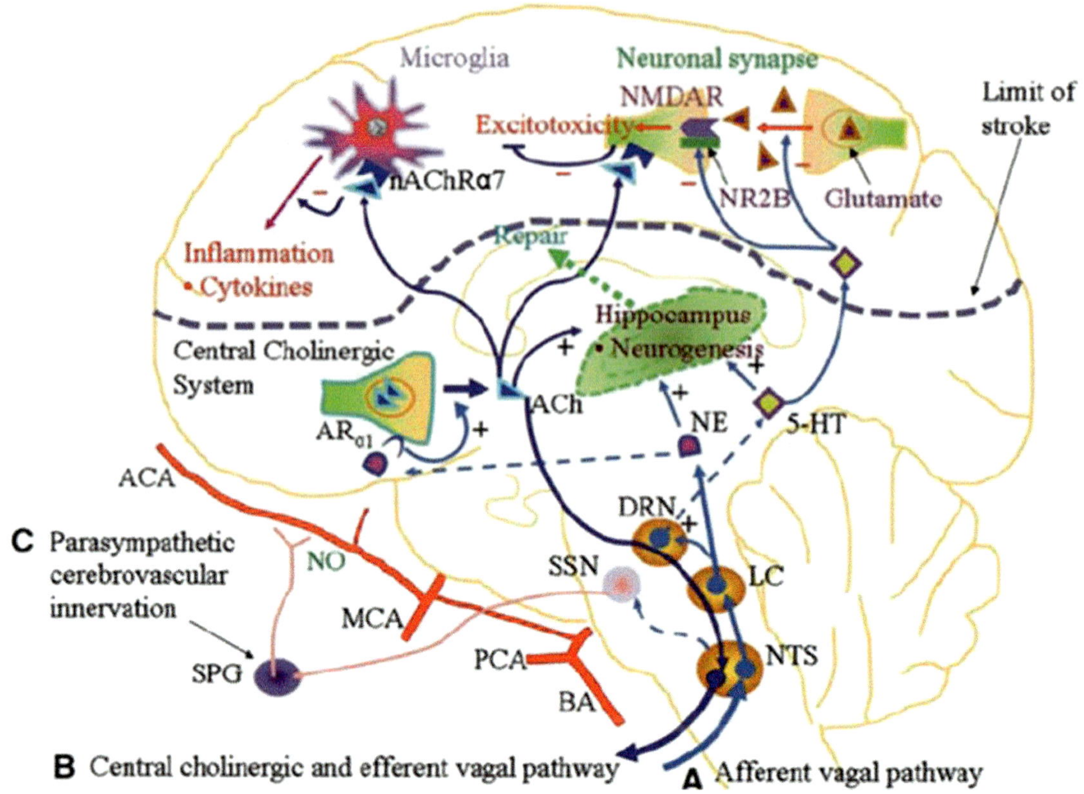


**Fig. 5.37** The neuroprotective mechanisms of the parasympathetic nervous system. (A) Afferent vagal pathway (represented by deep blue color): Afferent vagus nerve signals project to the dorsal vagal complex, where the majority of the fibers synapse on the nucleus tractus solitarius (NTS). Through the NTS projections to the locus coeruleus (LC), vagus nerve stimulation (VNS) causes the release of norepinephrine (NE). Norepinephrine subsequently stimulates the release of serotonin (5-hydroxytryptamine, 5-HT) from the dorsal raphe nucleus (DRN). Norepinephrine stimulates neurogenesis as well as excitation of cholinergic neurons leading to acetylcholine (ACh) release and inhibition of inflammation. 5-HT stimulates neurogenesis and suppresses excitotoxicity by inhibiting glutamate release and downregulating NR2B. (B) Central cholinergic and efferent vagal pathway (represented by dark blue color): The central cholinergic system releases ACh, which inhibits inflammation in the brain by activating *α* 7 nicotinic acetylcholine receptors (nAChR a 7), leading to suppression of cytokine release. The central cholinergic system also drives the cholinergic anti-inflammatory pathway systemically via the efferent vagus nerve. (C) Parasympathetic cerebrovascular innervation (represented by pink color): The sphenopalatine ganglion (SPG) receives preganglionic neurons from the superior salivatory nucleus (SSN). Postganglionic neurons from the SPG provide nitrergic innervation to the cerebral vasculature: anterior cerebral artery (ACA), middle cerebral artery (MCA), posterior cerebral artery (PCA), and basilar artery (BA). Through the release of nitric oxide (NO), stimulation of the SPG causes vasodilation and increased perfusion leading to neuroprotection. AR a 1, a 1-adrenergic receptor; NMDAR, N-methyl-D-aspartate receptor; "+" denotes stimulation; "–" denotes inhibition. (Republished with permission from SAGE Publications. Source: [292, 293])

gradual loss of homeostatic mechanisms associated with aging is, at least in part, due to an accumulation of oxidative damage [296–298]. Indeed, the "free radical theory of aging" is based on oxygen toxicity [296, 299]. Molecular oxygen is a biradical able to generate partially reduced molecules and then ROS. When all endogenous antioxidants are insufficient, ROS increases, altering the cell's normal redox state and, thus, provoking oxidative stress. High ROS levels cause toxic effects in the cell, because they are potentially detrimental for biological macromolecules, such as lipids, nucleic acids, and proteins (Fig. 5.39) [296, 301, 302].

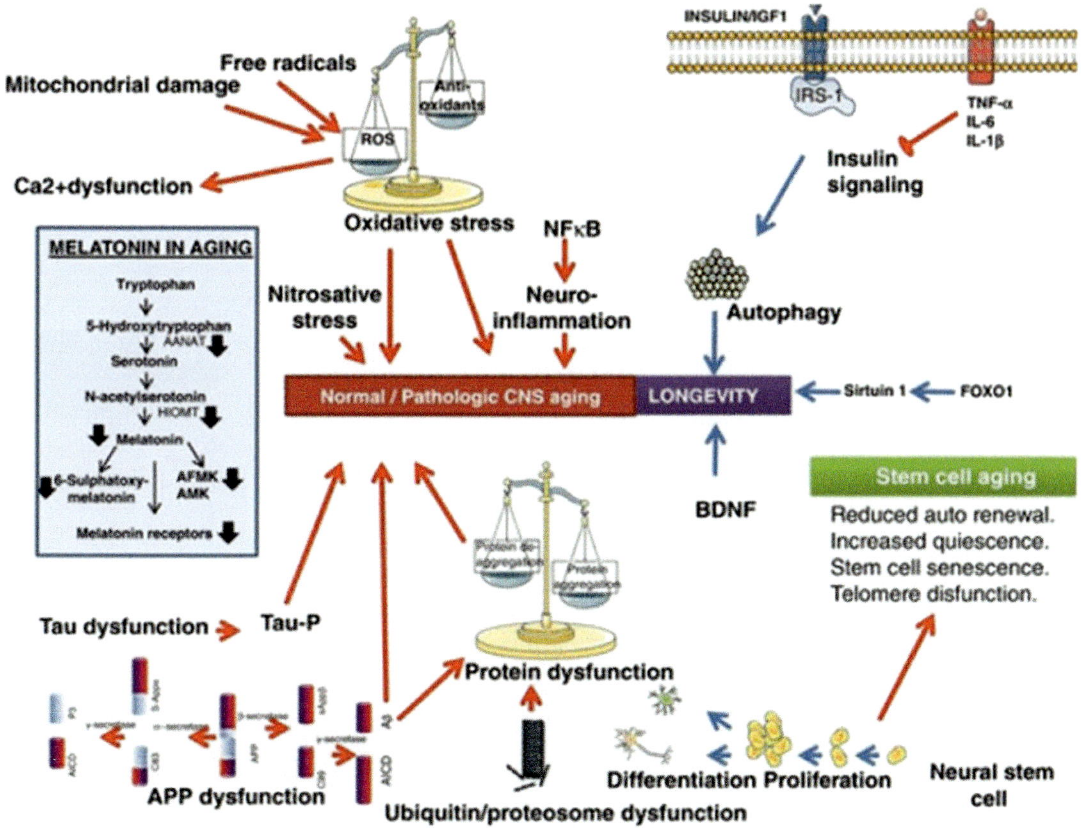


**Fig. 5.38** Mechanisms promoting normal and pathological central nervous system aging [23]. (Republished with permission from Springer International Publishing AG)

As a consequence of ROS accumulation causing oxidative stress, the imbalance of the normal redox state increases exponentially with age, paralleled by a remarkable decline of the cell repair machinery (Fig. 5.39) [303]. Oxidative stress contributes to the pathogenesis of several cardiovascular, pulmonary, and neuronal disorders common among elderly people, such as myocardial infarction, diabetes, atherosclerosis, COPD, or Alzheimer's disease [304–306]. Very recent studies indicated the multifactorial etiology of aging-associated diseases as related to both genetic and epigenetic changes due to oxidative stress [307]. Cardiac aging is characterized by cardiomyocyte cell death, hypertrophy, and fibrosis. Ischemia-reperfusion injury after acute myocardial infarction is a phenomenon strictly associated with oxidative stress damage [308] (Fig. 5.39).

Cardiovascular diseases are by far the leading cause of morbidity and mortality in industrialized nations [309]. Nowadays, due to remarkable progress in prevention and acute cardiac patient care, cardiovascular diseases manifest significantly later in life [309]. Therefore, the incidence of coronary artery disease, myocardial infarction, and heart failure, often strictly interconnected, increases almost exponentially with age [309]. Aging affects cardiovascular tissues, introducing typical markers: aged hearts show hypertrophy and fibrosis, whereas the aged vasculature is affected by arterial thickening and increased stiffness [310]. In this light, the health of cardiac and arterial systems is not mutually exclusive, as each system greatly affects the other [310]. For instance, an increase in arterial stiffness leads to compensatory mechanisms by the myocardium, which includes left ventricular hypertrophy and

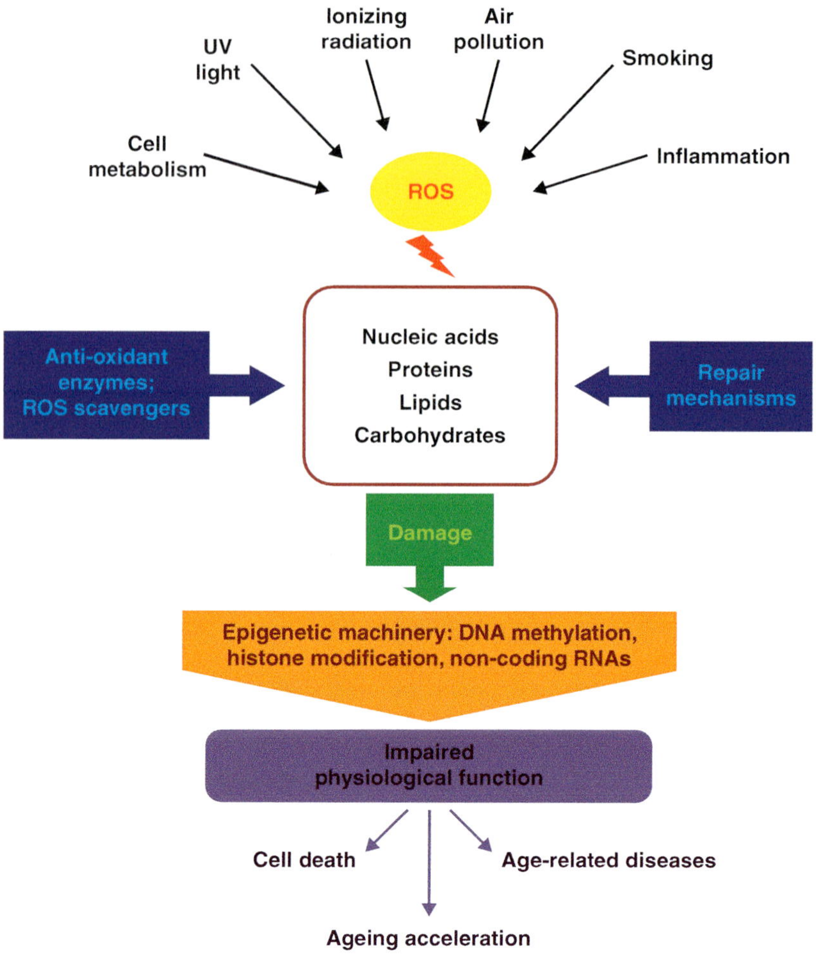


**Fig. 5.39** Oxidative stress and aging. See text for details. (Open Access, MDPI. Source: [300, 301])

fibroblast proliferation [311]. Physiological modifications may determine age-related pathophysiology, such as vascular dysfunction or insufficient vascular growth and remodeling. Heart fibrosis and hypertrophy induce slow propagation of electric impulse throughout the heart, modifying heart rate and the electrical impulse conduction, which increases the incidence of arrhythmias [312]. At the molecular level, aging is associated with changes in the activity of a series of enzymes necessary for cardiovascular homeostasis. For example, aged endothelial cells exhibit a decrease in eNOS activity and nitric oxide production [311].

ROS production increases during aging and determines oxidative stress, which might be responsible for cancer cells and senescence of endothelial cells [313]. Endothelial cell senescence is associated with endothelial dysfunction and vulnerability to atherosclerotic lesions. During aging, oxidative stress accumulates, paralleled with a decrease in nitric oxide production, which might be responsible of a process that "turns off" certain genes that promote aging, such as those involved in inflammation, in fat synthesis and storage, and in blood sugar management. This process facilitates the senescence-like phenotype of endothelial cells (Fig. 5.40). Statins, which induce eNOS activity via this process, may inhibit oxidative-dependent endothelial senescence [314].

In addition to the same endogenous oxidants as in the cardiovascular system, the lungs are constantly exposed to exogenous sources of oxidants. Some of the exogenous determinants of oxidation are air pollutants, noxious gases, and most commonly cigarette smoke [315, 316]. The accumula-

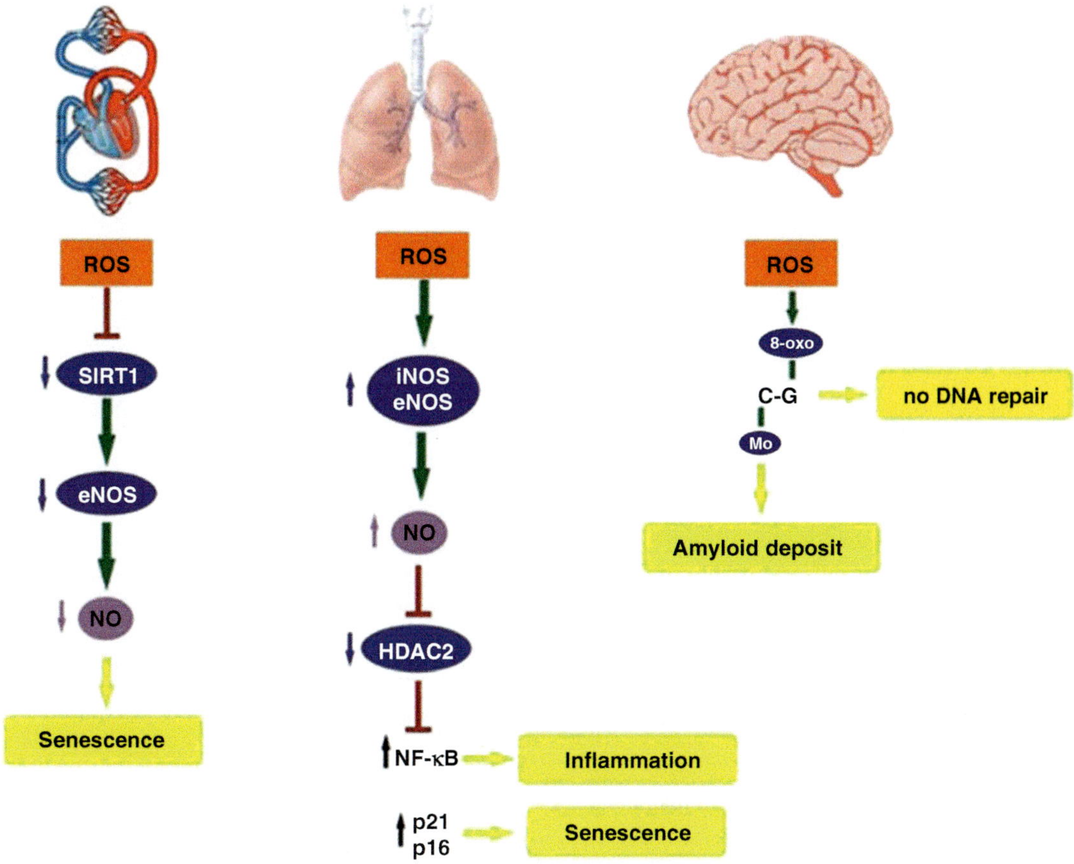


**Fig. 5.40** Oxidative stress, epigenetics and diseases. iNOS, inducible nitric oxide synthase; eNOS, endothelial nitric oxide synthase. See text for details. (Open Access, MDPI. Source: [292, 301])

tion of ROS directly impairs the function of lung cells, determining posttranslational modifications [315, 316]. COPD (see Fig. 5.21) manifests all posttranslational modification mechanisms. COPD is characterized by chronic low-grade systemic inflammation and premature aging, which determines the obstruction of lung airflow and decreases respiratory function [317]. Inflammation and cellular senescence in COPD are exacerbated by tobacco smoke, which accelerates or induces premature lung aging [317–319].

Cigarette smoke contains a number of free radicals and chemical compounds, representing the major source of inhaled RONS. Cigarette smoke is able to alter the intracellular balances of the DNA's histones, leading to a deregulated expression of pro-inflammatory genes [318, 319]. Cigarette smoke induces carbonyl stress and reduced nitric oxide production due to uncoupling of iNOS and eNOS. This enables pro-inflammatory genes [320–324] which may accelerate cellular senescence and pulmonary emphysema in COPD patients (Fig. 5.40).

As with the cardiovascular and respiratory systems, the nervous system is also vulnerable to oxidative stress. Although the brain holds high concentrations of lipids susceptible to peroxidation and uses high amounts of oxygen to produce energy, it has a relatively deficient antioxidant system [325]. Alzheimer's disease, the typical dementia form of aged people, is due to extracellular amyloid deposits and neurofibrillary tangles [326]. Oxidative DNA damage is now accepted as one of the earliest observable events in Alzheimer's disease. It can be detected in brains and in peripheral tissues of patients affected by mild cognitive impairment as well as at their late stages of Alzheimer's disease [326]. Astrocytes belonging to the hippocampus and cerebral cortex of Alzheimer's disease patients often demonstrate DNA double-strand breaks [327]. Late stages of Alzheimer's disease involve accumulation of oxidative DNA damage in aging brains (Fig. 5.40) [328].

"Healthy aging" is a result of the Mind-Body Program. It is why all six prongs are promoted, and they all support proper endothelial function, blood flow, and P&S nerve balance enabling proper P&S nerve function and control and coordination of all organs and systems of the body. Proper endothelial function, blood flow, and P&S nerve function require healthy levels of nitric oxide, omega-3 fatty acids, and antioxidants. All six prongs directly and indirectly support all three healthy levels, which slows the aging process of all cells throughout the body.

## Homocysteine

Excess homocysteine is contracted either genetically or through lifestyle influences, including low intakes of folate and vitamin $B_6$ [329]. Excess homocysteine decreases vascular reactivity, from atherosclerosis and thrombosis (Fig. 5.41), and is associated with heart disease and cardiovascular morbidity and mortality [330]. Folate and vitamin $B_6$ break down homocysteine (Fig. 5.42). Excess homocysteine activates enzymes which induce production of ROS which reduces nitric oxide bioavailability, including by accumulating ADMA (see Figs.4.27, 4.28, and 4.29). One path to ADMA is from homocysteine (Fig. 5.43). Homocysteine is elevated by oxidized LDL cholesterol. Homocysteine is a substance which is toxic to the blood vessel and endothelial cells if it is allowed to become elevated directly or indirectly by way of ADMA. Folic acid is important in reducing homocysteine levels [331]. Both pathways damage tissues. Homocysteine impairs medicines like statins

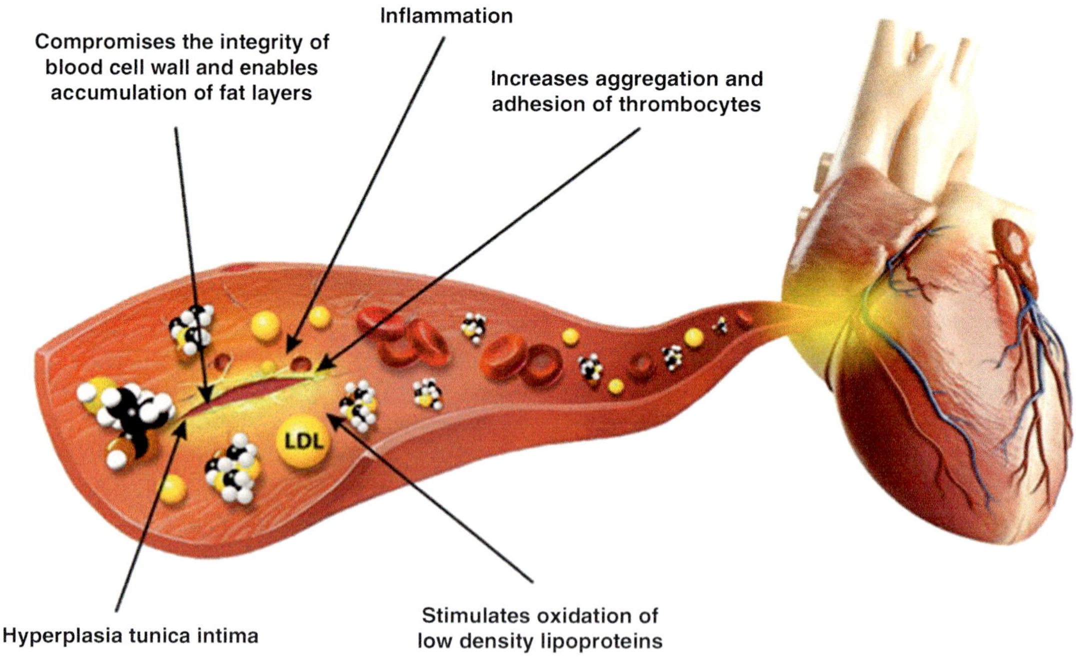


**Fig. 5.41** Excess homocysteine induces atherosclerosis through several mechanisms, including oxidation of LDL cholesterol, inflammation, and injury to the artery wall. (From Biomarkers in Cardiovascular Systems by Dr. Bibi Kulsoom, with permission. Source: http://elementswellness.com/homocysteine-and-your-heart/)

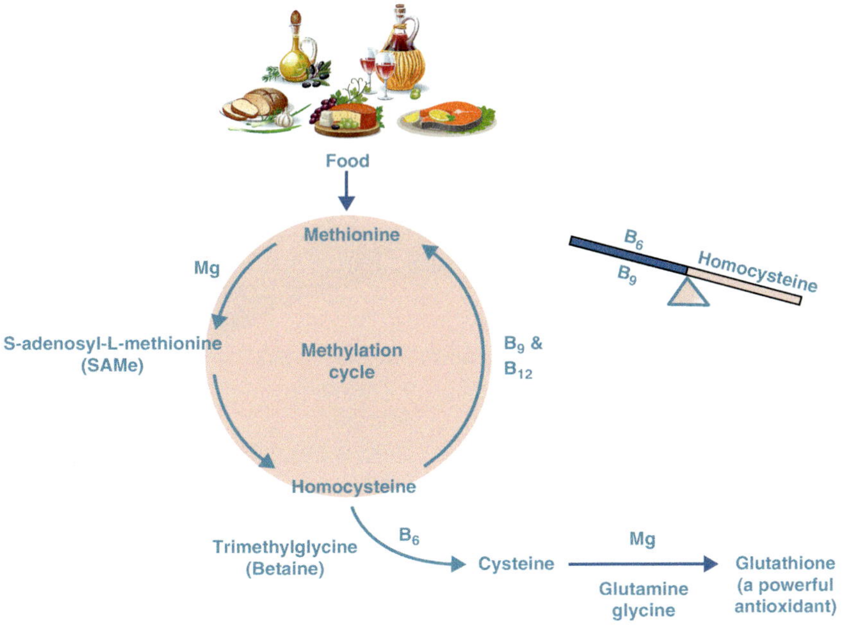


**Fig. 5.42** Methionine from protein-dense food is converted to homocysteine through S-adenosyl methionine (SAMe). Homocysteine is either broken down to cysteine by vitamin $B_6$ or returned to methionine by vitamin $B_{12}$ or folic acid. (Food icons from Shutterstock. Source: http://elementswellness.com/homocysteine-and-your-heart/)

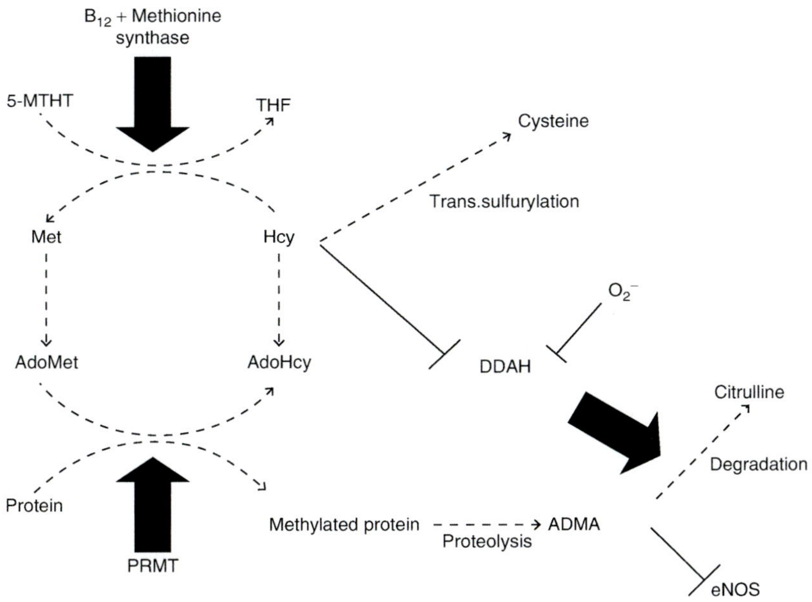


**Fig. 5.43** Intracellular synthesis and metabolism of homocysteine (Hcy) and asymmetric dimethylarginine (ADMA) and their biochemical link. Vitamin $B_{12}$ serves as a cofactor for the formation of methionine (Met) from homocysteine (Hcy) by methionine synthase using 5-methyl-tetrahydrofolate (5-MTHF), the dominant folate form in serum. S-adenosylmethionine (AdoMet) is the intermediate in this reaction and serves as the methyl donor to form S-adenosylhomocysteine (AdoHcy). Hcy is either re-methylated to Met or trans-sulfurated to cysteine. Asymmetric dimethylarginine (ADMA) is an endogenous competitive inhibitor of endothelial nitric oxide synthase (eNOS). ADMA is formed by methylation of arginine residues in proteins with protein methyltransferase (PRMT) and released after proteolysis. Metabolism of ADMA is mediated by dimethylarginine dimethylaminohydrolases (DDAHs), which are downregulated by reactive oxygen species and Hcy. (Open Access, Hindawi. Source: [132, 332])

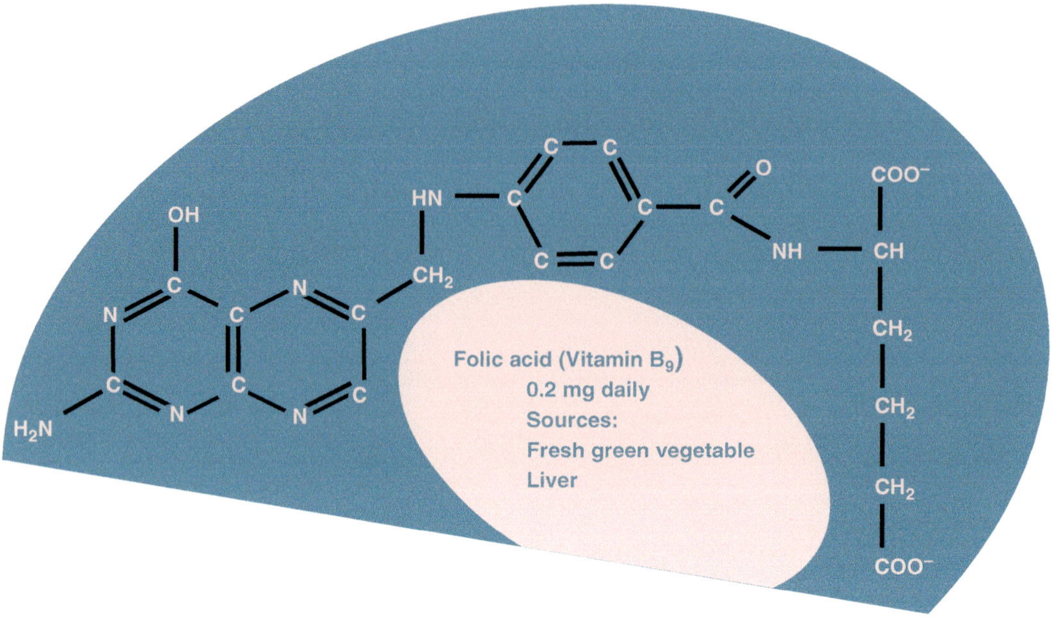


**Fig. 5.44** Structure and sources of folic acid (vitamin $B_9$). (Source: https://www.slideshare.net/drmustansar/folic-acid-b9)

from lowering cholesterol and raising nitric oxide levels by competing with L-arginine for the NOS enzyme. ADMA may also be generated (possibly from homocysteine) when there is an excess of nitric oxide in the presence of excess $Ca^{++}$, as when there is too much sheer stress from high, turbulent blood flow. Homocysteine is probably toxic to endothelial cells and is inhibited or lowered by folic acid. Homocysteine inhibits dimethylarginінase which degrades ADMA. This leaves ADMA available to uncouple eNOS and reduces nitric oxide production [332].

Folic acid (vitamin $B_9$; see Fig. 5.44) has been mentioned above. Nitric oxide is synthesized from L-arginine and oxygen by the enzyme NOS with BH4 as a cofactor. BH4 is synthesized from guanosine triphosphate (GTP) by GTP cyclohydrolase I and recycled from BH2 (7,8-dihydrobiopterin) by dihydrofolate reductase. Under conditions of low BH4 bioavailability, relative to NOS or BH2, oxygen activation is uncoupled from L-arginine oxidation, and NOS produces the superoxide $O_2^-$ instead of nitric oxide (Fig. 5.45) [333].

Homocysteine is an amino acid that is produced by the body by chemically altering adenosine (S-adenosyl methionine or SAMe; see Fig. 5.42). Excess homocysteine is associated with atherosclerosis (Fig. 5.41). Homocysteine levels in the blood are elevated for many reasons (see Fig. 5.46). These reasons can be divided into severe genetic causes and other milder causes. In the genetic condition, there is a deficiency in an important enzyme. In this rare and serious condition, there is a constellation of symptoms that include developmental delay, osteoporosis, visual abnormalities, formation of blood clots, and advanced atherosclerosis. This condition is mainly recognized in childhood. Milder genetic variations are more common causes of elevated homocysteine levels. In these conditions, the mediator molecules malfunction and are less efficient because of minor abnormalities in their structure. They also lead to elevation of homocysteine levels by slowing down the breakdown of homocysteine.

Excess homocysteine also affects the nervous system and mitochondria (see Fig. 5.47) [336]. Mild, yet abnormal, elevation in homocysteine levels (hyper-homocysteinemia) is common and seen in about 5–12% of the general population. In specific populations such as alcoholics (due to

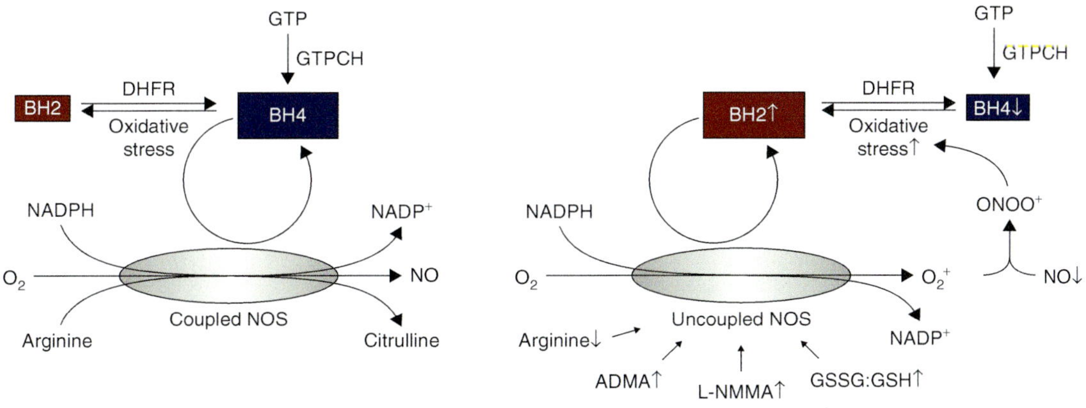


**Fig. 5.45** BH4 and the folate cycle. BH4 is synthesized from GTP and recycled from BH2 by the folate-based enzyme dihydrofolate reductase (DHFR). (Open Access, Springer Link. Source: [333]; http://www.beyondmthfr.com/mthfr-depression-folate-bh4-connection/)

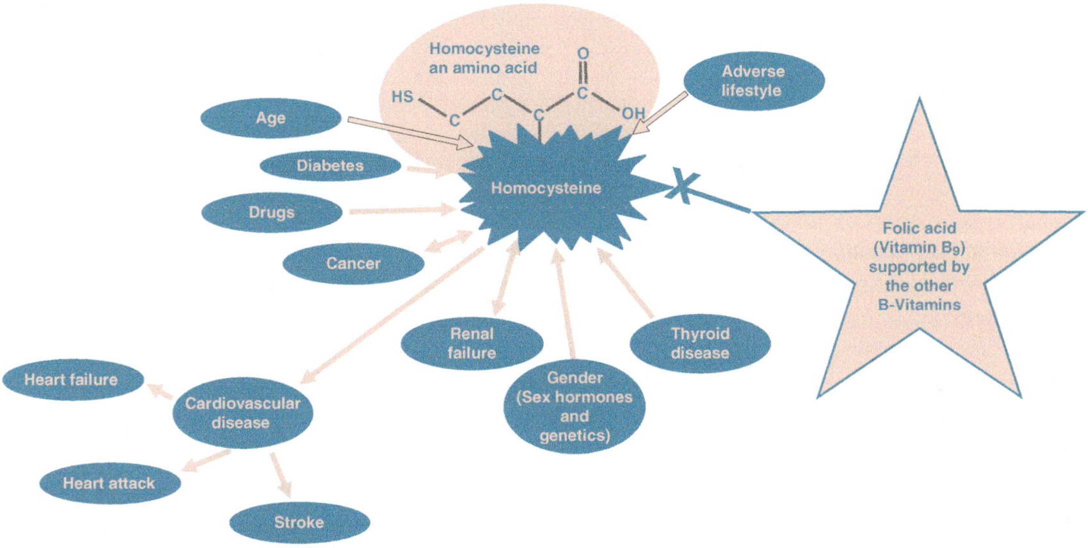


**Fig. 5.46** Causes of high homocysteine blood levels [334, 335]

poor vitamin intake) or patients with chronic kidney disease, this is often more common. The severe genetic form is rare (0.02%). Increasing folic acid intake, and thus decreasing homocysteine, decreases the risk of heart disease by 16%, blood clots in the legs by 25%, and stroke by 24% [361].

Many other observational studies have been performed to assess the effect of folate and the other B vitamins on heart disease. Most of these studies have concluded that oral intake of folate has been associated with lower risk of heart disease, possibly due to a lowering of homocysteine levels. The relation between oral intake of vitamins $B_{12}$ and $B_6$ and heart disease was not as obvious in many of these studies. However, in one study, it was concluded that even in people with elevated homocysteine levels due to genetic reasons, oral intake of folate and possibly other B vitamins was related with lower incidence of heart disease [334, 362].

Most of these data are obtained from observational studies rather than purely controlled scientific data. Despite these studies suggesting an

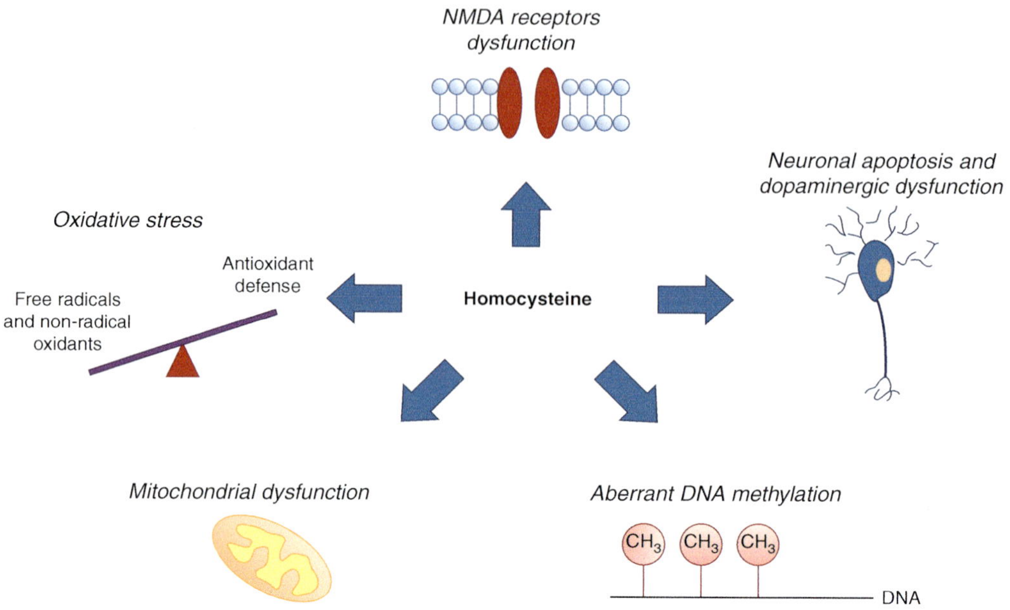


**Fig. 5.47** Mechanisms of homocysteine action as relevant to the nervous system. Homocysteine may interact with NMDA receptors altering glutamatergic transmission, exert toxic effects on dopaminergic neurons, initiate neuronal apoptosis, induce oxidative stress, lead to mitochondrial dysfunction, and influence DNA methylation altering gene expression. (Open Access, Frontiers in Behavioral Neuroscience. Source: [336])

association between the intake of these vitamins and the lower incidence of heart disease, there is no compelling clinical evidence to treat excess homocysteine levels in regard to prevention of heart disease, stroke, or blood clots [363]. As a result, homocysteine levels are not routinely measured in individuals with these problems. Kaplan-Meier survival rate curves for high and normal homocysteine levels [335] indicate that patients with excess homocysteine plasma levels demonstrate an average mortality rate greater than 15% higher, and nearly three 3 years shorter, than their normal homocysteine level counterparts. Folic acid and vitamins $B_6$ and $B_{12}$, when added to a diet, help to lower homocysteine levels and seem to reduce mortality risk.

## Folic Acid (Vitamin $B_9$)

A recent study shows the beneficial effects of folic acid in preventing vascular events [364]. The study is a sub-analysis of the China Stroke Primary Prevention Trial. A total of 10,789 Chinese hypertensive adults (mean age of 59.5 years), with no history of stroke or myocardial infarction, were randomly assigned to two equal and matched subpopulations: the experimental group were prescribed with 10 mg of enalapril and 0.8 mg of folic acid, and the control group were prescribed with 10 mg of enalapril with no folic acid. The result showed that patients with the lowest quartile of platelet count and lowest homocysteine levels (less than 15 mmol/L) had the lowest level of stroke, whereas those with high homocysteine levels (greater than 15 mmol/L) had the highest incidence of first stroke. Those individuals on folic acid treatment in the high-risk group, that is, those with low platelet and high homocysteine levels, had a 73% reduction in stroke with a hazard ratio of 0.27. There was no significant effect of folic acid on the low-risk group, that is, those patients with high platelets and low homocysteine levels. The authors go on to state that low platelet count levels may be a reflection, or marker, of endothelial dysfunction.

Methionine, an essential amino acid used in the biosynthesis of proteins, is also synthesized into homocysteine which is then synthesized into another amino acid, cysteine, via vitamin $B_6$. Cysteine, among other important roles, is synthesized into the powerful antioxidant glutathione. Too much homocysteine does not lead to more of the antioxidant glutathione but rather itself becomes a type of oxidant contributing to plaque formation, damaging the endothelium (see "Homocysteine"). Folic acid (folate) is important in brain and heart development and health, reducing the incidence of stroke and heart disease. It also plays a role in the endothelium, helping to maintain the necessary tight junctions that help to form both the blood-brain barrier, protecting the brain, and the endothelial barriers that protect the reproductive cells (sperm and eggs). As a result it is necessary for fertility in both men and women. In moderate doses folic acid may reduce the risk of many types of cancers [365, 366]. In excessive dose, it has been found to increase the risk in some cancers, especially prostate cancer [367, 368].

Folic acid supplementation is well known to lower homocysteine levels [369, 370]. The aforementioned China Stroke Study was the first randomized clinical trial to reveal that, among hypertensive populations without folic acid fortification, folic acid supplementation can reduce stroke by 21% on the average [371]. On a 4.2-year follow-up, the same study [364] revealed that folic acid supplementation can reduce first stroke by 73% among individuals with highest risk of first stroke (due to low platelet count and high homocysteine level). They conclude that this remarkable reduction in this subgroup supports the hypothesis and strengthens the biological plausibility of their findings.

Sub-analysis of the same study demonstrated that enalapril-folic acid therapy ($n = 7545$), compared with enalapril alone ($n = 7559$), can significantly delay the progression of chronic kidney disease (CKD) among patients with mild-to-moderate CKD [372]. They further go on to say that in addition to lowering homocysteine, folic acid may have other beneficial effects due to its multiple mechanisms of action. They state that it plays a role in DNA synthesis repair and methylation [373]. It is believed that folic acid maintains endothelial nitric oxide synthesis in its coupled state to favor generation of nitric oxide [1]. They go on to state that more folic acid can exert antioxidative [374] and anti-inflammatory [375] effects.

Folic acid is an important cofactor in many biochemical pathways, including as an antioxidant and anti-inflammatory agent. This data does suggest that it has important prophylactic effects on vascular events, and this may be because of its reduction of homocysteine in addition to antioxidant and anti-inflammatory effects. The latter effects serve those patients with autonomic dysfunction, promoting nervous system wellness, as small fiber disease is believed to be an oxidative stress phenomenon.

## Tryptophan

The kynurenine pathway of L-tryptophan metabolism produces several neuroactive and neuroprotective metabolites (see Fig. 5.48) [337]. L-tryptophan is an essential amino acid. Some of the neuroactive metabolites are serotonin and quinolinic acid. Serotonin in the brain regulates sleep and mood (anxiety and happiness). In the body, it helps to regulate bowel function, stimulate nausea, heal wounds (by facilitating local vasoconstriction and clotting), and maintain bone health (excessive levels may lead to osteoporosis). Quinolinic acid is a precursor to nicotine. Nicotine is a type of acetylcholine receptor on nerves which is prevalent in both the P&S nervous systems (see Fig. 5.49). Quinolinic acid is also a NMDA agonist and excitotoxin. As an excitotoxin, it is implicated in psychiatric disorders (i.e., anxiety-depression disorders and schizophrenia) and neurodegenerative processes in the brain. Quinolinic acid and kynurenic acid are mediators of neuronal dysfunction and nerve cell death in inflammatory brain diseases (e.g., abscess, meningitis, encephalitis, vasculitis) and demyelinating diseases (i.e., multiple sclerosis). Quinolinic acid is implicated in Alzheimer's, amyotrophic lateral sclerosis (ALS, possibly by targeting the associated neuron's mitochondria), brain ischemia, and Huntington's, Parkinson's, and HIV-associated neurocognitive disorder.

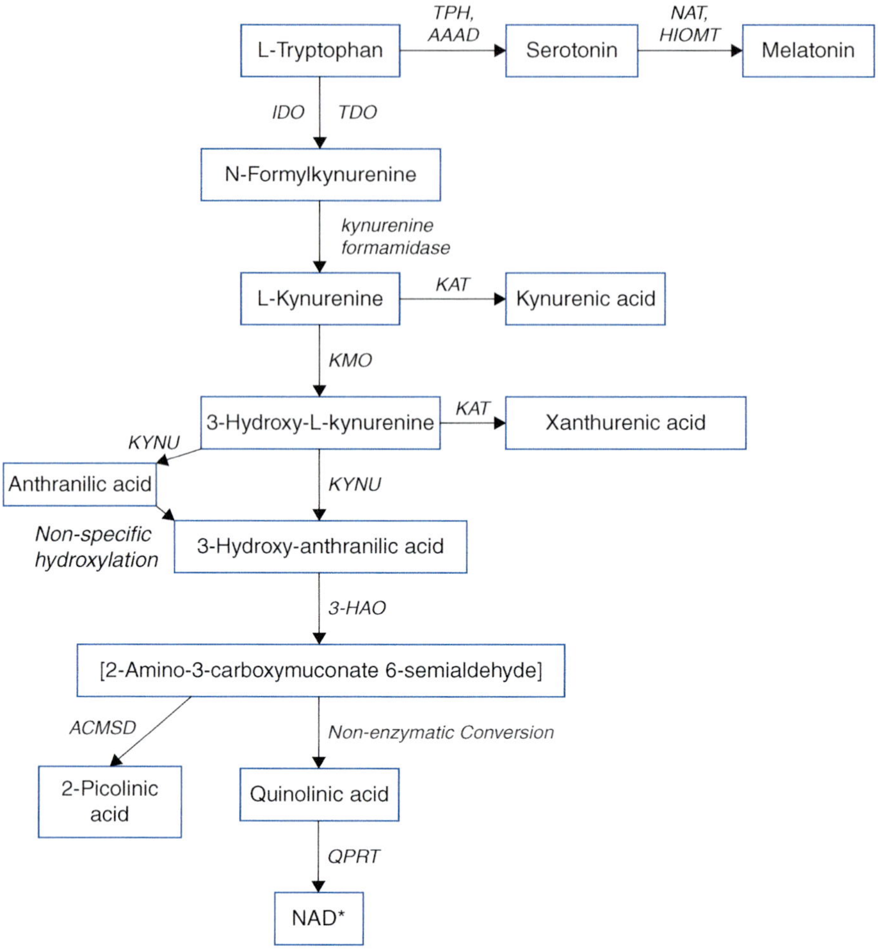


**Fig. 5.48** Tryptophan metabolism along the kynurenine pathway and serotonin pathway. Abbreviations: 3-HAO 3-hydroxy-anthranilate 3,4-dioxidase, AAAD aromatic L-amino acid decarboxylase, ACMSD α-amino-β-carboxymuconate-ε-semialdehyde decarboxylase, HIOMT hydroxyindole-O-methyltransferase, IDO indoleamine 2,3-dioxygenase, KAT kynurenine amino transferases I-III, KMO kynurenine 3-monooxygenase, KYNU kynureninase, NAT N-acetyltransferase, TDO tryptophan 2,3-dioxygenase, TPH tryptophan hydroxylase, QPRT quinolinic acid phosphoribosyl transferase, and $NAD^+$ nicotinamide adenine dinucleotide. (Open Access, Polish Physiological Society. Source: [337])

Within the brain, quinolinic acid is only produced by activated microglia and macrophages.

Serotonin and quinolinic acid play an important role in the pathophysiology of some of the inflammatory brain diseases listed above (Alzheimer's disease, Parkinson's disease, Huntington's disease, and AIDS-dementia complex and irritable bowel syndrome, schizophrenia, depression, epilepsy, and the aging process). Furthermore, Serotonin and quinolinic acid are often responsible for the altered functioning of the enteric nervous system. There is evidence that the kynurenine pathway is sensitive to changes in the concentration of many vitamins and minerals that play a crucial role as coenzymes and cofactors in the de novo synthesis of $NAD^+$ coenzyme, especially B vitamins, $Mn^{++}$, $Zn^{++}$, $Co^{++}$, $Cu^{++}$, $Mg^{++}$, and $Fe^{++}$. Collectively, B vitamins and some of these minerals are known as "kynurenines." Vitamin $B_6$ is the most crucial enzyme in L-tryptophan metabolism. Cofactor deficiencies influence the kynurenine pathway far more than kynurenine surpluses induced by supplements [337].

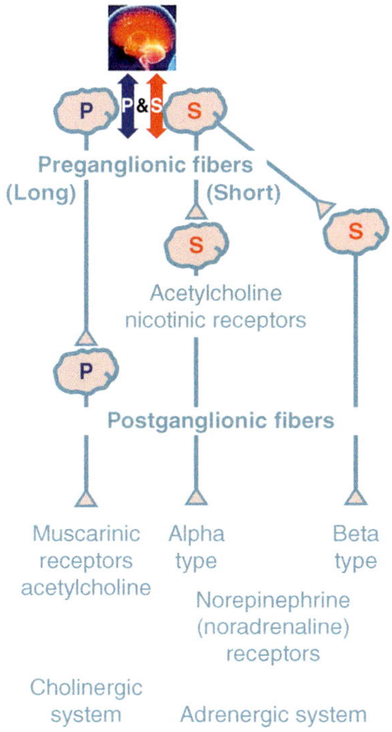


**Fig. 5.49** Position of nicotinic receptors in the P&S nervous systems. (Source: http://pharmacologycorner.com/acetylcholine-receptors-muscarinic-and-nicotinic/)

Catabolization of tryptophan leads to the production of NAD. As discussed in previous chapters, NAD is central to energy metabolism, serving as an essential coenzyme in glycolysis, the tricarboxylic acid (Krebs) cycle, the mitochondrial electron transport chain, and is central to the production of macromolecules, including nucleotides. NAD levels regulate sirtuin-mediated deacetylation, which modulates transcription factors and metabolic enzymes that promote mitochondrial oxidative function and enhance cell survival under stress conditions [376–378]. Sirtuin activity is required during embryogenesis and affects the fate of stem cells and progenitor cells; loss of activity causes multiple organ defects [379]. There is evidence that NAD deficiency impairs DNA repair [380] and may lead to congenital defects [381].

L-tryptophan deficiency has been shown to affect memory, dermatitis, depression, and anxiety. During dieting, L-tryptophan supplementation could prevent neuropsychiatric symptoms, including weight gain. From the description above, it is apparent that quinolinic acid, as an excitotoxin, contributes to oxidative stress, causing nerve and mitochondrial damage and inflammation. Serotonin, in excess, is also an oxidant: in the bones, it may lead to osteoporosis, and in the vasculature, vasoconstriction and clotting if prolonged. Adequate levels of vitamins and minerals help to minimize the oxidant effects of both neuroactive metabolites.

Melatonin responds to light (Fig. 5.50). In the brain, melatonin is the hormone that opposes and balances serotonin (Fig. 5.51), and when melatonin levels outside the brain are higher than serotonin, melatonin causes wakefulness.[13] In the brain, serotonin levels increase, and melatonin levels decrease, by about 10% around twilight to initiate the process of falling asleep, and the opposite occurs around daybreak to initiate the process of waking. In addition to helping to regulate the circadian rhythm, melatonin helps to regulate blood pressure. Outside the brain, melatonin causes skin pigmentation (including freckles). It acts as an antioxidant, primarily protecting nuclear and mitochondrial DNA.

Serotonin is an important neurotransmitter in the autonomic nervous system as well. Serotonin regulates gut secretion, motility, and sensation. It also influences the secretion of growth hormone from the pituitary. This causes the liver to produce insulin-like growth factor 1, which is necessary for development and growth. As mentioned above, melatonin has been shown to have great antioxidant properties and enhance mitochondrial function [24]. Ratio of serum products of the kynurenine pathway can affect the inflammatory status of the body. Studies have shown [382] that there is a protective effect of melatonin and L-tryptophan by reducing concentrations of pro-inflammatory factors such as Il-1, Il-6, and TNF-alpha.

[13] Melatonin, when taken as a supplement, cannot cross the blood-brain barrier. When the brain senses increased levels of melatonin outside the brain due to supplementation, it assumes more melatonin than needed is released. In response, the brain increases levels of available serotonin inside the brain to maintain the apparent proper balance. This then simulates the serotonin-melatonin balance of evening and helps to mediate the process of falling asleep.

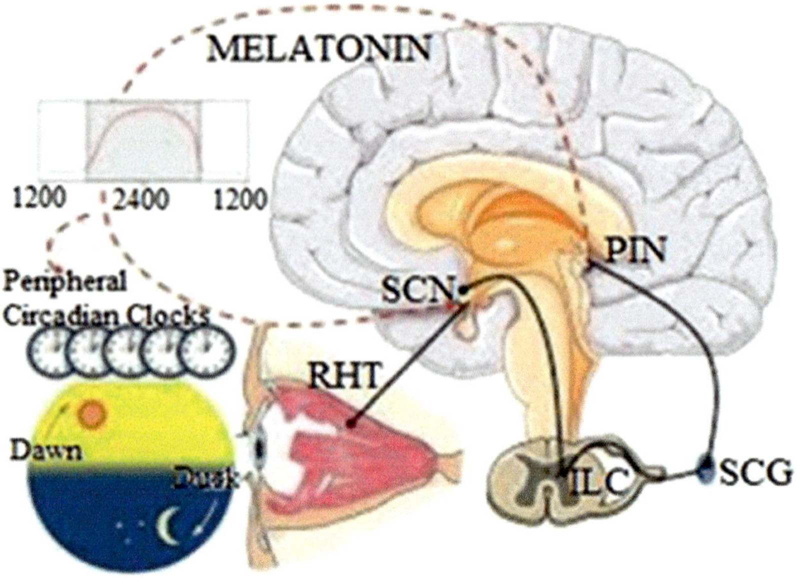


**Fig. 5.50** Control of melatonin synthesis by environmental light. Retinal ganglion cell receptors project via the retinohypothalamic tract (RHT) to the suprachiasmatic nuclei (SCN). From here, and through a multisynaptic pathway including the cervical sympathetics, pineal melatonin release is modulated. Melatonin both feeds back at the SCN and affects peripheral clocks. (Republished with permission from Springer International Publishing AG. Source: [23])

## Oxidative Stress and Autonomic Neuropathy, Type 2 Diabetes as a Model

All-cause mortality is greater than double for those diagnosed with type 2 diabetes and diabetic autonomic neuropathy (DAN) [383–396]. Oxidative stress is described as the mechanism related to autonomic injury found with DAN [397]. DAN often deteriorates to cardiovascular autonomic neuropathy (CAN) which, if left untreated, leads to sudden cardiac death [398]. Advanced autonomic dysfunction (AAD, similar to DAN in nondiabetics) demonstrates similar effects for nondiabetics, including oxidative stress as a mechanism and the progression to CAN [116]. Pathogenic mechanisms that have been implicated in diabetic neuropathy are (a) increased flux through the polyol pathway, leading to accumulation of sorbitol, a reduction in myoinositol, and an associated reduced $Na^+$-$K^+$-ATPase activity, and (b) endoneural microvascular damage and hypoxia due to nitric oxide inactivation by increased oxygen-free radical activity [399].

Diabetes affects all systems of the body and therefore is a model of chronic disease effects on the body. Hyperglycemia causes oxidative and nitrosative stress (abbreviated as oxidative stress) in the more sensitive tissues, including peripheral and central nerves, endothelial cells, immune cells, the microvasculature, and kidney filtration structures [340]. Hyperglycemia induces an increased presence of markers of oxidative stress, such as superoxide and peroxynitrite ions, and that antioxidant defense moieties are reduced in patients with diabetic peripheral neuropathy [400]. Therapies known to reduce oxidative stress are therefore recommended. ALA, through its multiple antioxidant properties, has long been found to slow, stay, and even reverse (for a time) the progression of DAN [401–405], as well as advanced autonomic dysfunction (AAD, similar to DAN, but in nondiabetics and without the insulin and glucose issues [personal communication, Colombo & DePace]). One of ALA's antioxidant properties is to increase reduced glutathione, another important endogenous antioxidant. Up to 600 mg ALA, depending on the severity, has been shown to improve neuropathic deficits. A leading therapy option [406] is the combination of ALA, omega-3 PUFA (see "Omega-3 Fatty Acids (Prong-1)"), and dihomo-gamma-linolenic acid (an omega-6 fatty acid [407]).

In diabetes, a contributor to oxidative stress is an excess of advanced glycation end products

(AGEs). AGEs are the result of nonenzymatic additions of glucose or other saccharides to proteins, lipids, and nucleotides. AGE generation leads to intra- and extracellular protein cross-linking and protein aggregation which alters intracellular signaling and gene expression, releases pro-inflammatory molecules, and results in an increased production of ROS (see Fig. 5.52) [338]. Compounds including vitamins $B_6$ and $B_{12}$ with the antioxidant ALA have helped reduce the production of ROS and the subsequent effects of AGE-induced oxidative stress.

Protein kinase C (PKC) activation is a critical step in the pathway to diabetic microvascular complications leading to cardiovascular disease [408]. It is activated by both hyperglycemia and disordered fatty-acid metabolism resulting in increased production of vasoconstrictive, angiogenic, and chemotactic cytokines including transforming growth factor β (TGF-β), VEGF, endothelin-1, and intercellular adhesion molecules.

There is evidence that oxidative stress leads to a deficiency of growth factors in diabetes, including nerve growth factor, as well as the dependent neuropeptides substance P and calcitonin gene-related peptide. These growth factors contribute to clinical perturbations in small-fiber function [409]. The pathogenesis of diabetic neuropathy includes loss of vasa nervorum, so it is likely that VEGF is involved [410]. In the pancreas, islet neogenesis-associated protein (INGAP) peptide comprises the core active sequence of INGAP, a pancreatic cytokine that induces new islet formation [411].

As with severe viral infections that can turn one's own immune system on one's (healthy) nerves, autoantibodies resulting from oxidative forces associated with diabetes have been implicated in both large fiber (sensory and motor) and small fiber (autonomic and pain fiber) neuropathies [340]. The viral coating of viruses and the myelin sheaths of nerves have a number of similarities attractive to the immune system [412]. Perhaps the clearest link between autoimmunity and neuropathy has been the demonstration of an 11-fold increase likelihood of chronic inflammatory demyelinating neuropathy, multiple motor polyneuropathy, and vasculitis in diabetes [413]. There may be selected cases, particularly those with autonomic neuropathy, with evidence of anti-neuronal, autoimmunity, and chronic inflammatory demyelinating neuropathy that may benefit from intravenous immunoglobulin or large-dose steroids [414].

DAN is a subset of diabetic neuropathy specific to the autonomic (P&S) nervous system(s) and is associated with all organ dysfunctions. As a result, DAN eventually causes dysfunction of every part of the body and has a significant nega-

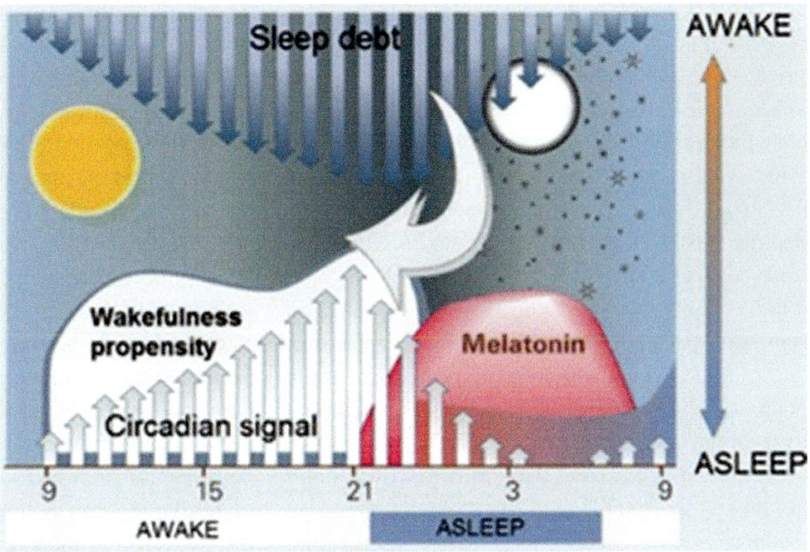


**Fig. 5.51** The evening rise in melatonin feeds back to inhibit the wakefulness-promoting effects of serotonin and the suprachiasmatic nuclei (SCN). (Republished with permission from Springer International Publishing AG. Source: [23])

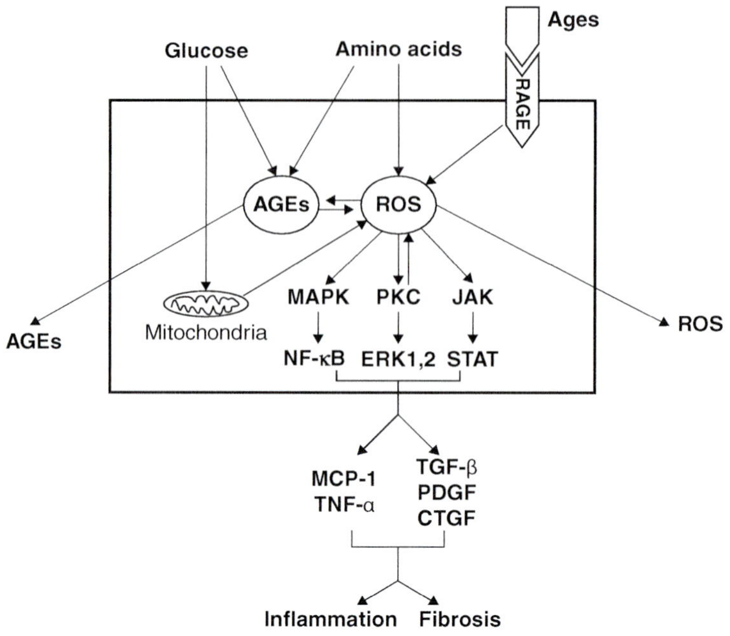


**Fig. 5.52** Cascade of events in cellular injury produced by AGE. Dietary protein is a source of preformed AGE and of amino acids that may form AGE in the circulation, kidney, and possibly other sites. Abbreviations: RAGE, receptor for AGE; ROS, reactive oxygen species; MAPK, mitogen-activated protein kinases; PKC, protein kinase C; JAK/STAT, Janus kinase/signal transducers and activators of transcription; ERK1,2, extracellular signal-regulated kinases 1 and 2; MCP-1, monocyte chemoattractant protein-1; CTGF, connective tissue growth factor. (Republished with permission from American Society of Nephrology. Source: [292, 338])

tive impact on quality and continuation of life [415]. The organ systems that most often exhibit prominent clinical autonomic signs and symptoms in diabetes include the pupils, sweat glands, genitourinary system, gastrointestinal tract, adrenal medullary system, and cardiovascular system. DAN does not include any sensory (e.g., pin prick, vibration, and pain) or motor dysfunctions. DAN involves lightheadedness (dizziness, arguably the worst of the symptoms), as well as nervous system dysfunction, vascular dysfunction, GI upset, blood pressure dysfunction, vision decline (faster than presbyopia), sex dysfunction, renal dysfunction, and heart disease. In fact, much of the sensory and motor dysfunction (including wound healing difficulties and amputation issues) is a function of poor autonomic nerve control of the vasculature, causing vascular dysfunction, leading to poor tissue perfusion, predisposing the patient to acquiring wounds and not having the sensation of the wound's existence (sensory nerves need blood also), facilitating infection (due to the poor perfusion and again without sensation), and ending in amputation. Clinical symptoms generally do not appear until long after the onset of diabetes. However, subclinical autonomic dysfunction can occur within a year of diagnosis in type 2 diabetes patients and within 2 years in type 1 diabetes patients [416].

Oxidative stress due to hyperglycemia significantly contributes to nerve damage. There is a component of the P&S branches of the autonomic nervous system that uses peptides as primary neurotransmitters. Like the enteric nervous system, some consider it a third component to the autonomic system: the neuropeptidergic system with its neurotransmitters substance P, vasoactive intestinal polypeptide, and calcitonin gene-related peptide, among others (Fig. 5.53). The neuropeptidergic system primarily subserves the glands of the endocrine system. Neuropeptidergic neurons are involved in DAN and the associated glandular disorders, including GI upset. This is the system that puts "butterflies" in the stomach

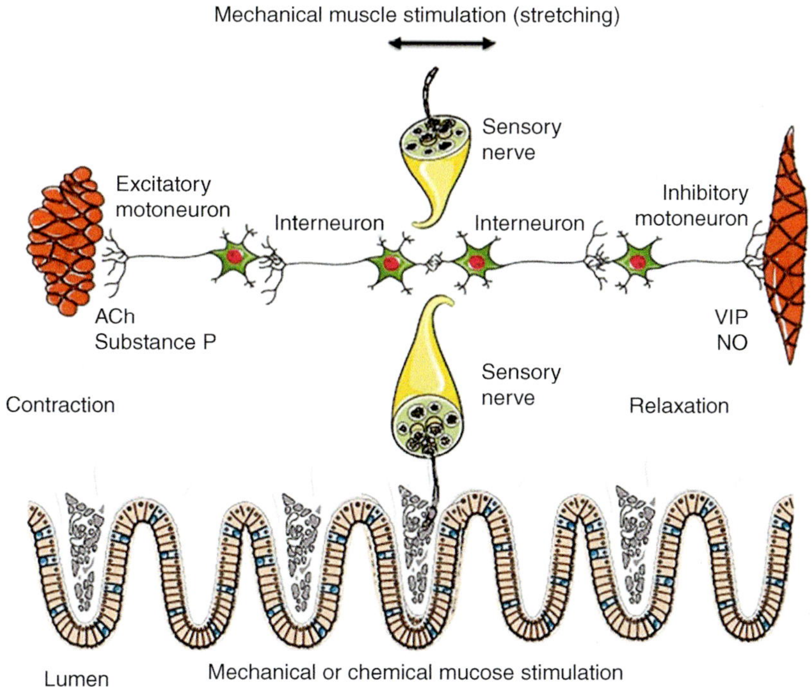


**Fig. 5.53** Peristaltic reflex of the small intestine. Enteric sensory nerves detect the chemical or mechanical stimulation of the mucosa or the stretching of the muscular layer. The signals are transmitted in an oral or anal direction by interneurons. Excitatory motor nerves release acetylcholine (Ach) and substance P, which cause muscle contractions on the oral side of the stimulus. Inhibitory motor nerves release vasoactive intestinal peptide (VIP) and nitric oxide (NO), which cause relaxation of the muscle on the anal side of the stimulus. (Republished with permission from Springer International Publishing AG. Source: [23])

when the sympathetics are stimulated in a way that is both emotional and stressful. Because the autonomic nervous system is "hidden" behind the organs, DAN remains among the least recognized and least understood disorders [340].

As mentioned above, oxidative stress leading to defective blood flow in the small capillary circulation is found with decreased responsiveness to mental arithmetic, cold pressor, handgrip, and heating [417]. The defect is associated with a reduction in the amplitude of vasomotion [418] due to autonomic dysfunction as a direct result of oxidative stress from hyperglycemia and resembles premature aging [419]. Similarly, there are differences in the glabrous and hairy skin circulations. In hairy skin, a functional defect is found prior to the development of (sensory-motor) neuropathy in nociceptive afferents [420] and is correctable with antioxidants [421]. Autonomic nerve dysfunction and neuropathy precede sensory-motor nerve dysfunction and neuropathy. The clinical counterpart is a dry cold skin due to autonomic dysfunction, leading to loss of sweating and development of fissures and cracks that are portals of entry for organisms, leading to infectious ulcers and gangrenes. Silent myocardial infarction, respiratory failure, amputations, and sudden death are hazards for the diabetic patients with CAN [422, 423].

CAN is late-stage autonomic dysfunction (neuropathy) and is characterized by very low parasympathetics, typically resulting in relatively high sympathetics (relative to the extant parasympathetics). In poorly controlled diabetic patients, this state is often reached 20 or more years ahead of "normal" aging subjects (see Fig. 5.35). This condition is possible from the oxidative stress induced by diabetes. For example, using cardiorespiratory-based P&S monitoring (ANSAR Medical Technologies, Inc.,

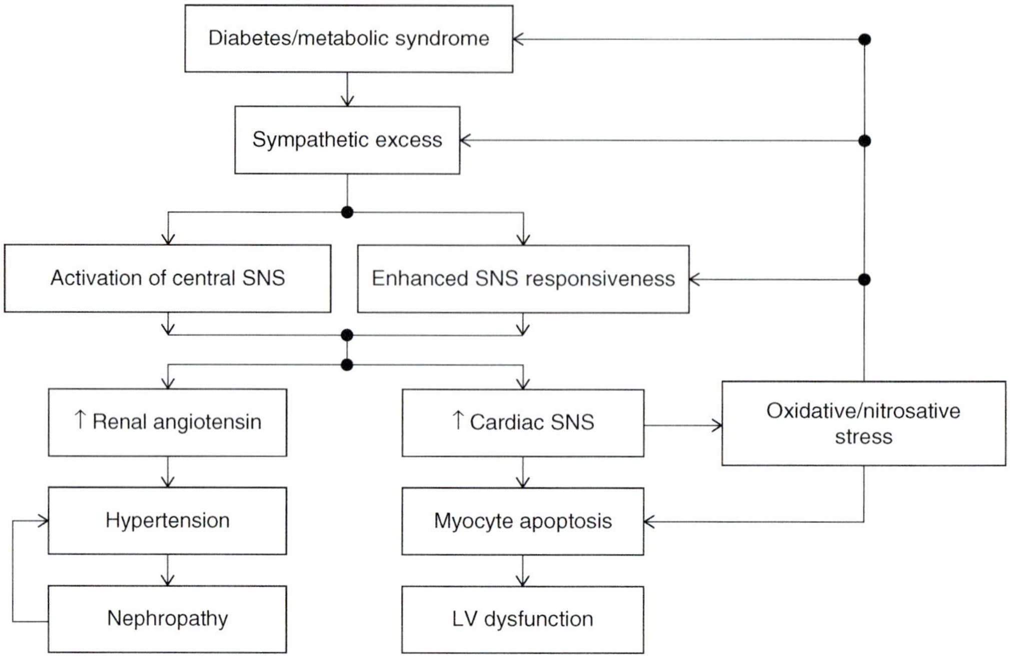


**Fig. 5.54** The role of sympathetic excess in chronic disease (using diabetes as the model). (Republished with permission from A.I. Vinik, MD, PhD. Adapted from [339, 340])

Philadelphia, PA) (now TMCAMS, Inc., Atlanta, GA), CAN is defined as the resting parasympathetic measure < 0.1 bpm$^2$. Typically in diabetics with CAN, the concurrent, independent, sympathetic measure would be relatively high, resulting in a sympathovagal balance (SB: the ratio of S/P at rest) > 3.0. A SB > 3.0 is (resting) sympathetic excess and is highly correlated with hypertension, heart disease, LV dysfunction, hyperhidrosis, and more (Fig. 5.54) [118]. The combination of CAN with high SB indicates high mortality risk from MACE.

The mortality for diabetic autonomic neuropathy has been estimated to be 44% within 2.5 years of diagnosing symptomatic autonomic neuropathy [424]. Meta-analysis data for the pooled prevalence rate risk for silent myocardial ischemia was 1.96, with 95% confidence interval of 1.53–2.51 ($p < 0.001$; $n = 1468$ total subjects). Thus, a consistent association between CAN and the presence of silent myocardial ischemia was shown (Fig. 5.55) [340].

The exact pathogenesis of CAN is complex and remains unclear [342–425], except that oxidative stress is involved (see Fig. 5.56). Most of the proposed mechanisms of neuronal injury are based on models of somatic rather than autonomic neuropathy. Although many of these mechanisms might be shared between autonomic and somatic neuropathies, differences do exist, as shown by the Steno-2 trial,[14] in which the multifactorial intervention (including intensive metabolic control and lifestyle changes) slowed the progression of autonomic but not somatic

[14] Steno-2 trial involved patients with T2DM and microalbuminuria. Intensive pharmacological intervention targeting hypertension, hyperlipidemia, and microalbuminuria, combined with behavioral treatment (exercise, diet, and smoking cessation), reduced the risk of autonomic neuropathy over the course of a 7.8-year follow-up. The risk for developing CAN was significantly lower on the intervention arm (49% in the intensive group vs. 65% in the conventional group; HR = 0.37; 95% CI, 0.18–0.79; $p = 0.002$). After a mean of 5.5 years following the end of the study, the same protective effect against the development of autonomic neuropathy persisted (RR = 0.53; 95% CI, 0.34–0.81; $p = 0.004$). There was also reduction in the risk for developing CVD (RR = 0.43; 95% CI, 0.19–0.94; $p = 0.04$) and overall mortality (RR = 0.54; 95% CI, 0.32–0.89; $p = 0.02$) in this study.

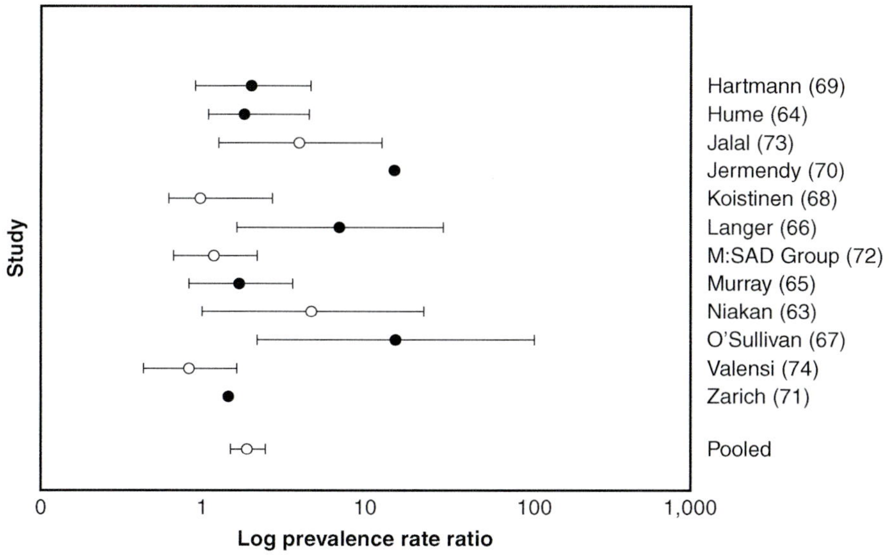


**Fig. 5.55** The association between CAN and silent myocardial infarction (using diabetes as the model). (Republished with permission from A.I. Vinik, MD, PhD. Adapted from [340, 341])

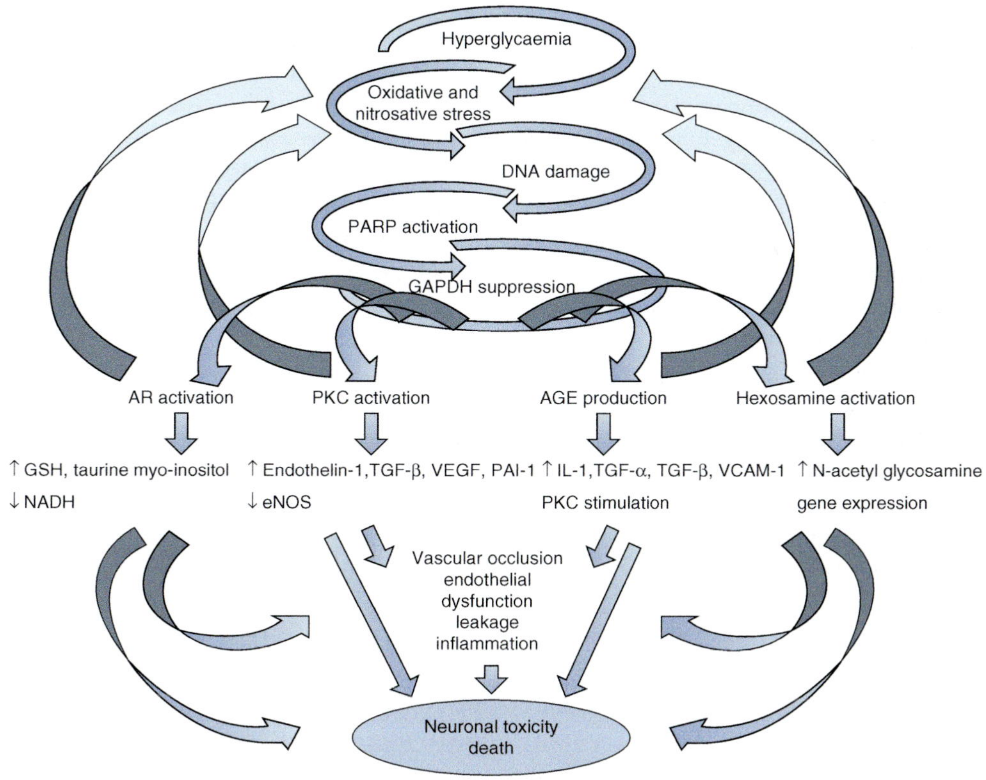


**Fig. 5.56** Hyperglycemia-induced neuronal ischemia, dysfunction, and death. Abbreviations: PKC protein kinase C, AGE advanced glycation end products, PARP poly ADP-ribose polymerase, GAPDH glyceraldehyde-3 phosphate dehydrogenase, GSH glutathione, NADH nicotinamide adenine dinucleotide, TGF-β transforming growth factor, VEGF vascular endothelial growth factor, PAI-1 plasminogen activator inhibitor-1, eNOS endothelial nitric oxide synthase, IL-1 interleukin 1, TNF-α, tumor necrosis factor-α, VCAM-1, vascular cell adhesion molecule 1. (Open Access, Baishideng Publishing Group Inc. Source: [342])

neuropathy [342]. The pathogenesis of CAN is likely to be multifactorial [427], involving several mechanisms and pathways. These mechanisms and pathways include oxidative and nitrosative stress [428]. These stresses lead to neuronal ischemia or direct neuronal dysfunction and death (see Fig. 5.56). These stresses also lead to endothelial dysfunction, which accelerates the progression of neuronal dysfunction and death due to neuronal ischemia. Neuronal axons are rich in mitochondria, which makes them particularly susceptible to the direct and indirect effects of oxidative and nitrosative stress [429].

As shown in Fig. 5.56, increased oxidative stress effects four pathways that contribute to glucose toxicity [430–433]. These different pathways can in return exacerbate oxidative stress and can induce changes in gene expression, transcription factors, diverse cellular products disrupting several cellular functions, and the communication between the cell and the surrounding matrix, all of which leads to neuronal dysfunction and death [434–436]. These pathways also result in impaired microvascular regulation and endothelial dysfunction by different mechanisms, leading to impairment of endothelial nitric oxide [437, 438]. This can lead to reduction of neurovascular perfusion, dysfunction, and cellular apoptosis [439].

Obstructive sleep apnea (OSA) is another possible factor in the development of CAN. OSA is very common in patients with diabetes and has been associated with increased sympathetic tone in patients without diabetes [440, 441]. The interrelationship between OSA and CAN is likely to be bidirectional. The intermittent hypoxia that occurs in OSA could lead to increased oxidative stress, nitrosative stress, and microvascular complications, which could lead to CAN [442]. CAN, from the perspective of a loss of parasympathetic activity [116], could lead to changes in upper airway tone. Changes in respiratory drive could predispose the patient to OSA [443, 444].

There are several proposed mechanisms for the development of diabetic cardiomyopathy. The parasympathetic denervation observed in the early stages of the disease leads to a dominant sympathetic tone [445], which promotes a cascade of intrinsic metabolic changes, including the release of high myocardial catecholamine levels and catecholamine toxicity [446, 447]. This catecholamine rise has been shown to induce mitochondrial uncoupling [448, 449], switching energy generation on a cardiac level from myocardial glucose to free fatty acids, which is considered an inefficient energy source [450], and therefore increases the oxygen demand [448, 449]. These alterations on the cardiac biochemical and cellular level lead ultimately to programmed cell death and fibrosis [451, 452], elevated oxygen consumption relevant to the cardiac work [453, 454], and finally, hypertrophy and remodeling of the left ventricle [455]. Crucial mediators in the above process are the mitochondrial ROS causing oxidative stress [456, 457], insulin resistance [458], and calcium-dependent apoptosis [456, 459, 460].

As mentioned above, the Steno-2 trial lifestyle changes (diet, physical exercise, and smoking cessation) have been shown to have a beneficial impact on the prevention, and progression, of CAN. Exercise is well known to have, perhaps, the greatest antioxidant effects. The benefit of lifestyle change was confirmed in the Diabetes Prevention Program: lifestyle modification demonstrated superior results in the improvement of autonomic dysfunction (assessed with HRV and QT indexes) as compared to the use of metformin or placebo [461]. Weight loss and dietary intervention accompanied [117] or not [462] by supervised training were associated with improvement on CAN indices. Aerobic training has also been shown to improve CAN, with some indication that mild physical exercise is recommended in less severe CAN cases. A recent review summarizing the evidence for the impact of lifestyle interventions on CAN has concluded that moderate endurance and aerobic exercise in both T1DM and T2DM improve HRV and cardiac autonomic function significantly, in favor of parasympathetic dominance, independent of BMI, glycemic or BP control, and duration of diabetes [463]. A minimum of 150 minutes of exercise per week is strongly recommended.

Recent developments in the understanding of how diabetes affects the enteric nervous system (considered by some as a part of the autonomic nervous system) has caused a paradigm shift in the thinking about gastrointestinal (GI) manifestations of diabetes [343]. Oxidative stress has been shown to play an important role in diabetes-induced apoptosis of enteric neurons. However, delivery of antioxidants by oral supplementation has not proved efficacious [464]. This calls for more research to find more creative approaches in delivering antioxidants to the enteric nervous system. Diabetes is known to change enteric microbiota. However, some species of gut microbiota can be used to decrease oxidative stress [465]. In addition to increased oxidative stress, change of the GI microenvironment also includes endothelial dysfunction (Fig. 5.57). A common hallmark of stress is stomach ulcers. Oxidative stress, through its effects on the P&S nervous systems, leads to stomach ulcers (see Fig. 5.58) [345].

## Antioxidant Balance

In general, with a proper antioxidant-oxidant balance, antioxidants sequester free radicals, including ROS and radical nitrogen species (RNS), and maintain them in a healthy mode. With healthy diet and exercise, antioxidants repair, remove, or prevent RONS damage. They add electrons to those and other free radicals, helping to prevent or repair mitochondrial dysfunction. Results from oxidative stress not balanced by an appropriate antioxidant environment can lead to chronic fatigue, fibromyalgia, migraines, neurodegenerative diseases, autonomic dysfunction, COPD, or atherosclerosis. ROS and RNS (RONS) are not always harmful. They are continually produced within the body as part of normal oxidative metabolism [466, 467]. Under the proper balanced anti-

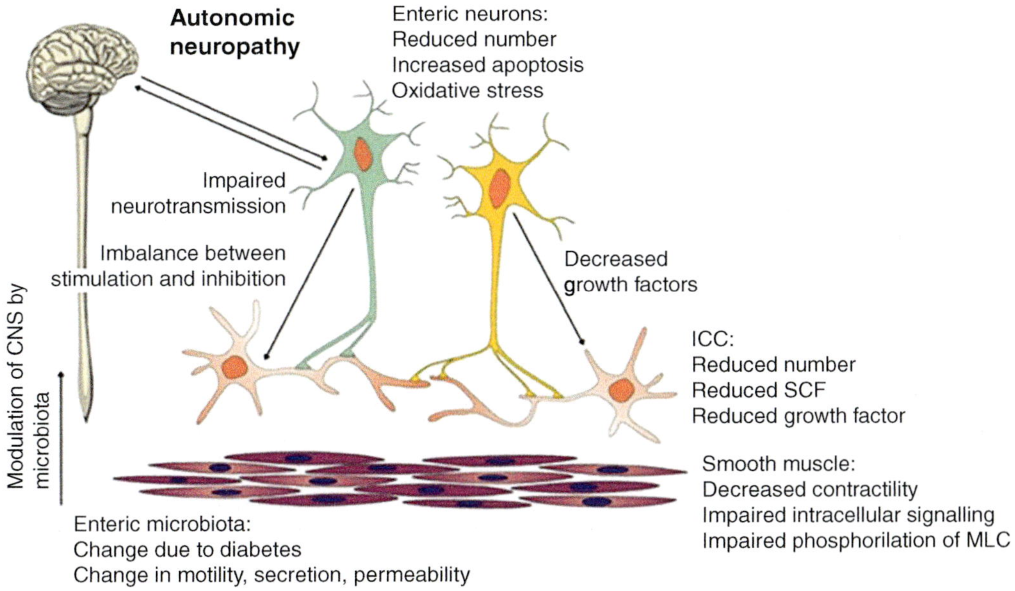


**Fig. 5.57** Potential mechanisms involving the enteric portion of the P&S nervous systems in impaired GI motility in diabetes. Mechanisms of GI enteric-autonomic neuropathy are complex and multifactorial, including oxidative stress and endothelial (nitric oxide) dysfunction. Autonomic neuropathy can affect both afferent and efferent connections between enteric and central nervous systems. Reduced number of enteric neurons is caused by increased oxidative stress and increased apoptosis. The number of interstitial cells of Cajal is also reduced, possibly due to lack of growth factors. The myopathic changes in smooth muscle and decreased contractility are due to impaired signaling (including nitric oxide signaling) pathways. Diabetes-induced changes in gut microbiota can modulate the CNS-gut interaction. Abbreviations: ICC interstitial cells of Cajal, SCF stem cell factor, MLC myosin light chain, DM diabetes mellitus, CNS central nervous system. (Republished with permission from Wiley Online Library. Source: [343])

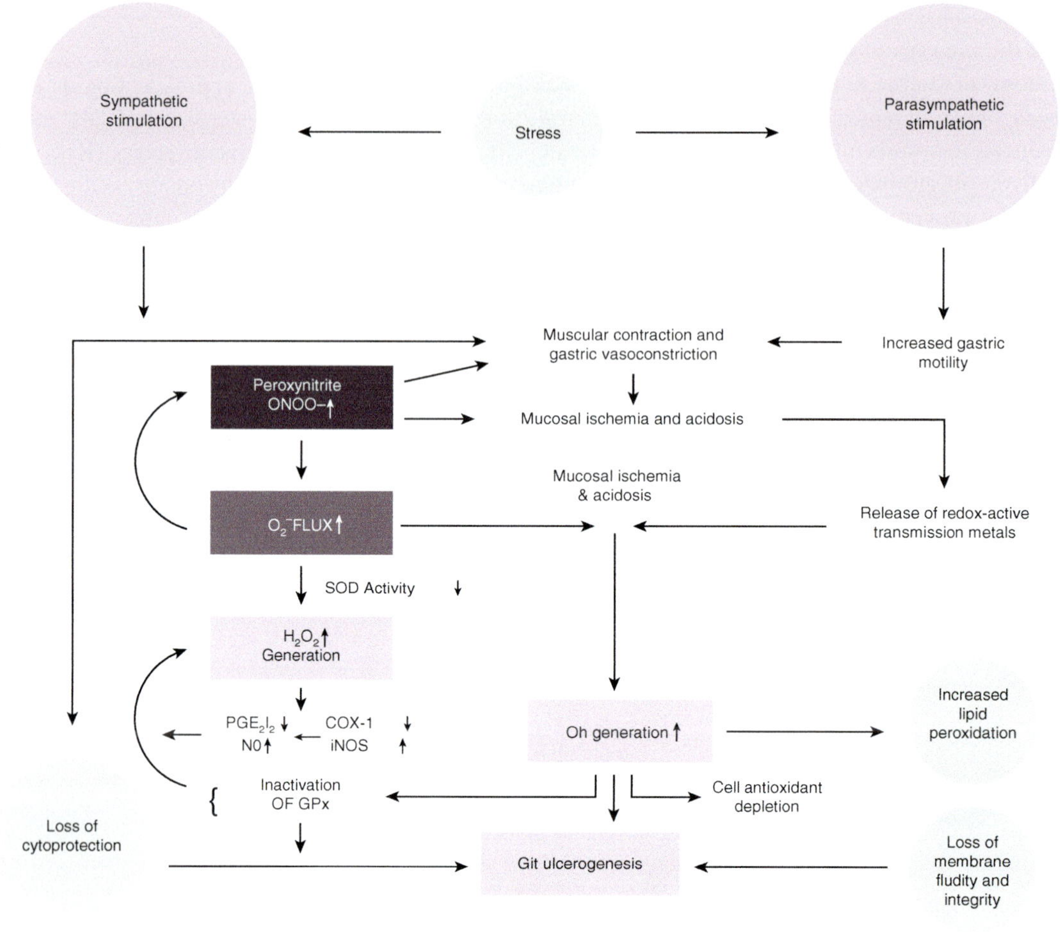


**Fig. 5.58** Oxidative stress and the involvement of both oxidative and nitrosative free radicals in the pathogenesis of ulcers in gastrointestinal tract (GIT) [344]. (Illustration by Elysian Creative Studio, www.elysiancreativestudio.com, Lizzy Colombo. Source: [345])

oxidant environment, not only do antioxidants themselves prevent, or repair, damage to tissues but so do RONS (see Fig. 5.59) [346]. RONS have a positive, physiological role in the protection against pathogens and in cell signaling [468] and act as intracellular messengers and are necessary for proper physiological function [469, 470].

Efficient antioxidant systems counteract the damaging action to cellular lipids, proteins, carbohydrates, and DNA [471] of the physiologically generated RONS when in high concentrations (Fig. 5.60) [472–474]. Endogenous antioxidants, in the human body, act through different types of mechanisms (Fig. 5.61) [347]. One example is reducing the ROS generation through chelating the metal ions (ferrum, copper, etc.) by specific or nonspecific proteins (ferritin, transferrin, albumin), so that these ions can no longer participate in redox reactions [475–479]. Another example is stopping the ROS formation chain reaction, generally via antioxidants with small molecular mass, such as reduced glutathione, vitamins E and C, uric acid, etc. [480, 481]. Another example is scavenging ROS with antioxidant enzymes such as SOD, catalase, glutathione peroxidase, glutathione reductase, etc. [474, 482]. Another example is repairing lesions caused by ROS via specific enzymes such as endonucleases, peroxidases, lipases, etc. [474].

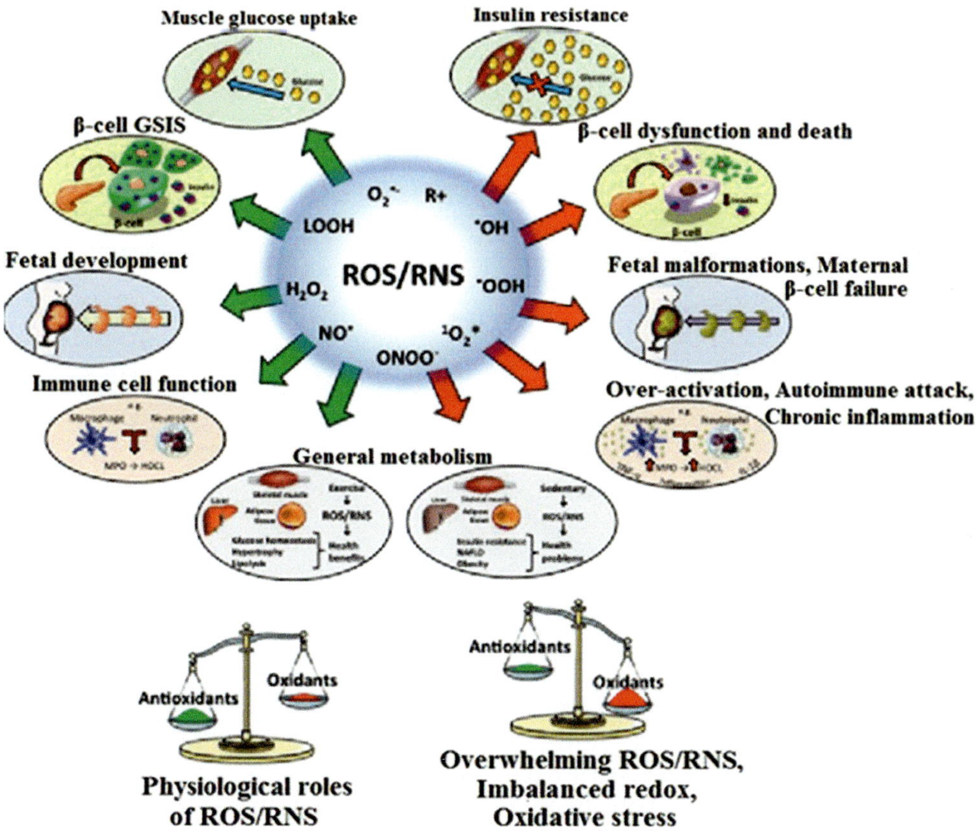


**Fig. 5.59** Radical oxygen or nitrogen species (ROS or RNS, respectively) are either healthful or harmful depending on local conditions. An appropriate antioxidant environment is necessary to maintain both ROS and RNS in their healthful modes. Abbreviations: GSIS glucose-stimulated insulin secretion. (Open Access, Biochemical Society, Portland Press. Source: [346])

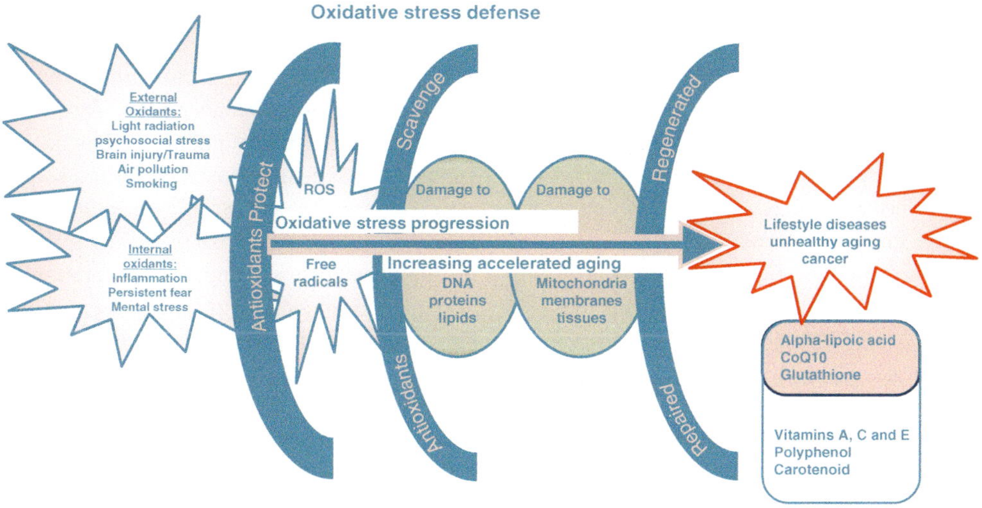


**Fig. 5.60** Defense against oxidative stress. Listed on the left is the progression from potential source of irritation to disease. Antioxidants, like those listed in the table (lower right), protect both at the chemical level (proteins or DNA) and the membrane level. (Source: http://www.cyclochem.com/cyclochembio/research_e/034.html)

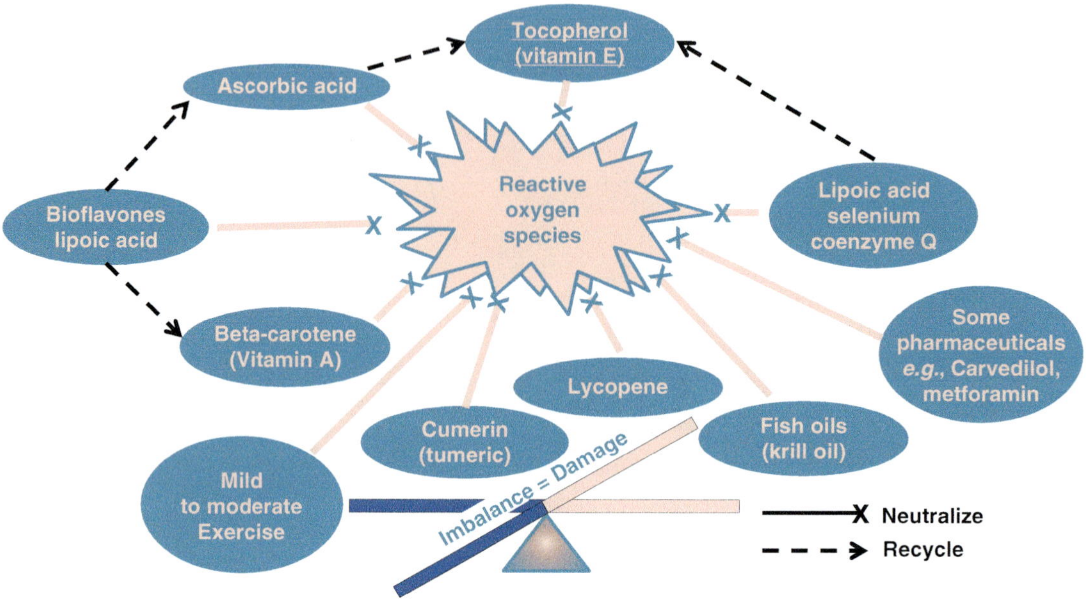


**Fig. 5.61** ROS neutralization by several biomolecules. (Source: [347])

These extensive antioxidant systems act differently to control the concentration of RONS, depending on their structure and properties, their hydrophilic or lipophilic character, and also their localization (intracellular or extracellular, such as in cell or organelle membranes, in the cytoplasm, etc.) [483]. These systems act synergistically and form a network which, when in balance, protects cells from the destructive action of RONS and keeps them in their constructive mode. Many of the different types and classifications of antioxidants are intrinsic to the body. Important antioxidants include bioflavonoids such as N-lipoic acid, ascorbic acid (vitamin C), tocopherol (vitamin E), selenium, and lycopene. Antioxidants act among each other to regenerate other antioxidants in a synergistic fashion. ALA and CoQ10 regenerate, or recycle, vitamins C and E and bioflavonoids and beta-carotene (see Fig. 5.3), thus amplifying not only its own antioxidant effects but those of the vitamins and flavonoids as well. Vitamin C also regenerates vitamin E (see Fig. 5.3) and ALA regenerates vitamin A (Fig. 5.62). ALA and CoQ10 are mitochondrial nutrients, arguably the most important, and are key in promoting adaptive responses to oxidative stress [468].

The antioxidant defense system is commonly divided into enzymatic (endogenous) and nonenzymatic (exogenous). Antioxidants are defined as a group of compounds characterized by their ability to be oxidized in place of other compounds present [484]. The main enzymatic antioxidants include SOD, catalase, and glutathione peroxidase. Vitamins A, C, and E, thiols, flavonoids, and ubiquinones represent the main nonenzymatic group, which can be obtained in a conventional diet and with supplementation. This demonstrates that antioxidant supplementation may result in an acute improvement in antioxidant-oxidant balance [485, 486].

Oxidant-antioxidant imbalance has been implicated in the pathogenesis of diseases affecting every organ system [487]. Data implicates a key role for ROS in signaling pathways important in multiple processes including proliferation, differentiation, immune function, and vaso-regulation. Examples include ROS and 4-hydroxy-2-nonenal-induced vascular cell proliferation and angiogenesis [488, 489], $H_2O_2$ regulation of bone marrow-derived stem and progenitor cell function [490], RONS regulation of neutrophil and monocyte function [491, 492], and ROS signaling that

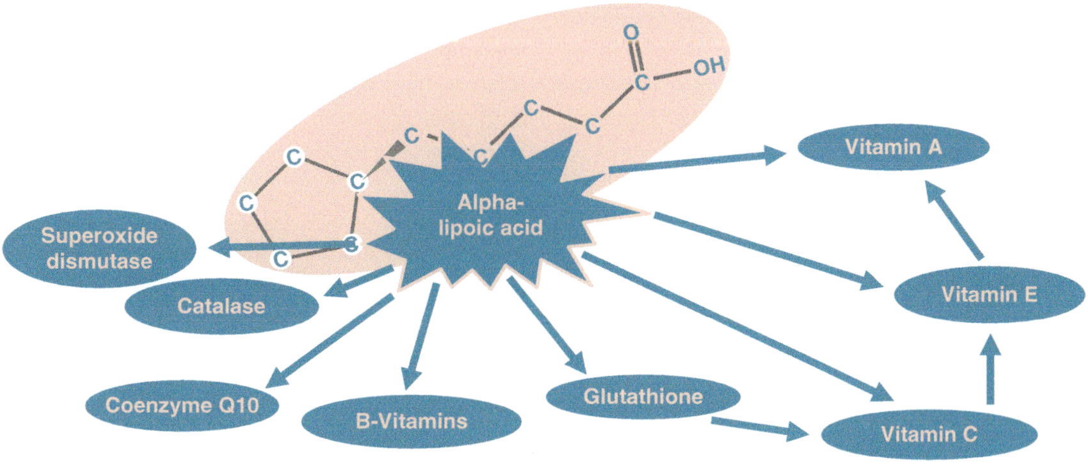


**Fig. 5.62** Alpha-lipoic acid and coenzyme Q10 are the most powerful and versatile antioxidant. They are designed to support P&S and mitochondrial health; they already exist within the nerves and mitochondria; and they recycle vitamins A and E. The preferred coenzyme Q10 is ubiquinol [28]. (Source: http://healthyprotocols.com/2_antioxidant.htm)

regulates pulmonary vessel tone, kinase-modulated vascular function, and mechanical stretch-induced vascular remodeling [493–495].

The pathophysiology of oxidative stress occurs when there is an imbalance in oxidant-antioxidant systems. While lipid peroxidation can be a marker of excess ROS production, oxidized lipids are also potent signaling molecules. Isoprostanes, for example, are by-products of membrane lipid peroxidation that provoke bronchoconstriction and airway hyper-responsiveness in asthma and powerful vasoconstriction in pulmonary arterial hypertension and acute lung injury [496, 497]. Certain highly reactive ROS are associated with indiscriminant oxidative or nitrosative stress, such as hydroxyl radical ($^{\bullet}HO$) or $ONOO^-$. In contrast, $H_2O_2$, $NO^{\bullet}$, and $O_2^{\bullet-}$ have relatively longer half-lives and specific cellular targets that enable them to function as signaling molecules. Sustained or increased production of these RONS promotes alterations in cell signaling responsible for disease progression. These species can regulate enzyme function, including kinases and phosphatases, G-protein or tyrosine kinase receptors, ion channel function, and transcription factors, resulting in an impact on numerous downstream pathways. RONS can directly modify reactive cysteine residues, which represent a major mechanism for redox-regulated signaling [498]. Posttranslational modifications include disulfide bond formation, reduction, oxidation, nitrosylation, and glutathionylation, which alter protein function. RONS usually have specific targets that are tightly regulated. The reactions are also usually rapid, reversible, and occur in specific tissue and cellular compartments.

An important factor which promotes oxidative processes is an increased core body temperature [499]. Physical exercise performed in the aerobic environment leads to considerable dehydration [500] and oxidative stress [501]. Both factors negatively impact the exercise efficiency. Furthermore passive body overheating also shifts the pro-antioxidant-oxidant balance toward oxidation [499]. Dehydration increases blood viscosity, reducing the cooling efficiency of the blood, causing more heat to be retained, increasing the potential for oxidation. While a couple of degrees increase in body core temperature may be healthy, too great an increase in body core temperature is not. It adds to oxidation ("burning") and inflammation.

From type 2 diabetes therapy research (using diabetes as a model of chronic disease), the use of ALA, also known as thioctic acid, improved CAN in a 4-month controlled randomized trial [502]. There is evidence that the vitamin E also improves HRV indices [503], further amplifying the effects of ALA. In a randomized controlled trial, vitamin E, when compared to placebo, managed to increase the R-R interval ($p < 0.05$) and the high frequency component of heart rate variability (HF; $p < 0.05$) in 50 type 2 diabetes patients over a period of 4 months [504].

In addition to its antioxidant properties, ALA has thiol-replenishing, redox-modulating properties [340]. There are two forms available: R-form and S-form. The R-form of ALA is the biologically active form and is produced naturally. The S-form is significantly less biologically active and is produced chemically. A number of studies show its favorable influence on microcirculation and reversal of symptoms of neuropathy [505–508]. A meta-analysis including 1258 patients from four randomized clinical trials concluded that 600 mg of I.V. ALA daily significantly reduced symptoms of neuropathy and improved neuropathic deficits [509]. The SYDNEY 2 trial showed significant improvement in neuropathic symptoms and neurologic deficits in 181 diabetic patients with three different doses of ALA compared to placebo over a 5-week period [403]. The result of the NATHAN study, which examined the long-term effects on electrophysiology and clinical assessments, showed that 4-year treatment with ALA in mild-to-moderate doses is well tolerated, slows the progression of neuropathy, and improves some neuropathic deficits and symptoms, but not nerve conduction [405]. However, nerve conduction typically measures the large A and B nerve fibers which are not the small C fibers of the P&S nerves.[15]

CoQ10 is a cofactor or coenzyme, not a vitamin. It is lipid soluble. It is produced and regenerated in the body. It sequesters active ROS, especially in mitochondria. It protects cell membranes and prevents lipid oxidation and, thereby, prevents atherosclerosis from propagating. It is beneficial to have a high concentration of CoQ10 in the blood. Unfortunately, its levels decline with age but may be replenished through supplements [510]. Higher levels of CoQ10 have been associated with reducing the risk of coronary artery disease and the potential of being cardioprotective, including lowering systolic blood pressure by as much as 17 mmHg and diastolic blood pressure by up to 10 mmHg without significant side effects [511, 512]. In the electron transport chain, where most ATP is made, CoQ10 limits the effects of mitochondrial electron leak and thereby mitochondrial damage and dysfunction. Increasing CoQ10 blood levels may prevent or treat skeletal myopathy as well as cardiomyopathy (skeletal myopathy is also known as statin myopathy), which occurs with patients consuming statins to lower cholesterol [513]. The reduced form of CoQ10, ubiquinol, is better absorbed and better utilized in this regard.

Also from type 2 diabetes therapy research [340], in addition to vitamins $B_6$ and $B_{12}$ with ALA, aldose reductase inhibitors (ARIs) reduce the flux of glucose through the polyol pathway, inhibiting tissue accumulation of the sugars sorbitol and fructose, reducing their free radical effects. In a 12-month study of zenarestat,[16] a dose-dependent improvement in sensory (large) nerve fiber density was shown [514]. In a 1-year trial of fidarestat[17] in Japanese diabetics with peripheral neuropathy, improvement of symptoms was shown [515]. A 3-year study of epalres-

[15]With nerve conduction velocity (NCV) studies, a very small electrical current is passed through the nerve bundle to determine conduction time. Of course, electricity takes the path of least resistance, meaning that it will preferentially flow through the large nerve fibers, not the small fibers. Therefore, NCV is a measure of large fibers, which are the sensory and motor fibers, not the P&S (or autonomic) nerve fibers. This is why vibration and pin prick tests are well correlated. In general, if the patient can feel the stimulus, it is not an autonomic test.

[16]Zenarestat (FK-366; FR-74366) is a powerful aldose reductase inhibitor which inhibits the metabolism of glucose by the polyol pathway, to slow or reduce progression of polyneuropathy. It was investigated as a treatment of diabetic neuropathy and cataract, but its development was terminated.

[17]Fidarestat (SNK-860) is a potent aldose reductase inhibitor under investigation for treatment of diabetic neuropathy. Fidarestat normalized the elevated sorbitol content of erythrocytes under fasting as well as postprandial conditions and possibly useful for both preventing and treating diabetic neuropathy.

tat[18] showed improved sensory nerve function, as measured by nerve conduction velocity, as well as vibration perception [516]. However, ARIs alone are proving insufficient and combinations of treatments may be needed [517], especially when treating quality of life symptoms (e.g., lightheadedness, GI and sleep disturbances, and sex dysfunction).

Protein kinase-C inhibitors (e.g., ruboxistaurin, a PKC-β inhibitor) in patients with less severe diabetic neuropathy (sural nerve action potential >0.5 μV) at baseline and clinically significant symptoms demonstrated a statistically significant improvement in symptoms and vibratory detection thresholds [518]. A smaller, single center study showed improvement in symptom scores, including autonomic-related endothelium-dependent skin blood flow measurements and quality of life scores in the ruboxistaurin-treated group [519]. These studies and the NATHAN studies have pointed out the change in natural history of diabetic neuropathy with the advent of therapeutic lifestyle change, statins, and ACE inhibitors, which have slowed the progression of neuropathy.

All in all, a proper antioxidant-oxidant balance (see insert, right) is required to restore and maintain health and wellness. In effect, this has been proven in the negative [520]. A systemic review and meta-analysis of randomized control trials concluded that there was no evidence to support the use of vitamin and antioxidant supplements for prevention of cardiovascular diseases. They based this conclusion on 2240 articles which used antioxidants or vitamins in conjunction with cardiovascular disease. After careful analysis, 50 trials were included for what they considered a high quality of 294,470 participants, with 156,663 in the intervention group and 137,850 in the control group. The mean age of the participants ranged from 49 to 82. Publication ranged from 1989 to 2012, spanning 23 years. The dose regimens used in each trial were vitamin A 10,000–25,000 units, vitamin $B_6$ at various doses three times a week, vitamin $B_{12}$ at various doses three times a week, vitamin C up to 1000 mg a day, vitamin D up to 1000 units daily or 100,000 units every 4 months, vitamin E up to 800 international units daily, beta-carotene up to 50 mg daily, folic acid up to 5 mg three times a week, and selenium. For the most part, these trials did not include CoQ10 and ALA. Thirty-nine trials used vitamin supplements only and 22 trials used the antioxidant supplements. In one trial, aspirin 325 mg was used and in only one trial CoQ10 is mentioned 100 mg a day, which is a low dose. No mention of ALA is listed. Omega-3 fatty acid at a ratio of 2:1 was mentioned in one trial. Therefore, these were predominantly trials involving only vitamins such as A, C, D, E, as well as B vitamins, beta-carotene, folic acid, and selenium.

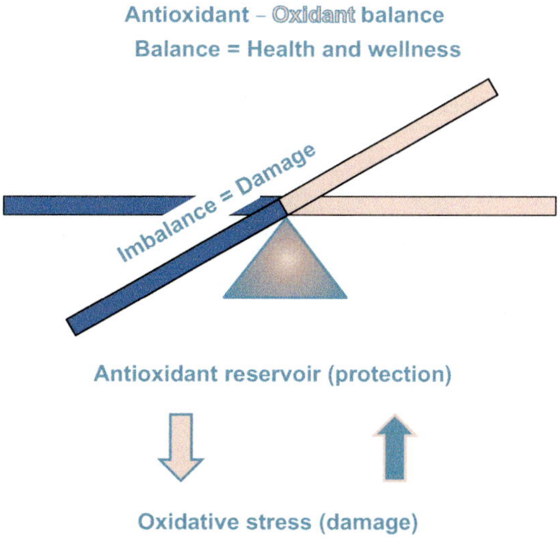


The fixed effects of the meta-analysis of all 50 trials did not show an association of reduced risk of cardiovascular disease. This data is in conflict with observational epidemiologic studies which have reported that intake of fruit and vegetables rich in vitamin and antioxidants is associated with a reduced risk of cardiovascular disease (see "Mediterranean Diet (Prong-4), Antioxidant Effects"). It was stated that this was the first trial

[18]Epalrestat is a noncompetitive and reversible aldose reductase inhibitor used for the treatment of diabetic neuropathy. Long-term treatment is well tolerated and can effectively delay the progression of diabetic neuropathy and ameliorate the associated symptoms of the disease, particularly in people with good glycemic control and limited microangiopathy.

that did a published comprehensive meta-analysis of high-quality randomized controlled trials [520]. It should be noted, however, that ALA and CoQ10 in combination with other supplements were not specifically studied in this meta-analysis. The missing ingredient is the recycling activities of ALA and CoQ10, as discussed above, amplifying their effects and those of the vitamins multiple times (see Fig. 5.3 and Fig. 5.62). Sufficient amounts of natural vitamins and antioxidants from fruits and vegetables are intrinsic to one's system, and their recycling causes their effective levels to be physiologic. It is not surprising, therefore, that synthetic vitamins such as A, E, C, and so forth have negative effects as they are not taken naturally and do not utilize cofactors such as these antioxidants. It is for this reason that using ALA, CoQ10, and a Mediterranean diet makes rational sense and has significant biological feasibility, especially in maintaining health and wellness in mitochondria and nerves, including P&S nerves (Fig. 5.63) [348].

Melatonin is selectively taken up by mitochondria and acts as a powerful antioxidant, regulating mitochondrial function (Fig. 5.64) [24, 349]. Melatonin is the pineal gland hormone and is a metabolic product of L-tryptophan (see Fig. 5.48). Melatonin increases the permeability of membranes and is the stimulator of antioxidant enzymes including superoxide dismutase, glutathione peroxidase, glutathione reductase, and catalase. It also acts as an inhibitor of lipoxygenase. Melatonin can cause resistance to oxidation damage by fixing the microsomal membranes. Melatonin has been shown to retard aging and inhibit neurodegenerative disorders, ischemia-reperfusion, septic shock, diabetes, cancer, and other complications related to oxidative stress by improving mitochondrial function [24].

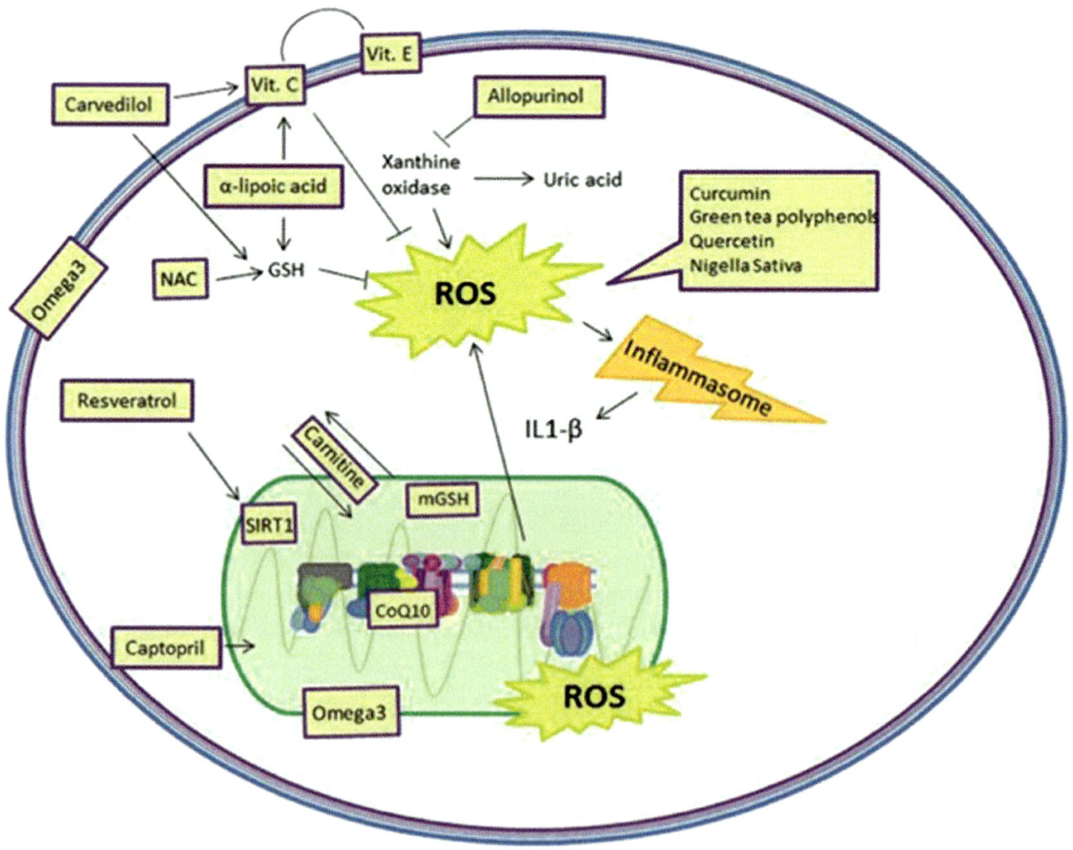


**Fig. 5.63** Functional sites of major antioxidant agents. (Open Access; Springer Nature, BMC. Source: [132, 348])

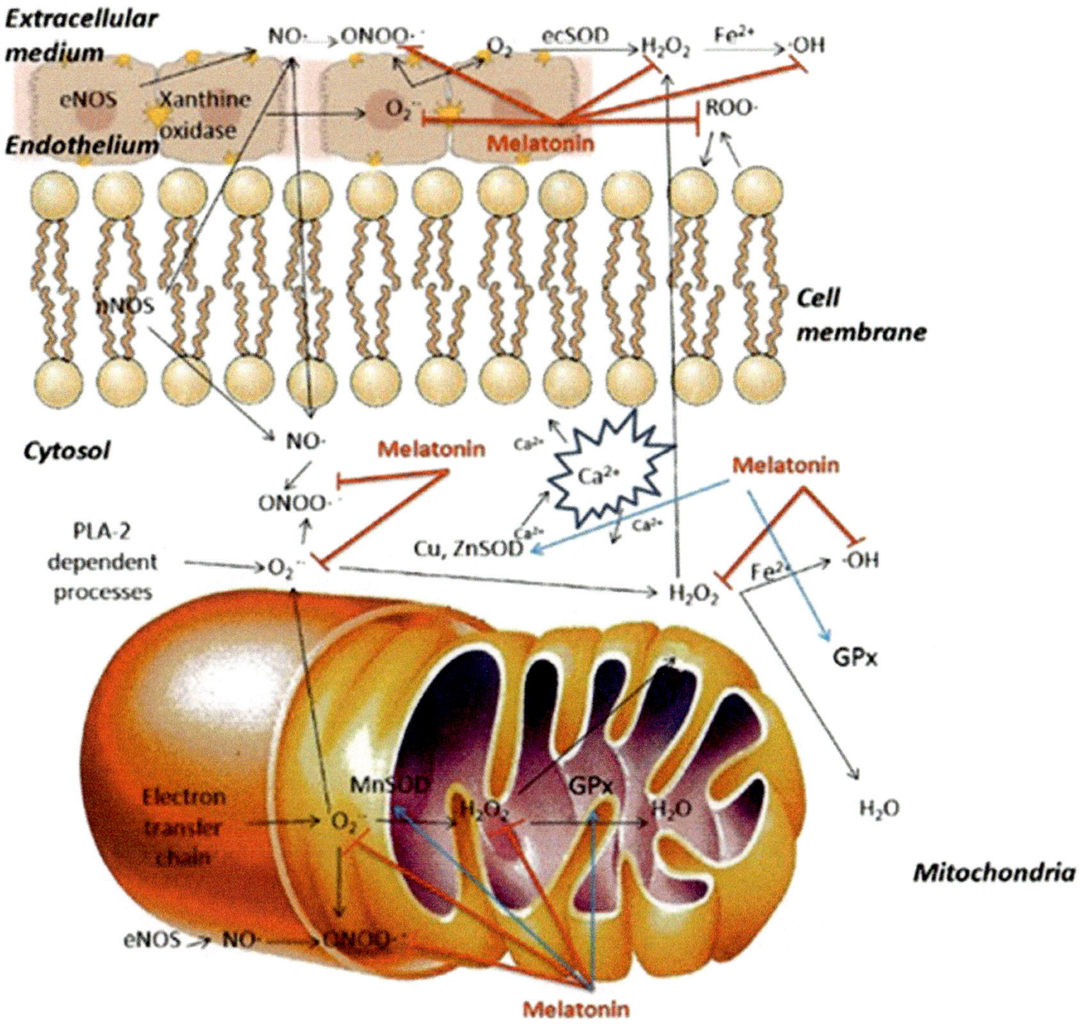


**Fig. 5.64** Melatonin's direct (red) an indirect effects (blue). In the endothelium, xanthine oxidase generates $O_2^{\bullet-}$. Melatonin is a scavenger of this ROS. In the extracellular medium and mitochondria, melatonin is a scavenger of $ONOO^-$ generated as a result of the availability of $NO^\bullet$ due to eNOS and nNOS activity. Furthermore, $O_2^{\bullet-}$ reactions with extracellular superoxide dismutase (ecSOD) gives rise to $H_2O_2$, which suffers a reduction with $Fe^{++}$ generating •OH. Melatonin neutralizes this ROS. Similar processes are observed in the cytosol and mitochondria with the action of MnSOD and Cu/ZnSOD. Glutathione peroxidase (GPx) reduces $H_2O_2$ to $H_2O$ and $O_2$. Melatonin has an indirect antioxidant effect by increasing the activities of the important antioxidant enzymes SOD and GPx. During ischemic-reperfusion injury, a depletion of ATP occurs, and an increase in cellular $Ca^{++}$ develops which augments oxidative stress and loss of mitochondrial function. Abbreviations: $O_2^{\bullet-}$ superoxide radical, •OH hydroxyl radical, $H_2O_2$ hydrogen peroxide, $NO^\bullet$ nitric oxide, $ROO^\bullet$ alkyl peroxyl radical, $ONOO^-$ peroxynitrite, eNOS endothelial nitric oxide synthase, iNOS inducible nitric oxide synthase, PLA-2 phospholipase A2. (Republished with permission from Springer Nature. Source: [292, 349])

Critically ill patients suffer from oxidative stress caused by RONS [521]. Although RONS are constantly produced under normal circumstances, critical illness can drastically increase their production. These patients have reduced plasma and intracellular levels of antioxidants and free electron scavengers or cofactors and decreased activity of the enzymatic system involved in ROS detoxification [522]. Sources of oxidative stress during critical illness include activation of phagocytic cells of the immune system, production of nitric oxide by the vascular endothelium, release of iron and copper ions and metalloproteins, and ischemia-reperfusion-induced tissue damage. The antioxidant-oxidant balance is of functional relevance during critical illness because it is involved in the pathogenesis of multiple organ failure [523–525]. RONS have been reported to trigger the release of cytokines from immune cells, activate inflammatory cascades, and increase the expression of adhesion molecules [526]. Inflammation and tissue injury result in an accumulation of granulocytes in organs, leading to greater generation of ROS, which further perpetuates or increases the inflammatory response and consequent tissue injury [527]. The critical condition of patients admitted to the ICU is associated with worsening oxidative stress. Intake of antioxidant vitamins below 66% of recommended daily allowance (RDA) and alteration in endogenous levels of substances with antioxidant capacity are related to redox imbalance in critically ill patients. Therefore, intake of antioxidant vitamins should be carefully monitored so that it is as close as possible to RDA [528, 529].

Administration of antioxidants and antioxidant vitamins at between 66% and 100% of RDA reduces the risk for oxidative stress by 94% [521]. Early antioxidant supplementation with vitamins C and E in surgical patients reduces the incidence of organ failure and shortens the ICU length of stay [530]. Critical care patients receiving dietary supplementation with antioxidant vitamins A, C, and E, compared with controls, reported higher plasma concentrations of vitamins A and E and LDL and greater resistance to LDL oxidation in the supplemented group [531]. However, they found no difference in clinical outcomes between vitamin-treated patients and control individuals. Again, this may be due to a lack of ALA or CoQ10. However, dietary supplementation with vitamins C and E for 10 days prevented lipid peroxidation and oxidative stress in critical care patients and significantly influenced their clinical outcome at 28 days [532].

Although oxygen is a prerequisite to life, at concentrations beyond the physiological limits, it may be hazardous to the cells. Since the lungs are directly exposed to very high amounts of oxygen, it is imperative for the organ to possess defenses against possible oxidative challenge. The lungs are therefore endowed with a battery of endogenous antioxidants [533]. Oxidant-antioxidant imbalance can lead to a variety of airway diseases, such as asthma, chronic obstructive pulmonary disease, and idiopathic pulmonary fibrosis. Antioxidant species help the lungs ward off the deleterious consequences of a wide variety of oxidants and RONS. The major nonenzymatic antioxidants of the lungs are glutathione, vitamins C and E, beta-carotene, and uric acid, and the enzymatic antioxidants are SOD, catalase, and peroxidases. These antioxidants are the first lines of defense against the oxidants and usually act at a gross level. Cellular redox chemistry has revealed the presence of certain specialized proteins such as peroxiredoxins, thioredoxins, glutaredoxins, heme oxygenases, and reductases, which are involved in cellular adaptation and protection against an oxidative assault. These molecules usually exert their action at a more subtle level of cellular signaling processes.

A goal is to have a positive antioxidant to oxidant balance. When there are too many prooxidants, there is tissue damage, and the seesaw tips toward the side of oxidative stress. When there is more defense or antioxidants, the seesaw will tip away from oxidative stress and toward host defense and protection of cells and membranes. Oxidative stress is a primary disorder that physicians seek to relieve. Especially in Prong-3, it targets oxidative stress with antioxidant approaches in the form of supplements. Oxidative stress was first coined by Helmut Sies (see photo insert, below) in 1985. While more sophisticated definitions of oxidative stress have evolved since the time of Dr. Sies, the basic definition for the purpose of this program will be adhered to. To summarize from above, moderate oxidative stress accelerates the aging process of senescence and promotes tumorigenesis. Overt oxidative stress causes apoptosis. Therefore, reducing oxidative stress has antiaging capabilities. Oxidative damage to lipids forms foam cells and begins the atherosclerotic process and causes it to propagate.

Therefore, reducing oxidative stress in lipids is extremely important in delaying or preventing atherosclerosis. In regard to lipid oxidation, lipid membranes get oxidized and promote cell death called lipid peroxidation. Fatty acids, which are polyunsaturated, are targets of ROS, especially the omega-6 fatty acid cell membranes [534].

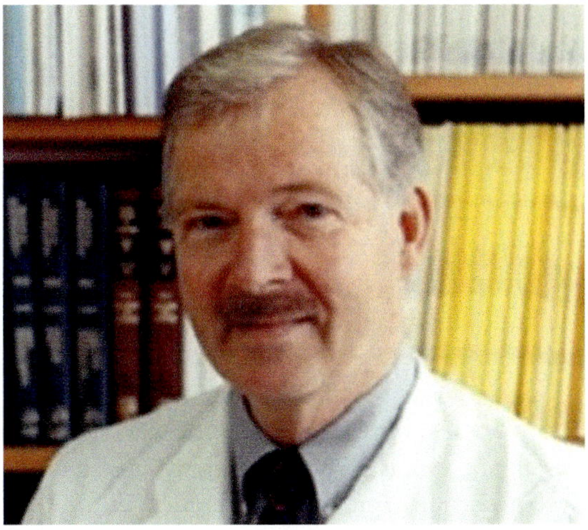

This is one reason why more omega-9 (such as the components of olive oil) and omega-3 (such as the components of fish oils) and not the components of omega-6 (which are seen in linoleic acid) are recommended. Vitamin E by itself does not prevent the formation of these oxidized lipids, and more than just vitamin E alone is required. Also, just lowering the LDL cholesterol particle count with statins, pharmacology, or other dietary measures will not prevent atherosclerosis if the oxidation of these lipids is also not prevented, even though they are in lower quantity. This is very important and this is why the Mind-Body Wellness Program highly recommends a multi-prong approach to possibly prevent or limit lipid oxidation. While the program endorses statins or other pharmacological agents to lower total LDL cholesterol, it also attempts to increase the oxidant balance and produce an antioxidant milieu with lifestyle changes and supplements [534].

Formation of free radicals from external sites such as UV radiation, inflammation from viruses and bacteria, and toxins such as cigarette smoking and ionizing radiation cause DNA damage and should be avoided. The key process involved with the function of antioxidants is that they donate electrons to free radicals. Free radicals (RONS) are in need of electrons because they may have an isolated electron or an electron shell which is unpaired. By providing an electron, the free radical is prevented from damaging other tissues by stealing electrons from these other tissues.

Virtually all diseases may be related to oxidative stress, including chronic fatigue, cancers, asthma, Parkinson's disease, blood vessel diseases, COPD, aging, hepatitis, macular degeneration, inflammatory bowel disease, kidney disease, skin disorders, Alzheimer's disease, diabetes, heart disease (including hypertension, atherosclerosis, and heart failure), migraine, fibromyalgia, and even autism. The simple aging process, along with anxiety, depression, attention deficit syndromes, and obsessive-compulsive behaviors, is found to be related to oxidative stress. In cardiovascular practice, all risk factors promote oxidative stress, including hypertension, diabetes, and smoking, as well as high homocysteine and high angiotensin II levels, which are powerful vasoconstrictors and produced in the bloodstream. To see an example of how oxidative stress causes progressive aging and tissue damage, consider an apple left in the open air which combines with oxygen, slowly shrivels up, deteriorates, shrinks, and becomes necrotic (see Fig. 2.26).

Chronic fatigue syndrome (CFS) is a very common ailment in primary practice. It consists of symptoms which last more than 6 months with at least four of the following: subjective memory impairment, tender lymph node, muscle pain, joint pain, headache, unrefreshing sleep, and post-exertional tiredness more than 24 hours. The vast majority of CFS patients (97%) may also have orthostatic dysfunction, a well-known autonomic dysfunction [116]. Orthostatic dysfunction is present when an individual upon standing has evidence of increased symptoms of lightheadedness (dizziness) or inability to focus or concentrate and has to sit down or lie down for relief. Orthostatic intolerance, orthostatic hypotension, and postural orthostatic tachycardia syndrome (POTS) are forms of orthostatic dysfunction [116]. Brain fog, near-fainting, and fainting are all parts of the spectrum of symptoms of orthostatic dysfunction. Orthostatic dysfunction, specifically orthostatic intolerance, and chronic fatigue syndrome are usually interrelated and involve mitochondrial dysfunction which is associated with autonomic dysfunction. Most forms of autonomic dysfunction are believed to be associated with mitochondrial dysfunction. The antioxidants CoQ10 and ALA which buffer free radicals are useful to treat chronic fatigue syndrome in patients with orthostatic intolerance. High-dose ALA [537] is also known to be a therapy for orthostatic dysfunction, especially orthostatic intolerance and orthostatic hypotension.

There are many triggers for autonomic dysfunction besides external toxins such as cigarette smoke or radiation. Emotional stress, viruses, and concussions can cause autonomic dysfunction, perhaps as a result of mitochondrial dysfunction. Fibromyalgia is a common syndrome and manifests as pain with tenderness in many joints, muscles, tendons, and tissues. Fibromyalgia may be reduced with CoQ10, which repairs mitochondrial membrane function and autonomic function. Autonomic dysfunction has also been linked to sleep problems, headaches, irritable bowel syndrome, depression, and anxiety [116]. The cause is often unknown. Triggers include physical and emotional stress. Individuals have abnormal pain responses. No virus has been identified that can cause fibromyalgia. It is often seen in women between the ages of 20 and 50. They may have chronic neck pain, chronic fatigue, and depression. The symptoms of fibromyalgia may mimic hypothyroidism, Lyme disease or various organic sleep disorders, and these other disorders need to be excluded. Fibromyalgia is also associated with orthostatic intolerance.

Orthostatic intolerance (OI) is a symptom. Orthostatic hypotension and orthostatic tachycardia are measureable components, namely, abnormal decreases in blood pressure with standing or abnormal increases in heart rate with standing, respectively [116]. Basically, orthostatic intolerance is defined when symptoms, when upright, are relieved by lying down. They are difficult to treat. Patient's underlying P or S nervous system dysfunction is targeted with pharmacology, lifestyle changes, volume changes, and also antioxidant approaches to treat these disorders [116], as the autonomic nervous system is closely linked to mitochondrial dysfunction.

A form of orthostatic hypotension is neurogenic orthostatic hypotension (NOH). NOH is caused by failure of the baroreceptor reflex usually as a result of neurologic intracellular α-synuclein production and aggregation [535], largely occurring in the dopaminergic neurons of the brainstem (e.g., substantia nigra), cerebellum, midbrain (e.g., hippocampus and thalamus), and neocortex. Alpha-synuclein is the major protein in Lewy bodies, which are pathological entities in autonomic diseases such as Parkinson's, multiple system atrophy, primary autonomic failure, and certain types of dementia, including Alzheimer's. NOH is a common and perhaps the most debilitating symptom in these diseases. With these diseases, α-synuclein accumulates in the presynaptic terminal, interfering with, or preventing, neurotransmitter release. Alpha-synuclein is highly expressed in neuronal mitochondria. It is localized in the inner membrane of mitochondria, associated with complex I activity of the mitochondrial respiratory chain. Mitochondrial alpha-synuclein may be a potential factor affecting mitochondrial function and predisposing some neurons to degeneration [536].

A similar process occurs in many other chronic diseases, such as diabetes, hypertension and cardiovascular diseases, and possibly dementia. Oxidative stress due to chronic disease leads to nerve dysfunction (including autonomic dysfunction and autonomic neuropathy), which leads to NOH. ALA suppresses α-synuclein accumulation in neurons, improving baroreceptor reflex, relieving NOH. This may be a more direct approach to NOH, rather than simply treating the symptoms of NOH with the commonly used medications

[537]. ALA suppresses neurologic intracellular accumulation of α-synuclein (the major cause of NOH) in many neurologic diseases [535, 538, 539]. It may suppress α-synuclein accumulation by preventing excess oxidation in neuronal mitochondria where α-synuclein is found on their inner membranes. Furthermore, ALA uniquely reduces resting hypertension and endothelial dysfunction, systemically [540–544].

With this additional information, a deeper understanding of orthostatic dysfunction has been developed (see Fig. 5.65). Orthostatic dysfunction is characterized by sympathetic withdrawal (SW) with postural change (i.e., standing). SW is an alpha-adrenergic, or alpha-sympathetic, dysfunction. OI is the primary and first clinical presentation. Postural orthostatic tachycardia syndrome (POTS) and neurogenic orthostatic hypotension (NOH) are more advanced forms of OI. POTS is typically found in younger women, a result of the fact that women tend to have smaller hearts, and increased heart rate is the primary means of providing the brain with more blood, but this method fails. NOH is found in older, sicker patients, who tend to have bigger hearts and in whom a drop in

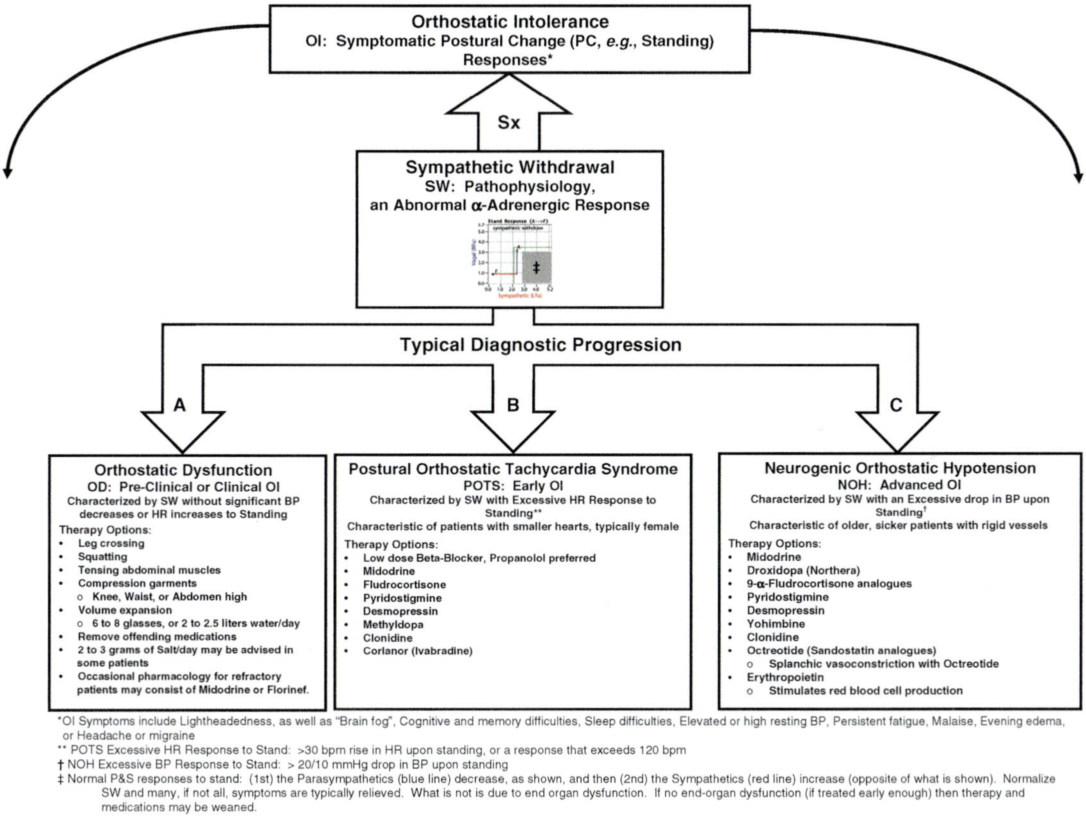


**Fig. 5.65** Orthostatic dysfunction is characterized by sympathetic withdrawal (SW) with postural change (i.e., standing). SW is an alpha-adrenergic or alpha-sympathetic dysfunction. Orthostatic intolerance (OI) is the primary and first clinical presentation. Postural orthostatic tachycardia syndrome (POTS) and neurogenic orthostatic hypotension (NOH) are more advanced forms of OI. POTS is typically found in younger women, a result of the fact that women tend to have smaller hearts and increased heart rate is the primary means of providing the brain with more blood, but this method fails. NOH is found in older, sicker patients, who tend to have bigger hearts and in whom a drop in pressure is the primary result leading to symptoms. (© DePace and Colombo, 2018)

pressure is the primary result leading to symptoms. Possible therapy options are presented in the figure.

As an autonomic dysfunction, orthostatic dysfunction is associated with migraine syndrome, sleep apnea, anxiety depression temperature dysregulation, chronic fatigue syndrome, gastroesophageal reflux, irritable bowel syndrome, tinnitus, syncope, and pre-fainting syndromes [116]. POTS is diagnosed as an increase in heart rate over 30 beats from lying to standing within 10 minutes and, for adolescents, more than a 40-beat rise. In diagnosing POTS, orthostatic hypotension (a drop in systolic blood pressure of 20 mm or a drop in diastolic blood pressure of 10 mm within 3 minutes of standing) has to be excluded before diagnosis. Symptoms of orthostatic intolerance in POTS patients last more than 6 months and are exacerbated by standing and are improved by lying down. Dehydration has to be excluded. These patients are often treated with increased salt and volume, compression stockings, eating smaller meals and fewer carbohydrates, avoiding caffeine, and various medications, of which midodrine is one of the key medications, if tolerated. An antioxidant cocktail, such as that discussed herein, is also recommended. This cocktail has proven empirically useful. Patients who faint or have syncope often demonstrate a vagal phenomenon, which is a form of autonomic dysfunction [116]. However, there are various forms of fainting which can be diagnostically worked-up with P&S Monitoring and treated, and, often times, these patients respond to antioxidant cocktails.

N-acetylcysteine (NAC) is a derivative of the amino acid cysteine. It is found in many over-the-counter nutritional supplements and has antioxidant properties. It is also used as an antidote for acetaminophen overdose and has been used with mixed results in protecting the kidneys from contrast-iodinated compounds prior to diagnostic testing in patients with renal disease or kidney disease. NAC has been used to treat various psychiatric diseases. It has also been used in drug addiction treatment. NAC has been demonstrated to work on multiple pathways implicated in psychiatric and neurological disorders which include oxidative stress, mitochondrial dysfunction, inflammatory mediators, neurotransmission, and neural plasticity (Fig. 5.66). NAC may help in the treatment of Alzheimer's disease and other neurodegenerative diseases, autism, adult attention deficit syndrome (ADHD), bipolar disorders, obsessive-compulsive disorder, and depressive disorders [350–353].

In regard to oxidative stress, it is known that the brain is uniquely vulnerable to RONS due to its high oxygen metabolism and limited ability to have antioxidants operative in neural tissue. There are protective antioxidant mechanisms such as SOD, catalase, glutathione reductase, and glutathione peroxidase (see Fig. 5.66). These neutralize RONS [540]. Reduction in glutathione has been shown in depression, schizophrenia, ADHD, and other brain disorders (this supports the role of an oxidative imbalance in psychiatric disorders [541, 542]), as well as autism, ADHD, certain cancers and autoimmune diseases, multiple sclerosis, and other neurodegenerative diseases [545–548]. Bioavailability of cysteine, which in high concentrations may cause cell death through oxidation, is a rate-limiting factor in the production of glutathione. As cysteine levels increase, more glutathione is needed (and produced) to ensure healthy levels of cysteine and minimize oxidative stress on cells to prevent cell damage and death which may underlie the brain diseases listed. Through diet and supplementation, maintaining healthy levels of glutathione with healthy levels of omega-3 fatty acids, cell damage may be repaired, minimizing the effects of the diseases listed.

Mitochondrial dysfunction has been shown in several psychiatric disorders to be important, including in bipolar disorder [549]. NAC has direct effects on mitochondrial function in different disorders. Since NAC is the precursor of intracellular antioxidant glutathione and is also a direct-acting free radical scavenger and antioxidant, it plays an important role in reducing oxidative stress. Too much glutamate (a precursor to glutathione) is associated with mood and anxiety disorders. Psychiatric disorders are also associated with derangements of inflammatory cytokines including IL-6, interferon, and tumor necrosis factor. NAC has anti-inflammatory prop-

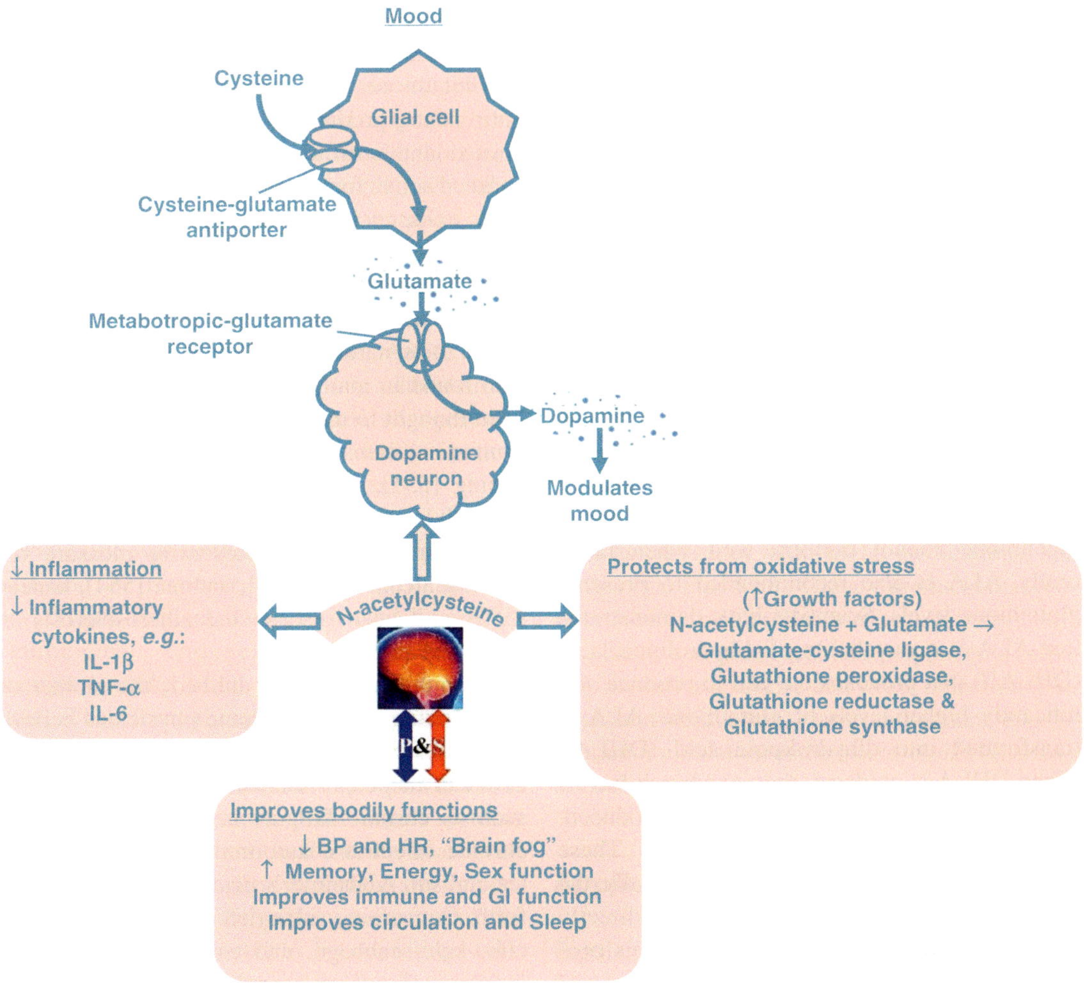


**Fig. 5.66** In the brain N-acetylcysteine has three functions: (1) it modulates neurotransmission of dopamine where cysteine enters a glial cell through a cysteine-glutamate antiporter, which releases glutamate to bind to a metabotropic-glutamate receptor on a dopamine neuron, which modulates dopamine release, thereby affecting mood; (2) it reduces inflammatory cytokines, including IL-1β, TNF-α, and IL-6; and (3) it protects from oxidative stress by interacting with glutamate to create glutamate-cysteine ligase, glutathione peroxidase, glutathione reductase, and glutathione synthase. All three functions lead to increased growth factors [350–353]. (Source: http://psycheducation.org/treatment/mood-stabilizers/n-acetyl-cysteine-nac/)

erties and directly inhibits inflammatory cytokines PNF alpha and IL-6 (Fig. 5.66). Through glutathione production, macrophages are impaired in the brain. In traumatic brain injury, NAC is as effective as an anti-inflammatory agent [550]. Cysteine lowers glutamate stimulation of neurons involved in mood and anxiety disorders to maintain health and wellness.

Glutathione (see Fig. 5.66) is an important antioxidant found in plants, animals, fungi, and bacteria. Glutathione is highest in freshly prepared meats as well as fruits and vegetables. A diet rich in fresh vegetables and fruits is associated with less DNA hypo-methylation, which is a factor in autism. Green tea has also been linked to increase glutathione levels in adults with metabolic syndrome. Some foods might help raise glutathione by increasing the levels of cysteine, an amino acid "building block" of glutathione. Cysteine is rich in high-protein foods such as meat, poultry, fish, eggs, and dairy, including goat's milk as well as cow's milk and associated body, especially the brain. Most of BH4 is produced by recycling BH2.

Major depression is associated with low plasma folate (vitamin $B_9$), particularly red cell folate, and low vitamin $B_{12}$ status. Low levels of vitamins $B_9$ and $B_{12}$ have been found in studies of depressive (including depression-anxiety) patients, and an association between depression and low levels of the two vitamins is found in studies of the general population. Low plasma or serum folate has also been found in patients with recurrent mood disorders treated by lithium. A link between depression and low folate has similarly been found in patients with alcoholism. The Hong Kong and Taiwan populations with traditional Chinese diets (rich in folate), including patients with major depression, have high serum folate concentrations. These countries have very low lifetime rates of major depression. Folate and vitamin $B_{12}$ are major determinants of one-carbon metabolism, in which S-adenosylmethionine (SAM) is formed. SAM donates methyl groups that are crucial for neurological function. Increased plasma homocysteine is a functional marker of both folate and vitamin $B_{12}$ deficiency. Increased homocysteine levels are found in depressive patients. Increased plasma homocysteine is associated with increased risk of depression. There is now substantial evidence of a common decrease in serum/red blood cell folate and serum vitamin $B_{12}$ and an increase in plasma homocysteine in depression. On the basis of current data, oral doses of both folic acid (800 μg daily) and vitamin $B_{12}$ (1 mg daily) should be tried to improve treatment outcome in depression-anxiety syndromes [557].

Many lines of evidence link bipolar disease to a fundamental abnormality in cellular energy generation [558], including mitochondrial dysfunction (see Fig. 5.67). Brain energy generation is increased in mania and decreased in depression. This is a critical finding [559], and there is corresponding evidence of an increased basal metabolic rate in mania and a higher maximum oxygen volume, independent of calorie intake [560]. Mitochondrial dysfunction in bipolar disease is further suggested by impaired brain energy metabolism, high rates of comorbidity of bipolar disease with mitochondrial diseases, the effects of mood stabilizers on mitochondria, increased mitochondrial DNA deletion in the neural tissue of bipolar disease patients, and the association of mitochondrial DNA mutations and polymorphisms with bipolar disease [561]. Changes in mitochondrial gene expression appear to be a critical component of the pathophysiology of bipolar disease [562].

Elevated basal intracellular calcium is documented in individuals with bipolar disease [357]. Increased glutamate receptor-mediated increases in calcium are also present, which ultimately alters neuroplasticity and may contribute to the excitotoxic processes reported in bipolar disease [354]. Studies have reported a reduction in the activity of complex I of the mitochondrial electron transport chain in bipolar disease, but not major depression [563]. Given the mitochondrial hypothesis of bipolar disease, it is of considerable interest that lithium increases the activity of mitochondrial complexes I/II and II/III in brain tissue [557]. Alterations in antioxidant enzymes have been reported in bipolar disease. For example, SOD activity is increased during the manic and depressed phases of bipolar disease, but not in normals. This is corroborated [558] in a report of increased SOD activity in unmedicated manic bipolar disease patients. Catalase activity was decreased in controls [564] and increased in unmedicated manic patients [565].

Interestingly, treating bipolar disease using the glutathione precursor and free radical scavenger NAC reduces depressive symptoms and improves functioning and quality of life. There are stage-dependent changes in oxidative parameters. The activity of glutathione reductase is increased in late-stage patients compared to early-stage patients and controls [563]. This stage-related change in oxidative biology may form part of the progressive failure of compensatory mechanisms over time and may in part underlie the phenomenology of the staging process. In contrast, studies have shown increased

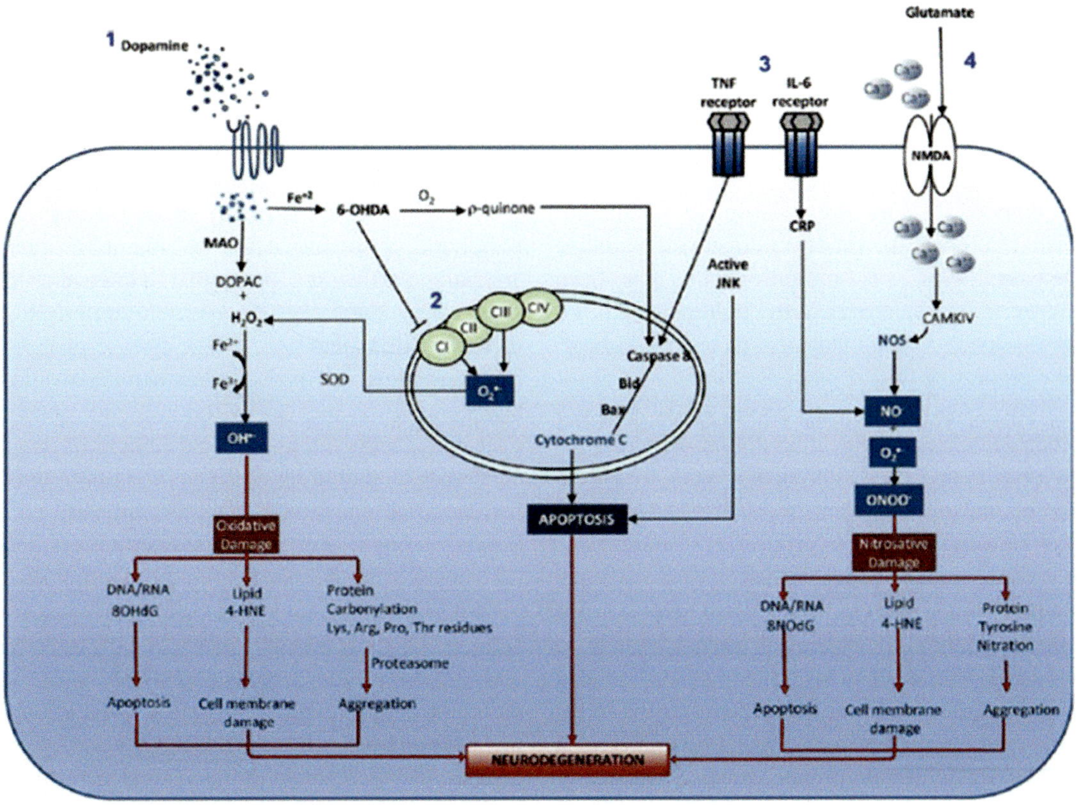


**Fig. 5.67** Potential contributing pathways involved in bipolar disorder. To date, a multitude of potential contributing factors implicated in bipolar disorder have been identified. These include alterations in dopamine, glutamate metabolism, and inflammation potentially leading to mitochondrial dysfunction and consequent increasing in apoptosis, cell membrane damage, and protein aggregation. Increased dopamine release leads to augmentation of the metabolization process. Dopamine can be metabolized via monoamine oxidase (MAO) or suffer auto-oxidation by reacting with iron ($Fe^{++}$). Dopamine reaction with MAO leads to increased ROS and $H_2O_2$ production [354]. (Republished with permission from Elsevier. Source: [355])

lipid peroxidation occurring as a result of uncompensated oxidative stress that is present independent of the phase of the illness [563, 565]. In addition, increased levels of lipid peroxidation were found in the cingulate cortex of patients with bipolar disease. Accumulation of oxidative damage is thought to lead to neuronal cell death by apoptosis or as a consequence of aggregation of oxidized proteins, which may result in impairment of mood-stabilizing mechanisms. Neurotrophins such as VEGF play a key role in neuronal survival and proliferation. Alterations in neurotrophins are well documented in bipolar disease and treatments. Of note, other neurotrophins have shown similar patterns in acute mood episodes [566].

Neuroprotection may be a viable and realistic goal in treating bipolar disease. There are two types of pathological processes amenable to intervention: (1) normal physiological processes that happen in excess, for example, excitotoxicity, pruning, or excessive apoptotic activity, and (2) the failure of trophic processes, such as reduced neurogenesis, senescence of progenitor cell generation, and differentiation, which can also be targeted. Such an approach would involve regulating the processes of growth, the regeneration, and the rescue of brain cells that may be at risk of damage or even death. Established mood stabilizers impact the pathways and mechanisms that are associated with neuroprogression in bipolar disease. For instance, lamotrigine, lithium, and valproic acid reduce oxidative stress [567], and atypical antipsychotics also reduce oxidative stress, not only via dopamine antagonism [357] but also via direct effects on oxidative defenses. NAC, as an antioxidant, has been shown to be efficacious in the treatment of bipolar disease [357] and may also have neuroprotective properties.

NAC is not only a precursor to the primary free radical scavenger, glutathione, but in addition has many other biological effects, including increasing glutamate in the nucleus accumbens and anti-inflammatory properties [568]. NAC reverses mitochondrial toxicity. For instance, menadione, a mitochondrial toxin that induces apoptosis through increased peroxide-induced oxidative stress, adversely affects mitochondrial function because it induces collapse of the mitochondrial inner transmembrane potential and a decrease in inner membrane mass. This toxicity is reversed by NAC [569].

## Application in Heart Failure

The mechanisms leading to heart failure are of multiple origins (see Fig. 5.68) [570]. These diseases result in a mismatch between the load applied to the heart and the energy needed for contraction. After initial insult, secondary mediators such as angiotensin II, norepinephrine, endothelin, and pro-inflammatory cytokines act directly on the myocardium or indirectly via changes in hemodynamic loading conditions to cause endothelial and myocardial dysfunction, cardiac and vascular remodeling with hypertrophy, fibrosis, cardiac dilation, and myocardial necrosis, leading eventually to heart failure. The adverse remodeling and increased peripheral resistance further aggravate heart failure.

Heart failure is a syndrome characterized initially by left ventricular dysfunction that triggers countermeasures aimed to restore cardiac output. These responses are compensatory at first, but eventually become part of the disease process itself, leading to a more rapid progression of cardiac failure. Among these responses is sympathetic activation that provides inotropic support to the failing heart, increasing stroke volume, and peripheral vasoconstriction to maintain mean arterial perfusion pressure. However, if unopposed, sympathetic activation continues in these functions and accelerates disease progression, affecting survival. Sympathetic activation has been attributed to withdrawal of normal restraining influences and enhancement of excitatory inputs, including changes in (1) peripheral baroreceptor and chemoreceptor reflexes, continuing to report insufficient perfusion pressures; (2) chemical mediators that control sympathetic outflow, including adrenal and cortisol responses; and (3) central integratory sites [571]. The latter includes associated parasympathetic dysfunction that typically precedes, and instigates, the offending sympathetic excess [116].

The interface between the sympathetic fibers and the cardiovascular system is formed by the adrenergic or sympathetic receptors. Dysregulation of cardiac β1-adrenergic receptor signaling and transduction are key features of heart failure progression. In contrast, cardiac β2-adrenergic receptors (primarily pulmonary) and α1-adrenergic receptors (primarily in the vasculature) typically continue to function normally and function in a compensatory fashion to maintain cardiac inotropy in a normal fashion, assuming a normal heart. When perfusion declines, the β2- and α-systems attempt to compensate and signal the β1 system to increase activity, which, in a failing heart, exacerbates the condition. β-Adrenergic (primarily β1) receptor blockers and the inhibitors of the renin-angiotensin-aldosterone axis form the mainstay of current medical management of chronic heart failure. Conversely, central sympatholytics have proved harmful, whereas central sympathomimetic inotropes are still used in selected patients with hemodynamic instability.

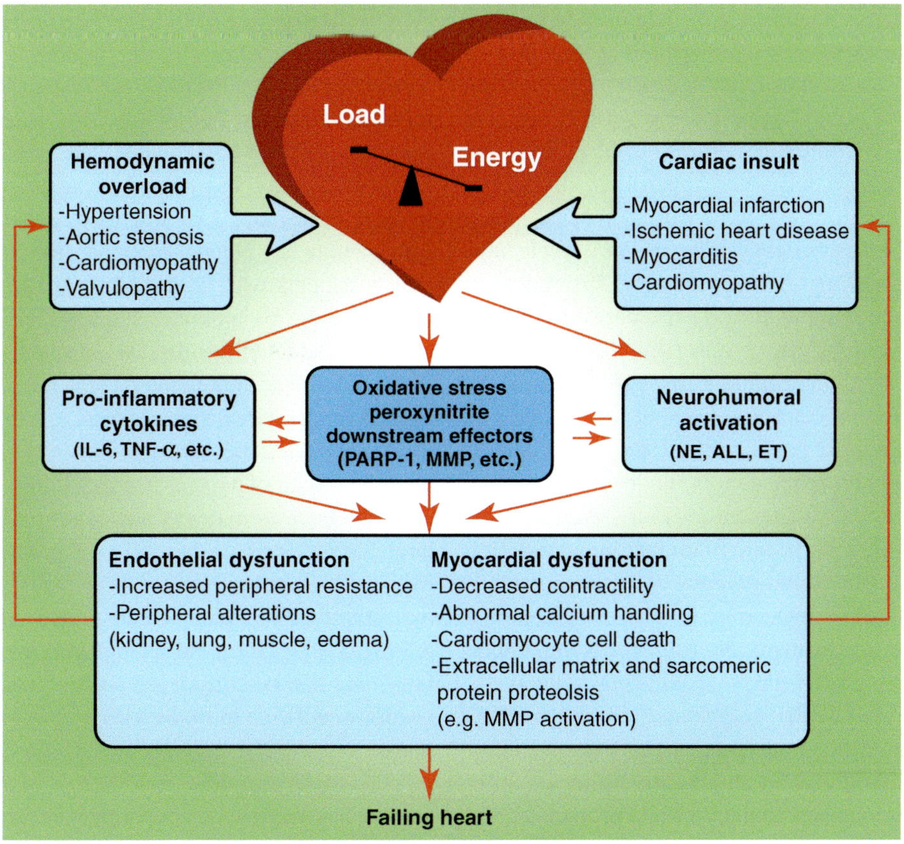


**Fig. 5.68** Progression of heart failure and the role of oxidative stress and peroxynitrite. The mechanisms leading to heart failure are of multiple origins and include acute and chronic ischemic heart disease, cardiomyopathies, myocarditis, pressure overload, and more. These diseases result in a mismatch between the load applied to the heart and the energy needed for contraction, leading to mechanoenergic uncoupling. After initial insult, secondary mediators such as angiotensin II (AII), norepinephrine (NE), endothelin (ET), pro-inflammatory cytokines [e.g., tumor necrosis factor-α (TNF-α) and interleukin 6 (IL-6), in concert with oxidative stress and peroxynitrite, activate downstream effectors (e.g., PARP-1 or MMPs)] act directly on the myocardium or indirectly via changes in hemodynamic loading conditions to cause endothelial and myocardial dysfunction, cardiac and vascular remodeling with hypertrophy, fibrosis, cardiac dilation, and myocardial necrosis, leading eventually to heart failure. The adverse remodeling and increased peripheral resistance further aggravate heart failure. Abbreviations: MMPs, matrix metalloproteinases; PARP-1, poly (ADP-ribose) polymerase [356, Fig. 3]. (Republished with permission from Elsevier. Source: [357])

Parasympathetic activation and its physiological effects are attenuated in heart failure [116, 572]. Data indicate that changes in vagus nerve control of heart rate become apparent at a very early developmental stage of left ventricular dysfunction, which may provide important prognostic information in patients at risk for developing progressive myocardial dysfunction [573]. In heart failure, vagal ganglionic transmission is reduced, muscarinic receptor density and composition are altered, and acetylcholinesterase activity is decreased. Left ventricular muscarinic stimulation has an independent negative lusitropic[21] (rate of myocardial relaxation or diastolic function; see insert [356], below) effect and

[21] In addition to sympathetic-adrenergic nerves, the heart is innervated by parasympathetic-cholinergic nerves derived from the vagus nerves. Acetylcholine (ACh) released by these fibers binds to muscarinic receptors in the cardiac muscle, especially at the SA and AV nodes that have a large amount of vagal innervation. ACh released by vagus nerve fibers binds to $M_2$ muscarinic receptors, a subclass of cholinergic receptors. This produces negative chronotropy and dromotropy in the heart, as well as negative inotropy and lusitropy in the atria (the negative inotropic and lusitropic effects of vagal stimulation are relatively weak in the ventricles).

antagonizes β-adrenergic stimulation [574]. Reduced vagus nerve control may be due to changes in presynaptic (ganglionic) function [565]. Abnormal baroreflex control of heart rate in patients with heart failure is well recognized. Evidence also exists for impairment of vagally mediated baroreflex bradycardia because vagal neurons with normal systolic pressure levels have a lower resting discharge rate [575]. Lack of sympathetic attenuation by the parasympathetic nervous system can be observed [116], which is caused by abnormalities in cardiopulmonary baroreceptors, central abnormalities, changes in the interactions between the P&S limbs, alterations at the nicotinic ganglionic level, or changes in the muscarinic receptors [576]. The lack of attenuation and chronic β-adrenergic stimulation leads to an enhanced potency of the negative inotropic effect of muscarinic agonists, suggesting a feedback mechanism altering parasympathetic influences [577]. P&S monitoring objectively and independently elucidates P&S activity, enabling earlier and more specific and patient-centric therapy plans, including earlier or more aggressive antioxidant and nitrate protocols.

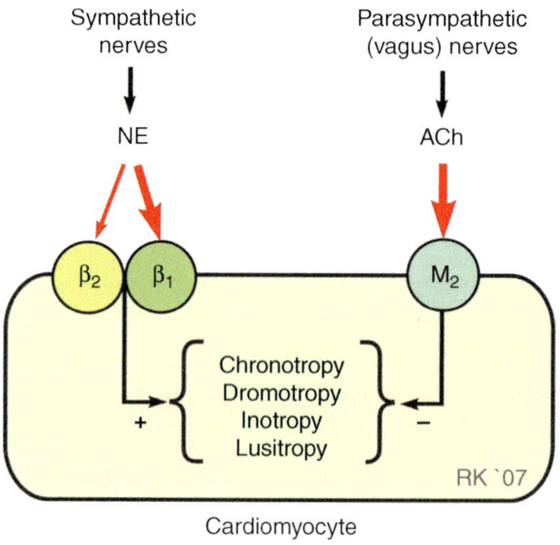


## Application in Fatty Liver Disease

Nonalcoholic fatty liver disease is considered the most prevalent form of chronic liver disease. It is associated with a significant lipid deposition in hepatocytes and characterized by persistent defects in hepatic enzymes. Although it presents histological features of alcohol-induced liver injury, it affects patients who drink little to no alcohol. To date, there are no approved drugs available to treat nonalcoholic fatty liver disease. Mechanisms leading to liver-fat accumulation include mitochondrial dysfunction and oxidative imbalance. Treatment of these underlying mechanisms may help to prevent the progression of hepatic steatosis [578].

Fatty liver is a reversible condition wherein large vacuoles of triglyceride fat accumulate in liver cells via the process of steatosis (i.e., abnormal retention of lipids within a cell; see Insert, below [579],[22]). Despite having multiple causes, fatty liver can be considered a single disease that occurs worldwide in those with excessive alcohol intake and the obese (with or without effects of insulin resistance). The condition is also associated with other diseases that influence fat metabolism [580]. When the process of fat metabolism is disrupted, the fat can accumulate in the liver in excessive amounts. The accumulation of fat in steatosis (alcoholic or nonalcoholic) may also be accompanied by a progressive inflammation of the liver (hepatitis), called steatohepatitis (see Insert, below[23]). Nonalcoholic fatty liver disease is commonly associated with metabolic syndrome (e.g., diabetes, hypertension, obesity, or dyslipidemia) but can also be due to any one of many causes [581, 582].

[22]Republished with permission from Oxford University Press.

[23]Adapted from Shutterstock Royalty-free stock vector images ID: 1030576897. Different stages of human liver illustration, by BlueRingMedia.

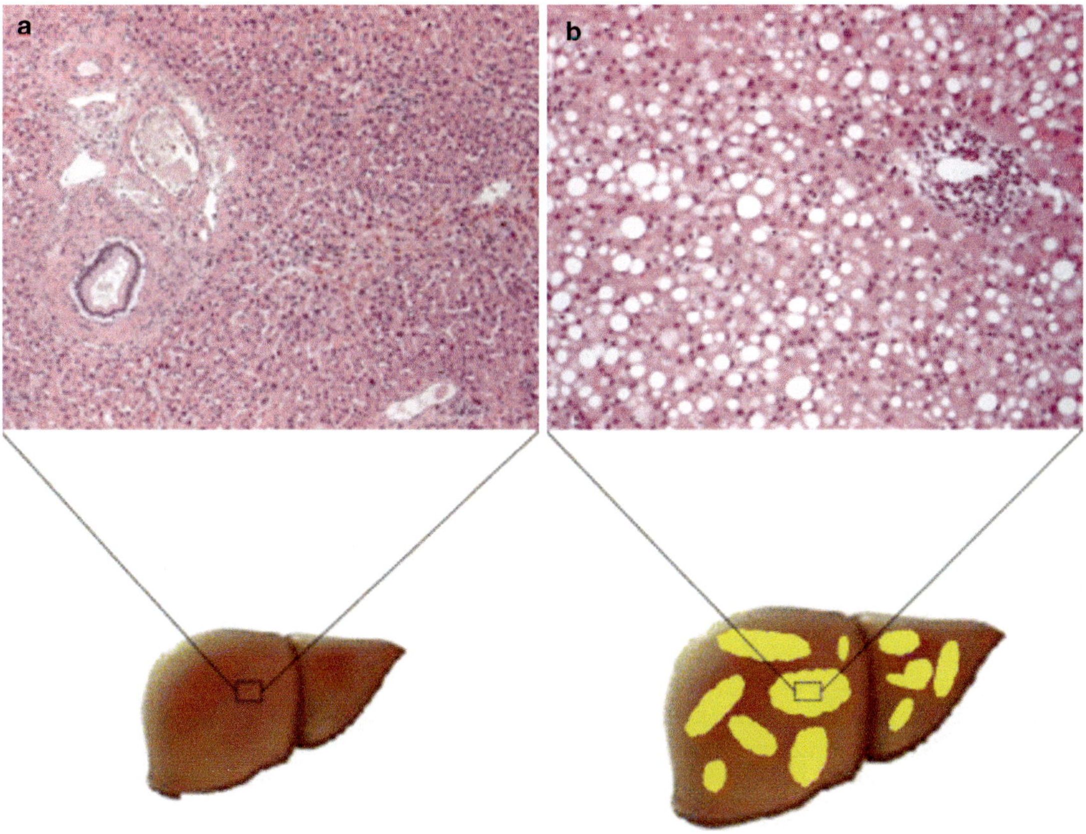


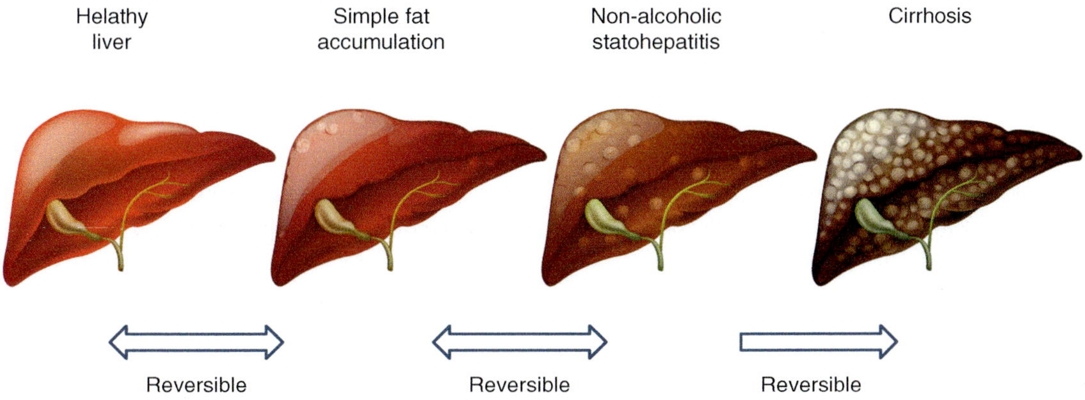


Initially, small fat vacuoles (liposomes) form around the nucleus of hepatocytes. The hepatocytes fill with multiple fat droplets that do not displace the centrally located nucleus. Eventually, the size of the vacuoles increases, pushing the nucleus to the periphery of the cell, giving characteristic signet ring appearance (macrovesicular fatty change). Large vacuoles may coalesce and produce fatty cysts, which are irreversible lesions. Macrovesicular steatosis is the most common form and is typically associated with diabetes, obesity, and corticosteroids.

Mechanisms leading to hepatic steatosis include defects in fatty acid metabolism which are responsible for pathogenesis of fatty liver disease. These defects may be due to (1) imbalances in energy consumption and its combustion, resulting in lipid storage, or (2) may be a consequence of peripheral resistance to insulin, whereby the transport of fatty acids from adipose tissue to the liver is increased [580, 583]. Impairment or inhibition of receptor molecules (PPAR-α, PPAR-γ, and SREBP1) that control the enzymes responsible for the oxidation and synthesis of fatty acids appears to contribute to fat accumulation. In addition, damage to mitochondria and other cellular structures further impairs cellular energy mechanisms. On the other hand, nonalcoholic fatty liver disease may begin as excess of unmetabolized energy in liver cells. Hepatic steatosis is considered reversible and to some extent nonprogressive if the underlying cause is reduced or removed.

Severe fatty liver is sometimes accompanied by inflammation, a situation referred to as steatohepatitis. Progression to nonalcoholic steatohepatitis depends on the persistence or severity of the inciting cause. The extent of inflammatory response varies widely and does not always correlate with the degree of fat accumulation. Steatosis (retention of lipid) and onset of steatohepatitis may represent successive stages in fatty liver disease progression [584]. Liver disease with extensive inflammation and a high degree of steatosis often progresses to more severe forms of the disease [359]. Hepatocyte ballooning and necrosis of varying degrees are often present at this stage. Liver cell death and inflammatory responses lead to the activation of hepatic stellate cells, which play a pivotal role in hepatic fibrosis. The extent of fibrosis varies widely. Perisinusoidal fibrosis is common, especially in adults, and predominates around the terminal hepatic veins [585]. The progression to cirrhosis may be influenced by the amount of fat and degree of steatohepatitis and by a variety of other sensitizing factors.

There is evidence that several classes of antioxidants may reverse fatty liver disease. These include polyphenols (i.e., resveratrol, quercetin, coumestrol, anthocyanins, epigallocatechin gallate, and curcumin), carotenoids (i.e., lycopene, astaxanthin, and fucoxanthin), and glucosinolates (i.e., glucoraphanin, sulforaphane, sinigrin, and allyl isothiocyanate). Given that there are no (currently) approved pharmaceuticals for fatty liver disease, antioxidants are a primary choice. Metformin and pioglitazone (off-label), statins (off-label), and vitamin E are agents that are currently found to be helpful in relieving and even reversing fatty liver.

Middle-aged and older adults who closely followed a Mediterranean-style diet for 6 years were at significantly lower risk of developing fatty liver disease than others in a large prospective study [586]. Over a median 6 years of follow-up, each one-standard-deviation rise in Mediterranean-style diet score (MDS) correlated with significantly decreased hepatic fat accumulation and a 26% lower odds of new-onset fatty liver disease (95% CI, 10–39%; p = 0.002) and with a significant increase in liver phantom ratio (0.57; 95% confidence interval, 0.27–0.86; p less than 0.001). This ratio signifies lower accumulation of liver fat. Similarly, every one-standard-deviation rise in the AHEI dietary score correlated with a 0.56 rise in liver phantom ratio (95% CI, 0.29–0.84; p less than 0.001) and with a 21% lower odds of incident fatty liver disease (95% CI, 5–35%; p = 0.02).

Individuals whose diets improved the most (those in the highest quartile of dietary score change) over time had about 80% less liver fat accumulate between baseline and follow-up compared with those whose diets worsened the most (those in the lowest quartile of dietary score change). Furthermore, relationship between diet and liver fat remained statistically significant (p = 0.02) even after accounting for changes in body mass index. The investigators also studied whether the presence of single nucleotide polymorphisms (SNPs) linked with NAFLD modified dietary effects. High genetic risk for NAFLD did not appear to lead to increased liver fat as long as diet improved or remained stable over time, they found. However, when diet worsened over time, high genetic NAFLD risk did correlate with significantly greater accumulation of liver fat (p less than 0.001).

## Application in Mast Cell Activation Syndrome and Food Allergies

Patients with mast cell disorders may or may not have true food allergies; however, most of these patients are triggered by high histamine foods. Many are triggered by pollen allergies or certain drugs that increase mast cells. These conditions involve mast cells not being "normal." Mast cell activation syndrome is an immunological condition in which mast cells (see Insert, below[24]) inappropriately and excessively release chemical mediators, resulting in a range of chronic symptoms, sometimes including anaphylaxis or near-anaphylaxis attacks [587–589]. Primary symptoms include cardiovascular, dermatological, gastrointestinal, neurological, and respiratory problems [588]. Unlike mastocytosis, where patients have an abnormally increased number of mast cells, patients with mast cell activation syndrome have a normal number of mast cells that do not function properly and are defined as "hyper-responsive" [588]. It is still a poorly understood condition. Mast cell activation syndrome is often found in patients with Ehlers-Danlos syndrome or postural orthostatic tachycardia syndrome (POTS) [590], both of which are P&S (autonomic) disorders. It is also found in subset groups of patients with common variable immunodeficiency [591] and Lyme disease [592]. Zyrtec, Zantac, and histamine blockers are first-line treatments, and P&S dysfunction therapy is also addressed.

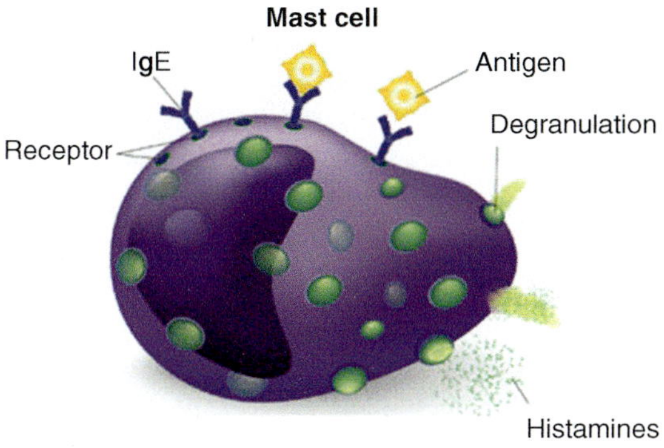


[24]Royalty free stock from https://www.123rf.com/photo_27277857_stock-vector-white-blood-cell-mast-cell-or-a-mastocyte-labrocyte-mast-cells-are-the-cells-responsible-for-causing.html

Mast cells are present in most tissues throughout the human body, especially connective tissue, skin, intestinal lining, cardiovascular system, nervous system, respiratory system, and reproductive organs (Fig. 5.69). They may have both positive and negative effects, either of which could potentially result from mast cell activation in the context of disease (Fig. 5.70) [358]. They are part of the allergic response designed to protect from threat and injury. When the body is exposed to a perceived threat, the mast cells secrete chemical mediators, such as histamine, interleukins, prostaglandins, cytokines, chemokine, and various other chemicals stored in the cytoplasm of the cell. These chemical messengers produce both local and systemic effects, such as increased permeability of blood vessels (inflammation and swelling), contraction of smooth muscle (stomach cramps and heart palpitations), and increased mucous production (congestion, sneezing, etc.). Historically, mast cells were only thought to be associated with allergic or anaphylactic responses. Now mast cells are known to have roles in immune activation, development of autoimmunity, and many other disorders, such as Ehlers-Danlos syndrome or POTS. The large increase in patients presenting with mast cell disorders may be, in part, due to more pervasive environmental toxins, molds, and chemicals.

Mast cells protect from injury and help the body to heal from wounds. Overactive mast cells are associated with a variety of serious symptoms, including skin rashes or hives, swelling or edema, flushing, itching, abdominal pain, nausea or vomiting, diarrhea, wheezing, shortness of breath, heart palpitations, anxiety, difficulty concentrating, headaches, brain fog, low blood pressure, and fatigue. Again, many of these are also associated with P&S dysfunction (Fig. 5.71). Mast cell activation syndrome can be classified as either (1) primary (clonal proliferation or mastocytosis, Fig. 5.72), (2) secondary (due to a specific stimulus), and (3) idiopathic (no identifiable cause).

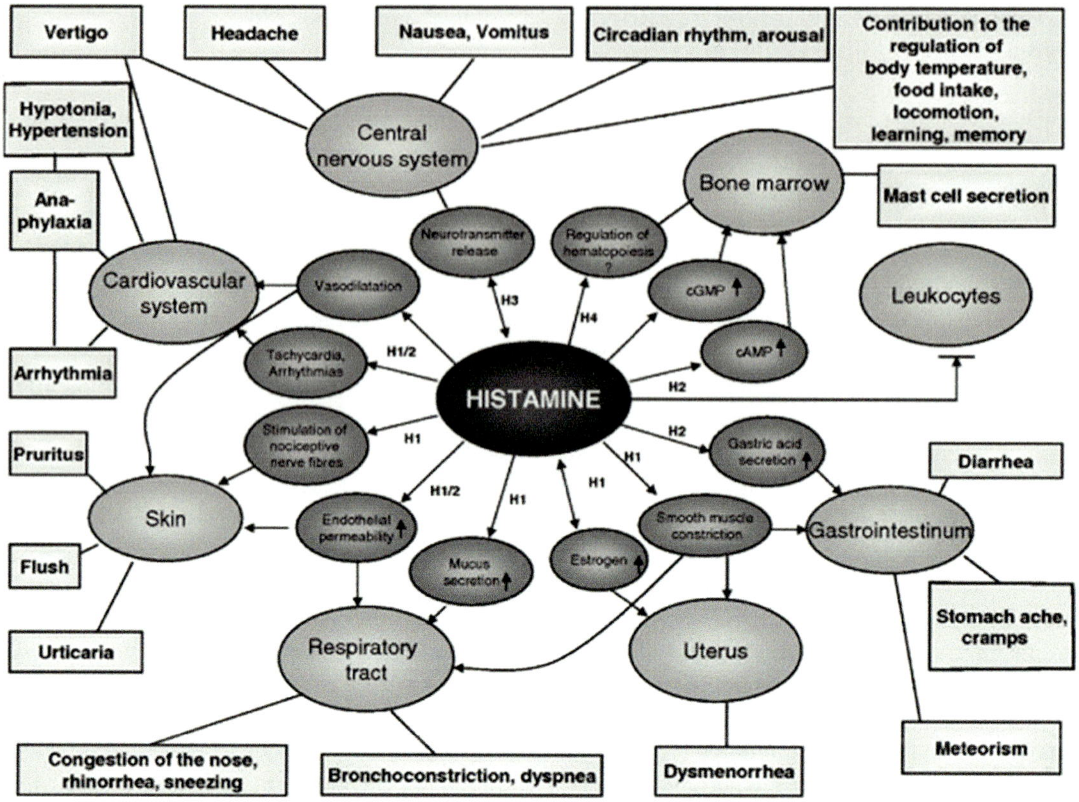


**Fig. 5.69** Mast cells release histamines as part of their defense against infection, allergens, and disease [61]. (Republished with permission from Oxford University Press. Source: https://www.jillcarnahan.com/2016/10/31/mast-cell-activation-syndrome-mcas-when-histamine-goes-haywire/)

## Preventing the Dark Side of Nitric Oxide

One way to keep nitric oxide from the dark side is to correct and maintain a proper cellular environment or milieu around nitric oxide. If there is an abundance of antioxidants, nitric oxide follows normal pathways and promotes health and wellness. Antioxidants sequester the oxidants, including ROS, preventing them from turning the nitric oxide into perinitrate, for example. Antidepressants, such as SSRIs like Prozac and Zoloft, will also (positively) modify the nitric oxide milieu and reduce oxidative stress. Immunosuppressants, corticosteroids, anti-tumor factor antibodies, and various metals also modify the milieu for the better by reducing oxidative stress.

Coenzyme Q10 (CoQ10) facilitates normal nitric oxide function by preventing it from being oxidized and becoming perinitrate and causing cell damage. CoQ10 buffers nitric oxide as it diffuses out of the endothelial cell and travels to the smooth muscle cell to relax it. Some studies have shown as much as a 17 mmHg drop in blood pressure is possible with CoQ10 via this pathway. CoQ10 supplementation is associated with significant improvement in endothelial function and helps to relieve endothelial dysfunction [593]. It is an excellent blood pressure lowering agent in

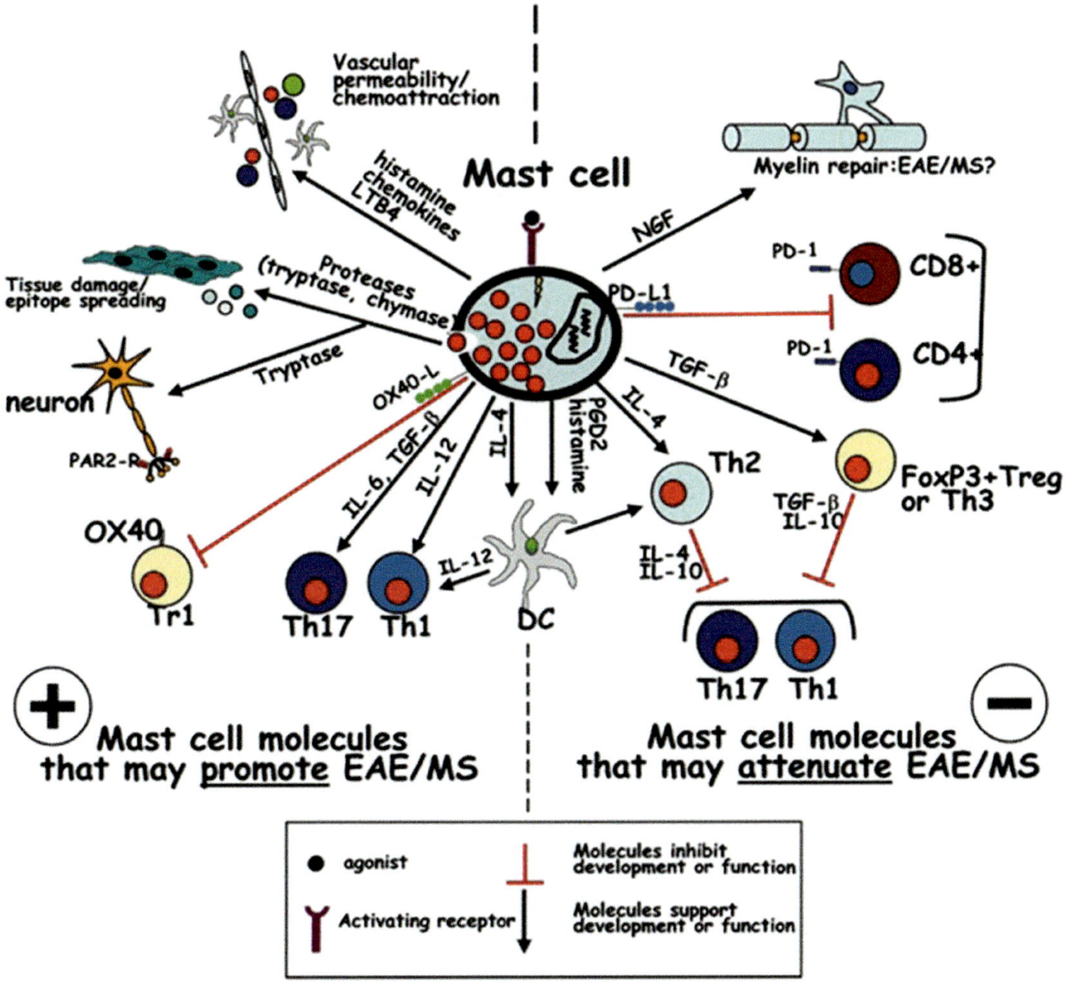


**Fig. 5.70** Mast cells can exert both positive and negative influences on the course of autoimmune diseases. Several variables can dictate the dominant influence mast cells can exert on immune cell function and ultimate tissue damage. Selective expression of mediators or cell surface immunomodulatory molecules, site variability of expression, and genetically determined heterogeneity in mast cell phenotypes all contribute to the quality of mast cell response in a given individual. From top left and counter clockwise: mast cell histamine, chemokines, and leukotrienes may enhance cellular trafficking into the CNS and permeation of the blood-brain barrier. Mast cell proteases can directly degrade tissue, causing direct damage, and may promote epitope spreading. The mast cell-specific protease tryptase has been shown to act directly on neuronal PAR-2 receptors to cause nerve excitability. Activation of PAR-2 receptors on other cells induces the production of pro-inflammatory mediators. Mast cells express cytokines that can directly promote Th1 (IL-12) and Th17 (IL-6 and TGF-β) cell differentiation or indirectly act on DCs through IL-4 to enhance IL-12 production and promote Th1 development. In contrast, mast cells may inhibit inflammation by enhancing Treg and Th3 cell development via the release of TGF-β (in the absence of IL-6) and skewing CD4+ cells toward a Th2 (via IL-4 release). Cytokine released by Treg cells block the development of a Th1 or Th17 response. Mast cell expression of PD-L1 may inhibit CD4+ and CD8+ cell responses, and the release of NGF could lead to repair in inflammatory CNS conditions like MS [358]. (© 2007. The American Association of Immunologists, Inc. Source: [359])

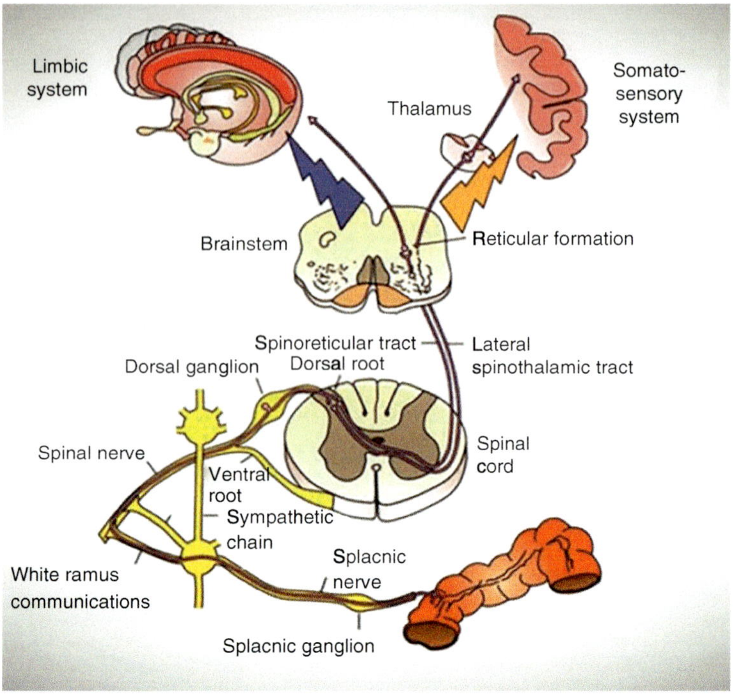


**Fig. 5.71** The somatosensory and limbic pathways for abdominal awareness. These connections underline the link between emotionality and digestive diseases. (Republished with permission from Springer International Publishing AG. Source: [23])

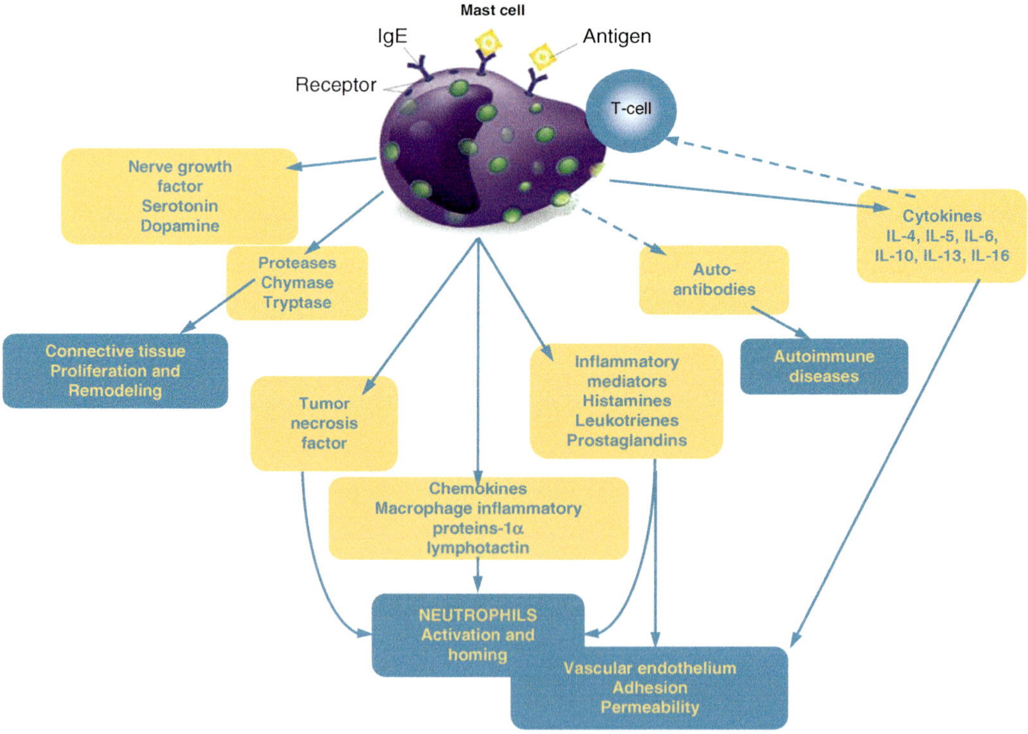


**Fig. 5.72** Mast cells are known to be the primary responders in allergic reactions, orchestrating strong responses to minute amounts of allergens. Several recent observations indicate that they may also have a key role in coordinating the early phases of autoimmune diseases, particularly those involving autoantibodies [358]. (Source: https://www.jillcarnahan.com/2016/10/31/mast-cell-activation-syndrome-mcas-when-histamine-goes-haywire/)

areas of low nitric oxide levels. Recall that CoQ10 is also very helpful in maintaining lipid health. According to previously referenced studies, these two properties, together, make CoQ10 especially useful in heart failure by keeping nitric oxide levels sufficiently high to promote health and wellness. In fact, CoQ10 buffers nitric oxide in all of its activities. Even though some of the studies are small, there is very favorable information on the effects of CoQ10 and nitric oxide in heart failure and other cardiac diseases [176–178] (see also the "Coenzyme Q10" section in this chapter), as well as Parkinson's disease (specifically the reduced form of CoQ10, ubiquinol-10, only [594]), migraines [595–597], depression [598–601], chronic fatigue [597, 598, 601], fibromyalgia [597] and other autonomic dysfunctions [602–604], and cognitive diseases [605] (see also references associated with the various functions of nitric oxide earlier in this chapter).

L-carnitine may increase nitric oxide signaling by improving endothelial function. Unfortunately, taking it orally has a poor bioavailability, but it does work. There is a glycine-type propionyl derivative of L-carnitine that has shown improved bioavailability in studies. They administered 26 athletic males 3–4 g a day and they exercised on a treadmill. The study showed that the subjects' nitric oxide levels improved, as did some antioxidant biomarkers measured in the blood called T-bars [606].

It is known that multiple or severe brain injury or trauma (traumatic brain injury, or TBI; e.g., secondary concussion syndrome) involves excess nitric oxide production leading to prolonged hyperactive microglia activity. In these patients, microglia turn from scavenging damaged or dead brain cells to attacking healthy brain cells. This condition also involves NMDA receptor hyperstimulation. NMDA glutamate receptors stimulate synthesis of nitric oxide in the brain. NMDA receptor overstimulation activates nNOS.[25] It has been observed that parasympathetic (cholinergic) excess (PE) is associated with TBI [personal communication, DePace and Colombo, Franklin Cardiovascular]. The symptoms of TBI, pain, anxiety, hypertension, left ventricular dysfunction, immune system depression, etc., are typically considered to be sympathetically mediated [607]. This apparent paradox is due to the fact that the above-referenced PE is always associated with sympathetic (adrenergic) excess (SE). Specifically, this is not a resting PE; it is a dynamic PE, recorded during a sympathetic challenge [608].

The parasympathetic nervous system is known to directly affect the immune system. Increases in both resting and dynamic parasympathetic activity increase immune responses. However, empirically, it has been found that dynamic PE is associated with prolonged immune responses inside the brain: microglial activation, possibly due to catecholaminergic prolonged, or over-, activation (sympathetic excess), secondary to PE. It is also associated with concurrent decreased immune responses outside the brain; the latter leads to increased incidences of pneumonia and death due to pneumonia [personal communication, Jean-François Pittet, MD, Univ. Alabama-Birmingham]. Bidirectional circuits link the CNS and the immune system (Fig. 5.73) [609]. The CNS communicates with the immune system to modulate its activity via sympathetic and parasympathetic, specifically vagus nerve innervation, catecholaminergic pathways, or neuropeptides and hormones. It seems as if, with brain injury, the immune system focuses on the brain, leaving the body vulnerable, thereby permitting infections to take hold in the lungs.

As a result of both autonomic branches being excessively high, there is a combination of symptoms from both branches. It is postulated that transient parasympathetic activity in the brain (see Fig. 5.74) promotes brain repair processes, including synaptic remodeling, beneficial neurochemical changes, decreased neurotoxicity, and decreased inflammation. However, chronic parasympathetic activity (prolonged dynamic PE) is associated with a reversal

[25] Selective inhibition of nNOS over related isoforms (eNOS and iNOS) is therapeutically desirable.

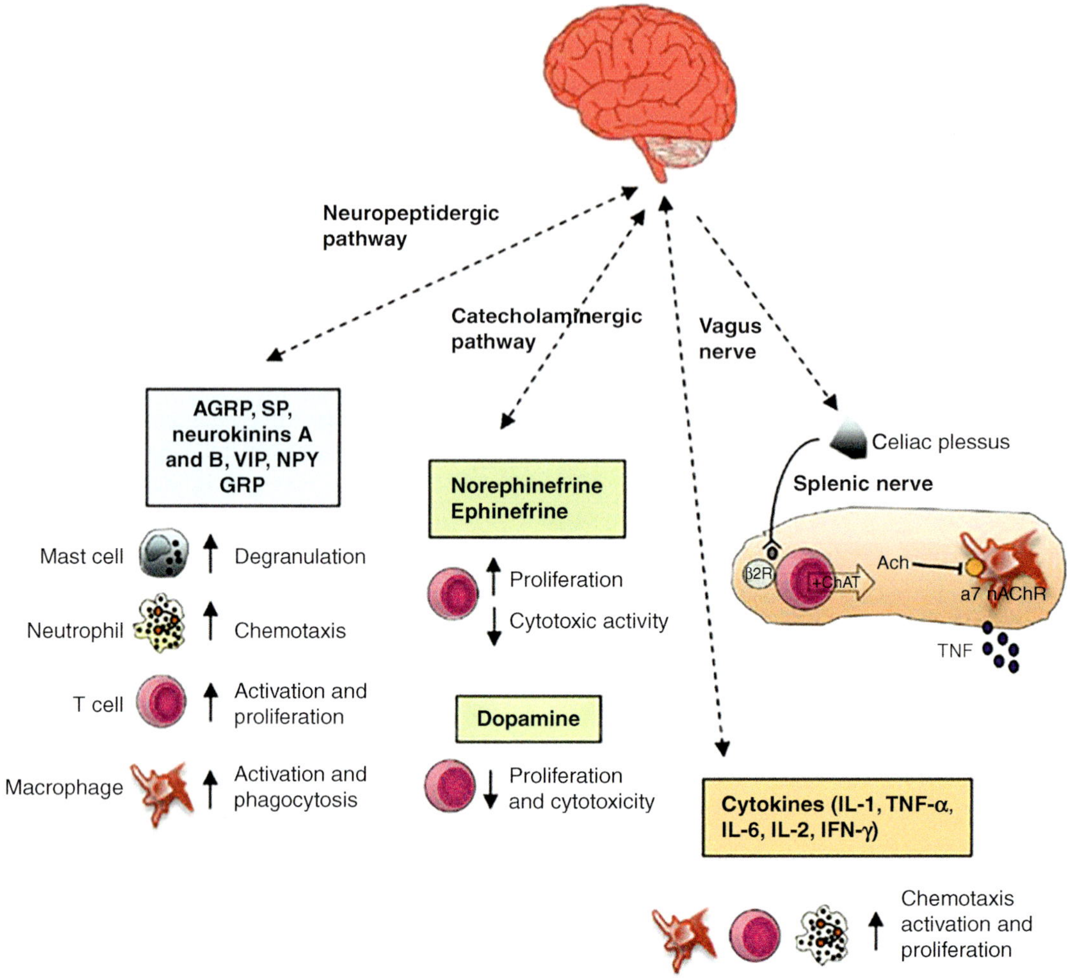


**Fig. 5.73** Bidirectional circuits link the CNS and the immune system. A schematic representation of the CNS-immune system crosstalk. The CNS can communicate with the immune system to modulate its activity, through different ways: the sympathetic and parasympathetic (specifically, vagus nerve) nervous system innervation, catecholaminergic pathway, or neuropeptide and hormone release. In this context, leptin modulates the immune system, by increasing the activation of T cells and decreasing Treg cell functions, thus representing a key player in the susceptibility to immune-mediated disorders (β2R, β2 receptor; α7 nAChR, α7 subunit of the nicotinic acetylcholine receptor). (Open Access, Frontiers in Immunology. Source: [360])

of microglia benefits, including CNS viral infections, AIDS-dementia complex, Alzheimer's disease, MS, and behavioral, memory, and cognitive dysfunctions due to secondary or higher TBI (including concussion) and stroke. The resulting microglial activity is a type of autoimmune response leading to neuronal cell death as a result of inflammation and oxidative stress. Again, treating (dynamic) PE as the primary autonomic dysfunction and, thereby, relieving many if not all of the symptoms of brain injury (when added to typical therapies for the specific type of brain injury) have been very successful, ostensibly by deactivating microglial and nitric oxide overproduction [personal communication, DePace and Colombo, Franklin Cardiovascular].

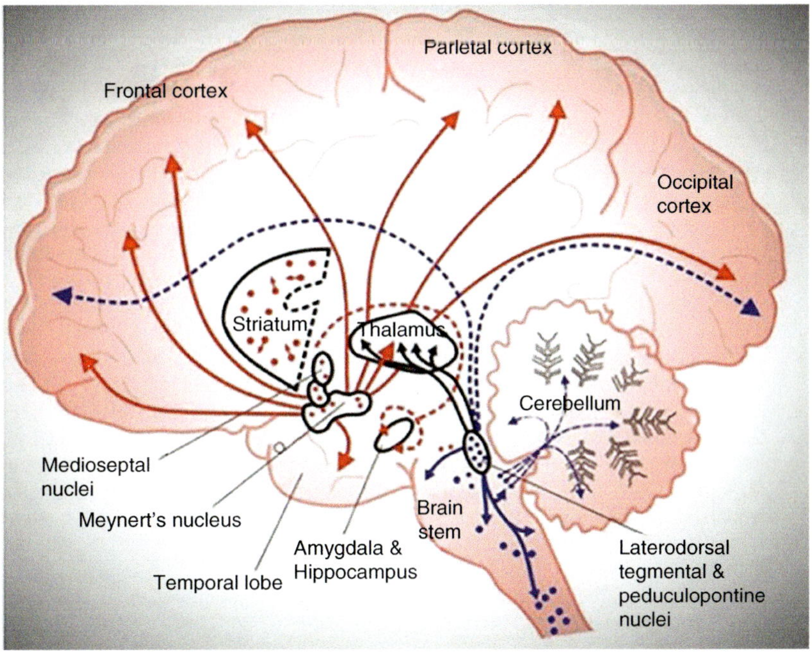


**Fig. 5.74** Principal cholinergic projections in the human brain. (Republished with permission from Springer International Publishing AG. Source: [23])

## References


1. Hensley K, Floyd RA, editors. Methods in biological oxidative stress. Methods in pharmacology and toxicology. Totowa: Humana Press; 2010.
2. Rahal A, Kumar A, Singh V, Yadev B, Tiwari R, Chakraborty S, Dhama K. Oxidative stress, Prooxidants, and antioxidants: The interplay. Biomed Res Int. 2014, Article ID 761264, 19 pages.
3. Nicolson G. Mitochondrial dysfunction and chronic disease: treatment with natural supplements. Altern Ther Health Med. 2014;20(Suppl 1):18–25.
4. Kroemer G, Galluzzi L, Brenner C. Mitochondrial membrane permeabilization in cell death. Physiol Rev. 2007;87(1):99–163. Review. https://doi.org/10.1152/physrev.00013.2006.
5. Parikh S, Goldstein A, Karaa A, Koenig MK, Anselm I, Brunel-Guitton C, Christodoulou J, Cohen BH, Dimmock D, Enns GM, Falk MJ, Feigenbaum A, Frye RE, Ganesh J, Griesemer D, Haas R, Horvath R, Korson M, Kruer MC, Mancuso M, McCormack S, Raboisson MJ, Reimschisel T, Salvarinova R, Saneto RP, Scaglia F, Shoffner J, Stacpoole PW, Sue CM, Tarnopolsky M, Van Karnebeek C, Wolfe LA, Cunningham ZZ, Rahman S, Chinnery PF. Patient care standards for primary mitochondrial disease: a consensus statement from the mitochondrial medicine society. Genet Med. 2017. https://doi.org/10.1038/gim.2017.107. [Epub ahead of print] Review.
6. Mammucari C, Gherardi G, Rizzuto R. Structure, activity regulation, and role of the mitochondrial calcium uniporter in health and disease. Front Oncol. 2017;7:139. https://doi.org/10.3389/fonc.2017.00139. eCollection 2017. Review.
7. Picca A, Lezza AMS, Leeuwenburgh C, Pesce V, Calvani R, Landi F, Bernabei R, Marzetti E. Fueling inflamm-aging through mitochondrial dysfunction: mechanisms and molecular targets. Int J Mol Sci. 2017;18(5). pii: E933. https://doi.org/10.3390/ijms18050933. Review.
8. Li R, Jia Z, Trush MA. Defining ROS in biology and medicine. Reactive oxygen species (Apex, NC). 2016;1(1):9–21. https://doi.org/10.20455/ros.2016.803.
9. Dizaj SM, Lotfipour F, Barzegar-Jalali M, Zarrintan MH, Adibkia K. Antimicrobial activity of the metals and metal oxide nanoparticles. Mater Sci Eng C Mater Biol Appl. 2014;44:278–84. https://doi.org/10.1016/j.msec.2014.08.031. Epub 2014 Aug 16. Review.
10. Vatansever F, de Melo WC, Avci P, Vecchio D, Sadasivam M, Gupta A, Chandran R, Karimi M, Parizotto NA, Yin R, Tegos GP, Hamblin MR. Antimicrobial strategies centered around reactive oxygen species – bactericidal antibiotics, photodynamic therapy, and beyond. FEMS Microbiol Rev. 2013;37(6):955–89. https://doi.org/10.1111/1574-6976.12026. Epub 2013 Jul 25. Review.
11. Brynildsen MP, Winkler JA, Spina CS, MacDonald IC, Collins JJ. Potentiating antibacterial activity by predictably enhancing endogenous microbial ROS production. Nat Biotechnol. 2013;31(2):160–5. https://doi.org/10.1038/nbt.2458. Epub 2013 Jan 6.

12. Dan Dunn J, Alvarez LA, Zhang X, Soldati T. Reactive oxygen species and mitochondria: a nexus of cellular homeostasis. Redox Biol. 2015;6:472–85. https://doi.org/10.1016/j.redox.2015.09.005. Epub 2015 Sept 10. Review.
13. D'Autréaux B, Toledano MB. ROS as signalling molecules: mechanisms that generate specificity in ROS homeostasis. Nat Rev Mol Cell Biol. 2007;8(10):813–24. Review.
14. Liou GY, Storz P. Reactive oxygen species in cancer. Free Radic Res. 2010;44(5):479–96. https://doi.org/10.3109/10715761003667554. Review.
15. Hafstad AD, Nabeebaccus AA, Shah AM. Novel aspects of ROS signalling in heart failure. Basic Res Cardiol. 2013;108(4):359. https://doi.org/10.1007/s00395-013-0359-8. Epub 2013 Jun 6. Review.
16. Zhang M, Shah AM. ROS signalling between endothelial cells and cardiac cells. Cardiovasc Res. 2014;102(2):249–57. https://doi.org/10.1093/cvr/cvu050. Epub 2014 Mar 3. Review.
17. Yuste JE, Tarragon E, Campuzano CM, Ros-Bernal F. Implications of glial nitric oxide in neurodegenerative diseases. Front Cell Neurosci. 2015;9:322. https://doi.org/10.3389/fncel.2015.00322. eCollection 2015. Review.
18. Frye RE, Rossignol DA. Mitochondrial dysfunction can connect the diverse medical symptoms associated with autism spectrum disorders. Pediatr Res. 2011;69(5 Pt 2):41R–7R. https://doi.org/10.1203/PDR.0b013e318212f16b. Review.
19. Meeus M, Nijs J, Hermans L, Goubert D, Calders P. The role of mitochondrial dysfunctions due to oxidative and nitrosative stress in the chronic pain or chronic fatigue syndromes and fibromyalgia patients: peripheral and central mechanisms as therapeutic targets? Expert Opin Ther Targets. 2013;17(9):1081–9. https://doi.org/10.1517/14728222.2013.818657. Epub 2013 Jul 9. Review.
20. Tanaka M, Tajima S, Mizuno K, Ishii A, Konishi Y, Miike T, Watanabe Y. Frontier studies on fatigue, autonomic nerve dysfunction, and sleep-rhythm disorder. J Physiol Sci. 2015;65(6):483–98. https://doi.org/10.1007/s12576-015-0399-y. Epub 2015 Sept 29. Review.
21. Van Cauwenbergh D, Nijs J, Kos D, Van Weijnen L, Struyf F, Meeus M. Malfunctioning of the autonomic nervous system in patients with chronic fatigue syndrome: a systematic literature review. Eur J Clin Investig. 2014;44(5):516–26. https://doi.org/10.1111/eci.12256. Review.
22. El-Hattab AW, Scaglia F. Mitochondrial cardiomyopathies. Front Cardiovasc Med. 2016;3:25. https://doi.org/10.3389/fcvm.2016.00025. eCollection 2016. Review.
23. Cardinali DP. Autonomic nervous system: basic and clinical aspects. Cham: Springer International Publishing AG; 2018.
24. Sharafati-Chaleshtori R, Shirzad H, Rafieian-Kopaei M, Soltani A. Melatonin and human mitochondrial diseases. J Res Med Sci. 2017;22:2. https://doi.org/10.4103/1735-1995.199092. eCollection 2017. Review.
25. Li S, Tan HY, Wang N, Zhang ZJ, Lao L, Wong CW, Feng Y. The role of oxidative stress and antioxidants in liver diseases. Int J Mol Sci. 2015;16(11):26087–124. https://doi.org/10.3390/ijms161125942. Review.
26. Martínez-Martínez LA, Mora T, Vargas A, Fuentes-Iniestra M, Martínez-Lavín M. Sympathetic nervous system dysfunction in fibromyalgia, chronic fatigue syndrome, irritable bowel syndrome, and interstitial cystitis: a review of case-control studies. J Clin Rheumatol. 2014;20(3):146–50. https://doi.org/10.1097/RHU.0000000000000089. Review.
27. Zsurka G, Kunz WS. Mitochondrial dysfunction and seizures: the neuronal energy crisis. Lancet Neurol. 2015;14(9):956–66. https://doi.org/10.1016/S1474-4422(15)00148-9. Review.
28. Murphy MP. Understanding and preventing mitochondrial oxidative damage. Biochem Soc Trans. 2016;44(5):1219–26. Review.
29. Li AN, Li S, Zhang YJ, Xu XR, Chen YM, Li HB. Resources and biological activities of natural polyphenols. Nutrients. 2014;6:6020–47.
30. Feng Y, Wang N, Ye X, Li H, Feng Y, Cheung F, Nagamatsu T. Hepatoprotective effect and its possible mechanism of Coptidis rhizoma aqueous extract on carbon tetrachloride-induced chronic liver hepatotoxicity in rats. J Ethnopharmacol. 2011;138:683–90.
31. Singal AK, Jampana SC, Weinman SA. Antioxidants as therapeutic agents for liver disease. Liver Int. 2011;31:1432–48.
32. Medina J, Moreno-Otero R. Pathophysiological basis for antioxidant therapy in chronic liver disease. Drugs. 2005;65:2445–61.
33. Kelly FJ. Oxidative stress: its role in air pollution and adverse health effects. Occup Environ Med. 2003;60:612–6. https://doi.org/10.1136/oem.60.8.612.
34. Al-Dalaen SM, Al-Qtaitat AI. Review article: oxidative stress versus antioxidants. Am J Biosci Bioeng. 2014;2(5):60–71.
35. Sindhi V, Gupta V, Sharma K, Bhatnagar S, Kumari R, Dhaka N. Potential applications of antioxidants – a review. J Pharm Res. 2013;7(9):828–835. ISSN 0974-6943. https://doi.org/10.1016/j.jopr.2013.10.001.
36. Villamena FA. Molecular basis of oxidative stress: chemistry, mechanisms, and disease pathogenesis. Hoboken: John Wiley & Sons, Inc.; 2013.
37. Carr AC, McCall MR, Frei B. Oxidation of LDL by myeloperoxidase and reactive nitrogen species: reaction pathways and antioxidant protection. Arterioscler Thromb Vasc Biol. 2000;20:1716–23.
38. Daugherty A, Dunn JL, Rateri DL, Heinecke JW. Myeloperoxidase, a catalyst for lipoprotein oxidation, is expressed in human atherosclerotic lesions. J Clin Invest. 1994;94:437–44.
39. Adly AAM. Oxidative stress and disease: an updated review. Res J Immunol. 2010;3:129–45.
40. Ho E, Karimi Galougahi K, Liu CC, Bhindi R, Figtree GA. Biological markers of oxidative stress: applica-

tions to cardiovascular research and practice. Redox Biol. 2013;1:483 91. https://doi.org/10.1016/j.redox.2013.07.006. Review.
41. Kirkman HN, Gaetani GF. Mammalian catalase: a venerable enzyme with new mysteries. Trends Biochem Sci. 2007;32(1):44–50. Epub 2006 Dec 8. Review.
42. Garrido N, Meseguer M, Simon C, Pellicer A, Remohi J. Pro-oxidative and anti-oxidative imbalance in human semen and its relation with male fertility. Asian J Androl. 2004;6(1):59–65.
43. Sonoda J, Pei L, Evans RM. Nuclear receptors: decoding metabolic disease. FEBS Lett. 2008;582(1):2–9.
44. Cai D. NFkappaB-mediated metabolic inflammation in peripheral tissues versus central nervous system. Cell Cycle. 2009;8:2542–8.
45. Lumeng CN, Saltiel AR. Inflammatory links between obesity and metabolic disease. J Clin Invest. 2011;121(6):2111–7.
46. Muriach M, Flores-Bellver M, Romero FJ, Barcia JM. Diabetes and the brain: oxidative stress, inflammation, and autophagy. Oxidative Med Cell Longev. 2014;2014:102158. https://doi.org/10.1155/2014/102158. Epub 2014 Aug 24. Review.
47. Cai D, Liu T. Inflammatory cause of metabolic syndrome via brain stress and NF-κB. Aging. 2012;4(2):98–115.
48. Zhang X, Zhang G, Zhang H, Karin M, Bai H, Cai D. Hypothalamic IKKbeta/NF-kappaB and ER stress link overnutrition to energy imbalance and obesity. Cell. 2008;135:61–73.
49. DeSouza CT, Araujo EP, Bordin S, et al. Consumption of a fat-rich diet activates a proinflammatory response and induces insulin resistance in the hypothalamus. Endocrinology. 2005;146(10):4192–9.
50. Belgardt BF, Mauer J, Wunderlich FT, et al. Hypothalamic and pituitary c-Jun N-terminal kinase 1 signaling coordinately regulates glucose metabolism. Proc Natl Acad Sci U S A. 2010;107(13):6028–33.
51. Ozcan U, Yilmaz E, Ozcan L, et al. Chemical chaperones reduce ER stress and restore glucose homeostasis in a mouse model of type 2 diabetes. Science. 2006;313(5790):1137–40.
52. Lin MT, Beal MF. Mitochondrial dysfunction and oxidative stress in neurodegenerative diseases. Nature. 2006;443(7113):787–95.
53. Brown MK, Naidoo N. The endoplasmic reticulum stress response in aging and age-related diseases. Front Physiol. 2012;3:263.
54. Cadenas E, Davies KJA. Mitochondrial free radical generation, oxidative stress, and aging. Free Radic Biol Med. 2000;29(3–4):222–30.
55. Hotamisligil GS. Endoplasmic reticulum stress and the inflammatory bas is of metabolic disease. Cell. 2010;140(6):900–17.
56. Tabas I, Ron D. Integrating the mechanisms of apoptosis induced by endoplasmic reticulum stress. Nat Cell Biol. 2011;13(3):184–90.
57. Meng Y, Yong Y, Yang G, et al. Autophagy alleviates neurodegeneration caused by mild impairment of oxidative metabolism. J Neurochem. 2013;126(6):805–18.
58. Rao RV, Ellerby HM, Bredesen DE. Coupling endoplasmic reticulum stress to the cell death program. Cell Death Differ. 2004;11(4):372–80.
59. Purkayastha S, Zhang G, Cai D. Uncoupling the mechanisms of obesity and hypertension by targeting hypothalamic IKK-beta and NF-kappaB. Nat Med. 2011;17:883–7.
60. Cullinan SB, Diehl JA. Coordination of ER and oxidative stress signaling: the PERK/Nrf2 signaling pathway. Int J Biochem Cell Biol. 2006;38(3):317–32.
61. Kar SK, Choudhury I. An empirical review on oxidative stress markers and their relevance in obsessive-compulsive disorder. Int J Nutr Pharmacol Neurol Dis. 2016;6:139–45.
62. Nisar A, Mamat AS, Hatim MI, Aslam MS, Muhammad MS. Identification of flavonoids (quercetin, gallic acid and rutin) from catharanthus roseus plant parts using deep eutectic solvent. Recent Adv Biol Med. 2017;3:1–6. https://doi.org/10.18639/RABM.2016.02.347628.
63. Halliwell B, Gutteridge J. Free radicals in biology and medicine. Oxford: Oxford University Press; 2007.
64. Powers SK, Jackson MJ. Exercise-induced oxidative stress: cellular mechanisms and impact on muscle force production. Physiol Rev. 2008;88(4):1243–76. https://doi.org/10.1152/physrev.00031.2007. Review.
65. Alam MN, Bristi NJ, Rafiquzzaman M. Review on in vivo and in vitro methods evaluation of antioxidant activity. Saudi Pharm J. 2013;21(2):143–52. https://doi.org/10.1016/j.jsps.2012.05.002. Epub 2012 Jun 15.
66. Davies MJ, Fu S, Wang H, Dean RT. Stable markers of oxidant damage to proteins and their application in the study of human disease. Free Radic Biol Med. 1999;27:1151–63.
67. Diplock AT. Introduction: markers of oxidative damage and antioxidant modulation. Free Radic Res. 2000;33(Suppl):S21–6.
68. Han D, Loukianoff S, McLaughlin L. Oxidative stress indices: analytical aspects and significance. In: Sen CK, Packer L, Hanninen O, editors. Handbook of oxidants and antioxidants in exercise. Amsterdam: Elsevier; 2000. p. 433–83.
69. Hwang ES, Kim GH. Biomarkers for oxidative stress status of DNA, lipids, proteins in vitro and in vivo cancer research. Toxicology. 2007;229:1–10.
70. Jones DP. Redefining oxidative stress. Antioxid Redox Signal. 2006;8:1865–79.
71. Lawson JA, Rokach J, FitzGerald GA. Isoprostanes: formation, analysis and use as indices of lipid peroxidation in vivo. J Biol Chem. 1999;274:24441–4.
72. Roberts LJ, Morrow JD. Measurement of F(2)-isoprostanes as an index of oxidative stress in vivo. Free Radic Biol Med. 2000;28:505–13.

73. Sachdev S, Davies KJ. Production, detection, adaptive responses to free radicals in exercise. Free Radic Biol Med. 2008;44:215–23.
74. Kasai H. Analysis of a form of oxidative DNA damage, 8-hydroxy-2′-deoxyguanosine, as a marker of cellular oxidative stress during carcinogenesis. Mutat Res. 1997;387:147–63.
75. Pillon NJ, Soulage CO. Chapter 19: lipid peroxidation by-products and the metabolic syndrome. In: Catala A, editor. Lipid peroxidation; 2012. https://doi.org/10.5772/46019
76. Cheng J, Wang F, Yu DF, Wu PF, Chen JG. The cytotoxic mechanism of malondialdehyde and protective effect of carnosine via protein crosslinking/mitochondrial dysfunction/reactive oxygen species/AMPK pathway in neurons. Eur J Pharmacol. 2011;650:184–94.
77. Long EK, Murphy TC, Leiphon LJ, Watt J, Morrow JD, Milne GL, Howard JRH, Picklo MJ. Trans-4-hydroxy-2-hexenal is a neurotoxic product of docosahexaenoic (22:6; n-3) acid oxidation. J Neurochem. 2008;105:714–24.
78. Bae EH, Cho S, Joo SY, Ma SK, Kim SH, Lee J, Kim SW. 4-Hydroxy-2-hexenalinduced apoptosis in human renal proximal tubular epithelial cells. Nephrol Dial Transplant. 2011;26:3866–73.
79. Uchida K, Shiraishi M, Naito Y, Torii Y, Nakamura Y, Osawa T. Activation of stress signaling pathways by the end product of lipid peroxidation. 4-hydroxy-2-nonenal is a potential inducer of intracellular peroxide production. J Biol Chem. 1999;274:2234–42.
80. Lee JY, Jung GY, Heo HJ, Yun MR, Park JY, Bae SS, Hong KW, Lee WS, Kim CD. 4-Hydroxynonenal induces vascular smooth muscle cell apoptosis through mitochondrial generation of reactive oxygen species. Toxicol Lett. 2006;166:212–21.
81. Pillon NJ, Croze ML, Vella RE, Soulère L, Lagarde M, Soulage CO. The lipid peroxidation by-product 4-hydroxy-2-nonenal (4-HNE) induces insulin resistance in skeletal muscle through both carbonyl and oxidative stress. Endocrinology. 2012;153:2099–111.
82. Luo J, Robinson JP, Shi R. Acrolein-induced cell death in PC12 cells: role of mitochondria-mediated oxidative stress. Neurochem Int. 2005;47:449–57.
83. Kostyuk V, Potapovich A, Cesareo E, Brescia S, Guerra L, Valacchi G, Pecorelli A, Raskovic D, De Luca C, Pastore S, Korkina L. Dysfunction of glutathione S-transferase leads to excess 4-hydroxy-2-nonenal and H2O2 and impaired cytokine pattern in cultured keratinocytes and blood of vitiligo patients. Antioxid Redox Signal. 2010. https://doi.org/10.1089/ars.2009.2976.
84. Curtis JM, Grimsrud PA, Wright WS, Xu X, Foncea RE, Graham DW, Brestoff JR, Wiczer BM, Ilkayeva O, Cianflone K, Muoio DE, Arriaga EA, Bernlohr DA. Downregulation of adipose glutathione S-transferase A4 leads to increased protein carbonylation, oxidative stress, and mitochondrial dysfunction. Diabetes. 2010;59:1132–42.
85. Furukawa S, Fujita T, Shimabukuro M, Iwaki M, Yamada Y, Nakajima Y, Nakayama O, Makishima M, Matsuda M, Shimomura I. Increased oxidative stress in obesity and its impact on metabolic syndrome. J Clin Invest. 2004;114:1752–61.
86. Wellen KE, Hotamisligil GS. Obesity-induced inflammatory changes in adipose tissue. J Clin Invest. 2003;112:1785–8.
87. Soares AF, Guichardant M, Cozzone D, Bernoud-Hubac N, Bouzaidi-Tiali N, Lagarde M, Geloen A. Effects of oxidative stress on adiponectin secretion and lactate production in 3T3-L1 adipocytes. Free Radic Biol Med. 2005;38:882–9.
88. Wang Z, Dou X, Gu D, Shen C, Yao T, Nguyen V, Braunschweig C, Song Z. 4-Hydroxynonenal differentially regulates adiponectin gene expression and secretion via activating PPARγ and accelerating ubiquitin-proteasome degradation. Mol Cell Endocrinol. 2012;349:222–31.
89. Trevisan M, Browne R, Ram M, Muti P, Freudenheim J, Carosella AM, Armstrong D. Correlates of markers of oxidative status in the general population. Am J Epidemiol. 2001;154:348–56.
90. Menon V, Ram M, Dorn J, Armstrong D, Muti P, Freudenheim JL, Browne R, Schunemann H, Trevisan M. Oxidative stress and glucose levels in a population-based sample. Diabet Med. 2004;21:1346–52.
91. Maxwell SR, Thomason H, Sandler D, Leguen C, Baxter MA, Thorpe GH, Jones AF, Barnett AH. Antioxidant status in patients with uncomplicated insulin-dependent and non-insulin-dependent diabetes mellitus. Eur J Clin Investig. 1997;27:484–90.
92. Dierckx N, Horvath G, van Gils C, Vertommen J, van de Vliet J, De Leeuw I, Manuel-y-Keenoy B. Oxidative stress status in patients with diabetes mellitus: relationship to diet. Eur J Clin Nutr. 2003;57:999–1008.
93. Kamenova P. Improvement of insulin sensitivity in patients with type 2 diabetes mellitus after oral administration of alpha-lipoic acid. Hormones (Athens). 2006;5:251–8.
94. Vincent HK, Bourguignon CM, Weltman AL, Vincent KR, Barrett E, Innes KE, Taylor AG. Effects of antioxidant supplementation on insulin sensitivity, endothelial adhesion molecules, and oxidative stress in normal-weight and overweight young adults. Metab Clin Exp. 2009;58:254–62.
95. Bashan N, Kovsan J, Kachko I, Ovadia H, Rudich A. Positive and negative regulation of insulin signaling by reactive oxygen and nitrogen species. Physiol Rev. 2009;89:27–71.
96. Adabag AS, Luepker RV, Roger VL, Gersh BJ. Sudden cardiac death: epidemiology and risk factors. Nat Rev Cardiol. 2010;7(4):216–25. https://doi.org/10.1038/nrcardio.2010.3.
97. Zimniak P. 4-Hydroxynonenal and fat storage: a paradoxical pro-obesity mechanism? Cell Cycle. 2010;9:3393–4.

98. Jacob S, Streeper RS, Fogt DL, Hokama JY, Tritschler HJ, Dietze GJ, Henriksen EJ. The antioxidant alpha-lipoic acid enhances insulin-stimulated glucose metabolism in insulin-resistant rat skeletal muscle. Diabetes. 1996;45:1024–9.
99. Ziegler D, Gries F. Alpha-lipoic acid and the treatment of diabetic peripheral autonomic cardiac neuropathy. Diabetes. 1997;46(Suppl 2):S62–6.
100. Prendergast JJ. Diabetic autonomic neuropathy: part 1. Early detection. Pract Diabetol. 2001;20(1):7–14.
101. Prendergast JJ. Diabetic autonomic neuropathy: part 2. Treatment. Pract Diabetol. 2001:30–6.
102. Ziegler D, Ametov A, Barinov A, Dyck PJ, Gurieva I, Low PA, Munzel U, Yakhno N, Raz I, Novosadova M, Maus J, Samigullin R. Oral treatment with alpha-lipoic acid improves symptomatic diabetic polyneuropathy: The SYDNEY 2 trial. Diabetes Care. 2006;29(11):2365–70.
103. Ametov AS, Barinov A, Dyck PJ, Hermann R, Kozlova N, Litchy WJ, Low PA, Nehrdich D, Novosadova M, O'Brien PC, Reljanovic M, Samigullin R, Schuette K, Strokov I, Tritschler HJ, Wessel K, Yakhno N, Ziegler D, SYDNEY Trial Study Group. The sensory symptoms of diabetic polyneuropathy are improved with alpha-lipoic acid. The SYDNEY trial. Diabetes Care. 2003;26(3):770–6.
104. Ziegler D, Low PA, Litchy WJ, Boulton AJM, Vinik AI, Freeman R, The NATHAN 1 Trial Group. Efficacy and safety of antioxidant treatment with α-lipoic acid over 4 years in diabetic polyneuropathy. Diabetes Care. 2011;34:2054–60.
105. Manning PJ, Sutherland WHF, Walker RJ, Williams SM, De Jong SA, Ryalls AR, Berry EA. Effect of high-dose vitamin E on insulin resistance and associated parameters in overweight subjects. Diabetes Care. 2004;27:2166–71.
106. Rudich A, Tirosh A, Potashnik R, Khamaisi M, Bashan N. Lipoic acid protects against oxidative stress induced impairment in insulin stimulation of protein kinase B and glucose transport in 3T3-L1 adipocytes. Diabetologia. 1999;42:949–57.
107. Maddux BA, See W, Lawrence JC Jr, Goldfine AL, Goldfine ID, Evans JL. Protection against oxidative stress-induced insulin resistance in rat L6 muscle cells by micromolar concentrations of alpha-lipoic acid. Diabetes. 2001;50:404–10.
108. Jungas T, Motta I, Duffieux F, Fanen P, Stoven V, Ojcius DM. Glutathione levels and BAX activation during apoptosis due to oxidative stress in cells expressing wild-type and mutant cystic fibrosis transmembrane conductance regulator. J Biol Chem. 2002;277:27912–8.
109. Dominy JE, Hwang J, Stipanuk MH. Overexpression of cysteine dioxygenase reduces intracellular cysteine and glutathione pools in HepG2/C3A cells. Am J Physiol Endocrinol Metab. 2007;293:E62–9.
110. Miyata T, Izuhara Y, Sakai H, Kurokawa K. Carbonyl stress: increased carbonyl modification of tissue and cellular proteins in uremia. Perit Dial Int. 1999;19(Suppl 2):S58–61.
111. Kirkham PA, Barnes PJ. Oxidative stress in COPD. Chest. 2013;144(1):266–73. https://doi.org/10.1378/chest.12-2664. Review.
112. Ziegler D, Gries F. Alpha-lipoic acid and the treatment of diabetic peripheral autonomic cardiac neuropathy. Diabetes. 1997;46(Suppl 2):S62–6.
113. Ziegler D, Ametov A, Barinov A, Dyck PJ, Gurieva I, Low PA, Munzel U, Yakhno N, Raz I, Novosadova M, Maus J, Samigullin R. Oral treatment with alpha-lipoic acid improves symptomatic diabetic polyneuropathy: the SYDNEY 2 trial. Diabetes Care. 2006;29(11):2365–70.
114. Ametov AS, Barinov A, Dyck PJ, Hermann R, Kozlova N, Litchy WJ, Low PA, Nehrdich D, Novosadova M, O'Brien PC, Reljanovic M, Samigullin R, Schuette K, Strokov I, Tritschler HJ, Wessel K, Yakhno N, Ziegler D, SYDNEY Trial Study Group. The sensory symptoms of diabetic polyneuropathy are improved with alpha-lipoic acid. The SYDNEY trial. Diabetes Care. 2003;26(3):770–6.
115. Ziegler D, Low PA, Litchy WJ, Boulton AJM, Vinik AI, Freeman R, The NATHAN 1 Trial Group. Efficacy and safety of antioxidant treatment with α-lipoic acid over 4 years in diabetic polyneuropathy. Diabetes Care. 2011;34:2054–60.
116. Colombo J, Arora RR, DePace NL, Vinik AI. Clinical autonomic dysfunction: measurement, indications, therapies, and outcomes. New York: Springer Science + Business Media; 2014.
117. Vinik A, Ziegler D. Diabetic cardiovascular autonomic neuropathy. Circulation. 2007;115:387–97.
118. Vinik AI, Maser RE, Nakave AA. Diabetic cardiovascular autonomic nerve dysfunction. US Endocr Dis. 2007;2:2–9.
119. Ali AM, Awad TG, Al-Adl NM. Efficacy of combined topiramate/thioctic acid therapy in migraine prophylaxis. Saudi Pharm J. 2010;18(4):239–43. https://doi.org/10.1016/j.jsps.2010.07.006. Epub 2010 Jul 30.
120. Mahboob A, Farhat SM, Iqbal G, Babar MM, Zaidi NU, Nabavi SM, Ahmed T. Alpha-lipoic acid-mediated activation of muscarinic receptors improves hippocampus- and amygdala-dependent memory. Brain Res Bull. 2016;122:19–28. https://doi.org/10.1016/j.brainresbull.2016.02.014. Epub 2016 Feb 18.
121. Logan AC, Wong C. Chronic fatigue syndrome: oxidative stress and dietary modifications. Altern Med Rev. 2001;6(5):450–9. Review.
122. Hiller S, DeKroon R, Hamlett ED, Xu L, Osorio C, Robinette J, Winnik W, Simington S, Maeda N, Alzate O, Yi X. Alpha-lipoic acid supplementation protects enzymes from damage by nitrosative and oxidative stress. Biochim Biophys Acta. 2016;1860(1 Pt A):36–45. https://doi.org/10.1016/j.bbagen.2015.09.001. Epub 2015 Sept 4.

123. Wollen KA. Alzheimer's disease: the pros and cons of pharmaceutical, nutritional, botanical, and stimulatory therapies, with a discussion of treatment strategies from the perspective of patients and practitioners. Altern Med Rev. 2010;15(3):223–44. Review.
124. Ajith TA, Padmajanair G. Mitochondrial pharmaceutics: a new therapeutic strategy to ameliorate oxidative stress in Alzheimer's disease. Curr Aging Sci. 2015;8(3):235–40. Review.
125. Li YH, He Q, Yu JZ, Liu CY, Feng L, Chai Z, Wang Q, Zhang HZ, Zhang GX, Xiao BG, Ma CG. Lipoic acid protects dopaminergic neurons in LPS-induced Parkinson's disease model. Metab Brain Dis. 2015;30(5):1217–26. https://doi.org/10.1007/s11011-015-9698-5. Epub 2015 Jun 19.
126. Zhao H, Zhao X, Liu L, Zhang H, Xuan M, Guo Z, Wang H, Liu C. Neurochemical effects of the R form of α-lipoic acid and its neuroprotective mechanism in cellular models of Parkinson's disease. Int J Biochem Cell Biol. 2017;87:86–94. https://doi.org/10.1016/j.biocel.2017.04.002. Epub 2017 Apr 6.
127. Zhao H, Zhao X, Liu L, Zhang H, Xuan M, Guo Z, Wang H, Liu C. Neurochemical effects of the R form of α-lipoic acid and its neuroprotective mechanism in cellular models of Parkinson's disease. Int J Biochem Cell Biol. 2017;87:86–94. https://doi.org/10.1016/j.biocel.2017.04.002. Epub 2017 Apr 6.
128. Namazi N, Larijani B, Azadbakht L. Alpha-lipoic acid supplement in obesity treatment: a systematic review and meta-analysis of clinical trials. Clin Nutr. 2017. pii: S0261-5614(17)30212-1. https://doi.org/10.1016/j.clnu.2017.06.002. [Epub ahead of print] Review.
129. DePace NL, Mears JP, Yayac M, Colombo J. Cardiac autonomic testing and diagnosing heart disease. "A clinical perspective.". Heart Int. 2014;9(2):37–44. https://doi.org/10.5301/heartint.5000218; published online 12/5/2014 12:29:58 PM.
130. DePace NL, Mears JP, Yayac M, Colombo J. Cardiac autonomic testing and treating heart disease. "A clinical perspective.". Heart Int. 2014;9(2):45–52. https://doi.org/10.5301/heartint.5000216; published online 11/19/2014 1:16:08 PM.
131. Sorescu D, Weiss D, Lassegue B, Clempus RE, Szocs K, Sorescu GP, Valppu L, Quinn MT, Lambeth JD, Vega JD, Taylor WR, Griendling KK. Superoxide production and expression of Nox family proteins in human atherosclerosis. Circulation. 2002;105:1429–35.
132. Ashar FN, Zhang Y, Longchamps RJ, Lane J, Moes A, Grove ML, Mychaleckyj JC, Taylor KD, Coresh J, Rotter JI, Boerwinkle E, Pankratz N, Guallar E, Arking DE. Association of mitochondrial DNA copy number with cardiovascular disease. JAMA Cardiol. 2017. https://doi.org/10.1001/jamacardio.2017.3683. [Epub ahead of print].
133. Förstermann U, Münzel T. Endothelial nitric oxide synthase in vascular disease: from marvel to menace. Circulation. 2006;113:1708–14.
134. Li H, Wallerath T, Münzel T, Förstermann U. Regulation of endothelial-type NO synthase expression in pathophysiology and in response to drugs. Nitric Oxide Biol Chem. 2002;7:149–64.
135. Drummond GR, Cai H, Davis ME, Ramasamy S, Harrison DG. Transcriptional and posttranscriptional regulation of endothelial nitric oxide synthase expression by hydrogen peroxide. Circ Res. 2000;86:347–54.
136. Riha RL, Diefenbach K, Jennum P, et al. Genetic aspects of hypertension and metabolic disease in the obstructive sleep apnoea-hypopnoea syndrome. Sleep Med Rev. 2008;12:49–63.
137. Goldbart AD, Row BW, Kheirandish-Gozal L, et al. High fat/refined carbohydrate diet enhances the susceptibility to spatial learning deficits in rats exposed to intermittent hypoxia. Brain Res. 2006;1090:190–6.
138. Somers VK, Mark AL, Abboud FM. Sympathetic activation by hypoxia and hypercapnia – implications for sleep apnea. Clin Exp Hypertens A. 1988;10(Suppl. 1):413–22.
139. Hedner J, Darpo B, Ejnell H, et al. Reduction in sympathetic activity after long-term CPAP treatment in sleep apnoea: cardiovascular implications. Eur Respir J. 1995;8:222–9.
140. Carlson JT, Hedner J, Elam M, et al. Augmented resting sympathetic activity in awake patients with obstructive sleep apnea. Chest. 1993;103:1763–8.
141. Narkiewicz K, Somers VK. Obstructive sleep apnea as a cause of neurogenic hypertension. Curr Hypertens Rep. 1999;1:268–73.
142. Lavie L, Lavie P. Molecular mechanisms of cardiovascular disease in OSAHS: the oxidative stress link. Eur Respir J. 2009;33:1467–84.
143. Tsuji H, Venditti FJ Jr, Manders ES, Evans JC, Larson MG, Feldman CL, Levy D. Reduced heart rate variability and mortality risk in an elderly cohort. The Framingham Heart Study. Circulation. 1994;90(2):878–83.
144. Vinik AI, Maser RE, Mitchell BD, Freeman R. Diabetic autonomic neuropathy. Diabetes Care. 2003;26(5):1553–79.
145. Maser R, Mitchell B, Vinik AI, Freeman R. The association between cardiovascular autonomic neuropathy and mortality in individuals with diabetes, a meta-analysis. Diabetes Care. 2003;26(6):1895–901.
146. DePace NL, Mears JP, Yayac M, Colombo J. Cardiac autonomic testing and diagnosing heart disease. "A clinical perspective". Heart Int. 2014;9(2):37–44. https://doi.org/10.5301/heartint.5000218; published online 12/5/2014 12:29:58 PM.
147. DePace NL, Mears JP, Yayac M, Colombo J. Cardiac autonomic testing and treating heart disease. "A clinical perspective". Heart Int. 2014;9(2):45–52. https://doi.org/10.5301/heartint.5000216; published online 11/19/2014 1:16:08 PM.
148. Bullinga JR, Alharethi R, Schram MS, Bristow MR, Gilbert EM. Changes in heart rate variability are correlated to hemodynamic improvement with chronic

CARVEDILOL therapy in heart failure. J Card Fail. 2005;11(9):693–9.
149. Fatoni C, Raffa S, Regoli F, Giraldi F, La Rovere MT, Prentice J, Pastori F, Fratini S, Salerno-Uriarte JA, Klein HU, Auricchio A. Cardiac resynchronization therapy improves heart rate profile and heart rate variability of patients with moderate to severe heart failure. J Am Coll Cardiol. 2005;46(10):1875–82.
150. Fathizadeh P, Shoemaker WC, Woo CCJ, Colombo J. Autonomic activity in trauma patients based on variability of heart rate and respiratory rate. Crit Care Med. 2004;32(5):1300–5.
151. Chen JY, Fung JW, Yu CM. The mechanisms of atrial fibrillation. J Cardiovasc Electrophysiol. 2006;17(Suppl 3):S2–7.
152. Copie X, Lamaison D, Salvador M, Sadoul N, DaCosta A, Faucher L, Legal F, Le Heuzey JY, VALID Investigators. Heart rate variability before ventricular arrhythmias in patients with coronary artery disease and an implantable cardioverter defibrillator. Ann Noninvasive Electrocardiol. 2003;8(3):179–84.
153. Alter P, Grimm W, Vollrath A, Czerny F, Maisch B. Heart rate variability in patients with cardiac hypertrophy – relation to left ventricular mass and etiology. Am Heart J. 2006;151(4):829–36.
154. Debono M, Cachia E. The impact of cardiovascular autonomic neuropathy in diabetes: is it associated with left ventricular dysfunction? Auton Neurosci. 2007;132(1–2):1–7.
155. Just H. Peripheral adaptations in congestive heart failure: a review. Am J Med. 1991;90:23S–6S.
156. Nakamura K, Matsumura K, Kobayashi S, Kaneko T. Sympathetic premotor neurons mediating thermoregulatory functions. Neurosci Res. 2005;51(1):1–8.
157. Manfrini O, Morgagni G, Pizzi C, Fontana F, Bugiardini R. Changes in autonomic nervous system activity: spontaneous versus balloon-induced myocardial ischemia. Eur Heart J. 2004;25(17):1502–8.
158. Clarke B, Ewing D, Campbell I. Diabetic autonomic neuropathy. Diabetologia. 1979;17:195–212.
159. Arora R. Recent insights into the role of the autonomic nervous system in the creation of substrate for atrial fibrillation. Implications for therapies targeting the atrial autonomic nervous system. Circ Arrhythm Electrophysiol. 2012;5:850–9.
160. Ng J, Villuendas R, Cokic I, Schliamser JE, Gordon D, Koduri H, Benefield B, Simon J, Murthy SN, Lomasney JW, Wasserstrom JA, Goldberger JJ, Aistrup GL, Arora R. Autonomic remodeling in the left atrium and pulmonary veins in heart failure: creation of a dynamic substrate for atrial fibrillation. Circ Arrhythm Electrophysiol. 2011;4:388–96.
161. Kishi T, Hirooks Y. Oxidative stress in the brain causes hypertension via sympathoexcitation. Front Physiol. 2012;17:335. https://doi.org/10.3389/fphys.2012.00335. eCollection 2012.
162. Kishi T, Hirooka Y, Sakai K, Shigematsu H, Shimokawa H, Takeshita A. Overexpression of eNOS in the RVLM causes hypotension and bradycardia via GABA release. Hypertension. 2001;38:896–901.
163. Patel K, Li YF, Hirooka Y. Role of nitric oxide in central sympathetic outflow. Exp Biol Med. 2001;226:814–24.
164. Noble A, Johnson R, Thomas A, Bass P. Arterial blood pressure. In: The cardiovascular system, systems of the body series. 2nd ed. Edinburgh: Elsevier; 2010.
165. Li DP, Chen SR, Pan HL. Nitric oxide inhibits spinally projecting paraventricular neurons through potentiation of presynaptic GABA release. J Neurophysiol. 2002;88:2664–74.
166. Garthwaite J. Concepts of neural nitric oxide-mediated transmission. Eur J Neurosci. 2008;27:2783–802.
167. Kimura Y, Hirooka Y, Sagara Y, Ito K, Kishi T, Shimokawa H, Takeshita A, Sunagawa K. Overexpression of inducible nitric oxide synthase in rostral ventrolateral medulla causes hypertension and sympathoexcitation via an increase in oxidative stress. Circ Res. 2005;96:252–60.
168. Oliveira-Sales EB, Colombari DSA, Davisson RL, Kasparov S, Hirata AE, Campos RR, Paton JFR. Kidney-induced hypertension depends on superoxide signaling in the rostral ventrolateral medulla. Hypertension. 2010;56:290–6.
169. Golbidi S, Frisbee JC, Laher XI. Chronic stress impacts the cardiovascular system: animal models and clinical outcomes. Review. Am J Physiol Heart Circ Physiol. 2015;308:H1476–98.
170. Gao L, Mao Q, Cao J, Wang Y, Zhou X, Fan L. Effects of coenzyme Q10 on vascular endothelial function in humans: a meta-analysis of randomized controlled trials. Atherosclerosis. 2012;221(2):311–6. https://doi.org/10.1016/j.atherosclerosis.2011.
171. Zhou M, Zhi Q, Tang Y, Yu D, Han J. Effects of coenzyme Q10 on myocardial protection during cardiac valve replacement and scavenging free radical activity in vitro. J Cardiovasc Surg. 1999;40(3):355–61.
172. Rosenfeldt F, Marasco S, Lyon W, Wowk M, Sheeran F, Bailey M, Esmore D, Davis B, Pick A, Rabinov M, Smith J, Nagley P, Pepe S. Coenzyme Q10 therapy before cardiac surgery improves mitochondrial function and in vitro contractility of myocardial tissue. J Thorac Cardiovasc Surg. 2005;129(1):25–32.
173. Mordente A, Martorana GE, Santini SA, Miggiano GA, Petitti T, Giardina B, Battino M, Littarru GP. Antioxidant effect of coenzyme Q on hydrogen peroxide-activated myoglobin. Clin Investig. 1993;71(8 Suppl):S92–6.
174. Folkers K, Littarru GP, Ho L, Runge TM, Havanonda S, Cooley D. Evidence for a deficiency of coenzyme Q10 in human heart disease. Int Z Vitaminforsch. 1970;40(3):380–90.
175. Folkers K, Vadhanavikit S, Mortensen SA. Biochemical rationale and myocardial tissue data on the effective therapy of cardiomyopathy with coenzyme Q10. Proc Natl Acad Sci U S A. 1985;82(3):901–4.

176. Mortensen SA. Overview on coenzyme Q10 as adjunctive therapy in chronic heart failure. Rationale, design and end-points of "Q-symbio" – a multinational trial. Biofactors. 2003;18(1–4):79–89.
177. Rosenfeldt F, Hilton D, Pepe S, Krum H. Systematic review of effect of coenzyme Q10 in physical exercise, hypertension and heart failure. Biofactors. 2003;18(1–4):91–100.
178. Sander S, Coleman CI, Patel AA, Kluger J, White CM. The impact of coenzyme Q10 on systolic function in patients with chronic heart failure. J Card Fail. 2006;12(6):464–72.
179. Kumar A, Singh RB, Saxena M, Niaz MA, Josh SR, Chattopadhyay P, Mechirova V, Pella D, Fedacko J. Effect of carni Q-gel (ubiquinol and carnitine) on cytokines in patients with heart failure in the Tishcon study. Acta Cardiol. 2007;62(4):349–54.
180. Hargreaves IP, Hargreaves AK. Coenzyme Q10 from fact to fiction. New York: Nova Science Publishers Inc; 2015. p. 67.
181. Morisco C, Trimarco B, Condorelli M. Effect of coenzyme Q10 therapy in patients with congestive heart failure: a long-term multicenter randomized study. Clin Investig. 1993;71(8 Suppl):S134–6.
182. Tarnopolsky MA, Beal MF. Potential for creatine and other therapies targeting cellular energy dysfunction in neurological disorders. Ann Neurol. 2001;49(5):561–74.
183. Matthews RT, Yang L, Browne S, Baik M, Beal MF. Coenzyme Q10 administration increases brain mitochondrial concentrations and exerts neuroprotective effects. Proc Natl Acad Sci U S A. 1998;95(15):8892–7.
184. Rustin P, von Kleist-Retzow JC, Chantrel-Groussard K, Sidi D, Munnich A, Rötig A. Effect of idebenone on cardiomyopathy in Friedreich's ataxia: a preliminary study. Lancet. 1999;354(9177):477–9.
185. Lodi R, Schapira AH, Manners D, Styles P, Wood NW, Taylor DJ, Warner TT. Abnormal in vivo skeletal muscle energy metabolism in Huntington's disease and dentatorubropallidoluysian atrophy. Ann Neurol. 2000;48(1):72–6.
186. Huntington Study Group. A randomized, placebo-controlled trial of coenzyme Q10 and remacemide in Huntington's disease. Neurology. 2001;57(3):397–404.
187. Sack MN, Fyhrquist FY, Saijonmaa OJ, Fuster V, Kovacic JC. Basic biology of oxidative stress and the cardiovascular system: part 1 of a 3-part series. J Am Coll Cardiol. 2017;70(2):196–211. https://doi.org/10.1016/j.jacc.2017.05.034.
188. Schaper J, Meiser E, Stämmler G. Ultrastructural morphometric analysis of myocardium from dogs, rats, hamsters, mice, and from human hearts. Circ Res. 1985;56(3):377–91.
189. Sack MN. Type 2 diabetes mitochondrial biology in the heart. J Mol Cell Cardiol. 2009;46:842–9.
190. Munzel T, Gori T, Keaney JF Jr, Macck C, Daiver A. Pathophysiologic role of oxidative stress in systolic and diastolic heart failure and the therapeutic implications. Eur Heart J. 2015;36:2555–64.
191. Sack MN. Mitochondrial depolarization in the role of uncoupling proteins and ischemia tolerance. Cardiovasc Res. 2006;72:210–9.
192. Oka T, Hikoso S, Yamaguchi G, et al. Mitochondrial DNA that escapes from autophagy cause inflammation and heart failure. Nature. 2012;485:251–5.
193. Blikseen M, Maierlo H, Omh IK, et al. Precirculating mitochondrial DNA after myocardial infarction. Int J Cardiol. 2012;158:132–4.
194. Okonko DO, Shah AM. Heart failure: mitochondrial dysfunction and oxidative stress in CHF. Nat Rev Cardiol. 2015;12(1):6–8. https://doi.org/10.1038/nrcardio.2014.189. Epub 2014 Nov 25.
195. Smith RA, Murphy MP. Animal and human studies with the mitochondria-targeted antioxidant MitoQ. Ann N Y Acad Sci. 2010;1201:96–103. https://doi.org/10.1111/j.1749-6632.2010.05627.x.
196. von Zglinicki T. Oxidative stress shortens telomeres. Trends Biochem Sci. 2002;27(7):339–44. PMID: 12114022.
197. Song Z, von Figura G, Liu Y, Kraus JM, Torrice C, Dillon P, Rudolph-Watabe M, Ju Z, Kestler HA, Sanoff H, Lenhard Rudolph K. Lifestyle impacts on the aging-associated expression of biomarkers of DNA damage and telomere dysfunction in human blood. Aging Cell. 2010;9(4):607–15. https://doi.org/10.1111/j.1474-9726.2010.00583.x. Epub 2010 Jun 17.
198. Njajou OT, Hsueh WC, Blackburn EH, Newman AB, Wu SH, Li R, Simonsick EM, Harris TM, Cummings SR, Cawthon RM, Health ABC study. Association between telomere length, specific causes of death, and years of healthy life in health, aging, and body composition, a population-based cohort study. J Gerontol A Biol Sci Med Sci. 2009;64(8):860–4. https://doi.org/10.1093/gerona/glp061. Epub 2009 May 12.
199. Ornish D, Lin J, Chan JM, Epel E, Kemp C, Weidner G, Marlin R, Frenda SJ, Magbanua MJ, Daubenmier J, Estay I, Hills NK, Chainani-Wu N, Carroll PR, Blackburn EH. Effect of comprehensive lifestyle changes on telomerase activity and telomere length in men with biopsy-proven low-risk prostate cancer: 5-year follow-up of a descriptive pilot study. Lancet Oncol. 2013;14(11):1112–20. https://doi.org/10.1016/S1470-2045(13)70366-8. Epub 2013 Sept 17.
200. Farzaneh-Far R, Lin J, Epel ES, Harris WS, Blackburn EH, Whooley MA. Association of marine omega-3 fatty acid levels with telomeric aging in patients with coronary heart disease. JAMA. 2010;303(3):250–7. https://doi.org/10.1001/jama.2009.2008.
201. Saliques S, Teyssier JR, Vergely C, Lorgis L, Lorin J, Farnier M, Donzel A, Sicard P, Berchoud J, Lagrost AC, Touzery C, Ragot S, Cottin Y, Rochette L, Zeller M. Circulating leukocyte telomere length and oxidative stress: a new target for statin therapy. Atherosclerosis. 2011;219(2):753–60. https://doi.

org/10.1016/j.atherosclerosis.2011.09.011. Epub 2011 Sept 16.

202. de Kreutzenberg SV, Ceolotto G, Cattelan A, Pagnin E, Mazzucato M, Garagnani P, Borelli V, Bacalini MG, Franceschi C, Fadini GP, Avogaro A. Metformin improves putative longevity effectors in peripheral mononuclear cells from subjects with prediabetes. A randomized controlled trial. Nutr Metab Cardiovasc Dis. 2015;25(7):686–93. https://doi.org/10.1016/j.numecd.2015.03.007. Epub 2015 Mar 24.
203. Cherkas LF, Hunkin JL, Kato BS, Richards JB, Gardner JP, Surdulescu GL, Kimura M, Lu X, Spector TD, Aviv A. The association between physical activity in leisure time and leukocyte telomere length. Arch Intern Med. 2008;168(2):154–8. https://doi.org/10.1001/archinternmed.2007.39.
204. Laimer M, Melmer A, Lamina C, Raschenberger J, Adamovski P, Engl J, Ress C, Tschoner A, Gelsinger C, Mair L, Kiechl S, Willeit J, Willeit P, Stettler C, Tilg H, Kronenberg F, Ebenbichler C. Telomere length increase after weight loss induced by bariatric surgery: results from a 10 year prospective study. Int J Obes. 2016;40(5):773–8. https://doi.org/10.1038/ijo.2015.238. Epub 2015 Nov 26.
205. Correia-Melo C, Hewitt G, Passos JF. Telomeres, oxidative stress and inflammatory factors: partners in cellular senescence? Longev Healthspan. 2014;3(1):1. https://doi.org/10.1186/2046-2395-3-1.
206. Bayne S, Liu JP. Hormones and growth factors regulate telomerase activity in ageing and cancer. Mol Cell Endocrinol. 2005;240(1–2):11–22.
207. Münzel T, Camici GG, Maack C, Bonetti NR, Fuster V, Kovacic JC. Impact of oxidative stress on the heart and vasculature: part 2 of a 3-part series. J Am Coll Cardiol. 2017;70(2):212–29. https://doi.org/10.1016/j.jacc.2017.05.035.
208. Maack C, Kartes T, Kilter H, et al. Oxygen free radical release in human failing myocardium is associated with increased activity of rac1-GTPase and represents a target for statin treatment. Circulation. 2003;108:1567–74.
209. Mollnau H, Oelze M, August M, et al. Mechanisms of increased vascular superoxide production in an experimental model of idiopathic dilated cardiomyopathy. Arterioscler Thromb Vasc Biol. 2005;25:2554–9.
210. Belch JJ, Bridges AB, Scott N, Chopra M. Oxygen free radicals and congestive heart failure. Br Heart J. 1991;65:245–8.
211. Heart Outcomes Prevention Evaluation Study Investigators. Effects of an angiotensin converting-enzyme inhibitor, ramipril, on cardiovascular events in high-risk patients. N Engl J Med. 2000;342:145–53.
212. Lonn E, Bosch J, Yusuf S, et al., HOPE and HOPE-TOO Trial Investigators. Effects of longterm vitamin E supplementation on cardiovascular events and cancer: a randomized controlled trial. JAMA. 2005;293:1338–47.
213. Förstermann U. Nitric oxide and oxidative stress in vascular disease. Pflugers Arch. 2010;459:923–39.
214. Förstermann U, Münzel T. Endothelial nitric oxide synthase in vascular disease: from marvel to menace. Circulation. 2006;113:1708–14.
215. Gryglewski RJ, Palmer RM, Moncada S. Superoxide anion is involved in the breakdown of endothelium-derived vascular relaxing factor. Nature. 1986;320:454–6.
216. Li H, Horke S, Förstermann U. Vascular oxidative stress, nitric oxide and atherosclerosis. Atherosclerosis. 2014;237:208–19.
217. Libby P. Interleukin-1 Beta as a target for atherosclerosis therapy: biological basis of CANTOS and beyond. J Am Coll Cardiol. 2017;70(18):2278–89. https://doi.org/10.1016/j.jacc.2017.09.028.
218. Ridker PM, Everett BM, Thuren T, MacFadyen JG, Chang WH, Ballantyne C, Fonseca F, Nicolau J, Koenig W, Anker SD, Kastelein JJP, Cornel JH, Pais P, Pella D, Genest J, Cifkova R, Lorenzatti A, Forster T, Kobalava Z, Vida-Simiti L, Flather M, Shimokawa H, Ogawa H, Dellborg M, Rossi PRF, Troquay RPT, Libby P, Glynn RJ, CANTOS Trial Group. Anti-inflammatory therapy with canakinumab for atherosclerotic disease. N Engl J Med. 2017;377(12):1119–31. https://doi.org/10.1056/NEJMoa1707914. Epub 2017 Aug 27.
219. Libby P. Inflammatory and immune mechanisms in atherogenesis. In: Leaf A, Weber P, editors. Atheroclerosis reviews. New York: Raven Press; 1990. p. 79–89.
220. Libby P, Ridker PM, Hansson GK. Inflammation in atherosclerosis: from pathophysiology to practice. J Am Coll Cardiol. 2009;54:2129–38.
221. Lichtman AH, Binder CJ, Tsimikas S, Witztum JL. Adaptive immunity in atherogenesis: new insights and therapeutic approaches. J Clin Invest. 2013;123:27–36.
222. Hansson GK, Libby P, Tabas I. Inflammation and plaque vulnerability. J Intern Med. 2015;278:483–93.
223. Libby P, Hansson GK. Inflammation and immunity in diseases of the arterial tree: players and layers. Circ Res. 2015;116:307–11.
224. Nus M, Mallat Z. Immune-mediated mechanisms of atherosclerosis and implications for the clinic. Expert Rev Clin Immunol. 2016;12:1217–37.
225. Weber C, Shantsila E, Hristov M, et al. Role and analysis of monocyte subsets in cardiovascular disease. Joint consensus document of the European Society of Cardiology (ESC) Working Groups "Atherosclerosis and Vascular Biology" and "Thrombosis.". Thromb Haemost. 2016;116:626–37.
226. Libby P. History of discovery: inflammation in atherosclerosis. Arterioscler Thromb. 2012; 32:2045–51.
227. Cook NR, Paynter NP, Eaton CB, et al. Comparison of the Framingham and Reynolds Risk scores for

global cardiovascular risk prediction in the multiethnic Women's Health Initiative. Circulation. 2012;125:1748–56, S1741–11.
228. Ridker PM. A test in context: high-sensitivity c-reactive protein. J Am Coll Cardiol. 2016; 67:712–23.
229. Ridker PM, Danielson E, Fonseca FA, et al. Rosuvastatin to prevent vascular events in men and women with elevated C-reactive protein. N Engl J Med. 2008;359:2195–207.
230. Schonbeck U, Libby P. Inflammation, immunity, and HMG-CoA reductase inhibitors: statins as antiinflammatory agents? Circulation. 2004;109:II18–26.
231. Ridker PM, Cannon CP, Morrow D, et al. C-reactive protein levels and outcomes after statin therapy. N Engl J Med. 2005;352:20–8.
232. Jain MK, Sangwung P, Hamik A. Regulation of an inflammatory disease: Kruppel-like factors and atherosclerosis. Arterioscler Thromb. 2014;34:499–508.
233. Libby P. The forgotten majority: unfinished business in cardiovascular risk reduction. J Am Coll Cardiol. 2005;46:1225–8.
234. Jernberg T, Asvold P, Henriksson M, Hjelm H, Thuresson M, Janzon M. Cardiovascular risk in post-myocardial infarction patients: nationwide real world data demonstrate the importance of a long-term perspective. Eur Heart J. 2015;36:1163–70.
235. Masoudi FA, Ponirakis A, de Lemos JA, et al. Trends in U.S. cardiovascular care: 2016 report from 4 ACC national cardiovascular data registries. J Am Coll Cardiol. 2017;69:1427–50.
236. Evrard SM, Lecce L, Michelis KC, Nomura-Kitabayashi A, Pandey G, Purushothaman KR, d'Escamard V, Li JR, Hadri L, Fujitani K, Moreno PR, Benard L, Rimmele P, Cohain A, Mecham B, Randolph GJ, Nabel EG, Hajjar R, Fuster V, Boehm M, Kovacic JC. Endothelial to mesenchymal transition is common in atherosclerotic lesions and is associated with plaque instability. Nat Commun. 2016;7:11853. https://doi.org/10.1038/ncomms11853.
237. Camici GG, Savarese G, Akhmedov A, Lüscher TF. Molecular mechanism of endothelial and vascular aging: implications for cardiovascular disease. Eur Heart J. 2015;36(48):3392–403. https://doi.org/10.1093/eurheartj/ehv587. Epub 2015 Nov 4. PMID: 26543043.
238. Lopaschuk GD, Ussher JR, Folmes CD, Jaswal JS, Stanley WC. Myocardial fatty acid metabolism in health and disease. Physiol Rev. 2010;90:207–58.
239. Niemann B, Rohrbach S, Miller MR, Newby DE, Fuster V, Kovacic JC. Oxidative stress and cardiovascular risk: obesity, diabetes, smoking, and pollution: part 3 of a 3-part series. J Am Coll Cardiol. 2017;70(2):230–51. https://doi.org/10.1016/j.jacc.2017.05.043.
240. Anderson EJ, Kypson AP, Rodriguez E, Anderson CA, Lehr EJ, Neufer PD. Substrate specific derangements in mitochondrial metabolism and redox balance in the atrium of the type 2 diabetic human heart. J Am Coll Cardiol. 2009;54:1891–8.
241. Brownlee M. Biochemistry and molecular cell biology of diabetic complications. Nature. 2001;414:813–20.
242. Salonen JT, Nyyssönen K, Tuomainen TP, et al. Increased risk of non-insulin dependent diabetes mellitus at low plasma vitamin E concentrations: a four year follow up study in men. BMJ. 1995;311:1124–7.
243. Itoh K, Mimura J, Yamamoto M. Discovery of the negative regulator of Nrf2, Keap1: a historical overview. Antioxid Redox Signal. 2010;13:1665–78.
244. Wegner M, Neddermann D, Piorunska-Stolzmann M, Jagodzinski PP. Role of epigenetic mechanisms in the development of chronic complications of diabetes. Diabetes Res Clin Pract. 2014;105:164–75.
245. Kayama Y, Raaz U, Jagger A, et al. Diabetic cardiovascular disease induced by oxidative stress. Int J Mol Sci. 2015;16:25234–63.
246. Aurich AC, Niemann B, Pan R, et al. Age dependent effects of high fat-diet on murine left ventricles: role of palmitate. Basic Res Cardiol. 2013;108:369.
247. Ghosh S, Rodrigues B. Cardiac cell death in early diabetes and its modulation by dietary fatty acids. Biochim Biophys Acta. 1761;2006:1148–62.
248. van de Weijer T, Schrauwen-Hinderling VB, Schrauwen P. Lipotoxicity in type 2 diabetic cardiomyopathy. Cardiovasc Res. 2011;92:10–8.
249. Niemann B, Chen Y, Teschner M, Li L, Silber RE, Rohrbach S. Obesity induces signs of premature cardiac aging in younger patients: the role of mitochondria. J Am Coll Cardiol. 2011;57:577–85.
250. The Heart Outcomes Prevention Evaluation Study Investigators. Vitamin E supplementation and cardiovascular events in high-risk patients. N Engl J Med. 2000;342:154–60.
251. Centers for Disease Control and Prevention (US), National Center for Chronic Disease Prevention and Health Promotion (US), Office on Smoking and Health (US). How tobacco smoke causes disease: the biology and behavioral basis for smoking- attributable disease: a report of the Surgeon General. Atlanta: Centers for Disease Control and Prevention; 2010. Available at: http://www.ncbi.nlm.nih.gov/books/NBK53014. Accessed 15 May 2017.
252. Cesaroni G, Forastiere F, Stafoggia M, et al. Long term exposure to ambient air pollution and incidence of acute coronary events: prospective cohort study and meta-analysis in 11 European cohorts from the ESCAPE project. BMJ. 2014;348:f7412.
253. Chen H, Goldberg MS, Burnett RT, Jerrett M, Wheeler AJ, Villeneuve PJ. Long-term exposure to traffic-related air pollution and cardiovascular mortality. Epidemiology. 2013;24:35–43.
254. Miller KA, Siscovick DS, Sheppard L, et al. Long-term exposure to air pollution and incidence of cardiovascular events in women. N Engl J Med. 2007;356:447–58.
255. Pope CA III, Verrier RL, Lovett EG, et al. Heart rate variability associated with particulate air pollution. Am Heart J. 1999;138:890–9.

256. Hoffmann B, Moebus S, Kröger K, et al. Residential exposure to urban air pollution, ankle brachial index, and peripheral arterial disease. Epidemiology. 2009;20:280–8.
257. Fowkes FG, Aboyans V, Fowkes FJ, McDermott MM, Sampson UK, Criqui MH. Peripheral artery disease: epidemiology and global perspectives. Nat Rev Cardiol. 2017;14:156–70.
258. Atkinson RW, Carey IM, Kent AJ, van Staa TP, Anderson HR, Cook DG. Long-term exposure to outdoor air pollution and incidence of cardiovascular diseases. Epidemiology. 2013;24:44–53.
259. Shah AS, Langrish JP, Nair H, et al. Global association of air pollution and heart failure: a systematic review and meta-analysis. Lancet. 2013;382:1039–48.
260. Shah AS, Lee KK, McAllister DA, et al. Short term exposure to air pollution and stroke: systematic review and meta-analysis. BMJ. 2015;350:h1295.
261. Stafoggia M, Cesaroni G, Peters A, et al. Long-term exposure to ambient air pollution and incidence of cerebrovascular events: results from 11 European cohorts within the ESCAPE project. Environ Health Perspect. 2014;122:919–25.
262. Low RB, Bielory L, Qureshi AI, Dunn V, Stuhlmiller DF, Dickey DA. The relation of stroke admissions to recent weather, airborne allergens, air pollution, seasons, upper respiratory infections, and asthma incidence, September 11, 2001, and day of the week. Stroke. 2006;37:951–7.
263. Raza A, Bellander T, Bero-Bedada G, et al. Short-term effects of air pollution on out-of hospital cardiac arrest in Stockholm. Eur Heart J. 2014;35:861–8.
264. D'Alessandro A, Boeckelmann I, Hammwhösner M, Goette A. Nicotine, cigarette smoking and cardiac arrhythmia: an overview. Eur J Prev Cardiol. 2012;19:297–305.
265. Baccarelli A, Martinelli I, Pegoraro V, et al. Living near major traffic roads and risk of deep vein thrombosis. Circulation. 2009;119:3118–24.
266. Messner B, Bernhard D. Smoking and cardiovascular disease: mechanisms of endothelial dysfunction and early atherogenesis. Arterioscler Thromb Vasc Biol. 2014;34:509–15.
267. Mills NL, Donaldson K, Hadoke PW, et al. Adverse cardiovascular effects of air pollution. Nat Clin Pract Cardiovasc Med. 2009;6:36–44.
268. Brook RD, Rajagopalan S. Particulate matter, air pollution, and blood pressure. J Am Soc Hypertens. 2009;3:332–50.
269. Liang R, Zhang B, Zhao X, Ruan Y, Lian H, Fan Z. Effect of exposure to PM2.5 on blood pressure: a systematic review and meta-analysis. J Hypertens. 2014;32:2130–40, discussion 2141.
270. Wauters A, Dreyfuss C, Pochet S, et al. Acute exposure to diesel exhaust impairs nitric oxide mediated endothelial vasomotor function by increasing endothelial oxidative stress. Hypertension. 2013;62:352–8.
271. Brook RD, Rajagopalan S, Pope CA III, et al. Particulate matter air pollution and cardiovascular disease: an update to the scientific statement from the American Heart Association. Circulation. 2010;121:2331–78.
272. Forbes LJ, Patel MD, Rudnicka AR, et al. Chronic exposure to outdoor air pollution and markers of systemic inflammation. Epidemiology. 2009;20:245–53.
273. Goodman JE, Prueitt RL, Sax SN, et al. Ozone exposure and systemic biomarkers: evaluation of evidence for adverse cardiovascular health impacts. Crit Rev Toxicol. 2015;45:412–52.
274. Yatera K, Hsieh J, Hogg JC, et al. Particulate matter air pollution exposure promotes recruitment of monocytes into atherosclerotic plaques. Am J Physiol Heart Circ Physiol. 2008;294:H944–53.
275. Bartoli CR, Wellenius GA, Coull BA, et al. Concentrated ambient particles alter myocardial blood flow during acute ischemia in conscious canines. Environ Health Perspect. 2009;117:333–7.
276. Campen MJ, Babu NS, Helms GA, et al. Nonparticulate components of diesel exhaust promote constriction in coronary arteries from ApoE_/_ mice. Toxicol Sci. 2005;88:95–102.
277. Cherng TW, Campen MJ, Knuckles TL, Gonzalez Bosc L, Kanagy NL. Impairment of coronary endothelial cell ETB receptor function after short-term inhalation exposure to whole diesel emissions. Am J Physiol Regul Integr Comp Physiol. 2009;297:R640–7.
278. Lemos M, Mohallen SV, Macchione M, et al. Chronic exposure to urban air pollution induces structural alterations in murine pulmonary and coronary arteries. Inhal Toxicol. 2006;18:247–53.
279. Brucker N, Moro AM, Charão MF, et al. Biomarkers of occupational exposure to air pollution, inflammation and oxidative damage in taxi drivers. Sci Total Environ. 2013;463–464:884–93.
280. Sørensen M, Daneshvar B, Hansen M, et al. Personal PM2.5 exposure and markers of oxidative stress in blood. Environ Health Perspect. 2003;111:161–6.
281. Li W, Wilker EH, Dorans KS, et al. Short-term exposure to air pollution and biomarkers of oxidative stress: the Framingham Heart Study. J Am Heart Assoc. 2016;5:e002742.
282. Bagryantseva Y, Novotna B, Rossner P Jr, et al. Oxidative damage to biological macromolecules in Prague bus drivers and garagemen: impact of air pollution and genetic polymorphisms. Toxicol Lett. 2010;199:60–8.
283. Ren C, Fang S, Wright RO, Suh H, Schwartz J. Urinary 8-hydroxy-20-deoxyguanosine as a biomarker of oxidative DNA damage induced by ambient pollution in the Normative Aging Study. Occup Environ Med. 2011;68:562–9.
284. Rossner P Jr, Rossnerova A, Sram RJ. Oxidative stress and chromosomal aberrations in an environmentally exposed population. Mutat Res. 2011;707:34–41.

285. Huang W, Wang G, Lu SE, et al. Inflammatory and oxidative stress responses of healthy young adults to changes in air quality during the Beijing Olympics. Am J Respir Crit Care Med. 2012;186:1150–9.
286. Pell JP, Haw S, Cobbe S, et al. Smoke-free legislation and hospitalizations for acute coronary syndrome. N Engl J Med. 2008;359:482–91.
287. Bondy SC, Campbell A, editors. Inflammation, aging, and oxidative stress. Oxidative stress in applied basic research and clinical practice. Cham: Springer International Publishing; 2016.
288. Vinik AI, Arora RR, Colombo J. Age matched attenuation of both autonomic branches in chronic disease: II. Diabetes mellitus. Cleveland Clinic Heart-Brain Summit, Cleveland Clinic Lou Ruvo Center for Brain Health, Las Vegas, 23–24 Sept 2010.
289. American Diabetes Association. Standards of medical care in diabetes – 2008. Diabetes Care. 2008;31(Suppl 1):S12–54.
290. American Diabetes Association. Standards of medical care in diabetes – 2013. Diabetes Care. 2013;36(Suppl 1):S11–66.
291. Umetani K, Singer DH, McCraty R, Atkinson M. Twenty-four hour time domain heart rate variability and heart rate: relations to age and gender over nine decades. J Am Coll Cardiol. 1998;31(3):593–601.
292. Maser R, Mitchell B, Vinik AI, Freeman R. The association between cardiovascular autonomic neuropathy and mortality in individuals with diabetes, a meta-analysis. Diabetes Care. 2003;26(6):1895–901.
293. Cheyuo C, Jacob A, Wu R, Zhou M, Coppa GF, Wang P. The parasympathetic nervous system in the quest for stroke therapeutics. J Cereb Blood Flow Metab. 2011;31(5):1187–95. https://doi.org/10.1038/jcbfm.2011.24. Epub 2011 Mar 2. Review.
294. Hayflick L. Biological aging is no longer an unsolved problem. Ann N Y Acad Sci. 2007;1100:1–13.
295. Kirkwood TB. Understanding the odd science of aging. Cell. 2005;120:437–47.
296. Beckman KB, Ames BN. The free radical theory of aging matures. Physiol Rev. 1998;78:547–81.
297. Lee CK, Klopp RG, Weindruch R, Prolla TA. Gene expression profile of aging and its retardation by caloric restriction. Science. 1999;285:1390–3.
298. Stadtman ER. Protein oxidation and aging. Science. 1992;257:1220–4.
299. Balaban RS, Nemoto S, Finkel T. Mitochondria, oxidants, and aging. Cell. 2005;120:483–95.
300. Olshansky B, Sabbah HH, Hauptman PJ, Colucci WS. Parasympathetic nervous system and heart failure. Circulation. 2008;118:863–871, originally published August 18, 2008. https://doi.org/10.1161/CIRCULATIONAHA.107.760405.
301. Cencioni C, Spallotta F, Martelli F, Valente S, Mai A, Zeiher AM, Gaetano C. Oxidative stress and epigenetic regulation in aging and age-related diseases. Int J Mol Sci. 2013;14(9):17643–63. https://doi.org/10.3390/ijms140917643. Review.
302. Haigis MC, Yankner BA. The aging stress response. Mol Cell. 2010;40:333–44.
303. Sohal RS, Weindruch R. Oxidative stress, caloric restriction, and aging. Science. 1996;273:59–63.
304. Davies KJ. Oxidative stress, antioxidant defenses, and damage removal, repair, and replacement systems. IUBMB Life. 2000;50:279–89.
305. Finkel T, Holbrook NJ. Oxidants, oxidative stress and the biology of aging. Nature. 2000;408:239–47.
306. Stadtman ER. Protein oxidation in aging and age-related diseases. Ann N Y Acad Sci. 2001;928:22–38.
307. Ben-Avraham D, Muzumdar RH, Atzmon G. Epigenetic genome-wide association methylation in aging and longevity. Epigenomics. 2012;4:503–9.
308. Boon RA, Iekushi K, Lechner S, Seeger T, Fischer A, Heydt S, Kaluza D, Treguer K, Carmona G, Bonauer A, et al. MicroRNA-34a regulates cardiac aging and function. Nature. 2013;495:107–10.
309. North BJ, Sinclair DA. The intersection between aging and cardiovascular disease. Circ Res. 2012;110:1097–108.
310. Oxenham H, Sharpe N. Cardiovascular aging and heart failure. Eur J Heart Fail. 2003;5:427–34.
311. Versari D, Daghini E, Virdis A, Ghiadoni L, Taddei S. The aging endothelium, cardiovascular risk and disease in man. Exp Physiol. 2009;94:317–21.
312. Strait JB, Lakatta EG. Aging-associated cardiovascular changes and their relationship to heart failure. Heart Fail Clin. 2012;8:143–64.
313. Ota H, Tokunaga E, Chang K, Hikasa M, Iijima K, Eto M, Kozaki K, Akishita M, Ouchi Y, Kaneki M. SIRT1 inhibitor, Sirtinol, induces senescence-like growth arrest with attenuated Ras-MAPK signaling in human cancer cells. Oncogene. 2006;25:176–85.
314. Ota H, Eto M, Kano MR, Kahyo T, Setou M, Ogawa S, Iijima K, Akishita M, Ouchi Y. Induction of endothelial nitric oxide synthase, SIRT1, and catalase by statins inhibits endothelial senescence through the Akt pathway. Arterioscler Thromb Vasc Biol. 2010;30:2205–11.
315. Rahman I, Marwick J, Kirkham P. Redox modulation of chromatin remodeling: impact on histone acetylation and deacetylation, NF-kappaB and pro-inflammatory gene expression. Biochem Pharmacol. 2004;68:1255–67.
316. Repine JE, Bast A, Lankhorst I. The oxidative stress study group. Oxidative stress in chronic obstructive pulmonary disease. Am J Respir Crit Care Med. 1997;156:341–57.
317. Tuder RM, Kern JA, Miller YE. Senescence in chronic obstructive pulmonary disease. Proc Am Thorac Soc. 2012;9:62–3.
318. Yao H, Rahman I. Role of histone deacetylase 2 in epigenetics and cellular senescence: implications in lung inflammaging and COPD. Am J Physiol Lung Cell Mol Physiol. 2012;303:L557–66.
319. Sundar IK, Yao H, Rahman I. Oxidative stress and chromatin remodeling in chronic obstructive pulmonary disease and smoking-related diseases. Antioxid Redox Signal. 2012;18:1956–71.

320. Adenuga D, Yao H, March TH, Seagrave J, Rahman I. Histone deacetylase 2 is phosphorylated, ubiquitinated, and degraded by cigarette smoke. Am J Respir Cell Mol Biol. 2009;40:464–73.
321. Marwick JA, Kirkham PA, Stevenson CS, Danahay H, Giddings J, Butler K, Donaldson K, Macnee W, Rahman I. Cigarette smoke alters chromatin remodeling and induces proinflammatory genes in rat lungs. Am J Respir Cell Mol Biol. 2004;31:633–42.
322. Moodie FM, Marwick JA, Anderson CS, Szulakowski P, Biswas SK, Bauter MR, Kilty I, Rahman I. Oxidative stress and cigarette smoke alter chromatin remodeling but differentially regulate NF-κB activation and proinflammatory cytokine release in alveolar epithelial cells. FASEB J. 2004;18:1897–9.
323. Rajendrasozhan S, Yang SR, Kinnula VL, Rahman I. SIRT1, an antiinflammatory and antiaging protein, is decreased in lungs of patients with chronic obstructive pulmonary disease. Am J Respir Crit Care Med. 2008;177:861–70.
324. Yang SR, Chida AS, Bauter MR, Shafiq N, Seweryniak K, Maggirwar SB, Kilty I, Rahman I. Cigarette smoke induces proinflammatory cytokine release by activation of NF-κB and posttranslational modifications of histone deacetylase in macrophages. Am J Physiol Lung Cell Mol Physiol. 2006;291:L46–57.
325. Kedar NP. Can we prevent Parkinson's and Alzheimer's disease? J Postgrad Med. 2003;49:236–45.
326. Coppede F, Migliore L. Evidence linking genetics, environment, and epigenetics to impaired DNA repair in Alzheimer's disease. J Alzheimers Dis. 2010;20:953–66.
327. Myung NH, Zhu X, Kruman II, Castellani RJ, Petersen RB, Siedlak SL, Perry G, Smith MA, Lee HG. Evidence of DNA damage in Alzheimer disease: phosphorylation of histone H2AX in astrocytes. Age. 2008;30:209–15.
328. Zawia NH, Lahiri DK, Cardozo-Pelaez F. Epigenetics, oxidative stress, and Alzheimer disease. Free Radic Biol Med. 2009;46:1241–9.
329. Rimm EB. Folate and vitamin B6 from diet and supplements in relation to risk of coronary heart disease among women. Bibl Nutr Dieta. 2001;55:42–5. Review.
330. Gupta A, Moustapha A, Jacobsen DW, Goormastic M, Tuzcu EM, Hobbs R, Young J, James K, McCarthy P, van Lente F, Green R, Robinson K. High homocysteine, low folate, and low vitamin B6 concentrations: prevalent risk factors for vascular disease in heart transplant recipients. Transplantation. 1998;65(4):544–50.
331. Rimm EB, Willett WC, Hu FB, Sampson L, Colditz GA, Manson JE, Hennekens C, Stampfer MJ. Folate and vitamin B6 from diet and supplements in relation to risk of coronary heart disease among women. JAMA. 1998;279(5):359–64.
332. Saito A, Kaseda R, Hosojima M, Sato H. Proximal tubule cell hypothesis for cardiorenal syndrome in diabetes. Int J Nephrol. 2010;2011:957164. https://doi.org/10.4061/2011/957164.
333. Alkaitis MS, Crabtree MJ. Recoupling the cardiac nitric oxide synthases: tetrahydrobiopterin synthesis and recycling. Curr Heart Fail Rep. 2012;9(3):200–10. https://doi.org/10.1007/s11897-012-0097-5. Review.
334. Clarke R, Bennett DA, Parish S, Verhoef P, Dötsch-Klerk M, Lathrop M, Xu P, Nordestgaard BG, Holm H, Hopewell JC, Saleheen D, Tanaka T, Anand SS, Chambers JC, Kleber ME, Ouwehand WH, Yamada Y, Elbers C, Peters B, Stewart AF, Reilly MM, Thorand B, Yusuf S, Engert JC, Assimes TL, Kooner J, Danesh J, Watkins H, Samani NJ, Collins R, Peto R, MTHFR Studies Collaborative Group. Homocysteine and coronary heart disease: meta-analysis of MTHFR case-control studies, avoiding publication bias. PLoS Med. 2012;9(2):e1001177. https://doi.org/10.1371/journal.pmed.1001177. Epub 2012 Feb 21.
335. Soinio M, Marniemi J, Laakso M, Lehto S, Rönnemaa T. Elevated plasma homocysteine level is an independent predictor of coronary heart disease events in patients with type 2 diabetes mellitus. Ann Intern Med. 2004;140:94–100.
336. Moustafa AA, Hewedi DH, Eissa AM, Frydecka D, Błażej M. Homocysteine levels in schizophrenia and affective disorders – focus on cognition. Front Behav Neurosci. 2014;8:343–55.
337. Majewski M, Kozlowska A, Thoene M, Lepiarczyk E, Grzegorzewski WJ. Overview of the role of vitamins and minerals on the kynurenine pathway in health and disease. J Physiol Pharmacol. 2016;67(1):3–19. Review.
338. Uribarri J, Tuttle KR. Advanced glycation end products and nephrotoxicity of high-protein diets. Clin J Am Soc Nephrol. 2006;1(6):1293–9. Epub 2006 Sept 27.
339. Ferrier DP. Biochemistry. 6th ed. Philadelphia: Lippincott, Williams & Williams, a Wolters Kluwer Business; 2014.
340. Vinik AI, Casellini C, Nakave A, Patel C. Diabetic neuropathies. Endotext.com. http://diabetesmanager.pbworks.com/w/page/17680180/Diabetic%20Neuropathies#Oxidativestress; Last edited by Rushakoff R. 2009.
341. DePace NL, Dowinsky SK, Sherman M. The heart repair manual. New York: WW Norton and Co; 1993.
342. Dimitropoulos G, Tahrani AA, Stevens MJ. Cardiac autonomic neuropathy in patients with diabetes mellitus. World J Diabetes. 2014;5(1):17–39. Published online Feb 15, 2014. https://doi.org/10.4239/wjd.v5.i1.17.
343. Yarandi S, Srinivasan S. Diabetic gastrointestinal motility disorders and the role of enteric nervous system: current status and future directions. Neurogastroenterol Motil. 2014;26(5):611–

24. Published online 2014 Mar 24. https://doi.org/10.1111/nmo.12330.
344. Konturek SJ, Konturek PC, Brzozowski T, Bubenik GA. Role of melatonin in upper gastrointestinal tract. J Physiol Pharmacol. 2007;58(Suppl 6):23–52. Review.
345. Czesnikiewicz-Guzik M, Konturek SJ, Loster B, Wisniewska G, Majewski S. Melatonin and its role in oxidative stress related diseases of oral cavity. J Physiol Pharmacol. 2007;58(Suppl 3):5–19. Review.
346. Newsholme P, Cruzat VF, Keane KN, Carlessi R, de Bittencourt PIH. Molecular mechanisms of ROS production and oxidative stress in diabetes. Biochem J. 2016;473(24):4527–50.
347. Ilie M, Margină D. Trends in the evaluation of lipid peroxidation processes. In: Catala A, editor. Lipid peroxidation, Ch 5; 2012. p. 111–30. http://www.intechopen.com/books/lipid-peroxidation
348. Granata S, Dalla Gassa A, Tomei P, Lupo A, Zaza G. Mitochondria: a new therapeutic target in chronic kidney disease. Nutr Metab (Lond). 2015;12:49. https://doi.org/10.1186/s12986-015-0044-z. eCollection 2015. Review.
349. Esteban Zubero E, García-Gil FA, López-Pingarrón L, Alatorre-Jiménez MA, Ramirez JM, Tan DX, García JJ, Reiter RJ. Melatonin role preventing steatohepatitis and improving liver transplantation results. Cell Mol Life Sci. 2016;73(15):2911–27. https://doi.org/10.1007/s00018-016-2185-2.
350. Bavarsad Shahripour R, Harrigan MR, Alexandrov AV. N-acetylcysteine (NAC) in neurological disorders: mechanisms of action and therapeutic opportunities. Brain Behav. 2014;4(2):108–22. https://doi.org/10.1002/brb3.208. Epub 2014 Jan 13. Review.
351. Berk M, Malhi GS, Gray LJ, Dean OM. The promise of N-acetylcysteine in neuropsychiatry. Trends Pharmacol Sci. 2013;34(3):167–77. https://doi.org/10.1016/j.tips.2013.01.001. Epub 2013 Jan 29. Review.
352. Dean O, Giorlando F, Berk M. N-acetylcysteine in psychiatry: current therapeutic evidence and potential mechanisms of action. J Psychiatry Neurosci. 2011;36(2):78–86. https://doi.org/10.1503/jpn.100057. Review.
353. Smaga I, Pomierny B, Krzyżanowska W, Pomierny-Chamioło L, Miszkiel J, Niedzielska E, Ogórka A, Filip M. N-acetylcysteine possesses antidepressant-like activity through reduction of oxidative stress: behavioral and biochemical analyses in rats. Prog Neuro-Psychopharmacol Biol Psychiatry. 2012;39(2):280–7. https://doi.org/10.1016/j.pnpbp.2012.06.018. Epub 2012 Jul 20.
354. Berk M, Kapczinski F, Andreazza AC, Deana OM, Giorlando F, Maes M, Yücelb M, Gama CS, Dodd S, Dean B, Magalhãesa PVS, Amminger P, McGorry P, Malhi GS. Pathways underlying neuroprogression in bipolar disorder: focus on inflammation, oxidative stress and neurotrophic factors. Neurosci Biobehav Rev. 2011;35:804–17.
355. Lott J. The mother of all antioxidants: how health gurus are misleading you and what you should know about glutathione. Archangel Ink; 2014.
356. Varga ZV, Giricz Z, Liaudet L, Haskó G, Ferdinandy P, Pacher P. Interplay of oxidative, nitrosative/nitrative stress, inflammation, cell death and autophagy in diabetic cardiomyopathy. Biochim Biophys Acta Mol basis Dis. 2015;1852(2):232–42. https://doi.org/10.1016/j.bbadis.2014.06.030.
357. Berk M, Bodemer W, van Oudenhove T, Butkow N. Dopamine increases platelet intracellular calcium in bipolar affective disorder and controls. Int Clin Psychopharmacol. 1994;9(4):291–3.
358. Christy AL, Brown MA. The multitasking mast cell: positive and negative roles in the progression of autoimmunity. J Immunol. 2007;179(5):2673–9.
359. Gramlich T, Kleiner DE, McCullough AJ, Matteoni CA, Boparai N, Younossi ZM. Pathologic features associated with fibrosis in nonalcoholic fatty liver disease. Hum Pathol. 2004;35(2):196–9.
360. Forester BP, Harper DG, Georgakas J, Ravichandran C, Madurai N, Cohen BM. Antidepressant effects of open label treatment with coenzyme Q10 in geriatric bipolar depression. J Clin Psychopharmacol. 2015;35(3):338–40. https://doi.org/10.1097/JCP.0000000000000326.
361. Wald DS, Wald NJ, Morris JK, Law M. Folic acid, homocysteine, and cardiovascular disease: judging causality in the face of inconclusive trial evidence. BMJ. 2006;333(7578):1114–7. Review.
362. Jenkins DJA, Spence JD, Giovannucci EL, Kim YI, Josse R, Vieth R, Blanco Mejia S, Viguiliouk E, Nishi S, Sahye-Pudaruth S, Paquette M, Patel D, Mitchell S, Kavanagh M, Tsirakis T, Bachiri L, Maran A, Umatheva N, McKay T, Trinidad G, Bernstein D, Chowdhury A, Correa-Betanzo J, Del Principe G, Hajizadeh A, Jayaraman R, Jenkins A, Jenkins W, Kalaichandran R, Kirupaharan G, Manisekaran P, Qutta T, Shahid R, Silver A, Villegas C, White J, Kendall CWC, Pichika SC, Sievenpiper JL. Supplemental vitamins and minerals for CVD prevention and treatment. J Am Coll Cardiol. 2018;71(22):2570–84. https://doi.org/10.1016/j.jacc.2018.04.020.
363. Abrahaham JM, et al. The homocysteine hypothesis: still relevant to the prevention and treatment of cardiovascular disease? Cleve Clin J Med. 2010;77(12):911–8.
364. Kong X, Huang X, Zhao M, Xu B, Xu R, Song Y, Yu Y, Yang W, Zhang J, Liu L, Zhang Y, Tang G, Wang B, Hou FF, Li P, Cheng X, Zhao S, Wang X, Qin X, Li J, Huo Y. Platelet count affects efficacy of folic acid in preventing first stroke. J Am Coll Cardiol. 2018;71(19):2136–46. https://doi.org/10.1016/j.jacc.2018.02.072.
365. Glynn SA, Albanes D. Folate and cancer: a review of the literature. Nutr Cancer. 1994;22(2):101–19. Review.
366. Common questions about diet and cancer: folate and folic acid. American Cancer Society. 2017. https://www.cancer.org/healthy/eat-healthy-get-active/

acs-guidelines-nutrition-physical-activity-cancer-prevention/common questions.html.
367. Wien TN, Pike E, Wisløff T, Staff A, Smeland S, Klemp M. Cancer risk with folic acid supplements: a systematic review and meta-analysis. BMJ Open. 2012;2(1):e000653. https://doi.org/10.1136/bmjopen-2011-000653. Print 2012.
368. Wang R, Zheng Y, Huang JY, Zhang AQ, Zhou YH, Wang JN. Folate intake, serum folate levels, and prostate cancer risk: a meta-analysis of prospective studies. BMC Public Health. 2014;14:1326. https://doi.org/10.1186/1471-2458-14-1326.
369. Stott DJ, MacIntosh G, Lowe GD, Rumley A, McMahon AD, Langhorne P, Tait RC, O'Reilly DS, Spilg EG, MacDonald JB, MacFarlane PW, Westendorp RG. Randomized controlled trial of homocysteine-lowering vitamin treatment in elderly patients with vascular disease. Am J Clin Nutr. 2005;82(6):1320–6.
370. Clarke R. Lowering blood homocysteine with folic acid-based supplements: meta-analysis of randomised trials. Indian Heart J. 2000;52(7 Suppl):S59–64.
371. Huo Y, Li J, Qin X, Huang Y, Wang X, Gottesman RF, Tang G, Wang B, Chen D, He M, Fu J, Cai Y, Shi X, Zhang Y, Cui Y, Sun N, Li X, Cheng X, Wang J, Yang X, Yang T, Xiao C, Zhao G, Dong Q, Zhu D, Wang X, Ge J, Zhao L, Hu D, Liu L, Hou FF, CSPPT Investigators. Efficacy of folic acid therapy in primary prevention of stroke among adults with hypertension in China: the CSPPT randomized clinical trial. JAMA. 2015;313(13):1325–35. https://doi.org/10.1001/jama.2015.2274.
372. Xu X, Qin X, Li Y, Sun D, Wang J, Liang M, Wang B, Huo Y, Hou FF, Investigators of the Renal Substudy of the China Stroke Primary Prevention Trial (CSPPT). Efficacy of folic acid therapy on the progression of chronic kidney disease: the renal substudy of the China stroke primary prevention trial. JAMA Intern Med. 2016;176(10):1443–50. https://doi.org/10.1001/jamainternmed.2016.4687.
373. Mandaviya PR, Stolk L, Heil SG. Homocysteine and DNA methylation: a review of animal and human literature. Mol Genet Metab. 2014;113(4):243–52. https://doi.org/10.1016/j.ymgme.2014.10.006. Epub 2014 Oct 14. Review.
374. Joshi R, Adhikari S, Patro BS, Chattopadhyay S, Mukherjee T. Free radical scavenging behavior of folic acid: evidence for possible antioxidant activity. Free Radic Biol Med. 2001;30(12):1390–9.
375. Zhao M, Chen YH, Dong XT, Zhou J, Chen X, Wang H, Wu SX, Xia MZ, Zhang C, Xu DX. Folic acid protects against lipopolysaccharide-induced preterm delivery and intrauterine growth restriction through its anti-inflammatory effect in mice. PLoS One. 2013;8(12):e82713. https://doi.org/10.1371/journal.pone.0082713. eCollection 2013.
376. Cantó C, Menzies KJ, Auwerx J. NAD(+) metabolism and the control of energy homeostasis: a balancing act between mitochondria and the nucleus. Cell Metab. 2015;22:31–53.
377. Huang J-Y, Hirschey MD, Shimazu T, Ho L, Verdin E. Mitochondrial sirtuins. Biochim Biophys Acta 2010;1804:1645–51.
378. Correia M, Perestrelo T, Rodrigues AS, et al. Sirtuins in metabolism, stemness and differentiation. Biochim Biophys Acta. 2017;1861(1 Pt A): 3444–55.
379. Cheng H-L, Mostoslavsky R, Saito S, et al. Developmental defects and p53 hyperacetylation in Sir2 homolog (SIRT1)-deficient mice. Proc Natl Acad Sci U S A. 2003;100:10794–9.
380. Kirkland JB. Niacin requirements for genomic stability. Mutat Res. 2012;733:14–20.
381. Shi H, Enriquez A, Rapadas M, Martin EMMA, Wang R, Moreau J, Lim CK, Szot JO, Ip E, Hughes JN, Sugimoto K, Humphreys DT, McInerney-Leo AM, Leo PJ, Maghzal GJ, Halliday J, Smith J, Colley A, Mark PR, Collins F, Sillence DO, Winlaw DS, Ho JWK, Guillemin GJ, Brown MA, Kikuchi K, Thomas PQ, Stocker R, Giannoulatou E, Chapman G, Duncan EL, Sparrow DB, Dunwoodie SL. NAD deficiency, congenital malformations, and niacin supplementation. N Engl J Med. 2017;377(6):544–52. https://doi.org/10.1056/NEJMoa1616361.
382. Celinski K, Konturek PC, Slomka M, Cichoz-Lach H, Brzozowski T, Konturek SJ, Korolczuk A. Effects of treatment with melatonin and tryptophan on liver enzymes, parameters of fat metabolism and plasma levels of cytokines in patients with non-alcoholic fatty liver disease – 14 months follow up. J Physiol Pharmacol. 2014;65(1):75–82.
383. Vinik AI, Maser RE, Nakave AA. Diabetic cardiovascular autonomic nerve dysfunction. US Endocr Dis. 2007;2:2–9.
384. Vinik A, Ziegler D. Diabetic cardiovascular autonomic neuropathy. Circulation. 2007;115:387–97.
385. Vinik AI, Freeman R, Erbas T. Diabetic autonomic neuropathy. Semin Neurol. 2003;23:365–72.
386. Vinik A, Erbas T, Pfeifer M, Feldman E, Stevens M, Russell J. Diabetic autonomic neuropathy. In: Zucchi SE, editor. The diabetes mellitus manual: a primary care companion to Ellenberg and Rifkin's. 6th ed. New York: McGraw Hill; 2004. p. 351.
387. Ziegler D, Low PA, Litchy WJ, Boulton AJM, Vinik AI, Freeman R, The NATHAN 1 Trial Group. Efficacy and safety of antioxidant treatment with α-lipoic acid over 4 years in diabetic polyneuropathy. Diabetes Care. 2011;34:2054–60.
388. Vinik AI, Maser RE, Ziegler D. Neuropathy. The crystal ball for cardiovascular disease. Diabetes Care. 2010;33(7):1688–90.
389. Vinik AI, Maser RE, Ziegler D. Autonomic imbalance: prophet of doom or scope for hope? Diabet Med. 2011;28:643–51.
390. Vinik AI. The conductor of the autonomic orchestra. Front Endocrinol. 2012;3(71):1–13.
391. Vinik AI, Nevoret ML, Casellini CM, Parson H. Diabetic neuropathy. Endocrinol Metab Clin N Am. 2013;42(4):747–87. https://doi.org/10.1016/j.ecl.2013.06.001. Review.

392. Maser RE, Mitchell BD, Vinik AI, et al. The association between cardiovascular autonomic neuropathy and mortality in individuals with diabetes: A meta-analysis. Diabetes Care. 2003;26:1895–901.
393. Vinik AI, Erbas T, Casellini CM. Diabetic cardiac autonomic neuropathy, inflammation and cardiovascular disease. J Diab Invest. 2013;4(1):4–18.
394. Vinik AI, Mehrabyan A. Diabetic neuropathies. Med Clin N Am. 2004;88:947–99.
395. Vinik AI, Strotmeyer ES, Nakave AA, Patel CV. Diabetic neuropathy in older adults. Clin Geriatr Med. 2008;24:407–35.
396. Vinik AI, Erbas T. Cardiovascular autonomic neuropathy: diagnosis and management. Curr Diab Rep. 2006;6:424–30.
397. Feldman EL. Oxidative stress and diabetic neuropathy: a new understanding of an old problem. J Clin Invest. 2003;111(4):431–3.
398. Tsuji H, Venditti FJ Jr, Manders ES, Evans JC, Larson MG, Feldman CL, Levy D. Reduced heart rate variability and mortality risk in an elderly cohort. The Framingham Heart Study. Circulation. 1994;90(2):878–83.
399. Vallianou N, Evangelopoulos A, Koutalas P. Alpha-lipoic acid and diabetic neuropathy. Rev Diabet Stud. 2009;6(4):230–6. https://doi.org/10.1900/RDS.2009.6.230. Epub 2009 Dec 30.
400. Ziegler D, Sohr CG, Nourooz-Zadeh J. Oxidative stress and antioxidant defense in relation to the severity of diabetic polyneuropathy and cardiovascular autonomic neuropathy. Diabetes Care. 2004;27:2178–83.
401. Ziegler D, Gries F. Alpha-lipoic acid and the treatment of diabetic peripheral autonomic cardiac neuropathy. Diabetes. 1997;46(Suppl 2):S62–6.
402. Prendergast JJ. Diabetic autonomic neuropathy: part 2. Treatment. Pract Diabetol. 2001:30–6.
403. Ziegler D, Ametov A, Barinov A, Dyck PJ, Gurieva I, Low PA, Munzel U, Yakhno N, Raz I, Novosadova M, Maus J, Samigullin R. Oral treatment with alpha-lipoic acid improves symptomatic diabetic polyneuropathy: The SYDNEY 2 trial. Diabetes Care. 2006;29(11):2365–70.
404. Ametov AS, Barinov A, Dyck PJ, Hermann R, Kozlova N, Litchy WJ, Low PA, Nehrdich D, Novosadova M, O'Brien PC, Reljanovic M, Samigullin R, Schuette K, Strokov I, Tritschler HJ, Wessel K, Yakhno N, Ziegler D, SYDNEY Trial Study Group. The sensory symptoms of diabetic polyneuropathy are improved with alpha-lipoic acid. The SYDNEY trial. Diabetes Care. 2003;26(3):770–6.
405. Ziegler D, Low PA, Litchy WJ, Boulton AJM, Vinik AI, Freeman R, The NATHAN 1 Trial Group. Efficacy and safety of antioxidant treatment with α-lipoic acid over 4 years in diabetic polyneuropathy. Diabetes Care. 2011;34:2054–60.
406. Serhiyenko VA, Serhiyenko AA. Diabetic cardiac autonomic neuropathy: do we have any treatment perspectives? World J Diabetes. 2015;6(2):245–58. https://doi.org/10.4239/wjd.v6.i2.245. Review.
407. Keen H, Payan J, Allawi J, Walker J, Jamal GA, Weir AI, Henderson LM, Bissessar EA, Watkins PJ, Sampson M, Gale EA, Scarpello J, Boddie HG, Hardy KJ, Thomas PK, Misra P, Halonen JP. Treatment of diabetic neuropathy with gamma-linolenic acid. Diabetes Care. 1993;16:8–15.
408. De Marchi E, Baldassari F, Bononi A, Wieckowski MR, Pinton P. Oxidative stress in cardiovascular diseases and obesity: role of p66Shc and protein kinase C. Oxidative Med Cell Longev. 2013;2013:564961. https://doi.org/10.1155/2013/564961. Epub 2013 Mar 27. Review.
409. Pittenger G, Vinik A. Nerve growth factor and diabetic neuropathy. Exp Diabesity Res. 2003;4:271–85.
410. Rivard A, Silver M, Chen D, Kearney M, Magner M, Annex B, Peters K, Isner JM. Rescue of diabetes-related impairment of angiogenesis by intramuscular gene therapy with adeno-VEGF. Am J Pathol. 1999;154:355–63.
411. Tam J, Rosenberg L, Maysinger D. INGAP peptide improves nerve function and enhances regeneration in streptozotocin-induced diabetic C57BL/6 mice. FASEB J. 2004;18:1767–9.
412. Milicevic Z, Newlon PG, Pittenger GL, Stansberry KB, Vinik AI. Anti-ganglioside GM1 antibody and distal symmetric "diabetic polyneuropathy" with dominant motor features. Diabetologia. 1997;40:1364–5.
413. Sharma K, Cross J, Farronay O, Ayyar D, Sheber R, Bradley W. Demyelinating neuropathy in diabetes mellitus. Arch Neurol. 2002;59:758–65.
414. Krendel DA, Costigan DA, Hopkins LC. Successful treatment of neuropathies in patients with diabetes mellitus. Arch Neurol. 1995;52:1053–61.
415. Vinik AI, Maser RE, Mitchell BD, Freeman R. Diabetic autonomic neuropathy. Diabetes Care. 2003;26(5):1553–79.
416. Pfeifer MA, Weinberg CR, Cook DL, Reenan A, Halter JB, Ensinck JW. Autonomic neural dysfunction in recently diagnosed diabetic subjects. Diabetes Care. 1984;7:447–53.
417. Stansberry KB, Hill MA, Shapiro SA, McNitt PM, Bhatt BA, Vinik AI. Impairment of peripheral blood flow responses in diabetes resembles an enhanced aging effect. Diabetes Care. 1997;20:1711–6.
418. Stansberry KB, Shapiro SA, Hill MA, McNitt PM, Meyer MD, Vinik AI. Impaired peripheral vasomotion in diabetes. Diabetes Care. 1996;19:715–21.
419. Stansberry KB, Hill MA, Shapiro SA, McNitt PM, Bhatt BA, Vinik AI. Impairment of peripheral blood flow responses in diabetes resembles an enhanced aging effect. Diabetes Care. 1997;20:1711–6.
420. Stansberry KB. Primary nociceptive afferents mediate the blood flow dysfunction in non-glabrous (hairy) skin of type 2 diabetes. Diabetes Care. 1999;22:1549–54.

421. Haak ES, Usadel KH, Kohleisen M, Yilmaz A, Kusterer K, Haak T. The effect of alpha-lipoic on the neurovascular reflex arc in patients with diabetic neuropathy assessed by capillary microscopy. Microvasc Res. 1999;58:28–34.
422. Ziegler D. Diabetic cardiovascular autonomic neuropathy: prognosis, diagnosis and treatment. Diabetes Metab Rev. 1994;10:339–83.
423. Valensi P. Diabetic autonomic neuropathy: what are the risks? Diabetes Metab. 1998;24:66–72.
424. Levitt NS, Stansberry KB, Wychanck S, Vinik AI. Natural progression of autonomic neuropathy and autonomic function tests in a cohort of IDDM. Diabetes Care. 1996;19:751–4.
425. Gaede P, Vedel P, Larsen N, Jensen GV, Parving HH, Pedersen O. Multifactorial intervention and cardiovascular disease in patients with type 2 diabetes. N Engl J Med. 2003;348:383–93.
426. Gaede P, Lund-Andersen H, Parving HH, Pedersen O. Effect of a multifactorial intervention on mortality in type 2 diabetes. N Engl J Med. 2008;358:580–91.
427. Edwards JL, Vincent AM, Cheng HT, Feldman EL. Diabetic neuropathy: mechanisms to management. Pharmacol Ther. 2008;120:1–34.
428. Vinik AI, Freeman R, Erbas T. Diabetic autonomic neuropathy. Semin Neurol. 2003;23:365–72.
429. Leinninger GM, Edwards JL, Lipshaw MJ, Feldman EL. Mechanisms of disease: mitochondria as new therapeutic targets in diabetic neuropathy. Nat Clin Pract Neurol. 2006;2:620–8.
430. Soriano FG, Virág L, Szabó C. Diabetic endothelial dysfunction: role of reactive oxygen and nitrogen species production and poly(ADP-ribose) polymerase activation. J Mol Med (Berl). 2001;79:437–48.
431. Obrosova IG, Julius UA. Role for poly(ADP-ribose) polymerase activation in diabetic nephropathy, neuropathy and retinopathy. Curr Vasc Pharmacol. 2005;3:267–83.
432. Yamagishi S, Uehara K, Otsuki S, Yagihashi S. Differential influence of increased polyol pathway on protein kinase C expressions between endoneurial and epineurial tissues in diabetic mice. J Neurochem. 2003;87:497–507.
433. Giacco F, Brownlee M. Oxidative stress and diabetic complications. Circ Res. 2010;107:1058–70.
434. Williams B, Gallacher B, Patel H, Orme C. Glucose-induced protein kinase C activation regulates vascular permeability factor mRNA expression and peptide production by human vascular smooth muscle cells in vitro. Diabetes. 1997;46:1497–503.
435. Russell JW, Sullivan KA, Windebank AJ, Herrmann DN, Feldman EL. Neurons undergo apoptosis in animal and cell culture models of diabetes. Neurobiol Dis. 1999;6:347–63.
436. Ramasamy R, Vannucci SJ, Yan SS, Herold K, Yan SF, Schmidt AM. Advanced glycation end products and RAGE: a common thread in aging, diabetes, neurodegeneration, and inflammation. Glycobiology. 2005;15:16R–28R.
437. Kolm-Litty V, Sauer U, Nerlich A, Lehmann R, Schleicher ED. High glucose-induced transforming growth factor beta1 production is mediated by the hexosamine pathway in porcine glomerular mesangial cells. J Clin Invest. 1998;101:160–9.
438. Wada R, Yagihashi S. Role of advanced glycation end products and their receptors in development of diabetic neuropathy. Ann N Y Acad Sci. 2005;1043:598–604.
439. Sayeski PP, Kudlow JE. Glucose metabolism to glucosamine is necessary for glucose stimulation of transforming growth factor-alpha gene transcription. J Biol Chem. 1996;271:15237–43.
440. Narkiewicz K, Somers VK. Sympathetic nerve activity in obstructive sleep apnoea. Acta Physiol Scand. 2003;177:385–90.
441. Bradley TD, Floras JS. Obstructive sleep apnoea and its cardiovascular consequences. Lancet. 2009;373:82–93.
442. Tahrani AA, Ali A, Raymond NT, Begum S, Dubb K, Mughal S, Jose B, Piya MK, Barnett AH, Stevens MJ. Obstructive sleep apnea and diabetic neuropathy: a novel association in patients with type 2 diabetes. Am J Respir Crit Care Med. 2012;186:434–41.
443. Ficker JH, Dertinger SH, Siegfried W, König HJ, Pentz M, Sailer D, Katalinic A, Hahn EG. Obstructive sleep apnoea and diabetes mellitus: the role of cardiovascular autonomic neuropathy. Eur Respir J. 1998;11(1):14–9.
444. Janovsky CC, Rolim LC, de Sá JR, Poyares D, Tufik S, Silva AB, Dib SA. Cardiovascular autonomic neuropathy contributes to sleep apnea in young and lean type 1 diabetes mellitus patients. Front Endocrinol (Lausanne). 2014;5:119. https://doi.org/10.3389/fendo.2014.00119. eCollection 2014.
445. Axelrod S, Lishner M, Oz O, Bernheim J, Ravid M. Spectral analysis of fluctuations in heart rate: an objective evaluation of autonomic nervous control in chronic renal failure. Nephron. 1987;45:202–6.
446. Felten SY, Peterson RG, Shea PA, Besch HR, Felten DL. Effects of streptozotocin diabetes on the noradrenergic innervation of the rat heart: a longitudinal histofluorescence and neurochemical study. Brain Res Bull. 1982;8:593–607.
447. Poulsen PL, Hansen KW, Mogensen CE. Increase in nocturnal blood pressure and progression to microalbuminuria in diabetes. N Engl J Med. 2003;348:260–24; author reply 260–24.
448. Hirabara SM, Silveira LR, Alberici LC, Leandro CV, Lambertucci RH, Polimeno GC, Cury Boaventura MF, Procopio J, Vercesi AE, Curi R. Acute effect of fatty acids on metabolism and mitochondrial coupling in skeletal muscle. Biochim Biophys Acta. 2006;1757:57–66.
449. Schrauwen P, Hoeks J, Hesselink MK. Putative function and physiological relevance of the mitochondrial uncoupling protein-3: involvement in fatty acid metabolism. Prog Lipid Res. 2006;45:17–41.
450. Collins-Nakai RL, Noseworthy D, Lopaschuk GD. Epinephrine increases ATP production in hearts

by preferentially increasing glucose metabolism. Am J Phys. 1994;267:H1862–71.
451. Francis GS. Diabetic cardiomyopathy: fact or fiction. Heart. 2001;85:247–8.
452. Frustaci A, Kajstura J, Chimenti C, Jakoniuk I, Leri A, Maseri A, Nadal-Ginard B, Anversa P. Myocardial cell death in human diabetes. Circ Res. 2000;87:1123–32.
453. Katz AM. Potential deleterious effects of inotropic agents in the therapy of chronic heart failure. Circulation. 1986;73:III184–90.
454. Eichhorn EJ, Bristow MR. Medical therapy can improve the biological properties of the chronically failing heart. A new era in the treatment of heart failure. Circulation. 1996;94:2285–96.
455. Yaplito-Lee J, Weintraub R, Jamsen K, Chow CW, Thorburn DR, Boneh A. Cardiac manifestations in oxidative phosphorylation disorders of childhood. J Pediatr. 2007;150:407–11.
456. Givertz MM, Sawyer DB, Colucci WS. Antioxidants and myocardial contractility: illuminating the "dark side" of beta-adrenergic receptor activation. Circulation. 2001;103:782–3.
457. Scacco S, Vergari R, Scarpulla RC, Technikova-Dobrova Z, Sardanelli A, Lambo R, Lorusso V, Papa S. cAMP-dependent phosphorylation of the nuclear encoded 18-kDa (IP) subunit of respiratory complex I and activation of the complex in serum-starved mouse fibroblast cultures. J Biol Chem. 2000;275:17578–82.
458. An D, Rodrigues B. Role of changes in cardiac metabolism in development of diabetic cardiomyopathy. Am J Physiol Heart Circ Physiol. 2006;291:H1489–506.
459. Iwai-Kanai E, Hasegawa K, Araki M, Kakita T, Morimoto T, Sasayama S. Alpha- and beta-adrenergic pathways differentially regulate cell type-specific apoptosis in rat cardiac myocytes. Circulation. 1999;100:305–11. Communal C, Singh K, Pimentel DR, Colucci WS. Norepinephrine stimulates apoptosis in adult rat ventricular myocytes by activation of the beta-adrenergic pathway. Circulation. 1998;98:1329–1334.
460. Communal C, Singh K, Pimentel DR, Colucci WS. Norepinephrine stimulates apoptosis in adult rat ventricular myocytes by activation of the beta-adrenergic pathway. Circulation. 1998;98:1329–34.
461. Carnethon MR, Prineas RJ, Temprosa M, Zhang ZM, Uwaifo G, Molitch ME. The association among autonomic nervous system function, incident diabetes, and intervention arm in the Diabetes Prevention Program. Diabetes Care. 2006;29:914–9.
462. Maser RE, Lenhard MJ. An overview of the effect of weight loss on cardiovascular autonomic function. Curr Diabetes Rev. 2007;3:204–11.
463. Voulgari C, Pagoni S, Vinik A, Poirier P. Exercise improves cardiac autonomic function in obesity and diabetes. Metabolism. 2013;62:609–21.
464. Golbidi S, Ebadi SA, Laher I. Antioxidants in the treatment of diabetes. Curr Diabetes Rev. 2011;7:106–25.
465. Rhee SH, Pothoulakis C, Mayer EA. Principles and clinical implications of the brain-gut-enteric microbiota axis. Nat Rev Gastroenterol Hepatol. 2009;6:306–14.
466. Finaud J, Lac G, Filaire E. Oxidative stress. Sports Med. 2006;36:327–58.
467. Powers SK, Talbert EE, Adhihetty PJ. Reactive oxygen and nitrogen species as intracellular signals in skeletal muscle. J Physiol. 2011;589:2129–38.
468. Silvestri S, Orlando P, Armeni T, Padella L, Brugè F, Seddaiu G, Littarru GP, Tiano L. Coenzyme Q10 and α-lipoic acid: antioxidant and pro-oxidant effects in plasma and peripheral blood lymphocytes of supplemented subjects. J Clin Biochem Nutr. 2015;57(1):21–6. Published online 2015 Apr 16. https://doi.org/10.3164/jcbn.14-130.
469. Dröge W. Free radicals in the physiological control of cell function. Physiol Rev. 2002;82:47–95.
470. Niess AM. Generation and disposal of reactive oxygen and nitrogen species. In: Mooren FC, Volker K, editors. Molecular and cellular exercise physiology. Champaign: Human Kinetics; 2005. p. 179–97.
471. Powers SK, Deruisseau KC, Quindry J, Hamilton KL. Dietary antioxidants and exercise. J Sports Sci. 2004;22:81–94.
472. Christofidou-Solomidou M, Muzykantov VR. Antioxidant strategies in respiratory medicine. Treat Respir Med. 2006;5(1):47–78. Review.
473. Halliwell B. Oxidative stress and neurodegeneration: where are we now? J Neurochem. 2006;97(6):1634–58. Review.
474. Sies H. Oxidative stress: oxidants and antioxidants. Exp Physiol. 1997;82(2):291–5. Review.
475. Aruoma OI, Halliwell B, Laughton MJ, Quinlan GJ, Gutteridge JM. The mechanism of initiation of lipid peroxidation. Evidence against a requirement for an iron(II)-iron(III) complex. Biochem J. 1989;258(2):617–20.
476. Elroy-Stein O, Bernstein Y, Groner Y. Overproduction of human Cu/Zn-superoxide dismutase in transfected cells: extenuation of paraquat-mediated cytotoxicity and enhancement of lipid peroxidation. EMBO J. 1986;5(3):615–22.
477. Freinbichler W, Colivicchi MA, Stefanini C, Bianchi L, Ballini C, Misini B, Weinberger P, Linert W, Vareŝlija D, Tipton KF, Della CL. Highly reactive oxygen species: detection, formation, and possible functions. Cell Mol Life Sci. 2011;68(12):2067–79. https://doi.org/10.1007/s00018-011-0682-x. Epub 2011 May 2. Review.
478. Halliwell B, Gutteridge JM. Role of iron in oxygen radical reactions. Methods Enzymol. 1984;105:47–56.
479. Velayutham M, Hemann C, Zweier JL. Removal of $H_2O_2$ and generation of superoxide radical: role of cytochrome c and NADH. Free Radic Biol Med.

2011;51(1):160–70. https://doi.org/10.1016/j.freeradbiomed.2011.04.007. Epub 2011 Apr 13.
480. Gordon MH. Significance of dietary antioxidants for health. Int J Mol Sci. 2012;13(1):173–9. https://doi.org/10.3390/ijms13010173. Epub 2011 Dec 23. Review.
481. Halliwell B. Reactive species and antioxidants. Redox biology is a fundamental theme of aerobic life. Plant Physiol. 2006;141(2):312–22.
482. Halliwell B. Phagocyte-derived reactive species: salvation or suicide? Trends Biochem Sci. 2006;31(9):509–15. Epub 2006 Aug 4. Review.
483. Powers SK, Lennon SL. Analysis of cellular responses to free radicals: focus on exercise and skeletal muscle. Proc Nutr Soc London. 1999;58:1025–33.
484. Seifried HE, Anderson DE, Fisher EI, Milner JA. A review of the interaction among dietary antioxidants and reactive oxygen species. J Nutr Biochem. 2007;18:567–79.
485. MacRae HS, Mefferd KM. Dietary antioxidant supplementation combined with quercetin improves cycling time trial performance. Int J Sport Nutr Exerc Metab. 2006;16:405–19.
486. Oh J, Shin Y, Yoon J, et al. Effect of supplementation with Ecklonia cava polyphenol on endurance performance of college students. Int J Sport Nutr Exerc Metab. 2010;20:72–9.
487. Villegas L, Stidham T, Nozik-Grayck E. Oxidative stress and therapeutic development in lung diseases. J Pulm Respir Med. 2014;4(4). pii: 194. Epub 2014 Jul 15.
488. Chapple SJ, Cheng X, Mann GE. Effects of 4-hydroxynonenal on vascular endothelial and smooth muscle cell redox signaling and function in health and disease. Redox Biol. 2013;1:319–31.
489. Ushio-Fukai M. VEGF signaling through NADPH oxidase-derived ROS. Antioxid Redox Signal. 2007;9:731–9.
490. Urao N, Ushio-Fukai M. Redox regulation of stem/progenitor cells and bone marrow niche. Free Radic Biol Med. 2013;54:26–39.
491. Baran CP, Zeigler MM, Tridandapani S, Marsh CB. The role of ROS and RNS in regulating life and death of blood monocytes. Curr Pharm Des. 2004;10:855–66.
492. Fialkow L, Wang Y, Downey GP. Reactive oxygen and nitrogen species as signaling molecules regulating neutrophil function. Free Radic Biol Med. 2007;42:153–64.
493. Birukov KG. Cyclic stretch, reactive oxygen species, and vascular remodeling. Antioxid Redox Signal. 2009;11:1651–67.
494. Frazziano G, Champion HC, Pagano PJ. NADPH oxidase-derived ROS and the regulation of pulmonary vessel tone. Am J Physiol Heart Circ Physiol. 2012;302:H2166–77.
495. Knock GA, Ward JP. Redox regulation of protein kinases as a modulator of vascular function. Antioxid Redox Signal. 2011;15:1531–47.
496. Janssen LJ. Isoprostanes and lung vascular pathology. Am J Respir Cell Mol Biol. 2008;39:383–9
497. Janssen LJ, Catalli A, Helli P. The pulmonary biology of isoprostanes. Antioxid Redox Signal. 2005;7:244–55.
498. Ckless K. Redox proteomics: from bench to bedside. Adv Exp Med Biol. 2014;806:301–17.
499. Matsuo M, Kaneko T. The chemistry of reactive oxygen species and related free radicals. In: Radak Z, editor. Free radicals in exercise and aging. Leeds: Human Kinetics; 2000. p. 1–34.
500. Sawka MN, Burke LM, Eichner ER, Maughan RJ, Montain SJ, et al. American College of Sports Medicine position stand. Exercise and fluid replacement. Med Sci Sports Exerc. 2007;39(2):377–90. PMID: 17277604.
501. Paik IY, Jeong MH, Jin HE, Kim YI, Suh AR, et al. Fluid replacement following dehydration reduces oxidative stress during recovery. Biochem Biophys Res Commun. 2009;383(1):103–7. https://doi.org/10.1016/j.bbrc.2009.03.135.
502. Ziegler D, Schatz H, Conrad F, Gries FA, Ulrich H, Reichel G. Effects of treatment with the antioxidant alpha-lipoic acid on cardiac autonomic neuropathy in NIDDM patients. A 4-month randomized controlled multicenter trial (DEKAN Study). Deutsche Kardiale Autonome Neuropathy. Diabetes Care. 1997;20:369–73.
503. Spallone V, Ziegler D, Freeman R, Bernardi L, Frontoni S, Pop-Busui R, Stevens M, Kempler P, Hilsted J, Tesfaye S, Low P, Valensi P; On Behalf of the Toronto Consensus Panel on Diabetic Neuropathy*. Cardiovascular autonomic neuropathy in diabetes: clinical impact, assessment, diagnosis, and management. Diabetes Metab Res Rev. 2011;27(7):639–53; Epub ahead of print.
504. Manzella D, Barbieri M, Ragno E, Paolisso G. Chronic administration of pharmacologic doses of vitamin E improves the cardiac autonomic nervous system in patients with type 2 diabetes. Am J Clin Nutr. 2001;73:1052–7.
505. Ametov AS, Barinov A, Dyck PJ, Hermann R, Kozlova N, Litchy WJ, Low PA, Nehrdich D, Novosadova M, O'Brien PC, Reljanovic M, Samigullin R, Schuette K, Strokov I, Tritschler HJ, Wessel K, Yakhno N, Ziegler D. The sensory symptoms of diabetic polyneuropathy are improved with alpha-lipoic acid: the SYDNEY trial. Diabetes Care. 2003;26:770–6.
506. Ruhnau KJ, Meissner HP, Finn R, Reljanovic M, Lobisch M, Schutte K, Nehrdich D, Tritschler H, Mehnert H, Ziegler D. Effects of 3-week oral treatment with the antioxidant thioctic acid (alpha-lipoic acid) in symptomatic diabetic polyneuropathy. Diabet Med. 1999;16(12):1040–3.
507. Ziegler D, Hanefeld M, Ruhnau KJ, Meissner HP, Lobisch M, Schutte K, Gries FA. Treatment of symptomatic diabetic peripheral neuropathy with the anti-oxidant alpha-lipoic acid. A 3-week multicentre

randomized controlled trial (ALADIN Study). Diabetologia. 1995;38:1425–33.
508. Reljanovic M, Reichel G, Rett K, Lobisch M, Schuette K, Moller W, Tritschler HJ, Mehnert H. Treatment of diabetic polyneuropathy with the antioxidant thioctic acid (alpha-lipoic acid): a two year multicenter randomized double-blind placebo-controlled trial (ALADIN II). Alpha Lipoic Acid in Diabetic Neuropathy. Free Radic Res. 1999;31(3):171–9.
509. Ziegler D, Nowak H, Kempler P, Vargha P, Low PA. Treatment of symptomatic diabetic polyneuropathy with the antioxidant alpha-lipoic acid: a meta-analysis. Diabet Med. 2004;21:114–21.
510. Mortensen SA, Rosenfeldt F, Kumar A, Dolliner P, Filipiak KJ, Pella D, Alehagen U, Steurer G, Littarru GP, Q-SYMBIO Study Investigators. The effect of coenzyme Q10 on morbidity and mortality in chronic heart failure: results from Q-SYMBIO: a randomized double-blind trial. JACC Heart Fail. 2014;2(6):641–9. https://doi.org/10.1016/j.jchf.2014.06.008. Epub 2014 Oct 1.
511. Rosenfeldt FL, Haas SJ, Krum H, Hadj A, Ng K, Leong JY, Watts GF. Coenzyme Q10 in the treatment of hypertension: a meta-analysis of the clinical trials. J Hum Hypertens. 2007;21(4):297–306. Epub 2007 Feb 8.
512. Rosenfeldt F, Hilton D, Pepe S, Krum H. Systematic review of effect of coenzyme Q10 in physical exercise, hypertension and heart failure. Biofactors. 2003;18(1–4):91–100. Review.
513. Deichmann R, Lavie C, Andrews S. Coenzyme q10 and statin-induced mitochondrial dysfunction. Ochsner J. 2010;10(1):16–21.
514. Greene DA, Arezzo JC, Brown MB. Effect of aldose reductase inhibition on nerve conduction and morphometry in diabetic neuropathy. Zenarestat Study Group. Neurology. 1999;53:580–91.
515. Hotta N, Toyota T, Matsuoka K, Shigeta Y, Kikkawa R, Kaneko T, Takahashi A, Sugimura K, Koike Y, Ishii J, Sakamoto N, The SNK-860 Diabetic Neuropathy Study Group. Clinical efficacy of fidarestat, a novel aldose reductase inhibitor, for diabetic peripheral neuropathy. Diabetes Care. 2001;24:1776–82.
516. Hotta N, Shigeta Y, Sakamoto N. Long-term effects of epalrestat, an aldose reductase inhibitor, on diabetic peripheral neuropathy: A 3-y multicenter comparative study, ARI-diabetes complications trial (ADCT) (abstract). Diabetes. 2005;54:A213.
517. Vinik AI, Mehrabyan A. Diabetic neuropathies. Med Clin North Am. 2004;88:947–99, xi.
518. Vinik AI, Bril V, Litchy WJ, Price KL, Bastyr EJ III. Sural sensory action potential identifies diabetic peripheral neuropathy responders to therapy. Muscle Nerve. 2005;32(5):619–25.
519. Casellini CM, Barlow PM, Rice AL, Casey M, Simmons K, Pittenger G, Bastyr EJ III, Wolka AM, Vinik AI. A 6-month, randomized, double-masked, placebo-controlled study evaluating the effects of the protein kinase C-{beta} inhibitor ruboxistaurin on skin microvascular blood flow and other measures of diabetic peripheral neuropathy. Diabetes Care. 2007;30:896–902.
520. Myung SK, Ju W, Cho B, Oh SW, Park SM, Koo BK, Park BJ. Efficacy of vitamin and antioxidant supplements in prevention of cardiovascular disease: systematic review and meta-analysis of randomised controlled trials. BMJ. 2013;346:f10. Published online 2013 Jan 18. https://doi.org/10.1136/bmj.f10
521. Abilés J, de la Cruz AP, Castaño J, Rodríguez-Elvira M, Aguayo E, Moreno-Torres R, Llopis J, Aranda P, Argüelles S, Ayala A, de la Quintana AM, Planells EM. Oxidative stress is increased in critically ill patients according to antioxidant vitamins intake, independent of severity: a cohort study. Crit Care. 2006;10(5):R146.
522. Therond P, Bonnefont-Rousselout D, Davit-Sparaul A, Conti M, Legrand A. Biomarkers of oxidative stress: an analytical approach. Curr Opin Clin Nutr Metab Care. 2000;3:373–84. https://doi.org/10.1097/00075197-200009000-00009.
523. Alonso de la Vega JM, Díaz J, Serrano E, Carbonell LF. Plasma redox status relates to severity in critically ill patients. Crit Care Med. 2000;28:1812–4. https://doi.org/10.1097/00003246-200006000-00021.
524. Motoyama T, Okamoto K, Kukita I, Hamaguchi M, Kinoshita Y, Ogawa H. Possible role of increase oxidant stress in multiple organ failure after systemic inflammatory response syndrome. Crit Care Med. 2003;31:1048–52. https://doi.org/10.1097/01.CCM.0000055371.27268.36.
525. Goode HF, Cowley HC, Walker BE, Howdle PD, Webster NR. Decreased antioxidant status and increased lipid peroxidation in patients with septic shock and secondary organ dysfunction. Crit Care Med. 1995;23:646–51. https://doi.org/10.1097/00003246-199504000-00011.
526. Grimble RF. Nutrition antioxidants and the modulation of inflammation theory and practice. New Horiz. 1994;2:175–85.
527. Hammerman C, Kaplan M. Ischemia and reperfusion injury. Clin Perinatol. 1998;25:757–77.
528. Yu BP. Cellular defenses against damage from reactive species. Physiol Rev. 1994;74:139–62.
529. Jeevanandam M, Begay CK, Shahbazian LM, Scott R, Petersen MD. Altered plasma cytokines and total glutathione levels in parenterally fed critically ill trauma patients with adjuvant recombinant human growth hormone therapy. Crit Care Med. 2000;28:324–9. https://doi.org/10.1097/00003246-200002000-00006.
530. Nathens AB, Neff MJ, Jurkavich GJ. Randomized, prospective trial of antioxidant supplementation in critically ill surgical patients. Ann Surg. 2002;236:814–22. https://doi.org/10.1097/00000658-200212000-00014.
531. Preiser JC, Gossum AV, Berré J, Vincent JL, Carpentier Y. Enteral feeding with a solution enriched with antioxidant vitamins A, C and E enhances the resistance to oxidative stress.

Crit Care Med. 2000;28:3828–32. https://doi.org/10.1097/00003246-200012000-00013.

532. Crimi E, Liguori A, Condorelli M, Cioffi M, Astuto M, Bontempo P, Pignalosa O, Viteri MT, Molinari AM, Sica V, et al. The beneficial effects of antioxidant supplementation in enteral feeding in critically ill patients: a prospective, randomized, double-blind, placebo-controlled trial. Anesth Analg. 2004;99:857–63. https://doi.org/10.1213/01.ANE.0000133144.60584.F6.
533. Rahman I, Biswas SK, Kode A. Oxidant and antioxidant balance in the airways and airway diseases. Eur J Pharmacol. 2006;533(1–3):222–39. Epub 2006 Feb 28. Review.
534. Spickett CM, Forman HJ, editors. Lipid oxidation in health and disease. Oxidative stress and disease. Boca Raton: CRC Press; 2015.
535. Freeman R, Abuzinadah A, Gibbons C, Jones P, Miglis M, Sinn,D. Orthostatic hypotension. J Am Coll Cardiol State Art Rev 2018; 22(7); 1294–1309.
536. Liu G, Zhang C, Yin J, Li X, Cheng F, Li Y, Yang H, Uéda K, Chan P, Yu S. Alpha-synuclein is differentially expressed in mitochondria from different rat brain regions and dose-dependently down-regulates complex I activity. Neurosci Lett. 2009;454(3):187–92. https://doi.org/10.1016/j.neulet.2009.02.056.
537. Murray GL, Colombo J. (R)alpha lipoic acid is a safe, effective pharmacologic therapy of chronic orthostatic hypotension associated with low sympathetic tone. Int J Angiol. 2019 (eFirst); 1. https://doi.org/10.1055/s-0038-1676957.
538. Zhang H, Jia H, Liu J, Ao N, Yan B, Shen W, Wang X, et al. Combined R-alpha-lipoic acid and acetyl-L-carnitine exerts efficient preventative effects in a cellular model of Parkinson's disease. J Cell Mol Med. 2010;14(1–2):215–25.
539. Biosa A, Outiero T, Bubacco L, Bisaglia M. Diabetes mellitus as a risk factor for Parkinson's disease: a molecular point of view. Mol Neurobiol. 2018;28:1025–9. https://doi.org/10.1007/s12035-018-1025-9.
540. Lee W, Kim S, Kim G, Han S, Won J, Jung C, et al. Alpha-lipoic acid activates dimethylaminohydrolase in cultured endothelial cells. Biochem Biophys Res Commun. 2010;398(4):653–8.
541. Goudy S, Regalia J, Cai F, Helke C. Alpha-lipoic acid treatment prevents the diabetes-induced attenuation of the afferent limb of the baroreceptor reflex in rats. Auton Neurosci. 2003;108(1–2):32–44.
542. Queiroz TM, Guimarães DD, Mendes-Junior LG, Braga VA. α-lipoic acid reduces hypertension and increases baroreflex sensitivity in renovascular hypertensive rats. Molecules. 2012;17(11):13357–67.
543. Mohammadi V, Khorvash F, Feizi A, Askari G. Does alpha-lipoic acid supplementation modulate cardiovascular risk factors in patients with stroke? A randomized, double-blind clinical trial. Int J Prev Med. 2018;9:34.
544. Tardif J, Rheaume E. Lipoic acid supplementation and endothelial function. Br J Pharmacol. 2008;153(8):1587–8.
545. Circu ML, Aw TY. Glutathione and apoptosis. Free Radic Res. 2008;42(8):689–706. https://doi.org/10.1080/10715760802317663. Review.
546. Franco R, Cidlowski JA. Apoptosis and glutathione: beyond an antioxidant. Cell Death Differ. 2009;16(10):1303–14. https://doi.org/10.1038/cdd.2009.107. Epub 2009 Aug 7. Review.
547. Circu ML, Aw TY. Glutathione and modulation of cell apoptosis. Biochim Biophys Acta. 2012;1823(10):1767–77. https://doi.org/10.1016/j.bbamcr.2012.06.019. Epub 2012 Jun 23. Review.
548. Franco R, Cidlowski JA. Glutathione efflux and cell death. Antioxid Redox Signal. 2012;17(12):1694–713. https://doi.org/10.1089/ars.2012.4553. Epub 2012 Jul 16. Review.
549. Konradi C, Eaton M, MacDonald ML, Walsh J, Benes FM, Heckers S. Molecular evidence for mitochondrial dysfunction in bipolar disorder. Arch Gen Psychiatry. 2004;61(3):300–8. Erratum in: Arch Gen Psychiatry. 2004 Jun;61(6):538.
550. Chen AT, Chibnall JT, Nasrallah HA. Placebo-controlled augmentation trials of the antioxidant NAC in schizophrenia: a review. Ann Clin Psychiatry. 2016;28(3):190–6.
551. Vavilin VA, Safronova OG, Manankin NA, Kaznacheeva LF, Lyakhovich VV. Glutathione-S-transferase polymorphism and clinical features of acute drug poisoning in children. Bull Exp Biol Med. 2005;139(4):431–3.
552. Morris G, Anderson G, Dean O, Berk M, Galecki P, Martin-Subero M, Maes M. The glutathione system: a new drug target in neuroimmune disorders. Mol Neurobiol. 2014;50(3):1059–84. https://doi.org/10.1007/s12035-014-8705-x. Epub 2014 Apr 22. Review.
553. Yeligar SM, Harris FL, Hart CM, Brown LA. Glutathione attenuates ethanol-induced alveolar macrophage oxidative stress and dysfunction by downregulating NADPH oxidases. Am J Physiol Lung Cell Mol Physiol. 2014;306(5):L429–41. https://doi.org/10.1152/ajplung.00159.2013. Epub 2014 Jan 17.
554. Kodama Y, Kishimoto Y, Muramatsu Y, Tatebe J, Yamamoto Y, Hirota N, Itoigawa Y, Atsuta R, Koike K, Sato T, Aizawa K, Takahashi K, Morita T, Homma S, Seyama K, Ishigami A. Antioxidant nutrients in plasma of Japanese patients with chronic obstructive pulmonary disease (COPD), asthma-COPD overlap syndrome, and bronchial asthma. Clin Respir J. 2015. https://doi.org/10.1111/crj.12436. [Epub ahead of print].
555. Vicentini GE, Fracaro L, de Souza SR, Martins HA, Guarnier FA, Zanoni JN. Experimental cancer cachexia changes neuron numbers and peptide levels in the intestine: partial protective effects after dietary supplementation with L-glutamine. PLoS One. 2016;11(9):e0162998. https://doi.org/10.1371/journal.pone.0162998. eCollection 2016.
556. Jason LA, Boulton A, Porter NS, Jessen T, Njoku MG, Friedberg F. Classification of myalgic

encephalomyelitis/chronic fatigue syndrome by types of fatigue. Behav Med. 2010;36(1):24–31. https://doi.org/10.1080/08964280903521370.
557. Mathew SJ. Treatment-resistant depression: recent developments and future directions. Depress Anxiety. 2008;25(12):989–92. https://doi.org/10.1002/da.20540.
558. Kato T, Kubota M, Kasahara T. Animal models of bipolar disorder. Neurosci Biobehav Rev. 2007;31(6):832–42. Epub 2007 Mar 27. Review.
559. Baxter LR Jr, Phelps ME, Mazziotta JC, Schwartz JM, Gerner RH, Selin CE, Sumida RM. Cerebral metabolic rates for glucose in mood disorders. Studies with positron emission tomography and fluorodeoxyglucose F 18. Arch Gen Psychiatry. 1985;42(5):441–7.
560. Caliyurt O, Altiay G. Resting energy expenditure in manic episode. Bipolar Disord. 2009;11(1):102–6. https://doi.org/10.1111/j.1399-5618.2008.00649.x.
561. Shao L, Martin MV, Watson SJ, Schatzberg A, Akil H, Myers RM, Jones EG, Bunney WE, Vawter MP. Mitochondrial involvement in psychiatric disorders. Ann Med. 2008;40(4):281–95. https://doi.org/10.1080/07853890801923753. Review. Erratum in: Ann Med. 2011 Jun;43(4):329.
562. Konradi C, Eaton M, MacDonald ML, Walsh J, Benes FM, Heckers S. Molecular evidence for mitochondrial dysfunction in bipolar disorder. Arch Gen Psychiatry. 2004;61(3):300–8. Erratum in: Arch Gen Psychiatry. 2004 Jun;61(6):538.
563. Andreazza AC, Kapczinski F, Kauer-Sant'Anna M, Walz JC, Bond DJ, Gonçalves CA, Young LT, Yatham LN. 3-Nitrotyrosine and glutathione antioxidant system in patients in the early and late stages of bipolar disorder. J Psychiatry Neurosci. 2009;34(4):263–71.
564. Maurer IC, Schippel P, Volz HP. Lithium-induced enhancement of mitochondrial oxidative phosphorylation in human brain tissue. Bipolar Disord. 2009;11(5):515–22. https://doi.org/10.1111/j.1399-5618.2009.00729.x.
565. Machado-Vieira R, Andreazza AC, Viale CI, Zanatto V, Cereser V Jr, da Silva Vargas R, Kapczinski F, Portela LV, Souza DO, Salvador M, Gentil V. Oxidative stress parameters in unmedicated and treated bipolar subjects during initial manic episode: a possible role for lithium antioxidant effects. Neurosci Lett. 2007;421(1):33–6. Epub 2007 May 22.
566. Rosa AR, Frey BN, Andreazza AC, Cereser KM, Cunha AB, Quevedo J, Santin A, Gottfried C, Gonçalves CA, Vieta E, Kapczinski F. Increased serum glial cell line-derived neurotrophic factor immunocontent during manic and depressive episodes in individuals with bipolar disorder. Neurosci Lett. 2006;407(2):146–50. Epub 2006 Sept 7.
567. Cui J, Shao L, Young LT, Wang JF. Role of glutathione in neuroprotective effects of mood stabilizing drugs lithium and valproate. Neuroscience. 2007;144(4):1447–53. Epub 2006 Dec 19.
568. Dodd S, Dean O, Copolov DL, Malhi GS, Berk M. N-acetylcysteine for antioxidant therapy: pharmacology and clinical utility. Expert Opin Biol Ther. 2008;8(12):1955–62. https://doi.org/10.1517/14728220802517901. Review.
569. Laux I, Nel A. Evidence that oxidative stress-induced apoptosis by menadione involves Fas-dependent and Fas-independent pathways. Clin Immunol. 2001;101(3):335–44.
570. Pacher P, Beckman JS, Liaudet L. Nitric oxide and peroxynitrite in health and disease. Physiol Rev. 2007;87(1):315–424. Review.
571. Triposkiadis F, Karayannis G, Giamouzis G, Skoularigis J, Louridas G, Butler J. The sympathetic nervous system in heart failure physiology, pathophysiology, and clinical implications. J Am Coll Cardiol. 2009;54(19):1747–62. https://doi.org/10.1016/j.jacc.2009.05.015. Review.
572. Olshansky B, Sabbah HN, Hauptman PJ, Colucci WS. Parasympathetic nervous system and heart failure: pathophysiology and potential implications for therapy. Circulation. 2008;118(8):863–71. https://doi.org/10.1161/CIRCULATIONAHA.107.760405. Review.
573. Kinugawa T, Dibner-Dunlap ME. Altered vagal and sympathetic control of heart rate in left ventricular dysfunction and heart failure. Am J Phys. 1995;268:R317–23.
574. Newton GE, Parker AB, Landzberg JS, Colucci WS, Parker JD. Muscarinic receptor modulation of basal and beta-adrenergic stimulated function of the failing human left ventricle. J Clin Invest. 1996;98:2756–63.
575. Zhao G, Shen W, Xu X, Ochoa M, Bernstein R, Hintze TH. Selective impairment of vagally mediated, nitric oxide-dependent coronary vasodilation in conscious dogs after pacing-induced heart failure. Circulation. 1995;91:2655–63.
576. Dibner-Dunlap ME, Thames MD. Control of sympathetic nerve activity by vagal mechanoreflexes is blunted in heart failure. Circulation. 1992;86:1929–34.
577. Eschenhagen T, Mende U, Nose M, Schmitz W, Scholz H, Schulte am Esch J, Sempell R, Warnholtz A, Wustel JM. Regulation and possible functional implications of G-protein mRNA expression in nonfailing and failing ventricular myocardium. Basic Res Cardiol. 1992;87:51–64.
578. Ferramosca A, Di Giacomo M, Zara V. Antioxidant dietary approach in treatment of fatty liver: new insights and updates. World J Gastroenterol. 2017;23(23):4146–57. https://doi.org/10.3748/wjg.v23.i23.4146.
579. Bhatia LS, Curzen NP. Non-alcoholic fatty liver disease: a new and important cardiovascular risk factor? Eur Heart J. 2012;33(10):1190–200. https://doi.org/10.1093/eurheartj/ehr453. Epub 2012 Mar 8.
580. Reddy JK, Rao MS. Lipid metabolism and liver inflammation. II. Fatty liver disease and fatty acid

oxidation. Am J Physiol Gastrointest Liver Physiol. 2006;290(5):G852–8.
581. Angulo P. Nonalcoholic fatty liver disease. N Engl J Med. 2002;346(16):1221–31.
582. Bayard M, Holt J, Boroughs E. Nonalcoholic fatty liver disease. Am Fam Physician. 2006;73(11):1961–8.
583. Medina J, Fernández-Salazar LI, García-Buey L, Moreno-Otero R. Approach to the pathogenesis and treatment of non-alcoholic steatohepatitis. Diabetes Care. 2004;27(8):2057–66.
584. Day CP, James OF. Steatohepatitis: a tale of two "hits"? Gastroenterology. 1998;114(4):842–5.
585. Zafrani ES. Non-alcoholic fatty liver disease: an emerging pathological spectrum. Virchows Arch. 2004;444(1):3–12.
586. Ma J, Hennein R, Liu C, Long MT, Hoffmann U, Jacques PF, Lichtenstein AH, Hu FB, Levy D. Improved diet quality associates with reduction in liver fat, particularly in individuals with high genetic risk scores for nonalcoholic fatty liver disease. Gastroenterology. 2018. pii: S0016-5085(18)30345-7. https://doi.org/10.1053/j.gastro.2018.03.038. [Epub ahead of print].
587. Valent P. Mast cell activation syndromes: definition and classification. Allergy. 2013;68(4):417–24.
588. Akin C, Valent P, Metcalfe DD. Mast cell activation syndrome: proposed diagnostic criteria. J Allergy Clin Immunol. 2010;126:1099–104.
589. Akin C. Mast cell activation syndromes presenting as anaphylaxis. Immunol Allergy Clin N Am. 2015;35(2):277–85.
590. Milner J. Research update: POTS, EDS, MCAS Genetics. Dysautonomia International Conference & CME. Washington, DC. Dysautonomia International Research Update: POTS, EDS, MCAS Genetics. Web; 2015.
591. Szczawinska-Poplonyk A. An overlapping syndrome of allergy and immune deficiency in children. J Allergy. 2012;2012:1–9.
592. Talkington J, Nickell SP. Borrelia burgdorferi spirochetes induce mast cell activation and cytokine release. Infect Immun. 1999;67(3):1107–15.
593. Gao L, Mao Q, Cao J, Wang Y, Zhou X, Fan L. Effects of coenzyme Q10 on vascular endothelial function in humans: a meta-analysis of randomized controlled trials. Atherosclerosis. 2012;221(2):311–6. https://doi.org/10.1016/j.atherosclerosis.2011.10.027. Epub 2011 Oct 25. Review.
594. Yoritaka A, Kawajiri S, Yamamoto Y, Nakahara T, Ando M, Hashimoto K, Nagase M, Saito Y, Hattori N. Randomized, double-blind, placebo-controlled pilot trial of reduced coenzyme Q10 for Parkinson's disease. Parkinsonism Relat Disord. 2015;21(8):911–6. https://doi.org/10.1016/j.parkreldis.2015.05.022. Epub 2015 May 29.
595. Butt JH, Franzmann U, Kruuse C. Endothelial function in migraine with aura – a systematic review. Headache. 2015;55(1):35–54. https://doi.org/10.1111/head.12494. Epub 2014 Dec 24. Review
596. Dalla Volta G, Carli D, Zavarise P, Ngonga G, Vollaro S. P026. Pilot study on the use of coenzyme Q10 in a group of patients with episodic migraine without aura. J Headache Pain. 2015;16(Suppl 1):A186. https://doi.org/10.1186/1129-2377-16-S1-A186.
597. Shoeibi A, Olfati N, Soltani Sabi M, Salehi M, Mali S, Akbari Oryani M. Effectiveness of coenzyme Q10 in prophylactic treatment of migraine headache: an open-label, add-on, controlled trial. Acta Neurol Belg. 2017;117(1):103–9. https://doi.org/10.1007/s13760-016-0697-z. Epub 2016 Sept 26.
598. Scapagnini G, Davinelli S, Drago F, De Lorenzo A, Oriani G. Antioxidants as antidepressants: fact or fiction? CNS Drugs. 2012;26(6):477–90. https://doi.org/10.2165/11633190-000000000-00000. Review.
599. Morris G, Anderson G, Berk M, Maes M. Coenzyme Q10 depletion in medical and neuropsychiatric disorders: potential repercussions and therapeutic implications. Mol Neurobiol. 2013;48(3):883–903. https://doi.org/10.1007/s12035-013-8477-8. Epub 2013 Jun 13. Review.
600. Maurya PK, Noto C, Rizzo LB, Rios AC, Nunes SO, Barbosa DS, Sethi S, Zeni M, Mansur RB, Maes M, Brietzke E. The role of oxidative and nitrosative stress in accelerated aging and major depressive disorder. Prog Neuro-Psychopharmacol Biol Psychiatry. 2016;65:134–44. https://doi.org/10.1016/j.pnpbp.2015.08.016. Epub 2015 Sept 6. Review.
601. Sanoobar M, Dehghan P, Khalili M, Azimi A, Seifar F. Coenzyme Q10 as a treatment for fatigue and depression in multiple sclerosis patients: a double blind randomized clinical trial. Nutr Neurosci. 2016;19(3):138–43. https://doi.org/10.1179/1476830515Y.0000000002. Epub 2015 Jan 20.
602. Salviati L, Trevisson E, Doimo M, Navas P. Primary coenzyme Q10 deficiency. In: Pagon RA, Adam MP, Ardinger HH, Wallace SE, Amemiya A, Bean LJH, Bird TD, Ledbetter N, Mefford HC, Smith RJH, Stephens K, editors. GeneReviews® [Internet]. Seattle: University of Washington; 2017. p. 1993–2017.
603. Mitsui J, Matsukawa T, Yasuda T, Ishiura H, Tsuji S. Plasma coenzyme Q10 levels in patients with multiple system atrophy. JAMA Neurol. 2016;73(8):977–80. https://doi.org/10.1001/jamaneurol.2016.1325.
604. Singh RB, Kartik C, Otsuka K, Pella D, Pella J. Brain-heart connection and the risk of heart attack. Biomed Pharmacother. 2002;56(Suppl 2):257s–65s.
605. Li Z, Wang P, Yu Z, Cong Y, Sun H, Zhang J, Zhang J, Sun C, Zhang Y, Ju X. The effect of creatine and coenzyme q10 combination therapy on mild cognitive impairment in Parkinson's disease. Eur Neurol. 2015;73(3–4):205–11. https://doi.org/10.1159/000377676. Epub 2015 Mar 10.

606. Atalay Guzel N, Erikoglu Orer G, Sezen Bircan F, Coskun Cevher S. Effects of acute L-carnitine supplementation on nitric oxide production and oxidative stress after exhaustive exercise in young soccer players. J Sports Med Phys Fitness. 2015;55(1–2):9–15. Epub 2014 Oct 7.
607. Lim HB, Smith M. Systemic complications after head injury: a clinical review. Anaesthesia. 2007;62(5):474–82. Review.
608. Tobias H, Vinitsky A, Bulgarelli RJ, Ghosh-Dastidar S, Colombo J. Autonomic nervous system monitoring of patients with excess parasympathetic responses to sympathetic challenges – clinical observations. US Neurology. 2010;5(2):62–6.
609. Procaccini C, Pucino V, De Rosa V, Marone G, Matarese G. Neuro-endocrine networks controlling immune system in health and disease. Front Immunol. 2014;5:143. https://doi.org/10.3389/fimmu.2014.00143. eCollection 2014. Review.

# Mediterranean Diet (Prong-4)

# 6

The fourth prong of the Mind-Body Wellness Program (Fig. 6.1) focuses on food! This is the first of the lifestyle prongs. Obviously, food is central to life. There are many sayings about food, ranging from the conservative (e.g., "eat to live, not live to eat") to the liberal (e.g., "eat what you want, you only live once"). It has been suggested that some who live in the more affluent countries and the more affluent areas of those countries live in a time of "food stress" (intake is greater than expenditure, rather than a more appropriate balance as depicted in the insert, right). When humans were "cave people," there was no fast food or processed food. Food was a local phenomenon. If it was not in season, it simply was not eaten. There were many fewer food allergies and food sensitives, because food lived in the same region as its consumers and was subject to the same conditions as the consumers. So the food carried allergens (in very small quantities) which "inoculated" the locals to the things people are now allergic to today. This causes many fewer allergies and promotes health and wellness. There was no refrigeration or even preservatives until salt was discovered. In fact, salt was an important discovery, as a preservative. The word "salary" is derived from the Latin word for salt (*salis*). Half of the Roman soldier's salary came in the form of salt, not coin. Have you ever noticed that cuisines from countries near the equator are significantly more spiced (not necessarily hot, but more highly flavored) than foods near the poles? Peoples nearer to the poles had natural refrigeration and were able to keep foods (especially meats) longer. Peoples nearer to the equator did not, and they needed to stretch the usability of foods. Therefore, they covered the early spoiled flavor with spices, before foods became rancid (poisonous).

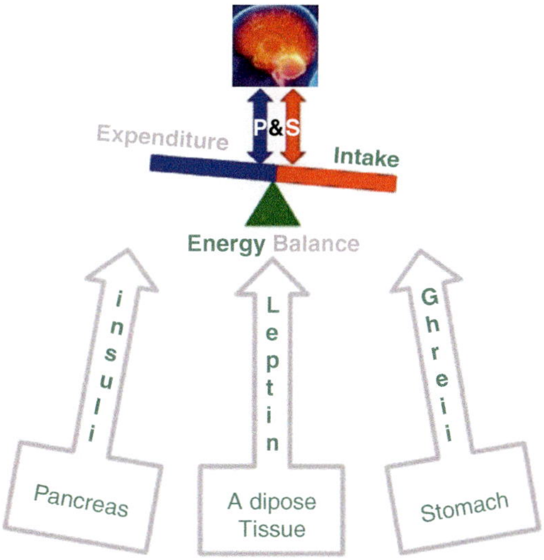


With technology "shrinking" the world, foods of all sources are readily available everywhere. More than ever, a saying accredited to Hippocrates is vital for health and wellness. "Let food be your medicine and let your medicine be your food." If one knows a little about the nutritional value of foods, including how cooking affects foods,



N. L. DePace, J. Colombo, *Clinical Autonomic and Mitochondrial Disorders*,
https://doi.org/10.1007/978-3-030-17016-5_6

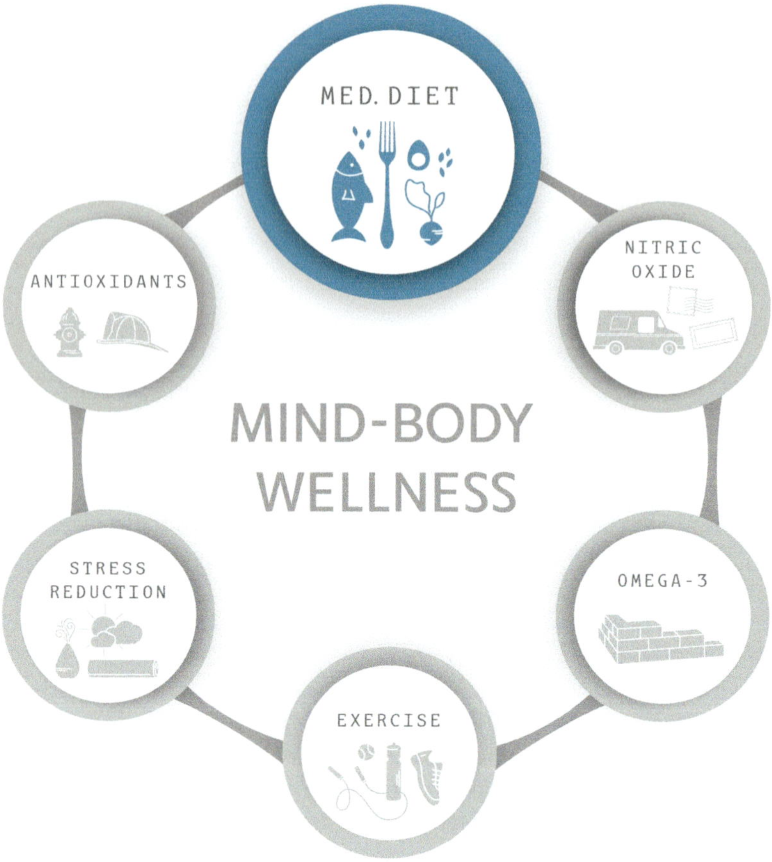


**Fig. 6.1** The Mind Body-Wellness Program – Mediterranean diet prong

Hippocrates' saying comes alive. For example, if there are women at the dinner table, adding some celery or spinach to their diet provides extra iron to their meal and helps replace that which may be lost once a month, helping them avoid fatigue and headache that may be associated with the loss of iron. If there are people at the table that are sad or depressed or anxious, green leafy vegetables and other foods rich in vitamins $B_6$ and $B_{12}$ and magnesium affect the parasympathetic nervous system to restore proper autonomic balance, thereby helping to elevate and stabilize mood disorders. An apple a day truly does keep the doctor away, including the trace levels of arsenic in apple seeds that are anticarcinogenic. Of course, all of these foods are better fresh, when picked ripe, and eaten ripe. "You are what you eat." Eating healthy is living healthy. If this is your lifestyle, then the occasional indulgence is easily tolerated by the body. As a good doctor once said, "if you do not eat the 'bad' things once in a while, how will your body 'know' what is 'good'?" The contrary is *absolutely* not true.

Now everything has changed. Many people eat without really thinking about it and spend as little time as possible cooking. A hectic morning may mean that they are worn out by lunchtime. This is exacerbated by no breakfast, a steady diet of preprocessed, high-glycemic foods with little nutritional value. Then lunch is all preprocessed: a can of soda and a fast-food "meal." In the evening, they are even more tired, and they have not even said "Hello" to their children. So dinner comes from a can, a box, or other fast-food or pre-prepared food source. Health has been relegated to a pill or a multivitamin. The hope is to make up for the American lifestyle of distilling the needed nutrients into pills. The American lifestyle is based on "fresh from the factory – 'natural' chemistry." A return to "'factory fresh' – from nature" – is strongly recommended.

The American lifestyle involves waking up and perking up with chemicals, relaxing, de-stressing, and going to sleep with chemicals, even making love, or having sex, with chemicals. Americans get sick, moat take more chemicals. The illness leads to additional symptoms and more chemicals. Please do not misinterpret; some of these chemicals are very important and potentially lifesaving. For example, before statins, certain types of atherosclerosis (e.g., patients with family histories of plaques near artery bifurcations) could not be treated with stents. They were walking heart attacks waiting to happen and no amount of exercise or doctors could stop the heart attack. However, at some point we need to stop and consider what all of these chemicals are doing to the body. Once a yearlong study (unpublished) was performed in a nursing home [personal communication, Dr. Colombo], and by balancing the patients' parasympathetic and sympathetic nervous systems, the patients' medication load was judiciously reduced from an average of 12–15 medications per week to 5–7 medications per week. By bringing their nervous systems into balance, several of the secondary symptoms were relieved, and the associated medications were no longer needed. The patients were suddenly more active and alert. This activity, and a proper diet, further reduced certain medications. Ultimately, grandchildren had their grandparents back, and the quality of life for all was significantly improved.

The average American does indeed believe that there is better living through chemistry. Food has become a medicine, in the shape of a pill. While this sounds like what Hippocrates said, unfortunately it is not anything like what he meant. The pill is now seen as a substitute, not as a supplement (as too many people glibly state without recognition). Most, if not all, people cannot eat enough, nor do they live in regions where times of the year provide enough, of the proper foods. Therefore, supplements are still needed. With age and bodies not producing or assimilating the necessary nutrients, supplements are still needed. However, they should not be the primary source, *only the supplementary source*.

The growth (as young people) and aging (as older people) processes were the original reasons for developing supplements. Then food became modernized and made convenient. Food is comprised of both macro- and micronutrients. Macronutrients constitute the majority of what is consumed: protein, carbohydrates, fat, alcohol, and fiber. These provide energy and the raw materials to adapt, grow, and heal. Micronutrients are found in very small amounts and include vitamins and minerals and other trace elements that are vital to health and wellness. Processing of foods to make them convenient tends to retain the macronutrients and dispose of, or destroy, the micronutrients. While this has become well known and recognized, as evidenced by the growing restaurant fad of "farm-to-table" (even if the "farm" is in a flower box in the back alley or is too many miles away), it still does not make up for what is disposed of in everything else. Now supplements are required by all, not just by children and the aged or sick.

The processing, pasteurizing, homogenizing, irradiating, ultra-preserving, etc., of the majority of the foods the average American eats are literally killing America, albeit slowly. It affects mental and nervous health, cardiovascular health, quality of life, and eventually mortality (continuation of life or longevity). Food is medicine, but like all medicines, not all are healthy for everyone. The rest of this chapter discusses the Mediterranean diet. My Sicilian great-grandmother helped to teach me to select the freshest foods to cook (even in the middle of Manhattan, in New York City) and to prepare it in a way to preserve the flavor and "value" (as she put it – meaning so much more than just flavor) of the food itself. In fact, the only times I was truly sick in my life were the times when I was not near a garden of my own (growing "organically" – not in the sense of what the government permits producers to claim as organic) or a local farmer I knew (farmer's markets are a real "windfall" – pun intended). Truly, the foods in this diet help establish and maintain health and wellness; however, the hidden benefit is in the fact that true adherence to this diet involves eating and cooking with fresh, whole, locally grown, unpreprocessed foods so that the nutrients and health benefits are preserved and ingested when consumed – and a little wine is enjoyed!

> Let food be your medicine and let medicine be your food. (Hippocrates, c.460 BC–c.377 BC)

The Mediterranean diet is probably the healthiest dietary pattern. It is the traditional diet from many of the countries that border the Mediterranean Sea, including Gibraltar, Spain, France, Monaco, Italy, Slovenia, Croatia, Bosnia, Herzegovina, Greece, and the Middle East. It is a plant-based diet where vegetables, fruits, and whole grains, along with legumes and nuts, are consumed in high amounts, with the "stars" of the diet being the olive, grape, and wheat (Fig. 2.32). It is interesting that these "stars" date back to antiquity: some of the oldest books of the Bible (Numbers 18:12 and Deuteronomy 7:13) reference "olive oil, new wine, and [whole] grain" as signs of love, wealth, peace offerings, and health and wellness.

> He will love you and bless you and ... bless the crops of your land – your grain, new wine and olive oil. (Deuteronomy 7:13, prior to 1406 BC)

The Mediterranean diet primarily consists of vegetables and olive oil with moderate protein. The primary protein source in the Mediterranean diet is fish, including shellfish. Red meat is consumed on a monthly basis. White meats are preferred and saturated fats are limited. Fish and shellfish are consumed on a weekly basis. Olive oil is the primary source of fat. Whole grains, fruits, vegetables, and nuts are typically natural and unprocessed. Dairy products, especially yogurt products, are used along with certain cheeses, such as goat cheese. Processed foods and foods that are high in sugars are eaten very infrequently, including desserts. From the grape, wine is the primary alcoholic beverage consumed. One glass of wine (5 oz) for women and up to two glasses for men (under age 65) is recommended.

Overall, the Mediterranean diet reduces the risk of oxidized LDL cholesterol ("ox-LDL," the cholesterol that turns "bad" in large amounts; see "Details of Oxidized LDL and Atherosclerosis Production"). Lower ox-LDL reduces or prevents atherosclerosis, which in turn reduces or prevents endothelial disease, which then reduces or prevents cardiovascular disease. The health benefits of the Mediterranean diet extend beyond just cardiovascular disease. It seems clear from the evidence that the Mediterranean diet is very healthy and may help prevent some of the world's leading killers, including cancer. It is obviously a much better option than the standard low-fat diet that is still being recommended all around the world [1]. The Mediterranean diet and cardiovascular disease and many more relationships will be discussed.

## Disease and the Mediterranean Diet

Numerous studies over several decades suggest that following the Mediterranean diet reduces the risk of all-cause mortality as well as cardiovascular disease, reduces the incidence of cancer (including breast cancer in women), improves cognitive health (including reducing the incidence of Parkinson's and Alzheimer's disease), and much more. The Mediterranean diet contains three to nine servings of vegetables, half to two servings of fruit, one to 13 servings of cereals, and up to eight servings of olive oil daily. It contains approximately 9300 kJ (approximately 2200 food calories), 37% as total fat, 18% as monounsaturated and 9% as saturated, and 33 g of fiber per day [2]. It typically consists of fish, monounsaturated fats from olive oil, fruits, vegetables, whole grains, legumes and nuts, and moderate amounts of wine. The Mediterranean dietary pattern, through a healthy profile of fat intake, low proportions of carbohydrates, low-glycemic index, and high content of dietary fiber, antioxidant compounds, and anti-inflammatories, reduces the risk of these pathologies. The inclusion of foods typical of the Mediterranean diet and greater adherence to this healthy pattern were related to a better nutrient profile, both in children and adults, with a lower prevalence of individuals showing inadequate intakes of micronutrients [3]. Overall, the Mediterranean diet was found to be a healthy dietary pattern in terms of morbidity and mortality [4].

The Mediterranean diet is one of the most, and best, studied diets. Comparisons between it and a low-fat diet, a low-carbohydrate diet, and the American Diabetes Association diet found the Mediterranean diet resulted in greater weight loss than the low-fat diet at ≥12 months but produced similar weight loss as other comparator diets. The Mediterranean diet was generally similar to comparator diets at improving other cardiovascular risk factor levels, including blood pressure and lipid levels in overweight or obese individuals trying to lose weight [5]. The Mediterranean diet has been shown to reduce the burden, or even prevent the development, of cardiovascular disease, breast cancer, depression, colorectal cancer, diabetes, obesity, asthma, erectile dysfunction, and cognitive decline. This diet is also known to improve surrogates of cardiovascular disease, such as waist-to-hip ratio, lipids, and markers of inflammation, as well as primary cardiovascular disease outcomes, such as death and events in both observational and randomized controlled trial data. These enhancements easily rival those seen with more established tools used to fight cardiovascular disease such as aspirin, beta-blockers, angiotensin-converting enzyme inhibitors, and exercise [6, 7].

Pooled analyses of individual components of the Mediterranean diet revealed that the protective effects of the diet appear to be most attributable to olive oil, fruits, vegetables, and legumes, but most effective when taken as a whole, together with exercise and stress reduction. An average reduced mortality risk of 40% for coronary heart disease, myocardial infarction, and stroke (MACE) incidence is associated with the diet [8]. After 2 years of follow-up, individuals assigned to a Mediterranean diet had more favorable changes in body weight, body mass index, systolic blood pressure, diastolic blood pressure, fasting plasma glucose, total cholesterol, and high-sensitivity C-reactive protein. The Mediterranean diet appears to be more effective than low-fat diets in inducing clinically relevant long-term changes in cardiovascular risk factors and inflammatory markers [9, 10].

The PREDIMED study was designed (see Fig. 6.2) to assess the long-term effects of the Mediterranean diet on individuals diagnosed with cardiovascular disease who were at high risk. Participants were randomly assigned to three diet groups: (1) Mediterranean diet supplemented with extra-virgin olive oil (EVOO), (2) Mediterranean diet supplemented with nuts, and (3) a control low-fat diet. Again, this time after 4.8 years (average), beneficial effects of the Mediterranean diet were reported regarding blood pressure, lipid profiles, lipoprotein particles, inflammation, oxidative stress, carotid atherosclerosis, and the expression of pro-atherogenic genes involved in vascular events and thrombosis. The study results demonstrate that a high-unsaturated fat and antioxidant-rich dietary pattern, such as the Mediterranean diet, help in the prevention of

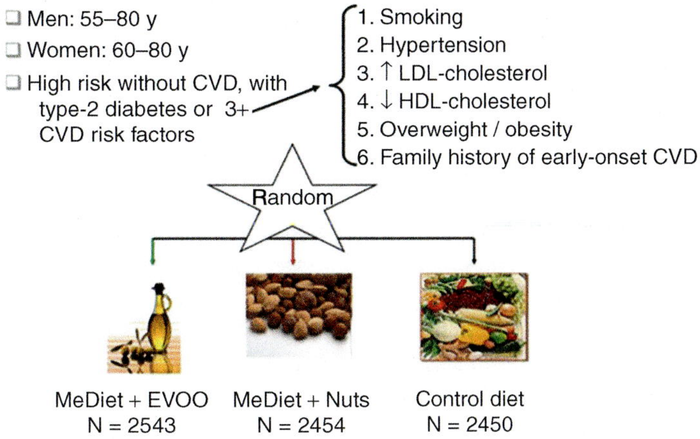


**Fig. 6.2** PREDIMED study design; see text. Abbreviations: CVD, cardiovascular disease; EVOO, extra-virgin olive oil; MeDiet, Mediterranean diet. (Republished with permission from Oxford Academic press. Source: [11])

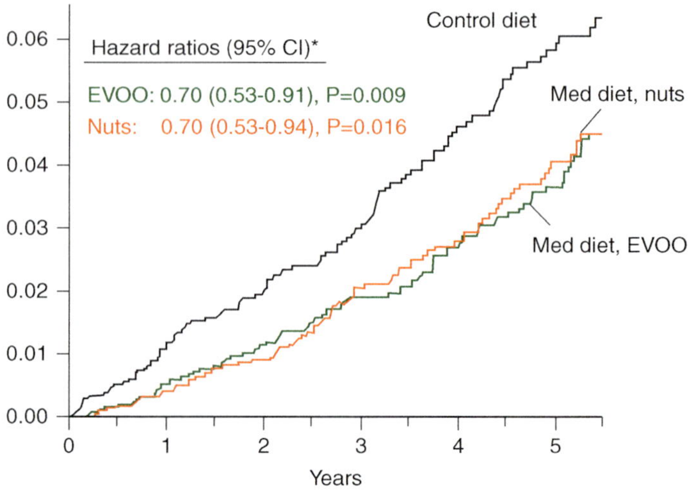


**Number at risk**

| | | | | | | |
|---|---|---|---|---|---|---|
| Control group | 2450 | 2268 | 2020 | 1583 | 1268 | 946 |
| MeDiet+EVOO | 2543 | 2486 | 2320 | 1987 | 1687 | 1310 |
| MeDiet+Nuts | 2454 | 2343 | 2093 | 1657 | 1389 | 1031 |

**Fig. 6.3** Incidence of cardiovascular disease by intervention group in the PREDIMED study; see text. Abbreviations: EVOO, extra-virgin olive oil; Med diet and MeDiet, Mediterranean diet. (Republished with permission from Oxford Academic press. Source: [11, 12, Fig. 2])

cardiovascular disease (see Fig. 6.3) [11, 12]. Both genetic and lifestyle factors contribute to individual-level risk of coronary artery disease. These factors were independently associated with susceptibility to coronary artery disease. Among participants at high genetic risk, a favorable lifestyle was associated with a nearly 50% lower relative risk of coronary artery disease than was an unfavorable lifestyle [13].

Low-fat diets (especially saturated fat) and diets rich in monounsaturated fats improve endothelial function [14]. The increased consumption of fat in the American diet has directly contributed to the growing burden of chronic disease. However, total fat intake does not predict change in body fat. Some foods previously relegated to the top of the pyramid because of high-fat content (nuts, full-fat yogurt) are associated with lower rates of weight gain than common high-carbohydrate foods (processed grains, potato products, sugary beverages) [15]. A positive and significant association was found between the Mediterranean diet and BP in adults [16]. Saturated fat and omega-6 polyunsaturated fat increase risk of coronary heart disease. Trans fats decreased coronary heart disease, but they did not significantly influence mortality risk [17].

The findings from the Lyon Diet Heart Study [18] illustrate the importance of a dietary pattern that emphasizes fruits, vegetables, breads and cereals, and fish, as well as alpha-linolenic acid (a Mediterranean-style diet). Risk factors beyond lipids and lipoproteins, which have historically been primary targets of intervention, have been implicated. Omega-3 fatty acids exert cardioprotective effects via multiple mechanisms: prevent arrhythmia, have anti-inflammatory properties, decrease synthesis of cytokines and mitogens, stimulate endothelial-derived nitric oxide, are antithrombotic, are prostaglandin and leukotriene precursors, and inhibit atherosclerosis (see "Omega-3 Fatty Acids (Prong-1)"). Therefore, it is possible that omega-3s account for the cardioprotective effect observed. The unprecedented reduction in coronary recurrence rates, despite the fact that lipid/lipoprotein risk factors were comparable, clearly points to other important risk factor modifications as major influences in the development of cardiovascular disease (Fig. 6.4). Notice the similarities between the PREDIMED study [12] (Fig. 6.3) and the primary prevention study [19] (Fig. 6.4), which are substantiated by the Lyon Diet Heart Study and the others included above.

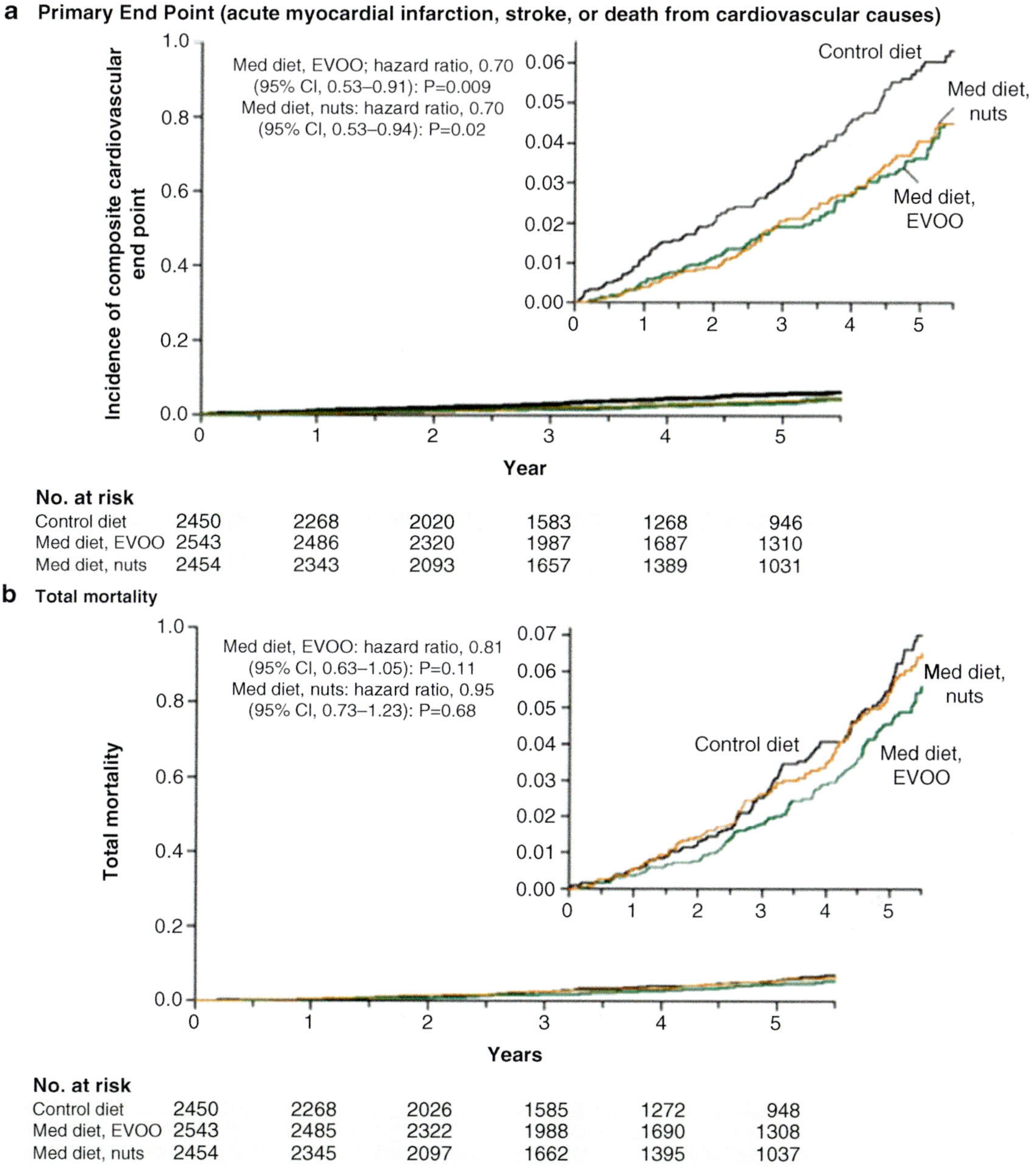


**Fig. 6.4** People age 55 to 80 who ate a Mediterranean diet including vegetables, fruits, and fish, supplemented with nuts or olive oils, were at lower risk of heart disease than people on a typical low-fat diet. Kaplan-Meier estimates of the incidence of outcome events in the total study population. Panel A shows the incidence of the primary end point (a composite of acute myocardial infarction, stroke, and death from cardiovascular causes), and Panel B shows total mortality. Hazard ratios were stratified according to center (Cox model with robust variance estimators). Abbreviations: CI, confidence interval; EVOO, extra virgin olive oil; and Med Mediterranean. (Republished with permission from Oxford Academic press. Source: [19])

Low-sodium, low-sodium with high-potassium, low-sodium with low-calorie, and low-calorie diets all led to significant systolic and diastolic BP reductions. In contrast, the Mediterranean diet led to a significant incremental reduction in diastolic but not systolic BP. Subgroup analysis also showed important variations in effectiveness based on duration, size, and participant demographics. Dietary modifications are associated with clinically meaningful, though variable, reductions in BP. Some diets are more effective than others and under different circumstances [20]. Another variation example is a Mediterranean diet with no restriction on fat intake may reduce the incidence of cardiovascular events, breast cancer, and type 2 diabetes [21]. These modifications are possible with the Mediterranean diet. Regardless, overall, greater adherence to a Mediterranean diet is associated with a significant improvement in health status, as seen by a significant reduction in overall mortality (9%), mortality from cardiovascular diseases (9%), incidence of or mortality from cancer (6%), and incidence of Parkinson's and Alzheimer's diseases (13%). A Mediterranean-like dietary pattern seems beneficial for primary prevention of major chronic diseases [22].

The Mediterranean diet was associated with better glycemic control and cardiovascular risk factors than control diets, including a lower-fat diet, suggesting that it is suitable for the overall management of type 2 diabetes [23]. Consumption of foods found in the Mediterranean diet improves cardio-metabolic health because of their rich composition of nutrients and phytochemicals and their synergizing effects on metabolic pathways [24, 25]. They reduce cardio-metabolic disease risk. The abundance of healthy, nutrient-dense foods that make up the plant-based diet determines its potential to beneficially influence metabolic pathways that lead to metabolic syndrome and type 2 diabetes, as well as other chronic conditions (Fig. 6.5) [24], and prevents these pathologies.

Adherence to a Mediterranean diet is associated with significant improvements in health status [26]. Greater adherence is associated with a significant reduction in the risk of diabetes (19%; moderate-quality evidence). Higher adherence to the Mediterranean diet was associated with 23% reduced risk of developing type 2 diabetes (combined relative risk for upper versus lowest available centile, 0.77; 95% CI, 0.66, 0.89). Subgroup analyses based on region, health status of participants, and number of confounders controlled showed similar results. Limitations include variations in Mediterranean diet adherence assessment tools, confounders' adjustment, duration of follow-up, and number of events with diabetes. The Mediterranean diet could, if appropriately adjusted to reflect local food availability and individual's needs, constitute a beneficial nutritional choice for the primary prevention of diabetes [27]. Two large prospective studies report a substantially lower risk (83% and 35%, respectively) of type 2 diabetes in healthy people or in post-infarct patients with the highest adherence to a Mediterranean diet [28].

The effects of a Mediterranean diet on indices of glycemic control in subjects with type 2 diabetes, as compared with other commonly used diets, showed improvement of fasting glucose and HbA1c levels that are greater with a Mediterranean diet and ranged from 7 to 40 mg/dl for fasting glucose and from 0.1 to 0.6% for HbA1c. No trial reported worsening of glycemic control with a Mediterranean diet. Two controlled trials in a secondary prevention setting demonstrated that post-infarct patients, including diabetic patients, had cardiovascular benefits from a Mediterranean diet. These data again suggest that adopting a Mediterranean diet may help prevent type 2 diabetes, as well as improve glycemic control and cardiovascular risk in persons with established diabetes [28]. The diet was significantly beneficial when the intervention was longer in duration, was conducted in Europe, used a behavioral technique, and was conducted using small groups.

The traditional Mediterranean diet had significant beneficial effects on four of the five metabolic risk factors. The diet demonstrated significant beneficial effects for waist circumference (>102 cm for men and > 88 cm for women), triglycerides (≥150 mg/dL), blood glucose (≥110 mg/dL), and systolic BP (≥130 mmHg).

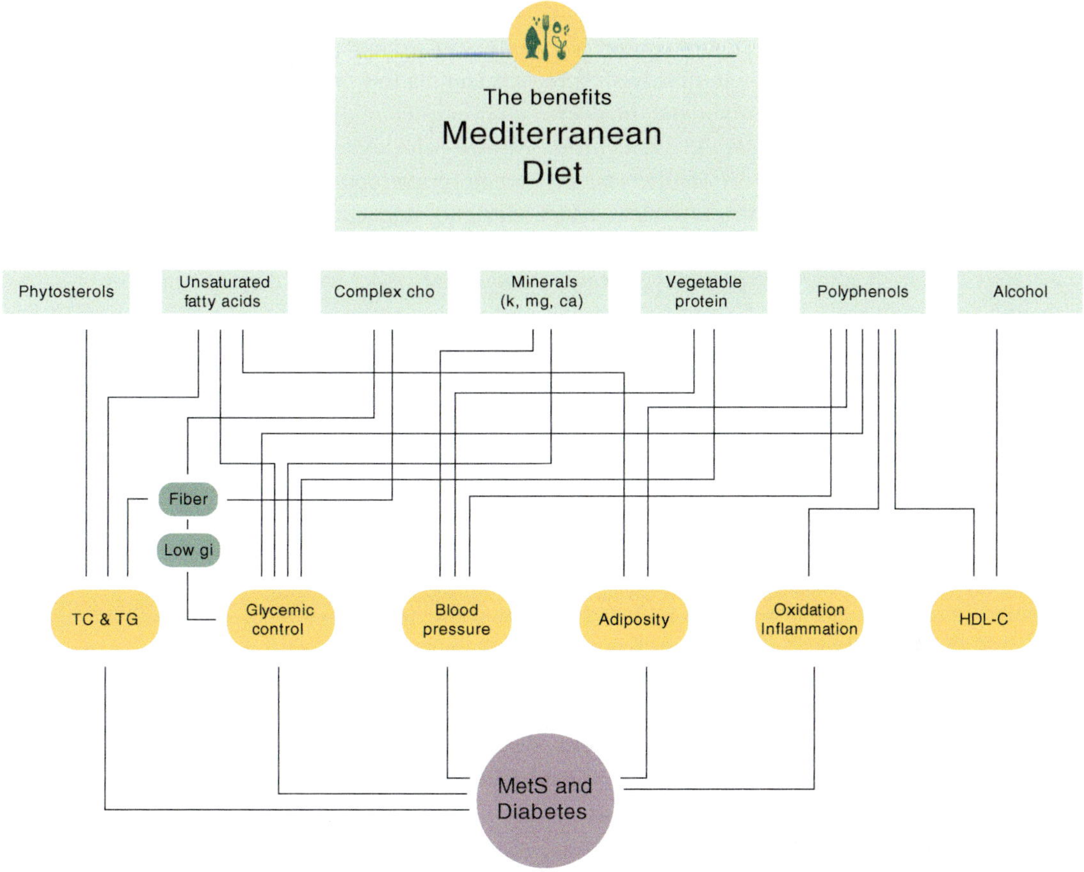


**Fig. 6.5** Abundant epidemiologic and clinical trial evidence supports the role of the Mediterranean diet (MedDiet) in the prevention and management of type 2 diabetes (T2DM) and metabolic syndrome (MetS). The main nutrients of the MedDiet are shown along with their principal biological targets (arrow connections). The net effects on intermediate markers of cardio-metabolic disease risk shown for these nutrients and their parent foods in clinical trials include the lowering of cholesterol and triglycerides (TGs), increased HDL cholesterol, improved glycemic control, decreased blood pressure, reduced adiposity, and antioxidant and anti-inflammatory actions. The overall result is reduced MetS and T2DM risk, as suggested for most of the MedDiet in observational cohort studies and the Prevención con Dieta Mediterránea trial. Abbreviations: CHO carbohydrate, EVOO extra-virgin olive oil, GI glycemic index, HDL-C HDL cholesterol, MedDiet Mediterranean diet, MetS metabolic syndrome, TC total cholesterol, Vegs, vegetables. (Illustration by Elysian Creative Studio, www.elysiancreativestudio.com, Lizzy Colombo. Source: Adapted from reference [24] with permission. [25])

The diet did not demonstrate significant benefit for HDL cholesterol (<40 mg/dL for men and <50 mg/dL for women) [29]. Metabolic syndrome is also characterized by abdominal obesity, dyslipidemia, elevated blood pressure, and impaired glucose tolerance, with increasing prevalence. The above findings are substantiated in other studies [30] which find that adoption of a Mediterranean dietary pattern, in addition to improving or preventing type 2 diabetes, was also associated with lower risk of, and the primary prevention of, metabolic syndrome, including prevalence and progression [31].

Beyond cardiovascular disease and its risk factors (e.g., diabetes), high adherence to a Mediterranean diet is significantly associated with lower risk of other chronic diseases and their mortality risk. High adherence to the diet reduced cancer risk and cancer mortality risk, with the greatest effect demonstrated for all-cause cancer mortality, followed in declining order by colorectal cancer, breast cancer, gastric cancer, prostate cancer, liver cancer, head and neck cancer, pancreatic cancer, and respiratory cancer. No significant association could be observed for esophageal, ovarian, endometrial, and bladder cancer. Among cancer survivors, the association between adherence to the highest Mediterranean diet category and risk of cancer mortality, and cancer recurrence, was not statistically significant. However, high adherence provides a prominent and consistent reduction in cancer mortality and risk of the types of cancer listed above [32]. Overall, high adherence to the diet helps with prevention and significantly reduces the risk of cancer incidence and thereby mortality [33].

A study [34] compared (1) incidence and mortality of all-cause cancer and (2) individual cancer risks for low- vs. high-risk groups and for the low-risk group vs. the nation. Low-risk men and women had healthy lifestyle patterns (e.g., followed a Mediterranean diet). High-risk subjects did not. The all-cause incidence and mortality risks demonstrate that 25% more women and 33% more men were diagnosed with cancer in the high-risk population as compared with the low-risk population. Mortality from all cancers is 48% higher in women and 44% higher in men for the high-risk population. The individual cancers in women and men were 82% and 78% higher for lung cancer, 29% and 20% higher for colon and rectal cancers, 30% and 29% higher for pancreatic cancer, and 36% and 44% higher for bladder cancer. Similar estimates were obtained for morbidity. For breast cancer (women only), incidence and mortality risks were 4% and 12% higher in the high-risk population, respectively. For fatal prostate cancer (men only), incidence is 21% higher. Substantially higher risks were obtained when the low-risk group was compared with the US population. For example, all-cancer risks in women and men are 41% and 63% higher, respectively. For colorectal cancer risks in women and men are 60% and 59% higher, respectively. Overall, a substantial cancer burden may be prevented through lifestyle modification. Primary prevention through healthy lifestyle patterns is helpful for cancer control.

For most epithelial cancers, risk decreased with adherence to types of Mediterranean diets. For digestive tract cancers, risks ranged between 15% and 40%. The diet provides a protective effect in women for breast, genital tract, urinary tract, and a few other epithelial cancers. Isolating components of the Mediterranean diet demonstrated an inverse relationship between fish, whole-grain foods, antioxidants, and other micronutrients and cancer risk. In contrast, subjects reporting frequent red meat intake showed increased risk for several common cancers. Whole-grain foods reduced risk of several types of cancer, particularly cancers of the upper digestive tract. In contrast, refined grains and, consequently, glycemic load and glycemic index were associated with increased risk of different types of cancer including, among others, breast and colorectal. Increased consumption of fruit, vegetables, olive oil, and other unsaturated fats and avoiding meat, refined carbohydrates, and saturated fats are shown to be the beneficial aspects of the Mediterranean diet [35].

Comparing a "healthy" (a type of Mediterranean diet), a "Western," and a "carbohydrate" diet in men with prostate cancer showed that the healthy pattern was not related to prostate cancer risk, while the Western pattern significantly increased it. The "carbohydrate" diet was positively associated with a higher risk of prostate cancer. A significant linear trend between the Western ($p = 0.011$) pattern, the carbohydrate ($p = 0.005$) pattern, and the increment of prostate cancer risk was observed [36]. In women, an inverse association between adherence to the Mediterranean diet and postmenopausal breast cancer (specifically, receptor-negative breast cancer) was demonstrated. This may have important implications for prevention because of the poorer prognosis of these breast cancer subtypes [37].

A healthy dietary pattern (i.e., Mediterranean diet, Nordic diet, Tibetan diet, and the dietary approaches to stop hypertension diet) is associated with significant reductions in inflammation as measured by C-reactive protein (CRP) [38]. In addition to CRP, other markers of inflammation were studied, including total adiponectin, high-molecular-weight adiponectin, tumor necrosis factor-α, adiponectin, leptin, resistin, and retinol-binding protein 4. No significant changes were found for all other biomarkers.

The Mediterranean diet (RR, 0.69; 95% CI, [0.57–0.84]; $P < 0.001$) and some of its components are related to decreased dementia, including unsaturated fatty acids (RR, 0.84; 95% CI, [0.74–0.95]; $P = 0.006$), antioxidants (RR, 0.87; 95% CI, [0.77–0.98]; $P = 0.026$), and vitamin B (RR, 0.72; 95% CI, [0.54–0.96]; $P = 0.026$). Increases in dementia are related to smoking (RR, 1.43; 95% CI, [1.15–1.77]; $P = 0.001$), low levels of vitamin D (RR, 1.52; 95% CI, [1.17–1.98]; $P = 0.002$), and ingestion of aluminum (RR, 2.24; 95% CI, [1.49–3.37]; $P < 0.001$). Low levels of vitamin D are also associated with cognitive decline. Findings indicate that the Mediterranean diet helps to prevent dementia [39]. Inflammation is associated with many pathologies, including dementia [40, 41]. Adherence to a Mediterranean diet has been associated with lower risk of various age-related diseases, including dementia. Higher adherence to Mediterranean diet was associated with better cognitive function, lower rates of cognitive decline, and reduced risk of Alzheimer's disease [42]. High compliance to the Mediterranean diet vs. a diet high in dairy and meat was compared. The Mediterranean diet is associated with a significant, and approximately linear, inverse relationship with the incident risk of cognitive disorders [43].

Studies of cognitive function (divided into domains of memory and executive function) [44] revealed a significant association between Mediterranean diet and older adults' episodic memory ($n = 25, 369$, $r = 0.01$, $P = 0.03$) and global cognition ($n = 41{,}492$, $r = 0.05$, $P \leq 0.001$), but not working memory ($n = 1487$, $r = 0.007$, $P = 0.93$) or semantic memory ($n = 1487$, $r = 0.08$, $P = 0.28$). The diet showed improvement in delayed recall ($n = 429$, $P = 0.01$), working memory ($n = 566$, $P = 0.03$), and global cognition ($n = 429$, $P = 0.047$), but not episodic memory ($n = 566$, $P = 0.15$), immediate recall ($n = 566$, $P = 0.17$), paired associates ($n = 429$, $P = 0.20$), attention ($n = 566$, $P = 0.69$), processing speed ($n = 566$, $P = 0.35$), or verbal fluency ($n = 566$, $P = 0.12$). The strongest evidence suggests a beneficial effect of the diet on older adults' global cognition [44].

Adherence to a Mediterranean-style diet has been suggested to have protective effects on bone health and decreases the incidence of bone fractures, especially the incidence of hip fractures as compared to all other types of fracture [45]. Adherence is associated with a higher mean bone mineral density as well [46]. It also demonstrates a consistent inverse relationship (protective) with asthma in children [47].

## Endothelial Function and the Mediterranean Diet

A variety of risk factors, including smoking, hypercholesterolemia, hyper-homocysteinemia, hypertension, and diabetes, adversely affect endothelial function. Diet factors in modulating endothelial function [48]. Dietary factors that influence endothelial function include omega-3 fatty acids, other fatty acids, antioxidants, folic acid (vitamin $B_9$) and vitamin $B_{12}$, L-arginine, soy proteins, and the Mediterranean diet. The Mediterranean diet facilitates the provision of these dietary factors.

Healthful levels of fatty acids are found in the Mediterranean diet, including high concentrations of omega-3s from oily fish and fish oil supplements; lower, healthful concentrations of omega-6s from vegetable oils; and high concentrations of omega-9s from olive oils. For example (from the "Omega-3 Fatty Acids (Prong-1)" chapter), after 4 months of treatment, the patients supplemented with omega-3 fatty acids had significantly improved endothelium-dependent vasodilation compared with control subjects. The chronic consumption of low-fat diets and Mediterranean-style diets improves endothelial function compared to a high-fat Western-type diet. With the exception of omega-3 fatty acids, acute or chronic high-fat meals induce a negative effect on endothelial function. This function is improved by the simultaneous administration of natural antioxidants such as red wine, fruits, and vegetables. Studies with fish oil further support the beneficial effects of these fatty acids on endothelial function and cardiovascular disease prevention.

High levels of antioxidants are found in fruits, especially citrus (e.g., vitamin C) and avocado (e.g., vitamin E); vegetables, especially olives and green leafy vegetables (e.g., vitamins A and E); certain tree nuts, including almonds, pine nuts, and hazelnuts (e.g., vitamin E); and yogurt and oily fishes (e.g., vitamin D). These vitamins may be supplemented. As discussed above, epidemiologic evidence links vitamins C and E with reduced risk of all-cause mortality and cardiovascular diseases by reducing the susceptibility of LDL oxidation and scavenging free radicals within the body. Vitamins C and E are found to have compounding reductions from supplementation of both, suggesting a synergistic effect. The most powerful antioxidants are alpha-lipoic acid (ALA) and CoQ10. ALA is found in the Mediterranean diet in yeast (from whole-grain breads), broccoli, spinach, and potatoes. However, ALA is best supplemented, as it only exists in the natural sources in very low amounts. CoQ10 is found in the Mediterranean diet in fatty fish, fish oils, peanuts, sesame seeds, and olive oils. There are additional antioxidants. Vitamins A, C, and E are potentiated (recycled) by ALA and CoQ10, which may contribute to their efficacy and significance, and the lack of ALA and CoQ10 may contribute to the lack of the vitamins' efficacy in some experiments.

The B vitamins (folic acid, aka $B_9$, and $B_{12}$) are primarily found in dark green leafy vegetables, avocado, and legumes. Folate intake caused significant mortality risk reduction from all causes and cardiovascular disease. The primary mechanism for the effect of folic acid is a reduction in plasma homocysteine which causes endothelial cell dysfunction. Folic acid has a beneficial effect on endothelial function as measured by flow-mediated vasodilation in healthy persons or patients with hyper-homocysteinemia. Folic acid's effects include antioxidant properties and help to increase nitric oxide production. In addition, folate and vitamin $B_{12}$ improve insulin resistance.

L-arginine is an essential amino acid found in the Mediterranean diet in pumpkin seeds, soybeans, and peanuts and in small concentrations in dairy products such as yogurt. L-arginine has been shown to have beneficial effect on endothelial function in patients with hypercholesterolemia or existing coronary artery disease. High consumption of nuts with high L-arginine content is associated with a significantly lower risk of chronic heart disease. L-arginine improves both endothelium-dependent vasodilation and abnormal interactions of vascular cells, platelets, and monocytes. L-arginine also shows beneficial effects in patients with dyslipidemia or cigarette smoking.

Dietary soy protein has several beneficial effects on cardiovascular health. It helps to reduce cholesterol and triglyceride concentrations. It has antioxidant properties. Together, these have direct beneficial effect on endothelial function. Cumulatively, the Mediterranean diet with moderate alcohol consumption, moderate to high physical activity levels, and non-smoking was associated with lower mortality rates from all causes, chronic heart disease, cardiovascular disease, cancer, and other causes during a 10-year follow-up. Most study findings demonstrate that diets rich in fats, red and processed meats, sweets, desserts, French fries, and refined grains cause endothelial cell dysfunction. Conversely, diets rich in fruits, vegetables, legumes, whole grains, fish, olive oil, L-arginine, folic acid, soy protein, antioxidants (vitamins C and E, beta-carotene, lutein, selenium), high-fiber diet, red wine, black/green tea, almonds, and walnuts improve endothelial cell function.

## Polyphenols and the Mediterranean Diet

Flavonoids and other polyphenols in foods such as red wine, tea, onions, garlic, apples, and other fruits are associated with reduced risk and often help slow or reverse endothelial dysfunction. Epidemiological data shows significant protective effects of polyphenols against atherosclerosis, oxidation of LDL cholesterol, cardiac events, and cancer (Fig. 6.6) [49]. Polyphenols are found largely in fruits, vegetables, cereals, and beverages. Fruits like grapes, apple, pear, cherries, and berries contain several hundred milligrams of polyphenols per 100 grams weight. Also, dry legumes and chocolate contain significant amount of polyphenols, as does red wine or tea and coffee. Studies have shown that polyphenols protect against development of cancer, osteoporosis, diabetes, cardiovascular disease, and neurodegenerative diseases [50, 51]. Olive oil is an excellent source of polyphenols.

All plant phenolic compounds arise from a common intermediate phenylalanine. Usually, there is one or more sugar residues linked to hydroxyl groups. Polyphenols are classified in different groups based on the number of phenol rings and their structural elements that bind these rings together. The main class includes Phenolic acids, flavonoids, stilbenes, and lignans (see insert below). Flavonoids are the most studied group. They have two aromatic rings bound together by three carbon atoms. Polyphenols give plants their color. The phenolic group in polyphenols can accept an electron to form relatively stable phenoxyl radicals by interrupting a chain of oxidation reaction in cellular compounds. They increase antioxidant capacity in foods and beverages and create reduced levels of oxidative damage to cellular DNA.

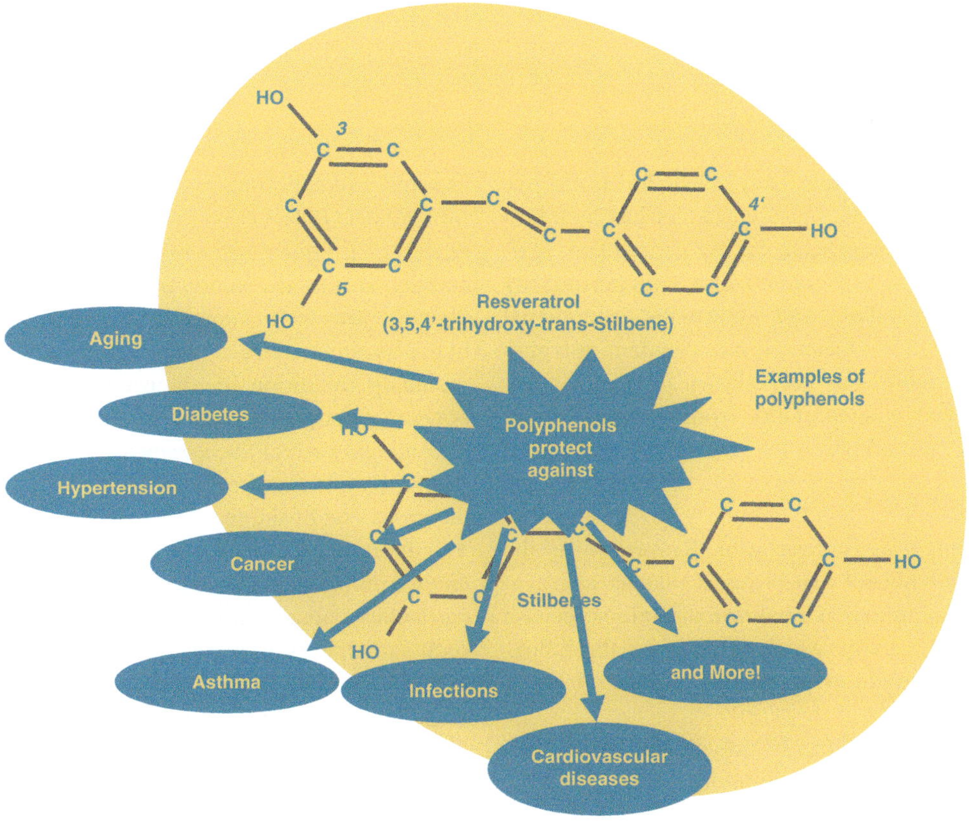


**Fig. 6.6** Pleiotropic health beneficial effects of dietary plant polyphenols. Polyphenols are naturally occurring compounds found largely in fruits, vegetables, cereals, and beverages. These molecules contribute to the bitterness, astringency of the food in which they are found. Researchers have found that these molecules are very good antioxidants and may neutralize the destructive reactivity of undesired reactive oxygen/nitrogen species produced as by-product during metabolic processes in the body. Epidemiological studies have revealed that polyphenols provide a significant protection against development of several chronic diseases as indicated. (Source: [49, Fig. 1]. Insert: Illustration by Elysian Creative Studio, www.elysiancreativestudio.com, Lizzy Colombo)

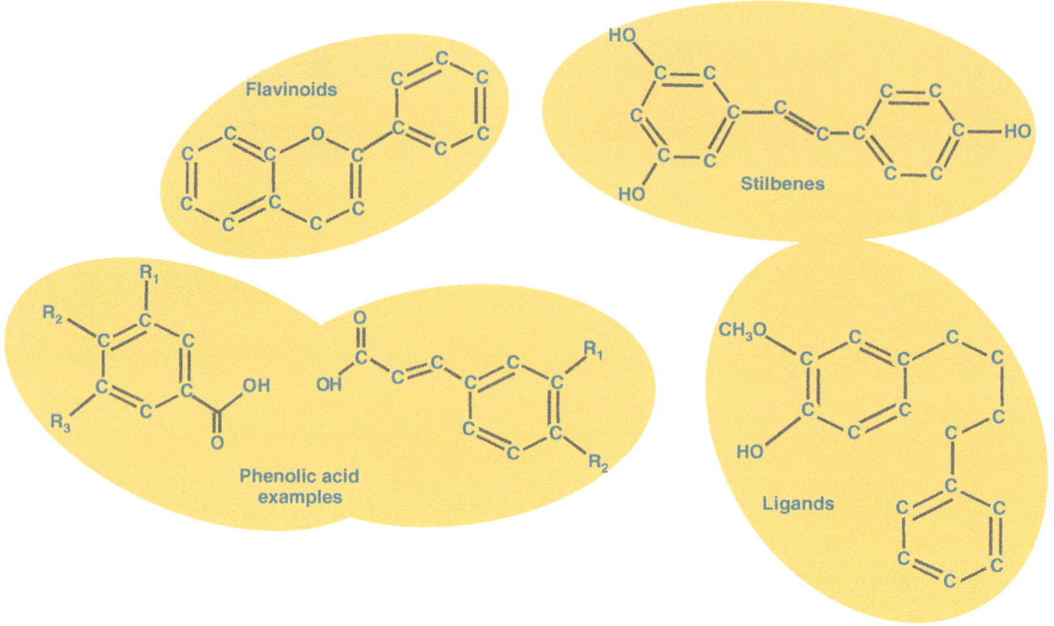


The polyphenols may also be protective against cardiovascular disease, not just by inhibiting oxidation of LDL but by antioxidant, antiplatelet, and anti-inflammatory properties, by increasing HDL, and improving endothelial function [52]. Quercetin, the abundant polyphenol in onions, has been shown to be adversely associated with mortality from coronary artery disease by inhibiting expression of metalloproteinase 1 and disruption of atherosclerotic plaque [52]. Black tea is a particularly strong polyphenol source, as is resveratrol. Resveratrol is the wine polyphenol that presents platelet aggregation via preferential inhibition of cyclooxygenase (COX 1) activity, which synthesizes thromboxane A2, an inducer of platelet aggregation and a vasoconstrictor [53].

Anticancer effects of polyphenols have been noted in various sites, including the mouth, stomach, duodenum, colon, liver, lung, mammary glands, and skin. Curcumin is also a polyphenol that had been tested and shows protective effects in some models against various cancers. It is believed that polyphenols influence the metabolism of pro-carcinogens by modulating the expression of cytochrome 450. Quercetin has been reported to possess anticancer properties, especially in experiments in mice by scavenging free radicals [54]. Onion polyphenols, especially quercetin, is known to possess strong antidiabetic activity. In fact the antidiabetic effects of polyphenols are well known. Polyphenols affect hypoglycemia through different mechanisms, including inhibition of glucose absorption and uptake by peripheral tissues.

Antiaging effects have been attributed to polyphenols, with the free radical oxidative stress theory as one of the most accepted mechanisms. The antioxidant capacity of plasma is related to dietary intake of antioxidants. Anthocyanins are particularly abundant in brightly colored foods such as berry fruits and grapes and grape seeds and are responsible for the color in those fruits. They have important anti-inflammatory and antioxidant effects and inhibit COX-1 and COX-2. Polyphenols are also beneficial in slowing the effects of aging on the nervous system. They cross the blood-brain barrier. Grape polyphenol has been studied as an antiaging agent and is believed to be beneficial in targeting the sirtuin class of NAD-dependent deacetylases. Resveratrol increases insulin sensitivity, decreases the expression of IGF-1, and increases AMP-activated protein kinase (AMPK) and peroxisome proliferator-activated receptor-c coactivator 1a (PGC-1a) activity.

Polyphenols demonstrate neuroprotective effects. It has been shown that people who drink three to four glasses of wine per day had an 80% decrease in symptoms of dementia and Alzheimer's disease compared to those who drank less or did not drink it at all [55]. Resveratrol is abundantly present in wine scavenges, $O_2^-$and $OH^-$in vitro, as well as lipid hydroperoxyl free radicals. It is an efficient antioxidant. Also, resveratrol has been shown to be protective against Parkinson's disease, a neurodegenerative disease of the substantia nigra [56]. Green tea has been shown to reduce the risk of developing Parkinson's disease via a pathway involving MAP kinases, which are fundamental for cell survival [57].

> … wine to gladden the heart of man, oil to make his face shine and bread to strengthen man's heart.
> (Psalm 104:15 (ESV), King David, c.979 BC)

## The Mediterranean Diet: What to Expect

In addition to its key components, the Mediterranean diet avoids (1) butter and margarine, which are replaced by olive and canola oils and nuts (to eliminate the saturated, trans, and hydrogenated fats), and (2) salt, which is replaced by herbs and spices. Fish is consumed at least twice a week, and frequent, moderate exercise is added. Elimination of saturated, trans, and hydrogenated fats is important because these contribute to heart disease. Olive oil is a mono-saturated fat which helps to reduce LDL. Extra-virgin and virgin olive oil are preferred since they are the least processed and contain the highest level of protective plant compounds that provide antioxidative effects. Canola oils and some nuts contain beneficial fats, including mono-saturated and polyunsaturated fats, and linoleic acid (a type of omega-3 fatty acid). Linoleic acid lowers triglycerides and blood clotting associated with sudden heart attacks, and it improves blood vessel health and helps to moderate BP. Linoleic acid is found in oily fishes, including mackerel, lake trout, herring, sardines, albacore tuna, and salmon.

Diet affects exercise. To optimize the efficacy of exercise, consume low-glycemic foods before and during exercise and high-glycemic food soon after exercise. Low-glycemic foods will release glucose more slowly and steadily, which will maximize performance and increase endurance. High-glycemic foods will cause a more rapid rise in blood glucose levels, helping energy recovery and speed postexercise recovery. Foods with a low-glycemic index, less than 55, include 100% stone-ground whole wheat or pumpernickel bread; oatmeal (rolled or steel-cut), oat bran, and muesli, quinoa; pasta, converted rice, barley, and bulgur wheat; sweet potato, corn, yam, lima/butter beans, peas, legumes, lentils, and chickpeas; skim milk and reduced-fat yogurt; and most fruits, non-starchy vegetables, and carrots. Foods with a high-glycemic index, greater than 70, include sugar; flour; rice; white potatoes; some fruits, including bananas, grapes, cherries, watermelon; raisins; many breakfast cereals, including puffed rice and corn flakes; bread; soda; and cookies and crackers.

An easy way to transition to the Mediterranean diet is to start by eating 7–10 servings of vegetables and fruits per day and switch to whole grains, including whole-grain cereals, rice, and pasta. Also, keep nuts, tahini, and natural peanut butter close for snacks. Then add one to two meals with fish per week. Avoid butter; instead use olive oil or canola oil. Avoid frying the fish, and use canola or olive oil in cooking, if necessary. Avoid red meat, sausage, bacon, and other fatty meats and high-fat dairy. For dairy (to ensure a source of calcium), consume low-fat dairy: 2% or less milk, low-fat cheese or ice cream, or fat-free yogurt.

With all of the fruits and vegetables included in the Mediterranean diet, plenty of antioxidants are consumed. Table 6.1 lists the 20 common foods with the most antioxidants.

**Table 6.1** Twenty common foods with the most antioxidants

| Rank | Food item | Serving size | Total antioxidant capacity per serving size |
|---|---|---|---|
| 1 | Small red bean (dried) | Half cup | 13,727 |
| 2 | Wild blueberry | 1 cup | 13,427 |
| 3 | Red kidney bean (dried) | Half cup | 13,259 |
| 4 | Pinto bean | Half cup | 11,864 |
| 5 | Blueberry (cultivated) | 1 cup | 9019 |
| 6 | Cranberry | 1 cup (whole) | 8983 |
| 7 | Artichoke (cooked) | 1 cup (hearts) | 7904 |
| 8 | Blackberry | 1 cup | 7701 |
| 9 | Prune | Half cup | 7291 |
| 10 | Raspberry | 1 cup | 6058 |
| 11 | Strawberry | 1 cup | 5938 |
| 12 | Red delicious apple | 1 whole | 5900 |
| 13 | Granny Smith apple | 1 whole | 5381 |
| 14 | Pecan | 1 ounce | 5095 |
| 15 | Sweet cherry | 1 cup | 4873 |
| 16 | Black plum | 1 whole | 4844 |
| 17 | Russet potato (cooked) | 1 whole | 4649 |
| 18 | Black bean (dried) | Half cup | 4181 |
| 19 | Plum | 1 whole | 4118 |
| 20 | Gala apple | 1 whole | 3903 |

Source: WebMD Public Information from the United States Department of Agriculture Reviewed by Charlotte E. Grayson Mathis, MD on April 01, 2005

An example of what might be eaten in a day:

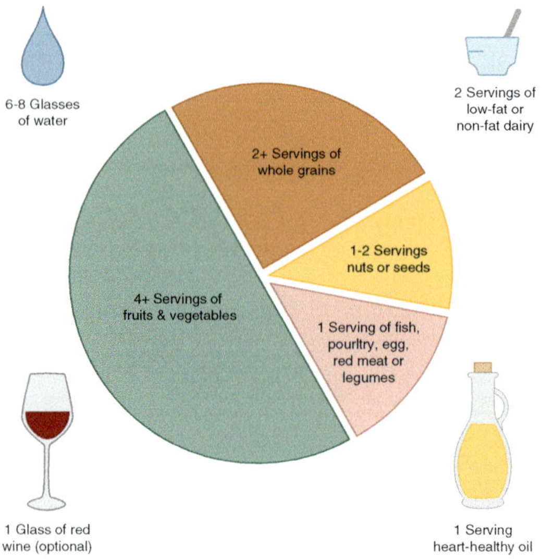


- *6–8, 8 oz glasses of water per day* to stay properly hydrated. This is of equal importance to the rest of the Mediterranean diet.
- *Breakfast*: a slice of sourdough bread with chopped tomatoes, red onion, and fresh herbs with crumbled feta and a drizzle of olive oil and balsamic vinegar. A slice of melon with tea or Greek coffee (or espresso) may be added.
- *Snack*: fresh fruit (pear, small bunch grapes, a couple of figs) or small handful of nuts (walnuts, almonds, or hazelnuts).
- *Lunch*: Mediterranean vegetable bake (briami) with small serving of rice.
- *Afternoon snack*: Greek plain natural yogurt drizzled with honey and a few crushed walnuts.
- *Dinner*: baked or grilled snapper (or other oily fish) with salad of fresh leafy greens drizzled with olive oil and lemon juice and a small glass of wine.
- *After dinner*: a small plate of fresh fruit to share (melon, grapes, figs, stone fruits).

## Health Benefits of Olive Oil

Olive oil is central to a healthy lifestyle, including the Mediterranean diet. Several sections of this book discuss the benefits of olive oil and its contents and the benefits of substituting olive oil for other types of less healthy fats. Olive oil, including its constituents, monounsaturated fats and antioxidants, helps to increase levels of omega-3 fatty acids and nitric oxide and reduces oxidative stress (the point of the first three prongs of the Mind-Body Wellness Program). Olive oil helps to maintain brain-heart health. The main health constituents of olive oil are its polyphenols. Polyphenols are micronutrients from plant-based foods, helping plants to defend against ultraviolet radiation and pathogens. Those contained in olive oil are estradiol, hydroxytamoxifen, oleuropein, and hydroxytyrosol (Fig. 6.7).

Estradiol in olives and olive oil is a phytosteroid. In humans, it is also a steroid that is converted to estrogen, the primary female sex hormone, and is important in the regulation of the estrous and menstrual cycles in the female reproductive system. Estradiol is essential for the

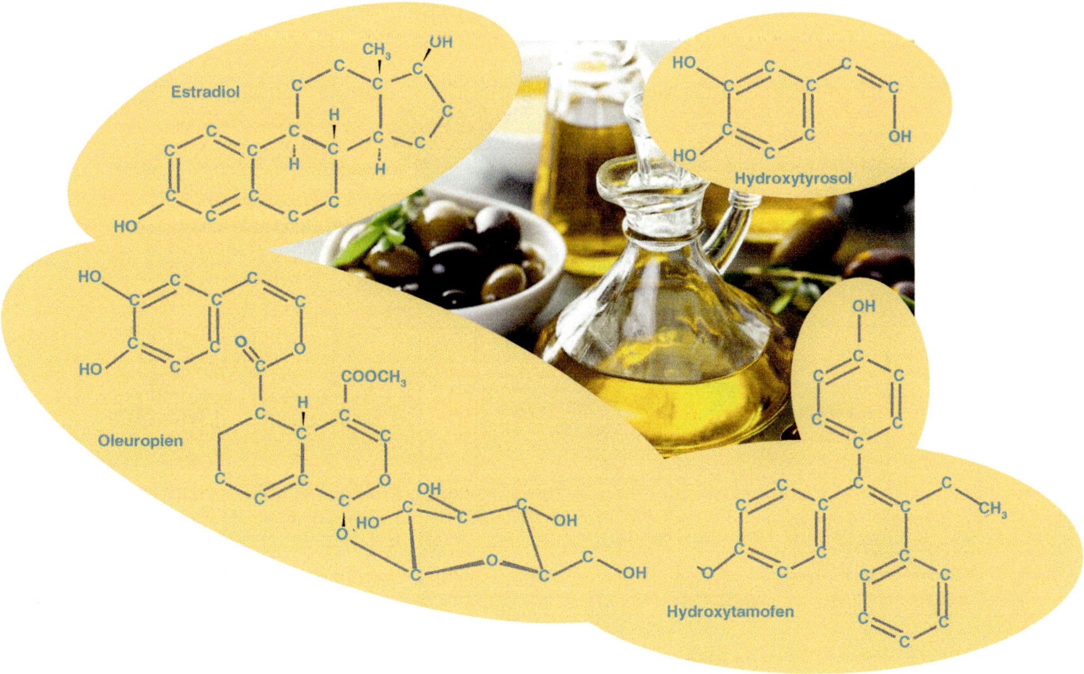


**Fig. 6.7** Olive oil polyphenols. (Adapted from Shutterstock Royalty-free stock illustration ID: 486373963, Olive oil in vintage bottles with black and green olives and leaves copyspace on rustic background, by Elena Veselova)

development and maintenance of female reproductive tissues such as the breasts, uterus, and vagina during puberty, adulthood, and pregnancy. While estrogen levels in men are lower compared to those in women, estrogens have essential functions in men. In both genders, it has important effects in many nonreproductive tissues, including the bone, fat, skin, liver, and brain. In women, estradiol is produced primarily in the follicles of the ovaries. In both genders, it is produced in endocrine (e.g., adrenal glands) and non-endocrine tissues, including fat, liver, breast, and neural tissues. Hydroxytamoxifen is a selective estrogen receptor modulator (antagonist) of the estrogen-related receptors. It has antitumor (breast cancer) effects as well as antiplatelet activities which are shown to reduce angiogenesis in tumors and, thereby, malignancy.

The main active constituents of olive oil include oleic acid and other phenolic constituents. The main phenolic compounds of olive oil are hydroxytyrosol and oleuropein. They give extra-virgin olive oil its bitter, pungent taste [58]. From oleic acid, oleuropein is produced and has pharmacological activities including antioxidant, anti-inflammatory, anti-atherogenic, anticancer activities, antimicrobial, and antiviral activities, as well as hypolipidemic and hypoglycemic effects [59]. The pharmacological properties of olive oil, the olive fruit, and its leaves have been recognized as important components of medicine and a healthy diet from the time before Hippocrates.

Hydroxytyrosol is a phenylethanoid, a type of phenolic phytochemical with antioxidant properties [60]. It is found in olive leaf and olive oil, in the form of its elenolic acid ester oleuropein and, especially after degradation, in its plain form. Hydroxytyrosol itself in pure form is a colorless, odorless liquid. The olives, leaves, and olive pulp contain large amounts of hydroxytyrosol compared to olive oil. However, it was found that black olives, such as common canned variety, containing iron(II) gluconate, contained little hydroxytyrosol, as iron salts are catalysts for its oxidation. Hydroxytyrosol helps to increase the antioxidant activities of catalase and superoxide dismutase, and as an anti-sclerotic, it helps to

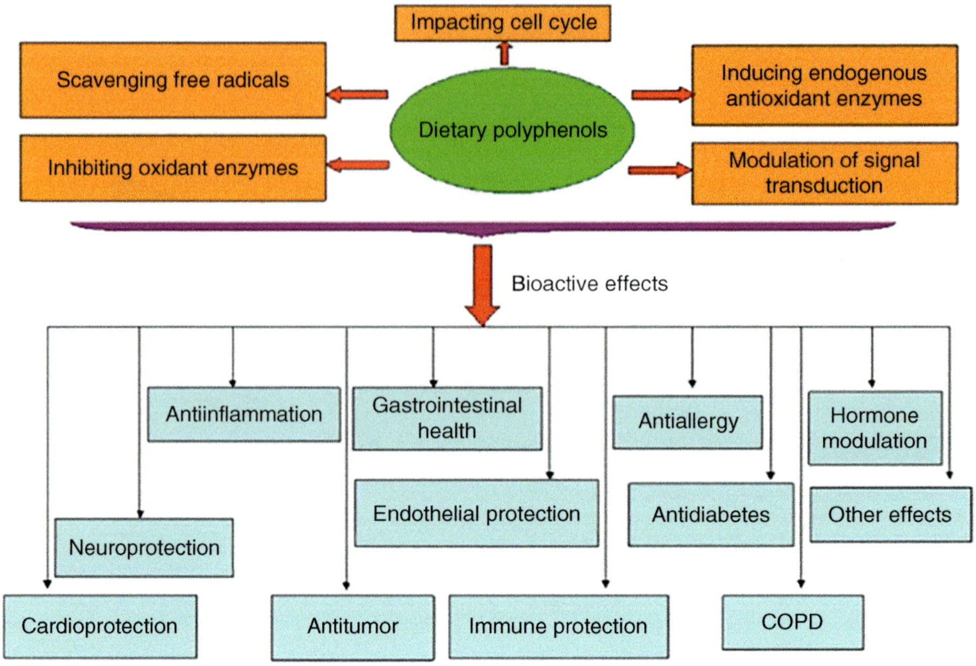


**Fig. 6.8** The bioactive effects of olive oil polyphenols [61, Fig. 2] (Open Acces, MDPI)

lower serum, total, and LDL cholesterol and slows the lipid peroxidation process [61].

The effects of these (dietary) polyphenols are summarized in Fig. 6.8. The primary bioactive effects include its antioxidant effects leading to healthy DNA repair, fewer mitochondria defects, and reduced aging factors (e.g., senescence-associated secretory phenotype or SASP) and inflammatory factors. Olive oil polyphenols also stabilize membranes (Fig. 6.9), prevent angiogenesis, and reduce inflammation. They are probiotic, acting as an antimicrobial. They improve endothelial function with antihypertensive properties [63].

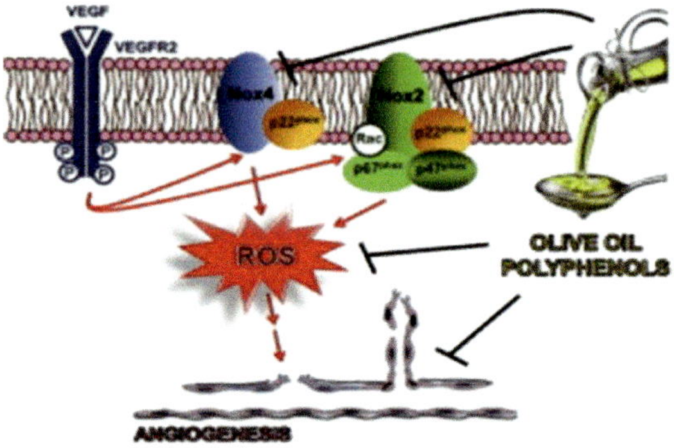


**Fig. 6.9** Olive oil polyphenols are antioxidant, anti-inflammatory, anti-sclerotic, and antihypertensive. Abbreviations: ROS, reactive oxygen species [62]. (Republished with permission from Elsevier. Source [63]

Stabilizing membranes with the omega-3 fatty acids promotes membrane health, helping them to be more flexible and resilient, and improves cellular signaling and membrane transport. Specifically from the olive oil polyphenols, the cis structure of oleic acid fits neatly into the phospholipid structure of biomembranes and alters receptor cites on the membrane surface to regulate blood pressure (Fig. 6.10) [64]. Oleic Acid (see insert below) from olive oil blocks the activity of the β-adrenoceptors to reduce BP. Olive oil also helps to maintain a healthy endothelium throughout the body. The endothelium is strategically located and is central to brain-heart health. It works to maintain healthy blood flow to nerves (including the brain) and the heart to help maintain their health. A healthy endothelium modulates both (1) circulating blood, by promoting healthy platelet function, coagulation, monocyte and leukocyte adhesion, and inflammation, and

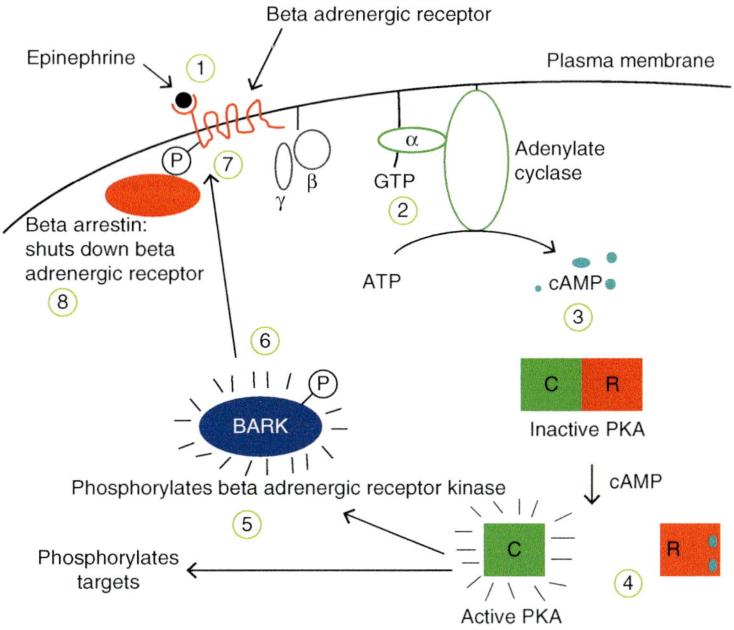


**Fig. 6.10** β-adrenergic signaling pathway. Epinephrine activates β-adrenoceptors, which in turn activate a G-protein. Lipid-protein interactions regulate the localization and activity of G-proteins and, therefore, cell signaling. G-proteins activate adenylyl cyclase that produce cAMP and activate PKA. Oleic acid from olive oil blocks the activity of the β-adrenoceptors to reduce blood pressure. (Republished with permission from Professor Pablo Vicente Escribá Ruiz, in memory of Dr. John E. Halver. Source: [64]. Insert: Illustration by Elysian Creative Studio, www.elysiancreativestudio.com, Lizzy Colombo)

(2) vascular smooth muscle cells, by promoting permeability, relaxing the contractile state, maintaining healthy proliferative (growth) and migratory response, and maintaining a healthy redox state. And as my great-grandmother used to say, it even keeps you regular.

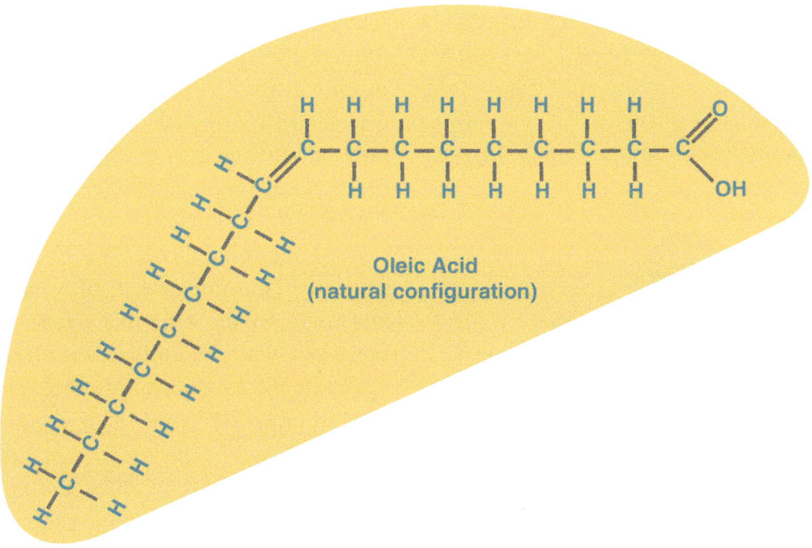


…oil to make his [Man's] face shine…

## The Power of the Grape

Grapes help to satisfy the Mediterranean diet recommendation of four or more servings of fruits and vegetables per day. Grapes can become wine, which at moderate levels (one to two 4 oz glasses per day) is also recommended with the Mediterranean diet. Grapes also offer additional benefits (see insert below). Like olives, grapes contain polyphenols. Grape polyphenols give grapes their color. Grape polyphenols are found in the skins and seeds of grapes. They function naturally as antioxidants (including to scavenge free radicals) and as an anti-atherosclerotic (keeping arteries more flexible). They help to maintain healthy platelet aggregation (anticlotting), stimulate nitric oxide production (reduce blood pressure), and more is being discovered. All of this benefits cardiovascular and nervous system health (the mind-body connection). Flavonoids are the largest and most studied subgroup of polyphenols. In grapes, flavonoids are particularly found in the skins and seeds. The skin has a high concentration of a class of flavonoids called anthocyanins, while the seeds contain flavanols, including proanthocyanidins. Grape juice has a greater polyphenol concentration than many other juices, including blueberry, cranberry, orange, pomegranate, and apple juices [65]. The antioxidant [66] and anticlotting [67, 68, 69] potential of red grape juice vs. red wine is about the same. The flavonoids in grape juice help manage the effects of LDL cholesterol, including protecting LDL cholesterol from oxidation [70, 71]. Purple grape juice (including red wine) polyphenols increases nitric oxide production, improves endothelial function, and reduces oxidation of LDLs, all helping to keep arteries more flexible (by promoting endothelial health). As a result, it is easier for arteries to dilate, improving circulation and reducing both systolic and diastolic blood pressure [72, 73], as well as nocturnal blood pressure [74], helping with coronary artery disease.

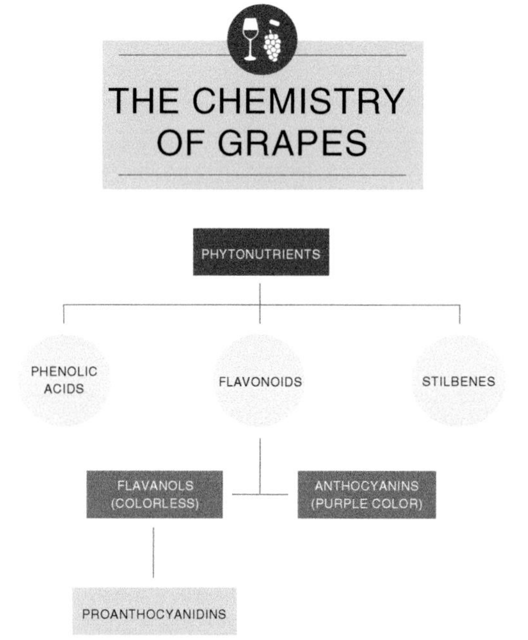


Poor nocturnal blood pressure control is an indicator of poor autonomic (P&S) control of the cardiovascular system which indicates risk of heart disease [75]. Improved endothelial health by grape juice consumption has been measured by enhanced flow-mediated dilation of the brachial artery [71, 76–78], including after cardiovascular disease is diagnosed. Grape polyphenols, proanthocyanidins, were identified as providing antiplatelet and anticlotting effects [79]. Epidemiological evidence on grape consumption and heart health, including the "French paradox," is outlined in a 2009 *Journal of Nutrition* article [75]. The paradox is based on the high level of cholesterol consumption (cheeses, butter, cream) and the low rate of heart disease attributed to the French national habit of moderate wine consumption. This review article supports the beneficial effects of grapes and grape polyphenols on cardiovascular health, including antioxidant effects, and effects on improved endothelial function, reduced platelet aggregation, and reduced systolic and diastolic blood pressure.

The health benefits of grape juice (including wine, especially red wine) may also include reducing blood glucose levels [80] and supporting cognitive [81–84] and immune health [85]. The cognitive benefit of grape juice and wine may be attributed to improved blood flow to the brain. As a component of the Mediterranean diet, wine (Fig. 6.11) helps slow and possibly even reverse age-related cognitive, including memory, decline. The immune health benefit may be attributed to the fact that grape juice contains vitamin C and the antioxidant effects of vitamin C. While the Mediterranean diet promotes higher consumption of fruits and vegetables, not all fruits and vegetables are created equally. Darker-colored fruits typically offer more phytonutrients than lighter options. Phytonutrients are plant compounds, like carotenoids, lycopene, resveratrol, and phytosteroids, found in plants, vegetables, tofu, and teas. Dark-skinned blue and purple fruits also have unique plant nutrients not found in many other colors of fruits and vegetables. Blue and purple fruits and vegetables account for about 3% of total produce intake, despite blue and purple fruits and vegetables being associated with healthier diets in both children and adults.

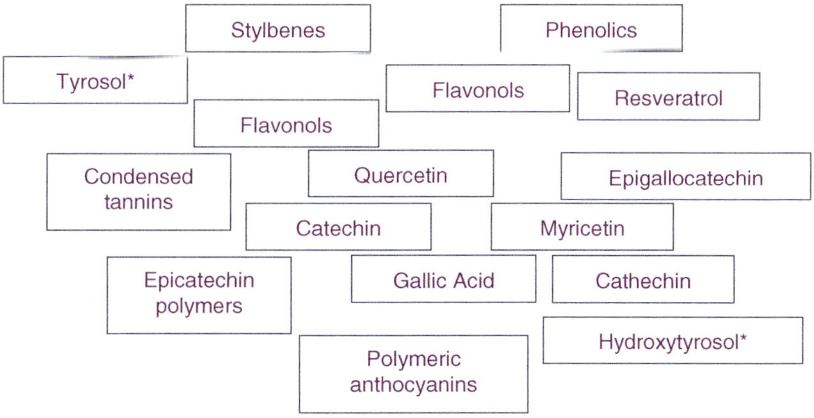


**Fig. 6.11** Main polyphenols in wine. *Polyphenols contained only in white wine [86, Fig. 8] (Open Access, InTech Open. Insert: Illustration by Elysian Creative Studio, www.elysiancreativestudio.com, Lizzy Colombo)

The most popular blue or purple fruits and vegetables are grapes, grape juice, raisins, blackberries, blueberries, plums, dried plums/prunes, eggplant, and purple cabbage.

...wine to gladden the heart of Man...

## The Incredible Whole Wheat Grain

The third "star" of the Mediterranean diet is wheat. The health benefits of wheat are now well known (see insert right). The benefits are due to the B vitamins (thiamin, folate, and vitamin $B_6$) and the minerals (magnesium, zinc, and manganese) it provides. Wheat is probably the most common cereal available worldwide and is even higher in demand in recent years due to its abundant health benefits. Over the years, it has shown itself to be one of the most successful and sustainable cereal crops in the world. It originated in Southwestern Asia, but today, it is grown in countless countries. Commonly, wheat cultivation is done at higher latitudes and is primarily used for baking bread products. Foods like bread, pasta, crackers, bagels, cakes, and muffins are just a few common examples of wheat sources.

Whole wheat is believed to be one of the most wholesome food items, and it ensures a diet rich in nutrients. Wheat is extremely beneficial for healthy living. It considerably lowers the hazards of heart diseases, owing to its comparatively low-fat content. It also regulates blood glucose levels in diabetic patients. Wheat is able to provide an immense energy source from all parts of the grain kernel, including the bran, germ, and endosperm. The nutrient value of wheat is retained even after processing it into flour. However, to receive the maximum benefit out of wheat products, it's advisable to choose those products that are made from whole wheat flour rather than the refined varieties.

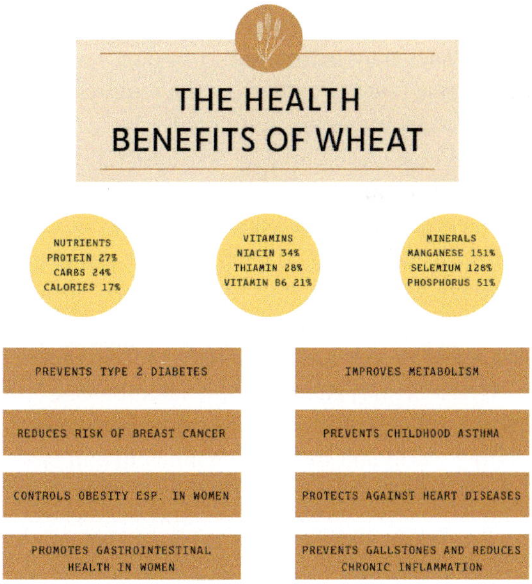


The health benefits of wheat greatly depend on the form in which it is consumed. Whole wheat is extremely nutritious. However, the benefits of wheat are reduced with bleached white flour which is obtained by processing only 60% of what may be extracted from the grain. In the

United States, most wheat products undergo this 60% extraction, as found in noodles, breads, and pasta, as well as in baked goods like rolls, biscuits, and cookies. In these foods, 40% of the original wheat grain was removed, including the outer brown layer, which contains the highly nutritious bran and the germ of the wheat grain. In the extraction process, more than half of the vitamins $B_1$, $B_2$, $B_3$, and E, calcium, phosphorus, folic acid, copper, zinc, iron, and fiber are lost. Purchasing 100% whole wheat products ensures that of all the nutrients of the bran and the germ are consumed, including the endosperm.

After personal experimentation in the kitchen, a mix of two-thirds bleached white flour to one-third whole wheat flour returns much of the nutrients lost in the processing. With this ratio of white to brown, most recipes for white flour (breads, rolls, biscuits, cookies, cakes, etc.) do not change, except (optional – personal preference) for perhaps a little more yeast, or chemical leavening, if a lighter product is desired. The two-thirds to one-third ratio may be used in noodles and pasta, as well as with rice, where a little more water may be desired to further soften the brown rice (since leavening is not required).

In recent years, the nutritional value of whole wheat is being recognized by consumers. Low-carb diets and an increase in the whole wheat cereal markets are prevalent around the world, especially in the Mediterranean. The wheat germ component of whole wheat is by itself a rich source of nutrients. Wheat germ has an abundance of vitamins and minerals, but it is particularly rich in vitamin E. Wheat germ is known to be a main source of the B complex vitamins in dietary structures throughout the world and includes vitamins like thiamin, folic acid, and vitamin $B_6$ and minerals like manganese, magnesium, and zinc. Wheat germ oil improves strength and may increase life span.

Wheat is rich in catalytic elements: mineral salts, calcium, magnesium, potassium, sulfur, chlorine, arsenic, silicon, manganese, zinc, iodide, copper, vitamin B, and vitamin E. This wealth of nutrients is why it is often used as a cultural base or foundation of nourishment. Issues like anemia, mineral deficiencies, gallstones, breast cancer, chronic inflammation, obesity, asthenia, tuberculosis, pregnancy problems, and breastfeeding problems are quickly improved by consuming whole wheat. It is also recommended to treat sterility. Since germinated wheat comprises two or three times more vitamin B than the common kind, the seeds are useful for treating gastrointestinal conditions, skin diseases, respiratory illnesses, and cardiovascular ailments. It is also known to help balance cholesterol levels and protect the heart.

Wheat has a natural ability to control weight in everyone, but this ability is more pronounced among women. The *American Journal of Clinical Nutrition* has shown through research that whole wheat, rather than its refined form, is a good choice for obese patients. Women who consumed whole wheat products over long periods showed considerably more weight loss than the other subjects. Whole grains like wheat are immensely effective on patients with metabolic disorders. Common types of metabolic syndromes include visceral obesity, also known as the "pear-shaped" body, high triglycerides, low levels of (protective) HDL cholesterol, and high blood pressure. It protects against all of these conditions. Foods made from refined grains not only tend to increase weight, but they also increase the hazards of insulin resistance. The whole grain requires burning more sugar to breakdown, thereby lower insulin requirements. Whole wheat bread and other fiber-rich foods are recommended. The majority of fiber works to help the digestive process in the body and improve the overall metabolism. Having a whole wheat diet is probably the most effective, quick, and enjoyable way to reduce metabolic syndrome but also to stay slim and healthy throughout life.

Wheat is rich in magnesium, which acts as a cofactor for more than 300 enzymes in the body. These enzymes are involved in the body's functional use of insulin and glucose secretion. Foods that contain whole grain by at least 51% weight are also low in saturated fat and cholesterol, causing lower risk of coronary ailments and certain types of cancer. Moreover, regular consumption of whole-grain wheat promotes healthy blood sugar control. Patients who suffer from diabetes are able to keep their sugar levels under control by replacing white rice with wheat in their diet, thereby lowering their triglycerides.

The betaine content of wheat is what aids in the prevention of chronic inflammation. Betaine is usually found in whole wheat, beets, and spinach. Betaine is any neutral chemical compound with a positively charged cationic functional group which bears no hydrogen atom and with a negatively charged functional group such as a carboxylate group which may not be adjacent to the cationic site (see insert below for an example).

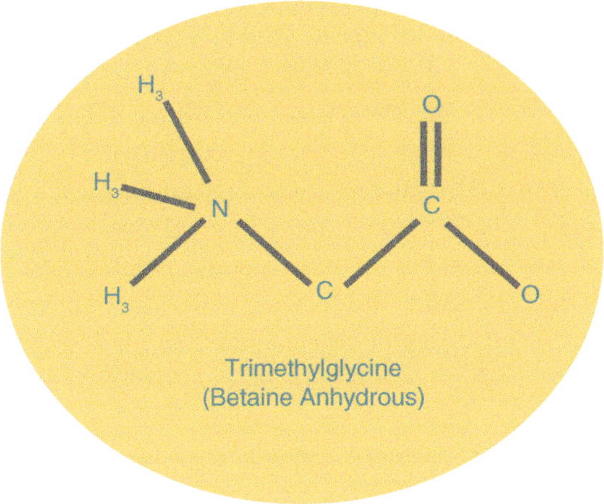


Historically, the term was reserved for trimethylglycine only. Biologically, betaine is involved in methylation reactions and detoxification of homocysteine. In biological systems, many naturally occurring betaines serve as organic osmolytes, substances synthesized or taken up from the environment by cells for protection against osmotic stress, drought, high salinity, or high temperature. Intracellular accumulation of betaines, non-perturbing to enzyme function, protein structure, and membrane integrity, permits water retention in cells, thus protecting from the effects of dehydration. It is also a methyl donor of increasingly recognized significance in biology. Inflammation is a key constituent in most types of rheumatic pains and also some rheumatic diseases. Thus, it is a good idea to eat healthy amounts of whole wheat food products that will actively reduce inflammation. Consumption of betaine affects a number of aspects in body chemistry that assures a lower risk of chronic inflammation and other ailments like osteoporosis, heart disease, Alzheimer's disease, cognitive decline, and type 2 diabetes.

In various surveys by the *American Journal of Gastroenterology*, it has been proven that breads and cereals made from whole wheat help women to avoid gallstones. Since whole wheat is rich in insoluble fiber, it assures a quick and smooth intestinal transit time and lowers the secretion of bile acids. Excessive bile acids are a major cause of gallstone formation. Moreover, a high intake of wheat increases insulin sensitivity and thereby lowers triglycerides or fat in the blood. Besides wheat, insoluble fiber is also ingested from the edible skins of fruits and certain vegetables like cucumbers, tomatoes, and squash, berries, apples, and pears. Beans also provide both insoluble and soluble fiber. All are recommended to be consumed as part of the Mediterranean diet.

Wheat is the most popular and easily available bulk laxative. Three cups of wheat consumption per day is enough to help an individual to live a long, healthy, and disease-free life. Maintaining a fiber-rich diet comprised of wheat breads and cereals that are high in bran reduces pain, flatulence, nausea, constipation, and distension. Diverticulitis often occurs due to inflammation with lower intestinal pains. This can also lead to chronic constipation and unnecessary straining, which can result in a sac or a pouch in the wall of the colon. Such cases can be easily dealt with naturally by keeping up with a fiber-rich diet and including whole wheat on a regular basis. However, like everything else in life, too much is not healthy either. Wheat contains oxalates, which are the naturally occurring substances in the body. Too much oxalate in bodily fluids can lead to crystallization, thereby causing gallstones, kidney stones, and gout.

Whole wheat acts as an anticarcinogenic agent, particularly in women. Wheat bran enhances the metabolic rate of estrogen. Excessive levels of estrogen may lead to breast cancer. To prevent this, whole wheat also contains lignans, which are phytonutrients acting as hormonelike substances. The lignans occupy the hormone receptors of the body, blocking the estrogen from binding and thereby being excessively active, reducing the risk of breast cancer. In total, whole wheat provides a balanced result. It provides the benefit as well as the limiter to keep the system in balance. In fact, most natural, unprocessed foods or nutraceuticals which offer health benefits also, in the same product, provide buffers to prevent the health benefit from becoming unhealthy. (Remember the example of oxygen: too little causes low energy, not healthy, and too much burns or oxidizes, and destroys, also not healthy; only just enough is needed to be healthy and well.) Approximately 30 grams of whole wheat consumed per day is recommended, especially for pre-menopausal women. This amount has been found to reduce the risks of breast cancer by up to 41% compared with equivalent amounts of other forms of fiber. Another anticarcinogenic activity of wheat bran is to reduce the risks of colon cancer. Wheat bran considerably reduces bile acid secretion and bacterial enzymes in the stool, which reduces this risk.

Mediterranean-style diets of whole grains and fish has been found to lower the risk of childhood asthma by up to 50% [87]. A study shows that considerably increased whole wheat in the diets of children and mothers on special diets high in fish and whole grains reduced the possibility of becoming asthmatic by almost 66%. Bronchial hyper-responsiveness is the key factor that encourages asthma. This condition is characterized by the narrowing of the airways and increased sensitivity. Children who eat wheat and fish in high amounts do not suffer from such ailments. Magnesium and vitamin E provided by wheat also contribute in reducing the problem of asthma. However, in some cases, wheat consumption may be harmful for asthma patients, since wheat also happens to be a food allergen closely linked with asthma. Complete examination and diagnosis of all possible allergies is recommended. Note that wheat allergies, like many food allergies, are due to the fact that much of the wheat (food) that is eaten is not grown local to the consumer; therefore, there is no immunity built up to the allergens that are causing the unhealthy condition. The natural ecosystem is not able to function.

Plant lignans, mentioned above, are converted by responsive flora in the intestines into mammalian lignans. One of these lignans is called enterolactone, which protects against breast and other hormone-dependent cancers and also heart disease. Note that whole wheat is not the only source of lignans; nuts, seeds, and berries are also rich sources of plant lignans, as well as various other vegetables, fruits, and beverages like coffee, tea, and wine. All are components recommended in a Mediterranean-style diet. As mentioned above, whole wheat's ability to protect against heart disease is based on its antioxidant and cholesterol-balancing effects. Specifically, given these effects, lignans from whole wheat together with a balanced Mediterranean diet help to prevent, or work to reduce the effects of, heart disease and brain trauma by reducing obesity, high blood pressure, and high LDL cholesterol and slowing the progression of atherosclerosis by reducing the oxidation of LDLs, thereby reducing the frequency of heart attacks and strokes. The effectiveness of pharmaceuticals for heart disease, such as ACE inhibitors and β-blockers, are significantly enhanced by whole wheat and other whole grains as part of the Mediterranean diet, and they have less of an impact on the rest of the body's systems due to their balanced composition.

...and bread to strengthen man's heart.

## Resveratrol

Resveratrol (see insert below for an example) is a stilbenoid, a type of natural phenol, and a phytoalexin produced by several plants. The "French paradox" showed a correlation between red wine intake and low mortality due to coronary heart diseases. The red wine substance resveratrol was claimed to play a key role. As a result, resveratrol may be the most investigated plant secondary metabolite. Resveratrol demonstrates antioxidant and other healthful properties [88]. While studies continue into the biological activities of one function or compound at a time, the holistic benefits of the Mediterranean diet and the benefits of many "natural" remedies continue to demonstrate that nature is multivariate. It is important to know the effect of a single molecule. However, the effect of any one molecule is modulated by its carrying matrix, its bioavailability, and its synergies with other molecules. This is the balance in nature mentioned above. This balance automatically buffers and protects [89].

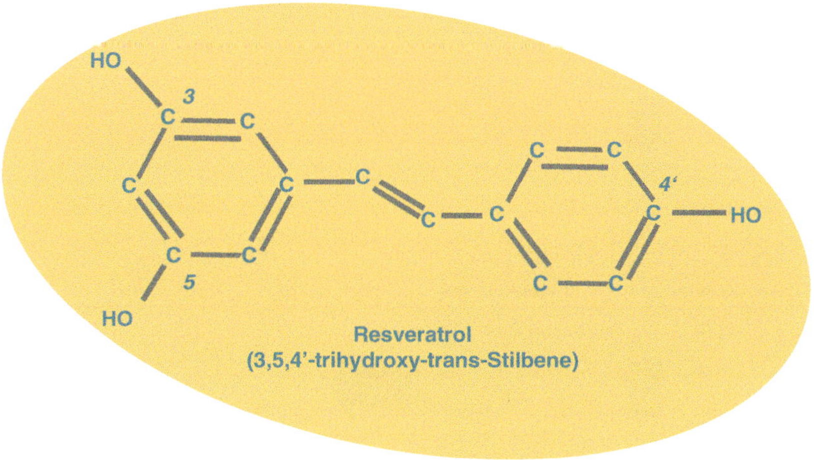


Sources of resveratrol in food include the skin of grapes, blueberries, raspberries, and mulberries. The levels of resveratrol found in food vary considerably, even in the same food from season to season and batch to batch. Red wine contains between 0.2 and 5.8 mg/l resveratrol, depending on the grape variety [90]. Red wine contains more resveratrol than white wine because red wine is fermented together with the grape skins, whereas white wine is fermented after grape skins have been removed. The composition of wine is different from that of grapes since the extraction of resveratrol from grapes depends on the duration of the skin contact, and the resveratrol 3-glucosides are in part hydrolyzed, yielding both *trans*- and *cis*-resveratrol (see Table 6.2). Ounce for ounce, peanuts have about 25% as much resveratrol as red wine [89]. Peanuts, especially sprouted peanuts, have a content similar to grapes in a range of 2.3–4.5 µg/g and 11.7–25.7 µg/g before sprouting and after sprouting, respectively, depending upon the variety and source location. Mulberries (especially the skin) are a source of as much as 50 micrograms of resveratrol per gram dry weight (see Table 6.3).

**Table 6.2** Resveratrol concentrations in wine and grape juice

| Beverage | Resveratrol (mean/range) (mg/150 ml) |
|---|---|
| Red wine | 0.27/0–2.78 |
| Rose wine | $0.12/5.00e^{-03}$–0.29 |
| White wine | 0.04/0.00–0.17 |
| Sparkling wine | $9.00e^{-03}/8.00e^{-03}$–$1.00e^{-02}$ |
| Green grape juice | $5.08e^{-03}$/0.00–$1.00e^{-02}$ |

Source: Wikipedia

**Table 6.3** Resveratrol concentrations in selected foods

| Food | Serving | Total resveratrol (mg) |
|---|---|---|
| Peanuts (raw) | 1 cup (146 grams) | 0.01–0.26 |
| Peanut butter | 1 cup (258 grams) | 0.04–0.13 |
| Red grapes | 1 cup (160 grams) | 0.24–1.25 |
| Cocoa powder | 1 cup (200 grams) | 0.28–0.46 |

Source: [90], Wikipedia

A concern regarding resveratrol is its lack of bioavailability in the body and therefore what else it might do in the body. What is known is that resveratrol will modify LOX-1, the oxidized LDL cholesterol receptor that enables the progression of atherosclerosis. Resveratrol (1) increases endothelial nitric oxide expression, (2) induces the superoxide SOD enzymes which are protective and antioxidant, (3) decreases the activity of NADPH oxidase, (4) decreases the expression of inflammatory NF-kB, (5) inhibits COX-1, and (6) reduces smooth muscle cell migration by reducing angiotensin II (Fig. 6.12). Resveratrol's effect as an anti-inflammatory enhances immune response and endothelial function [91]. In fact, the strength of the Mediterranean diet regarding atherosclerosis may be the use of the grape. The grape is a crucial ingredient with

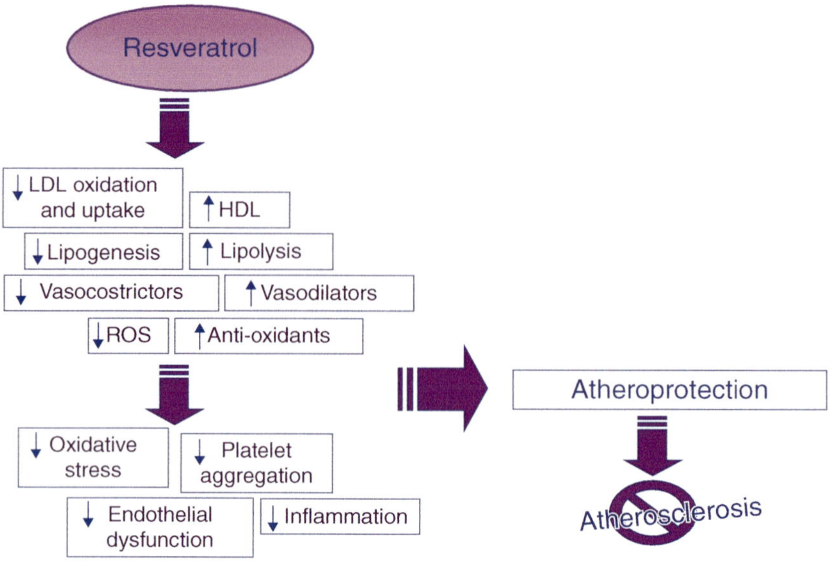


**Fig. 6.12** Main athero-protective mechanisms exerted by resveratrol [86, Fig. 6] (Open Access, InTech Open)

its source of resveratrol to decrease LOX-1 mediation and modulate LOX-1 to oxidize LDL if not taken up in the scavenger cells. Resveratrol has emerged in recent years as a compound conferring strong protection against metabolic, cardiovascular, and other age-related complications, including neurodegeneration and cancer. This has generated the notion that resveratrol treatment acts as a calorie-restriction mimetic, possibly helping to manage metabolic disorders [92, 93].

Resveratrol activates AMPK in various tissue cells (Fig. 6.13) [93]. For example, activating AMPK stimulates hepatic fatty acid oxidation. There are data linking resveratrol for being protective in patients with mitochondrial disorders [95–97] and neurological dysfunction [98–102], although this has been controversial. However, despite numerous studies, it is still inconclusive whether consuming this phenol can extend life expectancy or have anticancer effects. It was once thought that the benefit of red wine on heart disease, the so-called French paradox, was due to the effects of resveratrol. However, the benefit of grape consumption and wine is probably multifactorial and not restricted just to this natural phenol [103].

## Antioxidant Effects

Many components of the Mediterranean diet provide or promote antioxidant effects. However, grapes, oranges, and blueberries, which are some of the best food sources of antioxidants, are not enough; not enough foods are able to be consumed without increasing the risks antioxidants are meant to decrease. As modeled by type 2 diabetes (see "Oxidative Stress and Autonomic Neuropathy, Type II Diabetes as a Model") and demonstrated in the Steno-2 trial and Diabetes Prevention Program, lifestyle changes have been shown to have a beneficial impact on the prevention, and progression, of CAN. Lifestyle changes include diet, physical exercise, and smoking cessation. Physical exercise is known to have, perhaps, the greatest antioxidant effects. Lifestyle modification demonstrated superior results in the improvement of autonomic dysfunction (assessed with HRV and QT indexes) as compared to the use of metformin or placebo. Weight loss and dietary intervention accompanied by supervised training were associated with improvement on CAN indices. Aerobic training has also been shown to improve CAN, with some indication

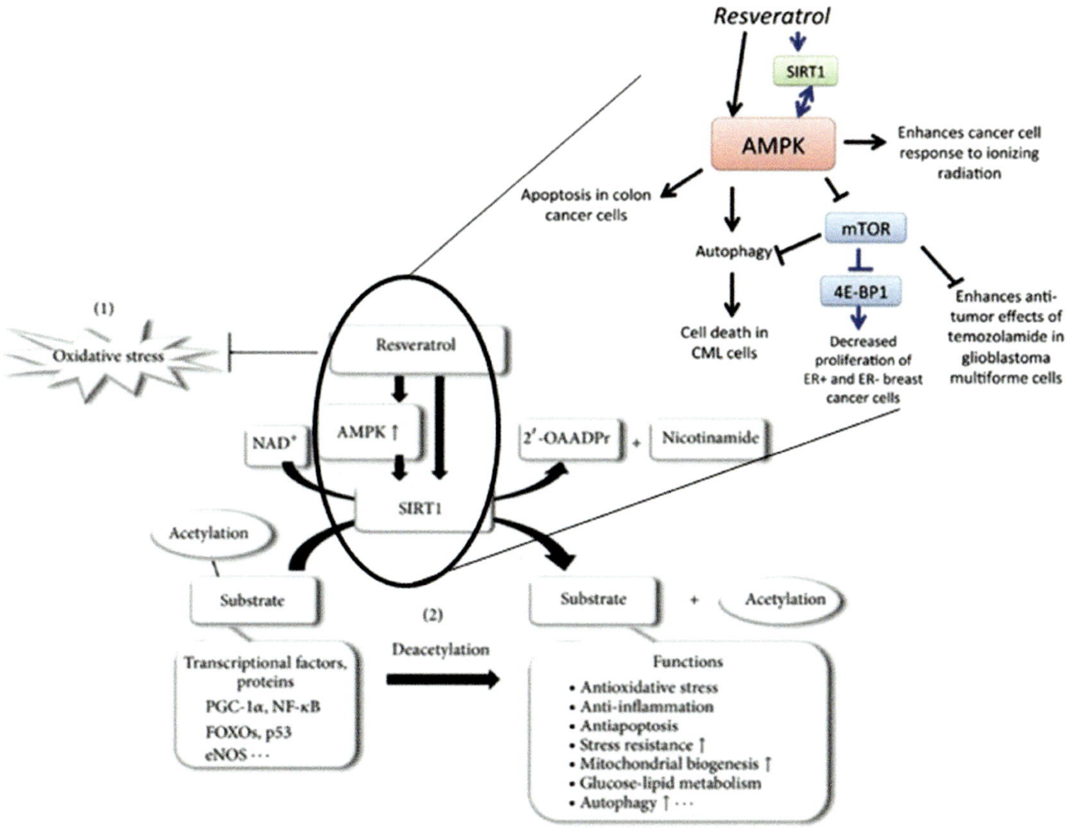


**Fig. 6.13** Proposed mechanisms by which resveratrol exerts cyto-protection. (1) Resveratrol attenuates oxidative stress. (2) Resveratrol activates SIRT1, which is an $NAD^+$ -dependent deacetylase, directly or indirectly via AMPK activation. SIRT1 plays an important role in the regulation of oxidative stress, inflammation, apoptosis, stress resistance, mitochondrial biogenesis, autophagy, and glucose-lipid metabolism, via the deacetylation of many substrates. (Source: https://www.hindawi.com/journals/omcl/2013/568093/fig1/). **Insert**: Schematic representation of AMPK-dependent anticancer effects of resveratrol. Activation of AMPK by resveratrol leads to apoptosis of cancer cells and enhancement of cancer cell response to ionizing radiation and autophagy. Main: [94] (Open Access, Hindawi). Insert: [93, Fig. 3] (Open Access, Frontiers in Oncology). Source: [93]

that mild physical exercise is recommended in less severe CAN cases. A recent review summarizing the evidence for the impact of lifestyle interventions on CAN has concluded that moderate endurance and aerobic exercise in both type 1 and type 2 diabetes (considered to be a model of chronic disease on the autonomic nervous system) improve HRV and cardiac autonomic function significantly, in favor of healthy levels of parasympathetic dominance (known to be cardioprotective), independent of BMI, glycemic or BP control, and duration of diabetes [104].

Diets rich in fruits and vegetables reduce blood pressure (BP) and atherosclerosis and thereby the risk of adverse cardiovascular events. In addition to resveratrol, polyphenols (Fig. 6.14) and flavonoids (Fig. 6.15, see also insert below) are also strong antioxidants and have significant effects as anti-atherosclerotics. Certain vegetables possess a high nitrate content. The dietary nitrate load also prevented endothelial dysfunction induced by an acute ischemic insult and significantly attenuated platelet aggregation. Interruption of the salivary conversion of nitrate to nitrite (facilitated by bacterial anaerobes situated on the surface of the tongue) prevented the rise in plasma nitrite, blocked the decrease in BP, and abolished the inhibitory effects on platelet aggregation, con-

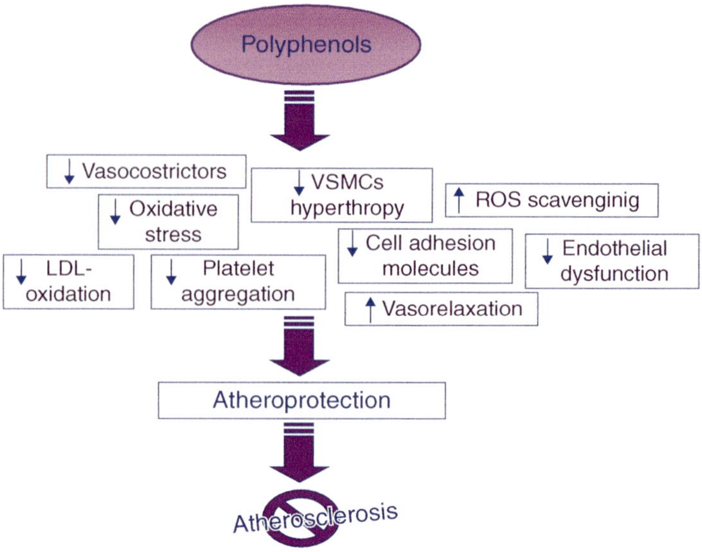


**Fig. 6.14** Polyphenols act as antioxidants and help as an anti-sclerotic [86, Fig. 5] (Open Access, InTech Open)

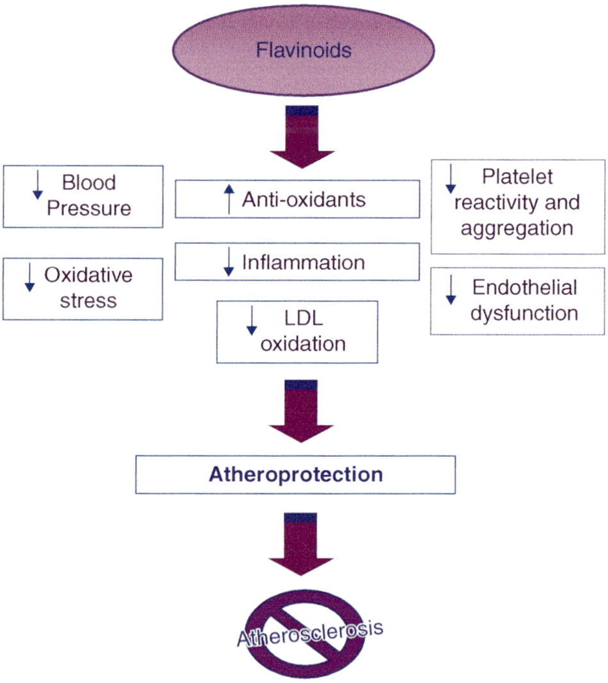


**Fig. 6.15** Flavonoids act as antioxidants and help as an anti-sclerotic [86, Fig. 7] (Open Access, InTech Open. Insert: Photo from: pixabay.com at https://www.pexels.com/photo/brown-loft-bread-in-white-textile-on-beige-table-162440/)

firming the vaso-protective nature of nitrite converted from the ingested nitrate. Findings suggest that dietary nitrate, in part, underlies the beneficial effects of a vegetable-rich diet [105].

It is estimated that if an individual increases fruit and vegetable intake to 600 grams daily, the worldwide burden of atherosclerotic disease could be reduced by 31% for ischemic heart disease and 19% for ischemic stroke [106]. Folic acid treatment decreased the risk of cardiovascular disease by 15% in patients with end-stage renal disease and advanced chronic kidney disease [107]. Folic acid supplements with B vitamins have potential benefits, including lower homocysteine levels and the prevention of stroke [108]. A meta-analysis [109] reviewed 200 epidemiological studies. The majority showing a protective effective increase in fruit and vegetable intake concludes that high content of polyphenolic antioxidants in fruits and vegetables is probably the main factor responsible for the beneficial effects for cancer and cancer prevention.

Wine is allowed and 4–6 ounces is usually consumed with dinner. The benefit of wine over other sources of alcohol is the fact that it is absorbed slowly because it is (1) often eaten with meals, which (2) causes a sustained level of alcohol in the blood, and (3) it is rich in flavonoids which produce antioxidants, as discussed.

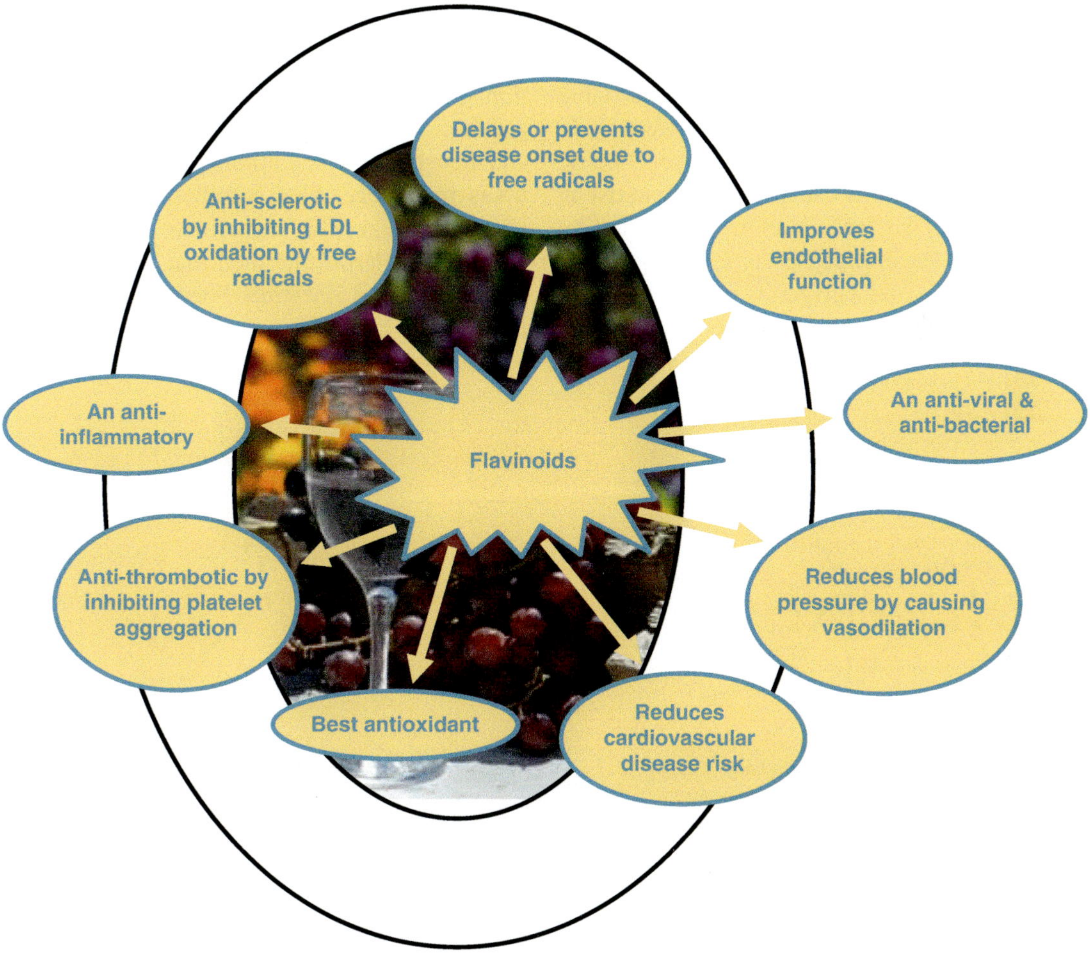


The Mediterranean diet is also associated with a non-sedentary lifestyle. Physical activity, preferably a moderate level of daily exercise, and the Mediterranean diet are complimentary. Physical exercise is an additional prong (#5: see "Exercise (Prong-5)"). Exercise is arguably the strongest of all antioxidants. Exercise raises core body temperature which is like the passive immune response of a fever, reducing the need for the immune system to involve oxidants in neutralizing pathogens. It increases circulation to all areas of the body helping to passively remove wastes and contaminants, increase oxygen supplies to all areas of the body, boost active immune responses, and much more.

## Mediterranean Diet Summary

In summary, the Mediterranean diet utilizes "good" fats (actually good levels of all fats). These include omega-3 fatty acids which are seen in fish oil products and omega-9 fatty acids which are seen in the high content of monounsaturated fatty acids found in virgin and extra-virgin olive oils. Also in the diet, there is a high consumption of dietary fiber with a low-glycemic index and low-glycemic load. Glycemic load refers to the type of sugars that are consumed and how they influence insulin secretion. For example, table sugar or sucrose is the most common sweetener. It is composed of glucose and fructose. Glucose is absorbed by the blood and leads to rapid rise in blood sugar, whereas fructose only slightly affects blood sugar. Glucose has a glycemic index of 100. Fructose has a glycemic index of only 19. Sucrose, a table sugar, has a glycemic index of 68. The higher the glycemic index, the worse the health effect for the body. Fructose is found in all fruits and in honey. It is 30% sweeter than ordinary sugar and is healthier because it has a lower-glycemic index. It is obtained in fruits that are consumed in the Mediterranean diet.

Lactose is a milk sugar and is found in milk and other dairy products. It has a glycemic index of 46. Yogurt is a preferred dairy product and a source of lactose in the Mediterranean diet, which is its main component. Actually in yogurt, the lactose has been broken down by fermentation (see insert below); as a result these products are more digestible. The bacteria are probiotic and beneficial. In addition, prebiotic (dietary) fibers from vegetables, legumes, oats, and barley are nondigestible ingredients that are found in the Mediterranean diet that stimulate the growth of good intestinal flora (e.g., *E.coli*, in moderate or normal amounts).

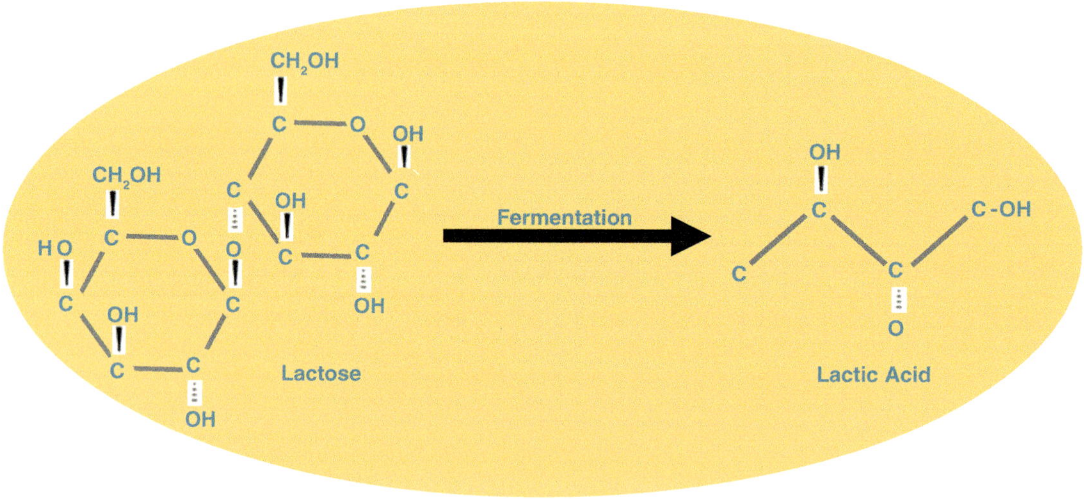


Maltose (see insert below) or malt sugar has one of the highest glycemic indices (105–110) since it is composed of two glucose molecules. It is found, for example, in beer. Therefore, beer is limited or omitted in the Mediterranean diet. Beer is not good for individuals who are overweight. Regarding sugars in general, in a 2000-calorie diet, no more than 1½ oz or 50 g of added sugar per day is recommended. Store-bought fruit juices are not recommended, as a 7 oz glass can contain up to 20 g of sugar, whereas 3 oz of whole strawberries contains just 5 g of natural sugar. Whole strawberries also have dietary fiber and vitamin C.

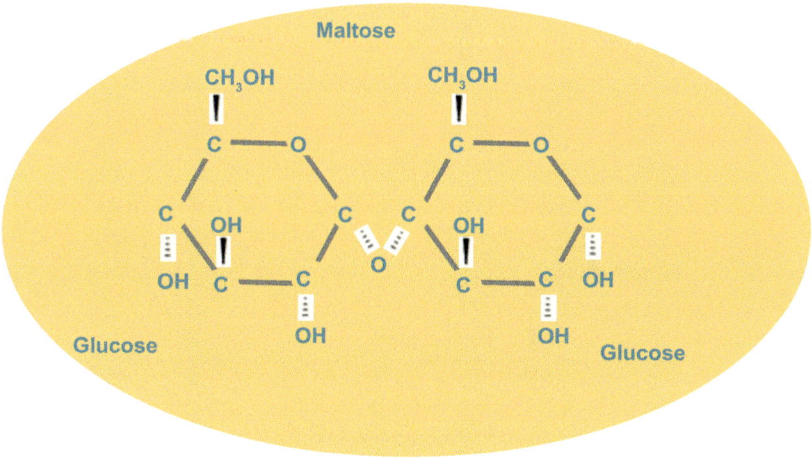


In the Mediterranean diet, starches include pasta made from durum wheat and certain types of rice including brown, basmati, and long-grain rice. These have a lower-glycemic index than white flour, which is why they are preferred. However, they are rich in carbohydrates and are limited to some degree in the Mediterranean diet, because excess carbohydrates are converted in the body to fat. Also, stone-ground whole wheat flour is healthier than ordinary white flour, again due to a lower-glycemic index and the high content of dietary fiber. The Mediterranean diet uses a minimum of white flour.

The Mediterranean diet has many anti-inflammatory and antioxidant effects which have already been discussed in the prongs on fish oil and antioxidants such as omega-3 fatty acids, alpha-lipoic acid, and coenzyme Q10.

Endothelial cells, as mentioned, form a monolayer of cells important for smooth muscle function and vascular tone in all of the blood vessels of the body. They cause nitric oxide to be secreted and blood vessels to dilate. The endothelium produces not only nitric oxide but other vasodilating substances such as endothelium-derived hyperpolarizing factor (Fig. 6.16) [110] and beneficial prostacyclin ($PGI_2$; see Fig. 6.16). These counteract the constricting substances that are produced by the endothelial cells which are known as thromboxane A2 and endothelin-1. Endothelial function can be measured with an ultrasound technique known as the brachial vasodilator response to reactive hyperemia after inflating a blood pressure cuff and then releasing it. The increase in blood flow provides an indication of the reserve of the endothelial cells in producing nitric oxide and some of the other vasodilating properties [111]. Endothelial cells also form the barriers that protect the reproductive organs (surrounding the ovaries and testes, protecting and nourishing the gametes) and the brain (the blood-brain barrier, protecting and nourishing the brain).

In the Mind-Body Wellness Program, all components enhance endothelial function, increase the production of nitric oxide, and dilate the blood vessels. This has been documented in many studies involving brachial vasodilator responses. As discussed throughout the book, these include long-chain omega-3 fatty acids (prong-1), nitric oxide and L-arginine and related compounds (prong-2), antioxidants, folic acid, vitamin D and vitamin B12 (prong-3), the Mediterranean diet (prong-4), exercise (prong-5), and stress reduction (prong-6). Overall, the program recommends the Mediterranean diet with moderate alcohol consumption, moderate to high physical activity levels, and no smoking (better lifestyle). This is because the program in its entirety is associated with lower mortality from all types of coronary heart disease, cardiovascular disease (including stroke), and cancer, even after 10 years of prolonged follow-up studies. This highlights the beneficial effects of keeping the endothelial cells healthy and producing healthy amounts of nitric oxide.

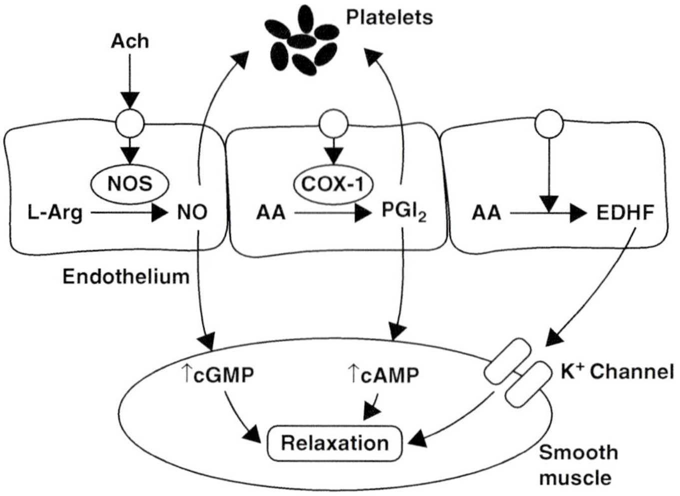


**Fig. 6.16** Some mechanisms of endothelium-dependent relaxation. Nitric oxide (NO) is produced by nitric oxide synthase (NOS) from the amino acid L-arginine (l-Arg). Nitric oxide diffuses to vascular muscles where it activates soluble guanylate cyclase, causing increased production of guanosine 3′,5′-cyclic monophosphate (cGMP), which results in relaxation. Prostacyclin ($PGI_2$) is normally produced by cyclooxygenase-1 (COX-1) from arachidonic acid (AA). $PGI_2$ diffuses to vascular muscle where it activates adenylate cyclase, causing increased production of adenosine 3′,5′-cyclic monophosphate (cAMP), which results in relaxation. Endothelium-derived hyperpolarizing factor (EDHF) is probably a product of AA metabolism. EDHF diffuses to vascular muscle where it activates potassium ($K^+$) channels. Increased activity of potassium channels produces hyperpolarization and relaxation of vascular muscle. Abbreviation: ACh, acetylcholine. (Republished with permission from The American Physiological Society. Source: [110])

However, no one component of the Mind-Body Wellness Program alone stands out. In essence, the Mediterranean diet acts in a team effort just as an American football team requires all components such as a great coach, offensive line, defensive line, quarterback, running backs, receivers, and so forth, all components working in conjunction to produce the desired effect, namely, winning the ball game. A win is longevity with good health.

There are many definitions of the Mediterranean diet. Perhaps the specific diet that was followed in Crete was the most beneficial. However, most of the Southern European countries that border the Mediterranean have healthy lifestyles and diets with chief components that have been outlined above. Unfortunately, people from Mediterranean countries have strayed from tradition and are beginning to consume sugared soft drinks, sweets, hidden saturated fats in bakery products, and snacks and use refined flour and processed foods. This is a less healthy diet.

Numerous studies, including epidemiological, observational, and randomized studies, have shown that Mediterranean diet is associated with lower instances of mortality from all causes as listed above. Studies have also shown beneficial effects on cognitive behavior in patients who have followed the Mediterranean diet and perhaps decreased incidence of dementia, including Alzheimer's disease. Again, the first of these significant studies was the Seven Countries Study, which began in the early 1970s and demonstrated that the diets of individuals in regions such as Southern Italy had lower cardiac event rates than those in Northern Italy or other countries remote from the Mediterranean basin. More recently, studies such as the PREDIMED study, which included almost 7500 individuals at high risk for cardiovascular disease, showed that a Mediterranean diet, whether enhanced with added extra-virgin oil or nuts, performed better than a low-fat controlled diet.

The risk of heart attack, stroke, and death was reduced by approximately 30% in the Mediterranean diet groups [12]. Analyses showed that levels of oxidized LDL cholesterol decreased with the diet, but not the low-fat control group. Incidence of type 2 diabetes was also decreased. Other studies such as the Lyon Diet Heart Study (a secondary prevention study), which included a Mediterranean-type diet supplemented with an omega-rich margarine and was compared to a prudent Western diet, had a 70% less likely incidence of heart attack or dying from heart disease. These were individuals who already had a heart attack.

Other large studies subsequently showed the benefit of the Mediterranean diet in primary prevention. The Mediterranean diet reduced the incidence of metabolic syndrome by (1) improving endothelial function, (2) decreasing inflammation, and (3) decreasing insulin resistance. Also, weight loss was greater in the diet than low-fat diets. Studies have shown greater blood pressure lowering effects and reduced triglycerides and serum lipids with the Mediterranean diet vs. low-fat diets.

Prediabetic or insulin-resistant patients are often started on medications such as metformin in an attempt to delay the need for further drug treatment of type 2 diabetes. The above studies also show that the Mediterranean diet may delay or prevent the need for drugs in patients with newly diagnosed type 2 diabetes [25, 28, 112, 113–114].

The Mediterranean diet is known as a stress-reducing diet [1, 4, 6, 9, 11–12, 16, 18, 19, 23, 25, 28, 115–116]. Certain foods consumed, such as those with high-glycemic loads, can actually increase stress by producing extra insulin when a rapid rise in blood sugar occurs. Blood sugar falls quickly after a high-glycemic load and produces postprandial hypoglycemia or low blood sugar. These are stresses on the body, especially on the parasympathetic and sympathetic nervous systems and thereby the cardiovascular system. This has been linked to higher incidences of heart attacks and vascular events, including stroke. By limiting obesity and frequent insulin peaks and valleys, the Mediterranean diet reduces stress, including by promoting a better pattern of cortisol secretion [117, 118]. Elevated cortisol increases appetite and craving for sugar and high-glycemic foods. It is said that foods that are rich in both carbohydrates and fat have a calming or antidepressant effect. Unfortunately, stress and high cortisol levels cause people to seek foods with high-glycemic indices leading to high insulin levels, increasing abdominal fat, and higher risk of diabetes, heart disease, and cancer. The Mediterranean diet, because of its omega-3 content with fish, has anticlotting properties and may prevent thrombosis by reducing or preventing stress-induced oxidation of LDLs (see "Details of Oxidized LDL and Atherosclerosis Production"). Also, the antioxidant properties of the diet have been thought to delay aging since oxidative stress does promote the aging process and senescence.

The Mediterranean diet is very similar to the traditional Japanese diet, and a new trend toward a "Japomediterranean" diet is now in vogue and includes olive oil, wine, fish, nuts, beans, seeds, soy, vegetables, fruits, bread, rice, seaweed, dairy products, and mushrooms. The Japanese diet has also been shown to have beneficial effects, similar to the Mediterranean diet [119, 120]. Aspects of the Japanese diet are promoted because Japanese traditional diets share a number of features of Mediterranean diets including seafood, beans, vegetables, fruits, and grains that are seen mutually in both diets. However, the dietary consumption of alcohol is different. Wine is used in the Mediterranean diet and sake in the Japanese diet, which is made from rice or corn. For the most part, the Mediterranean and Japanese diet have low-glycemic loads which contribute to decrease risk of cardiovascular disease, some cancers, most chronic diseases, and less oxidative stress.

As discussed, the Mediterranean diet has been associated with decreased risk of developing cognitive disorders. It may well be the best modality to preventing or slowing down the development of dementia such as Alzheimer's disease even more than pharmaceuticals. Further research is ongoing.

The Mediterranean diet is associated with a reduced risk of cancer incidents and mortality [121], including in the elderly [122]. The diet is associated with decreased epithelial cancers, digestive and laryngeal tract cancers, and upper airway digestive tract cancers [123]. In women, it has a protective effect against cancers of their genital and urinary tracts and other epithelial neoplasm [124, 125]. In contrast, refined grains and the consequently high-glycemic loads were associated with increased risks of cancers.

In the coming years, predicted death rates because of cancer will further decline, but the overall number of cases will increase, mostly as a consequence of an aging population. A target for cancer prevention will remain a healthy diet and control of obesity in addition to a decrease in smoking. A healthy diet is the traditional Mediterranean diet (based on high consumption of plant foods and cereals, olive oil as the main (added) fat, low intake of red meat, and moderate consumption of wine). The Mediterranean diet is associated with a reduced risk of cancer, in addition to cardiovascular disease. Cancer prevention is associated with a balanced ratio of omega-6 to omega-3 fatty acids and high amounts of fiber, antioxidants, and polyphenols found in fruit, vegetables, olive oil, and wine of the Mediterranean diet. This includes the "Mediterranean way of drinking," that is, regular, moderate consumption of wine mainly with food. This pattern of drinking increases longevity; reduces the risk of cardiovascular disease, stroke, and dementia; and does not appreciably influence the overall risk of cancer. However, heavy alcohol drinking is associated with digestive, upper respiratory tract, liver, and breast cancers; therefore, avoidance or restriction of alcohol consumption to two drinks/day for men and one drink/day for women is a global public health priority [126].

Interestingly, endometrial cancer has been associated with dietary fat intake and is not protected by the Mediterranean diet [127]. However, strict adherence to the Mediterranean diet was not observed. Regardless, the study found that to reduce the risk of endometrial cancer, a plant-based diet low in calories from fat is recommended. This diet is rich in legumes, fiber, whole grains, vegetables, and fruits. Therefore for females, close physician supervision is recommended as to what aspects of the Mediterranean diet the individual should follow, especially if they are at risk for cancers such as endometrial cancer. Since none of these studies have been double blinded, completely controlled trials, one cannot state with certainty that the Mediterranean diet will prevent certain types of cancers or even all cancers. However, dietary patterns emphasizing the consumption of fruits, vegetables, whole grains, legumes, nuts, seeds, and low-fat dairy products are highly recommended for most people, especially those at risk for cancer [128].

Extra-virgin olive oil is a beneficial fatty acid which contains modest amounts of vitamin E and vitamin K [129]. It is replete with numerous, and excellent, antioxidants. It contains a monounsaturated fat called oleic acid which reduces inflammation, including markers such as CRP. It may beneficially affect certain genes which are linked to cancer. Also, monounsaturated fats in extra-virgin olive oil are resistant to high heat, making it a healthy choice when used in cooking. Olive oil is the only source of monounsaturated fat associated with a reduced risk of stroke and heart disease by preventing LDL cholesterol from becoming oxidized, improving endothelial function, and improving clotting (see "Details of Oxidized LDL and Atherosclerosis Production"). It has also been shown to lower blood pressure and may reduce the need for blood pressure medicines. Olive oil has not been shown to increase weight and may actually cause weight loss. Olive oil combined with the Mediterranean diet may have significant beneficial effects on cognitive health, including dementia and Alzheimer's disease.

The Mediterranean diet includes healthy fats which are omega-3 and omega-9 (virgin olive oil). Specifically, it uses mostly "good" fats and very few of the so-called "bad" fats or saturated fats within the diet. However, no more than 35% of the daily recommended calories are from fat. Low saturated fats are preferred than saturated fats. Carbohydrates with a low-glycemic index are used. Foods are not processed. High fiber and high antioxidant levels are employed. As the Mediterranean diet is an excellent diet for weight loss, oftentimes, women are limited to 1500 calories a day and men 1800 calories a day. The goal of the Mediterranean diet is to lower the omega-6 to omega-3 ratio for any given cholesterol level: lower this ratio to as close to 1 as possible (the Western diet is usually 10:1) to obtain the associated protection from coronary heart disease. Similar to LDL as compared HDL, too much Omega-6 fatty acids have detrimental effects, whereas (like HDLs) more omega-3s have protective effects in the body.

A healthy ratio of Omega-3 to Omega-6 is important for wellness, just as a healthy ratio of HDL to LDL.

Vegetables commonly used in the Mediterranean diet include tomatoes, cucumbers, onions, carrots, lettuce, bell peppers, cabbage, squash, parsley, chives, zucchini, and garlic. Spices are also used. While cinnamon (without the sugar) is not considered a key spice in the Mediterranean diet, it is an extremely useful spice for antioxidant and insulin sensitivity affects. Sweet potatoes are also seen in the Mediterranean diet to some degree. In the Japomediterranean diet, coriander is also used. Uncooked red beets are highly recommended in as high quantities as possible because they are an excellent source of inorganic nitrates which promote nitric oxide production (see "Beet Root Powder").

Fruits used in the Mediterranean diet include figs and grapes. Other fruits often seen are apples, bananas, oranges, lemons, grapefruit, watermelon (an excellent source of citrulline) clementine, cantaloupe, strawberries (an excellent source of fiber), kiwi, plums, apricots, peaches, and pears. Grapes are a key component of the Mediterranean diet. Polyphenols are naturally sourced in the skin and seeds of grapes. Polyphenols act as antioxidants to sequester many free radicals which may be harmful. They are a subtype of phytonutrients and there are a large number of flavonoids found in vegetables, teas, wines, and various juices, as well as fruits.

Curcumin, primarily from turmeric, decreases LOX-1 expression (preventing oxidized LDL from binding), decreases the expression of scavenger receptors and macrophages, decreases the inflammatory NK-kB, and decreases angiotensin-mediated upregulation of LOX-1. Flavonoids, commonly used in the Mediterranean diet, also decrease ox-LDL and ox-LDL-induced endothelial nitric oxide. By preventing these decreases, flavonoids help to decrease superoxide production. Superoxides are another type of free radical. As mentioned above, another common natural substance which will modify LOX-1 is resveratrol, which is found in grapes, peanuts, mulberries, and red wine.

LOX-1 regulates LDL function. Natural LOX-1 modulators in addition to curcumin (aka, turmeric) are flavonoids and resveratrol, which are provided through the Mediterranean diet, especially by drinking small amounts of red wine (one to two glasses per day). Other (inducing) therapies to treat heart diseases, including atherosclerosis-induced diseases that have indirect effects on LOX-1 expression, are aspirin, statins, and oral hypoglycemic agents. They may beneficially negate and therefore decrease inflammation in atherosclerosis. Curcumin, or turmeric, reduces angiotensin to mediate cardiomyocyte (heart muscle cell) growth via LOX-1 inhibition [130]. Excessive cardiomyocyte growth can lead to heart failure or cardiomyopathy.

A strong antioxidant environment limits the amount of ox-LDL. In the future, negating the effects of the LOX-1 receptor is expected to be extremely important. While gene models and monoclonal antibodies to LOX-1 are being developed, there are natural mechanisms such as flavonoids, turmeric, and resveratrol to use in the interim. The latter can be seen in the Mediterranean diet. Limiting LOX-1 activation may be another advantage of drinking red wine.

Legumes such as white and red beans, fava beans, lima beans, split peas, chick peas, lentils of all types, and black-eyed peas are often seen in the Mediterranean diet. Grains, such as breads with whole wheat or rye, are often used. Rice such as basmati, brown, and wild is preferred. Wheat pasta is also used. Bulgur and barley are very healthy grains.

It should be stressed that the Mediterranean diet is much more than a simple diet. It is a lifestyle change. Physical activity and low-stress environments are often inherently associated with this diet. The Mediterranean diet, by nature of its association with healthy lifestyle changes and healthy dietary patterns, lowers cancer risk, heart disease risk, obesity, diabetes, and other chronic diseases and promotes weight loss. It is, in essence, a "more holistic fulfillment of healthy living" (see insert below, compared with "paleo" and "clean eating" diets). Analyses of which component of the Mediterranean diet is most important found none. In addition, the Mediterranean diet, in randomized controlled studies, observational studies, and meta-analyses, has been shown beneficial in both primary and secondary prevention of cardiovascular disease [9, 10, 17–22].

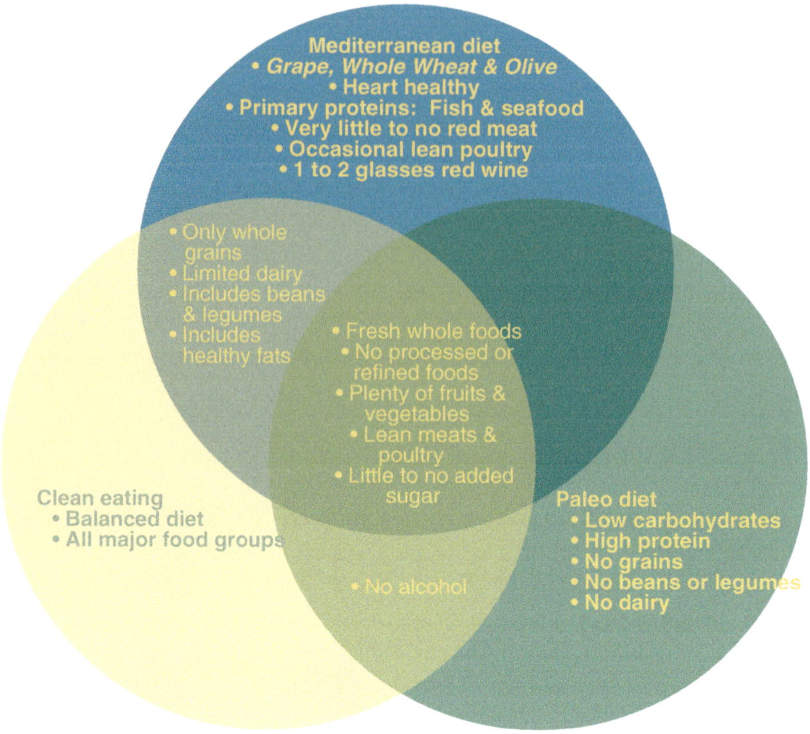


The Mediterranean diet also improves exercise capacity. In regard to lipids, it has been shown to reduce LDL, triglycerides, and total cholesterol levels and increase HDL[1] levels, but more importantly, it reduces the LDL oxidation levels. In essence, the Mediterranean diet reduces oxidative stress. It does this by improving antioxidant capacity, reducing ROS, and reducing isoprostane substances, which are harmful. When one looks at various measures to reduce cardiac risk such as aspirin, beta-blockers, cholesterol-lowering medications such as statins, and medicines to block the angiotensin receptor pathway (ACE inhibitors and angiotensin receptor blockers), one sees that the Mediterranean diet has a risk ratio reduction equivalent to, if not better than, those risk factors. Perhaps the only risk reduction factor that may be comparable to the Mediterranean diet in potency is smoking cessation, if one is a smoker. Other cardioprotective activities shown to reduce cardiac risk with favorable risk ratios such as moderate alcohol intake, physical activity, and omega-3 fatty acids are actually components of the Mediterranean diet.

Not all plant-based foods are equally healthy. Diets that adhere to (1) whole grains as the main form of carbohydrates, (2) unsaturated fats as the predominant form of dietary fat, and (3) an abundance of fruits and vegetables and adequate omega-3 fatty acid intake are the only diets that reduce the effects of, or prevent, chronic diseases.

Olive oil stabilizes membranes, reduces inflammation, and acts as an antioxidant and a probiotic by being antimicrobial. It has antihypertensive properties. Eating about two tablespoons or 23 g of olive oil a day is recommended, for it may reduce the risk of coronary heart disease due to the monounsaturated fats present in olive oil.

The Mediterranean diet may improve cognitive function and is demonstrated to reduce coronary heart disease, hypertension, diabetes,

[1] Cholesterol balance is the "good" to "bad" lipoprotein balance (HDL to LDL). The body does need a very little, relatively speaking, of the "bad" cholesterol (LDL), or fat, for normal nerve function. While this is not a specific target, it is a benefit.

dyslipidemia, metabolic syndrome, and diabetes. Higher adherence to the Mediterranean diet improves insulin sensitivity and decreases oxidative stress. It has been shown to improve basic proteins such as neurotrophins which protect neurons and has been associated with decreases of the inflammatory protein CRP. Interleukin levels are also reduced. All of these inflammatory molecules have been shown to be detrimental to human cells, including brain cells, and may underlie increased cognitive impairment.

Evidence suggests that adopting the Mediterranean diet may actually help prevent type 2 diabetes. It improves the glycemic control in patients with established diabetes by increasing sensitivity. The Mediterranean diet is a good diet for those with busy lives. Today in America, people think they are too busy to stop and eat healthy. Fast foods, pizza, soft drinks, and other dietary products taken on the run are almost always bad choices. Americans would rather ingest a pill to receive the proper antioxidants and nutrients that are inherent in the Mediterranean diet. However, taking a magic pill in the morning is not the answer and would not replace a good healthy diet with associated lifestyle factors.

## Alcohol Consumption

A large study analyzed alcohol consumption to all-cause cardiovascular and cancer-related mortality in US adults [131]. Interestingly, this very sophisticated and well-done statistical study was from China in collaboration with researchers at the University of Texas. In this study, the abstinence bias was accounted for. This means that individuals stopped drinking many times because of chronic illnesses or because of health factors. The conclusion (Fig. 6.17) was that light to moderate alcohol intake might have a protective effect on all-cause and cardiovascular-type mortality in the US adults. Heavy or binge drinking was associated with increased risk of all-cause and cancer-specific mortality but not cardiac disease.

While large amounts of polyphenols from heavy alcohol consumption might have a protective effective on the cardiovascular system (albeit less protection than moderate drinking), heavy alcohol consumption is *not* advised since the increased risk of other causes of death outweighs the benefits.

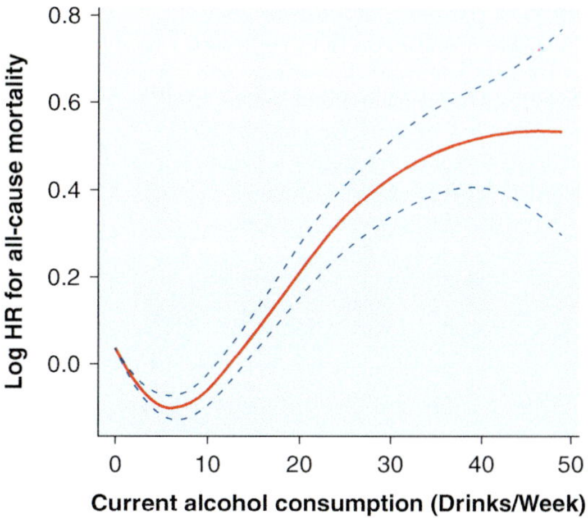


**Fig. 6.17** Alcohol consumption and all-cause mortality risk in US adults. (Republished with permission from Elsevier. Source: [131])

This epidemiological study confirmed the results of many studies that there is a J-shaped curve with alcohol consumption. It appears that no drinking or heavy drinking or even binge drinking increased cardiac mortality compared to light or moderate drinking. More than three drinks a day qualifies as heavy drinking. Therefore, one to two drinks a day is the recommended limit. If patients are not drinking, do not encourage them to start, since they can easily get excessive in time and go over the three-drink limit. However, there have been data in the past that patients that have a small amount of alcohol intake do better than people who do not drink at all in perspective studies.

A strong editorial review of this study gave the following recommendations:

1. Regular or moderate alcohol consumption protects against fatal and nonfatal cardiovascular disease and all-cause mortality both in healthy adults and individuals with cardiovascular disease.
2. There is a J-shaped curve with alcohol consumption and dose-effect relationships.

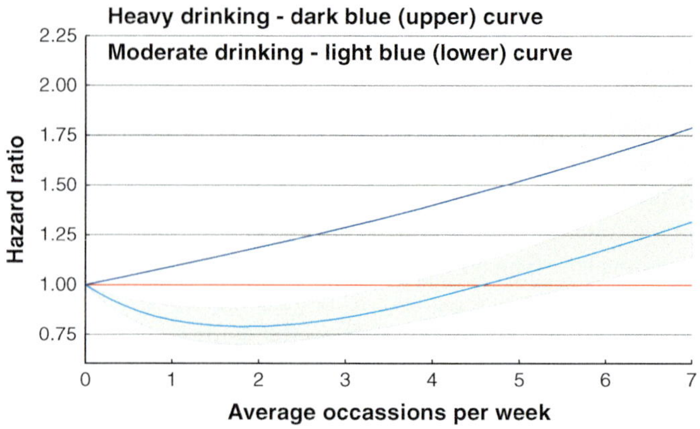


**Fig. 6.18** Alcohol consumption and all-cause mortality risk. Mortality risk by frequency of heavy (5+ drinks) and non-heavy (<5 drinks) drinking occasions per week. Hazard ratio, with 95% CI, is plotted separately for each population (Wiley Online Library) [133]. (Republished with permission from Wiley Online Library)

3. For light to moderate levels of alcohol consumption, the risk of some cancers such as breast and colorectal might be increased very little and probably does not make clinical relevance, and each individual should look at their genetic background and other risk factors before drinking alcohol in light quantities. Most all cancers are not increased with light alcohol consumption.
4. Lifetime alcohol abstainers should not start drinking for health reasons only, but should be encouraged to adopt healthy lifestyles. These authors recommend regular physical activity, no smoking, weight control, and dietary habits such as the Mediterranean diet as the collective key to wellness.
5. The net effect of excessive or regular binge alcohol use is detrimental to human organs and functions as a major public health and social problem.

There are many reasons why alcohol may be beneficial in light to moderate quantities. It can increase the "good," HDL cholesterol. It encourages fibrinolysis and reductions in plasma viscosity, making the blood less thick. Fibrinogen concentrations are also reduced. Platelets do not aggregate, preventing clot formation. As stated above, compared with lifetime abstainers, those who were light or moderate alcohol consumers were at reduced risk of mortality from all cause and cardiovascular disease [131]. This was supported in an editorial that reiterated the fact that a J-shaped curve characterizes the association between the amount of alcohol consumed and risk of cardiovascular disease. It is quite evident that light to moderate intake of alcohol is associated with lower rates of all-cause cardiovascular mortality, whereas heavy drinking and binge drinking increased the risk of all-cause and cancer mortality, but not cardiovascular.

Others [132, 133] (Fig. 6.18) emphasize the importance of the "J-curve." It is recommended that younger people should not expect any substantial benefit from moderate drinking; however, for most older people, the overall benefit of light drinking, especially with cardiovascular risks, clearly outweighs the possibility of any cancer risks. For a young woman with no coronary risk factors, the breast cancer data suggests limited alcohol intake to very modest amounts, but postmenopausal woman should consider the overall health advantage of choosing a drink of moderate alcohol since there was a question of little increased risk of breast cancer.

## References


1. Gunnars K. 5 Studies on the Mediterranean diet – does it really work? https://authoritynutrition.com/5-studies-on-the-mediterranean-diet
2. Davis C, Bryan J, Hodgson J, Murphy K. Definition of the Mediterranean diet; a literature review. Nutrients. 2015;7(11):9139–53. https://doi.org/10.3390/nu7115459. Review.
3. Castro-Quezada I, Román-Viñas B, Serra-Majem L. The Mediterranean diet and nutritional adequacy: a review. Nutrients. 2014;6(1):231–48. https://doi.org/10.3390/nu6010231. Review.

4. Sofi F, Macchi C, Abbate R, Gensini GF, Casini A. Mediterranean diet and health status: an updated meta-analysis and a proposal for a literature-based adherence score. Public Health Nutr. 2014;17(12):2769–82. https://doi.org/10.1017/S1368980013003169. Epub 2013 Nov 29. Review.
5. Mancini JG, Filion KB, Atallah R, Eisenberg MJ. Systematic review of the Mediterranean diet for long-term weight loss. Am J Med. 2016;129(4):407–415.e4. https://doi.org/10.1016/j.amjmed.2015.11.028. Epub 2015 Dec 22. Review.
6. Widmer RJ, Flammer AJ, Lerman LO, Lerman A. The Mediterranean diet, its components, and cardiovascular disease. Am J Med. 2015;128(3):229–38. https://doi.org/10.1016/j.amjmed.2014.10.014. Epub 2014 Oct 15. Review.
7. Liyanage T, Ninomiya T, Wang A, Neal B, Jun M, Wong MG, Jardine M, Hillis GS, Perkovic V. Effects of the Mediterranean diet on cardiovascular outcomes-a systematic review and meta-analysis. PLoS One. 2016;11(8):e0159252. https://doi.org/10.1371/journal.pone.0159252. eCollection 2016. Review.
8. Grosso G, Marventano S, Yang J, Micek A, Pajak A, Scalfi L, Galvano F, Kales SN. A comprehensive meta-analysis on evidence of Mediterranean diet and cardiovascular disease: are individual components equal? Crit Rev Food Sci Nutr. 2017;57(15):3218–32. https://doi.org/10.1080/10408398.2015.1107021.
9. Nordmann AJ, Suter-Zimmermann K, Bucher HC, Shai I, Tuttle KR, Estruch R, Briel M. Meta-analysis comparing Mediterranean to low-fat diets for modification of cardiovascular risk factors. Am J Med. 2011;124(9):841–51.e2. https://doi.org/10.1016/j.amjmed.2011.04.024.
10. Satija A, Bhupathiraju SN, Spiegelman D, Chiuve SE, Manson JE, Willett W, Rexrode KM, Rimm EB, Hu FB. Healthful and unhealthful plant-based diets and the risk of coronary heart disease in U.S. adults. J Am Coll Cardiol. 2017;70(4):411–22. https://doi.org/10.1016/j.jacc.2017.05.047.
11. Ros E, Martínez-González MA, Estruch R, Salas-Salvadó J, Fitó M, Martínez JA, Corella D. Mediterranean diet and cardiovascular health: teachings of the PREDIMED study. Adv Nutr. 2014;5(3):330S–6S. https://doi.org/10.3945/an.113.005389. Print 2014 May. Review.
12. Estruch R, Ros E, Salas-Salvadó J, Covas MI, Corella D, Arós F, Gómez-Gracia E, Ruiz-Gutiérrez V, Fiol M, Lapetra J, et al. Primary prevention of cardiovascular disease with a Mediterranean diet. N Engl J Med. 2013;368:1279–90.
13. Khera AV, Emdin CA, Drake I, Natarajan P, Bick AG, Cook NR, Chasman DI, Baber U, Mehran R, Rader DJ, Fuster V, Boerwinkle E, Melander O, Orho-Melander M, Ridker PM, Kathiresan S. Genetic risk, adherence to a healthy lifestyle, and coronary disease. N Engl J Med. 2016;375(24):2349–58. Epub 2016 Nov 13.
14. Fuentes F, López-Miranda J, Sánchez E, Sánchez F, Paez J, Paz-Rojas E, Marín C, Gómez P, Jimenez-Perepérez J, Ordovás JM, Pérez-Jiménez F. Mediterranean and low-fat diets improve endothelial function in hypercholesterolemic men. Ann Intern Med. 2001;134(12):1115–9.
15. Ludwig DS. Lowering the bar on the low-fat diet. JAMA. 2016;316(20):2087–8. https://doi.org/10.1001/jama.2016.15473.
16. Nissensohn M, Román-Viñas B, Sánchez-Villegas A, Piscopo S, Serra-Majem L. The effect of the Mediterranean diet on hypertension: a systematic review and meta-analysis. J Nutr Educ Behav. 2016;48(1):42–53.e1. https://doi.org/10.1016/j.jneb.2015.08.023. Epub 2015 Oct 21. Review.
17. Wang Q, Afshin A, Yakoob MY, Singh GM, Rehm CD, Khatibzadeh S, Micha R, Shi P, Mozaffarian D, Global Burden of Diseases Nutrition and Chronic Diseases Expert Group (NutriCoDE). Impact of non-optimal intakes of saturated, polyunsaturated, and trans fat on global burdens of coronary heart disease. J Am Heart Assoc. 2016;5(1). pii: e002891. https://doi.org/10.1161/JAHA.115.002891.
18. Kris-Etherton P, Eckel RH, Howard BV, St Jeor S, Bazzarre TL; Nutrition Committee Population Science Committee and Clinical Science Committee of the American Heart Association. AHA Science Advisory: Lyon Diet Heart Study. Benefits of a Mediterranean-style, National Cholesterol Education Program/American Heart Association Step I Dietary Pattern on Cardiovascular Disease. Circulation. 2001;103(13):1823–5. http://circ.ahajournals.org/content/103/13/1823.long
19. Estruch R, Ros E, Salas-Salvadó J, Covas MI, Corella D, Arós F, Gómez-Gracia E, Ruiz-Gutiérrez V, Fiol M, Lapetra J, Lamuela-Raventos RM, Serra-Majem L, Pintó X, Basora J, Muñoz MA, Sorlí JV, Martínez JA, Martínez-González MA, PREDIMED Study Investigators. Primary prevention of cardiovascular disease with a Mediterranean diet. N Engl J Med. 2013;368(14):1279–90. https://doi.org/10.1056/NEJMoa1200303. Epub 2013 Feb 25. Erratum in: N Engl J Med. 2014 Feb 27;370(9):886.
20. Gay HC, Rao SG, Vaccarino V, Ali MK. Effects of different dietary interventions on blood pressure: systematic review and meta-analysis of randomized controlled trials. Hypertension. 2016;67(4):733–9. https://doi.org/10.1161/HYPERTENSIONAHA.115.06853. Epub 2016 Feb 22. Review.
21. Bloomfield HE, Koeller E, Greer N, MacDonald R, Kane R, Wilt TJ. Effects on health outcomes of a Mediterranean diet with no restriction on fat intake: a systematic review and meta-analysis. Ann Intern Med. 2016;165(7):491–500. https://doi.org/10.7326/M16-0361. Epub 2016 Jul 19. Review.
22. Sofi F, Cesari F, Abbate R, Gensini GF, Casini A. Adherence to Mediterranean diet and health status: meta-analysis. BMJ. 2008;337:a1344. https://doi.org/10.1136/bmj.a1344. Review.
23. Esposito K, Maiorino MI, Bellastella G, Chiodini P, Panagiotakos D, Giugliano D. A journey into a Mediterranean diet and type 2 diabetes: a sys-

tematic review with meta-analyses. BMJ Open. 2015;5(8):e008222. https://doi.org/10.1136/bmjopen-2015-008222. Review.
24. Ros E, Hu FB. Consumption of plant seeds and cardiovascular health: epidemiologic and clinical trial evidence. Circulation. 2013;128:553–65.
25. Salas-Salvadó J, Guasch-Ferré M, Lee CH, Estruch R, Clish CB, Ros E. Protective effects of the Mediterranean diet on type 2 diabetes and metabolic syndrome. J Nutr. 2016. pii: jn218487. [Epub ahead of print] Review.
26. Schwingshackl L, Missbach B, König J, Hoffmann G. Adherence to a Mediterranean diet and risk of diabetes: a systematic review and meta-analysis. Public Health Nutr. 2015;18(7):1292–9. https://doi.org/10.1017/S1368980014001542. Epub 2014 Aug 22. Review.
27. Koloverou E, Esposito K, Giugliano D, Panagiotakos D. The effect of Mediterranean diet on the development of type 2 diabetes mellitus: a meta-analysis of 10 prospective studies and 136,846 participants. Metabolism. 2014;63(7):903–11. https://doi.org/10.1016/j.metabol.2014.04.010. Epub 2014 Apr 24. Review.
28. Esposito K, Maiorino MI, Ceriello A, Giugliano D. Prevention and control of type 2 diabetes by Mediterranean diet: a systematic review. Diabetes Res Clin Pract. 2010;89(2):97–102. https://doi.org/10.1016/j.diabres.2010.04.019. Epub 2010 May 23. Review.
29. Garcia M, Bihuniak JD, Shook J, Kenny A, Kerstetter J, Huedo-Medina TB. The effect of the traditional Mediterranean-style diet on metabolic risk factors: a meta-analysis. Nutrients. 2016;8(3):168. https://doi.org/10.3390/nu8030168. Review.
30. Godos J, Zappalà G, Bernardini S, Giambini I, Bes-Rastrollo M, Martinez-Gonzalez M. Adherence to the Mediterranean diet is inversely associated with metabolic syndrome occurrence: a meta-analysis of observational studies. Int J Food Sci Nutr. 2017;68(2):138–48. https://doi.org/10.1080/09637486.2016.1221900. Epub 2016 Aug 25. Review.
31. Esposito K, Kastorini CM, Panagiotakos DB, Giugliano D. Mediterranean diet and metabolic syndrome: an updated systematic review. Rev Endocr Metab Disord. 2013;14(3):255–63. https://doi.org/10.1007/s11154-013-9253-9. Review.
32. Schwingshackl L, Hoffmann G. Adherence to Mediterranean diet and risk of cancer: an updated systematic review and meta-analysis of observational studies. Cancer Med. 2015;4(12):1933–47. https://doi.org/10.1002/cam4.539. Epub 2015 Oct 16. Review.
33. D'Alessandro A, De Pergola G, Silvestris F. Mediterranean diet and cancer risk: an open issue. Int J Food Sci Nutr. 2016;67(6):593–605. https://doi.org/10.1080/09637486.2016.1191444. Epub 2016 Jun 2. Review.
34. Song M, Giovannucci E. Preventable incidence and mortality of carcinoma associated with lifestyle factors among white adults in the United States. JAMA Oncol. 2016;2(9):1154–61. https://doi.org/10.1001/jamaoncol.2016.0843.
35. La Vecchia C. Mediterranean diet and cancer. Public Health Nutr. 2004;7(7):965–8. Review.
36. Fabiani R, Minelli L, Bertarelli G, Bacci S. A western dietary pattern increases prostate cancer risk: a systematic review and meta-analysis. Nutrients. 2016;8(10). pii: E626. Review.
37. van den Brandt PA, Schulpen M. Mediterranean diet adherence and risk of postmenopausal breast cancer: results of a cohort study and meta-analysis. Int J Cancer. 2017;140(10):2220–31. https://doi.org/10.1002/ijc.30654. Epub 2017 Mar 5.
38. Neale EP, Batterham MJ, Tapsell LC. Consumption of a healthy dietary pattern results in significant reductions in C-reactive protein levels in adults: a meta-analysis. Nutr Res. 2016;36(5):391–401. https://doi.org/10.1016/j.nutres.2016.02.009. Epub 2016 Feb 22. Review.
39. Cao L, Tan L, Wang HF, Jiang T, Zhu XC, Lu H, Tan MS, Yu JT. Dietary patterns and risk of dementia: a systematic review and meta-analysis of cohort studies. Mol Neurobiol. 2016;53(9):6144–54. https://doi.org/10.1007/s12035-015-9516-4. Epub 2015 Nov 9.
40. Stephan BCM, Harrison SL, Keage HAD, Babateen A, Robinson L, Siervo M. Cardiovascular disease, the nitric oxide pathway and risk of cognitive impairment and dementia. Curr Cardiol Rep. 2017;19(9):87. https://doi.org/10.1007/s11886-017-0898-y. Review.
41. Cuello AC. Early and late CNS inflammation in Alzheimer's disease: two extremes of a continuum? Trends Pharmacol Sci. 2017. pii: S0165-6147(17)30144-X. https://doi.org/10.1016/j.tips.2017.07.005. [Epub ahead of print] Review.
42. Lourida I, Soni M, Thompson-Coon J, Purandare N, Lang IA, Ukoumunne OC, Llewellyn DJ. Mediterranean diet, cognitive function, and dementia: a systematic review. Epidemiology. 2013;24(4):479–89. https://doi.org/10.1097/EDE.0b013e3182944410. Review.
43. Wu L, Sun D. Adherence to Mediterranean diet and risk of developing cognitive disorders: an updated systematic review and meta-analysis of prospective cohort studies. Sci Rep. 2017;7:41317. https://doi.org/10.1038/srep41317.
44. Loughrey DG, Lavecchia S, Brennan S, Lawlor BA, Kelly ME. The impact of the Mediterranean diet on the cognitive functioning of healthy older adults: a systematic review and meta-analysis. Adv Nutr. 2017;8(4):571–86. https://doi.org/10.3945/an.117.015495. Print 2017 Jul. Review. PMID: 28710144.
45. Kunutsor SK, Laukkanen JA, Whitehouse MR, Blom AW. Adherence to a Mediterranean-style diet and incident fractures: pooled analysis of observational evidence. Eur J Nutr. 2017; https://doi.org/10.1007/s00394-017-1432-0.
46. Malmir H, Saneei P, Larijani B, Esmaillzadeh A. Adherence to Mediterranean diet in relation

to bone mineral density and risk of fracture: a systematic review and meta-analysis of observational studies. Eur J Nutr. 2017. https://doi.org/10.1007/s00394-017-1490-3.
47. Papamichael MM, Itsiopoulos C, Susanto NH, Erbas B. Does adherence to the Mediterranean dietary pattern reduce asthma symptoms in children? A systematic review of observational studies. Public Health Nutr. 2017;14:1–13. https://doi.org/10.1017/S1368980017001823.
48. Sainani GS. Role of diet, exercise and drugs in modulation of endothelial cell dysfunction. J Assoc Physicians India. 2012;60:14–9.
49. Pandey KB, Rizvi SI. Plant polyphenols as dietary antioxidants in human health and disease. Oxidative Med Cell Longev. 2009;2(5):270–8. https://doi.org/10.4161/oxim.2.5.9498. Review.
50. Graf BA, Milbury PE, Blumberg JB. Flavonols, favonones, flavanones and human health: epidemiological evidence. J Med Food. 2005;8:281–90.
51. Arts ICW, Hollman PCH. Polyphenols and disease risk in epidemiologic studies. Am J Clin Nutr. 2005;81:317–25.
52. García-Lafuente A, Guillamón E, Villares A, Rostagno MA, Martínez JA. Flavonoids as anti-inflammatory agents: implications in cancer and cardiovascular disease. Inflamm Res. 2009;58:537–52.
53. Pirola L, Frojdo S. Resveratrol: one molecule, many targets. IUBMB Life. 2008;60:323–32.
54. Kamaraj S, Vinodhkumar R, Anandakumar P, Jagan S, Ramakrishnan G, Devaki T. The effects of quercetin on antioxidant status and tumor markers in the lung and serum of mice treated with benzo(a)pyrene. Biol Pharm Bull. 2007;30:2268–73.
55. Scarmeas N, Luchsinger JA, Mayeux R, Stern Y. Mediterranean diet and Alzheimer disease mortality. Neurology. 2007;69:1084–93.
56. Aquilano K, Baldelli S, Rotilio G, Ciriolo MR. Role of nitric oxide synthases in Parkinson's disease: a review on the antioxidant and anti-inflammatory activity of polyphenols. Neurochem Res. 2008;33:2416–26.
57. Rossi L, Mazzitelli S, Arciello M, Capo CR, Rotilio G. Benefits from dietary polyphenols for brain aging and Alzheimer's disease. Neurochem Res. 2008;33:2390–400.
58. Kiritsakis A. Olive oil- from the tree to the table. 2nd ed. Trumbull: Food and Nutrition Press, Inc; 1998. p. 006611.
59. Visioli F, Poli A, Gall C. Antioxidant and other biological activities of phenols from olives and olive oil. Med Res Rev. 2002;22(1):65–75.
60. Baldioli M, Servili M, Perretti G, Montedoro GF. Antioxidant activity of tocopherols and phenolic compounds of virgin olive oil. J Am Oil Chem Soc. 1996;73(11):1589–93.
61. Han X, Shen T, Lou H. Dietary polyphenols and their biological significance. Int J Mol Sci. 2007;8(9):950–88. https://doi.org/10.3390/i8090950. Review.
62. Calabriso N, Massaro M, Scoditti E, D'Amore S, Gnoni A, Pellegrino M, Storelli C, De Caterina R, Palasciano G, Carluccio MA. Extra virgin olive oil rich in polyphenols modulates VEGF-induced angiogenic responses by preventing NADPH oxidase activity and expression. J Nutr Biochem. 2016;28:19–29. https://doi.org/10.1016/j.jnutbio.2015.09.026.
63. Estruch R, Ros E, Salas-Salvadó J, Covas MI, Corella D, Arós F, Gómez-Gracia E, Ruiz-Gutiérrez V, Fiol M, Lapetra J, Lamuela-Raventos RM, Serra-Majem L, Pintó X, Basora J, Muñoz MA, Sorlí JV, Martínez JA, Martínez-González MA, PREDIMED Study Investigators. Primary prevention of cardiovascular disease with a Mediterranean diet. N Engl J Med. 2013;368(14):1279–90. https://doi.org/10.1056/NEJMoa1200303. Epub 2013 Feb 25. Erratum in: N Engl J Med. 2014 Feb 27;370(9):886.
64. Escribá PV, Halver JE. How Oleic acid in olive oil reduces blood pressure. www.pitt.edu/~super4/33011-34001/33541.ppt
65. Seeram NP, Aviram M, Zhang Y, Henning SM, Feng L, Dreher M, Heber D. Comparison of antioxidant potency of commonly consumed polyphenol-rich beverages in the United States. J Agric Food Chem. 2008;56(4):1415–22.
66. Durak I, Avci A, Kacmaz M, Büyükkoçak S, Cimen MY, Elgün S, Oztürk HS. Comparison of antioxidant potentials of red wine, white wine, grape juice and alcohol. Curr Med Res Opin. 1999;15(4):316–20.
67. Keevil JG, Osman HE, Reed JD, Folts JD. Grape juice, but not orange juice or grapefruit juice, inhibits human platelet aggregation. J Nutr. 2000;130(1):53–6.
68. Folts JD. Antithrombotic potential of grape juice and red wine for preventing heart attacks. Pharm Biol. 1998;36(Supplement 1):21–7.
69. Freedman JE, Parker C 3rd, Li L, Perlman JA, Frei B, Ivanov V, Deak LR, Iafrati MD, Folts JD. Select flavonoids and whole juice from purple grapes inhibit platelet function and enhance nitric oxide release. Circulation. 2001;103(23):2792–8.
70. O'Byrne DJ, Devaraj S, Grundy SM, Jialal I. Comparison of the antioxidant effects of Concord grape juice flavonoids alpha-tocopherol on markers of oxidative stress in healthy adults. Am J Clin Nutr. 2002;76(6):1367–74.
71. Stein JH, Keevil JG, Wiebe DA, Aeschlimann S, Folts JD. Purple grape juice improves endothelial function and reduces the susceptibility of LDL cholesterol to oxidation in patients with coronary artery disease. Circulation. 1999;100(10):1050–5.
72. Park YK, Kim JS, Kang MH. Concord grape juice supplementation reduces blood pressure in Korean hypertensive men: double-blind, placebo controlled intervention trial. Biofactors. 2004;22(1–4):145–7.
73. Mark D, Maki K. Concord grape juice reduces blood pressure in men with high systolic blood pressure. Experimental biology. San Diego. 11–15 Apr 2003.
74. Dohadwala MM, Hamburg NM, Holbrook M, Kim BH, Duess M, Levit A, Titas M, Chung WB, Vincent FB, Caiano T, Frame AA, Keaney JF Jr, Vita JA. Effects of Concord grape juice on ambulatory

blood pressure in prehypertension and stage 1 hypertension. Am J Clin Nutr. 2010;91(5):1052–9.
75. Dohadwala MM, Vita JA. Grapes and cardiovascular disease. J Nutr. 2009;139(9):1788S–93S.
76. Chou EJ, Keevil JG, Aeschlimann S, Wiebe DA, Folts JD, Stein JH. Effect of ingestion of purple grape juice on endothelial function in patients with coronary heart disease. Am J Cardiol. 2001;88(5):553–5.
77. Anselm E, Chataigneau M, Ndiaye M, Chataigneau T, Schini-Kerth VB. Grape juice causes endothelium-dependent relaxation via a redox-sensitive Src- and Akt-dependent activation of eNOS. Cardiovasc Res. 2007;73(2):404–13.
78. Fitzpatrick DF, Hirschfield SL, Coffey RG. Endothelium-dependent vasorelaxing activity of wine and other grape products. Am J Physiol Heart Circ Physiol. 1993;265(34):H774–8.
79. Albers AR, Varghese S, Vitseva O, Vita JA, Freedman JE. The antiinflammatory effects of purple grape juice consumption in subjects with stable coronary artery disease. Arterioscler Thromb Vasc Biol. 2004;24(Nov):e179–80.
80. Vislocky LM, Fernandez MLF. Biomedical effects of grape products. Nutr Rev. 2010;68(11):656–70.
81. Krikorian R, Nash TA, Shidler MD, Shukitt-Hale B, Joseph JA. Concord grape juice supplementation improves memory function in older adults with mild cognitive impairment. Br J Nutr. 2010;103(5):730–4.
82. Shukitt-Hale B, Carey A, Simon L, Mark DA, Joseph JA. Effects of Concord grape juice on cognitive and motor deficits in aging. Nutrition. 2006;22(3):295–302.
83. Ho L, Ferruzzi MG, Janle EM, Lobo J, Chen TY, Talcott ST, Simon J, Wu QL, Wang J, Cheng A, Weaver CM, Percival SS, Pasinetti GM. Bioavailability of grape-derived polyphenolics and implications in Alzheimer's disease prevention and therapy. Presented at Experimental Biology; 2010 Apr 24–28; Anaheim;2010.
84. Joseph JA, Shukitt-Hale B, Casadesus G. Reversing the deleterious effects of aging on neuronal communication and behavior: beneficial properties of fruit polyphenolic compounds. Am J Clin Nutr. 2005;81(1 Suppl):313S–6S.
85. Lipson SM, Cohen P, Zhou J, Burdowski A, Stotzky G. Cranberry cocktail juice, cranberry concentrates, and proanthocyanidins reduce reovirus infectivity titers in African green monkey kidney epithelial cell cultures. Mol Nutr Food Res. 2007;51(6):752–8.
86. Rodella LF, Favero G. Atherosclerosis and current anti-oxidant strategies for atheroprotection. Curr Trends Atherogenesis. 2012 (InTech, Open Access). https://doi.org/10.5772/53035.
87. Mallol J, Crane J, von Mutius E, Odhiambo J, Keil U, Stewart A, ISAAC Phase Three Study Group. The International Study of Asthma and Allergies in Childhood (ISAAC) phase three: a global synthesis. Allergol Immunopathol (Madr). 2013;41(2):73–85. https://doi.org/10.1016/j.aller.2012.03.001. Epub 2012 Jul 6.
88. Fremont L. Biological effects of resveratrol. Life Sci. 2000;66(8):663–73.
89. Khakimov B, Engelsen SB. Resveratrol in the foodomics era: 1:25,000. Ann N Y Acad Sci. 2017. https://doi.org/10.1111/nyas.13425. [Epub ahead of print] Review.
90. Higdon J, Drake VJ, Steward WP. Resveratrol. Corvallis: Micronutrient Information Center. Linus Pauling Institute, Oregon State University; 2016.
91. Schwager J, Richard N, Widmer F, Raederstorff D. Resveratrol distinctively modulates the inflammatory profiles of immune and endothelial cells. BMC Complement Altern Med. 2017;17(1):309. https://doi.org/10.1186/s12906-017-1823-z.
92. Kulkarni SS, Cantó C. The molecular targets of resveratrol. Biochim Biophys Acta. 2015;1852(6):1114–23. https://doi.org/10.1016/j.bbadis.2014.10.005. Epub 2014 Oct 12. Review.
93. Kim I, He YY. Targeting the AMP-activated protein kinase for cancer prevention and therapy. Front Oncol. 2013;3:175. https://doi.org/10.3389/fonc.2013.00175. eCollection 2013.
94. Kitada M, Koya D. Renal protective effects of resveratrol. Oxid Med Cell Longev. 2013;2013, Article ID 568093, 7 pages. https://doi.org/10.1155/2013/568093.
95. Wang S, Wang J, Zhao A, Li J. SIRT1 activation inhibits hyperglycemia-induced apoptosis by reducing oxidative stress and mitochondrial dysfunction in human endothelial cells. Mol Med Rep. 2017;16(3):3331–8. https://doi.org/10.3892/mmr.2017.7027. Epub 2017 Jul 17.
96. Teixeira J, Chavarria D, Borges F, Wojtczak L, Wieckowski MR, Karkucińska-Wieckowska A, Oliveira PJ. Dietary polyphenols and mitochondrial function: role in health and disease. Curr Med Chem. 2017. https://doi.org/10.2174/0929867324666170529101810. [Epub ahead of print].
97. Yousuf S, Atif F, Ahmad M, Hoda N, Ishrat T, Khan B, Islam F. Resveratrol exerts its neuroprotective effect by modulating mitochondrial dysfunctions and associated cell death during cerebral ischemia. Brain Res. 2009;1250:242–53. https://doi.org/10.1016/j.brainres.2008.10.068. Epub 2008 Nov 11.
98. Bhandari R, Kuhad A. Resveratrol suppresses neuroinflammation in the experimental paradigm of autism spectrum disorders. Neurochem Int. 2017;103:8–23. https://doi.org/10.1016/j.neuint.2016.12.012. Epub 2016 Dec 23.
99. Hermann DM, Zechariah A, Kaltwasser B, Bosche B, Caglayan AB, Kilic E, Doeppner TR. Sustained neurological recovery induced by resveratrol is associated with angioneurogenesis rather than neuroprotection after focal cerebral ischemia. Neurobiol Dis. 2015;83:16–25. https://doi.org/10.1016/j.nbd.2015.08.018. Epub 2015 Aug 24.

100. Pang C, Cao L, Wu F, Wang L, Wang G, Yu Y, Zhang M, Chen L, Wang W, Lv W, Chen L, Zhu J, Pan J, Zhang H, Xu Y, Ding L. The effect of trans-resveratrol on post-stroke depression via regulation of hypothalamus-pituitary-adrenal axis. Neuropharmacology. 2015;97:447–56. https://doi.org/10.1016/j.neuropharm.2015.04.017. Epub 2015 Apr 29.
101. Zhang F, Wang H, Wu Q, Lu Y, Nie J, Xie X, Shi J. Resveratrol protects cortical neurons against microglia-mediated neuroinflammation. Phytother Res. 2013;27(3):344–9. https://doi.org/10.1002/ptr.4734. Epub 2012 May 14.
102. Anekonda TS. Resveratrol – a boon for treating Alzheimer's disease? Brain Res Rev. 2006;52(2):316–26. Review.
103. Ferrières J. The French paradox: lessons for other countries. Heart. 2004;90(1):107–11.
104. Voulgari C, Pagoni S, Vinik A, Poirier P. Exercise improves cardiac autonomic function in obesity and diabetes. Metabolism. 2013;62:609–21.
105. Webb AJ, Patel N, Loukogeorgakis S, Okorie M, Aboud Z, Misra S, Rashid R, Miall P, Deanfield J, Benjamin N, MacAllister R, Hobbs AJ, Ahluwalia A. Acute blood pressure lowering, vasoprotective, and antiplatelet properties of dietary nitrate via bioconversion to nitrite. Hypertension. 2008;51(3):784–90. https://doi.org/10.1161/HYPERTENSIONAHA.107.103523. Epub 2008 Feb 4.
106. Lock K, Promerleau J, Causer L, Altman DR, McKee M. The global burden of disease attributable to low consumption of fruit and vegetables: implications for the global strategy of diet. Bull World Health Organ. 2005;83:100–8.
107. Quin X, Huo Y, Langman CB, Hou F, Chen Y, Matossin D, et al. Folic acid therapy and cardiovascular disease in end-stage renal disease or advanced chronic kidney disease: a metaanalysis. Clin J Am Soc Nephrol. 2011;6:482–8.
108. Lee M, Hong KS, Chang SC, Saver JL. Efficiency of homocysteine lowering therapy with folic acid and stroke prevention: a metaanalysis. Stroke. 2010;41:1205–12.
109. Potter JD. Cancer prevention: epidemiology and experiment. Cancer Lett. 1997;114(1–2):7–9.
110. Faraci FM, Heistad DD. Regulation of the cerebral circulation: role of endothelium and potassium channels. Physiol Rev. 1998;78(1):53–97.
111. Rubinshtein R, Kuvin JT, Soffler M, Lennon RJ, Lavi S, Nelson RE, Pumper GM, Lerman LO, Lerman A. Assessment of endothelial function by non-invasive peripheral arterial tonometry predicts late cardiovascular adverse events. Eur Heart J. 2010;31(9):1142–8. https://doi.org/10.1093/eurheartj/ehq010. Epub 2010 Feb 24.
112. Mita T, Watada H, Ogihara T, Nomiyama T, Ogawa O, Kinoshita J, Shimizu T, Hirose T, Tanaka Y, Kawamori R. Eicosapentaenoic acid reduces the progression of carotid intima-media thickness in patients with type 2 diabetes. Atherosclerosis. 2007;191(1):162–7. Epub 2006 Apr 17.
113. Wu JH, Micha R, Imamura F, Pan A, Biggs ML, Ajaz O, Djousse L, Hu FB, Mozaffarian D. Omega-3 fatty acids and incident type 2 diabetes: a systematic review and meta-analysis. Br J Nutr. 2012;107(Suppl 2):S214–27. https://doi.org/10.1017/S0007114512001602. Review.
114. Brinton EA, Ballantyne CM, Bays HE, Kastelein JJ, Braeckman RA, Soni PN. Effects of icosapent ethyl on lipid and inflammatory parameters in patients with diabetes mellitus-2, residual elevated triglycerides (200–500 mg/dL), and on statin therapy at LDL-C goal: the ANCHOR study. Cardiovasc Diabetol. 2013;12:100. https://doi.org/10.1186/1475-2840-12-100. Erratum in: Cardiovasc Diabetol. 2015 Jul–Aug;9(4):618.
115. Menotti A, Puddu PE. How the Seven Countries Study contributed to the definition and development of the Mediterranean diet concept: a 50-year journey. Nutr Metab Cardiovasc Dis. 2015;25(3):245–52. https://doi.org/10.1016/j.numecd.2014.12.001. Epub 2014 Dec 12.
116. Nanri A, Mizoue T, Shimazu T, Ishihara J, Takachi R, Noda M, Iso H, Sasazuki S, Sawada N, Tsugane S, Japan Public Health Center-Based Prospective Study Group. Dietary patterns and all-cause, cancer, and cardiovascular disease mortality in Japanese men and women: the Japan public health center-based prospective study. PLoS One. 2017;12(4):e0174848. https://doi.org/10.1371/journal.pone.0174848. eCollection 2017.
117. Benbaibeche H, Haffaf el M, Kacimi G, Oudjit B, Khan NA, Koceïr EA. Implication of corticotropic hormone axis in eating behaviour pattern in obese and type 2 diabetic participants. Br J Nutr. 2015;113(8):1237–43. https://doi.org/10.1017/S0007114515000549. Epub 2015 Mar 18.
118. García-Prieto MD, Tébar FJ, Nicolás F, Larqué E, Zamora S, Garaulet M. Cortisol secretary pattern and glucocorticoid feedback sensitivity in women from a Mediterranean area: relationship with anthropometric characteristics, dietary intake and plasma fatty acid profile. Clin Endocrinol. 2007;66(2):185–91.
119. Kanauchi M, Kanauchi K. Development of a Mediterranean diet score adapted to Japan and its relation to obesity risk. Food Nutr Res. 2016;60:32172. https://doi.org/10.3402/fnr.v60.32172. eCollection 2016.
120. Zhang R, Wang Z, Fei Y, Zhou B, Zheng S, Wang L, Huang L, Jiang S, Liu Z, Jiang J, Yu Y. The difference in nutrient intakes between Chinese and Mediterranean, Japanese and American diets. Nutrients. 2015;7(6):4661–88. https://doi.org/10.3390/nu7064661.
121. Verberne L, Bach-Faig A, Buckland G, Serra-Majem L. Association between the Mediterranean diet and cancer risk: a review of observational studies. Nutr Cancer. 2010;62(7):860–70. https://doi.org/10.1080/01635581.2010.509834. Review.

122. Tyrovolas S, Panagiotakos DB. The role of Mediterranean type of diet on the development of cancer and cardiovascular disease, in the elderly: a systematic review. Maturitas. 2010;65(2):122–30. https://doi.org/10.1016/j.maturitas.2009.07.003. Epub 2009 Aug 4. Review.
123. Pelucchi C, Bosetti C, Rossi M, Negri E, La Vecchia C. Selected aspects of Mediterranean diet and cancer risk. Nutr Cancer. 2009;61(6):756–66. https://doi.org/10.1080/01635580903285007. Review.
124. La Vecchia C. Mediterranean diet and cancer. Public Health Nutr. 2004;7(7):965–8. Review.
125. La Vecchia C. Estrogen and combined estrogen-progestogen therapy in the menopause and breast cancer. Breast. 2004;13(6):515–8. Review.
126. Giacosa A, Barale R, Bavaresco L, Gatenby P, Gerbi V, Janssens J, Johnston B, Kas K, La Vecchia C, Mainguet P, Morazzoni P, Negri E, Pelucchi C, Pezzotti M, Rondanelli M. Cancer prevention in Europe: the Mediterranean diet as a protective choice. Eur J Cancer Prev. 2013;22(1):90–5. https://doi.org/10.1097/CEJ.0b013e328354d2d7. Review.
127. Dalvi TB, Canchola AJ, Horn-Ross PL. Dietary patterns, Mediterranean diet, and endometrial cancer risk. Cancer Causes Control. 2007;18(9):957–66. Epub 2007 Jul 19.
128. Kontou N, Psaltopoulou T, Panagiotakos D, Dimopoulos MA, Linos A. The Mediterranean diet in cancer prevention: a review. J Med Food. 2011;14(10):1065–78. https://doi.org/10.1089/jmf.2010.0244. Epub 2011 Jun 11. Review.
129. Sacchi R, Paduano A, Savarese M, Vitaglione P, Fogliano V. Extra virgin olive oil: from composition to "molecular gastronomy". Cancer Treat Res. 2014;159:325–38. https://doi.org/10.1007/978-3-642-38007-5_19. Review.
130. Kang BY. Curcumin reduces angiotensin to mediated cardiomyocyte growth via LOX-1 inhibition. J Cardiovasc Pharmacol. 2010;55:417–24.
131. Xi B, Veeranki SP, Zhao M, Ma C, Yan Y, Mi J. Relationship of alcohol consumption to all-cause, cardiovascular, and cancer-related mortality in U.S. adults. J Am Coll Cardiol. 2017;70(8):913–22. https://doi.org/10.1016/j.jacc.2017.06.054.
132. de Gaetano G, Costanzo S. Alcohol and health: praise of the J curves. J Am Coll Cardiol. 2017;70(8):923–5. https://doi.org/10.1016/j.jacc.2017.07.710.
133. Plunk AD, Syed-Mohammed H, Cavazos-Rehg P, Bierut LJ, Grucza RA. Alcohol consumption, heavy drinking and mortality: re-thinking the J-shaped curve. Alcohol Clin Exp Res. 2014;38(2):471–8. https://doi.org/10.1111/acer.12250.

# Exercise (Prong-5) 7

The fifth prong of the Mind-Body Wellness Program focuses on exercise (Fig. 7.1). "Exercise" is not a bad word! It does not have to be drudgery. Perhaps a better description is "active lifestyle," which may include exercise (in the sense of the current vernacular), but it should reflect the lifestyle of people before automobiles, elevators, television remotes, and cell phones. It can be a single (preferably daily) acute bout of physical exertion or muscular activity that expends energy above one's basal or resting level [1]. Exercise can also be a daylong habit of activity, included but not limited to household chores, taking the stairs, shopping, gardening, walking, and playing with children. The physiologic and psychologic benefits of exercise are numerous. It is better than any supplement or pill available. It is probably better than any combination of supplements or pills or possibly even pharmacological agents. In fact, as mentioned throughout the book, exercise with supplements, etc., including diet which supports exercise, is the best combination for minimizing morbidity risk, which optimizes quality and continuation of life, and minimizes mortality risk, which optimizes longevity and minimizes the impact of disease if and when it happens. It does so many beneficial things to the body (Fig. 7.2):

- *Happier Moods* from the release of endorphins in the brain and other brain chemicals that elevate mood. Regular physical activity (3–5 times a week for 30–60 each time) reduces risk of depression.
- *Reduced Pain.* Endorphins are natural pain killers and can help to provide temporary pain relief.
- *Immune Health.* From two aspects of exercise: (1) physical activity raises the body's core temperature, simulating a fever (20 minutes or more of exercise, three or more times per week, helps to prevent disease before it starts); (2) exercise, as stated above, is arguably the strongest antioxidant available (see "The Importance of Antioxidants" in Chap. 2) and provides all of the benefits detailed in the Chap.5, including defeating (promoting the oxidation of) all types of infections: viral, bacterial, fungal, mold, etc.
- *Better Sleep Quality.* Five or 6 hours after workout, the decreased body core temperature signals the body to sleep, promoting less time to fall asleep and sounder sleep cycles, resulting in more restorative sleep and less daytime drowsiness. Also, less weight may mean less risk of sleep apnea and snoring.
- *Improved Concentration and Creativity.* Exercise increases circulation, thereby increasing tissue oxygenation and removal of wastes from throughout (detoxifies) the body. In the brain, this improves function, including concentration, creativity, and productivity. In addition to an improved cardiovascular system, the endorphins released stimulate the mind for more creative thoughts.



N. L. DePace, J. Colombo, *Clinical Autonomic and Mitochondrial Disorders*,
https://doi.org/10.1007/978-3-030-17016-5_7

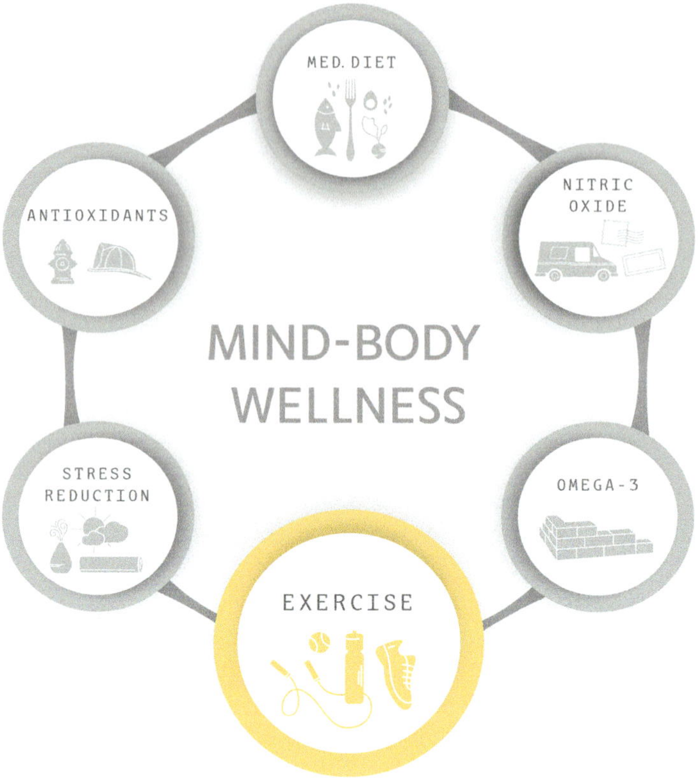


**Fig. 7.1** The mind body-wellness program – exercise prong. (Illustration by Elysian Creative Studio, www.elysiancreativestudio.com, Lizzy Colombo)

- *Reduce Stress Levels and Anxiety*. "Too busy" is a common excuse to skip a workout, but physical activity actually helps alleviate stress and promotes productivity. Exercise increases the body's ability to handle stress. It produces higher levels of norepinephrine, a chemical that regulates areas of the brain that send stress signals. The more the body is trained with the healthy physical stresses of mild to moderate exercise, the better the body responds to emotional stress.
- *Maintain Mental Fitness*. Through aging, brainpower decreases and the brain actually grows smaller. Mental decline can start as early as 24 years of age. Elderly who exercise show less brain shrinkage than those who do not. Exercise may also reverse brain shrinkage. Regular physical activity (3–5 times a week for 30–60 minutes) helps maintain or sharpen thinking, learning, and judgment skills with age and increases memory by increasing the volume of gray matter in the brain.
- *Parasympathetic and Sympathetic (P&S) Nervous Systems*. The P&S (autonomic) nervous systems control and coordinate all of the organs and "involuntary" functions of the body. A proper balance is needed, both at rest and during activity. Note, sleeping is an activity and so is sitting at a desk and working, but sitting watching television is not. Exercise by itself can balance the P&S nervous systems better than any supplement or diet alone. Again, the best is when exercise and diet and the rest of the Mind-Body Wellness Program are taken together! Establishing and maintaining P&S balance should always be a goal, and exercise is an excellent adjunct to pharmacology and other lifestyle measures, including diet in this regard.
- *Stress Reduction*. Exercise reduces stress, reducing cortisol levels (as mentioned above), psychosocial stress, anxiety, depression (as mentioned above), and fatigue. It reduces oxidative stress, improving endothelial function, increasing nitric oxide production and the numbers of mitochondria for more energy.

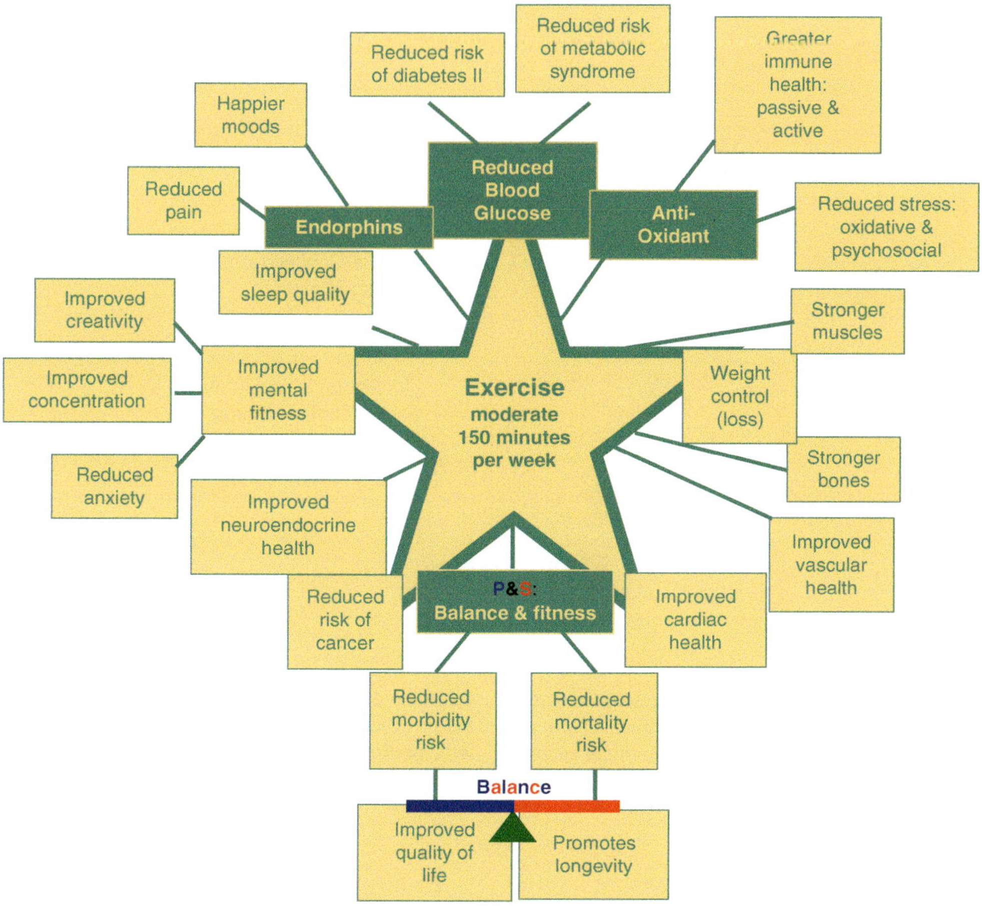


**Fig. 7.2** Exercise does many beneficial things to the body

- *Heart and Vascular Health.* Physical activity engages the entire body, and a healthier cardiovascular system means the heart is better able to circulate blood to all parts of the body, including in older individuals. Heart disease and stroke are two of the leading causes of death in the United States. Following physician recommendations and getting at least 150 minutes a week (2½ hours) of moderate-intensity activity reduces the risk for these diseases. The more exercise, the more that risk is reduced. Regular physical activity improves almost all cardiac risk factors, including by increasing HDL cholesterol, lowering LDL cholesterol (clears arteries), lowering blood pressure, increasing cardiovascular fitness, and making the blood less prone to thrombosis or clotting, not only around the heart but also in the brain. Greater blood flow to the brain underlies the brain function improvements mentioned above, including restorative sleep, improves mood, reduces depression, helps clear "brain fog," and improves cognitive abilities and perhaps memory.
- *Neuroendocrine Health.* Exercise reduces cortisol release for better neuroendocrine balance (Fig. 7.3). It helps to keep insulin levels healthy and increases insulin sensitivity. It boosts sex hormones. It helps to maintain healthy thyroid and hypothyroid hormone levels, including levels of growth hormones, which in adults helps with healing and repair.
- *Weight Control (Loss).* Diet and physical activity play a critical role in weight management. Weight gain occurs when the calories burned, including those burned during physical activity, are less than the calories consumed. The amount of physical activity

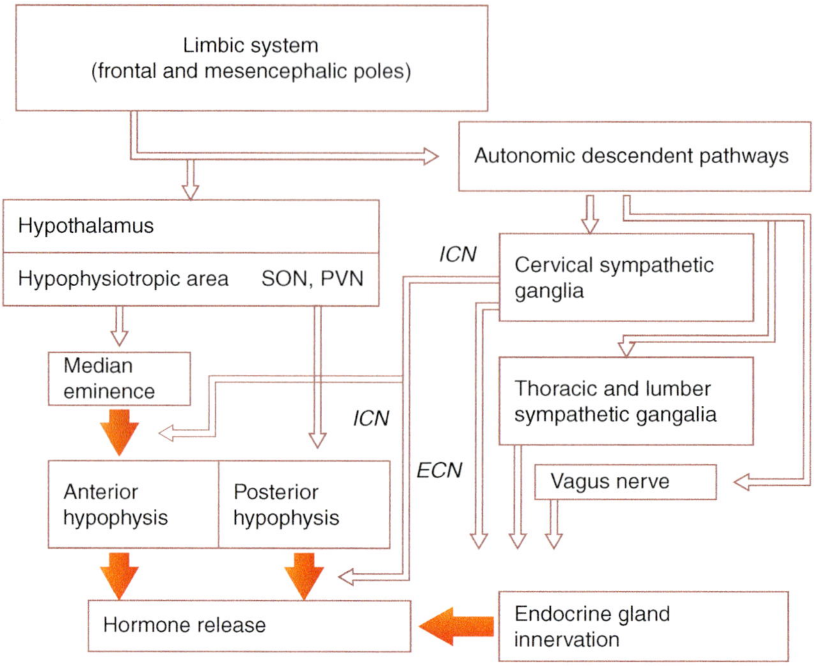


**Fig. 7.3** Nerves innervating endocrine glands constitute alternative pathways through which the brain communicates with the glands. Depicted is the hierarchical and parallel organization of neurohormonal pathways. Abbreviations: ICN Internal Carotid Nerve, ECN External Carotid Nerve, SON Supraoptic Nucleus, PVN Paraventricular Nucleus [ [2], Fig. 3.30]. (Republished with permission from Springer International Publishing AG. Insert: Illustration by Elysian Creative Studio, www.elysiancreativestudio.com, Lizzy Colombo)

required for weight management varies greatly, depending on metabolism (genetics), age (including stage of development), environment, and more. Physical activity can help with weight loss as well as weight maintenance. Establishing and maintaining a healthy weight requires both regular physical activity and a healthy eating plan.

- *Reduced Risk of Type 2 Diabetes and Metabolic Syndrome.* Regular physical activity reduces risk of developing type 2 diabetes and metabolic syndrome. Metabolic syndrome includes a combination of (1) too much fat around the waist, (2) high blood pressure, (3) low HDL cholesterol, (4) high triglycerides, or (5) high blood sugar. Lower rates of these conditions are seen with 120–150 minutes (2–2½ hours) a week of at least moderate-intensity aerobic activity. The more exercise, the more the risk is reduced. Regular physical activity also helps control blood glucose levels and can reverse type 2 diabetes and metabolic syndrome.
- *Reduced Cancer Risk.* Regular physical activity reduces risk of cancers as compared with people who do not exercise regularly. Physically active people have a lower risk of colon cancer. Physically active women have a lower risk of breast cancer. Regular physical activity reduces risk of endometrial and lung cancer and improves quality of life. Cancer survivors who exercise regularly have improved quality of life and physical fitness over those who do not.
- *Strengthen Bones and Muscles.* Bones and joints, as well as muscles, change with activity level and age. They also need more protection with age. Physical activity strengthens them, which protects bones and joints. Strong and healthy bones, joints, and muscles promote an active lifestyle. Adding a proper diet ensures the necessary micronutrients to maintain bone, joint, and muscle health. Physical activity of at least a moderately intense level slows the loss of bone density that comes with age. Altogether, exercise helps to reduce the risk of

falling in elderly, either due to fewer leg bone fractures or improved muscle strength. Hip fracture is a serious health condition that often negatively affects quality of life, especially for older adults (e.g., climbing stairs, grocery shopping, or playing with the grandchildren). However, 2–5 hours of at least moderate-intensity aerobic activity each week lowers risk of hip fracture.

- Regular physical activity reduces risk of developing, and helps to manage, arthritis and other joint disorders. For arthritis, 2–2½ hours a week of moderate-intensity, low-impact activity improves the ability to manage pain and do everyday tasks and improves quality of life, not just from the pain but also in terms of range of motion [3].
- Muscle-strengthening activities help increase or maintain muscle mass and strength. Gradually increasing the amount of weight and number of repetitions provides even more benefits, including endurance, no matter the age. Regular physical activity helps to return and improve quality of life and reduces morbidity risk (including dizziness and lightheadedness, thereby reducing fall risk) and mortality risk, at any age.
- *Promotes Longevity* (*Promotes Living Longer*). Exercise alone has never been proven to increase longevity. However, by reducing mortality risk, increasing the antioxidant milieu, boosting immune activity, reducing stress (including pain), and maintaining nervous system and cardiovascular health (establishing and maintaining P&S balance and mitochondrial health in support of wellness), a patient's natural longevity is promoted or preserved. Only a few lifestyle choices have as large an impact on health as physical activity. People who are physically active for about 7 hours a week have a 40% lower risk of dying early than those who are active for less than 30 minutes a week; and this activity does not have to be vigorous; moderate-intensity is sufficient. Everyone may gain the health benefits of physical activity. Age, ethnicity, shape, or size does not matter. One hundred and fifty minutes of moderate exercise per week (approximately 21 minutes per day) is routinely advocated for patients.

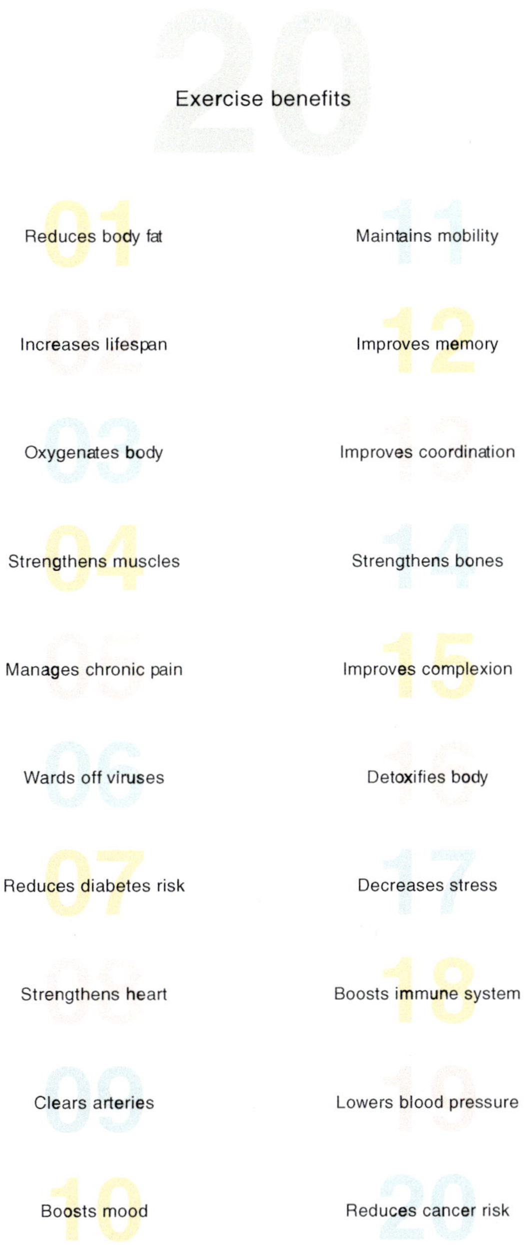


- *Caution*: As always, an exercise regimen should be started under close physician supervision. The wrong types of exercise may do more harm than good, including increasing body fat (and thereby weight), fatigue, and pain due to the fact that the body is programmed to overreact to stresses. Under these conditions, the body sees exercise as stress and works to protect itself against the stress.

With certain diseases (e.g., some arrhythmias, diabetes, stroke or aneurysm risk, or heart disease), the wrong type of exercise may also lead to heart attack, stroke, or sudden death. It is best to start slow and build up and always listen to your body. Until endurance is built, recommended goals may not be reached for a while. This is not bad; keep at it until the goals are reached. The health benefits of physical activity far outweigh the risks of getting hurt.

As with a pure Mediterranean diet, strict compliance with the recommended 150 minutes of exercise per week is not required to get beneficial effects. Smaller amounts of exercise are helpful, just not as much [4].

## Exercise and the Nervous System

The lack of exercise may place a patient on an accelerated track to autonomic neuropathy (see Fig. 7.4). As mentioned in the "Oxidative Stress in Cardiovascular Diseases" section (Chap. 2), the Rostral Ventrolateral Medulla (RVLM) is a brain stem nucleus that receives a wide variety of inputs, including cardiovascular and exercise-related inputs from both central and peripheral sources (see Fig. 7.5). It regulates sympathetic control over baroreceptor reflex and thereby blood pressure and hypertension. The RVLM and its outputs are also effected by exercise; as a result, it mediates the blood pressure effects of exercise and inactivity [6, 7].

The RVLM provides the mechanism whereby physical inactivity independently contributes to the development of cardiovascular diseases and disorders that are becoming epidemic in the United States. The lack of normal, healthy, and regular exercise-related input (e.g., at least 30 minutes of moderate exercise a day) is associated with deleterious changes in the structure and function of RVLM neurons. These changes result in heightened sympathetic outflow and end-organ damage, including the vasculature, nerves, heart, and kidneys [9].

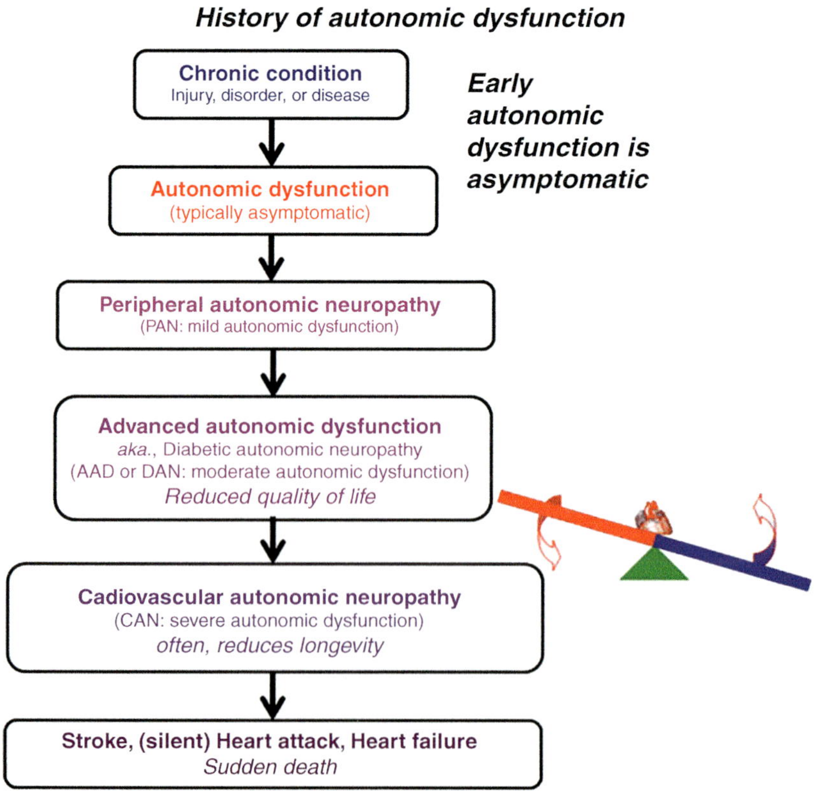


**Fig. 7.4** The history of autonomic dysfunction. Early autonomic dysfunction (characterized as parasympathetic and sympathetic imbalance) may be asymptomatic for years. In many diseases, PAN, AAD or DAN, and early CAN may also be asymptomatic. Autonomic neuropathy is often characterized by sympathetic excess (the red side of the "see-saw" is high relative to the blue, parasympathetic, side). The initial chronic condition may also be due to (hereditary) autonomic dysfunction (imbalance). See text for details [5].

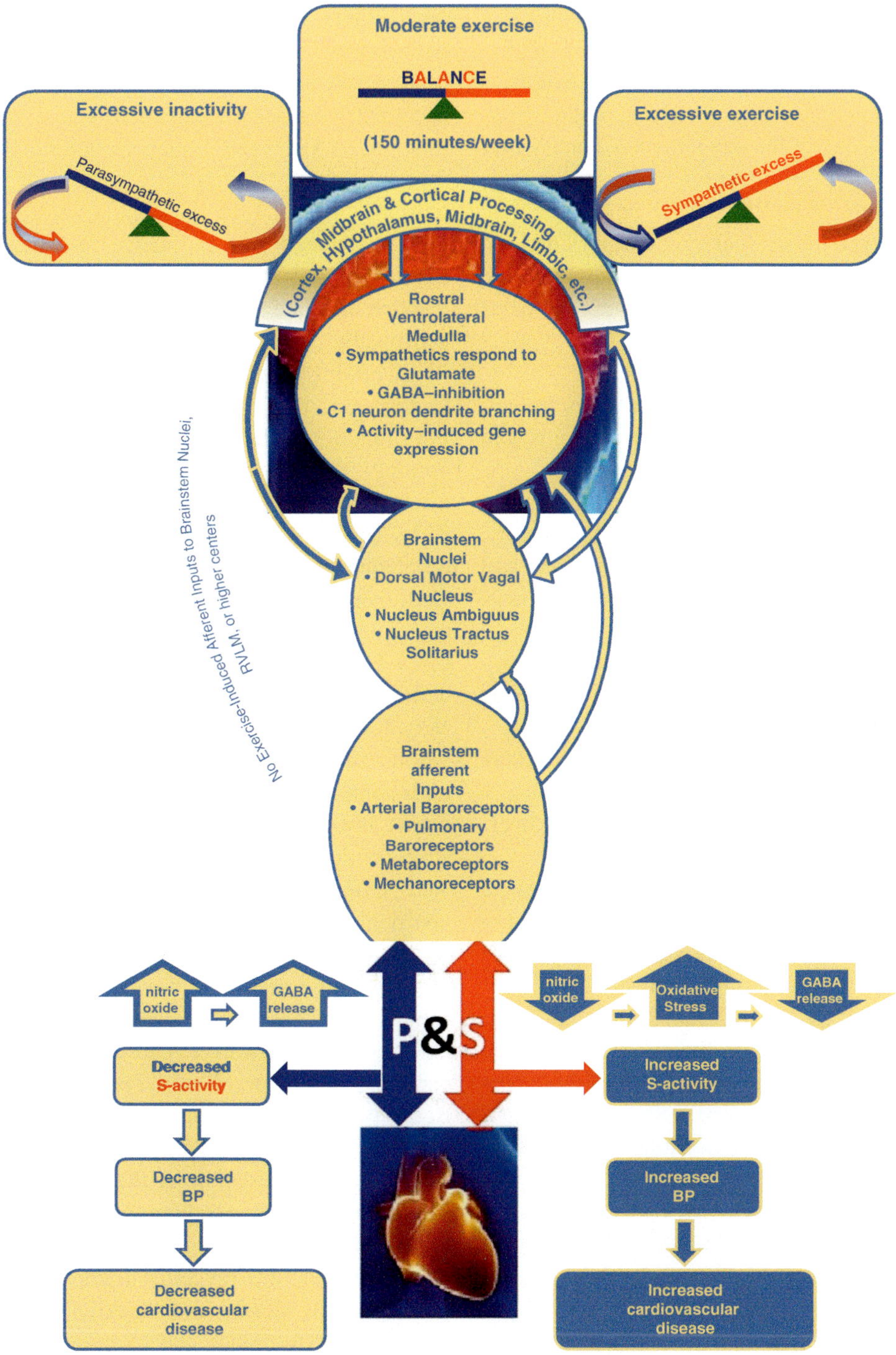


**Fig. 7.5** The effect of chronic exercise and chronic inactivity on the rostral ventrolateral medulla (RVLM), sympathetic nerve activity (SNA), and cardiovascular (CV) disease. The schematic depicts the RVLM as a key brain region in the integration of exercise-related input including peripheral and central afferents. Chronic exercise (*left*, dark arrows) vs. chronic inactivity (*right*, light arrows) produce central nervous system alterations that have opposite effects on BP and CV disease. With chronic inactivity, changes at the level of the RVLM seem to strengthen mechanisms of SNA. Significant neuroplasticity at the level of the RVLM explains exaggerated SNA observed in sedentary humans. Associated nitric oxide involvement is indicated by light arrows (lower left) and dark arrows (lower right), respectively; see also Fig. 5.27 [6]. (Figure modified from [7]. Source: [8])

This problem is not resolved with medication. Half of patients prescribed three or more antihypertensive medications are still hypertensive [10]. There is no magic pill that can replace exercise. This is one of the dangers of sedentary lifestyle, including eliminating recess from grade schools (leading to ADD/ADHD, anxiety/depression, obesity, fatigue, weak immune systems, and even poor grades). High blood pressure and hypertension that results from chronic high BP is a common cause of diseases of the:

- Vasculature – atherosclerosis, arteriosclerosis, aneurysms, and possibly varicose veins and peripheral artery disease
- Nervous system, including the brain – tension headaches, some types of migraines, anxiety, sleep apnea and other sleep disorders, and P&S dysfunction leading to autonomic neuropathy, cognitive difficulties, "brain fog," attention disorders, stroke, and sudden death
- Heart – cardiomyopathy, heart failure, heart attack, and sudden death
- Kidneys – renal hypertension and kidney failure
- Upper and lower GI systems – GERD, diverticulitis, and irritable bowel syndrome
- Other systems – diabetes, insulin resistance, metabolic syndromes, retinal damage, skin and complexion disorders, obesity, some types of cancers, and possibly sex dysfunction

Prolonged periods of inactivity (even with 20 minutes of moderate exercise in a day) promote sympathetic excess (SE). SE promotes high BP and insulin resistance, leading to fat buildup, oxidative stress, and inflammation. Inactivity, thereby, causes the above cascade of diseases, many of which have compounding effects on the others. Too much sitting significantly increases morbidity and mortality risk and accelerates aging and death. (There is a reason why hypertension is called the "silent killer," and "Sitting is the new Smoking.") Persistent SE increases baroreceptor reflex, which increases BP, which causes hypertension. SE with Hypertension accelerates the onset of the above diseases. SE also accelerates the onset of P&S dysfunction. Even as the sympathetics decline, they typically remain stronger than the parasympathetics, resulting in high sympathovagal balance (SB). High SB accelerates the onset of advanced autonomic dysfunction (AAD, which is diabetic autonomic neuropathy, if in a diabetic), which increases morbidity risk and the presentation of the symptoms associated with the above cascade of diseases (Fig. 7.4).

Note how late in the progression of autonomic neuropathy do symptoms present (see Fig. 7.6). At this point in time, in the progression of P&S (autonomic) decline, up to 80% of a patient's P&S function is lost; and the decline *was asymptomatic*! This is why a habit of regular (at least moderate) exercise is necessary, starting from an early age [5]. Ultimately, high SB and high BP accelerate the onset of the final stage of aging: Cardiovascular Autonomic Neuropathy (CAN) and its associated mortality risk (see Fig. 7.6). CAN is end-stage autonomic neuropathy. It is defined as very low parasympathetic activity. Very low parasympathetic activity is very dangerous (remember the sympathetics are typically high compared with the parasympathetics at this point). It means that the parasympathetics are not strong enough to prevent a sympathetically mediated ventricular tachy-rhythm from becoming ventricular fibrillation and sudden death [5].

A habit of healthy and regular exercise (started at an early age, see Fig. 7.7) will prevent many of the diseases that have become epidemic in the United States. However, exercise alone is not enough. Remember, all of the parts of the Mind-Body Wellness Program are needed and work together. As mentioned in the last chapter, diet affects exercise. To optimize the efficacy of exercise, consume low-glycemic foods before and during exercise and high-glycemic food soon after exercise. Low-glycemic foods will release glucose more slowly and steadily, which will maximize performance and increase endurance. High-glycemic foods will cause a more rapid rise in blood glucose levels, helping energy recovery and speed post-exercise recovery [11].

The following foods have a low-glycemic index, less than 55: 100% stone-ground whole wheat or pumpernickel bread; oatmeal (rolled or

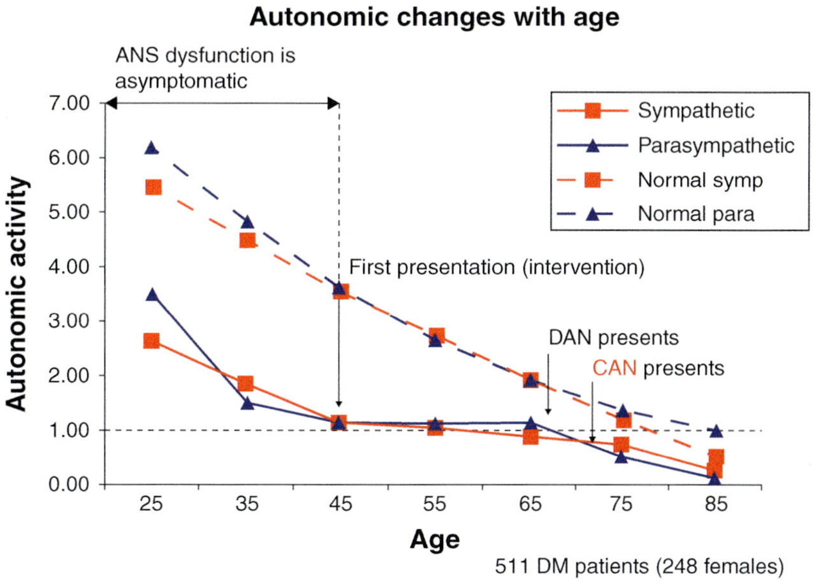


**Fig. 7.6** Age-matched comparison between normal subjects' (broken lines) and patients' (solid lines) resting P&S (blue and red, respectively) responses. Chronic disease accelerates P&S decline and predisposes sympathetic excess. (Republished with permission from Springer. Source: [5, Fig. 12.2])

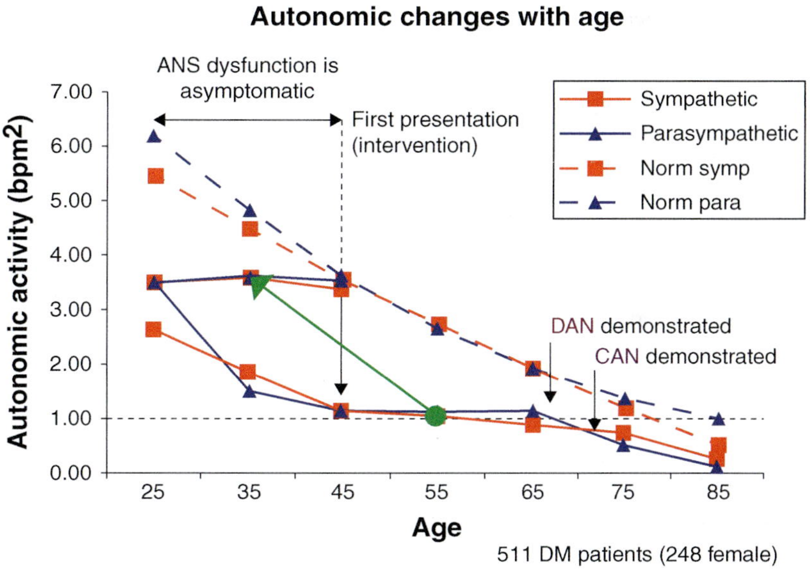


**Fig. 7.7** The flat portions of the patients' P&S curves in Fig7.6 are the responses to the patients complying with therapy, including exercise and other lifestyle modifications. As shown here, with early intervention, the "flat portion" can be realized earlier in life, returning patients to the normal subjects' path, preserving quality of life and minimizing morbidity and mortality risk. (Republished with permission from Springer. Source: [5, Fig. 12.3])

steel-cut), oat bran, muesli, and quinoa; pasta, converted rice, barley, and bulgur wheat; sweet potato, corn, yam, lima/butter beans, peas, legumes, lentils, and chickpeas; skim milk and reduced-fat yogurt; and most fruits, non-starchy vegetables, and carrots. Foods with a high-glycemic index, greater than 70, include sugar; flour; rice; white potatoes; some fruits, including bananas, grapes, cherries, and watermelon; raisins; many breakfast cereals, including puffed rice and corn flakes; bread; soda; and cookies and crackers (see also "The Mediterranean Diet: What To Expect").

## Antioxidant Effects

As mentioned above, the Steno-2 Trial lifestyle changes (diet, physical exercise, and smoking cessation) have been shown to have a beneficial impact on the prevention, and progression, of CAN. Exercise is well known to have, perhaps, the greatest antioxidant effects. The benefit of lifestyle change was confirmed in the Diabetes Prevention Program: lifestyle modification demonstrated superior results in the improvement of autonomic dysfunction (assessed with HRV and QT indexes) as compared to the use of metformin or placebo [12]. Weight loss and dietary intervention accompanied, [13] or not [14], by supervised training was associated with improvement on CAN indices. Aerobic training has also been shown to improve CAN, with some indication that mild physical exercise is recommended in less severe CAN cases. A recent review summarizing the evidence for the impact of lifestyle interventions on CAN has concluded that moderate endurance and aerobic exercise in both type 1 and type 2 diabetes mellitus improve HRV and cardiac autonomic function significantly, in favor of parasympathetic dominance, independent of BMI, glycemic or BP control, and duration of diabetes [15].

Exercise improves blood flow and nerve function and reduces atherosclerosis. Exercise promotes antioxidant activities [16], including the scavenging of ROS, thereby preventing the conversion of nitric oxide to peroxynitrite which increases nitric oxide levels, which inhibits LDL oxidation and leukocyte adhesion. In this way, it may augment statins as measured by improved flow-mediated brachial artery dilation greater than with statins alone [17]. Overall, it is all about balance. Antioxidant-oxidant balance is a dynamic balance established under conditions of homoeostasis between free radicals that are created (e.g., by exercise) and those consumed (scavenged) [18, 19]. This definition concerns cells, body fluids, and organs or organ systems. Antioxidant balance may be permanently affected by dynamic changes due to physiological (physical exercise) or pathological factors (illness, presence of xenobiotics, or UV radiation) [18].

Physical exercise of great intensity (that which is too strenuous as compared to the individual's level of conditioning) involves muscle damage, which in part is caused by free radicals that contribute to a more intensive lipid peroxidation [20]. Exercise-induced oxidative damage depends on exercise intensity and duration [21, 22]. In the active muscle, oxidative stress is generated when aerobic metabolism is increased due to the production of ROS and reactive nitrogen species [18, 23].

As stated above, an important factor which perturbs antioxidant balance is an increased core body temperature [24]. Physical exercise performed in the aerobic environment leads to considerable dehydration [25] and oxidative stress [26]. Both factors negatively impact the exercise efficiency. Both passive and active overheating of core body temperature disturbs antioxidant balance to oxidation [24]. If exercise is excessive, or too stressful, then the antioxidant balance shifts to oxidation. Initially, athletes have higher antioxidant level and lower plasma peroxidation level compared to untrained men. With exercise, the untrained also acquire higher antioxidant levels, in a dose-dependent fashion. Once trained, athletes and the newly trained demonstrate higher antioxidant balance than those who did not exercise. Oxidative stress differs depending on the environment. For example, thermal stress: physical exercise at elevated ambient temperature caused lower antioxidant levels compared to sauna bathing, which caused higher levels of antioxidants.

Yoga (Fig. 7.8) seems to increase heart rate variability, a measure of vagus nerve tone [27] (more variability indicates more parasympathetic activity). The vagus nerve plays an important role in all aspects of health. Yoga can stimulate the vagus nerve by movement, chanting, and breathing exercises. Vagus nerve stimulation increases gamma-aminobutyric acid (GABA) inside the brain and the rest of the parasympathetic nervous system. GABA is the main inhibitory neurotransmitter in the brain, reducing neuronal excitability throughout the central nervous system. It is specifically associated with neuronal circuits that control fear and anxiety which results from over-excitation of these central nerves. Less stress helps dilate blood vessels and improves blood flow and endothelial function, reducing hypertension and risk for atherosclerosis and cardiovascular disease. Outside the central nervous system, the parasympathetic nervous system control of the immune system includes antioxidant effects.

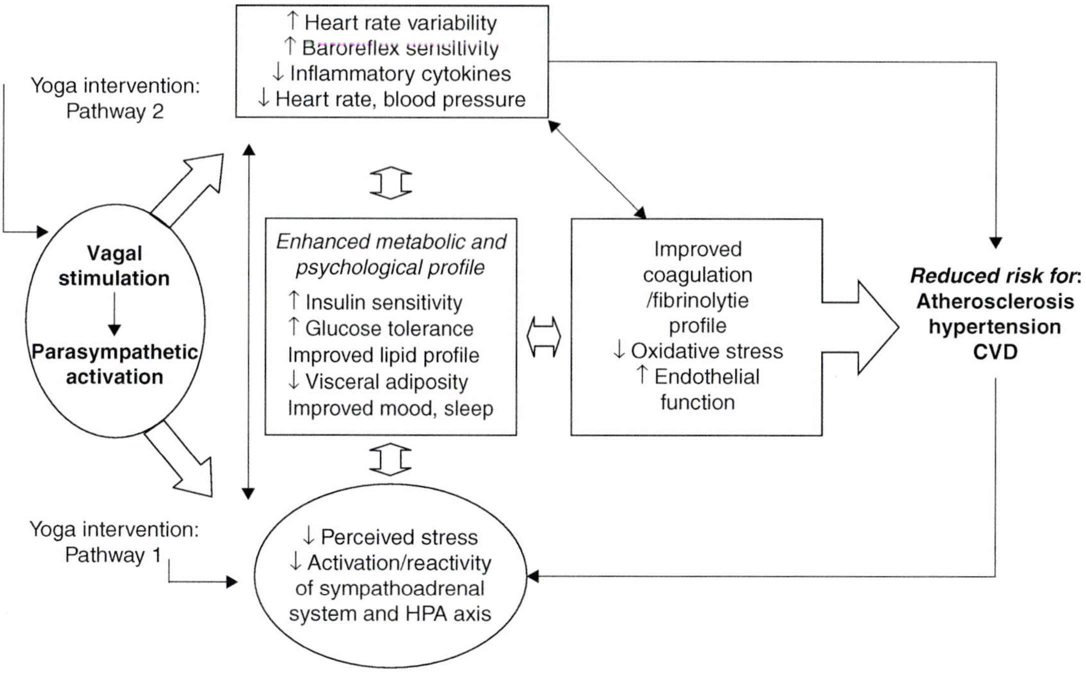


**Fig. 7.8** Pathways by which yoga may decrease cardiovascular risk. (Open Access, Wolters Kluwer Health, IJPM. Source: [27] and https://selfhacked.com/blog/health-benefits-yoga/)

## Exercise and Endothelial Function

Mitochondria are benefitted by regular physical exercise through nitric oxide antioxidation. Mitochondrial biogenesis and gene expression improves with exercise, increasing mitochondrial size and number. The expression of endothelial NOS and other molecular mediators increases, which increases nitric oxide levels (Fig. 7.9). Another major mediator is heat shock proteins (HSP, Figs. 4.30 and 4.31). HSP causes proper folding and configuration of proteins and transports proteins across membranes. It helps refold proteins damaged in response to stress, not just heat stress but cold exposure, UV light stress, hypoxia, toxins, infection, and inflammation.

Exercise training increases vascular sheer stress, which exerts its beneficial effects on endothelial function by activation of several signal transduction pathways [29]. HSPs are present in mast cells, including endothelial cells, and play an important role in cellular homeostasis and cell protection from damage in response to stress stimuli [30]. Exercise is a physiological stimulus factor of HSP [30–32].

The number of blood vessels (via Vascular Endothelial Growth Factor (VEGF, Fig. 4.17) induced angiogenesis) and the volumes of the vessels increase in muscles with exercise, which also increases endothelial volume, which also increases nitrous oxide levels. As a result, exercise augments blood flow and laminar sheer stress, which helps to prevent, and reduce, atherosclerosis. Exercise training increases capillary density and the capillary-to-fiber ratio in skeletal muscles [33]. Various angiogenetic factors, such as VEGF and Fibroblast Growth Factor (FGF), which play an important role in angiogenesis, are catalyzed by exercise [34].

Regular physical exercise decreases nitric oxide inactivation by augmenting the antioxidant system, by promoting superoxide dismutase (SOD) and glutathione peroxidase (GPs), and by attenuating nicotinamide adenine dinucleotide phosphate (NADH/NADPH) oxidase activity (see Fig. 4.28), all leading to an increase in nitric

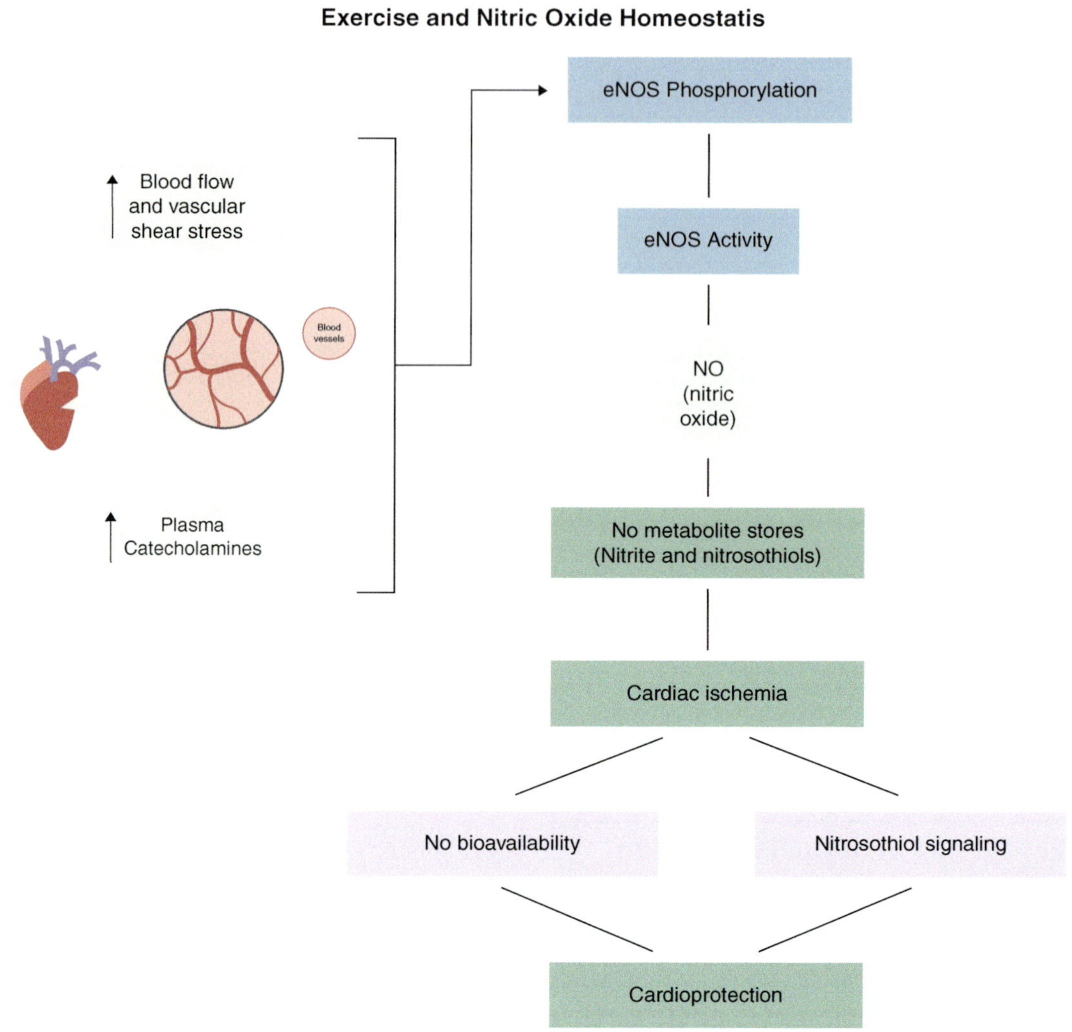


**Fig. 7.9** Schematic diagram highlighting the effects of exercise on nitric oxide homeostasis. Abbreviations: NO, nitric oxide; eNOS, endothelial NO synthase. See text for details. (Illustration by Elysian Creative Studio, www.elysiancreativestudio.com, Lizzy Colombo. Source: [28])

oxide levels throughout the body [35–38]. Long-term exercise significantly reduces plasma Norepinephrine concentrations in patients with hypertension [29]. This reduction plays an important role in the protection of the endothelium, leading to augmented Acetylcholine-stimulated nitric oxide release in hypertensive patients. In other words, regular exercise augments endothelial function through a decrease in vasoconstrictors. (Acetylcholine is the parasympathetic neurotransmitter, working in opposition to the sympathetic system, helping to lower the stress response from the sympathetic system.) Exercise causes healthy levels of blood pressure, lipid metabolism, glucose metabolism, body weight, vascular shear stress, neurohormonal release, and antioxidant balance [39–42]. It upregulates the immune system, including pathways that promote anti-inflammatory action. All this slows the progression of autonomic neuropathy, which reduces morbidity and mortality risk, including cardiovascular mortality [43].

Other endothelium-dependent vasodilators, such as prostaglandins and endothelium-derived hyperpolarizing factor (EDHF), also contribute to exercise-induced vasodilation [44]. Both angiotensin-type antihypertensives (ACE-Is and ARBs) exert a positive effect on vascular endothelial function independent of their antihypertensive effects [45]. ARBs protect endothelium by reduction of the activity of the nitric oxide antagonist Endothelin-1 [46]. Statin therapy improves prognosis in patients at risk for cardiovascular disease [47]. Statins upregulate activation of eNOS and thus improve endothelial cell function [48]. Exercise augments statins activity.

The generated nitric oxide can either be used immediately to induce vasodilatation in an effort to match blood flow to metabolic demands or be metabolized into nitrite and nitrosothiols (Fig. 7.9). This conceivably would continue with each passing exercise period, resulting in elevated steady-state levels of the metabolites in the heart. Increasing these stores before myocardial ischemia is important because nitric oxide bioavailability is dampened during ischemia. Therefore, the stored nitrite can be reduced to nitric oxide during myocardial ischemia by either acid reduction or by any of the identified nitrite reductases. Additionally, nitrosothiols can act to protect proteins during the early oxidative burst of reperfusion and then act as a redox-sensitive nitric oxide donor later. The increased nitric oxide from either nitrite or nitrosothiols can then protect the heart against ischemic injury by any of its known cardio-protection actions [28].

Activation of the $\beta_1$-adrenergic receptor ($\beta_1$-AR) results in increased heart rate, cardiac stroke work, and cardiac output to meet the demands placed on the heart during strenuous exercise (Fig. 7.10). Furthermore, during exercise, sympathetic stimulation via the $\beta_3$-adrenergic receptor ($\beta_3$-AR), and perhaps the $\beta_2$-adrenergic receptor ($\beta_2$-AR), leads to the activation of eNOS, resulting in an increase in the production of nitric oxide. One of the primary mechanisms related to activation of eNOS is its concomitant phosphorylation. Together, this results in robust activation of eNOS with increased generation of nitric oxide. The increase in nitric oxide can then again protect the heart against ischemic injury [28].

The benefit of regular exercise depends on the type and intensity of the exercise. Daily exercise such as walking, jogging, yoga, cycling, or swimming lowers blood pressure and offers the rest of the benefits listed above. As introduced above, exercise that is too strenuous for the individual's conditioning increases oxidative metabolism and produces a prooxidant environment. Regular moderate exercise (that is not too strenuous compared to the individual's conditioning) promotes an antioxidant state and preserves endothelial function. It is clinically important to select the appropriate intensity, duration, frequency, and kind of exercise. As always, new exercise regimens should be started under close physician supervision [49, 50]. Thus exercise may have a beneficial effect on the progression of P&S dysfunction and the development of cardiovascular disease through preserving endothelial function [43]. In fact, it may also be preventative if started early enough, before the onset of P&S dysfunction (which can start as early as the second decade of life) [5].

## Exercise and Physical Activity

As mentioned above, "exercise" is not a dirty word! Think of exercise or physical activity as in the time before automobiles, elevators, television remotes, and cell phones. As with the Mediterranean diet, physical activity was simply part of life. Even riding a horse requires a greater energy level than at rest. Many of the diseases that are "epidemic" in the world were only found in the wealthy and ruling class, those who could afford carriages to ride in and servants to do their "leg-work." The "upper class" stopped their physical exertion, changed their diets, and, under the delusion of "refinement" and "propriety," adopted much more stressful lifestyles. In fact, obesity was a sign of status. Only those who could afford it were obese. Today, most of society is based on the automobile. In fact, the newer cities are designed to sprawl to enable the automobile. The older cities, built before the automobile, were designed so that the residents could reach their common destinations (grocery, butcher,

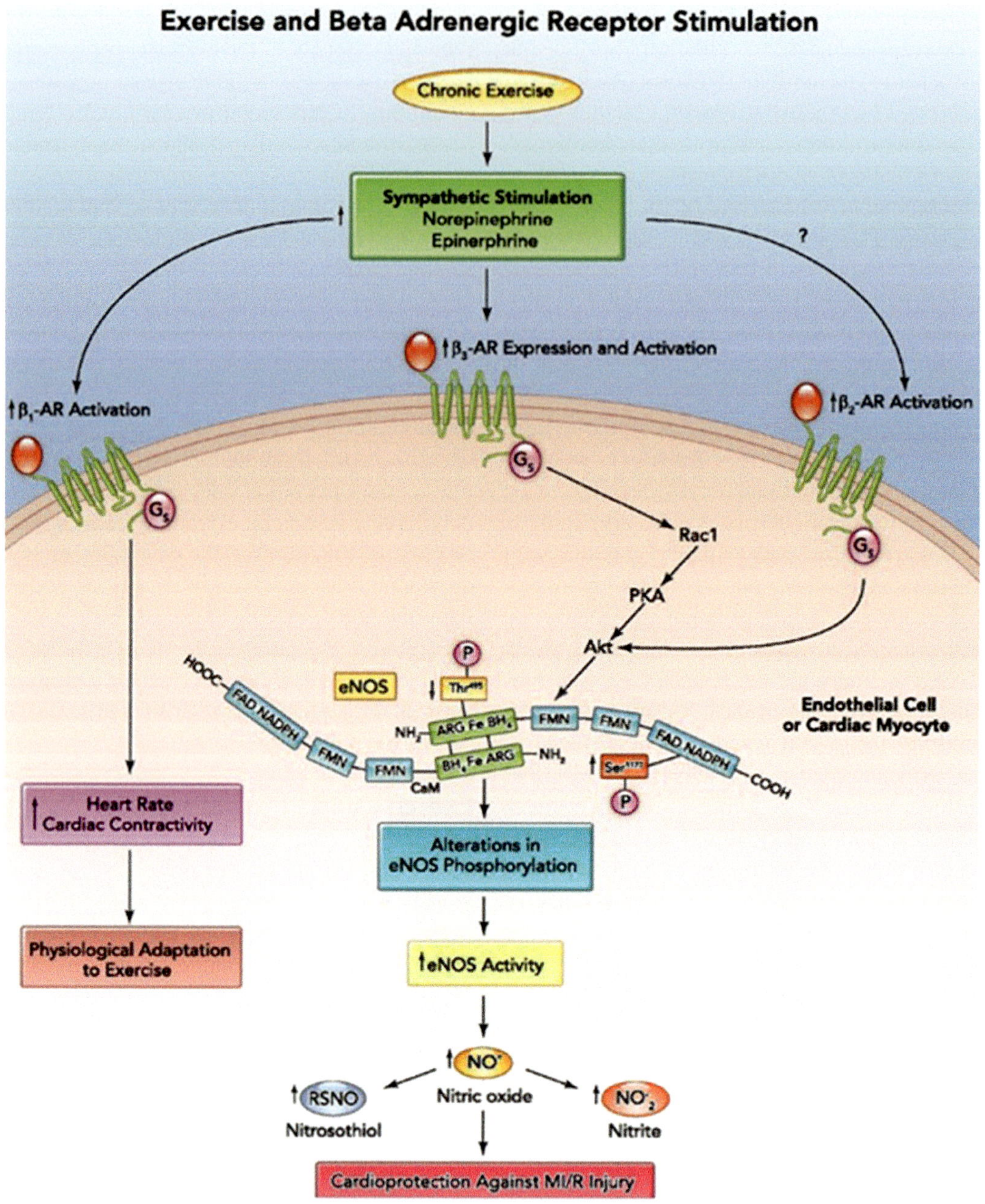


**Fig. 7.10** Schematic diagram highlighting the activation of eNOS via β-adrenergic receptor stimulation. See text for details. (Republished with permission from The American Physiological Society. Source: [28, Fig. 2]. Insert: Open Access; Elsevier, Cell Metabolism)

church, physician, etc.), in a reasonable amount of time, by walking.

An active lifestyle (which involves physical activity) may be just as healthful as more modern lifestyles that include (planned) exercise. Exercise sessions are usually planned out and structured with a goal to improve and maintain physical fitness. It usually, but not always, involves voluntary muscle movement. Physical activity is activity where the goal is different from exercise but also requires expending energy and often provides health benefits. If one walks from the parking lot to the job site, that is physical activity. But if one goes to a park or track and walks around at a predetermined heart rate or time schedule, this is more consistent with exercise. Therefore, exercise is a type of physical activity which has a more specific goal or focus.

Exercise can be aerobic or anaerobic. It can also be continuous, dynamic, rhythmical, static, or a resistance exercise. Oftentimes, it is a combination of different modalities and involves muscle action. Exercise intensity and exercise duration are important variables. Oftentimes, a physician or an exercise trainer, depending on the patient's level of fitness and health, will prescribe a program. When individuals have certain physical restrictions, oftentimes, they may need to be monitored more carefully. For example, cardiac patients, post-heart attack, are often monitored in a cardiac rehabilitation program with a monitor while exercising 3 times a week for 12 weeks as prescribed by their cardiologist and supervised by trained nurses. Healthy individuals are recommended to partake in 150 minutes per week of moderate activity or exercise, cumulative. Young adults and adolescence may require up to 60 minutes a day; children even more for healthy development of muscles and bones. Individuals with chronic illnesses who are restricted may only be able to do a certain amount and not reach these duration goals.

The common goal of exercise is to maintain or lose weight and strengthen the functional capacity of the heart and lungs. In most people, exercise makes the heart function more efficiently.[1] Increasing heart and lung capacity is well known to decrease the risk of heart disease [51–55] and is now also associated with reduced risk of dementia, including Alzheimer's disease [56–59]. For example, patients with myocardial infarction, heart failure, valve replacement, hypertension, pulmonary hypertension, COPD, and of course diabetes can increase their oxygen consumption with exercise. It causes a reduction in heart rate and blood pressure and improvement in blood lipid profile and sense of well-being. By reducing heart rate at rest and submaximal workloads, exercise can protect against cardiac arrhythmias.

People with valvular heart disease can improve the working capacity of their skeletal muscles and be able to perform daily activities better with an exercise program. Even chronic heart failure can improve, with improvement of skeletal muscle metabolism and distribution of blood throughout the body to various tissues. Individuals with peripheral vascular disease with claudication and inability to walk far can begin increasing their exercise duration and distance. Exercise has been shown to be an effective treatment in hypertension and reducing the rise in blood pressure over time and reduces both the resting systolic and diastolic blood pressure.

Exercise can also improve bone health and increase bone mineral density [60–62]. In individuals with arthritis, it improves fitness, decreases joint swelling and pain, and can improve osteoporosis and slow down the age-related decrease in bone mass [63, 64]. In various neurodegenerative diseases, exercise increases strength and functional capacity and can improve physical fitness and functional performance in these individuals [56]. Exercise has been shown to be important in reducing emotional outbursts, creates a sense of well-being, and can alleviate depression and anxiety symptoms [65–68]. In individuals who have insomnia or disorders associated with poor sleep, exercise can improve sleep quality and energy levels of the individuals [69, 70].

Exercise can prevent premature death and is effective in combatting coronary heart disease [71–77]. Exercise is effective in stroke prevention [78, 79], primarily through reducing high blood pressure and lowering atherosclerotic plaque and blood clots. It also has beneficial effects on lipids, especially high triglycerides and

[1] The most notable exception is hypertrophic cardiomyopathy patients who express the recessive gene, in whom the heart muscle thickens with exercise, reducing stroke volume and ejection fraction, leading to heart attack or sudden death. Normally, the heart muscle does not thicken with exercise or stress, like skeletal muscles, but still gets stronger.

low HDL [80–82]. Exercise is important in treatment of type 2 diabetes and metabolic syndrome and preventing worsening or even emergence of these syndromes [70, 80, 83–85]. Exercise has been shown to have health benefits in colon cancer [86, 87], breast cancer in women [88, 89], and prostate cancer in men [90]. Exercise can also prevent weight gain and may affect weight loss, especially when combined with reduced calorie diets. Importantly, because of its favorable effects on bone structure, it can prevent falls, especially in geriatric patients [91–93]. Including the effects of exercise on depression and anxiety and related disorders by improving aerobic fitness and muscle strength in general, exercise improves one's ability to function on a daily basis.

Exercise has also been shown to improve the immune system [94–96], including autonomic regulation of the immune system [97]. Moderate aerobic exercise has been shown to increase the number, and activity, of white blood cells, such as neutrophils, which protect against bacterial infections [98, 99]. Exercise increases phagocytic activity and secretion of cytokines which fight infection and inflammation and are secreted by macrophages in the body [100]. Exercise can increase the number of B and T cells, which are immune-regulating cells in the body [101]. Natural killer cells and macrophages are important cells in the immune system's defense against the spread of malignancies. Moderate exercise can increase the activity of natural killer cells as well as increase macrophage activity [102].

In association with leisure time, physical activity was associated with a lower risk of 13 cancers, including esophageal, lung, kidney, gastric cardiac, endometrial, myeloid leukemia, myeloma, colon, rectal, bladder, and breast [103]. Interestingly, alone leisure time activity is associated with higher risk of malignant melanoma and prostate cancer. Smoking is shown to modify the association of lung cancer but no other smoking-related cancers. Lifestyle factors are important for cancer development, and a substantial cancer burden may be prevented through lifestyle modifications which include 75 rigorous intensity or 150 minutes of moderate-intensity exercise per week [104] among other lifestyle changes such as no smoking, moderate alcohol drinking, or an ideal weight with BMI of 18.5–27.5 [105].

Studies state that moderate activities are comparable to walking briskly, for women as well as men, and across many disease states [106, 107]. The Surgeon General with the National Institutes of Health [108], the American Heart Association [109], a joint Centers for Disease Control and Prevention, and American College of Sports Medicine consensus [110, 111] all agreed that the benefits of moderate exercise generally occur by engaging in at least 30 minutes of modest activity on most, preferably all, days of the week. Walking briskly was defined as a pace that is about 3–4 miles per hour for about 30 minutes. "Activities" can include any other form of occupational or recreational activity that is dynamic in nature and of similar intensity, such as yard work, household tasks, cycling, and swimming. This amount of exercise equates to approximately five to seven 30-minute sessions per week at an intensity equivalent to 3–6 times the resting metabolic rate (approximately 70 calories per hour), or approximately 600–1200 calories expended per week [112]. The Surgeon General and organizations listed above all corroborate that the benefits on cardiovascular risk factors are:

- Increase in exercise tolerance
- Reduction in body weight
- Reduction in blood pressure
- Reduction in bad (LDL and total) cholesterol
- Increase in good (HDL) cholesterol
- Increase in insulin sensitivity

They all agree that there are a number of physiological benefits of exercise. The two examples they offer are (1) improvements in muscular function and strength and (2) improvement in the body's ability to take in and use oxygen (maximal oxygen consumption or aerobic capacity). As the ability to transport and use oxygen improves, regular daily activities can be performed with less fatigue. This is particularly important for patients with cardiovascular and pulmonary disease, whose exercise capacity is typically lower than that of healthy individuals. There is also evidence that exercise training improves the capacity of the blood vessels to dilate in response to exercise or hormones, consistent with better vascular wall function and an improved ability to provide oxygen to the muscles during exercise. Studies measuring muscular strength and flexibility before and after exercise programs suggest that there are improvements in nerve (brain) and bone health and ability to perform daily activities, as well as a lower likelihood of developing back pain and of disability, particularly in older age groups.

The Surgeon General and organizations listed above all state that every American adult should participate in 30 minutes or more of moderate-intensity activity on most and probably all days of the week. This includes taking the stairs instead of elevators, doing house work or gardening, even a half hour or more a day on your feet cooking meals for your family, and other activities that are considered part of an active lifestyle, not just what is typically considered exercise. During exercise, it is true there is a transient risk of having heart-related complications such as a heart attack or cardiac arrhythmia. Patients should always get clearance from a physician before undertaking any exercise. Patients should continue to work with a physician to increase exercise levels to reach the moderate levels recommended. In reality, however, the majority of heart attacks, approximately 90%, occur in a resting state and not during physical activity. Initially, it was thought that if over the age of 45 with two more risk factors for heart disease, patients should consult their physician before starting any type of exercise program. As stated above, it is now strongly recommended that all patients should consult with their physicians even in the absence of other risk factors. The issue is that the latest mortality risk measure is cardiovascular autonomic neuropathy (CAN) as documented by P&S monitoring. As demonstrated in the ACCORD study [113, 114], CAN is asymptomatic at first, and the first symptoms may be sudden death. Physicians are able to determine CAN risk and what levels of exercise are beneficial. Depending on medical history (i.e., diabetes, hypertrophic cardiomyopathy, etc.), CAN is possible even before age 45.

To specify the benefits listed above, moderate exercise promotes skeletal muscle hypertrophy and hyperplasia, increases flow through blood vessels, increases insulin sensitivity and mitochondrial biogenesis, and increases adipose "browning" [115]. Exercise can increase cardiac cell growth and can have cardio-protective effects against ischemic injury. It is believed that exercise improves the calcium handling of the myocardium [116].[2] In fact, the genetics underlying calcification of arteries may be reversed with exercise [117]. It has been shown that exercise can increase blood vessel angiogenesis, including in the heart. While thickening of the heart may be pathological or detrimental in conditions like hypertension, there is a beneficial increase in heart muscle growth supporting cardiac remodeling. In individuals who exercise regularly, the heart has considerable plasticity. Exercise training promotes efficient glucose and fatty acid handling and mitochondrial biogenesis.

As one ages, autonomic and mitochondrial dysfunction becomes more evident, and this is linked to many disease processes (including those which include fatigue, including persistent fatigue and chronic fatigue syndrome). Exercise is one of the few proven methods of improving autonomic balance and mitochondrial function and decreasing the burden of autonomic and mitochondria dysfunction which are not healthy. Patients with mitochondrial disorders have a low maximal oxygen uptake, which can lead to exercise intolerance and

[2] The United States, arguably, has the highest incidence of arterial calcification. This is due to ubiquitous pasteurization. Pasteurization, while mainly beneficial, also extracts vitamin K2. Vitamin K2, specifically long-chain vitamin K2, is a cofactor that clears the liver and enters the blood stream with lipoproteins (LDLs, HDLs, and triacylglycerol-rich lipoproteins) where it helps to collect calcium from arteries and other soft tissue and redistribute it to the bones, teeth, and other hard tissue. In western cultures, unpasteurized hard cheeses are the best source of long-chain vitamin K2, but still only provide small amounts. Other unpasteurized dairy products also provide long-chain vitamin K2. Since significant quantities of cheeses are required to provide vitamin K2 benefit, there is a risk of atherosclerosis as well; however, small amounts of red wine (one to two servings) often help to reduce atherosclerotic risk.

fatigue and interfere with daily living activities (quality of life). This interference is compounded by the quality of life deficits associated with autonomic dysfunction, including digestive and sleep disorders, bladder, bowel, and sex dysfunction, dizziness, and high BP.

Resistant exercises can increase strength, and endurance exercise can improve exercise tolerance as well as biochemical enzyme activity [118]. All in all, exercise counteracts (slows) the negative effects of aging. Aging is associated with oxidative stress mainly due to what is termed "leaky mitochondria," where partial reduction of the oxygen in the electron transport chain generates free radicals and ROS (see "The Importance of Antioxidants"). This causes damage of mitochondrial membrane lipids, reducing energy production and adversely affecting P&S nerve function. Electron escape from the mitochondrion is a pathological process and leads to progressive mitochondrial dysfunction and creates a vicious cycle with increasing ROS generation. Exercise has been shown to upregulate mitochondrial NADH cytochrome C reductase and other important enzymes in the electron transport chain, neutralizing excess oxidants. Regular exercise also increases activity of beneficial antioxidant enzymes such as Superoxide Dismutase (SOD) in the brain, enhancing the cellular repair process.

Combining the information from the previous chapters: increasing ROS production occurs in skeletal muscles and other organs such as the heart and brain (nervous system). Aging also reduces protein synthesis which limits antioxidant defenses and repair capabilities. Aging is associated with progressive loss of muscle mass and strength (a condition known as sarcopenia). This increases muscle injury. Injured muscles will release inflammatory molecules. This leads to reduced physical activity and increased adiposity. Increasing fat cell accumulation is a state of low-grade and chronic inflammation, and many inflammatory cytokines such as TNF-α and interleukin 6 (IL-6) are increased and circulate. CRP is increased as well. There are also higher inflammatory cell counts, such as neutrophils and myocytes. An important transcription factor known as nuclear factor kappa B (NF-kB) is also released during oxidative stress.

The good news is that regular exercise interrupts this process and may reverse it, for a time, slowing the aging process. Regular exercise reduces the level of systemic inflammation and markers such as CRP, IL-6, and TNF-α, both in young and old. In the brain, exercise increases the content of Brain Derived Neurotrophic Factor (BDNF) which is very important in higher cognitive function. Reduced systemic inflammation is especially true in exercise associated with weight loss. Again, obesity is associated with chronic inflammation, especially adipose tissue that is visceral fat deposits where macrophages are trapped and significant inflammatory molecules are produced. Exercise induces the release of adiponectin for adipose tissue which exerts an anti-inflammatory and antioxidant effect. Adiponectin is a protein hormone which regulates glucose levels and fatty acid oxidation (breakdown) in adipose tissue. It is inversely related to body mass index. Adiponectin decreases glycogenesis and increases glucose uptake, oxidation of lipids, triglyceride clearance, promotes weight loss, protects against endothelial dysfunction, decreases (TNF-α), and is inversely associated with obesity.

Exercise inhibits the infiltration of macrophages into adipose tissue and switches them from a more inflammatory type to a less inflammatory type. In addition to supporting passive immune responses (e.g., short-term increases in body temperature, simulating fever), exercise also regulates the immune system and activates the adaptive components with suppression of inflammation. This involves regulating T and B cells. By stimulating mitochondrial biogenesis and enhancing mitochondrial oxidative capacity, exercise lessens mitochondrial aging and interrupts the viscous cycle of oxidative damage.

Being sedentary increases risk; it is considered a cardiac risk factor. Individuals who are moderately active with exercise but who sit significant periods of time have more risk than individuals who are moderately active with exercise who do not sit for significant periods of time. Reduced stress, especially decreasing psychosocial stress and chronic mental stress, may be another cardio-protective mechanism of regular exercise. Even in more elderly and frail patients, getting them to walk more each day is recommended. To help them meet the exercise recommendations, it is suggested that they buy a pedometer and track the number of steps that they walk a day. Two thousand steps are equivalent to one mile. The goal is to get as many patients as possible to walk 6000 steps, or 3 miles, a day and to build up to that if need be in a prescription exercise formula.

As stated in Chap. 5, AMP-activated protein kinase (AMPK) improves the health of mitochondria (see insert, right [119]). It is a fuel-sensing enzyme that is present in most all the cells of the body. The AMPK system acts as a sensor of cellular energy status and is conserved in most of the cells of the body. It is activated by an increase in the cellular ratio of the concentrations of AMP to ATP. This ratio is usually altered when metabolic stresses interfere with the production of the energy molecule ATP, especially when there is a shortage of glucose or oxygen. A typical example of this is a lack of blood supply to an organ, which causes ischemia or lack of oxygen. Also, active muscle contraction, especially when vigorous, can accelerate ATP consumption which activates the AMPK system (Fig. 7.11).

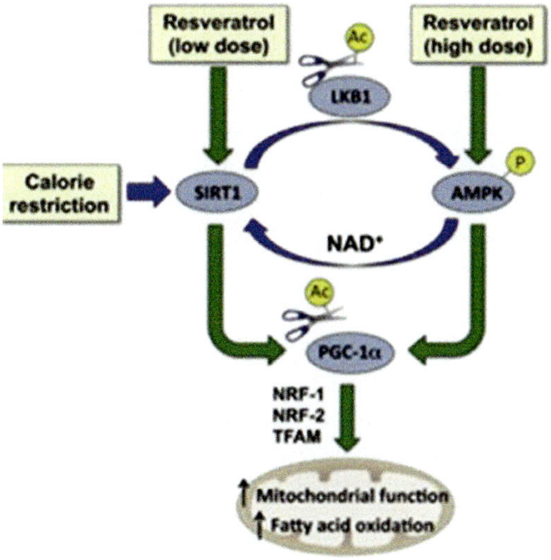


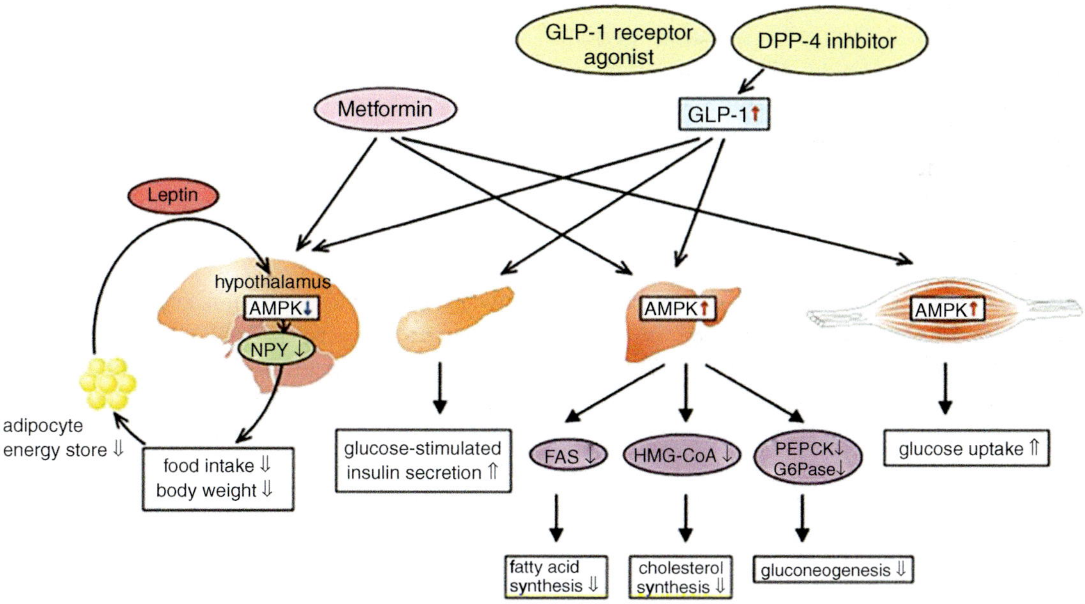


**Fig. 7.11** Metformin and glucagon-like peptide-1 (GLP-1) inhibit adenosine monophosphate-activated protein (AMPK) in the hypothalamus and activate AMPK in peripheral tissues. Hypothalamic AMPK activity is suppressed by leptin. Through metformin, low glucose-induced AMPK phosphorylation is inhibited, and the mRNA expression of neuropeptide Y is suppressed in the hypothalamus. In peripheral tissues, activated AMPK inhibits 3-hydroxy-3-methylglutaryl-coenzyme A and suppresses fatty acid synthase expression, resulting in a decrease in fatty acid and cholesterol synthesis. AMPK also controls hepatic gluconeogenesis by inhibiting phosphoenolpyruvate carboxykinase and glucose-6-phosphatase. Additionally, metformin stimulates AMPK in muscle and induces glucose uptake. (Republished with permission from Wolters Kluwer Health, Medknow. Source: [120])

Because exercise is involved in activating the AMPK enzyme pathway [59], many of the therapeutic benefits of regular physical activity may occur through this pathway, including for specific disease disorders such as metabolic syndrome, type 2 diabetes, and Alzheimer's disease. When AMPK is activated by stresses such as actively contracting muscles in exercise, or a lack of blood supply due to low oxygen, many biochemical reactions occur. These reactions underlie the functions of the mitochondria, the production of blood vessels (angiogenesis), the control of food intake, and whole-body energy as governed by the hypothalamus. AMPK is a key factor in the regulation of the myocardial metabolism in response to ischemia, pressure overload, and heart failure, and regulation of mitochondrial function after ischemia/reperfusion [121].

At the cellular level in the periphery of the body, AMPK activation counteracts the adverse effects of metabolic syndrome, which includes insulin resistance and inflammation from lipid deposits in tissues. AMPK enzyme activation increases fatty acid oxidation and glucose uptake by muscle cells. It (normally) decreases protein synthesis during muscle contraction. Regular exercise decreases inflammation and increases the blood thinning property of the blood stream (aka increased fibrinolytic activity). Long-term exercise training, up to 12 weeks, increases AMPK concentrations and its effects. Inactivity is associated with decreased activation of AMPK-mediated effects [122]. This may be the mechanism behind the link between chronic inactivity and increased risk of type 2 diabetes, coronary heart disease, Alzheimer's disease, and various cancers such as colon and liver cancer.

Metabolic syndrome is a constellation of findings which involves central obesity, especially around the abdomen, high blood sugar, hypertension, and high triglycerides along with low HDL levels. These patients have insulin resistance which is pro-inflammatory. It is also a procoagulant state. With increases in inflammatory markers such as IL-6, (TNF-$\alpha$), and plasminogen-activator inhibitor (PAI), patients with metabolic syndrome have higher risk of atherosclerosis, type 2 diabetes, non-alcoholic fatty liver disease, various cancers, and Alzheimer's or Parkinson's disease. These disorders are not seen as frequently in people who exercise regularly.

Interestingly, treatment with diabetic drugs such as metformin or thiazolidinediones diminishes systemic insulin resistance similar to exercise. These medicines can actually activate the AMPK enzyme system in human muscles (Fig. 7.11) [120]. It is not surprising that a medicine such as metformin has shown decreased incidence of large vessel disease by 39% [123] when used as isolated therapy in type 2 diabetics in the United Kingdom Prospective Diabetes Study (UKPDS) and also a 35% [124] decrease in cancer prevalence in patients treated with metformin for many years. This suggests AMPK may even be a tumor suppressor. This may explain why regular exercise is known to protect against atherosclerosis and various types of cancers, including cancer of the breast, colon, and prostate.

A protein or histone known as SIRT1 (Fig. 7.12) has been linked to longevity when associated with caloric restriction [125]. SIRT1 may function by activating the AMPK enzyme system. Resveratrol (found naturally in grapes, see "Resveratrol" in Mediterranean Diet "(Prong-4)", Chap. 6) activates AMPK [125]. Dietary, behavioral, and pharmacologic inputs converge on cAMP-AMPK-SIRT1 signaling to produce metabolic benefits. Resveratrol inhibits PDEs, leading to increased cAMP levels, Epac1 activation, elevated intracellular calcium, and AMPK activation. Calorie restriction and other behavioral inputs also activate AMPK. Downstream of AMPK, an increase in $NAD^+$ levels leads to SIRT1 activation, which promotes beneficial metabolic changes primarily through deacetylation and activation of PGC-1a. In a parallel pathway, increased cAMP levels activate PKA, which directly phosphorylates and activates SIRT1. SIRT1 activation by either pathway, as well as potential activation of other $NAD^+$-dependent enzymes, can lead to numerous physiologic outputs.

It has been suggested that AMPK activation may be important in the circulatory system by increasing endothelial nitric oxide synthase activity (Fig. 7.13) [126], thereby increasing nitric

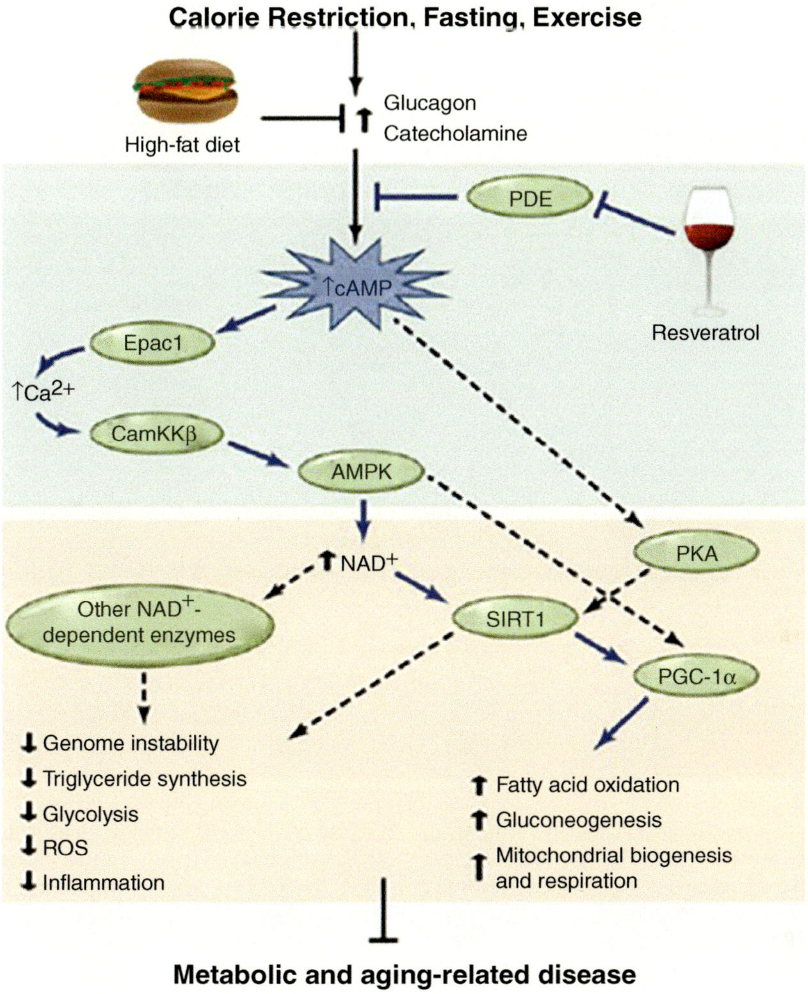


**Fig. 7.12** Dietary, behavioral, and pharmacologic inputs converge on cAMP-AMPK-SIRT1 signaling to produce metabolic benefits. Resveratrol inhibits PDEs, leading to increased cAMP levels, Epac1 activation, elevated intracellular calcium, and AMPK activation. Calorie restriction and other behavioral inputs also activate AMPK. Downstream of AMPK, an increase in $NAD^+$ levels, leads to SIRT1 activation, which promotes beneficial metabolic changes. Blue box (top) highlights current findings; orange box (bottom) highlights pathway components previously identified that reside downstream of the current, as well as some of the reported and theoretical outputs of the signaling pathways detailed above. Blue arrows indicate the current, proposed, linear pathway; dashed lines indicate molecular connections previously reported. Abbreviations: PDE, phosphodiesterase; cAMP, cyclic AMP; Epac1, cAMP-regulated guanine nucleotide exchange factor 1; CamKKb, calcium/calmodulin-dependent kinase kinase beta; AMPK, AMP-activated protein kinase; PKA, protein kinase A; $NAD^+$, nicotinamide adenine dinucleotide; PGC-1a, peroxisome proliferator-activated receptor gamma coactivator-1 alpha; ROS, reactive oxygen species [125]. (Republished with permission from Elsevier)

oxide levels to increase blood flow, especially to tissues deprived of oxygen during exercise. Exercise increases both AMPK and nitric oxide. Increasing AMPK activity has been seen in single bouts of exercise or extended durations of training and appears to enhance mitochondrial capacity and biogenetics. With long-term exercise, AMPK may have a significant role in stimulating new blood vessel growth to provide increased blood supply to trained muscles.

Aging induces endothelial dysfunction by increasing oxidative stress and inflammation.

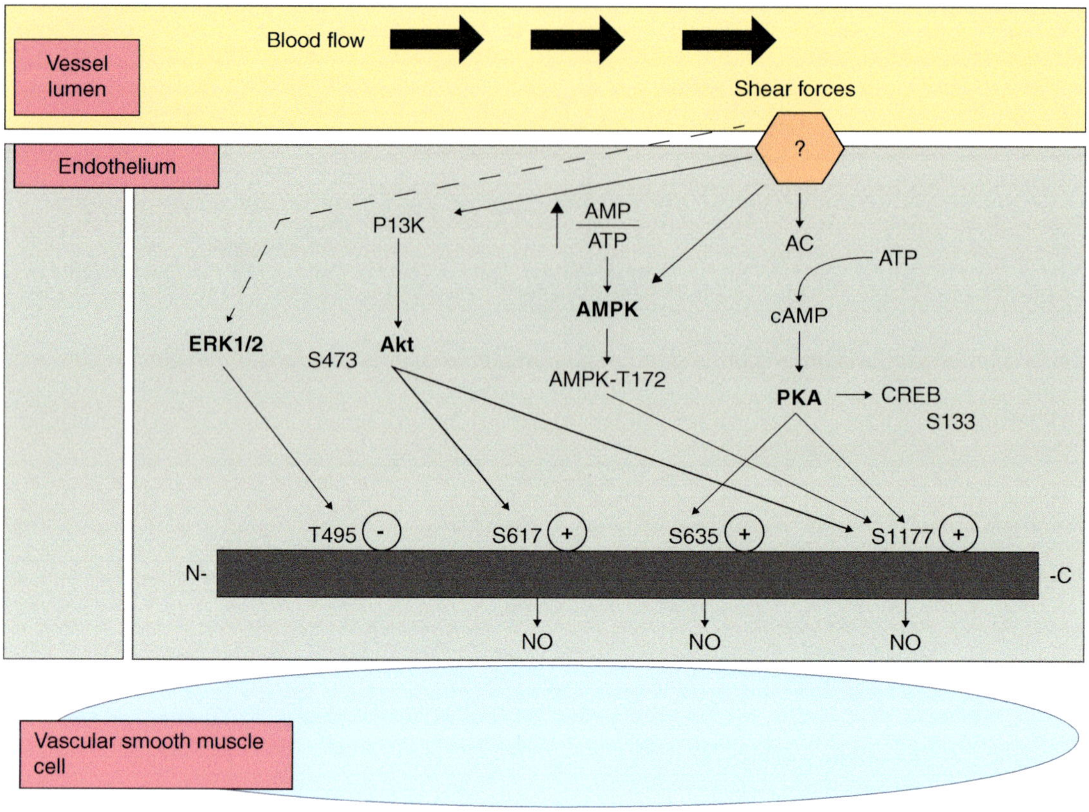


**Fig. 7.13** Proposed regulation of endothelial nitric oxide synthase (eNOS) phosphorylation by Akt, AMPK, PKA, and ERK 1/2 after stimulation of unidentified shear force receptor(s) by exercise-induced increases in blood flow. Abbreviations: (?), unidentified shear force receptor; PI3K, phosphatidyl-inositol-3-kinase; Akt, Akt/protein kinase B; AC, adenylate cyclase; cAMP, cyclic adenosine monophosphate; ATP, adenosine triphosphate; PKA, protein kinase A; AMP, adenosine monophosphate; AMPK, adenosine monophosphate-activated protein kinase; CREB, cyclic AMP response element binding protein; ERK, extracellular signal-regulated kinases 1 and 2; NO, nitric oxide; (+), positive regulatory phosphorylation sites, e.g., serine (S) 617, S635, S1177; (−), negative regulatory phosphorylation site, e.g., threonine (T) 495. Continuous lines/arrows indicate increased activation; dotted line/arrow indicates activation that is dependent upon duration of stimulation. (Republished with permission from John Wiley and Sons. Source: [126])

Excessive superoxide ($O_2^-$) production is one pathway. Superoxide production may be modulated by nicotinamide adenine dinucleotide phosphate (NADPH) oxidase, Superoxide Dismutase (SOD), uncoupling of endothelial nitric oxide synthase (eNOS), and other mechanisms (e.g., dysfunctional mitochondria). Excessive superoxide leads to peroxynitrite formation ($ONOO^-$) and protein oxidation (Nitrotyrosine), as well as activation of nuclear factor-B (NF-κB) and induction of inflammatory cytokines. All of this contributes to cell death and thereby the aging effect. Exercise blocks oxidative stress and inflammation (Fig. 7.14) [127]. For example, aging increases the risk of CVDs (including atherosclerosis) through the development of arterial dysfunction through both endothelial dysfunction and stiffening of arteries (see Fig. 2.28). With exercise as a lifestyle modification, preferably with proper diet stress reduction, age-related arterial dysfunction may be prevented or reversed [128].

Aging induces arterial stiffness, in part, via structural changes to the arterial wall. Oxidative stress and inflammation involving excessive superoxide ($O_2^{-}$) production and inflammatory cytokines mediate increases in collagen deposition,

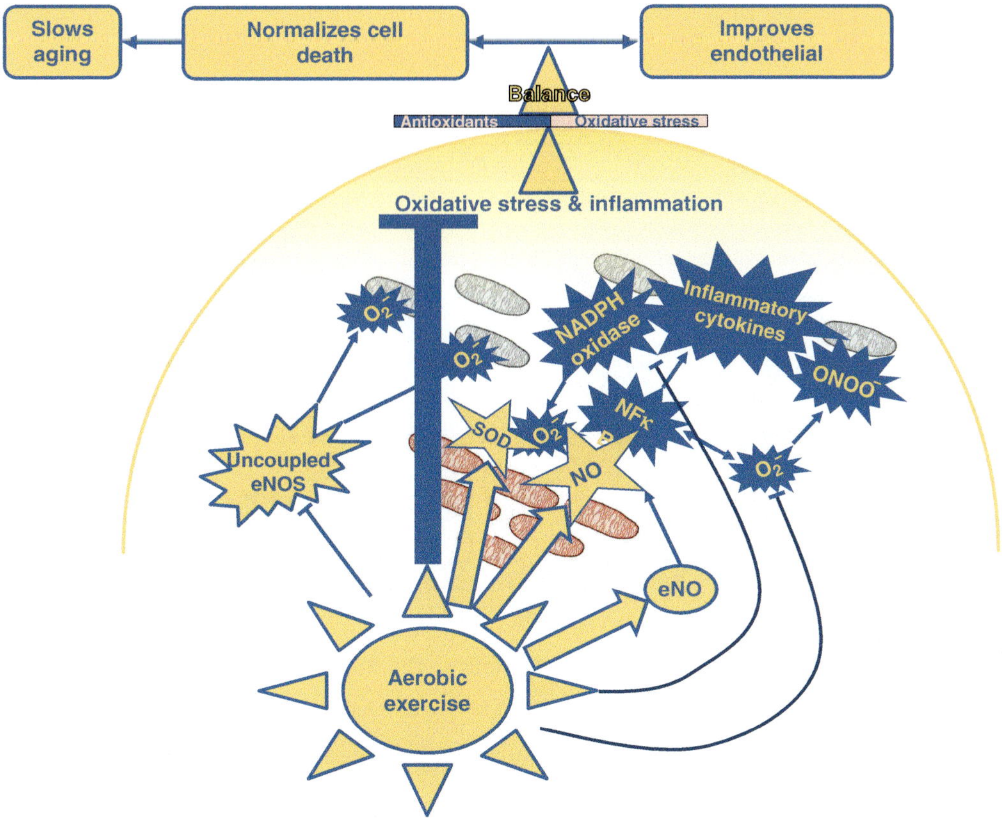


**Fig. 7.14** Effects of aging and exercise on endothelial function [127]. Exercise reduces stress and inflammation [128]. (Figure adapted from [127, Fig. 9])

fragmentation of elastin, protein oxidation (Nitrotyrosine), and formation of Advanced Glycation End Products (AGEs). Exercise inhibits or reverses these age-related changes, resulting in suppression of arterial stiffening (Fig. 7.15) [128].

Aging leads to endothelial dysfunction mediated by vascular oxidative stress and inflammation. Excessive $O_2^-$ production, modulated by NADPH oxidase, SOD, uncoupling of endothelial nitric oxide (NO) synthase (eNOS), and other mechanisms (e.g., dysfunctional mitochondria), is a central mediator of these events. Excessive $O_2^-$ causes peroxynitrite ($ONOO^-$) formation and protein oxidation (Nitrotyrosine), as well as the activation of NF-κB and induction of inflammatory cytokines. Exercise blocks oxidative stress and inflammation, preventing or relieving endothelial dysfunction (Fig. 7.14) [128].

Aerobic exercise protects against arterial dysfunction not only by directly lowering traditional risk factors [e.g., (LDL)] but also by inducing "resistance" against currently existing harmful levels of risk factors (Fig. 7.16) [128].

Exercise and other evidence-based complementary strategies (e.g., healthy dietary intake or nutraceuticals) that induce some of the protective effects of exercise by increasing nitric oxide levels and antioxidant defenses include (1) SOD, (2) lowering $O_2^-$ production, e.g., by inhibiting NADPH oxidase, (3) and reducing inflammation, i.e., by activating NF-κB and inflammatory cytokines, serve to preserve vascular function with aging (Fig. 7.17) [128].

In summary, much of the beneficial effects of exercise may be mediated through the AMPK system, which acts as a "sensory receptor" of cellular energy status. Long-term benefit from activating this system with habitual exercise may result in better insulin sensitivity, fluidity of the vascular system, and decrease in inflam-

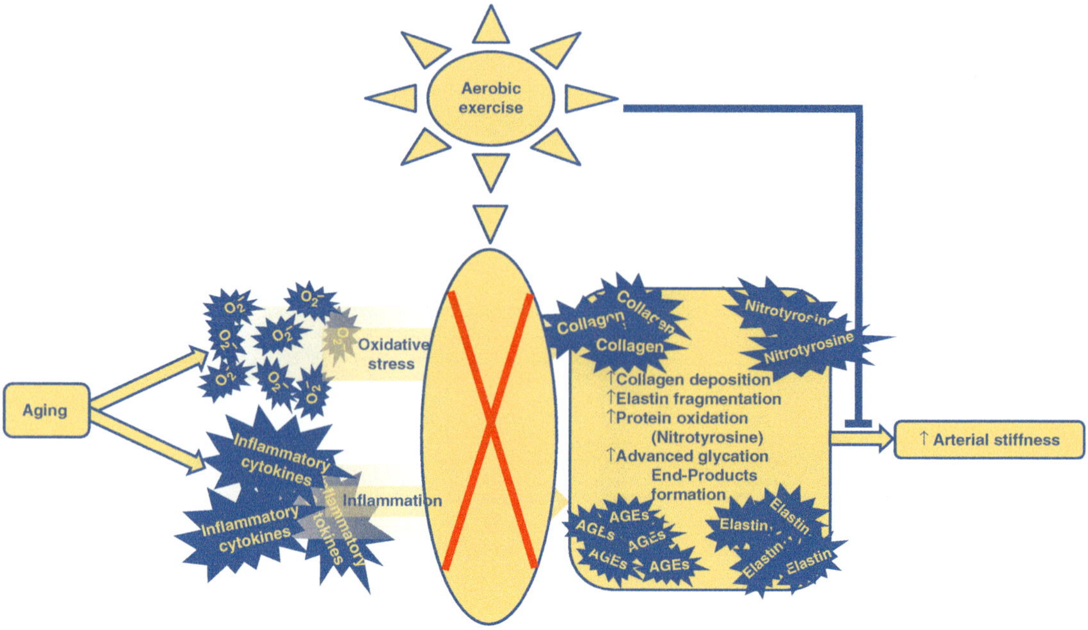


**Fig. 7.15** Effects of aging and aerobic exercise on arterial stiffness. Exercise reduces stress and inflammation. (Adapted from [128, Fig. 3])

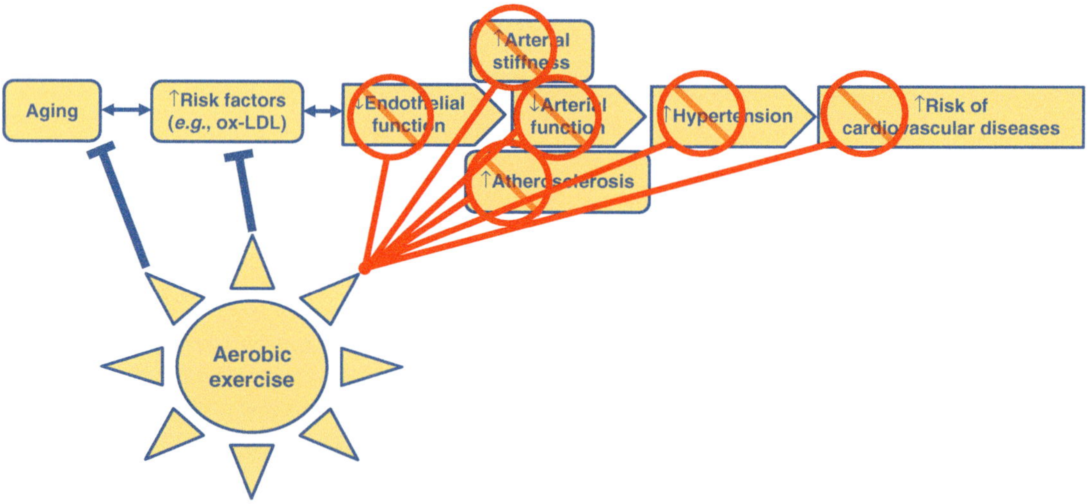


**Fig. 7.16** Aging, aerobic exercise, and adverse risk factors lead to CVD. Exercise blocks the risk factors. (Adapted from [128, Fig. 5])

mation. The converse is that sedentary people have a lack of AMPK activation, and this may have long-term consequences for mitochondrial functions and lead to cellular dysfunction and significant disease activity. Decreased AMPK activity in the hypothalamus may increase sympathetic nervous system activity, which may also be harmful, by amplifying stress levels and inflammation. Exercise, both short- and long-term, has significant beneficial effects on the

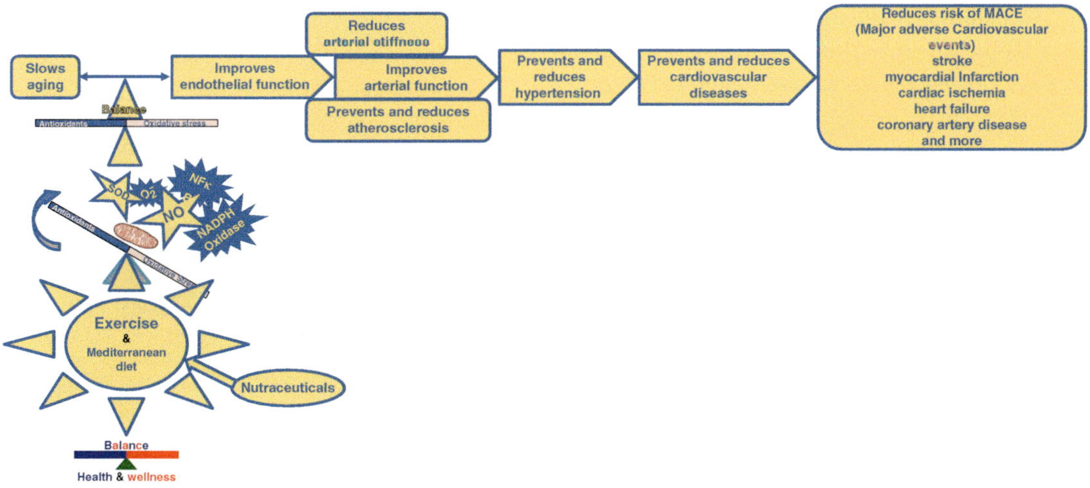


**Fig. 7.17** Aging, aerobic exercise, and other healthy lifestyle strategies, like exercise and diet, establish and maintain a balance between antioxidants and the combination of free radicals and ROS tipped toward the antioxidants (a healthy balance) that blocks the aging process. (Adapted from [128, Fig. 6])

human body including the blood vessels, blood flow, stress, sympathetic activity, and at the cellular level with the mitochondria.

As stated in Chap. 5, exercise boosts cysteine and glutathione (GSH) levels. N-acetyl cysteine (NAC) is a derivative of the amino acid cysteine. It is found in many over-the-counter nutritional supplements and has antioxidant properties. It has been used in several studies to treat various psychiatric diseases. It has also been used in drug addiction treatment. NAC has been considered in treatment of Alzheimer's disease and other neurodegenerative diseases, autism, adult attention deficit syndrome (ADHD), bipolar disorders, obsessive-compulsive disorder, and depressive disorders. NAC seems to work on multiple pathways implicated in psychiatric and neurological disorders which include oxidative stress, mitochondrial dysfunction, inflammatory mediators, neurotransmission, and neural plasticity [116, 129, 130].

NAC provides cysteine, based on a rate-limiting amino acid in GSH production. GSH reduces superoxide radical into hydrogen peroxide which then gets neutralized to water by catalase activity. The so-called cysteine-cysteine cycle serves as a direct free radical scavenger system. NAC has direct effects on mitochondrial function in different disorders. Since NAC is the precursor of the intracellular antioxidant GSH and is also a direct-acting free radical scavenger and antioxidant, it plays an important role in reducing oxidative stress and inflammation, including inflammatory cytokines associated with psychiatric disorders and traumatic brain injury. NAC is associated with reduced lung inflammation, by suppressing inflammatory markers, helping with respiratory disorders. By way of cysteine, exercise increases NAC production. NAC is often added to the supplement recommendations (ALA, CoQ10, L-carnitine) for patients with emotional upset and anxiety disorders.

GSH is an important antioxidant found in plants, animals, fungi, and bacteria. It is capable of preventing damage from reactive oxidant species. It is a tripeptide which contains cysteine and glycine. The ratio of reduced-GSH to oxidized-GSH within cells is a very important measure of cellular oxidative stress. GSH is one of the major endogenous antioxidants produced by cells. It maintains antioxidants such as vitamin C and vitamin E in their reduced active form. It also regulates nitric oxide cycle. It is used for biochemical reactions such as DNA synthesis and repair. It has important functions in iron metabolism and has roles in cell cycle and cell death. Exercise promotes the benefits of GSH.

As mentioned above, GSH has been dubbed "the mother of all antioxidants." Some physicians believe that in functional medicine, GSH levels are deficient in people with most chronic diseases, such as chronic fatigue, heart disease, cancer, chronic infections, autoimmune disease, diabetes, autism, Alzheimer's disease, asthma, and so forth. Consuming sulfa-rich foods such as broccoli, kale, cabbage, and cauliflower may help increase GSH production. Exercise boosts GSH levels and improves immune system. NAC has been used for years as a means of potentially boosting GSH levels.

NAC treatment improves depression and depression-anxiety symptoms, as assessed by Montgomery-Asberg Depression Rating Scale and Hamilton Depression Rating Scale when compared to placebo (SMD = 0.37; 95% CI = 0.19–0.55; $P < 0.001$). Subjects receiving NAC had better depressive symptoms scores on the Clinical Global Impressions-Severity of Illness scale at follow-up than subjects on placebo (SMD = 0.22; 95% CI = 0.03–0.41; $P < 0.001$). In addition, global functionality was better in NAC than in placebo conditions. There were no changes in quality of life. With regard to adverse events, only minor adverse events were associated with N-acetylcysteine (OR = 1.61; 95% CI = 1.01–2.59; $P = 0.049$). Administration of NAC ameliorates depressive symptoms, improves functionality, and shows good tolerability [131].

## References


1. Plowman SA, Smith DL. Exercise physiology: for health, fitness, and performance. Philadelphia: Lippincott, Williams and Wilkins; 2014.
2. Cardinali DP. Autonomic nervous system: basic and clinical aspects. Cham: Springer International Publishing AG; 2018.
3. Potteiger JA. ACSM's introduction to exercise science. Philadelphia: Lippincott, Williams and Wilkins; 2014.
4. Williams KA, Patel H. Healthy plant-based diet: what does it really mean? J Am Coll Cardiol. 2017;70(4):423–5.
5. Colombo J, Arora RR, DePace NL, Vinik AI. Clinical autonomic dysfunction: measurement, indications, therapies, and outcomes. New York: Springer Science + Business Media; 2014.
6. Mischel NA, Subramanian M, Dombrowski MD, Llewellyn-Smith IJ, Mueller PJ. Inactivity-related neuroplasticity in brainstem control of sympathetic outflow: unraveling underlying molecular, cellular, and anatomical mechanisms. Am J Physiol Heart Circ Physiol. 2015;309:H235–43. https://doi.org/10.1152/ajpheart.00929.2014. Epub 2015 May 8.
7. Mueller PJ. Physical (in)activity-dependent alterations at the rostral ventrolateral medulla: influence on sympathetic nervous system regulation. Am J Physiol Regul Integr Comp Physiol. 2010;298:R1468–74.
8. Lott J. The mother of all antioxidants: how health gurus are misleading you and what you should know about glutathione. Archangel Ink; 2014.
9. Fisher JP, Young CN, Fadel PJ. Central sympathetic overactivity: maladies and mechanisms. Auton Neurosci. 2009;148:5–15.
10. Go AS, Mozaffarian D, Roger VL, et al. Executive summary: heart disease and stroke statistics – 2013 update: a report from the American Heart Association. Circulation. 2013;127:143–52.
11. Lindberg FA. The GI Mediterranean diet: the glycemic index-based life-saving diet of the Greeks. Berkley: Ulysses Press; 2009.
12. Carnethon MR, Prineas RJ, Temprosa M, Zhang ZM, Uwaifo G, Molitch ME. The association among autonomic nervous system function, incident diabetes, and intervention arm in the Diabetes Prevention Program. Diabetes Care. 2006;29:914–9.
13. Vinik A, Ziegler D. Diabetic cardiovascular autonomic neuropathy. Circulation. 2007;115:387–97.
14. Maser RE, Lenhard MJ. An overview of the effect of weight loss on cardiovascular autonomic function. Curr Diabetes Rev. 2007;3:204–11.
15. Voulgari C, Pagoni S, Vinik A, Poirier P. Exercise improves cardiac autonomic function in obesity and diabetes. Metabolism. 2013;62:609–21.
16. Matsuo M, Kaneko T. The chemistry of reactive oxygen species and related free radicals. In: Radak Z, editor. Free radicals in exercise and aging. Leeds: Human Kinetics; 2000. p. 1–34.
17. Sudano I, Spreker LE, Hermam F, Flammer A, Corti R, Noli G, et al. Protection of endothelial function targets for nutritional and pharmacologic intervention. J Cardiovasc Pharmacol. 2006;47(suppl 2):S136–50.
18. Powers SK, Jackson MJ. Exercise-induced oxidative stress: cellular mechanisms and impact on muscle force production. Physiol Rev. 2008;88:1243–76.
19. Zembroń-Łacny A, Szyszka K, Hübner-Woźniak E. The pro-antioxidant-oxidant balance in the blood of middle – distance runners. Biol Sport. 1998;16:51–9.
20. Alessio HM, Hagerman AE, Fulkerson BK, Ambrose J, Rice RE, et al. Generation of reactive oxygen species after exhaustive aerobic and isometric exercise. Med Sci Sports Exerc. 2000;32(9):1576–81.
21. Goto C, Higashi Y, Kimura M, Noma K, Hara K, et al. Effect of different intensities of exercise on endothelium-dependent vasodilation in humans: role of endothelium-dependent nitric oxide and oxidative stress. Circulation. 2003;108(5):530–5.

22. Knez WL, Jenkins DG, Coombes JS. Oxidative stress in half and full ironman triathletes. Med Sci Sports Exerc. 2007;39(2):283–8.
23. Pilch W, Szygula Z, Tyka AK, Palka T, Tyka A, Cison T, Pilch P, Teleglow A. Disturbances in pro-antioxidant-oxidant balance after passive body overheating and after exercise in elevated ambient temperatures in athletes and untrained men. PLoS One. 2014;9(1):e85320. https://doi.org/10.1371/journal.pone.0085320. eCollection 2014.
24. Matsuo M, Kaneko T. The chemistry of reactive oxygen species and related free radicals. In: Radak Z, editor. Free radicals in exercise and aging. Leeds: Human Kinetics; 2000. p. 1–34.
25. Sawka MN, Burke LM, Eichner ER, Maughan RJ, Montain SJ, et al. American College of Sports Medicine position stand. Exercise and fluid replacement. Med Sci Sports Exerc. 2007;39(2):377–90. PMID: 17277604.
26. Paik IY, Jeong MH, Jin HE, Kim YI, Suh AR, et al. Fluid replacement following dehydration reduces oxidative stress during recovery. Biochem Biophys Res Commun. 2009;383(1):103–7. https://doi.org/10.1016/j.bbrc.2009.03.135.
27. Sengupta P. Health impacts of yoga and pranayama: a state-of-the-art review. Int J Prev Med. 2012;3(7):444–58.
28. Calvert JW, Lefer DJ. Role of β-adrenergic receptors and nitric oxide signaling in exercise-mediated cardioprotection. Physology. 2013;28(4):216–24. https://doi.org/10.1152/physiol.00011.2013.
29. Traub O, Berk BC. Laminar shear stress: mechanisms by which endothelial cells transducer an atheroprotective force. Arteroscler Thromb Vasc Biol. 1998;18:677–85.
30. Garcia-Cardenia G, Fan R, Shah V, Sorrentino R, Cinno G, Papapetriopoulas A, Sessa WC. Dynamic activation of endothelial nitric oxide synthase by Hsp90. Nature. 1998;392:821–4.
31. Fleming I, Busse R. Signal transduction of eNOS activation. Cardiovasc Res. 1999;43:532–41.
32. Russell KS, Haynes MP, Caulin-Glaser T, Rosneck J, Sessa WC, Bender JR. Estrogen stimulates heat shock protein 90 binding to endothelial nitric oxide synthase in human vascular endothelial cells. Effects on calcium sensitivity and NO release. J Biol Chem. 2000;275:5026–30.
33. Hudicka O, Brown M, Egginton S. Angiogenesis in skeletal and cardiac muscle. Physiol Rev. 1992;72:369–417.
34. Lee JS, Feldman AM. Gene therapy for therapeutic myocardial angiogenesis a promising synthesis of two emerging technologies. Nat Med. 1998;4:739–42.
35. Dijhorst-Oci LT, Stores ES, Koomans HA, Rabelink TJ. Acute simultaneous stimulation of nitric oxide and oxygen radicals by angiotensin II in humans in vivo. J Cardiovasc Pharmacol. 1999;33:420–4.
36. Romero JC, Reckelhoff JE. Role of angiotensin and oxidative stress in essential hypertension. Hypertension. 1999;34:943–9.
37. Cai H, Harrison DG. Endothelial dysfunction in cardiovascular diseases: the role of oxidant stress. Circ Res. 2000;87:840–4.
38. Sowers JR. Hypertension angiotensin II and oxidative stress. N Engl J Med. 2002;346:1999–2001.
39. Martin JE, Dubbert PM, Cushman WC. Controlled trial of aerobic exercise in hypertension. Circulation. 1990;81:1560–7.
40. Wood PD, Statanick ML, Williams PT, Haskell WL. The effects on plasma lipoproteins of a prudent weight-reducing diet with or without exercise in overweight men and women. N Engl J Med. 1991;325:461–6.
41. Arakawa K. Antihypertensive mechanism of exercise. J Hypertens. 1993;11:223–9.
42. Paffenbarger RS, Hyde RT, Wing AL, et al. The association of changes in physical-activity level and other lifestyle characteristics with mortality among men. N Engl J Med. 1993;328:538–45.
43. Higashi Y, Yoshizumi M. Exercise and endothelial function: role of endothelium derived nitric oxide and oxidative stress in healthy subjects and hypertensive patients. Pharmacol Ther. 2004;102:87–96.
44. Griffin KL, Laughlin MH, Parker JL. Exercise training improves endothelium-mediated vasorelaxation after chronic coronary occlusion. J Appl Physiol. 1999;87:1948–56.
45. Mancini GB, Henry GC, Macaya C, O'Neil BJ, Pucilo AL, Carere RG, et al. Angiotensin-converting enzyme inhibition with quinapril improves endothelial vasomotor dysfunction in patients with coronary artery disease. The TREND (Trial on Reversing Endothelial Dysfunction) study. Circulation. 1996;94:258–65.
46. Ghadoni L, Virdis A, Magagna A, Taddei S, Salvetti A. Effects of the angiotensin II type 1 receptor blocker candesartan on endothelial function in patients with essential hypertension. Hypertension. 2000;35:501–6.
47. The long term intervention with Pravastatin in ischaemic Disease (LIPID) Study Group. Prevention of cardiovascular events and death with pravastatin in patients with coronary heart disease and a broad range of mitral cholesterol levels. N Engl J Med. 1998;339:1349–57.
48. Fryer LG, Hajduch E, Rencurel F, Salt IS, Hundal HS, Hardie DG, et al. Activation of glucose transport by AMP-activated protein kinase via stimulation of nitric oxide synthase. Diabetes. 2000;49:1978–85.
49. Abraham P, Saumet JL, Chevalier JM. External iliac artery endofibrosis in athletes. Sports Med. 1997;24:221–6.
50. Bergholm R, Makimattila S, Valkomen M, Liu ML, Lahdempera S, Taskinen MR, Sovijarvi A, Malmberg P, Yki-Jarvinen H. Intense physical training decreases circulating antioxidants and endothelium-dependent vasodilation in vivo. Atherosclerosis. 1999;145:341–9.
51. Nichols S, Gleadall-Siddall DO, Antony R, Clark AL, Cleland JGF, Carroll S, Ingle L. Estimated peak functional capacity: an accurate method for assessing change in peak oxygen consumption after cardiac

rehabilitation? Clin Physiol Funct Imaging. 2017. https://doi.org/10.1111/cpf.12468.
52. Palermo P, Corrà U. Exercise prescriptions for training and rehabilitation in patients with heart and lung disease. Ann Am Thorac Soc. 2017;14(Supplement_1):S59–66. https://doi.org/10.1513/AnnalsATS.201702-160FR.
53. Abdul-Jawad Altisent O, Puri R, Regueiro A, Chamandi C, Rodriguez-Gabella T, Del Trigo M, Campelo-Parada F, Couture T, Marsal JR, Côté M, Paradis JM, DeLarochellière R, Doyle D, Mohammadi S, Dumont E, Rodés-Cabau J. Predictors and association with clinical outcomes of the changes in exercise capacity after transcatheter aortic valve replacement. Circulation. 2017;136(7):632–43. https://doi.org/10.1161/CIRCULATIONAHA.116.026349. Epub 2017 Jun 6.
54. Talwar A, Sahni S, Verma S, Khan SZ, Dhar S, Kohn N. Exercise tolerance improves after pulmonary rehabilitation in pulmonary hypertension patients. J Exerc Rehabil. 2017;13(2):214–7. https://doi.org/10.12965/jer.1732872.436. eCollection 2017 Apr. PMID: 28503536.
55. Cheng ST, Wu YK, Yang MC, Huang CY, Huang HC, Chu WH, Lan CC. Pulmonary rehabilitation improves heart rate variability at peak exercise, exercise capacity and health-related quality of life in chronic obstructive pulmonary disease. Heart Lung. 2014;43(3):249–55. https://doi.org/10.1016/j.hrtlng.2014.03.002. Epub 2014 Mar 29. PMID: 24685394.
56. Karssemeijer EGA, Aaronson JA, Bossers WJ, Smits T, Olde Rikkert MGM, Kessels RPC. Positive effects of combined cognitive and physical exercise training on cognitive function in older adults with mild cognitive impairment or dementia: a meta-analysis. Ageing Res Rev. 2017. pii: S1568-1637(17)30114-9. https://doi.org/10.1016/j.arr.2017.09.003. [Epub ahead of print] Review.
57. Ebrahimi K, Majdi A, Baghaiee B, Hosseini SH, Sadigh-Eteghad S. Physical activity and beta-amyloid pathology in Alzheimer's disease: a sound mind in a sound body. EXCLI J. 2017;16:959–72. https://doi.org/10.17179/excli2017-475. eCollection 2017. Review. PMID: 28900376.
58. Cheng ST. Cognitive reserve and the prevention of dementia: the role of physical and cognitive activities. Curr Psychiatry Rep. 2016;18(9):85. https://doi.org/10.1007/s11920-016-0721-2. Review.
59. Richter EA, Ruderman NB. AMPK and the biochemistry of exercise: implications for human health and disease. Biochem J. 2009;418(2):261–75. https://doi.org/10.1042/BJ20082055. Review.
60. Segev D, Hellerstein D, Dunsky A. Physical activity – does it really increase bone density in postmenopausal women? A review of articles published between 2001–2016. Curr Aging Sci. 2017. https://doi.org/10.2174/1874609810666170918170744.
61. Swedish Council on Health Technology Assessment. Osteoporosis – prevention, diagnosis and treatment: a systematic review [Internet]. Stockholm: Swedish Council on Health Technology Assessment (SBU); 2003.
62. Senderovich H, Tang H, Belmont S. The role of exercises in osteoporotic fracture prevention and current care gaps. Where are we now? Recent updates. Rambam Maimonides Med J. 2017;8(3). https://doi.org/10.5041/RMMJ.10308. Review.
63. Loeser RF, Beavers DP, Bay-Jensen AC, Karsdal MA, Nicklas BJ, Guermazi A, Hunter DJ, Messier SP. Effects of dietary weight loss with and without exercise on interstitial matrix turnover and tissue inflammation biomarkers in adults with knee osteoarthritis: the Intensive Diet and Exercise for Arthritis trial (IDEA). Osteoarthr Cartil. 2017. pii: S1063-4584(17)31107-X. https://doi.org/10.1016/j.joca.2017.07.015.
64. Feldman BM. Exercise as medicine for children with arthritis. J Rheumatol. 2017;44(8):1103–5. https://doi.org/10.3899/jrheum.170461.
65. Gordon BR, McDowell CP, Lyons M, Herring MP. The effects of resistance exercise training on anxiety: a meta-analysis and meta-regression analysis of randomized controlled trials. Sports Med. 2017. https://doi.org/10.1007/s40279-017-0769-0. [Epub ahead of print] Review.
66. Yeh HP, Stone JA, Churchill SM, Brymer E, Davids K. Physical and emotional benefits of different exercise environments designed for treadmill running. Int J Environ Res Public Health. 2017;14(7). pii: E752. https://doi.org/10.3390/ijerph14070752.
67. Awick EA, Ehlers DK, Aguiñaga S, Daugherty AM, Kramer AF, McAuley E. Effects of a randomized exercise trial on physical activity, psychological distress and quality of life in older adults. Gen Hosp Psychiatry. 2017. pii: S0163-8343(17)30101-9. https://doi.org/10.1016/j.genhosppsych.2017.06.005. [Epub ahead of print].
68. Hearing CM, Chang WC, Szuhany KL, Deckersbach T, Nierenberg AA, Sylvia LG. Physical Exercise for treatment of mood disorders: a critical review. Curr Behav Neurosci Rep. 2016;3(4):350–9. https://doi.org/10.1007/s40473-016-0089-y. Epub 2016 Oct 14.
69. Kovacevic A, Mavros Y, Heisz JJ, Fiatarone Singh MA. The effect of resistance exercise on sleep: a systematic review of randomized controlled trials. Sleep Med Rev. 2017. pii: S1087-0792(16)30152-6. https://doi.org/10.1016/j.smrv.2017.07.002. [Epub ahead of print] Review.
70. S Delevatti R, Schuch FB, Kanitz AC, Alberton CL, Marson EC, Lisboa SC, Pinho CDF, Bregagnol LP, Becker MT, Kruel LFM. Quality of life and sleep quality are similarly improved after aquatic or dry-land aerobic training in patients with type 2 diabetes: a randomized clinical trial. J Sci Med Sport. 2017. pii: S1440-2440(17)31029-0. https://doi.org/10.1016/j.jsams.2017.08.024. [Epub ahead of print].
71. Koo P, Gjelsvik A, Choudhary G, Wu WC, Wang W, McCool FD, Eaton CB. Prospective association of physical activity and heart failure hospitalizations among black adults with normal ejection frac-

tion: The Jackson Heart Study. J Am Heart Assoc. 2017;6(9). pii: e006107. https://doi.org/10.1161/JAHA.117.006107.

72. Torell MF, Strömsöe A, Zagerholm E, Herlitz J, Claesson A, Svensson L, Börjesson M. Higher survival rates in exercise-related out-of-hospital cardiac arrests, compared to non-exercise-related – a study from the Swedish Register of Cardiopulmonary Resuscitation. Eur J Prev Cardiol. 2017;1:2047487317729251. https://doi.org/10.1177/2047487317729251.
73. Maessen MF, Eijsvogels TM, Stevens G, van Dijk AP, Hopman MT. Benefits of lifelong exercise training on left ventricular function after myocardial infarction. Eur J Prev Cardiol. 2017;1:2047487317728765. https://doi.org/10.1177/2047487317728765.
74. Campkin LM, Boyd JM, Campbell DJT. Coronary artery disease patient perspectives on exercise participation. J Cardiopulm Rehabil Prev. 2017;37(5):305–14. https://doi.org/10.1097/HCR.0000000000000195.
75. Nichols S, Gleadall-Siddall DO, Antony R, Clark AL, Cleland JGF, Carroll S, Ingle L. Estimated peak functional capacity: an accurate method for assessing change in peak oxygen consumption after cardiac rehabilitation? Clin Physiol Funct Imaging. 2017. https://doi.org/10.1111/cpf.12468.
76. Piña IL, Apstein CS, Balady GJ, Belardinelli R, Chaitman BR, Duscha BD, Fletcher BJ, Fleg JL, Myers JN, Sullivan MJ, American Heart Association Committee on exercise, rehabilitation, and prevention. Exercise and heart failure: a statement from the American Heart Association Committee on exercise, rehabilitation, and prevention. Circulation. 2003;107(8):1210–25. Review.
77. Myers J. Cardiology patient pages. Exercise and cardiovascular health. Circulation. 2003;107(1):e2–5.
78. Tinlin L, Fini N, Bernhardt J, Lewis LK, Olds T, English C. Best practice guidelines for the measurement of physical activity levels in stroke survivors: a secondary analysis of an observational study. Int J Rehabil Res. 2017. https://doi.org/10.1097/MRR.0000000000000253.
79. Oberlin LE, Waiwood AM, Cumming TB, Marsland AL, Bernhardt J, Erickson KI.Effects of physical activity on poststroke cognitive function: a meta-analysis of randomized controlled trials. Stroke. 2017. pii: STROKEAHA.117.017319. https://doi.org/10.1161/STROKEAHA.117.017319.
80. Yfanti C, Tsiokanos A, Fatouros IG, Theodorou AA, Deli CK, Koutedakis Y, Jamurtas AZ. Chronic eccentric exercise and antioxidant supplementation: effects on lipid profile and insulin sensitivity. J Sports Sci Med. 2017;16(3):375–82. eCollection 2017 Sept.
81. Mendes R, Sousa N, Reis VM, Themudo-Barata JL. Implementing low-cost, community-based exercise programs for middle-aged and older patients with type 2 diabetes: what are the benefits for glycemic control and cardiovascular risk? Int J Environ Res Public Health. 2017;14(9). pii: E1057. https://doi.org/10.3390/ijerph14091057. PMID: 28902144.
82. Miele EM, Headley SAE, Germain M, Joubert J, Herrick S, Milch C, Evans E, Cornelius A, Brewer B, Taylor B, Wood RJ. High-density lipoprotein particle pattern and overall lipid responses to a short-term moderate-intensity aerobic exercise training intervention in patients with chronic kidney disease. Clin Kidney J. 2017;10(4):524–31. https://doi.org/10.1093/ckj/sfx006. Epub 2017 Mar 27. PMID: 28852492.
83. Villafaina S, Collado-Mateo D, Fuentes JP, Merellano-Navarro E, Gusi N. Physical exercise improves heart rate variability in patients with type 2 diabetes: a systematic review. Curr Diab Rep. 2017;17(11):110. https://doi.org/10.1007/s11892-017-0941-9. Review.
84. Ostman C, Smart NA, Morcos D, Duller A, Ridley W, Jewiss D. The effect of exercise training on clinical outcomes in patients with the metabolic syndrome: a systematic review and meta-analysis. Cardiovasc Diabetol. 2017;16(1):110. https://doi.org/10.1186/s12933-017-0590-y. PMID: 28854979.
85. Myers J, Atwood JE, Froelicher V. Active lifestyle and diabetes. Circulation. 2003;107(19):2392–4.
86. Brown JC, Zemel BS, Troxel AB, Rickels MR, Damjanov N, Ky B, Rhim AD, Rustgi AK, Courneya KS, Schmitz KH. Dose-response effects of aerobic exercise on body composition among colon cancer survivors: a randomised controlled trial. Br J Cancer. 2017. https://doi.org/10.1038/bjc.2017.339.
87. Brown JC, Troxel AB, Ky B, Damjanov N, Zemel BS, Rickels MR, Rhim AD, Rustgi AK, Courneya KS, Schmitz KH. Dose-response effects of aerobic exercise among colon cancer survivors: a randomized phase II trial. Clin Colorectal Cancer. 2017. pii: S1533-0028(16)30168-2. https://doi.org/10.1016/j.clcc.2017.06.001.
88. Hartman SJ, Nelson SH, Myers E, Natarajan L, Sears DD, Palmer BW, Weiner LS, Parker BA, Patterson RE. Randomized controlled trial of increasing physical activity on objectively measured and self-reported cognitive functioning among breast cancer survivors: the memory & motion study. Cancer. 2017. https://doi.org/10.1002/cncr.30987.
89. Livsey L, Lewis K. Breast cancer survivors' perceptions of participating in a supervised exercise intervention: an exploratory review of the literature. Women Health. 2017. https://doi.org/10.1080/03630242.2017.1372844.
90. Vashistha V, Singh B, Kaur S, Prokop LJ, Kaushik D. The effects of exercise on fatigue, quality of life, and psychological function for men with prostate cancer: systematic review and meta-analyses. Eur Urol Focus. 2016;2(3):284–95. https://doi.org/10.1016/j.euf.2016.02.011. Epub 2016 Mar 9. Review.
91. Daly RM. Exercise and nutritional approaches to prevent frail bones, falls and fractures: an update. Climacteric. 2017;20(2):119–24. https://doi.org/10.1080/13697137.2017.1286890. Epub 2017 Feb 8. Review.

92. Greenway KG, Walkley JW, Rich PA. Impact exercise and bone density in premenopausal women with below average bone density for age. Eur J Appl Physiol. 2015;115(11):2457–69. https://doi.org/10.1007/s00421-015-3225-6. Epub 2015 Aug 1.
93. Fuchs RK, Kersh ME, Carballido-Gamio J, Thompson WR, Keyak JH, Warden SJ. Physical activity for strengthening fracture prone regions of the proximal femur. Curr Osteoporos Rep. 2017;15(1):43–52. https://doi.org/10.1007/s11914-017-0343-6. Review.
94. Turner JE, Brum PC. Does regular exercise counter T cell immunosenescence reducing the risk of developing cancer and promoting successful treatment of malignancies? Oxidative Med Cell Longev. 2017;2017:4234765. https://doi.org/10.1155/2017/4234765. Epub 2017 Jul 2. Review.
95. Hojman P. Exercise protects from cancer through regulation of immune function and inflammation. Biochem Soc Trans. 2017;45(4):905–11. https://doi.org/10.1042/BST20160466. Epub 2017 Jul 3. Review.
96. Gustafson MP, DiCostanzo AC, Wheatley CM, Kim CH, Bornschlegl S, Gastineau DA, Johnson BD, Dietz AB. A systems biology approach to investigating the influence of exercise and fitness on the composition of leukocytes in peripheral blood. J Immunother Cancer. 2017;5:30. https://doi.org/10.1186/s40425-017-0231-8.
97. Ackland GL, Minto G, Clark M, Whittle J, Stephens RCM, Owen T, Prabhu P, Del Arroyo AG. Autonomic regulation of systemic inflammation in humans: a multi-center, blinded observational cohort study. Brain Behav Immun. 2017. pii: S0889-1591(17)30398-7. https://doi.org/10.1016/j.bbi.2017.08.010.
98. Jafariyan S, Monazzami A, Nikosefat Z, Nobahar M, Yari K. Inflammatory and immune responses to a 3-day period of downhill running in active females. Cell Mol Biol (Noisy-le-Grand). 2017;63(7):76–83. https://doi.org/10.14715/cmb/2017.63.7.13.
99. Bartlett DB, Shepherd SO, Wilson OJ, Adlan AM, Wagenmakers AJM, Shaw CS, Lord JM. Neutrophil and monocyte bactericidal responses to 10 weeks of low-volume high-intensity interval or moderate-intensity continuous training in sedentary adults. Oxidative Med Cell Longev. 2017;2017:8148742. https://doi.org/10.1155/2017/8148742. Epub 2017 Jun 1.
100. Clark LV, Buckland M, Murphy G, Taylor N, Vleck V, Mein C, Wozniak E, Smuk M, White PD. Cytokine responses to exercise and activity in patients with chronic fatigue syndrome: case control study. Clin Exp Immunol. 2017. https://doi.org/10.1111/cei.13023.
101. Monteiro Junior RS, de Tarso Maciel-Pinheiro P, da Matta M, Portugal E, da Silva Figueiredo LF, Terra R, Carneiro LSF, Rodrigues VD, Nascimento OJM, Deslandes AC, Laks J. Effect of exercise on inflammatory profile of older persons: systematic review and meta-analyses. J Phys Act Health. 2017;3:1–24. https://doi.org/10.1123/jpah.2016-0735.
102. Zimmer P, Schenk A, Kieven M, Holthaus M, Lehmann J, Lövenich L, Bloch W. Exercise induced alterations in NK-cell cytotoxicity – methodological issues and future perspectives. Exerc Immunol Rev. 2017;23:66–81.
103. Moore SC, Lee IM, Weiderpass E, Campbell PT, Sampson JN, Kitahara CM, Keadle SK, Arem H, Berrington de Gonzalez A, Hartge P, Adami HO, Blair CK, Borch KB, Boyd E, Check DP, Fournier A, Freedman ND, Gunter M, Johannson M, Khaw KT, Linet MS, Orsini N, Park Y, Riboli E, Robien K, Schairer C, Sesso H, Spriggs M, Van Dusen R, Wolk A, Matthews CE, Patel AV. Association of leisure-time physical activity with risk of 26 types of cancer in 1.44 million adults. JAMA Intern Med. 2016;176(6):816–25. https://doi.org/10.1001/jamainternmed.2016.1548.
104. O'Donovan G, Lee IM, Hamer M, Stamatakis E. Association of "weekend warrior" and other leisure time physical activity patterns with risks for all-cause, cardiovascular disease, and cancer mortality. JAMA Intern Med. 2017;177(3):335–42. https://doi.org/10.1001/jamainternmed.2016.8014.
105. Song M, Giovannucci E. Preventable incidence and mortality of carcinoma associated with lifestyle factors among white adults in the United States. JAMA Oncol. 2016;2(9):1154–61. https://doi.org/10.1001/jamaoncol.2016.0843.
106. Manson JE, Hu FB, Rich-Edwards JW, Colditz GA, Stampfer MJ, Willett WC, Speizer FE, Hennekens CH. A prospective study of walking as compared with vigorous exercise in the prevention of coronary heart disease in women. N Engl J Med. 1999;341(9):650–8.
107. Hu FB, Sigal RJ, Rich-Edwards JW, Colditz GA, Solomon CG, Willett WC, Speizer FE, Manson JE. Walking compared with vigorous physical activity and risk of type 2 diabetes in women: a prospective study. JAMA. 1999;282(15):1433–9.
108. US Public Health Service, Office of the Surgeon General. Physical activity and health: a report of the surgeon general. Atlanta: US Department of Health and Human Services, Centers for Disease Control and Prevention, National Center for Chronic Disease Prevention and Health Promotion; 1996.
109. Fletcher GF, Balady GJ, Amsterdam EA, et al. Exercise standards for testing and training: a statement for healthcare professionals from the American Heart Association. Circulation. 2001;104:1694–740.
110. Pate RR, Pratt MP, Blair SN, et al. Physical activity and public health: a recommendation from the Centers for Disease Control and Prevention and the American College of Sports Medicine. JAMA. 1995;273:402–7.
111. American College of Sports Medicine. Guidelines for exercise testing and prescription. 6th ed. Baltimore: Lippincott Williams & Wilkins; 2000.

112. Myers J. Cardiology patient pages. Exercise and cardiovascular health. Circulation. 2003;107(1):c2–5.
113. Pop-Busui R, Evans GW, Gerstein HC, Fonseca V, Fleg JL, Hoogwerf BJ, Genuth MS, Grimm RH, Corson MA, Prineas R, The ACCORD Study Group. Effects of cardiac autonomic dysfunction on mortality risk in the action to control cardiovascular risk in diabetes (ACCORD) trial. Diabetes Care. 2010;33:1578–84.
114. Vinik AI, Maser RE, Ziegler D. Neuropathy. The crystal ball for cardiovascular disease. Diabetes Care. 2010;33(7):1688–90.
115. Dinas PC, Valente A, Granzotto M, Rossato M, Vettor R, Zacharopoulou A, Carrillo AE, Davies NA, Gkiata P, Jamurtas AZ, Koutedakis Y, Metsios GS, Flouris AD. Browning formation markers of subcutaneous adipose tissue in relation to resting energy expenditure, physical activity and diet in humans. Horm Mol Biol Clin Invest. 2017. pii: /j/hmbci.ahead-of-print/hmbci-2017-0008/hmbci-2017-0008.xml. https://doi.org/10.1515/hmbci-2017-0008.
116. Høydal MA, Stølen TO, Kettlewell S, Maier LS, Brown JH, Sowa T, Catalucci D, Condorelli G, Kemi OJ, Smith GL, Wisløff U. Exercise training reverses myocardial dysfunction induced by CaMKIIδC overexpression by restoring Ca2+ homeostasis. J Appl Physiol (1985). 2016;121(1):212–20. https://doi.org/10.1152/japplphysiol.00188.2016. Epub 2016 May 26.
117. Khera AV, Emdin CA, Drake I, Natarajan P, Bick AG, Cook NR, Chasman DI, Baber U, Mehran R, Rader DJ, Fuster V, Boerwinkle E, Melander O, Orho-Melander M, Ridker PM, Kathiresan S. Genetic risk, adherence to a healthy lifestyle, and coronary disease. N Engl J Med. 2016;375(24):2349–58. Epub 2016 Nov 13.
118. Nicolson GL. Mitochondrial dysfunction and chronic disease: treatment with natural supplements. Integr Med (Encinitas). 2014;13(4):35–43.
119. Price NL, et al. SIRT1 is required for AMPK activation and the beneficial effects of resveratrol on mitochondrial function. Cell Metab. 2012;15(5):675–90. https://doi.org/10.1016/j.cmet.2012.04.003.
120. Nakano M, Inui A. Metformin and incretin-based therapies up-regulate central and peripheral Adenosine monophosphate-activated protein affecting appetite and metabolism. Indian J Endocrinol Metab. 2012;16(Suppl S3):529–31.
121. Carling D, Viollet B. Beyond energy homeostasis: the expanding role of AMP-activated protein kinase in regulating metabolism. Cell Metab. 2015;21(6):799–804. https://doi.org/10.1016/j.cmet.2015.05.005. Review.
122. Towler MC, Hardie DG. AMP-activated protein kinase in metabolic control and insulin signaling. Circ Res. 2007;100(3):328–41. Review.
123. UK Prospective Diabetes Study (UKPDS) Group. Intensive blood-glucose control with sulphonylureas or insulin compared with conventional treatment and risk of complications in patients with type 2 diabetes (UKPDS 33). Lancet. 1998;352:837–53.
124. Ruiter R, Visser LE, van Herk-Sukel MP, Coebergh JW, Haak HR, Geelhoed-Duijvestijn PH, Straus SM, Herings RM, Stricker BH. Lower risk of cancer in patients on metformin in comparison with those on sulfonylurea derivatives: results from a large population-based follow-up study. Diabetes Care. 2012;35(1):119–24. https://doi.org/10.2337/dc11-0857. Epub 2011 Nov 18.
125. Tennen RI, Michishita-Kioi E, Chua KF. Finding a target for resveratrol. Cell. 2012;148(3):387–9. https://doi.org/10.1016/j.cell.2012.01.032.
126. Zhang QJ, McMillin SL, Tanner JM, Palionyte M, Abel ED, Symons JD. Endothelial nitric oxide synthase phosphorylation in treadmill-running mice: role of vascular signalling kinases. J Physiol. 2009;587(Pt 15):3911–20. https://doi.org/10.1113/jphysiol.2009.172916. Epub 2009 Jun 8.
127. Seals DR, Edward F. Adolph Distinguished Lecture: the remarkable anti-aging effects of aerobic exercise on systemic arteries. J Appl Physiol. 2014;117(5):425–39. https://doi.org/10.1152/japplphysiol.00362.2014.
128. Santos-Parker JR, LaRocca TJ, Seals DR. Aerobic exercise and other healthy lifestyle factors that influence vascular aging. Adv Physiol Educ. 2014;38(4):296–307. https://doi.org/10.1152/advan.00088.2014.
129. Berk M, Malhi GS, Gray LJ, Dean OM. The promise of N-acetylcysteine in neuropsychiatry. Trends Pharmacol Sci. 2013;34(3):167–77. https://doi.org/10.1016/j.tips.2013.01.001. Epub 2013 Jan 29. Review.
130. Dean O, Giorlando F, Berk M. N-acetylcysteine in psychiatry: current therapeutic evidence and potential mechanisms of action. J Psychiatry Neurosci. 2011;36(2):78–86. https://doi.org/10.1503/jpn.100057. Review.
131. Fernandes BS, Dean OM, Dodd S, Malhi GS, Berk M. N-acetylcysteine in depressive symptoms and functionality: a systematic review and meta-analysis. J Clin Psychiatry. 2016;77(4):e457–66. https://doi.org/10.4088/JCP.15r09984.

# 8 Psychosocial Stress Reduction (Prong-6)

What is the dreadful thing that is never wanted, is never invited, but visits too many on a daily basis? Although it is accepted and patients learn to live with it, it negatively affects mood, concentration, families, sleep, and even love lives. Worst of all, it can affect health. Studies have shown that it can even shorten life. Have you guessed it yet? … *Stress*. Stress is accepted as part of daily life. Unfortunately, there is no easy way to stay away from stress or keep it out of the lives of patients. However, a tested, tried, non-pharmaceutical method to help reduce stress and mitigate its effects is presented herein.

This prong focuses on stress reduction, specifically psychosocial stress (Fig. 8.1). Oxidative stress reduction discussed above is stress at the cellular and system level. Psychosocial stress and other stresses, such as from environmental, temperature, exercise, and other factors, are whole body stresses. These "whole body" stresses are the stresses that will be discussed in this chapter. "Whole body" stressors produce cognitive, emotional, physiological, and behavioral changes that can be detrimental to both physical and psychological health and well-being. They typically involve the central nervous system, P&S nervous systems, immune system, and endocrine system [1]; and secondarily, the cardiovascular system. In the past decade, more and more individuals experience psychosocial stress on a daily basis. Heavy workloads, job insecurity, and living in poverty are circumstances that can result in chronically increased stress, which in turn can lead to chronic psychological disorders such as depression. Stress and depression lead to inflammation. Besides the heavy psychological burden, chronic stress is also associated with an increased risk of cardiovascular disease, which is exacerbated by inflammation [2]. Individuals with increased stress perception have a substantially higher prevalence of myocardial infarction [3–15] and stroke [16].

1. Stress is a threatened homeostasis.
2. Homeostasis is mediated, primarily, through the P&S nervous systems. During stressful situations there is increased activity in the P&S nervous systems (a little stress for a short while is healthy; too much stress or stress for too long is not healthy).
3. Stress reactions invariably cause sympathetic activation increasing HR & BP (again, a little stress and, therefore, a little sympathetic activation for a short while are healthy; too much sympathetic activation or prolonged sympathetic activation is not healthy).
4. A properly functioning vagus nerve and parasympathetic system[1] relieve stress and reduce sympathetic activity.
5. A properly functioning vagus nerve helps to prevent prolonged stress responses, thereby normalizing or increasing immune responses

[1]The Vagus Nerve is approximately 70% of the parasympathetic nervous system.



N. L. DePace, J. Colombo, *Clinical Autonomic and Mitochondrial Disorders*,
https://doi.org/10.1007/978-3-030-17016-5_8

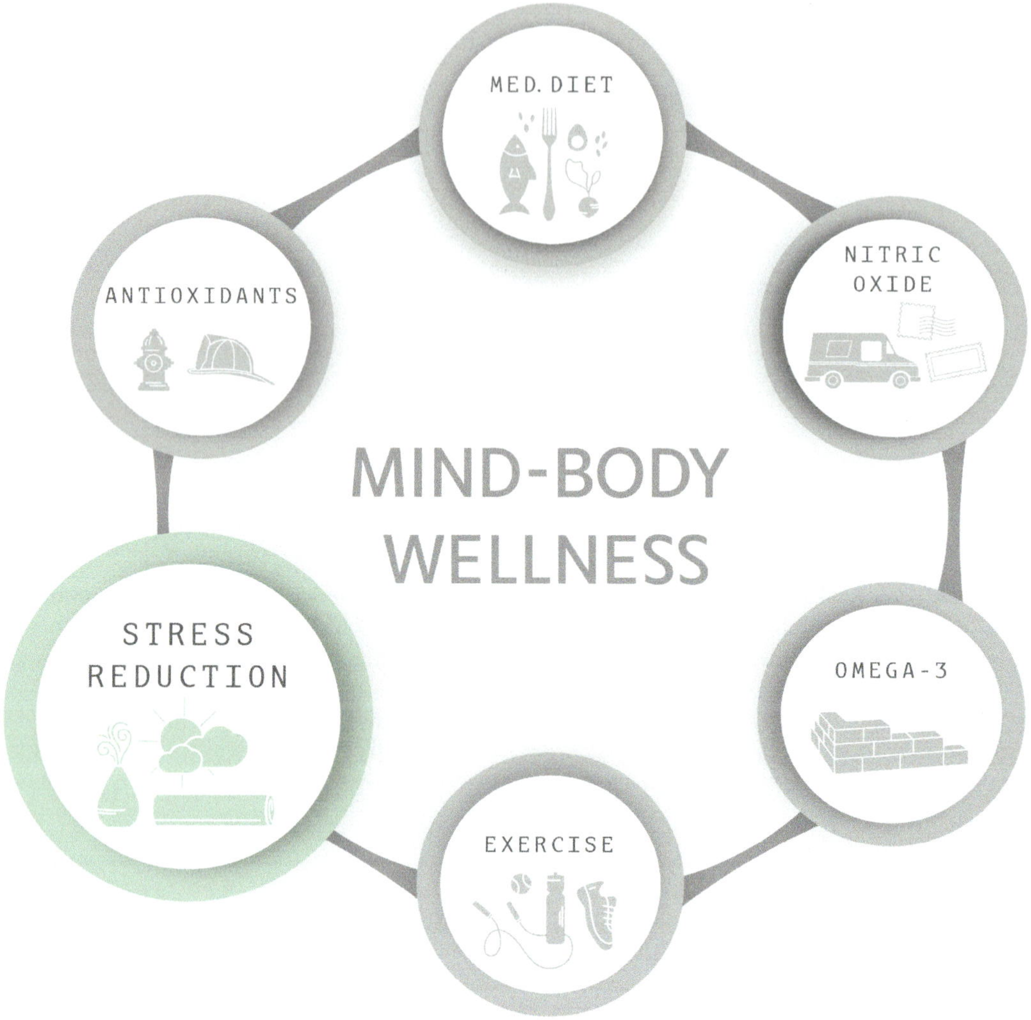


**Fig. 8.1** The (FC) Mind-Body Wellness Program – psychosocial stress reduction prong. (Illustration by Elysian Creative Studio, www.elysiancreativestudio.com, Lizzy Colombo)

and decreasing inflammation or terminating prolonged inflammation (a little inflammation for a short while is healthy; too much inflammation or prolonged inflammation is not healthy).

6. Stress-induced, prolonged sympathetic activity increases inflammation (again a little sympathetic activation for a short while is healthy; too much sympathetic activation or prolonged sympathetic activation is not healthy).
7. As stress rises so cortisol rises, via sympathetic activity which drives cortisol release.
8. Prolonged or excessive stress causes parasympathetic excess (PE, the body's protec-

tive system goes into "overdrive"). PE causes excessive immune responses (not healthy). There is a "hidden," dynamic PE[2] which typically causes secondary sympathetic excess (SE), which in turn causes excessive, or excessively extended, conditions including #2, #3, #6, and above.

9. Ongoing stress leads to chronic oxidative stress (stress at the cellular level) and organ dysfunction.
10. Stress-induced P&S activation is linked to myocardial infarction – global analysis from the INTERHEART study.
11. Acute stress can cause plaque rupture and heart attack.
12. In acute stress, sympathetic activity increases, epinephrine and cortisol rise, vagus nerve (parasympathetic) activity decreases, and angiotensin-renin activity increases.
13. Chronic stress increases appetite, increases sympathetic activity, and leads to visceral obesity, metabolic syndrome, and diabetes; also it is pro-thrombotic; an example is job stress.

All P&S dysfunctions are P&S imbalances, and actually there are two general types of imbalances: a resting imbalance and a dynamic or challenge imbalance. The typical imbalance is a resting imbalance and is due to the fact that the P nervous system (the majority of which, outside the central nervous system, is the vagus nerve) is a longer and a more exposed portion of the autonomic nervous system (ANS) and therefore more vulnerable to insult or attack. P&S balance then suffers, and the P nervous system declines faster than the S nervous system. Ultimately this is like the "brakes" failing faster than the "accelerator" on a car. The problem is that once the "brakes" inside fail, they cannot be replaced. This progression includes (1) peripheral autonomic neuropathy (PAN, or peripheral autonomic dysfunction[3]), (2) advanced autonomic dysfunction (AAD, indicating increased morbidity risk – the risk of more secondary symptoms) or diabetic autonomic neuropathy (DAN, which is AAD with the complications of abnormal insulin and blood glucose levels due to diabetes), and finally (3) cardiovascular autonomic neuropathy (CAN, indicating increased mortality risk – the risk of sudden death or other major adverse cardiac event, aka MACE, including heart attack or stroke). See Fig. 7.4 and insert below [18].

[2]The standard belief is that an increase in one branch of the autonomic nervous system is accompanied by a decrease in the other branch. In this way balance and homeostasis is maintained. Unfortunately, this assumption only holds in truly healthy individuals. Unprovoked parasympathetic excess (PE) during sympathetic stimulation is abnormal. This dynamic PE is "hidden" behind a sympathetic excess that is secondary to the PE. As a result, the symptoms masquerade as if they were generated by a primary sympathetic excess (SE). However, when treated as a primary SE, the patients do not respond as expected. When they are treated for a primary PE, they do improve. An example of such a patient is a patient with both depression (from PE) and hypertension (from SE). These patients tend to not be stable, because by treating the patient with direct or indirect sympathetic blockade (i.e., antihypertensives), more of the extant sympathetic control over the PE is blocked, the body is still demanding its blood, and not all sympathetic channels are being blocked; therefore, the body finds a way to defeat the antihypertensive, and the blood pressure increases after all [17]. (See "Dynamic Parasympathetic Excess" below.)

[3]At this stage "neuropathy" is a misnomer and has led to the misperception that P&S imbalance cannot be treated. As a result many people have suffered unnecessarily. "Neuropathy" implies "dead nerves." The nerves are not dead, just damaged, and they can be healed and their function normalized for their age. This is why "dysfunction" is the preferred term.

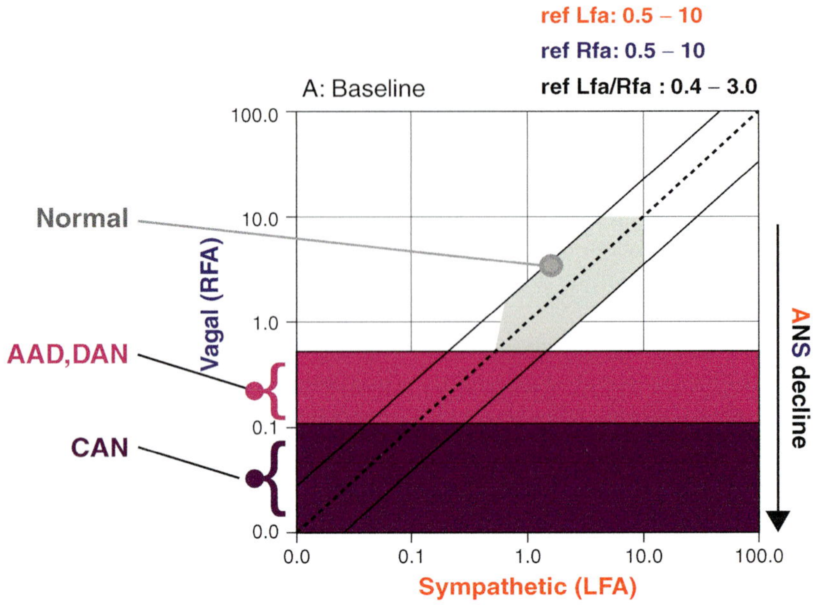


Insert: Republished with permission from Springer

Many types of P&S dysfunctions are reversible, assuming no end-organ damage or dysfunction. Psychosocial stress is one such P&S dysfunction. Unfortunately it is a complex P&S dysfunction, which is why it manifests in many forms across the typical patient population. However, there are some general similarities. The two main generalities are a (1) challenge, primary PE with (2) a secondary SE. The parasympathetics are the protective branch, and in anxiety and stress patients, the parasympathetics are excessively activated (PE). This in turn causes a SE. (Again, the parasympathetics set the threshold around which the sympathetics react. Therefore the PE, by raising the threshold, forces the SE.[4]) PE alone is not necessarily bad until it causes a secondary SE. While PE is trying to protect the system, the resultant is a SE that causes palpitations and all of the symptoms of anxiety, ADD/ADHD, PTSD, depression/anxiety syndromes, and other labile or difficult to control or unexplained conditions or disorders. Some types of P&S dysfunctions are temporary and may recover over time, such as functional CAN (CAN that is reversed with therapy, as opposed to structural CAN that is not reversed with therapy). Identification and treatment is therefore important. Some types of P&S dysfunction cannot recover completely, but can recover only partially. Ultimately, all that may be done is to delay continued deterioration of P&S nerve fibers (in effect delay the aging effect). Delay is facilitated by establishing and maintaining proper P&S balance for the individual. This balance may be achieved with several measures, including diet, exercise, supplements, and stress reduction; such as with the Mind-Body Wellness program.

[4]A good analogy is your car. When stopped at a red light, you have your foot on the brakes. When the light turns green, the first thing you do is take your foot off the breaks. Even before you step on the accelerator, the car is moving, accelerating. Then you step on the accelerator and move faster. Acceleration is facilitated by releasing the brakes. The same happens in the body. However, if you do not take your foot off the brakes and step on the accelerator, you still go, but it takes you longer to get to speed, or you have to step on the accelerator harder, over-revving the engine. The condition of keeping your foot on the brakes is like PE with SE.

## Hypothalamus-Pituitary-Adrenal Axis Connects Brain and Body

There are three stages to the acute stress response. First, the stressor is detected with sensory organs. The second stage is the stress response: defense or escape. The third stage is when the acute becomes chronic. If the stressor cannot be avoided and it persists, then the third stage is entered, a state of exhaustion ensues (Fig. 8.2) [20]. Stress responses are coordinated by autonomic nervous system and the hypothalamus-pituitary-adrenal axis (Fig. 8.3) [22]. The hypothalamic-pituitary-adrenal axis underlies the fight-or-flight response via a hormonal

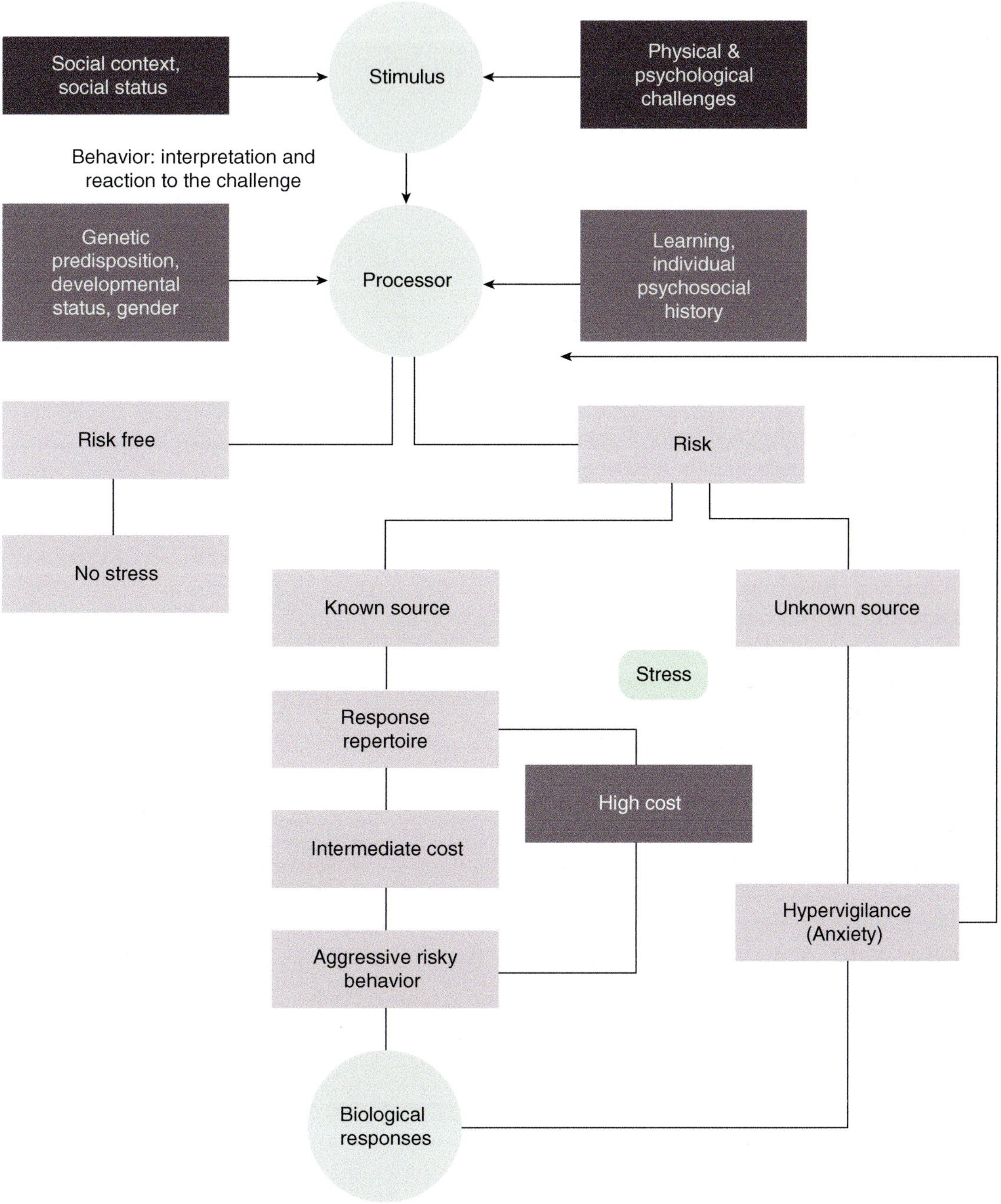


**Fig. 8.2** Behavioral and biological aspects of the defense behavior. The sequence of phenomena follows exposure to a novel situation. Strategies are of two types, high or low energy level. The objective is adaptation. If adaptation does not occur, the stress reaction appears, with stimulation of the pituitary-adrenal axis [19]. (Illustration by Elysian Creative Studio, www.elysiancreativestudio.com, Lizzy Colombo)

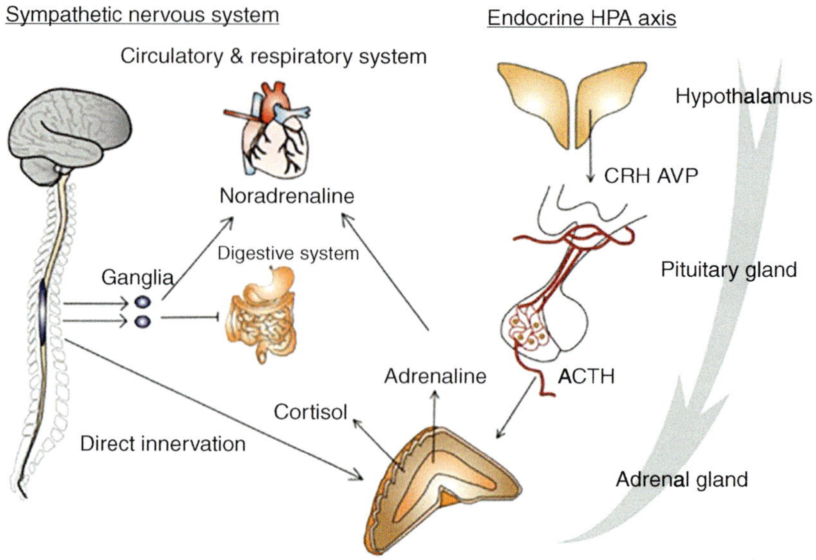


**Fig. 8.3** Human stress response pathways operating through the autonomic nervous system and the endocrine system. The neural and hormonal signals interact and complement each other through the regulatory action of the hypothalamus-pituitary-adrenal axis (HPA axis). Abbreviations: ACTH adrenocorticotropic hormone, AVP arginine/vasopressin, CRH corticotrophin-releasing hormone [21]. (Open Access, MDPI)

cascade of catecholamines and corticoid hormones. The stress response starts with the activation of the sympathetic system. The sympathetics stimulate the adrenal medulla to release adrenaline and noradrenaline. These two forms of adrenaline (aka epinephrine[5]) increase heart rate and vasoconstriction. Concurrently, the paraventricular nucleus (PVN) neurons in the hypothalamus release corticotrophin-releasing hormone (CRH) and arginine/vasopressin (AVP), stimulating the anterior pituitary gland. In response, the pituitary secretes adrenocorticotropic hormone (ACTH), which acts on the adrenal cortex to release glucocorticoids (such as cortisol), mobilizing energy reserves (i.e., glycogenolysis in the liver) to support the defense response (fight or flight, Fig. 8.4) [23].

Glucocorticoids also cause catecholamine to be released from the adrenal medulla. Concurrently, adrenaline activates a release of glucagon by the pancreas to further increase the catabolism of glycogen in the liver and raise glucose concentration in the blood. Other hormones such as cytokines or endogenous opioids may also be produced or released, depending on the nature, duration, and intensity of the stressor,

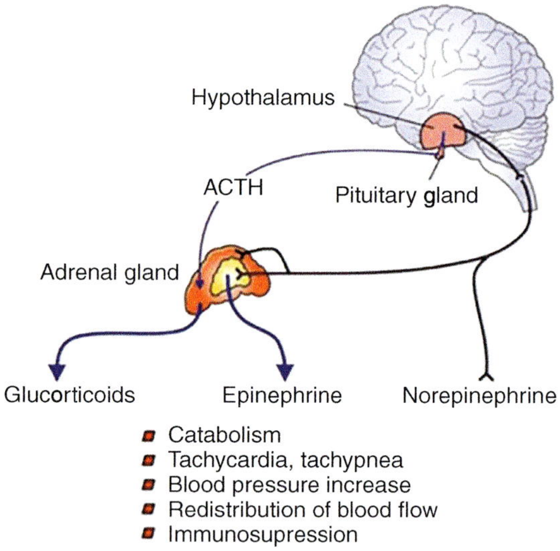


**Fig. 8.4** Pituitary release of ACTH activates adrenal sympathetic nerves to support defense behavior (fight or flight) [19, Fig. 5.12]. (Republished with permission from Springer International Publishing AG)

to act in diverse ways to limit the degree of tissue damage. In this way, stress responses can vary depending on the type and duration of the stressor. Under chronic stress, the immune system, metabolic pathways, and cognitive processes in the organism gradually weaken until exhaustion and failure are reached [20, 24]. For example, repetitive hypothalamus-pituitary-

[5]Epinephrine and adrenaline are the same chemical, discovered at the same time (1904) by two different researchers, one in the US and one in England. The US named the chemical "epinephrine" and the British named the chemical "adrenaline."

adrenal activation resulting in an excess of glucocorticoids in the blood can lead to metabolic diseases such as metabolic syndrome or type 2 diabetes [25, 26].

Strong emotional and mental stresses are now recognized as playing a significant role in severe and fatal ventricular arrhythmias. The mechanisms include central processing at the cortical and brain stem level, the autonomic nerves, and the electrophysiology of the heart (Fig. 8.10, below) [27]. This is part of the mind-body and brain-heart connection. These mechanisms include regulatory processes which incorporate interactive feedforward and feedback mechanisms, and must be considered together, intact. These mechanisms underlie the colloquial beliefs that people may "die of fright" or are "worried to death." Strong emotions, as evidenced by the epidemic-like prevalence of the diagnosis of anxiety clogging emergency rooms, may precipitate arrhythmias which may turn malignant and lead to sudden cardiac death (Fig. 8.10).

Anxiety and other emotions and stress, immediate, remembered, and imagined, also affect other systems of the body, including the immune system. For example, "puppy love" or "stage fright" responses, including flushing, cold sweat, "jitters," rapid breathing and pulse, "butterflies" in the stomach (see Fig. 5.70), and the need to evacuate bladder (Fig. 8.5) or bowels (Fig. 8.6), are caused by the CNS communicating via brain stem nuclei through the P&S nervous systems to the viscera (see insert, right). A bidirectional communication exists between the CNS and the immune system. The P&S nervous systems, through neurotransmitters and neuropeptides, work in parallel with the hypothalamic-pituitary-adrenal axis (Fig. 8.7) through the actions of glucocorticoids to modulate inflammatory events. The immune system, through the action of cytokines and other factors, in turn, activates the central nervous system to orchestrate negative feedback mechanisms that keep the immune response in check. Disruption of these interactions has been associated with a number of syndromes including inflammatory, autoimmune, and cardiovascular diseases, metabolic and psychiatric disorders, and the development of shock.

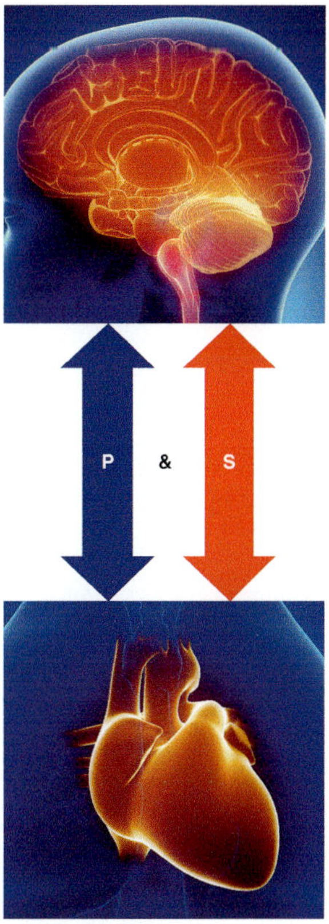


Insert: Reproduced with permission – Brain: Adapted from Shutterstock Royalty-free stock illustration ID: 133874900, Female brain x-ray anatomy, by CLIPAREA l Custom media. Heart: Adapted from Shutterstock Royalty-free stock illustration ID: 82159072, Human heart with thorax, by CLIPAREA)

Disruption of the hypothalamic-pituitary-adrenal axis can lead to increased mortality. Another branch of the hypothalamic-pituitary-adrenal axis is the hypothalamic-pituitary-gonadal axis, which plays an important part in regulating immunity through the secretion of sex hormones. Estrogen and testosterone modulate the immune system (Fig. 8.7) [28]. Progesterone is well known to be crucial for reproductive organ development and maintenance of pregnancy. It also has a role as an important immune regulator. Glucocorticoids and Progesterone modulate inflammatory and infectious disease responses. Glucocorticoids play a crucial role in regulating the immune response, from initial activation to eventual suppression and restoration of homeostasis. As a result of the complexity of neuroendocrine-immune interactions, no single event that changes glucocorticoid and progesterone receptor activity

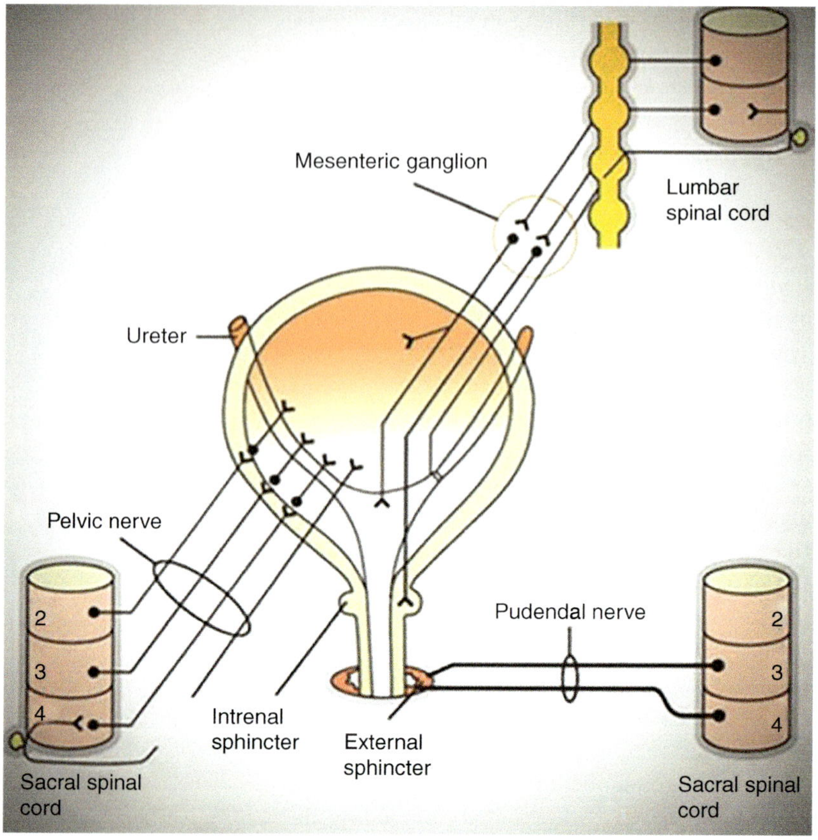


**Fig. 8.5** Bladder innervation. Parasympathetic innervation stimulates the detrusor via sacral spine S2–S4, whereas sympathetic (mesenteric ganglion from the lumbar spine) innervation inhibits the detrusor and stimulates the trigone. The external sphincter receives somatic innervation through the pudendal nerve (the somatic pathway) [19, Fig. 3.20]. (Republished with permission from Springer International Publishing AG)

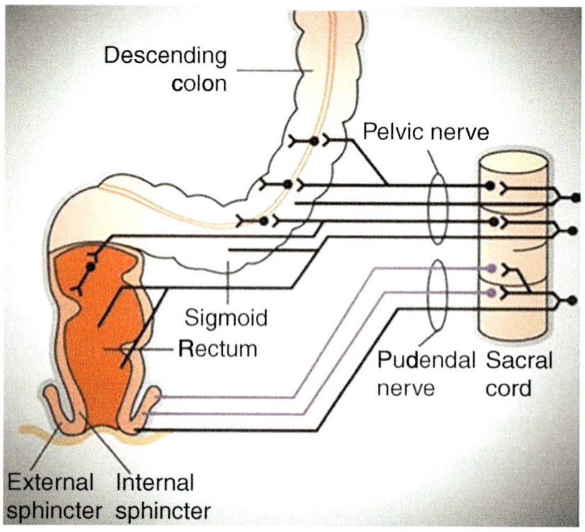


**Fig. 8.6** Bowel innervation. The external anal sphincter is under voluntary control, whereas the internal anal sphincter is under parasympathetic control. The internal sphincter is relaxed by rectal distension [19, Fig. 3.22]. (Republished with permission from Springer International Publishing AG

may be fully responsible for the development, and progression, of disease. Dysregulation of glucocorticoid and progesterone activity contribute to the development of autoimmune and inflammatory diseases [28].

Crosstalk between the neuroendocrine and immune systems can also result in production of factors by the nervous and endocrine systems that alter immune cell function and subsequent modulation of immune responses against infectious agents and other pathogens (Fig. 8.8). Continued exposure to these factors is also known to increase susceptibility to, and severity of, disease. Neuroendocrine factors are thought to play a major role in gender-specific differences in development of certain disorders, including autoimmune and inflammatory diseases that have a two- to tenfold higher incidence in females. Neuroendocrine factors can affect immune cells at the level of gene transcription but have also

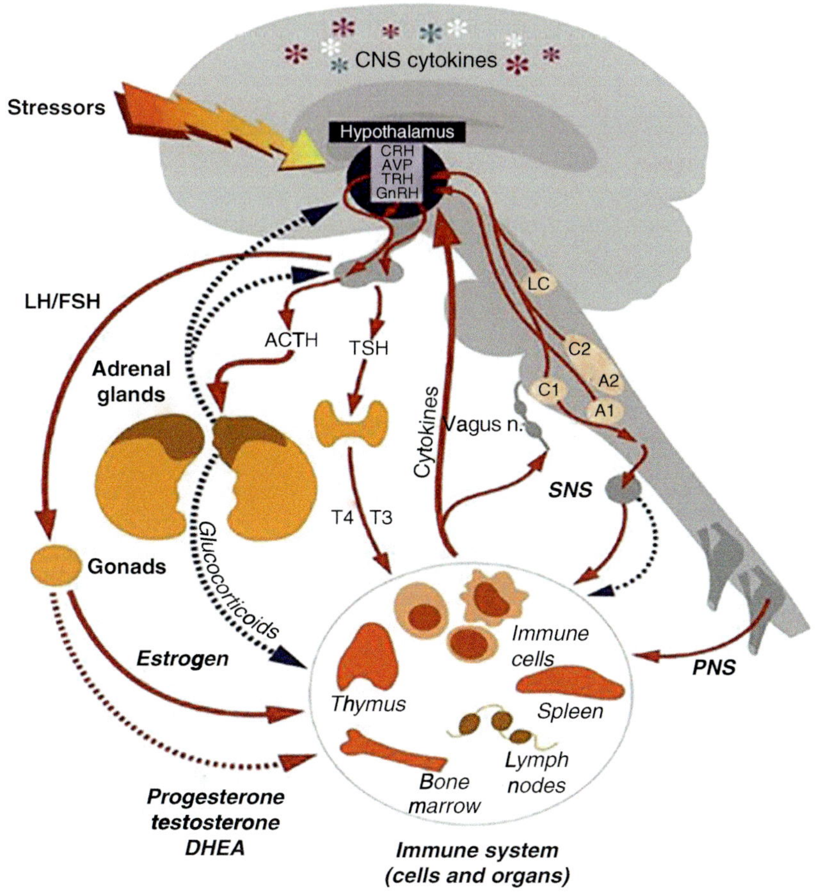


**Fig. 8.7** Bidirectional communication between the hypothalamic-pituitary axes, the P&S nervous systems, and the immune system. Hormones released by the adrenals and gonads, such as glucocorticoids and progesterone, respectively, work in parallel with neurotransmitters and neuropeptides to regulate the immune system. In turn, cytokine signaling provides stimulus or feedback to the hypothalamus to regulate the hormonal and neuronal response. Abbreviations: Broken lines represent negative regulatory pathways; solid lines represent positive regulatory pathways, A1, C1, A2, and C2, brain stem adrenergic nuclei, ACTH adrenocorticotrophic hormone, AVP arginine vasopressin, CRH corticotrophin-releasing hormone, DHEA dehydroepiandrosterone, FSH follicle-stimulating hormone, GnRH gonadotropin-releasing hormone, LC locus coeruleus, LH luteinizing hormone, PNS peripheral nervous system, SNS sympathetic nervous system, T3 triiodothyronine, T4 thyroxine, TRH thyrotropin-releasing hormone, TSH thyroid-stimulating hormone, vagus n. vagus nerve [28]. (Open Access, Society for Leukocyte Biology

been shown to modify immune cell activity by interacting with intracellular molecules. This results in a modified ability of these cells to mount a potent immune response [29].

Of course, reducing stress is the best way to reduce or prevent the effects of stress, including neurological, immune, cardiovascular, GI, psychiatric, inflammatory, and oxidative stress-related disorders. As discussed, exercise is best means of reducing stress and its effects when stress cannot be avoided. Antioxidants and anti-inflammatories, through diet and supplements, may also help to reduce the effects of stress.

## The Nervous System's Brain-Body Connections

The nervous system is often said to be infinitely complex; however, basic knowledge of human neuroscience is all that is necessary to understand how stress affects almost every aspect of the

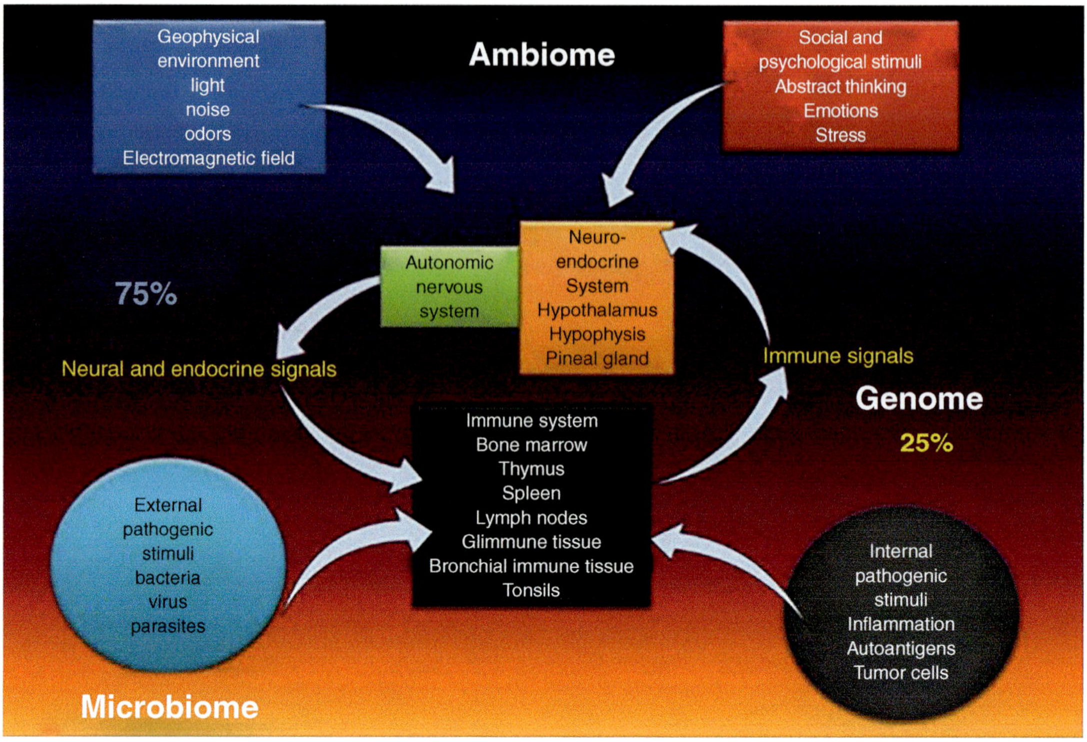


**Fig. 8.8** The nervous system communicates within the immune system via two pathways: (1) through the P&S systems, which innervates the lymph nodes, thymus, spleen, and bone marrow, and (2) through the neuroendocrine system (hypothalamus-pituitary axis and pineal gland), via the secretion of pituitary, adrenocortical, thyroid, and gonadal hormones and melatonin, thus modulating the immune response. The various cytokines initiate the communication governed by hypothalamic neurons and mediated primarily through the P&S systems. The ambiome is defined as the set of non-genetic, changing elements that surround the individual and that contribute to the development and building of the human being and therefore the state of health or the appearance of disease. The ambiome is part of the biopsychosocial-ecological reality of the individual from which the Microbiome has been extracted. The microbiome defines the set of microorganisms that are normally located in different places in the human body, in particular the digestive tract (see Fig. 3.11) [19, Fig. 1.6]. (Republished with permission from Springer International Publishing AG)

body. The brain's connection to the entire body is made up of three essential biologic "circuits":

1. *The spinal cord* is responsible for sending signals to and from the brain that involve sensation, skeletal muscle contraction, and reflexes of skeletal muscles. The ability to walk or run and the subsequent feeling of soreness in the calves and quads is mediated by electrical signals within the spinal cord.
2. *The sympathetic chain* is responsible for facilitating the proverbial "fight-or-flight" response. This neurologic "wiring" is the conduit by which the brain tells the eyes to dilate, the heart to beat faster, breathing to get rapid and shallow, skin to sweat, and redirects blood flow from the stomach and intestines to better supply the muscles that may be used to fight or to run away. If the "fight-or-flight" state persists for longer than a few minutes, it becomes difficult to focus on any one task.
3. *The parasympathetic nervous system as mediated by the vagus nerve*. Everyone would agree that situations that trigger intense sympathetic chain activation can feel decidedly unpleasant. Now, let's not get unnerved yet (no pun intended), because the third brain-body connection is carried out by the vagus nerve, which serves as the corollary[6] to sympathetic chain activation. It delivers signals that slow

[6]Yes, "corollary." The P&S nervous systems do not always work in opposition. In fact, they tend to be more synergistic, rather than oppositional.

heart rate and breathing and that rebalances blood flow, etc. This system is activated when a human is in a relaxed, contented state.

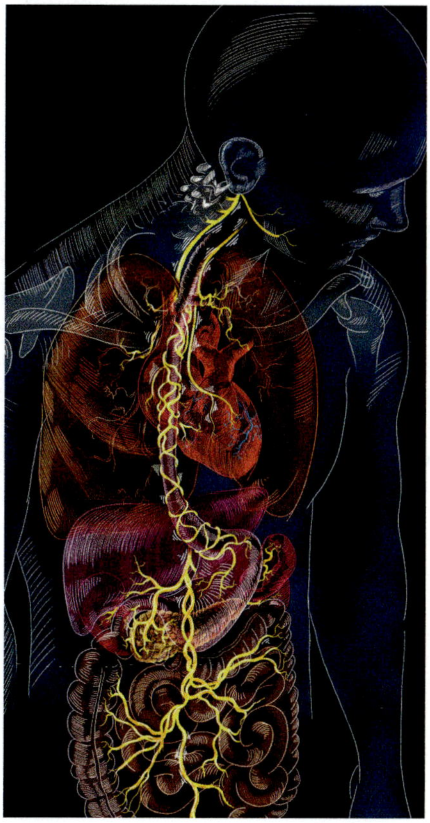

Insert: Adapted with permission from Nicolle Rager Fuller: Vagus nerve anatomy, illustration C037/4895, from https://www.sciencephoto.com/media/887799/view

In normal, non-stressful situations, the parasympathetic system (via the vagus nerve) keeps the sympathetic system in balance. Many people, especially Americans, suffer from a constant baseline of stress because their parasympathetic system is dominated by an overactive sympathetic system. This imbalance has been hypothesized to be a result of society's high expectation for achievement, communication, financial pressures, compounded by marital and social discord, or simply attributable to one's genetic makeup, or a combination of the above. Nonetheless, as innovative creatures, and over thousands of years, man has tried just about everything to achieve the reduction of anxiety and improve calmness, mood, focus, and sleep.

→*The right cerebral hemisphere* is associated with (1) holistic processing of multisensory input; (2) visual spatial skills; (3) memory stored in auditory, visual, and spatial modes; (4) remembering nonverbal material; and (5) color discrimination.

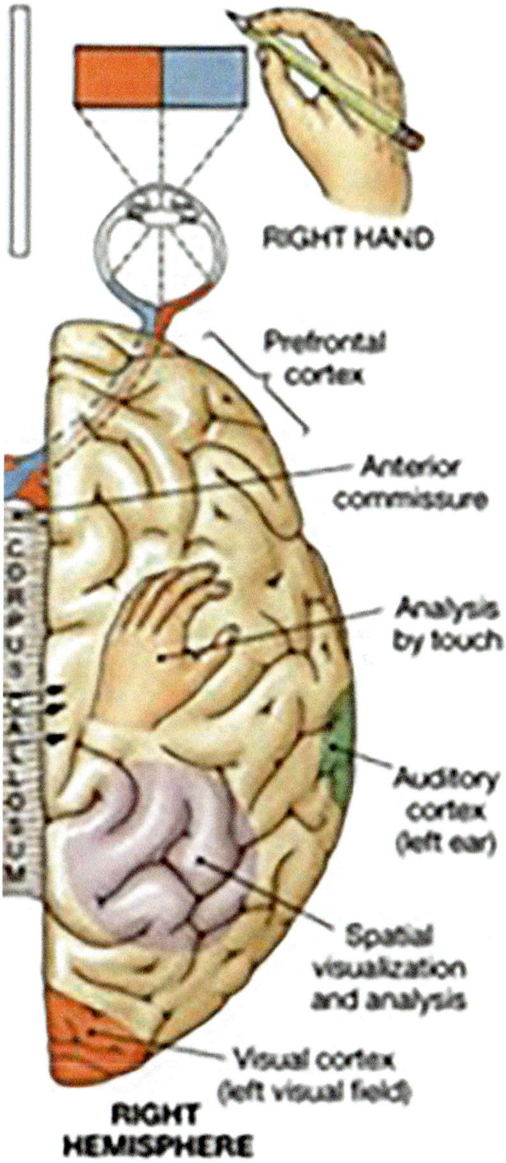


Modified with permission from C. Jones, 21 Jul 14, http://www.glooo.co.uk/blog/targetaudience-know/

←*The left cerebral hemisphere* is associated with (1) analytic and sequential thinking; (2) language, mathematics, abstraction, and reasoning; (3) ability to name objects and their attributes; and (4) memory stored in language format.

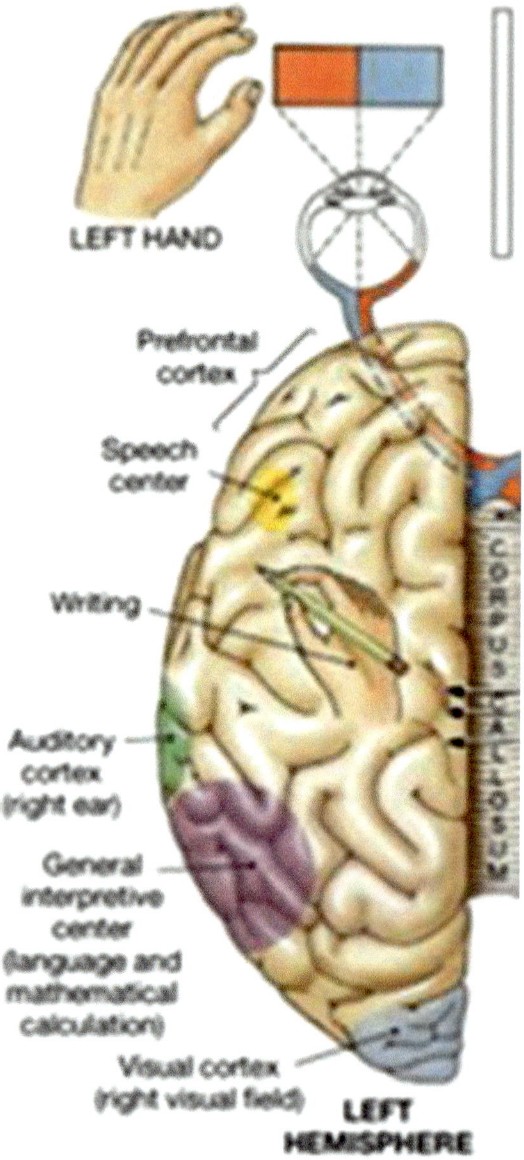


↓*The limbic system* consists of the hypothalamus, cingulated gyrus, amygdala, hippocampus, mammillary bodies, and septum. It influences endocrine and P&S nervous systems. It is connected with the brain's pleasure center (the nucleus accumbens), thereby mediating sexual arousal and the "high" from natural and chemical activities and agents. The limbic system mediates emotion through the hippocampus and stores, consolidates, and transitions short- to long-term memory. It is connected to the prefrontal cortex and is thereby related to the pleasure obtained from solving problems, etc. Stimulation of specific areas of this system can also lead to feelings of dread and anxiety and can also result in violent behaviors, including attack, defense, and explosive and emotional speech, in other words, anger.

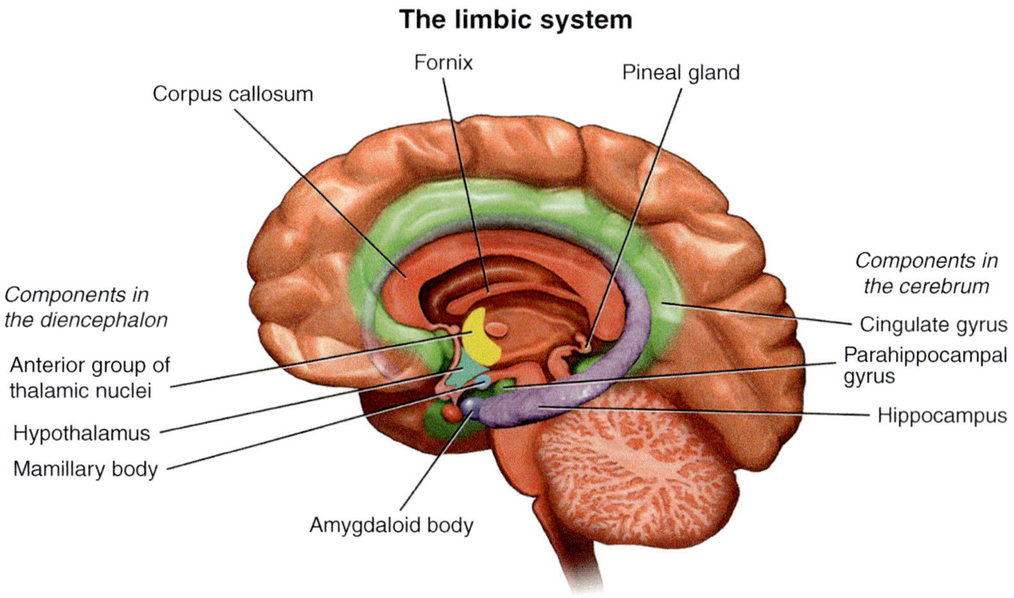


Modified with permission from Bruce Blaus: Blausen.com staff (2014); "Medical gallery of Blausen Medical 2014." WikiJournal of Medicine 1 (2). https://doi.org/10.15347/wjm/2014.010. ISSN 2002-4436. (Blausen 0614 LimbicSystem.png, 11 Feb 14); Open Access, InTech Open)

The amygdala stores emotional memory. It is involved in the sense of smell, especially as it relates to memory and the sense of danger. It sends impulses to the midbrain (e.g., for sensory integration) and brain stem (e.g., including medullary P&S nuclei), which results in the release of adrenaline and noradrenaline which may act as stress hormones. It seems to be the core of social networking and organizes and appraises history and previous interpersonal encounters. As a result, it seems to be the source of prejudice, gender bias, and "love at first sight." It colors sensory information with emotion. Psychosocial stress activates metabolic activity in the amygdala which is associated with the development of cardiovascular disease independent of traditional risk factors [16].

The hypothalamus connects the cortex to the basal ganglia, thalamus, midbrain, pons, medulla (e.g., including P&S nuclei), and spinal cord. It regulates the functioning of the pituitary gland and controls (1) autonomic nerve function and (2) major endocrine effects (e.g., water balance, appetite, and sex drive). The septal nuclei play a role in reward and reinforcement and are considered a pleasure zone. They also play a role in social behavior (play), especially in females.

The hypothalamus and amygdala include projections to the medullary brain stem P&S nuclei, thereby modulating cardiac, respiratory, vomiting, and vasomotor centers. Through these projections, the medulla mediates P&S and involuntary activities, e.g., ventilation, plasma pH, HR, and BP. BP is mediated via vasoconstriction, baroreceptor activation, the vasomotor center, and sympathetic drive (in reverse order). In the brain stem, the nucleus tractus solitarius (NTS), nucleus ambiguus (NA), and dorsal motor vagal (DMV) nucleus are important structures involved in efferent and afferent vagal (parasympathetic) activity. The nucleus of the solitary tract is a site of integration of both the afferent and efferent neural regulation of the cardiorespiratory as well as the immune systems [30, 31]. The lateral hypothalamus (lat HT) and the amygdala with the basolateral nucleus (BL) generate inhibitory control over parasympathetic structures in the brain stem during stressful events and in anxiety. To provide balance, the medial prefrontal cortex (mPFC) and the orbitofrontal cortex (OFC) facilitate vagal output and inhibit the rostral ventrolateral medulla (RVLM; see also Fig. 7.5) ([32]; (−) indicates primarily inhibitory influences; (+) indicates primarily facilitatory influences).

Vagus nerve and sympathetic nerve connections to the major organs are depicted in the insert below [33]. Finally, emotions, including anxiety, depression, anger, and love, effect thoracic and visceral organs via projections from the DMV and NA, primarily via the vagus nerve, and the projections from the NTS and RVLM, primarily via the sympathetic chain (see insert, next page).

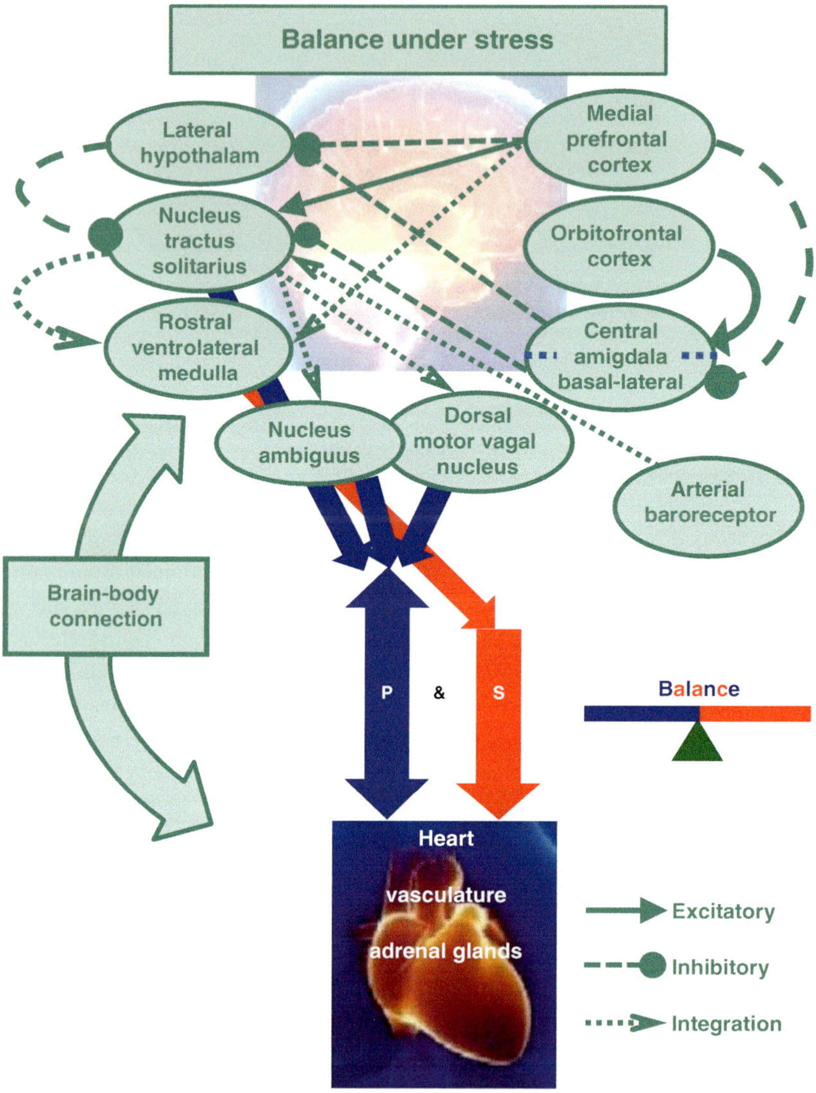

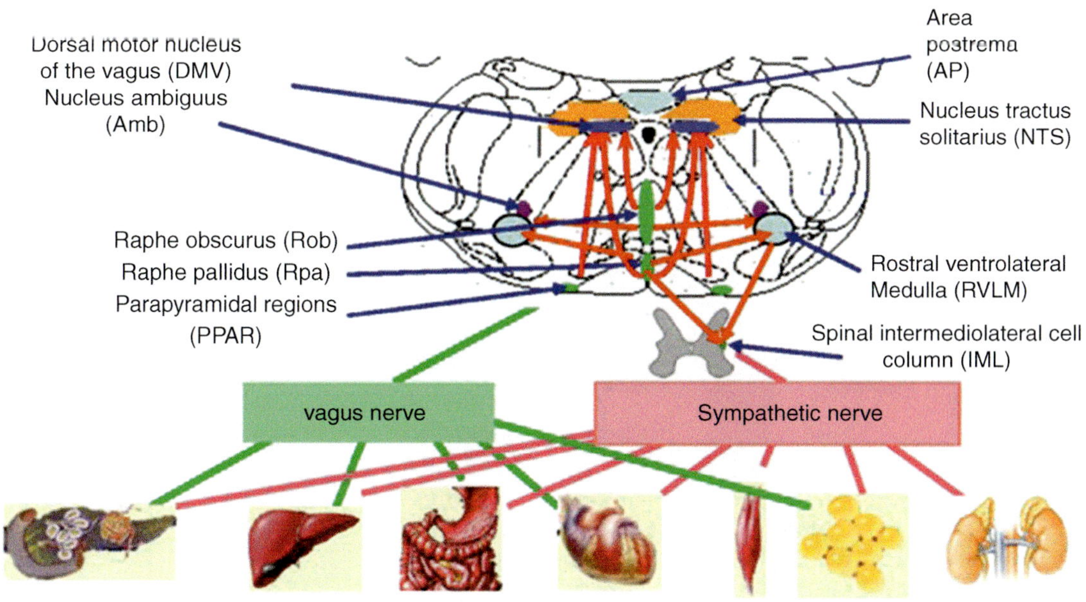


## Modulation of Parasympathetic and Sympathetic Input to the Heart

Evidence suggests that the right cerebral hemisphere is predominantly concerned with negative emotion and reactionary, sympathetic activity, whereas the left hemisphere is predominantly concerned with positive emotion and parasympathetic activity (Fig. 8.9) [34]. The parasympathetics establish the baseline around which the sympathetics react. P&S projections from the brain stem to the heart are mainly ipsilateral. There is also some degree of lateralization of the distribution of the right and left autonomic nerves on the heart. These considerations form the basis for the laterality hypothesis [35]: central neural nuclei project, via the brain stem and P&S nerves, asymmetrically on the heart. This asymmetric and inhomogeneous activation of the myocardium can become pro-arrhythmic when P&S balance is disturbed: too high, indicating sympathetic excess potentially leading to tachycardia and arrhythmia, or too low, indicating parasympathetic excess potentially leading to bradycardia and arrhythmia [36, 37].

Again, the cardiovascular consequences of chronic psychological stress have known secondary effects on cardiac function with documented pathophysiological mechanisms that more directly target cardiac performance. One example is stress-induced cardiomyopathy, including Takotsubo syndrome [38] and "Broken Heart" syndrome. All three refer to a transient left ventricular dysfunctional syndrome wherein physical or emotional stress has a major role in its pathogenesis [39, 40]. Even though many of its clinical and laboratory signs (such as chest pain, shortness of breath, and electrocardiographic and angiographic features) resemble acute coronary symptoms, atherosclerosis has no role in the pathophysiology [41]. Clinical presentation mimics acute coronary syndrome or myocardial infarction, however, during angiography, ventricular apical ballooning without significant coronary obstruction is evident.

Perimenopausal women have an extra susceptibility to Takotsubo syndrome, probably because of the role of estrogen deficiency as a participating factor in the pathogenesis. Other suggested mechanisms include acute catecholamine surges, abnormal coronary vessel reactivity that reduces myocardial microperfusion, impaired myocardial metabolism, viral infection, and endothelial dysfunction. Sympathetic excess (SE) is associated with early post-stress measurements of plasma catecholamines in afflicted patients. Evidence for a therapeutic and prophylactic role of sympathetic

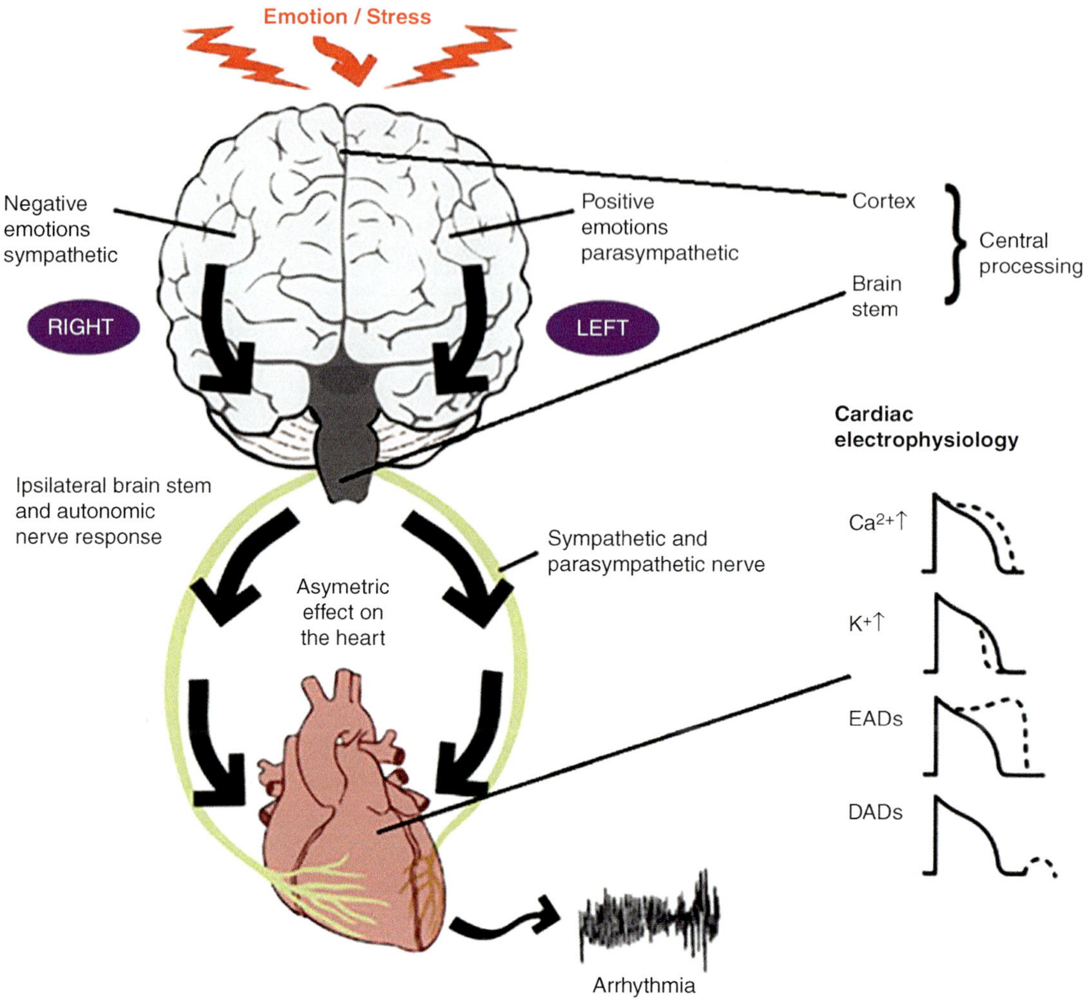


**Fig. 8.9** The right cerebral hemisphere predominantly processes negative emotion and sympathetic activity. The left hemisphere predominantly processes positive emotion and parasympathetic activity. P&S nerve traffic from the brain to the heart is mainly ipsilateral between the brain stem and heart. There is also some degree of lateralization of the distribution of the right and left autonomic nerves on the heart. This is the basis for the asymmetric central neural processing on the heart and the induction of inhomogeneous repolarization and pro-arrhythmic mechanisms [27, Fig. 2] (Open Access, Frontiers in Physiology)

blockade also highlights the role of autonomic imbalance [42]. High levels of catecholamines reduce coronary flow in the microcirculation leading to myocardial stunning [43, 44]. A higher density of adrenergic (sympathetic) receptors in apical regions of the heart has been suggested to account, in part, for ventricular dysfunction and apical ballooning [45].

Feelings of tension, frustration, and sadness double the risk of myocardial infarction in patients with coronary artery disease [46]. In 98 young patients (ages 38–60) with myocardial infarction who underwent three, single-photon, emission-computed tomography imaging (SPECT) tests at rest, those with higher levels of anger, either in reaction to an environmental stimulus or as a chronic personality character, were more prone to myocardial ischemia when exposed to mental stress [47]. Similar findings were made in an earlier 14-year study of 1328 patients with coronary heart disease where there was an inverse relationship between the degree of hostility (measured by the Cook-Medley hostility scale) and survival rates in subjects below 61 years of age [48].

In addition to ischemia, which can trigger cardiac arrhythmias, psychological stress destabilizes the myocyte membrane [49]. SE and catecholamine surges are implicated in the arrhythmogenic effects of emotional disturbance [50, 51]. Increases in catecholamine levels during human emotional turmoil are correlated with changes in HR, systolic BP, and repolarization indexes (T-wave amplitude, T-wave area, and T-wave alternans, which is a periodic beat-to-beat variation in the amplitude or shape of the ECG and is an indicator of those at high risk of developing potentially fatal cardiac arrhythmias). Ventricular parasympathetic nerves are known to have protective effect against ventricular arrhythmias [52]. It is thought that decreased parasympathetic activity (such as found in cardiovascular autonomic neuropathy) during psychological stresses (e.g., anxiety, rage, anger) would facilitate ventricular arrhythmias [53]. It should be pointed out that the situation is likely more complicated than merely considering the balance of the P&S neural regulation of cardiac function and electrical activity. For example, the role of temporal and spatial activation of various components of the P&S systems is heretofore unclear. However, evidence from the lab, with the discovery of a dynamic parasympathetic excess (PE; see "Dynamic Parasympathetic Excess"), provides an explanation for depression (the PE attribute) with a (secondary) SE that drives the ventricular dysfunction [17]. Emotions result from complex responses to external (or internal) stimuli, which activate various loci in the brain asymmetrically [54, 55], resulting in impulses that are transferred ipsilaterally and stimulate autonomic ganglions in a spatially inhomogeneous manner to elicit appropriate responses [56]. This brain-cardiovascular cross talk with its anatomical and physiological variations could partially account for the range of responses to stress in different people. Normalizing resting and dynamic P&S balance helps to maintain normal emotional responses.

## Hematologic Consequences of Stress

Disturbances in hemostasis are an important consideration in the pathogenesis of stress-induced cardiovascular disease. The balance between procoagulant and anticoagulant factor is a constantly changing process that is often skewed in many pathological conditions. Enhanced prothrombotic states have long been described in the fight-or-flight response [56]. This primitive response protects animals from hemorrhage in cases of accidental trauma. However, repetitive and prolonged stress in association with endothelial dysfunction outweighs the counteracting anticoagulant system and can potentially lead to thrombus formation [57, 58]. Heightened coagulation is linked to stress-induced, adverse cardiovascular disease.

The brain's perception and interpretation of a stressful situation is likely to initiate hypercoagulopathy. Hemodynamic parameters, catecholamine levels, and D-dimer changes all correlate with stress appraisal; moreover, anticipation of a higher amount of stress or a more challenging situation induced greater levels of fibrin turnover [59]. The relationship between stress perception and coagulation cascade, as a risk factor for cardiovascular disease, has also been confirmed by studies showing higher serotonin sensitivity of platelets in depressed and anxious individuals [60, 61]. Both human platelet serotonin uptake sites and brain serotonin transporter proteins originate from the same gene [62], suggesting an active interplay between the brain and blood coagulation system mediated by serotonin [63]. Age, gender, integrity of cardiovascular system, and socioeconomic status are participating factors in this interplay, as the elderly [64], males [65], those with lower socioeconomic status [65], and also those with a history of coronary heart disease or hypertension [66, 67] are at increased risk for having a higher procoagulant activity for extended periods of time. Inversely, a state of happiness blunts the stress-induced fibrinogen response, irrespective of age, gender, socioeconomic status, body mass, and smoking [68].

Another explanation for a heightened coagulatory status could be SE [69]. There is a solid body of evidence that support this notion. For instance, infusion of adrenaline increases blood levels of factor VIII, von Willebrand factor antigen, tissue type plasminogen activator, and platelet levels within 15–40 min. Platelets and endothelial adrenoceptors have essential roles in these reactions [70]. Stimulation of endothelial β-receptors releases factor VIII, von Willebrand factor, and tissue plasminogen activator. Catecholamines also adjust coagulation by affecting hepatic clearance of these factors [70, 71]. Chemical sympathetic blockade with 6-hydroxydopamine prevents stress-induced pro-thrombotic enhancement [72].

Increased ratio of blood cells and macromolecules to plasma volume (hemoconcentration) is another potential participant that hastens stress-induced pro-coagulatory status [73]. The resultant excess viscosity increases endothelial shear stress and raises the probability of rupturing atherosclerotic plaques [73]. SE of any type is also implicated as a major cause, since the increased systolic and diastolic BP resulting from SE causes plasma to move from the intravascular space, while there is retention of blood cells and proteins in the vascular lumen [74]. This phenomenon could occur during stress-induced hypercoagulopathy, although de novo synthesis or activation of coagulation factors cannot be ruled out [74].

Cortisol levels are the most reliable indicators of hypothalamic-pituitary-adrenal (HPA) activity and have been measured in urine, saliva, serum, and hair [75]. There is an abrupt surge in the plasma cortisol levels following acute stress, which then returns to baseline values after removal of stress [76]. Intense chronic stressful conditions abolish physiological diurnal variations of cortisol secretion and lead to a high-steady-state value [77]. Assessment of salivary cortisol is arguably the most useful method to measure stress levels since it represents 70% of free (unbound form) plasma cortisol levels and is not influenced by salivary volume and flow [78]. Salivary production is controlled by the autonomic nervous system; the amount and composition of saliva is expected to change during the course of psychological disturbances. Sampling of saliva does not induce pain or stress, and because of the stability of cortisol in saliva, samples can be kept at room temperature for up to 4 weeks [79]. Transfer of cortisol from blood to saliva is a fast process (2–3 min); therefore, this method can detect acute variations in blood levels and circadian rhythm [79].

Inflammatory cytokines such as IL-6, TNF-α, and CRP have been used as nonspecific markers of stress in epidemiologic studies. Inflammation is mediated by the autonomic nervous system. Many adverse effects of psychological disorders, including endothelial dysfunction and an overactivity of the inflammatory systems, have been related to alterations to the circulating profile of cytokines [80, 81]. For instance, early childhood abuse in girls increases the risk of diabetes and cardiovascular diseases, possibly through immune and chronic inflammatory dysregulation associated with SE [82]. Increased levels of erythrocyte sedimentation ratio and CRP, as nonspecific markers of systemic inflammation, occur in depressed patients [83]. In a study of 199 women at different stages of breast cancer, 10 weeks of cognitive behavioral stress management downregulated anxiety-induced expression of pro-inflammatory cytokines in circulating leukocytes [84].

The exact mechanism(s) and source(s) of cytokine production during stressful situations remain to be elucidated. One proposed mechanism is suppression or dysregulation of the parasympathetic nervous system. Stimulation of the efferent branch of the vagus nerve diminishes cytokine production from macrophages and other immune cells via stimulation of nicotinic receptors. This anti-inflammatory effect of acetylcholine may be blunted in stressed people who have sympathetic overactivity [85]. Another putative mechanism is the stimulatory role of angiotensin II on immune cells leading to the production of inflammatory mediators [86, 87]. Some evidence reiterates the critical role of adipose tissue in the induction of inflammation; this raises the possible role of adipose tissue as an important source of pro-inflammatory cytokines in depression [88].

As mental stress boosts the pro-inflammatory state, one can expect a skew in the oxidative-antioxidant balance that favors the generation of free radicals. For instance, increased levels of homocysteine and CRP (two markers of inflammation) during psychological stresses escalate the production of ROS [89, 90]. Psychological stress also activates NF-κB, which in turn induces a pro-oxidative state [91]. Mental stress activated NF-κB within 10 min in a group of healthy volunteers; this stimulation was proportional to the levels of stress hormones (cortisol, catecholamines, etc.) released and returned to basal levels within 60 min after removal of stress [92]. Increased oxidative stress augmented sensitivity to lipid oxidation and elevated plasma antioxidant status [93]. Stress reduces social interaction and enhances anxiety-originated behavior in the submissive individual. Similarly, heroin addiction and deafness also reduces social interaction which is associated with increased morbidity and mortality risk including increased MACE (i.e., myocardial infarction, sudden cardiac death, and stroke) risk.

## Emotion and Sudden Arrhythmic Death

There is documented evidence of people dying almost immediately following highly charged emotional events [94, 95]. Population studies have shown an increase in the incidence of sudden death at times of heightened psychological stress such as natural disasters or wars [96–99]. Studies show that emotion influences the ease of arrhythmia induction and termination [100] and of ventricular repolarization known to be important in arrhythmogenesis [101–105]. It is generally considered that both the spatial and temporal patterns of P&S inputs to the heart together with altered myocardial electrophysiology due to disease are risk factors. These P&S inputs are influenced by, and convey, central neural processing of emotions [106, 107] (Fig. 8.10).

Considering the brain and heart as an interactive unit, emotional generation of ventricular arrhythmias is due to (1) the electrophysiological changes occurring in the myocardium as a result of P&S nerve stimulation, (2) the modulatory role of P&S nerves which attempt to balance each other, and (3) central neural processing of emotional input and afferent input from the heart and vasculature. Sympathetic nerve stimulation acting through β-adrenergic receptors influences the heart, including an increase in inward $Ca^{++}$ current ($I_{ca}$; see insert below [27, Fig. 3]) and a decrease in outward potassium ($K^{-}$) current ($I_k$), thereby tending to lengthen and shorten action potential duration and refractoriness, respectively. Sympathetic stimulation favors the formation of both early after depolarizations (EAD) and delayed after depolarizations (DAD). These effects may be pro-arrhythmic as a result of triggered activity or modulation of refractoriness (Fig. 8.9).

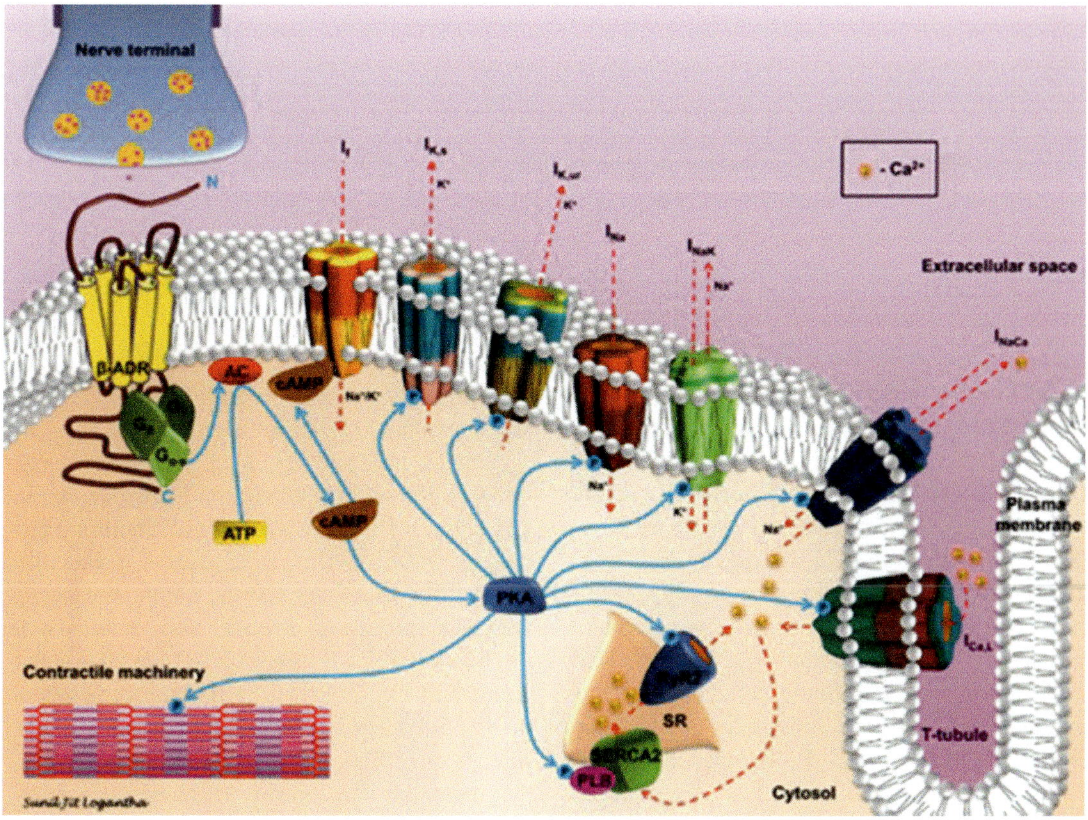


Insert: Open Access, Frontiers in Physiology

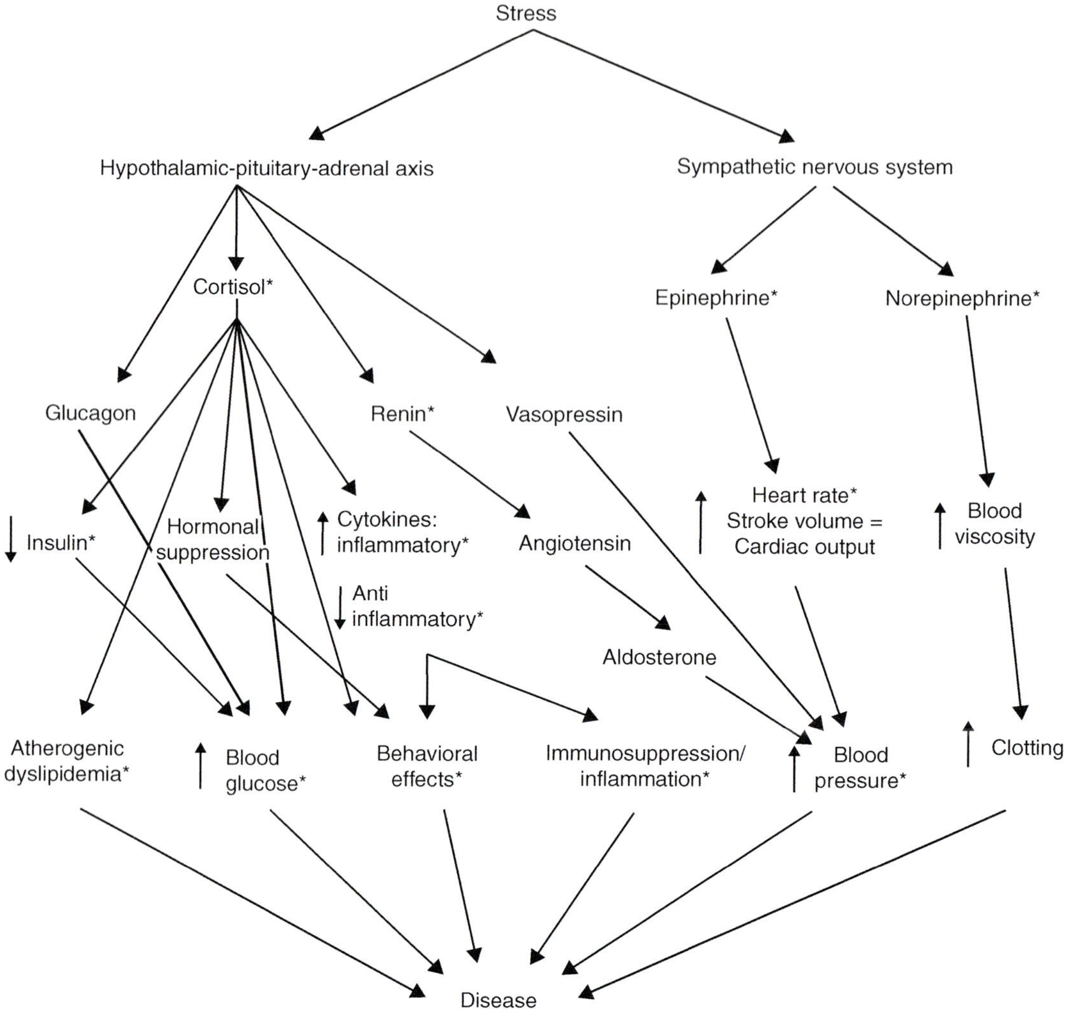


**Fig. 8.10** The impact of stress on the hypothalamic-pituitary-adrenal (HPA) axis and the sympathetic nervous system. *Yoga has been shown to have significant beneficial effects in these items [108] (Open Access, International Journal of Preventative Medicine)

Historically, it has been believed that enhanced sympathetic stimulation is pro-arrhythmic, while enhanced parasympathetic activity is protective [109, 110]. These are generally correct for resting measures of P&S activity and corroborated by others more recently [111–113] (e.g., Fig. 8.11). Depressed parasympathetic activity is the definition of CAN and is a risk factor for ventricular fibrillation and sudden death [37, 52–114, 115]. The clinical anti-arrhythmic benefits of stellate ganglion section and β-adrenergic blockade are well known [116, 117]. P&S balance is not a simple see-saw effect as co-activation also occurs [118–120] and often underlies difficult to manage conditions, as well as anxiety, ADD/ADHD, and unexplained arrhythmia or seizure [18].

A wide range of asymmetric behavior exists between left and right cerebral hemispheres [35, 121] (Fig. 8.10). Lateralization of emotional processing in the cortex is conveyed ipsilaterally through the brain stem to the autonomic nerves which in turn are distributed asymmetrically in the heart (Figs. 8.12 and 8.13 [122] for sympathetic and Fig. 8.14 [123] for parasympathetic innervation). An increase in the naturally occurring spatial inhomogeneity of repolarization facilitates the development of reentrant arrhythmias [124]. The autonomic nerves from the left

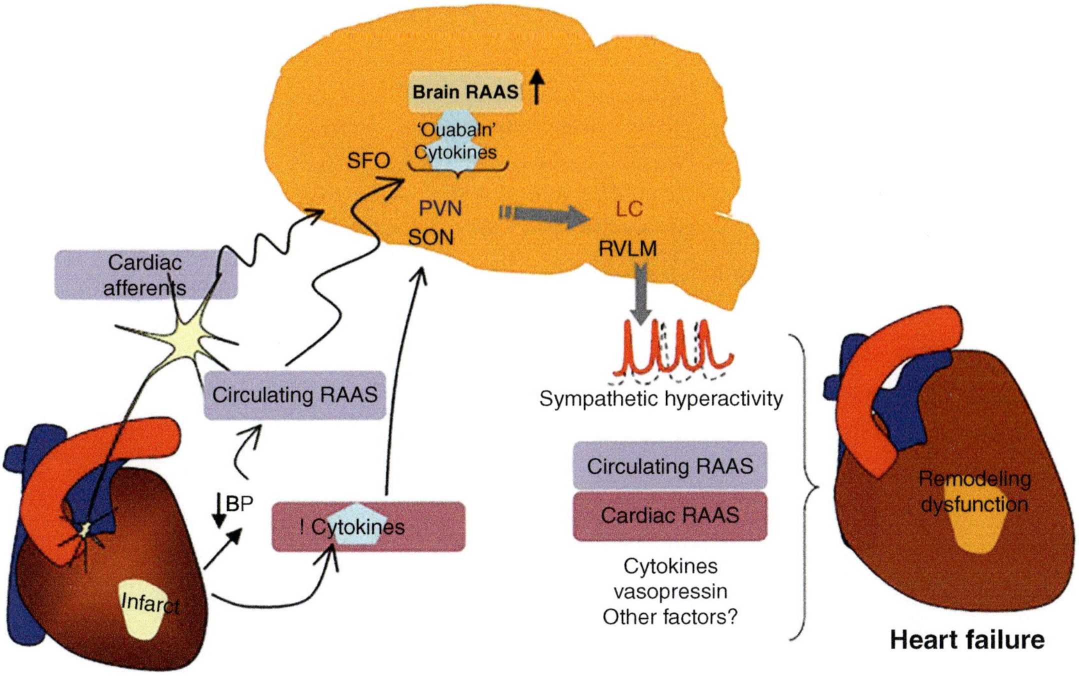


**Fig. 8.11** Brain mechanisms contributing to sympathetic hyperactivity and heart failure. Mechanisms leading to post MI activation of the central nervous system, the major systems and nuclei activated in the CNS, and the subsequent activation of peripheral mechanisms contributing to progressive cardiac remodeling and dysfunction are depicted [112]. Abbreviations: LC locus coeruleus, PVN paraventricular nucleus, RAAS renin-angiotensin-aldosterone system, RVLM rostral ventrolateral medulla, SFO subfornical organ, SON supraoptic nucleus. (Republished with permission from American Heart Association, Circulation Research)

and right cortical hemispheres are asymmetrically distributed over the ventricles. Functional autonomic asymmetry exists in response to selective autonomic nerve stimulation, with a trend for left-sided neural innervation of the posteroinferior aspect and left ventricle and right-sided neural innervation of the anterior aspect and right ventricle, albeit with substantial overlap [125–127]. Stimulation of individual stellate ganglion nerve branches selectively influences specific regions of the myocardium [128]. Nerves which have been interrupted by ischemia or infarction may undergo nerve sprouting, resulting in patchy areas of hyperinnervation [129–131]. These processes promote electrophysiological inhomogeneity as a result of inhomogeneous autonomic effects and facilitate arrhythmogenesis.

Several reflexes exist which regulate autonomic efferent input to the heart in response to afferent information from mechano- or chemoreceptors in the myocardium, thoracic blood vessels, and lungs. In general, high SB,[7] which indicates a relative, resting, sympathetic excess (SE), is a pro-arrhythmic state, whereas low SB, which indicates a relative, resting, parasympathetic excess (PE), may also be a resting state that is pro-arrhythmic. In patients at risk for arrhythmia due to heart disease or cardiovascular autonomic neuropathy (CAN), low-normal SB, a parasympathetic dominant state (but not excessive) is a resting state that is known to be anti-arrhythmic (protective of the heart) [18, 37–52, 132]. In other words, too much parasympathetic activity (low SB or PE) promotes arrhythmia, whereas a proper amount of parasympathetic activity (low-normal SB) is protective and promotes wellness.

[7] Sympathovagal balance is the ratio of resting sympathetic activity to resting parasympathetic activity (SB = S/P). High SB indicates a resting sympathetic excess (SE, relative to resting parasympathetic activity). Low SB indicates a resting parasympathetic excess (PE, relative to resting sympathetic activity).

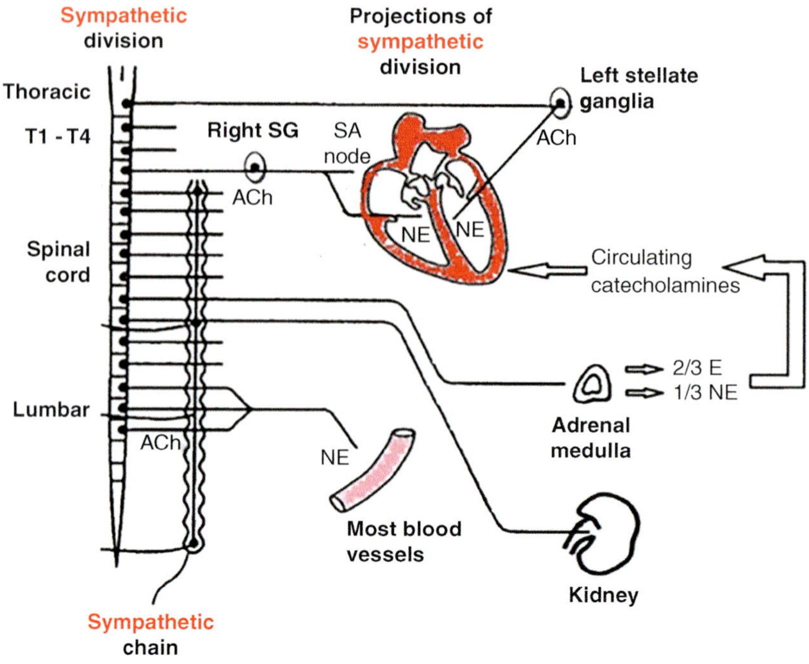


**Fig. 8.12** Cardiac sympathetic control [122] (see Fig. 8.13, below, for details of left and right stellate cardiac innervation). Abbreviations: ACh acetylcholine, E epinephrine, NE norepinephrine, SG stellate ganglion

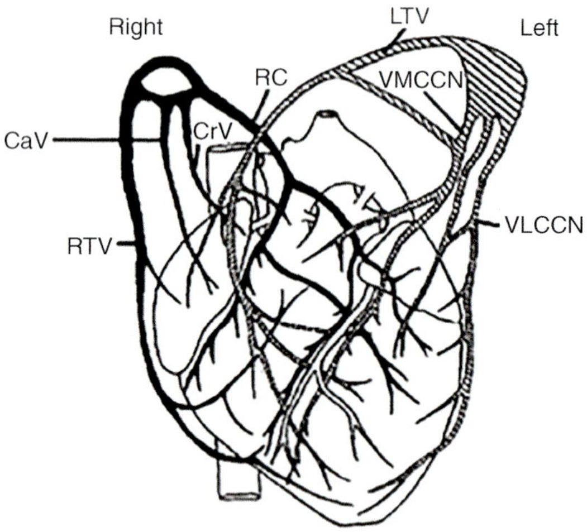


**Fig. 8.13** Sympathetic stellate control of the heart [122]. Abbreviations: CaV caudovagal N., CrV craniovagal N., LTV left thoracic vagus N., RC recurrent cardiac N., RTV right thoracic vagus N., VLCCN ventrolateral cervical cardiac N., VMCCN ventromedial cervical cardiac N. (Republished with permission from American Heart Association, Circulation Research)

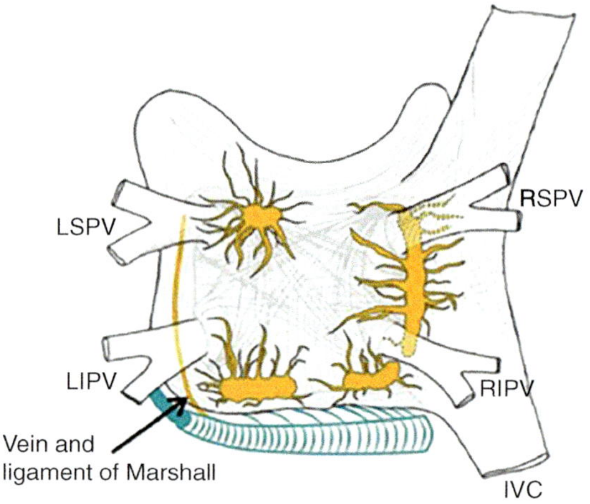


**Fig. 8.14** Purported parasympathetic innervation of the heart [123]. Abbreviations: IVC inferior vena cava, LIPV left inferior pulmonary vein, LSPV left superior pulmonary vein, RIPV right inferior pulmonary vein, RSPV right superior pulmonary vein. (Republished with permission from Elsevier)

As indicated, these are all resting states. In the dynamic states, P&S dysfunction is also pro-arrhythmic. If there is a dynamic autonomic imbalance, arrhythmia may be induced. Dynamic SEs are well known as pro-arrhythmic, as well as pro-stroke and pro-aneurism states. Dynamic PEs may also be pro-arrhythmic states and tend to occur postprandially, in preparation for sleep, or after exercise (especially in the shower, as compounded by the stimulus of heated water). There is also a hidden, dynamic PE. It is hidden behind a sympathetic challenge. It results in a SE that is pro-arrhythmic, as above; however, typically, these cases include both SE symptoms (high BP) and PE symptoms (with depression). When these cases are treated as a primary sympathetic excess, the patient does not respond as expected (seems to be non-compliant) and becomes more unstable in their response to disease. However, when treated as a primary PE and PE is normalized, the patient stabilizes, then it follows that SE is normalized, and the arrhythmia risk is reduced, along with lower BPs and HRs. This progression is natural, often without the need of further (SE) therapy. Since the parasympathetics set the response threshold for the sympathetics, by reducing the (dynamic) PE, the threshold is reduced, and the sympathetic response is thereby normalized and prevented from becoming excessive (SE) and a "trigger" for arrhythmia.

A mechanism for sympathetic stimulation turning pro-arrhythmic is through the stimulation of β-adrenergic receptors. This pathway in fact provides many pro-arrhythmic mechanisms. For example, the baroreflex [see insert below, 133] is mediated through the sympathetic nervous system and modulates sympathovagal balance (SB) and the net autonomic input to the heart. Baroreflex is typically in response to central pressure or volume changes, leading to deformation of the aortic and carotid baroreceptors, and is a means of maintaining homeostasis. As another example, mechanical or chemical stimulation of the posteroinferior aspect of the left ventricle may result in enhanced parasympathetic activity, while stimulation of the anterior aspect may induce enhanced sympathetic activity [134–136]. Afferent-efferent feedback loops interact with the vasomotor center in the medulla oblongata and higher brain centers. In patients with heart disease, mental and physical stress caused a right-lateralized shift in dorsal pons and midbrain activity [137] associated with enhanced sympathetic drive to the heart and potentially pro-arrhythmic changes in cardiac repolarization. This explains a stress-related lateralized relay between cortex and heart.

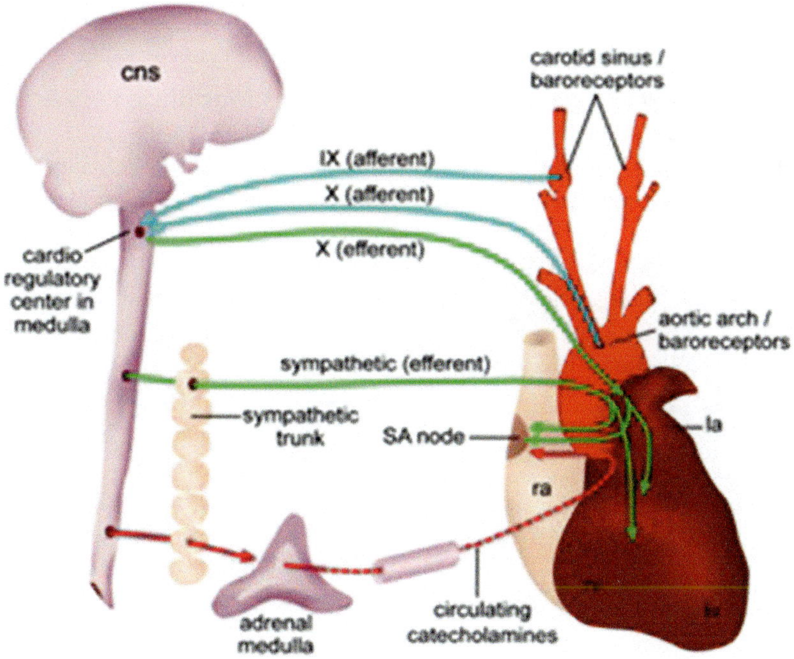

The atria are richly innervated by ganglionic plexi and sympathovagal nerve tracts. Pulmonary vein activity responsible for triggering and potentially maintaining atrial fibrillation (AFib) can be increased by both vagal (parasympathetic) and sympathetic stimulation [138]. For example, vagally mediated AFib usually occurs at night during a period of bradycardia. In response to the bradycardia, the sympathetics are activated which may lead to AFib as a result of increased pulmonary vein ectopic firing. Vagus nerve projections (see insert, right) from the hypothalamus area of the brain to the heart, diaphragm, and viscera subserve atria and visceral activity. It wraps around the heart and solar plexus center and is very involved with feelings and thinking. Healing and even learning are extraordinarily difficult when the vagus nerve is disturbed. Clinically, stress (a sympathetic stimulus[8]) has been shown to be associated with an increased incidence of lone AFib, when in combination with increased caffeine consumption (also a sympathetic stimulus) and a type A personality (a state of sympathetic dominance, typically indicated as a high SB) [139–141]. For example, recent stress, high coffee intake, and obesity (another possible high SB condition) were associated with greater risk of AFib. The three conditions each cause a possible sympathetic dominance, compounding each other, so that the net is a sympathetic excess (SE) state that is pro-arrhythmic. Type A individuals are more likely to be hypercholesterolemic and have high levels of circulating catecholamines with diminished mononuclear leukocyte β-adrenergic receptor function. This creates a pro-arrhythmic autonomic milieu (high SB). In vulnerable atria, this is itself a trigger, particularly if there has been a degree of electrophysiological remodeling in the myocardium following prolonged episodes of AFib with resultant shortening of action potential duration and fibrosis to maintain reentrant wavelet activity.

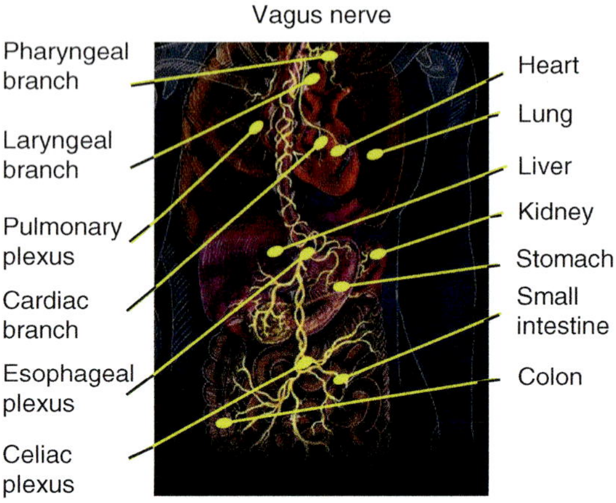


Insert: Open Access, Springer Link; Adapted with permission from Nicolle Rager Fuller: Vagus nerve anatomy, illustration C037/4895, from https://www.sciencephoto.com/media/887799/view; Open Access, Elsevier

## Emotions Modulate P&S Activity

Emotions impact the P&S and, thereby, arrhythmogenesis in several ways including altered SB, alterations in the spatial distribution of autonomic input to the heart, and by causing coronary arterial vasoconstriction and ischemia. It is a popular belief that increased emotional stress equates with adrenaline release and sympathetic activation. However, this is an oversimplification, and some emotions appear to be associated with parasympathetic activity (i.e., "Broken Heart" syndrome). The issue of whether different emotions are associated with different patterns of autonomic activity and different cortical representations is an ongoing debate [142, 143]. Anger is the most common emotion precipitating ventric-

[8]Chronic stress is a chronic sympathetic stimulus and results in high SB, indicating resting sympathetic dominance, potentiating a pro-arrhythmic state. Acute stress is an acute sympathetic stimulus that does not result in long-term high SB, indicating chronic SE. However, the acute sympathetic stimulus can be "the straw that broke the camel's back" and may trigger an arrhythmia if SB is high to begin with, due to other reasons (i.e., diabetes, sleep apnea, hypertension, anxiety, etc.).

ular arrhythmia [144, 145]. For example, in patients with cardioverter defibrillators (ICD), the state of anger occurred significantly more frequently in periods prior to ICD shocks than during control periods. In contrast, this was not observed for the incidence of anxiety, worry, sadness, happiness, feeling in control, or being interested. The greater arrhythmogenic effect of anger could be due to either engaging specific properties of the autonomic nerves [146–150] or simply due to eliciting a greater arousal response.

Anger and other stresses are associated with both increased plasma catecholamines [151] and decreased vagal activity [152]. Episodes of anger promote greater increases in sympathetic activity compared with other emotions [149, 150]. Anger-induced T-wave alternans (see insert, below [145]) in laboratory testing in patients with implantable cardiac devices are found to be predictive of future arrhythmic events, suggesting that emotion-induced repolarization instability is one mechanism linking emotion and sudden death [105]. Anger-triggered ventricular arrhythmias in patients with ICDs are more likely to be pause dependent and polymorphic, suggesting that anger may create a substrate for more disorganized rhythms [153]. Even anger recall in patients mainly with cardioverter defibrillators during noninvasive electrophysiology studies can make ventricular arrhythmias easier to induce and more difficult to terminate [100].

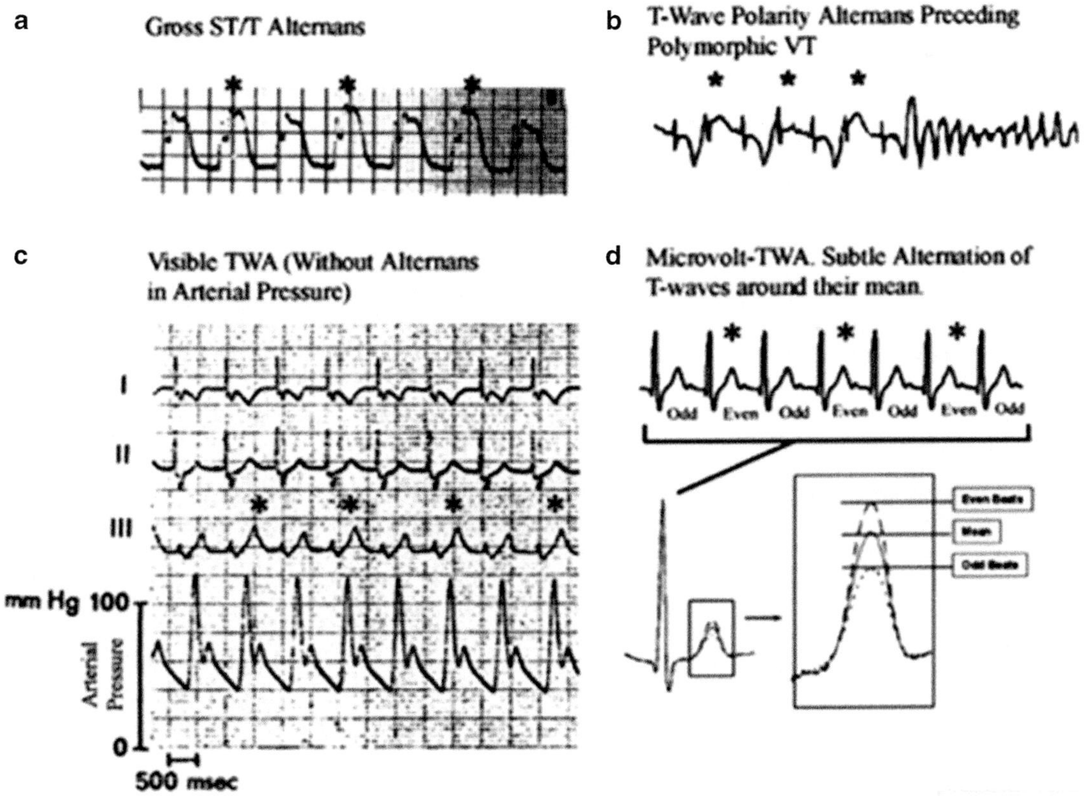

Using the high-frequency component (HF-HRV) as a measure of parasympathetic activity, anger recall was associated with an increase in resting HR, but no change in resting HF-HRV, suggesting a relative increase in resting sympathetic activity[9]. In contrast fear, happiness, and sadness were associated with an increase in resting HR but a decrease in resting HF-HRV, suggesting an overall decrease in resting parasympathetic activity, or an increase in SB. This is in keeping with a reduction in resting vagal tone reported in patients with panic attacks [154]. A reduction in resting vagal tone causes an increase in sympathovagal balance which is a relative increase in resting sympathetic tone. More recently, P&S monitoring[10] has shown that panic attacks (anxiety) are also associated with a dynamic PE in response to (a sympathetically mediated) stress (either Valsalva or stand challenge in the P&S clinical study[11]) [18].

Early studies using ambulatory ECG recordings reported substantial increases in HR during a range of real-life stressful situations: road car driving induced HRs in the region of 90–100 bpm, the more intense mental challenge of public speaking induced HRs in the region of 130 bpm, and the extreme stresses of parachute jumping and racing car driving induced HRs between 140 and 180 bpm [155]. These observations are in accord with the popular belief that mental stress is associated with increases in HR. However, subjects undergoing dental procedures or watching violence on movies have been shown to develop HR slowing despite feeling highly stressed, with concomitant increases in circulating levels of catecholamines [155]. These observations are associated with a complex interplay between the P&S nervous systems in response to different types of emotional input, including the possibility of an underlying ("hidden") PE causing a simultaneous, secondary SE. This apparent dichotomy is well documented and explained by P&S monitoring. Some of the mechanisms involved in stress-induced cardiovascular adverse effects are summarized in Fig. 8.15 [156].

## Stress, Emotions, the Vagus Nerve, and Inflammation

Higher cortical centers that mediate emotions involve brain stem P&S centers (e.g., nucleus tractus solitarius; see Fig. 8.16 [157]) that project P&S nerves to the heart, immune system (mediating inflammation[12]; see insert below [158, Fig. 2]), and elsewhere (e.g., GI system, which is

[9]Even with the assumptions and approximations required by HRV (alone) analyses, in the cases of angry patients, the changes in the HF-HRV term is likely to be an indicator of relative changes in parasympathetic activity. The reason is that anger tends to cause an increased respiratory rate, which may be assumed to be high enough to cause the parasympathetic activity to be fully represented by the HF-HRV term, leaving no parasympathetic activity to be represented by the LF-HRV term. It is an indication of relative changes because the HF-HRV term still includes "noise."

[10]P&S monitoring is a spectral analysis, signal processing technique that enables independent, simultaneous measurements of both P&S nervous systems' activities, without the assumptions and approximations required by HRV (alone) analyses [18].

[11]The Valsalva challenge is a series of short Valsalva maneuvers that are each kept to less than or equal to 15 seconds to prevent the parasympathetic cascade that is the hallmark of long Valsalva maneuvers. As taught in medical school, long Valsalva maneuvers are strong parasympathetic stimuli, which they absolutely are, but if terminated prior to 15 seconds or so, they remain only (net) sympathetic stimuli.

The stand challenge is a net sympathetic stimulus, where the parasympathetics normally decrease and then the sympathetics normally increase.

[12]Like oxygen and water, inflammation is beneficial to the body in appropriate amounts. Acute inflammation helps with the immune and healing (repair) processes. Chronic inflammation, however, is never good. Chronic inflammation is acute inflammation that lasts too long or is not deactivated by the parasympathetics.

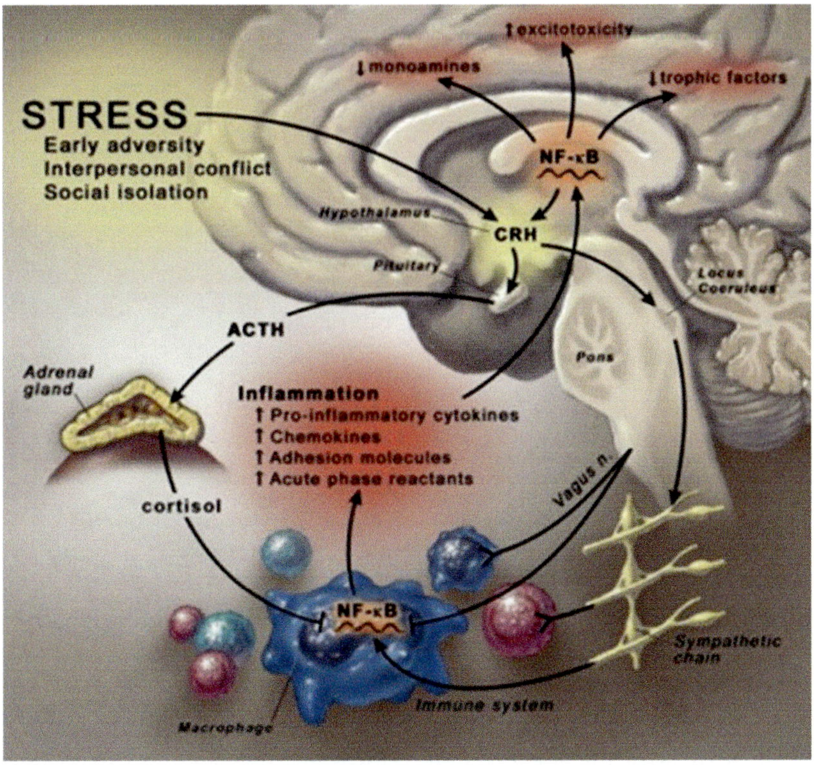


the projection responsible for "butterflies" in the stomach during certain emotions). Inflammation is intimately connected to all the major diseases of the current era, reducing QoL, shortening lives, and causing pain on a persistent daily basis (including the various forms of arthritis) [159, 160]. The vagus nerve, connecting the brain to the body, is an anti-inflammatory neural circuit that mediates the body's cytokine production and thereby inflammatory response. The parasympathetics set the metabolic threshold around which the sympathetics respond. In this way, the sympathetics modulate the inflammatory responses as part of an immune or injury response. Persistently and abnormally elevated parasympathetic activity during the stress response may maintain persistently elevated sympathetic responses, prolonging the inflammatory response. If parasympathetic, and thereby sympathetic, responses become chronically elevated, then the beneficial, acute inflammatory response becomes chronic and harmful, compounded by "cytokine storms" which may also increase mortality risk. If the injury is in the brain, chronic inflammation in the brain diverts immune resources from the body, putting the body at risk, thereby raising mortality risk. Breathing exercises, yoga, and emotional and mental frameworks (including both positive and negative states of mind) influence the immune system via the vagus nerve (and thereby influencing the rest of the organs and systems of the body).

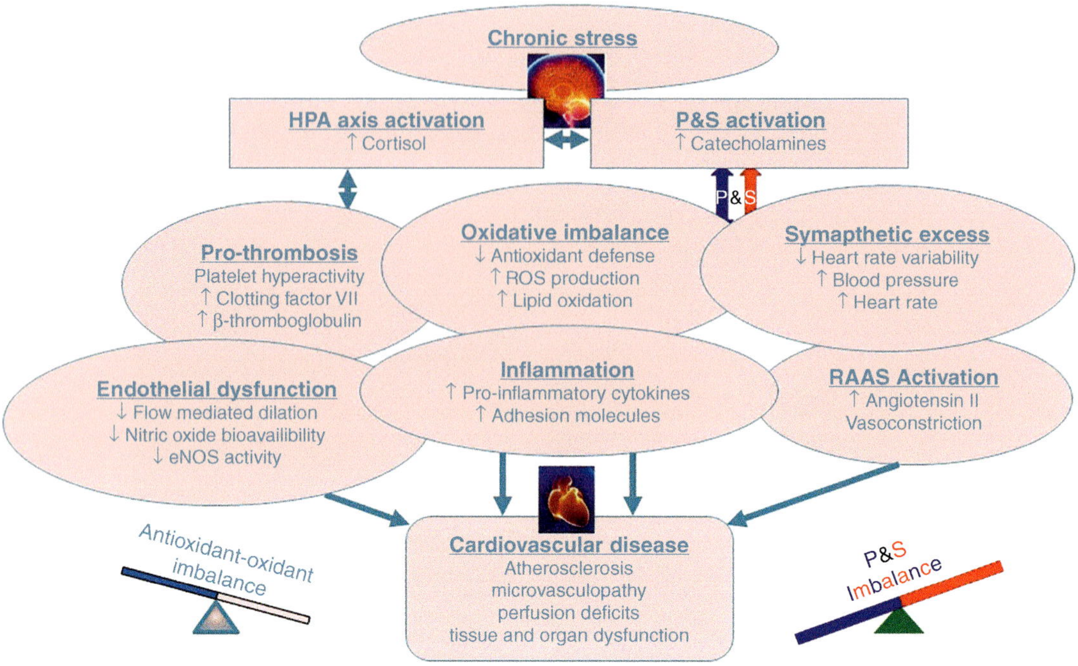


**Fig. 8.15** Figure 5.28 is repeated here for convenience. Some of the mechanisms involved in stress-induced cardiovascular adverse effects. Note that many of these mechanisms involve the other prongs of the Mind-Body Program and are the reasons why no one prong is superior or inferior to the others. All are needed, working together to maintain health and wellness. To that end psychosocial stress reduction and stress reduction in general are therapies that are included in the Program. In the figure above, while they are shown as separate systems, the adrenal part of the HPA axis is associated with the sympathetic nervous system, the RAAS system is a component of the sympathetic nervous system, and inflammation and oxidative stress are direct consequences of sympathetic activation. Of course, prolonged sympathetic activation turns these helpful processes into harmful processes. Abbreviations: HPA hypothalamic-pituitary-adrenal, RAAS renin-angiotensin-aldosterone system, ROS reactive oxygen species, eNOS endothelial nitric oxide (NO) synthase [156])

Regardless of the location, vagally mediated acetylcholine (which has a role in learning and memory, including "gut brain" learning and memory) mediates inflammation. The abnormal vagal (or parasympathetic) state is outlined above. Under normal, healthy, and well conditions, increases in vagal activity decrease sympathetic activity, thereby reducing or ending the immune response and vice versa. Reducing or ending the immune response by lowering sympathetic activity also reduces stress and relaxes the body and the mind. The "inflammatory reflex" is a neurological mechanism involving the vagus nerve which senses inflammation and transmits this information to the brain stem. The brain stem in turn transmits, via the vagus efferents, information to the spleen (where pro-inflammatory cytokine production is inhibited) and white blood cells (lymphocytes or T cells) (Fig. 8.16). Splenic lymphocytes (T cells) also produce acetylcholine, further reducing the production of pro-inflammatory cytokines by activating macrophages. Acetylcholine from splenic lymphocytes interacts with α7-nicotinic acetylcholine receptors expressed on cytokine producing macrophages. Intracellular signal transduction through this receptor inhibits the activity of nuclear factor-κB to suppress cytokine production.

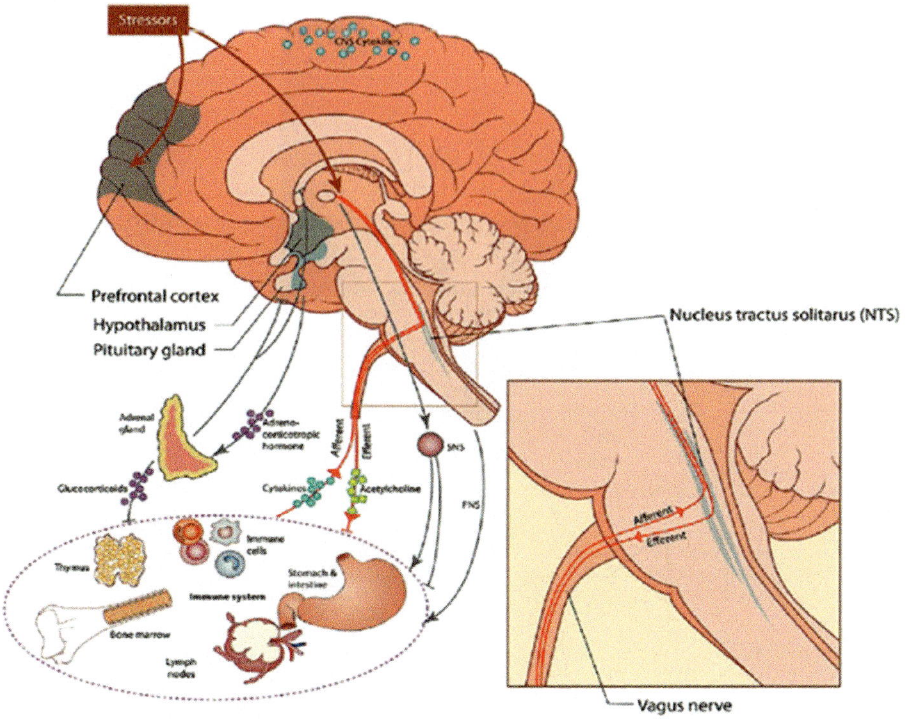


**Fig. 8.16** Connections of brain stem P&S centers [157] (Open Access, Elsevier). (See text for details)

Upregulated sympathetic activity opposes the (normal) action of the vagus in the spleen perpetuating the production and release of pro-inflammatory cytokines. This contributes to a significant pathogenic role for inflammation in the development and progression of the leading causes of morbidity and mortality in Western societies, including heart disease, cancer, stroke, diabetes, and sepsis. Inflammation accelerates deposition of atherosclerotic plaques leading to myocardial and cerebral infarction, mediates insulin resistance, stimulates tumor growth, and causes organ damage in lethal sepsis. Therefore, without the influence of the vagus, cytokines are produced in much larger quantities in response to infections and injury. Regardless of the method (conscious or subconscious), stimulation of the vagus controls the activation of circulating immune cells as well as production of cytokines.

The dangers of uncontrolled inflammation are inherent in the molecular activity of cytokines. Maintenance of health and wellness requires tight control over the steps leading to the production and release of cytokines. As discussed in the omega-3 chapter of this book (Chap. 3), cardiovascular disease (the Western world's greatest mortality risk) is a result of atherosclerosis. Atherosclerosis is, in part, controlled by the action of cytokine-produced C-reactive protein (CRP). As discussed in the Exercise chapter (Chap. 7), there is an inverse relationship between inflammation as measured by CRP levels and physical activity levels. Further, P&S levels, as measured by heart rate variability (HRV), have a direct relationship with CRP (see insert, below) [18]. Typically, the most physically active people demonstrate the lowest CRP and highest HRV.

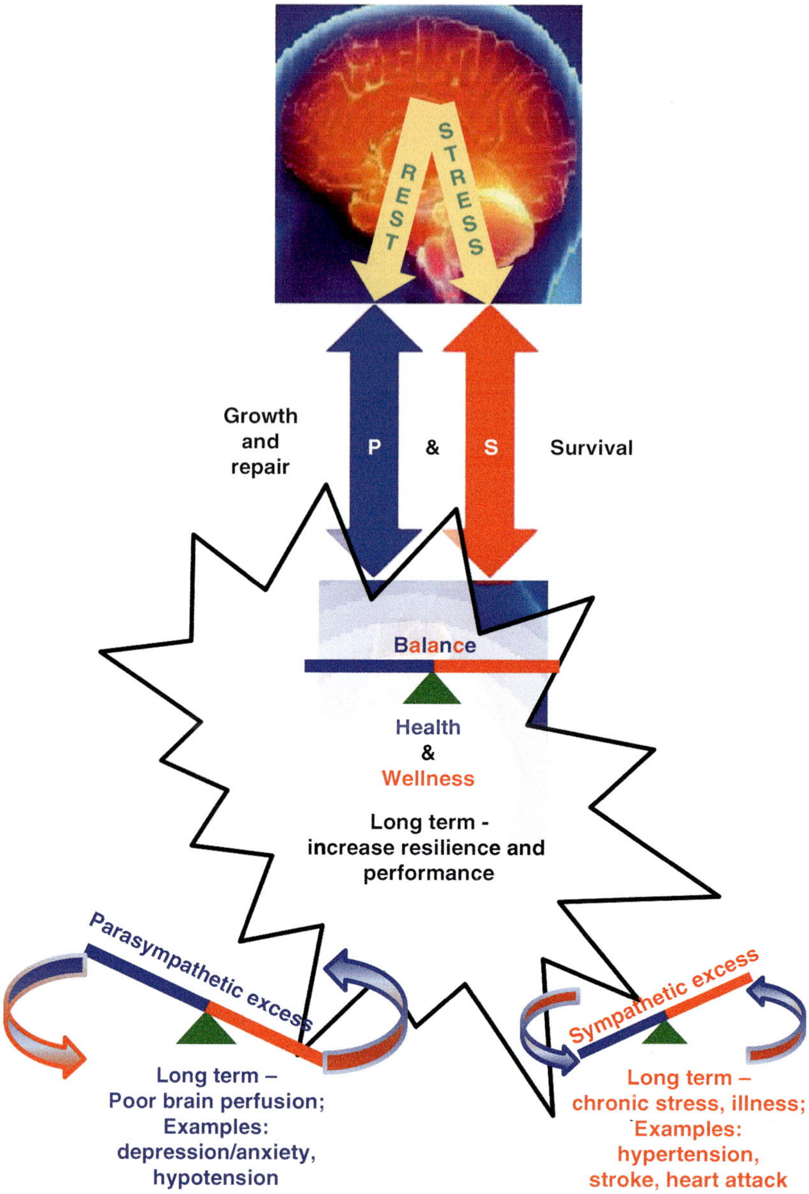


## Lateralization of Emotions and P&S Responses

As mentioned above, the left and right halves of the forebrain are associated with different emotions [34] (positive emotions with the left and negative emotions with the right hemisphere). Specific neural pathways seemed to be used for particular emotions. For example, dysregulation in the amygdala, hippocampus, and Brodmann areas 9 and 45 are associated with increased anxiety and sympathetic activation [137, 161–164]. A similar lateralization is also described for the cortical control of the heart [165]. Sympathetic effects predominantly arise from the right hemisphere, and parasympathetic effects predominantly arise from the left hemisphere [166]. Together, these similar lateralizations suggest a neuroanatomical basis for the different emotional influences known to effect cardiovascular function and other organ systems. They may also be associated with cardiovascular dysfunction, even before, and possibly compounded by, P&S dysfunction.

The sympathetics uniquely control the vasculature. (Parasympathetic control is indirectly mediated through its influence on the sympathetics.) Severe or fatal ventricular arrhythmias are often due to ischemic heart disease, usually coronary artery disease. Mental stress, known be a cause of SE, may induce ischemia as a result of epicardial or microvascular constriction together with an increased oxygen demand [167–170]. Also, mental stress may aggravate the effects of ischemia on vasoconstriction superimposed on already insufficient perfusion.

A persistent finding in patients with depression is the elevation of corticotrophin-releasing hormone (CRH) and arginine-vasopressin neurons in the paraventricular nucleus (PVN) in comparison to control subjects [171, 172]. Unrestrained CRH synthesis in the central nucleus of the amygdala (CeA) may produce dysregulation of the hypothalamic-pituitary-adrenal axis (see insert below [19]), which is associated with many of the behavioral, physiological, and reproductive consequences associated with stress-related disorders. In fact, this may underlie the "Broken Heart" syndrome, where depression may cause sudden death [173] or possibly may severely depress the immune system to enable a simple cold to be life-threatening, what is commonly known as "giving up the desire to live" (see insert, next page [174]).

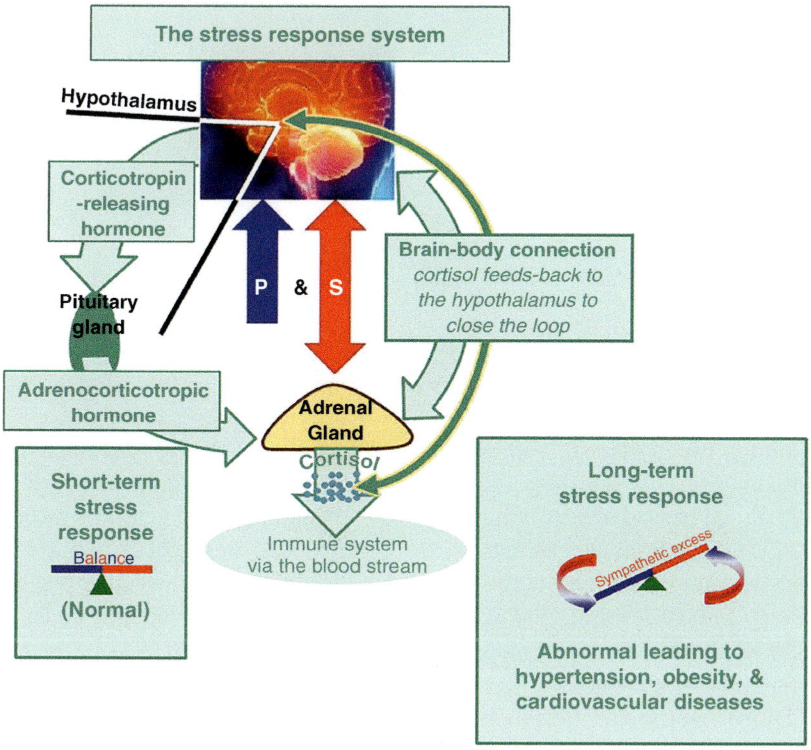

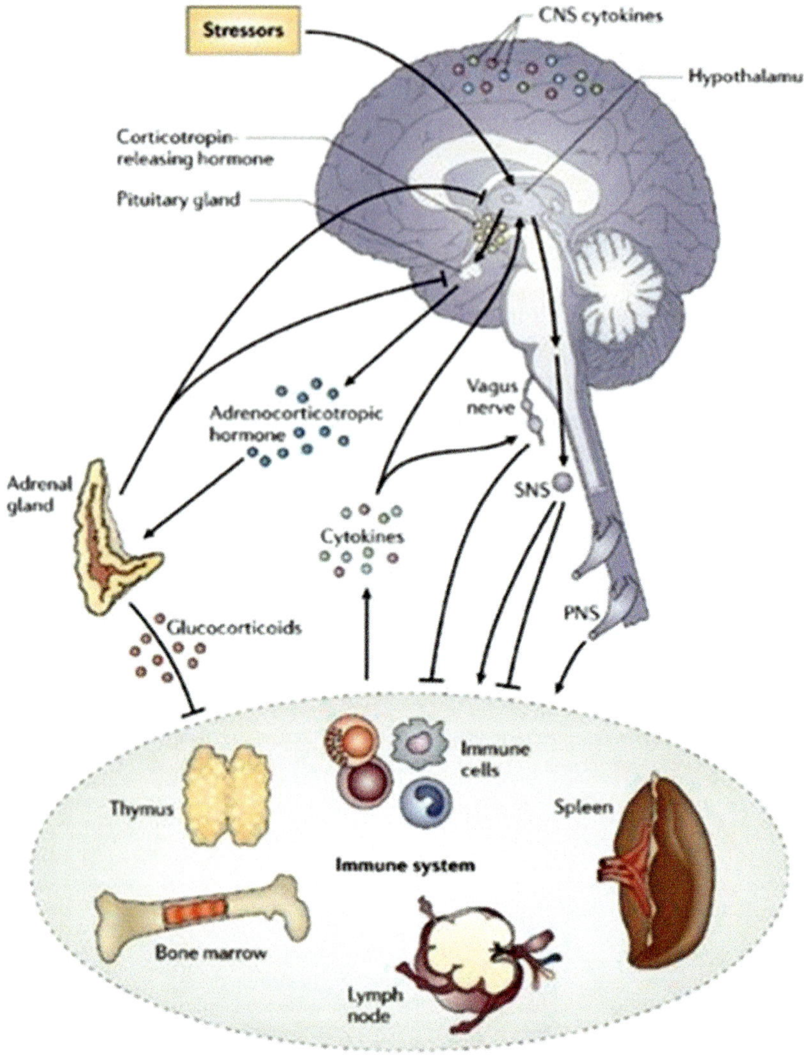


Insert: Reproduced with permission from Elsevier; Open Access, Springer Nature, Nature Reviews, Immunology

An association between stressful life conditions and arrhythmic events has been demonstrated recently in subjects demonstrating long QT intervals [175]. Symptomatic patients with long QT syndrome had experienced more stressful life conditions, and the level of vital exhaustion as a measure of chronic stress was more than three times higher among patients with long QT syndrome with arrhythmic events than in asymptomatic long QT syndrome patients.

Even though there is little doubt about the increased activity of the P&S nervous systems during stressful situations, it remains unclear how this eventually manifests in endothelial dysfunction – the start of atherosclerosis which is a beginning of cardiovascular disease. Sympathetic nervous system overactivity, elicited by lower body negative pressure simulating the stress of hypovolemia, reduced flow-mediated dilation [176], a measure of the body's stress response [177]. This response was blocked by intra-arterial phentolamine, an α-1, sympathetic antagonist, demonstrating the role of α-adrenergic receptors [178]. This result was confirmed in healthy young adults in whom the negative effect of mental stress on endothelial function was simulated and confirmed by propranolol and neurogenic blockade (β-sympathetic antagonists), but not by phentolamine [179]. These results demonstrate the role of the sympathetic nervous system in angiogenesis due to stress-induced endothelial dysfunction [180–182].

Excessive sympathetic activity (sympathetic excess or SE) occurs during chronically stressful conditions. The α-sympathetic system primarily causes vasoconstriction of the peripheral vasculature increasing BP. The β-1, sympathetic system primarily increases HR, which indirectly further increases BP, and the β-2, sympathetic system primarily causes vasodilation of the core vasculature and bronchodilation; the former also further increases BP by increasing blood volume in and around the heart. Exposure to chronic, repetitive ("habituated") stress upregulates catecholamine production, facilitating SE [183]. Note SE is in response to habituated stressors: repeated exposure to the same stressors. SE is not elicited by novel stressors. However, individuals who already demonstrate elevated, systemic sympathetic activity due to a history of chronic stress habituate to the repetition of a novel stressor faster, and the initial sympathetic response to the novel stressor is typically exaggerated due to the higher baseline established by that individual's history. Again, chronic SE harms the cardiovascular system in different ways. First, the continuous pressor effects of released catecholamines may counteract vasodilatory effects of nitric oxide and can also accelerate the atherosclerotic process [184–186]. As discussed, excessive (prolonged) nitric oxide levels cause the opposite reaction to normal nitric oxide levels (turning it to an oxidative stressor), and in addition to that which was discussed in the nitric oxide chapter (Chap. 4), nitric oxide may also be involved in triggering catecholamine surges in chronic stress [187, 188].

Another possible (and parallel) mechanism of SE is activation of the renin-angiotensin-aldosterone system (RAAS). Angiotensin II, a potent vasoconstrictor, can harm endothelial cells independently of its pressor effect [189]. For example, increased cellular lipid peroxidation [190] and reduced cholesterol efflux [191] in macrophages and scavenger cells lead to accelerated foam cell formation and a hastened atherosclerotic process. Angiotensin II stimulates uptake of oxidized LDL by macrophages, possibly mediated by IL-6 [192]. Margination, adhesion, and translocation of leukocytes, all prerequisites for atherosclerosis, are enhanced by angiotensin II type 1 receptors (AT1Rs) [193–196]. Angiotensin II also promotes the expression and production of adhesive and pro-inflammatory molecules (vascular cell adhesion protein 1, intercellular adhesion molecule 1, monocyte chemoattractant protein-1, macrophage inflammatory protein-1α, and IL-8) on the endothelial and vascular smooth muscle cells [197–202]. Angiotensin II affects vascular smooth muscle signal transduction and several growth factors (transforming growth factor-β, platelet-derived growth factor, and basic fibroblast growth factor) that stimulate smooth muscle proliferation [203]. Central and peripheral blockade of AT1Rs with Candesartan provides cardiovascular benefits in addition to modifying responses to psychological stress [204–206]. In addition, Candesartan abolished hormonal and sympathetic responses mediated by the HPA axis under stress while also reducing anxiety and protecting against gastric ulceration [207]. Despite the consequences of activation of AT1Rs by angiotensin II, angiotensin II also activates another counter-regulatory mechanism: angiotensin II type 2 (AT2)/Mas receptors. The type 2 receptors have beneficial effects during stressful situations. They downregulate sympathetic nervous activity during stressful conditions, providing the cardioprotective effects of angiotensin II [208, 209].

## The Brain-Heart Connection

The brain-heart connection is, in part, based on specific cortical representations of emotions mediated through autonomic reflexes to influence the physiology of the myocardium (see Fig. 8.17). Feedback mechanisms from the heart to brain play a significant modulatory role, particularly in pathological conditions, not only of the heart but

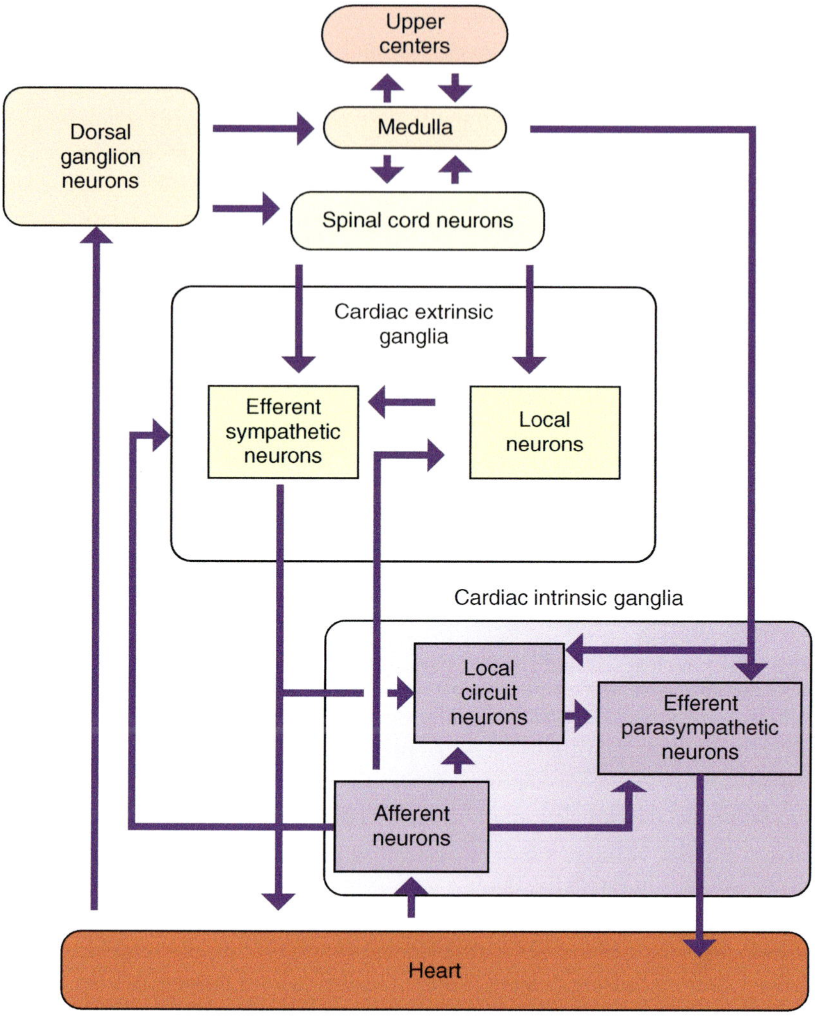


**Fig. 8.17** Schematic representation of the extrinsic and intrinsic innervation of the heart [19, Fig. 4.11]. (Republished with permission from Springer International Publishing AG)

of all organs and organ systems. The brain-heart connection is the core of the mind-body connection.

Many diseases are not optimally managed. Using hypertension (Fig. 8.18) again as an example, hypertension is one of the most diagnosed diseases in the world, and over 40% are poorly managed, if at all. Among all of its known damaging, cardiovascular, cerebrovascular, renal, and other end-organ effects, hypertension is a known risk factor for dementia in middle-aged patients. It is associated with cognitive impairment, stroke, and brain atrophy. While hypertension is more common in men than in women, women who develop hypertension in their 40s are up to 73% more likely to suffer from dementia later in life than their normotensive counterparts [211]. However, men in similar states do not demonstrate any increased risk. Risk of end-organ damage and development of cardiovascular disease linked to high BP is consistently higher in women.

This study of 5646 younger adults (an "early adulthood" stage with an average age of 33 years and a "mid-adulthood" stage with an average age of 44 years) tallied a total of 532 dementia cases over the course of their 15-year follow-up period – 298 in women and 234 in men [211]. Only 15% of the original population died without a dementia diagnosis. In both men and women, neither hypotension, prehypertension, nor hypertension was associated with an increased dementia risk in early adulthood. In

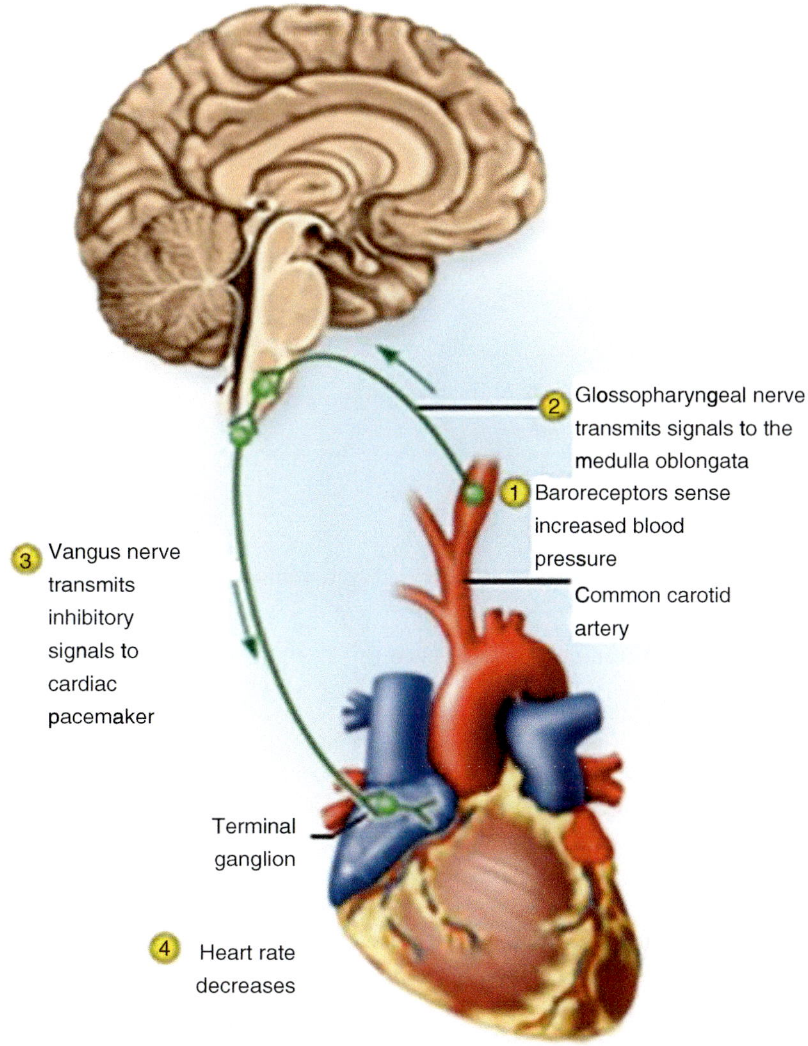


**Fig. 8.18** Visceral reflex to high BP. High BP is detected by arterial stretch receptors (1), which sends their signals to the CNS via afferent neurons (2), then efferent signals (3) travel to the heart (4), and heart slows, reducing BP. This is an example of a homeostatic negative feedback loop (2 – 3 – 4 – 1). The glossopharyngeal nerve transmits signals to medulla oblongata. Baroreceptors sense increased BP in the common carotid artery. The vagus transmits inhibitory signals to the cardiac pacemaker in the terminal ganglion which decreases HR [210, Fig. 15.1]. (© The McGraw-Hill Companies, Inc.; republished with permission)

midlife, an elevated dementia risk was connected only to hypertension. Mid-adulthood saw a 65% increased risk in hypertensive women. Hypertensive women in their 30s did see a 31% increased risk of dementia; those numbers don't differ largely from counterparts with normotensive blood pressure.

Hypertension is highly associated with stroke. An estimated 60% of all first strokes are permanently incapacitating or cause death. Reducing the stress underlying high BP, underlying hypertension, relieves hypertension, which reduces stroke risk factors and which reduces the occurrence of stroke. Often stroke precipitates brain injury, and for those who survive, it leaves them with cognitive or functional deficits. The unfortunate fact about stroke is that an estimated 80% of all first strokes are due to risk factors that can be changed, such as high BP! As a result, many efforts have been made to prevent, screen for, and treat these risk factors. The problem goes back to the fact that high BP is silent ("the silent killer"). It does not hurt until it is too late. Frequent BP checks and wellness visits and preventative measures such as exercise, proper diet, and stress reduction are essential to prevent the ravages of high BP. The effects of stress, including through high BP, affect all aspects of life, see the insert below. Stress management, as recommended herein, helps to relieve these effects and restore quality of life.

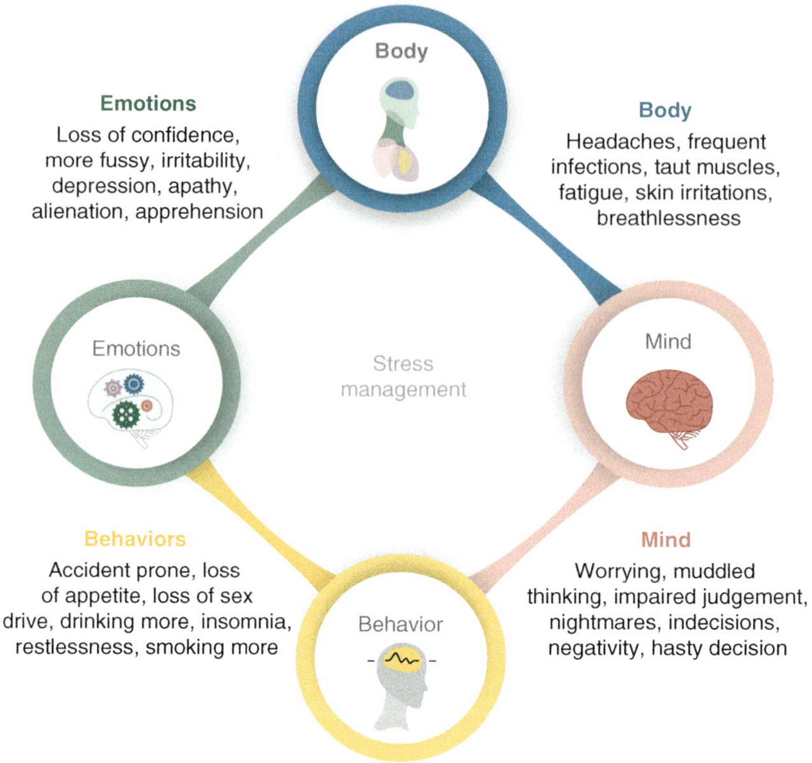


Insert: Illustration by Elysian Creative Studio, www.elysiancreativestudio.com, Lizzy Colombo; Adapted with permission from Nicolle Rager Fuller: Vagus nerve anatomy, illustration C037/4895, from https://www.sciencephoto.com/media/887799/view

Despite educational and prevention efforts, stroke patients are increasingly demonstrating one or more risk factors [212]. A study of more than 900,000 cases of ischemic stroke from 2004 and 2014 found a total of 92.5% of patients had at least one risk factor, and most of the risk factors increased in prevalence as the study progressed. Yet there was a widespread increase in the number of stroke patients with one or more risk factors by the end of the study. These alarming findings support the call for further action to develop more effective methods to prevent and control these risk factors to reduce stroke risk [213]. The study found that:

- The proportion of patients with at least one risk factor grew from 88% in 2004 to 95% in 2014.
- The proportion of patients with multiple risk factors also increased over time.
- Nearly half (49%) of Hispanic stroke patients had diabetes, compared to 44% of African-Americans and 30% of Caucasians.
- From 2004 to 2014, the prevalence of high BP (73–84%), high cholesterol (29–59%), and diabetes (31–38%) all increased.
- The number of stroke patients who smoked or abused drugs increased annually by 5–7%, respectively, over the course of the study.

As indicated in these examples, the brain may influence the body and vice versa. Chronic stress, including psychosocial stress, often develops hypertension in these patients through a chronic increase in (resting) sympathetic activity (the body's stress response), which chronically increases baroreceptor reflex which, in turn, raises resting blood pressure. Attempting to normalize (resting) sympathetic activity in these cases is made more difficult in the face of the fact that chronic sympathetic overactivation depletes the parasympathetic nervous system, including vagus nerve activity. Again, relieving or reducing the stress is the best therapy. In lieu of reducing stress, normalizing both resting and dynamic P&S balance help to minimize stress responses. At the very least, normalizing systolic and diastolic BP helps to minimize the effects of stress on the brain, heart, vasculature, kidneys, and other organs.

## Dentistry Is Also Connected

Many are unaware of the complexity and significance of how the temporomandibular joint (TMJ), cervical spine, and the P&S nervous systems are interrelated. The TMJ moves about 2000 times in 24 hours (estimated to be the body's most active joint). The major function of the spine is to support the head. The P&S nerves that travel through the vertebrae of the cervical spine serve all of the body's organs, so any disruption may result in serious illness, disability, and even early death. As result of psychosocial stress, several common TMJ disorders present. TMJ disorders involve the muscles that move the jaw and can involve the jaw joints as well. Many people with psychosocial stress will clench their jaw or grind their teeth more than a healthy person. Two major causes of TMJ dysfunction are extensive clenching or grinding of teeth.

The trigeminal or fifth cranial nerve feeds information from all of the jaw movement muscles, joints, a portion of the throat, ears, back of the eye sinus cavities, and the side of the head directly into the limbic system of the brain. The fifth nerve is the communications center for all pain arising in the neck, head, jaw, eyes, ears, sinuses, and the cervical spine. These facts help explain why temporomandibular dysfunction (TMD) can have such a wide effect on the jaw, head, and neck and can be attributed to headaches and also explain how dysfunction of jaw muscles and joints could amplify problems in the limbic system. As discussed above, the limbic system is directly connected with the P&S nervous systems, thereby transmitting the pain and stress to the viscera, including the heart. Note pleasing touches of the head and neck (i.e., gentle and loving caresses) are also transmitted to the viscera via the P&S with an opposite effect.

Symptoms of TMD can present with or without joint noise and can be accompanied by a restricted mandibular range of motion. Pain is usually localized in the muscles of mastication, the accessory muscles of mastication in the posterior cervical area, the TMJ joints, and the area of the ears. Not only may this pain be transmitted to the P&S as additional stress via the limbic system; TMD may cause sleep disorders (i.e., obstructive sleep apnea). When breathing is obstructed, there is an additional stress that is transmitted to the P&S, which is well known to increase risk of developing high BP, high cholesterol, diabetes, heart attack, stroke, and metabolic disorders.

Psychosocial stress can slowly cause spinal misalignment over time. The pain and dysfunction of the TMJ modifies how the individual carries her/his head and the balance in the strength of the muscles of the cervical spine misalign the spine, enabling the nerves projecting through that spine, including P&S nerves, to be impinged. This is especially true for the parasympathetic nervous system, of which the primary projections of the vagus nerve into the chest and upper abdomen pass out of the cervical spine. Spinal misalignment often happens so slowly, in fact, that an individual will perceive the misalignment and associated discomfort to be normal until it becomes too disabling or painful. Any incoming nociceptive stimuli through C1, C2, or C3 (facets, discs, and muscles), as well as the vertebral and Dural arteries, can cause the neurological pain. Altered neuromusculoskeletal function caused by imbalance to the upper cervical structure causes noxious stimuli often resulting in headache.

Neuromuscular dental techniques, as well as atlas/axis balancing (as needed), are an effective combination for correction of biomechanical imbalances. A wide range of symptoms, including cervicogenic pain, migraines, disc compressions, craniofacial imbalances, neuropathies, palsies, fibromyalgia, Meniere's syndrome, and tinnitus, are effectively managed by elimination of neuromuscular imbalances. Without relief, symptoms can lead to long-term exhaustion, fatigue, and sleep disorders. Memory loss and cognitive problems may also arise. Feelings of irritability and restlessness from the body's stress response rise in response to the lack of proper breathing. Many people with TMJ (with or without knowledge or symptoms and with or without sounds such as clicking, popping, and grating) also complain of chronic headaches, morning headaches, limited mandibular movements or locking open/closed, dizziness, ear fullness or pain with no apparent other etiology, facial pain, neck pain or stiffness, loud snoring, unrefreshing sleep, dry mouth upon awakening, chest retraction in young children during sleep (chest pulls in), high BP, overweight, irritability, personality change, depression, difficulty concentrating, excessive perspiring during sleep, heartburn, insomnia, frequent nocturnal urination (nocturia), restless sleep, nocturnal snorting, gasping, choking (may wake self-up), rapid weight gain, and confusion upon awakening. These complaints may be taken as possible early indicators of TMD. With TMJ, cervical spine, and P&S nervous systems so complexly interrelated, it is critical for healthcare providers to work together to identify the signs early and relieve the symptoms, even before pain and dysfunction present, including by reducing or relieving the psychosocial stress itself.

## The Vagus Nerve

The vagus nerve (see insert below) is approximately 75% of the parasympathetic nervous system outside the brain. Vagus means "wandering" in Latin. The vagus nerve has outposts in nearly every organ and a direct line into the brain stem. About 80% of its nerve fibers signal information from the body to the brain. The remaining 20% signal the body from the brain. Doctors have long exploited the nerve's influence on the brain to combat epilepsy and depression. Electrical stimulation of the vagus (aka vagus nerve stimulation or VNS), through a surgically implanted device, has already been approved by the US FDA as a therapy for patients who do not find relief from existing treatments. Researchers are considering stimulating different branches of the vagus nerve to improve treatments for a myriad of conditions, including high BP, chronic pain, anxiety, heart disease, autoimmune inflammatory diseases like rheumatoid arthritis, and inflammatory bowel disorders such as Crohn's disease, gastroparesis, chronic, severe migraine, and more.

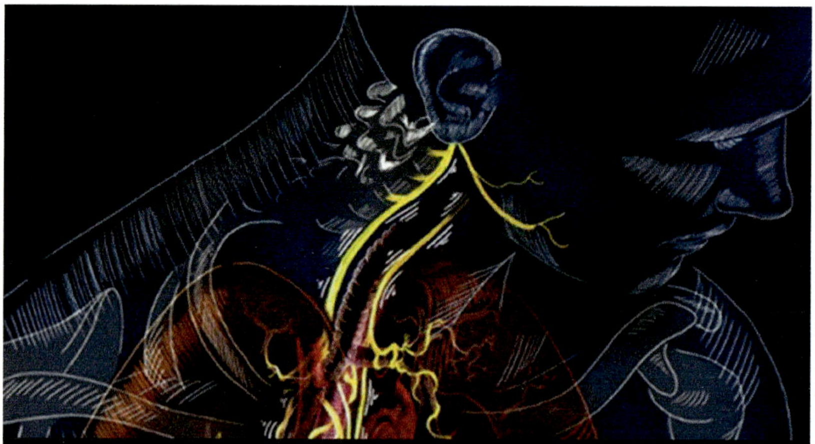

**WHAT NERVE** The vagus nerve's path from brain to heart and other organs was detailed by the Greek anatomist Galen, a leading physician of the Roman Empire in the second century.

Insert: Adapted with permission from Nicolle Rager Fuller: Vagus nerve anatomy, illustration C037/4895, from https://www.sciencephoto.com/media/887799/view

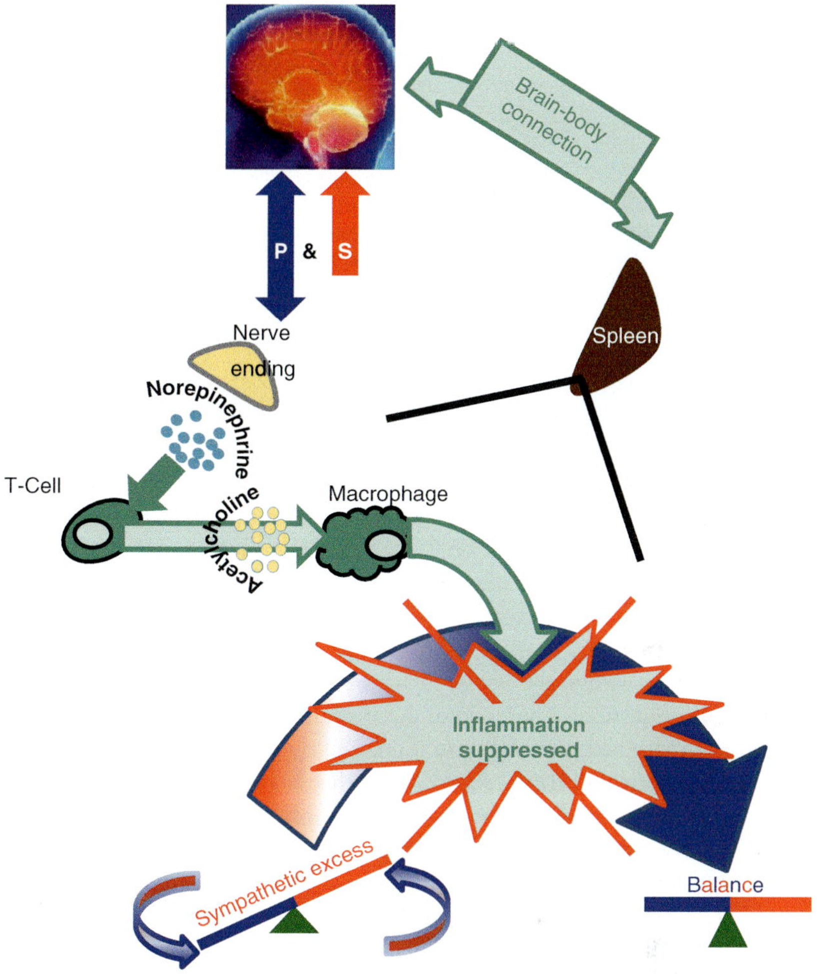


**Fig. 8.19** The vagus nerve detects inflammation or infection in the body and relays signals from the brain stem along its efferent fibers. This signal prompts other nerves to release norepinephrine, which makes immune T cells in the spleen release the chemical acetylcholine to depress inflammation via macrophages [214–216]. (Source: K. Tracey/Feinstein Instit. for Med. Research)

Arguably the most important function of the vagus nerve is to relieve stress. The nerve branches into two parts in the neck (see insert below) and innervates most of the organs in the chest and abdomen, including the heart, lungs, liver, stomach, pancreas, kidneys, intestines, bladder, sex organs, and rectum. It controls a vast range of bodily functions including digestion, heart rate, blood pressure, inflammation and immunity (Fig. 8.19), sweating, and the gag reflex. It has control over a variety of hormones in addition to acetylcholine and norepinephrine and more. Clinical experience has shown that reducing excessive vagus nerve activity reduces the amount of hormone replacement therapy needed for hypothyroidism, estrogen, and progesterone-related difficulties (i.e., "hot flashes," night sweats, mood disorders, and depression), growth hormones, and insulin. However, these benefits are only possible if the associated gland is still functional. Via the vagus, the body responds to feelings, both physical and emotional. When people are tense, HR increases, breathing quickens, and the stomach is in knots. The vagus nerve is sending information up to the brain that the body is in distress. When the body is relaxed, HR slows, breathing deepens, the stomach is soft, and all this information signals to the brain that all is well.

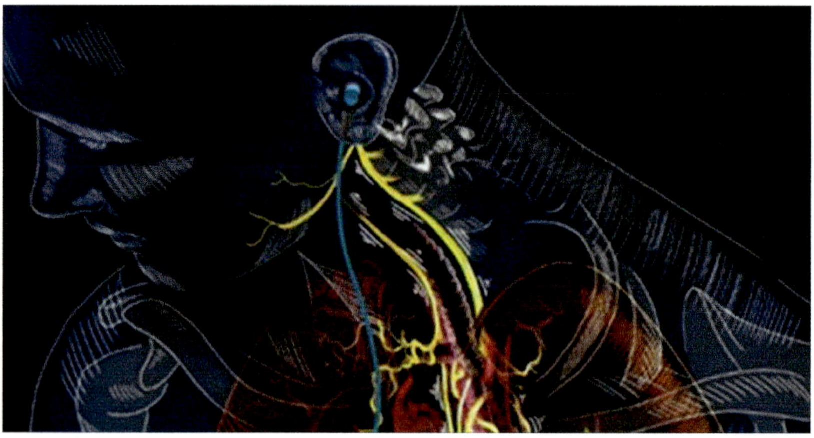

When something is wrong, the sympathetic nervous system becomes more active to manage the stress. When all is well, the vagus nerve, and the rest of the parasympathetic nervous system, becomes more active to manage the rest and relax response. Under stress, the vagus is suppressed. As a result, digestion is hampered, the immune system is suppressed, the ability to think clearly dwindles, and HR and BP increase. All of this is fine for a short period of time, such as when chased down a dark alley by the proverbial saber-toothed tiger. However, when it continues over an extended period of time, it starts to have some seriously negative effects, including reducing the ability to heal and stay healthy and well, let alone function at optimum performance levels.

Eventually, people may habituate to this cascade of harmful hormones and even get "addicted" to the chemicals of stress. As a result, it is impossible to truly relax, and patients enter survival mode. For example, when trying to meditate, one simply cannot close their eyes to focus on relaxing; or when on vacation, one takes half the time to relax and then starts to stress over the return, so they never actually relax. However, it is possible to self-stimulate the vagus nerve.

Stimulating the vagus decreases sympathetic activity [217], thereby indirectly slowing HR, dilating blood vessels to reduce BP, reducing insulin levels, etc. This organically helps to relieve hypertension, heart failure, certain types of arrhythmias, diabetes, and more, including intractable hiccups. At the same time, the vagus directly increases immune responses, decreases inflammation (Fig. 8.20 [214–216]) and oxidation, increases detoxification, increases the motility of the gastrointestinal system, etc. Overall, the net result is to promote a happier mood, improved cognitive function, improved sex function, more restful sleep, improved social interactions, reduced sweating, more patience, less irritability, and fewer poor decisions. It is possible to stimulate the vagus nerve with:

- *Breathing* – On average, six (6) breaths per minute (10 seconds per breath, with 5 seconds for inhalation and 5 seconds for exhalation, in a relaxed attitude[13]) is the optimal stimulus for the human vagus nerve. As the depth and rate of breathing are controlled to this level (aka stomach breathing), the patient is gently instructed to focus on relaxing to maintain this stimulus as a vagal (parasympathetic) stimulus.
- *Positive thoughts, including gratitude* – This stimulates the "happy centers" of the brain. These are located in and around the limbic system in the midbrain and brain stem. As a bonus, these centers are also involved in learning and memory. These "happy thoughts" improve the ability to learn and remember. It

[13]The same six breathes per minute in a stressed or hyper-state is known as hyperventilation and is neither relaxing nor an optimal stimulus for the parasympathetic or vagus nerves.

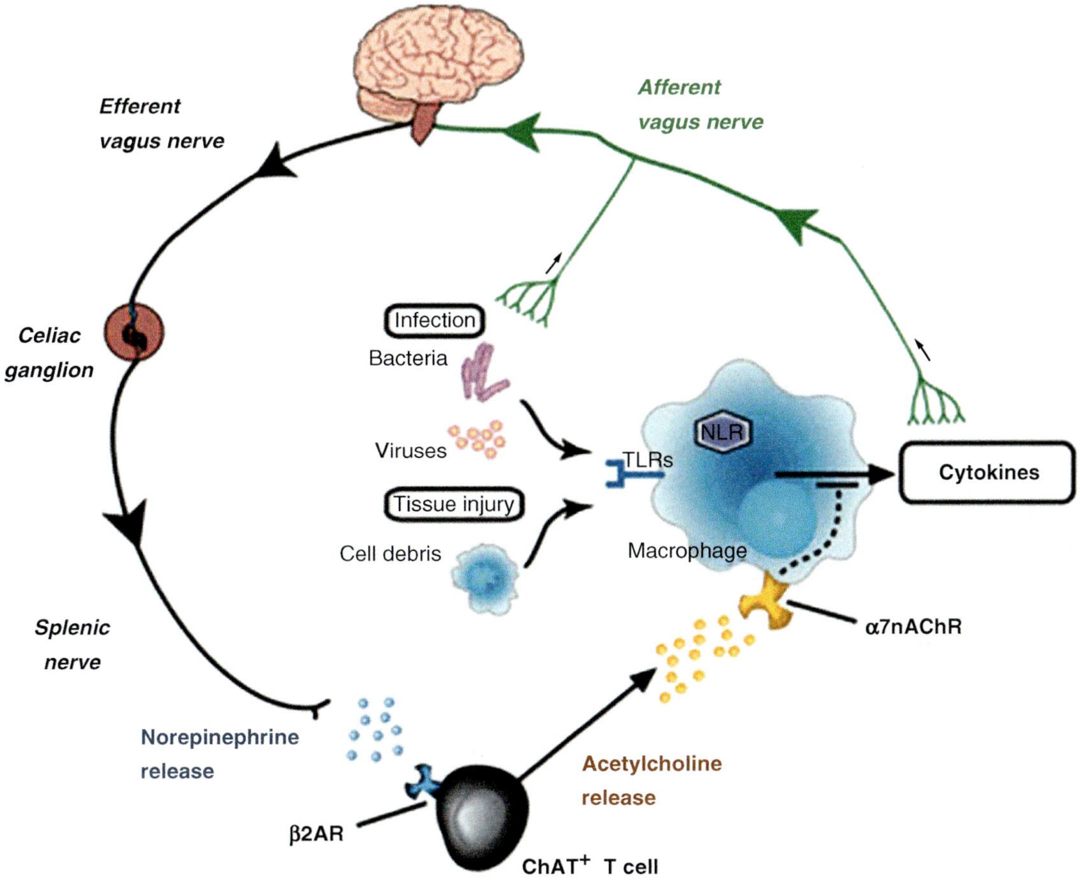


**Fig. 8.20** The inflammatory reflex is a process which links the immune and nervous systems together where the nervous system helps regulate the inflammatory process. The vagus nerve senses the presence of inflammatory cytokines and, upon stimulation, sends a signal to the brain that relays the message to the celiac ganglion where parasympathetic nerve fibers meet sympathetic fibers. The sympathetic fibers trigger the spleen to release T cells that release acetylcholine to dampen inflammation by signaling macrophages to reduce pro-inflammatory cytokine output and increase anti-inflammatory cytokine output. Patients with non-resolving inflammation, such as those with autoimmune diseases, obesity, and type 2 diabetes, have impaired vagus nerve function that prevents resolution of their inflammation [218, Fig. 2]. (Republished with permission from The American Physiological Society. Source: http://synergyhw.blogspot.com/2015/05/acetylcholine-and-adrenal-function-is.html)

is the reason why people, especially children, express joy in learning something new! Furthermore, when people choose to not be a victim, but rather choose to believe that everything happens for a reason and that that reason provides an opportunity to grow, people are more self-confident and self-assured, promoting an improved quality of life and slowing the aging processes (including oxidation and inflammation), which also promotes increased mitochondrial activity, thereby increasing energy levels.

- *Exercise – Again, "exercise" is not a dirty word!* Exercise stimulates the vagus nerve to provide the benefits listed above. Furthermore, in addition to stimulating the vagus nerve into releasing acetylcholine into all of the organs, exercise releases endorphins which further reduce inflammation and also reduce the perception of pain. Less pain also enhances mood, sleep, and many of the benefits listed above.
- *Spending time with loved ones and good friends* – This stimulates higher cortical

centers in the brain, helping to share burdens and off-load stress, which feeds down to the limbic system and then the vagus nerve. Often, this time is spent around good food and drink, furthering the ability to reduce stress.

Regarding VNS (see Fig. 8.21), there is a lot left to learn. While studies continue to explore its broad potential, much about the vagus remains a mystery. In some cases, it's not yet clear exactly how the nerve exerts its influence, and researchers are still figuring out where and how to best apply electricity. Stimulation of the vagus prompts release of acetylcholine. Acetylcholine, a neurotransmitter-like norepinephrine, is able to prevent inflammation. It has profound control over HR and BP. Patients with heart failure tend to have less active vagus nerves (in other words, CAN; see "Oxidative Stress in Cardiovascular Diseases," Chap. 5). Trying to correct the problem with electrical stimulation (VNS) is possible and is being researched [219–224]. However, all the results thus far are preliminary. The studies that have been finished to date are relatively small. VNS is being tried in atrial fibrillation to augment or replace current therapies that include drugs that alter heart rhythm (to reduce, or relieve, the fibrillation) or thin the blood (to prevent the associated blood clots). VNS is especially hopeful in patients for whom current therapies do not work or respond with difficult side effects, including heart failure [225], atrial fibrillation [214, 226], epilepsy [227, 228], depression [229, 230], memory loss [231], headaches [232], and diabetes [233]. Again, VNS is still in its infancy, and clinical applications haven't been adequately tested.

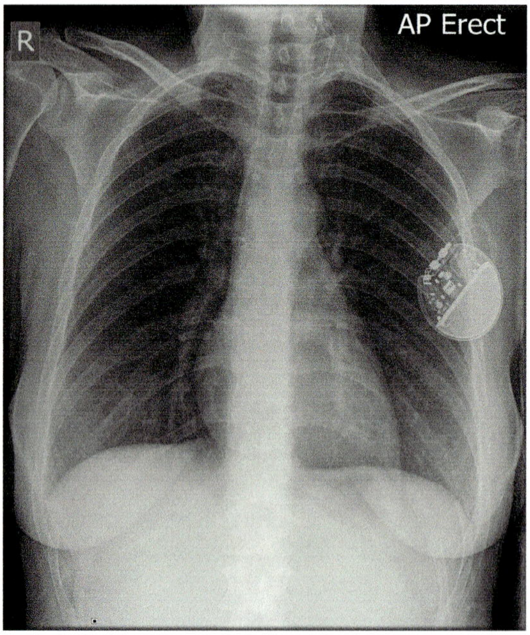


**Fig. 8.21** Implanted vagus nerve stimulators send electricity from a generator in the chest to the nerve in the neck. (This case is courtesy of Dr. Ian Bickle, Radiopaedia.org, rID: 56361 (Copyright Clearance Center))

Research continues into the best method to apply the electrical stimulation of VNS [234]. If possible, surgery to implant the device may be avoided. In the ear, tiny projections of vagus fibers run close to the surface of the skin, primarily under the tragus (in the ear, white dots, see insert, next page). While a number of skeptics remain, there is ancient anecdotal evidence for this as a potential. The anecdotal evidence is based on the ancient Eastern art of Acupuncture. The acupuncture meridians mostly overlay the paths of the vagus nerve, including in the ear. VNS is being studied with the approach through the tragus [235–237]. The ear isn't the only non-surgical target. There are devices that can stimulate the vagus nerve when placed on the throat [237, 238]. The device was initially tested to reduce asthma symptoms, given the vagus nerve's anti-inflammatory action. During testing, patients reported that their headaches were disappearing. The device is being investigated to treat chronic cluster headaches, severe headache attacks that can come and go for over a year, again, especially for those for whom pharmaceutical therapies have not helped. Ultimately, the decision between implanted and handheld may be reduced to patient compliance. Implanted devices may be forgotten and have high rates of compliance, handhelds have the potential to also be forgotten, and compliance is compromised.

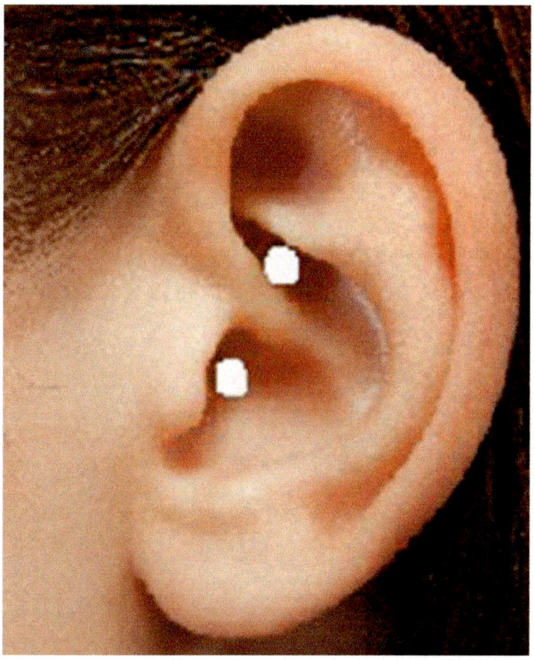

Insert: Adapted from Shutterstock Royalty-free stock illustration ID: 78186766, Human ear closeup, by Ninell

Regardless, this sector of medicine while promising is still a long way off, and the fundamental questions of exactly where to place a device and how much of a stimulus to deliver are still being researched. The vagus nerve's multitasking, two-way nature makes it a challenge to fully understand and control. Stimulating one branch to effect one target organ often causes multiple effects in other branches and therefore other organs. While this is necessary under normal conditions to have a balanced and coordinated response to (external or internal) stimuli, from a therapeutic perspective, it is often the case where only the target organ is dysfunctional and the other organs effected do not need to be stimulated to help relieve the patient of their symptoms. As a result, overstimulation occurs, and additional symptoms or disorders are created.

As with medication, vagal nerve stimulation can be much like the nursery rhyme: "I know an old lady that swallowed a fly, …, then she swallowed a spider to catch the fly, …, then a cat to catch the spider, …, then a dog …," and so on. The question is where does it stop? The best remedy, when possible, is to go back to the source and simply prevent the flies from being swallowed or at the very least remove the fly that was swallowed and remove the source. Once the source is relieved, then the rest can be relieved or eliminated. This is wellness and what is support with lifestyle and supplement recommendations.

The intensity of electrical current, duration of stimulation, and each patient's health status could all affect the results of VNS therapy for the individual. Furthermore, these issues are not constant, which means VNS cannot be assumed to be constant and remain effective. Widespread effect, such as suppressing inflammation caused by the immune system, could even be harmful to some patients. The good news is that the branches of the vagus nerve themselves may help the situation. While you may think of them as wires, this model only goes so far. In fact, from the point of view of VNS, they are less like wires and more like resistors. They organically limit the amount of electricity that they will conduct (due to the existence of electrical potential thresholds, the thresholds above which electrical activity will generate action potentials on the nerves), and the electricity they conduct is lost over relatively short lengths of nerve (subthreshold, excitatory, or inhibitory potentials, which, if they do not add up in time and space to exceed the threshold, are lost, and no action potential is generated; see Fig. 8.22 [239]). There is also a fatigue phenomenon, where excessive (in time or amplitude) stimulation will cause an imbalance in the ion distribution across the nerve membrane and no potentials are formed, effectively blocking the stimulus. Everyone's specific vagal anatomy is different, and knowledge of the individual's vagus nerve map is important to know what is being stimulated. All of these limitations may help to direct and guide VNS to target only the branch(es) and therefore only the dysfunctional end organ, preventing overstimulation of other, healthier organs. Using direct or transcutaneous stimulation of the vagus nerve has not only demonstrated scientifically proven positive effects on a plethora of conditions, but it also confers a continuum of benefits by balancing one's nervous system, promoting innumerable wellness benefits. Overall, and with these issues in mind,

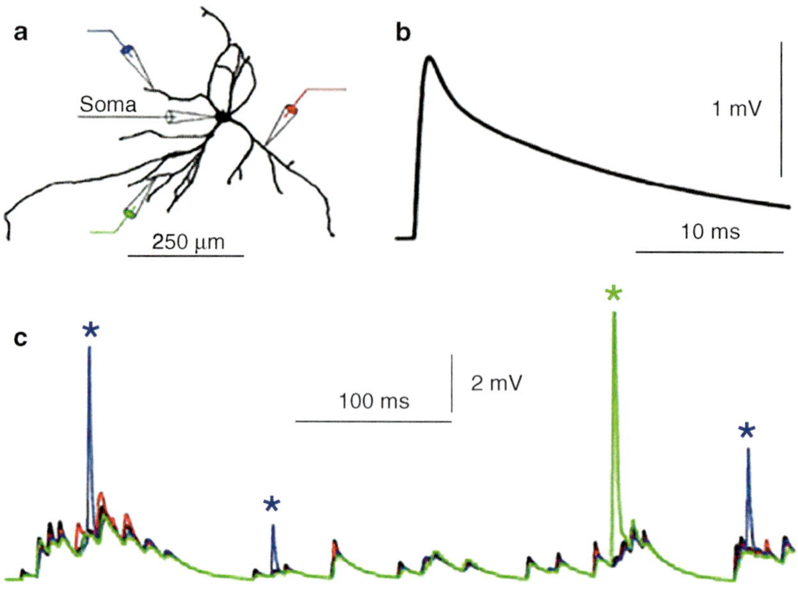


**Fig. 8.22** Simulation of electrical activity in nerves. Recorded simultaneously from different somato-dendritic locations. (**a**): a sketch of the neuron with the approximate placement of the recording electrodes (red, blue, black, and green). (**b**): an example time course of a (subthreshold, excitatory postsynaptic) potential elicited and recorded at the nerve cell body. (**c**): superimposed recordings from the recording electrodes [239, Fig. 6]. (Republished with permission from The American Physiological Society)

VNS has a long way to go before its promised, general effects are available and its potential for tremendous precision is realized.

## The Brain-Gut Connection

The impact of stress, anxiety, and affective disorders on the gastrointestinal (GI) tract is poorly understood and may in part explain the lack of effective therapeutic approaches to treat many GI disorders such as irritable bowel syndrome (IBS). In the brain, the amygdala is an important structure for regulating anxiety with the central nucleus of the amygdala facilitating the activation of the hypothalamic-pituitary-adrenal axis (see Fig. 8.3) and the P&S nervous systems in response to stress. Chronic stress enhances amygdala activity and promotes neural plasticity throughout the amygdaloid complex. This portion of the emotional brain has direct influence on the regulation of enteric function (Fig. 8.23) [240].

## Dynamic Parasympathetic Excess

The standard belief is that an increase in one branch of the autonomic nervous system is accompanied by a decrease in the other branch. In this way, balance and homeostasis is maintained. Unfortunately, this assumption only holds in truly healthy individuals. Unprovoked parasympathetic excess (PE) during sympathetic stimulation is abnormal. This dynamic PE (PE) is "hidden" behind a sympathetic excess (SE) that is secondary to the PE. As a result, the symptoms masquerade as if they were generated by a primary SE. However, when treated as a primary SE, the patients do not respond as expected. When they are treated for a primary PE, they do improve. An example of such a patient is a patient with both depression (from PE) and hypertension (from SE). These patients tend to not be stable, because by treating the patient, more of the extant sympathetic control over the PE is blocked, the body is still demanding its blood, and not all sympathetic channels are being blocked; there-

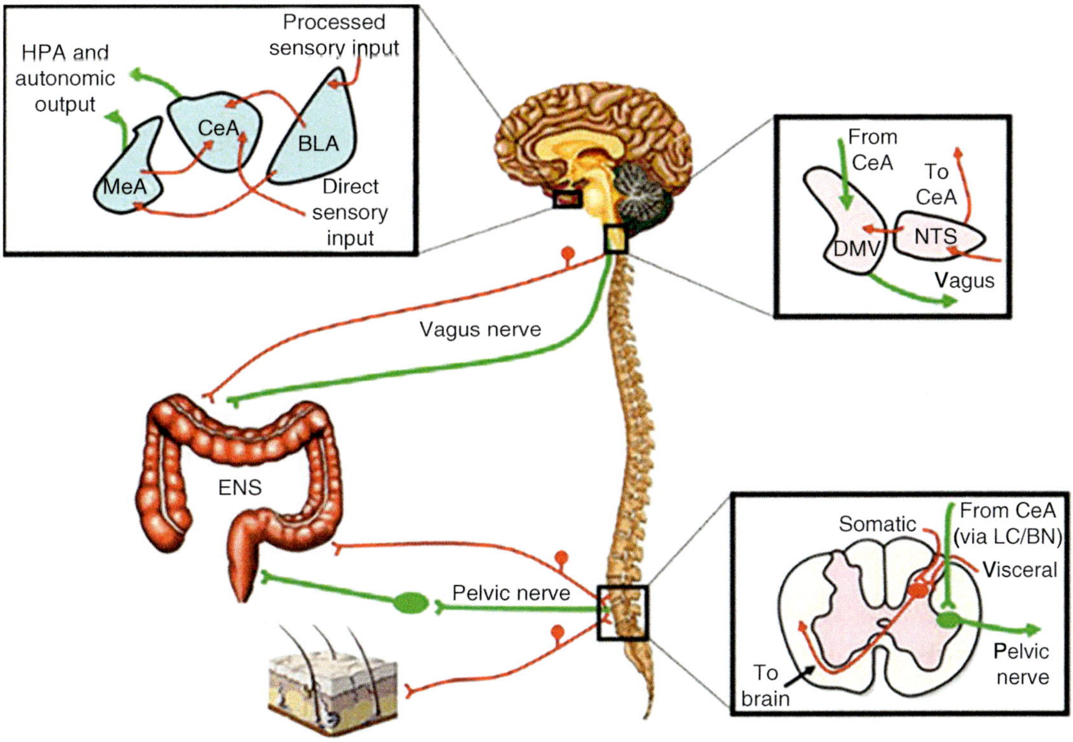


**Fig. 8.23** Hypothesized pathways representing the primary amygdala-peripheral interactions. Sensory-motor interactions between the amygdala and proximal colon are mediated by the vagus nerve and the nuclei of the dorsal vagal complex. The amygdala also influences distal colonic motility through the pelvic nerve via the LC/BN complex, while convergence of visceral and somatic afferents occurs in the lumbosacral spinal cord. Red represents afferent pathways, and green depicts efferent connections. BLA basolateral nucleus of the amygdala, BN Barrington's nucleus, CeA central nucleus of the amygdala, DMV dorsal motor nucleus of the vagus, ENS enteric nervous system, HPA hypothalamic-pituitary-adrenal, LC locus coeruleus, MeA medial nucleus of the amygdala, NTS nucleus of the solitary tract [240]. (Open Access, Frontiers in Neuroscience)

fore, the body finds a way to defeat the antihypertensive, and BP increases after all [17].

PE can only be detected with a device that independently and simultaneously measures P&S activity, in all physiologic states. The only mathematical means of measuring P&S activity simultaneously and independently is with two independent measures of the autonomic nervous system, such as heart beat and respiratory activity. The only capable device, documented by the FDA as a cardiorespiratory monitor and not just an EKG, is the ANX 3.0 from ANSAR Medical Technologies, Inc., Philadelphia, PA, USA (now TMCAMS, Inc., Atlanta, GA). PE during physiological challenges – Valsalva or postural change from the clinical autonomic test – is independent of the clinical state of the patient. PE (whether Valsalva or stand) is associated with the following:

> difficult to control BP, blood glucose, or hormone level (*e.g.*, thyroid, estrogen, and growth hormones), difficult to describe pain syndromes (including CRPS and Fibromyalgia), difficult to manage weight-loss, unexplained arrhythmia (palpitations) or seizure, symptoms of depression or anxiety, PTSD, fatigue, exercise intolerance, general malaise, sex dysfunction, sleep or GI disturbance, lightheadedness, cognitive dysfunction or "brain fog," or frequent headache or migraine.

The clinical P&S (or TMCAMS) test includes three dynamic challenges that simulate common, daily activities: deep breathing challenge (which stimulates the parasympathetic nervous system), Valsalva challenge (which stimulates the sympathetic nervous system), and the postural change or stand challenge (which stimulates both the P&S systems and tests the coordination between the P&S systems). Dynamic balances by definition require one branch to be significantly higher than the other, but there are limits, both lower and upper limits to how much higher (see insert below [18, Figs. 10.4, 10.5, and 10.6]).

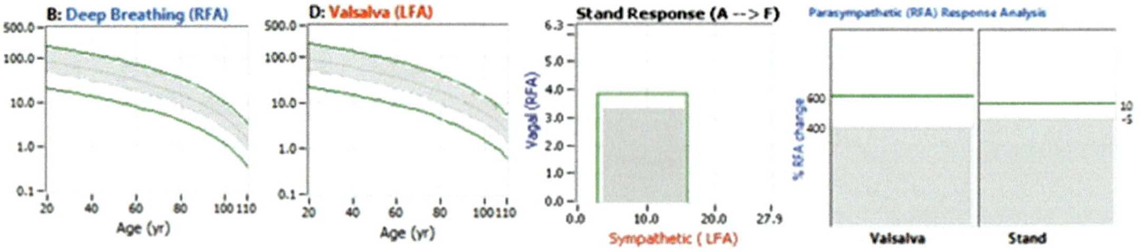


Insert: Adapted with permission from Springer

Dynamic imbalances contribute significantly to quality of life (QoL) dysfunctions, as well as PAN and AAD (or DAN). Even though the primary issue in CAN is minimizing the risk of MACE, once CAN is minimized by normalizing P&S balance (sympathovagal balance), normalizing remaining dynamic imbalances may help to improve QoL. Oftentimes, when P&S dysfunction is secondary to a disease entity, the autonomics will improve when the underlying disease is treated and improved. When causes of P&S dysfunction cannot be identified, the condition is called idiopathic. In many instances, treatment can improve the symptoms and abnormalities. There may be no cure, but treatment often improves QoL. In these cases, the goal of therapy, including lifestyle changes (exercise and proper diet) is to have more better days than bad days oftentimes in treating patients with these illnesses.

PE with stand may also mask sympathetic withdrawal, the P&S condition that underlies orthostatic dysfunction. However, even with all of this, patients demonstrated normal resting HR and BP and no other apparent causes for their symptoms. For this, they are eventually referred to psych-eval. Valsalva SE is considered secondary to Valsalva PE. Establishing PE may help clarify a diagnosis when patients demonstrate multiple seemingly contradictory symptoms (e.g., hypertension with depression) and provide a more integrated approach to therapy. In pain management, PE may differentiate chronic regional pain syndrome (CRPS, formerly RSD). PE appears to be involved in depression-anxiety syndromes, fibromyalgia, chronic fatigue syndromes, and metabolic syndrome. To treat, consider titrating low-dose anticholinergic therapy to treat the PE, history dependent. If PE and SE exist concurrently, the double cocktail, carvedilol, has been found to treat both. PE is common in post-concussion or brain injury patients and may explain the symptoms that manifest even some time after the injury or event. Treating PE and establishing and maintaining proper SB will help to also treat the concussion.

Patients apparently born with dynamic PE (there seems to be a hereditary trait to autonomic dysfunction) tend to start out with lower HRs and BPs and are slower to excite. For example, these individuals are slower to "break a sweat" when exercising and are more likely to be relatively calm during a near-accident, responding as if everything is in slow motion, and only become anxious after the danger has passed. If these individuals remained this way, they would likely outlive those who are more excitable. However, a significant insult to the body, including pregnancy in women, reverses this trend, and the dynamic parasympathetic excess (PE) carries a secondary sympathetic excess (SE), which leads to less stable physiologic conditions that accelerates autonomic decline, increasing morbidity and mortality risk, and the decline in quality of life and longevity. The associations of PE & SE with oxidative stress, inflammation, and endothelial dysfunction and their association with psychosocial stress indicate that relieving PE can reduce stress, which reduces oxidation, inflammation, and endothelial dysfunction. As a result, reducing stress, including PE, is in itself an antioxidant. Like exercise, which is arguably the most powerful antioxidant, reducing stress is arguably the second most powerful antioxidant.

There are many treatment modalities to help relieve the symptoms of stress, including prophylactic therapies that seem to help reduce the symptoms of singular, anticipated stressors such as public speaking [241]. This study demonstrated that a mixture of 3 g/day of each of L-lysine and L-arginine taken for 10 days prior to a public speaking event by subjects with high anxiety traits resulted in enhanced adrenocorticotropic hormone, cortisol, adrenaline, and noradrenaline levels and galvanic skin responses during stress compared to those in placebo-treated group. However, increases in the heart rate and blood pressure in response to public speaking task were not influenced by amino acid treatment. Perhaps this suggests that the higher cortical constructs amplifying hormonal stress responses were treated, while the more basal neurological reflex responses to stress were maintained and still protecting the individual.

The fact that HR and BP responses where not modified by treatment demonstrates that only the symptoms of stress were reduced by that treatment modality. This exemplifies the effects of most anxiolytics. The experiences with stress, and the associated anxiety and cardiovascular disorder that result from stress, demonstrate that at the core of the excessive stress response is a form of depression, measured as PE. Causing, in part, and compounding the depression is the poor brain perfusion also caused by PE. Depression is a common and debilitating condition, which is often treated with antidepressants. Depression increases the risk of adverse cardiovascular outcomes two- to fourfold over cardiac patients who are not depressed [242]. Yet controversy still exists as to whether use of antidepressants, particularly selective serotonin reuptake inhibitors (SSRIs), increases or reduces the risk [243, 244]. This is important because antidepressants are one of the most commonly prescribed types of drug worldwide, and their use is increasing, especially the use of SSRIs due to their minimal effect on BP as compared with the other types of antidepressants [245–247].

The heretofore inability to directly measure parasympathetic activity has perpetuated the controversy over antidepressants. Included in this controversy is the joint statement from the American Heart Association and the American College of Cardiologists in 2008 stating that there is no statistically significant evidence that standard therapy for heart failure (triple adrenergic blockade) is inducing depression in some patients. This statement refers back to the Val-HeFT studies in the 1990s suggesting that approximately 35% of heart failure patients were over blocked, thereby inducing depression and elevating risk of MACE [248]. P&S monitoring is now able to directly measure parasympathetic activity, identify these 35% greater risk patients, and prevent excessive sympathetic blockade, thereby reducing their risk and improving patient outcomes [249].

Direct measures of parasympathetic activity have also helped to discover that SSRIs may also be the antidepressant with the weakest effect on the P&S nervous systems. This provides rationale as to why the cardiologists prefer SSRIs over the other antidepressants: SSRIs do not increase BP as much as the others because it does not affect parasympathetic activity significantly, which means that sympathovagal balance is not greatly affected, which means that the relative sympathetic activity in these patients is not significantly affected, and with little sympathetic effect, baroreceptor reflex is not effected, which means BP is not affected. However, neither is the depression and its comorbidities (e.g., sleep and cognitive difficulties, "brain fog," GI upset, etc.) significantly affected because the PE is not significantly affected. So without a direct parasympathetic measure, the typical reaction is to titrate higher the dose of SSRI or add another antidepressant, furthering the suicide and other risks made well known by all of the antidepressant commercials.

These patients are often switched to another antidepressant (as opposed to adding another), and almost always their dose is significantly reduced even to the minimum available. Remember, the P&S nervous systems are like a pendulum. A pendulum is not corrected with a sledge hammer. Rather, it takes multiple, *gentle* nudges to correct a pendulum. This is the rationale for very-low-dose antidepressants, what is called low-dose anticholinergic therapy, such as 10.0 mg nortriptyline, a day at dinner. At these levels, patients report sleeping better within about 2 weeks and after 6–9 months at the earliest (typically no more than 18 months), when the PE is relieved, weaning the patients from the antidepressant is then considered, assuming they have not already self-weaned. Even though antidepressants carry the well-known side effects, and the non-SSRI types have a significant effect on blood pressure, these effects are at the high, clinical doses recommended by the manufacturer. At the very low doses suggested for autonomic therapy, the effect on blood pressure is minimal, and at worst transient, for once P&S balance is restored, high blood pressure is also relieved. However, if high blood pressure is a significant concern, and any risk of increase is potentially dangerous, consider switching to or titrating carvedilol in place of the anticholinergic. Carvedilol is a double cocktail, in the face of autonomic dysfunction (high blood pressure and depression definitely indicate autonomic dysfunction – both P&S are high), which treats both blood pressure and depression by treating both P&S [18].

These findings are corroborated by the drug safety communication issued by the USFDA in 2011, stating that citalopram should not be prescribed at doses greater than 40 mg per day, based on findings of QT interval prolongation [250]. The European Medicines Agency issued a similar safety warning in 2011. Further studies have reported QT interval prolongation with citalopram and also with escitalopram [251, 252]. QT interval prolongation is a result of PE and can lead to arrhythmias including potentially fatal torsade de pointes [253]. If SSRIs are effective anticholinergics, even indirectly, they should have relieved PE, and therefore prolonged QT interval should not present. While SSRIs are indeed safe, in that they do not significantly increase BP or the occurrence of arrhythmia or MACE [254], they also do not significantly affect PE and therefore only mask the symptoms of depression, forcing long-term use.

## Some Comments on Adrenal Fatigue

The adrenal glands produce a variety of hormones that are essential to life, including cortisol (the stress hormone) and aldosterone (a fluid balance hormone), as well as adrenaline (the stress response hormone). The medical term adrenal *insufficiency* (Addison's disease) refers to inadequate production of one or more of these hormones as a result of an underlying disease. Signs and symptoms of adrenal *insufficiency* may include fatigue, body aches and weakness, unexplained weight loss, low BP, light-headedness or dizziness upon standing, loss of body hair, skin discoloration (hyperpigmentation), and loss of menstrual periods in women. Furthermore, Addison's disease is rare. If there is fatigue related to hormones, it's more likely to be a thyroid problem or diabetes rather than an adrenal issue.

Adrenal fatigue is a term applied to a collection of nonspecific symptoms, such as body aches, sleep disturbances, fatigue (including trouble getting out of bed and chronic tiredness, even after rising in the morning), nervousness, "brain fog" (including trouble thinking clearly or finishing tasks), and digestive problems, all thought to be caused by poorly working adrenal glands in people who are under mental, emotional, or physical stress. This is the basis for the confusion. The similarities between the two lists of symptoms lead people to misinterpret the differences. In a 2016 publication, a systematic search was performed at PubMed, MEDLINE (Ensco), and Cochrane databases, from the beginning of the data until April 22, 2016. The keywords that were searched were "adrenal" + "fatigue," "adrenal" + "burnout," "adrenal" + "exhaustion," "hyponatremia," "burnout" + "cortisol," "fatigue" + "cortisol," "clinical" + "burnout," "cortisol" + "vitality," "adrenal" + "vitality," and "cortisol" + "exhaustion." Eligibility criteria were (1) articles written in English, (2) cortisol profile and fatigue or energy status as the primary outcome, (3) tests performed for evaluating the adrenal axis, (4) the absence of corticosteroid therapy influence, and (5) the absence of confounding diseases. From 3470 articles found, 58 studies fulfilled the criteria: 33 studies involved healthy individuals and 25 studies involved symptomatic patients. The results are an almost systematic finding of conflicting results derived from most of the study methods utilized, regardless of the validation and the quality of tests performed. Some limitations of the review include (1) heterogeneity of the study design, (2) the descriptive nature of most studies, (3) the poor-quality assessment of fatigue, (4) the use of an unsubstantiated methodology in terms of cortisol assessment (not endorsed by endocrinologists), (5) false premises leading to an incorrect sequence of research direction, and (6) inappropriate/invalid conclusions regarding causality and association between different information. This systematic review proves that there is no substantiation that "adrenal fatigue" is an actual medical condition. Therefore, adrenal fatigue is still a myth [255].

While the term "adrenal fatigue" often shows up in popular health books and on alternative medicine websites, it isn't an accepted medical diagnosis. Adrenal insufficiency can be diagnosed by blood tests and special stimulation tests that show inadequate levels of adrenal hormones. Proponents of the adrenal fatigue diagnosis claim this is a mild form of adrenal insufficiency caused by chronic stress. The unproven theory behind adrenal fatigue is that the adrenal glands are unable to keep pace with the demands of perpetual fight-or-flight arousal. As a result, they can't produce quite enough of the hormones needed to feel good. Further, they claim that existing blood tests, according to this theory, aren't sensitive enough to detect such a small decline in adrenal function, but the body is. The problem is that the adrenals are still producing the hormones! Yes, it's very frustrating to have persistent symptoms that cannot be readily explained. But accepting a medically unrecognized diagnosis could be worse. Unproven remedies for so-called adrenal fatigue may leave patients feeling more sick or lead to other disorders that are caused by the therapy, while the real cause, such as depression or fibromyalgia, continues to take its toll.

Some doctors say these symptoms can be due to other health problems. Robert Vigersky, MD, a physician familiar with P&S monitoring and a past president of the Endocrine Society, says the symptoms are very common in people in general. Though people often blame their hormonal glands, such as the adrenals or thyroid, for their tiredness, Vigersky says in many cases, fatigue is due to common problems such as poor sleep habits, poor diet, stress at work or home, and depression. All of these can affect energy level without involving adrenal glands. Fatigue is also a symptom of many diseases such as anemia, arthritis, diabetes, and heart failure. In these cases and more, "adrenal fatigue" has been questioned. These patients have been tested with P&S monitoring, and some form of PE has been found in every case [Personal communication, Drs. DePace and Colombo]. As stated above, PE is known to underlie diseases such as depression and fibromyalgia. With fatigue or any other symptom that is thought to be associated with "adrenal fatigue," proper testing is recommended. A primary care doctor may check for common illnesses that cause fatigue. If a hormone-related problem does not exist, then perhaps an endocrinologist is needed. Endocrinologists may do a variety of tests to check hormone levels. If a diagnosis of Addison's disease (adrenal insufficiency) is made, then the doctor will be able to document that the adrenal glands do not make enough hormones. Unlike adrenal fatigue, this lack of hormones will be detected by blood tests and recognized by other physicians. In most cases of this disease, the adrenal glands have been damaged by the immune system, from diseases like tuberculosis, cancer (such as lymphoma), and AIDS.

Be cautious with unproven treatments. According to the Endocrine Society, some supplements sold for adrenal health may be harmful. Some of these contain extracts of human hormone glands, which can lead to an excess amount of that hormone which may cause real disorders or diseases. Instead of these potentially harmful supplements, consider a change in lifestyle and the safe and medically proven supplements, for example:

1. Eat plenty of fruits and vegetables, eat more fish (or at least take fish oil supplements to get more *omega-3 fatty acids*), and avoid junk food (a description of the *Mediterranean diet*).
2. Get enough sleep and *exercise* regularly.
3. Reduce stress (both *oxidative stress* with antioxidants and *psychosocial stress*).
4. Increase energy levels with *nitric oxide supplements*.

## Reducing Stress Is an Antioxidant

As stated previously, stress is a state of threatened homeostasis (Fig. 8.24). The human body attempts to adapt to stress. It is difficult to control this stress with pharmacology alone. Simply removing one's self from what is considered a stressful environment is not always the answer. Many medicines that are used to alleviate stress have toxic side effects which include habituation. Also, a resistance to mediations can occur in time (tachyphylaxis), which often occurs with chronic use of medicines to treat emotional stress. Biological stress exerts a complex interaction of hemodynamic, inflammatory, neural, humeral, and hemostatic changes that account for the increased incidence of myocardial infarction and coronary atherosclerosis.

Stress effects the mind-body connection. Stress adversely affects the P&S nervous systems. It impairs vagal (parasympathetic) tone which is protective [52], increases cortisol levels which can promote stress further; increases the adrenal medullary system in general, producing more catecholamines, which raises HR and BP; and increases oxidative stress and mitochondrial dysfunction. All of these directly or indirectly increase sympathetic tone, and prolonged sympa-

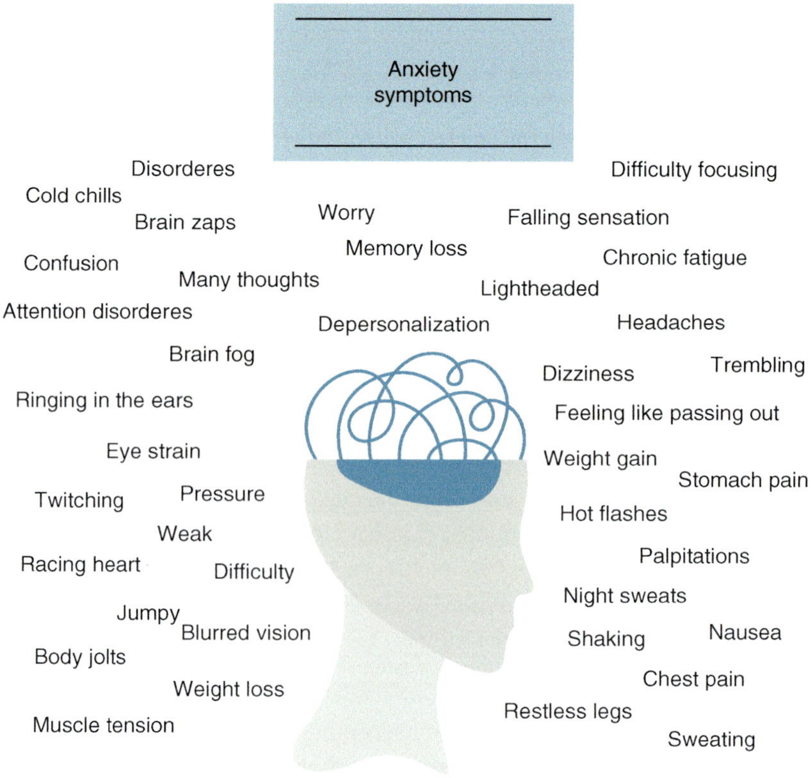


**Fig. 8.24** Symptoms and perceptions of anxiety. (Illustration by Elysian Creative Studio, www.elysiancreativestudio.com, Lizzy Colombo)

thetic tone is known to lead to cardiovascular disease, including heart attack and stroke. Many patients have complained of unresolved stress, even after medication and therapy. They have been found with atypical P&S coordination that is perpetuated or made worse by traditional therapies (e.g., a "hidden" PE that occurs during a sympathetic challenge such as stress [17]). For proper therapy, titrated to the individual, a P&S test is first required (typical autonomic testing will not reveal this condition).

Summarizing from above, physiological effects of stress include an increased cholesterol and fatty acid level in the body for energy production system. BP is increased with increasing stress. Inflammation is a response to stress. Local inflammation may cause redness, swelling, heat, and pain in joints. Ongoing stress perpetuates inflammation and may cause the blood to clot faster and form more blood clotting elements. Psychosocial stress increases production of blood sugar for energy and increases stomach acids and gastric secretion (Fig. 8.25) which may promote gastric and esophageal irritation (GERD). Also, increasing stress can decrease protein synthesis and intestinal movement. It may also impair immune responses and cause the allergic response system to be depressed. A faster

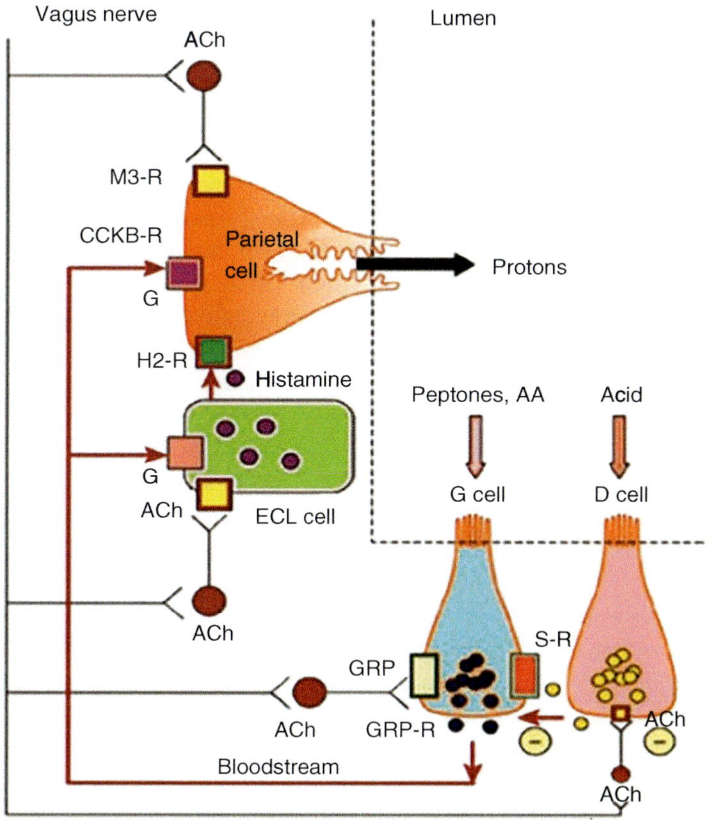


**Fig. 8.25** Regulation of gastric acid secretion by nerves and hormones. During the cephalic phase of digestion, vagal cholinergic nerves stimulate directly the parietal cells and induce histamine release from enterochromaffin-like cells (ECLs), which also stimulates parietal cells. Vagal fibers also release gastrin-releasing peptide (GRP) in the antrum to induce gastrin (G cells), which through the bloodstream induces histamine release and stimulates the parietal cells. During the gastric phase of digestion, food in the stomach causes local reflexes that stimulate the secretion of gastrin. Acidification of the gastric antrum stimulates somatostatin release (D cells), which inhibits the release of gastrin and this acid secretion. Vagal stimulation inhibits somatostatin release [19, Fig. 3.25]. (Republished with permission from Springer International Publishing AG)

heart beat and faster respiration are often consequences of stress effects on the autonomic nervous system, increasing metabolism.

The known association between psychological stress and cardiovascular risk factors was significantly emphasized in the famous INTERHEART study which gave a global analysis of psychological stress and myocardial infarction [256]. Holter monitors and ambulatory BP monitoring have been used to assess stress such as at the workplace, which may also reduce heart rate variability (HRV, a measure of autonomic activity) [257, 258]. Epidemiological studies have also been important in emphasizing the relationship and cause of psychosocial stress and cardiac disease.

Acute stress can trigger plaque rupture. Acute stress prepares biological organisms for fight-or-flight defense mechanisms [259]. With acute stress, both (1) norepinephrine (aka noradrenaline) is released from the autonomic nervous systems fibers and (2) adrenaline (epinephrine) from the adrenal glands. Norepinephrine stimulates alpha-1 and beta-1 receptors and epinephrine alpha-2 and beta-2 receptors. Catecholamines are rapidly cleared from the plasma with a half-life of several minutes; however, sympathetic norepinephrine undergoes rapid uptake back into the nerve and is much shorter acting. Stress may increase HR by activating sympathetic nerves but also by inhibiting the parasympathetic-vagal nerve which acts as a brake on the sinus node. HR per se is not a good indicator of cardio-sympathetic activity but HRV, that is, the variability of HR, is.

During acute stress with a defense reaction, there is sympathetic activation of most of the organs in the body, and epinephrine and cortisol are secreted, and the renin-angiotensin system is activated. There is withdrawal of vagus or parasympathetic input, which increases the HR along with sympathetic activation. BP is elevated. Stress raises the HR by increasing cardio-sympathetic nerves and decreasing vagal input and may be a stimulus for arrhythmias and cause ischemia. This can increase plaque rupture in patients who are vulnerable with plaques which are unstable. Low HRV can also increase cardiovascular risk [260, 261].

The hypothalamic-pituitary-adrenal axis is very important in coordinating the stress response. Glucocorticoids are major components of the stress systems and affect many different systems. They can attenuate inflammation, cellular proliferation, and tissue repair processes. Prolonged responses of stress result in various endocrine, autoimmune, metabolic, and psychiatric changes which can increase morbidity and mortality from cardiovascular disease. These include stress-induced hypercortisolism and central obesity, which is a component of metabolic syndrome. Visceral obesity is a sequelae of stress because of chronic cortisol elevations. Chronic stress increases appetite, increases sympathetic system activation, and increases the hypothalamic-pituitary-adrenal axis which increases cortisol. This leads to visceral obesity, metabolic syndrome, and insulin resistance, and eventually diabetes. Endothelial damage and atherosclerosis with its inherent risk of cardiovascular events and mortality can ensue. Lifestyle changes along with pharmacology and appropriate antioxidant balance are very important in controlling this.

It therefore appears that stress of an acute nature predominantly affects the P&S systems with sympathetic activity and the hypothalamic-pituitary-adrenal (HPA) axis secondarily, whereas chronic stress prominently affects the HPA axis with chronic cortisol elevation and its adverse consequences and the P&S secondarily. In the latter, the P&S must adapt to the chronic situation. Stress can also affect the hemostasis of the blood system. This can activate platelets and cause blood to coagulate more easily. Heart attacks are often caused by atherosclerotic plaque ruptures due to inflammatory weakening of a fibrous cap over a plaque. Endothelial dysfunction may promote thrombus and clot formation. Therefore, platelets and coagulation seem to contribute to accelerated atherosclerosis [262].

Job stress has been associated with a prothrombotic state with elevated fibrinogen in factor VII and reduced fibrinolytic activity [263]. During acute stress, the sympathetic-adrenal system may be involved in hemostatic changes, whereas the HPA axis and vagal function seem more important in modulating hemostatic activity during chronic stress. While vacations are highly recommended to remove the individual from job stress to relax, there are those who simply cannot relax. In some of these cases, the vacation itself becomes a stress. Reducing stress depends as much on the individual as it does the stressor.

Perhaps the epitome of abnormal stress responses is PTSD. In these cases, the stress has been internalized, and there is no escaping. Current research in PTSD has suggested several mechanisms of how this increased cardiovascular disease. PTSD is strongly associated with other psychiatric disorders including anxiety and depression, which have been shown to predict future cardiovascular events, even when controlling for conventional cardiovascular risk factors and symptoms of depression and anxiety [264, 265]. In PTSD, there is evidence of high cortisol levels and peripheral adrenergic activity [266]. It is believed that sympathetic overactivity in increased norepinephrine levels may promote pro-inflammatory and procoagulant changes which contribute to ongoing inflammation and hypercoagulable states. This may be exacerbated by the dynamic PE discussed above [17]. This can promote clot formation and plaque ruptures and myocardial infarction. There is also low (resting) vagal tone in PTSD, and, in this case, the protective mechanism or braking mechanism is being nullified [267, 268]. In addition, research [18] has shown that the low resting vagal tone enabling a resting sympathetic excess (SE) is exacerbated by a dynamic vagal, or parasympathetic, excess (PE) that further amplifies the SE. As described above, the dynamic PE introduces the depression that is characteristic of PTSD, and both forms of SE (resting and dynamic) lead to the stress and chronic stress-related symptoms characteristic of PTSD. PTSD occurs in a sizable portion of patients after myocardial infarction. It can adversely affect their prognosis. It promotes inflammation and hypercoagulability. It adversely affects the P&S nervous systems. It promotes endothelial dysfunction and low-grade inflammation. Further research is needed in this area.

Stressors produce cognitive, emotional, psychological, and behavioral changes that can be harmful to one's physical and psychological well-being. Psychosocial stress may be characterized as depression with anxiety (Fig. 8.24). Abnormal cognitive changes include worry and loss of concentration, memory loss, especially short-term memory loss, and an inability to make decisions. People can also have acute mental status changes. Emotional changes may include anxiety, apprehension, irritation, anger, shame, guilt, depression, and other negative emotions.

Not just the central and P&S nervous systems but the immune and endocrine systems may be affected by stress. Dry throat and mouth, trembling and muscle tension, cold hands and feet, headaches, fatigue, frequent illness, and weakness may all be manifestation of chronic ongoing stress. Stress may adversely affect people's relationships with others and their ability to perform at work. Stress may also exacerbate asthma conditions and other chronic lung conditions including reactive airway disease. Menstrual disorders may present and may worsen with stress as in recurrent vaginal infections in women. Impotence and premature ejaculation may be evidence of stress in men. Skin rashes, eczema, and psoriasis may become worse. Diseases of the digestive tract such as gastritis and esophagitis may be worsened. Also, stomach ulcers may be produced. Irritable bowel syndrome is a common manifestation of ongoing stress. Stress affecting the musculoskeletal system may cause neck and shoulder pain (aka "Coat Hanger" pain) and a fibromyalgia-type syndrome with musculoskeletal aches. Stress may also exacerbate low back pain. Stress has even been associated with hair loss and baldness. Stress, if it is acute, may cause a shock-like state to the heart muscle and a condition called Takotsubo cardiomyopathy. It may also cause restriction of arteries, including arterial spasm. When it occurs in the coronary arteries, it may cause severe chest pain or heart attacks.

Chronic stress predisposes individuals and makes them more susceptible to infections. Immune function is depressed. People with chronic stress have been known to be predisposed to pulmonary embolism after long trips presumably because of increased clotting propensity.

There may be an increase in viral cancers with stress. Ongoing psychosocial stress may be a trigger for autoimmune diseases, migraines, obsessive-compulsive behavior, posttraumatic stress, insomnia, depression, irritable bowel syndrome, reflux esophagitis, and substance abuse. Skin rashes, hives, and ectopic dermatitis worsen with stress. Some authorities believe that degenerative neurological disorders like Parkinson's disease will worsen with psychosocial stress.

One adverse effect of chronic stress is that increased cortisol causes greater sensitization of the rewards center and stimulates pleasurable behavior, which may cause individuals to seek drugs or excessive intake of palatable foods which are high in fat and high in sugar. By increasing palatable food, another source of visceral fat accumulation is provided, and this mechanism creates central, leptin, and insulin resistance. Elevated BP and arrhythmias are found to be more difficult to treat when individuals are exposed to chronic psychosocial stress. Only after this stress is ameliorated or reduced are these abnormalities easier to control. Serum lipid levels seem to also be difficult to control in individuals with psychosocial stress, especially high triglyceride and low HDL levels. Some of this may be a reflection of diet noncompliance during times of stress. Of course, obesity and weight gain are promoted during high levels of psychosocial stress. Therefore, obtaining ideal weight or ideal BMI is very difficult with ongoing chronic stress. It is thought that high emotional stress may also be linked to promotion of ROS and increased oxidative stress states.

Identifying stress and stress management are crucial components of wellness. Unfortunately, it is difficult to monitor stress and quantitate it. A stress questionnaire was developed in the book, *The Heart Repair Manual*, published by W.W. Norton in 1992. There are many questionnaires that have been proposed to test for stress. The P&S test quantifies the effects of stress on the nervous system to help determine how to treat. There are many modalities to lower stress, in addition to pharmaceuticals, nutraceuticals, and supplements. These include:

1. Meditation or prayer[14] [269–274]
2. Progressive relaxation techniques[15]
3. Biofeedback or neurofeedback techniques[16] (see "Neurofeedback," Chap. 9)
4. Acupuncture
5. Massage
6. Deep breathing exercises
7. Cognitive behavior therapy
8. Exercise
9. Yoga
10. Tai chi

P&S monitoring and the Mind-Body Wellness Program help individuals identify and treat the factors contributing to chronic psychosocial stress and encourage these individuals to seek stress reduction modalities they are most comfortable with pursuing and complying with, whether it be a form of meditation, yoga, exercise, or biofeedback. Tranquilizers, such as benzodiazepine, are strongly discouraged. Yet they are not discouraged in cognitive behavioral therapy and pharmacotherapy, especially under the guidance of a psychiatrist. However, with the use

[14] Meditation or prayer has been demonstrated to reduce stress by increasing parasympathetic activity (reducing or normalizing sympathovagal balance).

[15] A method of deep muscle relaxation based on the premise that muscle tension is the body's physiological response to anxiety-provoking thoughts and that muscle relaxation blocks anxiety. Therapy focuses on tightening and relaxing specific muscle groups in sequence. It's also known as progressive muscle relaxation which teaches you how to relax your muscles through a two-step process. First, particular muscle groups in your body are systematically put under tension, such as your neck and shoulders. Next, the tension is released and should be more relaxed. Whether reducing muscle tension is a result of relaxation or a cause of relaxation is unknown. Little, if any, rigorous research has been performed in this area. However, the time spent relaxing, which is well known to increase parasympathetic activity, has been demonstrated to reduce stress by increasing parasympathetic activity (reducing or normalizing sympathovagal balance). See "Meditation or Prayer" above.

[16] Biofeedback uses HR, for example, as a means of training the nervous system to relax. Neurofeedback uses EEG waves (from your brain) as a means of training the nervous system to relax. Neurofeedback requires trained healthcare professionals to train the patient and interpret and assess the outcomes. Biofeedback does not.

of very-low-dose tricyclics, SNRIs, or SSRIs, in conjunction with P&S monitoring and hemodynamic results including HR and BP and exercise testing, replacement therapy may be tailored. Of course, the twofold basis to all of this is (1) the three supplements to "heal the foundation," with (2) the three lifestyle changes, including stress reduction, to keep the foundation strong.

## References


1. Harrington R. Stress, health & well-being: thriving in the 21st century. Belmont: Wadsworth Cengage Learning; 2013.
2. Hjemdahl P, Rosengren A, Steptoe A, editors. Stress and cardiovascular disease. London: Springer-Verlag; 2012.
3. Bot I, Kuiper J. Stressed brain, stressed heart? Lancet. 2017;389(10071):770–1. https://doi.org/10.1016/S0140-6736(17)30044-2. Epub 2017 Jan 12.
4. Chi JS, Kloner RA. Stress and myocardial infarction. Heart. 2003;89(5):475–6.
5. Pignalberi C, Patti G, Chimenti C, Pasceri V, Maseri A. Role of different determinants of psychological distress in acute coronary syndromes. J Am Coll Cardiol. 1998;32(3):613–9.
6. Yusuf S, Hawken S, Ounpuu S, Dans T, Avezum A, Lanas F, McQueen M, Budaj A, Pais P, Varigos J, Lisheng L, INTERHEART Study Investigators. Effect of potentially modifiable risk factors associated with myocardial infarction in 52 countries (the INTERHEART study): case-control study. Lancet. 2004;364(9438):937–52.
7. Ohlin B, Nilsson PM, Nilsson JA, Berglund G. Chronic psychosocial stress predicts long-term cardiovascular morbidity and mortality in middle-aged men. Eur Heart J. 2004;25(10):867–73.
8. Tofler GH, Stone PH, Maclure M, Edelman E, Davis VG, Robertson T, Antman EM, Muller JE. Analysis of possible triggers of acute myocardial infarction (the MILIS study). Am J Cardiol. 1990;66(1):22–7.
9. Brezinka V, Kittel F. Psychosocial factors of coronary heart disease in women: a review. Soc Sci Med. 1996;42(10):1351–65. Review.
10. Gonzales TK, Yonker JA, Chang V, Roan CL, Herd P, Atwood CS. Myocardial infarction in the Wisconsin Longitudinal Study: the interaction among environmental, health, social, behavioural and genetic factors. BMJ Open. 2017;7(1):e011529. https://doi.org/10.1136/bmjopen-2016-011529.
11. Bunker SJ, Colquhoun DM, Esler MD, Hickie IB, Hunt D, Jelinek VM, Oldenburg BF, Peach HG, Ruth D, Tennant CC, Tonkin AM. "Stress" and coronary heart disease: psychosocial risk factors. Med J Aust. 2003;178(6):272–6. Review.
12. Kuper H, Adami HO, Theorell T, Weiderpass E. Psychosocial determinants of coronary heart disease in middle-aged women: a prospective study in Sweden. Am J Epidemiol. 2006;164(4):349–57. Epub 2006 Jun 20.
13. Welin C, Lappas G, Wilhelmsen L. Independent importance of psychosocial factors for prognosis after myocardial infarction. J Intern Med. 2000;247(6):629–39.
14. Rosengren A, Hawken S, Ounpuu S, Sliwa K, Zubaid M, Almahmeed WA, Blackett KN, Sitthi-amorn C, Sato H, Yusuf S, INTERHEART investigators. Association of psychosocial risk factors with risk of acute myocardial infarction in 11119 cases and 13648 controls from 52 countries (the INTERHEART study): case-control study. Lancet. 2004;364(9438):953–62.
15. Smyth A, O'Donnell M, Lamelas P, Teo K, Rangarajan S, Yusuf S, INTERHEART Investigators. Physical activity and anger or emotional upset as triggers of acute myocardial infarction: The INTERHEART study. Circulation. 2016;134(15):1059–67.
16. Tawakol A, Ishai A, Takx RA, Figueroa AL, Ali A, Kaiser Y, Truong QA, Solomon CJ, Calcagno C, Mani V, Tang CY, Mulder WJ, Murrough JW, Hoffmann U, Nahrendorf M, Shin LM, Fayad ZA, Pitman RK. Relation between resting amygdalar activity and cardiovascular events: a longitudinal and cohort study. Lancet. 2017;389(10071):834–45. https://doi.org/10.1016/S0140-6736(16)31714-7. Epub 2017 Jan 12.
17. Tobias H, Vinitsky A, Bulgarelli RJ, Ghosh-Dastidar S, Colombo J. Autonomic nervous system monitoring of patients with excess parasympathetic responses to sympathetic challenges – clinical observations. US Neurol. 2010;5(2):62–6.
18. Colombo J, Arora RR, DePace NL, Vinik AI. Clinical autonomic dysfunction: measurement, indications, therapies, and outcomes. New York: Springer Science + Business Media; 2014.
19. Cardinali DP. Autonomic nervous system: basic and clinical aspects. Cham: Springer International Publishing AG; 2018.
20. Selye H. The stress of life. 2nd ed. New York: McGraw-Hill; 1956.
21. Even N, Devaud JM, Barron A. General stress responses in the honey bee. Insects. 2012;3:1271–98. https://doi.org/10.3390/insects3041271.
22. Ulrich-Lai YM, Herman JP. Neural regulation of endocrine and autonomic stress responses. Nat Rev Neurosci. 2009;10:397–409.
23. Bamberger CM, Schulte HM, Chrousos GP. Molecular determinants of glucocorticoid receptor function and tissue sensitivity to glucocorticoids. Endocr Rev. 1996;17:245–61.
24. McEwen BS. The neurobiology of stress: from serendipity to clinical relevance. Brain Res. 2000;886:172–89.
25. Chrousos GP. Stress and disorders of the stress system. Nat Rev Endocrinol. 2009;5:374–81.

26. Stratakis CA, Chrousos GP. Neuroendocrinology and pathophysiology of the stress system. Ann N Y Acad Sci. 1995;771:1–18.
27. Taggart P, Lambiase P. Anger, emotion, and arrhythmias: from brain to heart. Front Physiol. 2011;19(2):67–72.
28. Tait AS, Butts CL, Sternberg EM. The role of glucocorticoids and progestins in inflammatory, autoimmune, and infectious disease. J Leukoc Biol. 2008;84(4):924–31. https://doi.org/10.1189/jlb.0208104.
29. Butts CL, Sternberg EM. Neuroendocrine factors alter host defense by modulating immune function. Cell Immunol. 2008;252(1–2):7–15.
30. Thayer JF, Loerbroks A, Sternberg EM. Inflammation and cardiorespiratory control: the role of the vagus nerve. Respir Physiol Neurobiol. 2011;178(3):387–94. https://doi.org/10.1016/j.resp.2011.05.016. Epub 2011 May 27. Review.
31. Felton DL. Neural influence on immune responses: underlying suppositions and basic principles of neural-immune signaling. Prog Brain Res. 2000;122:381–9.
32. Bär K-J, Boettger MK, Berger S, Baier V, Sauer H, Yeragani VK, Voss A. Decreased baroreflex sensitivity in acute schizophrenia. J Appl Physiol. 2007;102(3):1051–6.
33. Hong Y. Sympathovagal imbalance in type 2 diabetes – role of brainstem thyrotropin-releasing hormone. In: Masuo K, editor. Type 2 diabetes. IntechOpen. https://doi.org/10.5772/56541.
34. Craig AD. Forebrain emotional asymmetry: a neuroanatomical basis? Trends Cogn Sci. 2005;9:566–71.
35. Lane RD, Jennings JR. Hemispheric asymmetry, autonomic asymmetry and the problem of sudden death. In: Davidson RJ, Hugdahl K, editors. Brain asymmetry. Cambridge, MA: The MIT Press; 1995. p. 271–304.
36. DePace NL, Mears JP, Yayac M, Colombo J. Cardiac autonomic testing and diagnosing heart disease. "A clinical perspective". Heart Int. 2014;9(2):37–44. https://doi.org/10.5301/heartint.5000218; published online 12/5/2014 12:29:58 PM.
37. DePace NL, Mears JP, Yayac M, Colombo J. Cardiac autonomic testing and treating heart disease. "A clinical perspective". Heart Int. 2014;9(2):45–52. https://doi.org/10.5301/heartint.5000216; published online 11/19/2014 1:16:08 PM.
38. Akashi YJ, Goldstein DS, Barbaro G, Ueyama T. Takotsubo cardiomyopathy: a new form of acute, reversible heart failure. Circulation. 2008;118:2754–62.
39. Nalivaiko E. Animal models of psychogenic cardiovascular disorders: what we can learn from them and what we cannot. Clin Exp Pharmacol Physiol. 2011;38:115–25.
40. Pelliccia F, Greco C, Vitale C, Rosano G, Gaudio C, Kaski JC. Takotsubo syndrome (stress cardiomyopathy): an intriguing clinical condition in search of its identity. Am J Med. 2014;127:699–704.
41. Terefe YG, Niraj A, Pradhan J, Kondur A, Afonso L. Myocardial infarction with angiographically normal coronary arteries in the contemporary era. Coron Artery Dis. 2007;18:621–6.
42. Pelliccia F, Greco C, Vitale C, Rosano G, Gaudio C, Kaski JC. Takotsubo syndrome (stress cardiomyopathy): an intriguing clinical condition in search of its identity. Am J Med. 2014;127:699–704.
43. Kurisu S, Sato H, Kawagoe T, Ishihara M, Shimatani Y, Nishioka K, Kono Y, Umemura T, Nakamura S. Tako-tsubo-like left ventricular dysfunction with ST-segment elevation: a novel cardiac syndrome mimicking acute myocardial infarction. Am Heart J. 2002;143:448–55.
44. Sharkey SW, Lesser JR, Zenovich AG, Maron MS, Lindberg J, Longe TF, Maron BJ. Acute and reversible cardiomyopathy provoked by stress in women from the United States. Circulation. 2005;111:472–9.
45. Mori H, Ishikawa S, Kojima S, Hayashi J, Watanabe Y, Hoffman JI, Okino H. Increased responsiveness of left ventricular apical myocardium to adrenergic stimuli. Cardiovasc Res. 1993;27:192–8.
46. Gullette EC, Blumenthal JA, Babyak M, Jiang W, Waugh RA, Frid DJ, O'Connor CM, Morris JJ, Krantz DS. Effects of mental stress on myocardial ischemia during daily life. JAMA. 1997;277:1521–6.
47. Pimple P, Shah A, Rooks C, Bremner JD, Nye J, Ibeanu I, Murrah N, Shallenberger L, Kelley M, Raggi P, Vaccarino V. Association between anger and mental stress-induced myocardial ischemia. Am Heart J. 2015;169:115–21.
48. Boyle SH, Williams RB, Mark DB, Brummett BH, Siegler IC, Barefoot JC. Hostility, age, and mortality in a sample of cardiac patients. Am J Cardiol. 2005;96:64–6.
49. Reich P, DeSilva RA, Lown B, Murawski BJ. Acute psychological disturbances preceding life-threatening ventricular arrhythmias. JAMA. 1981;246:233–5.
50. Lampert R, Shusterman V, Burg MM, Lee FA, Earley C, Goldberg A, McPherson CA, Batsford WP, Soufer R. Effects of psychologic stress on repolarization and relationship to autonomic and hemodynamic factors. J Cardiovasc Electrophysiol. 2005;16:372–7.
51. Lampert R. Anger and ventricular arrhythmias. Curr Opin Cardiol. 2010;25:46–52.
52. Curtis BM, O'Keefe JH. Autonomic tone as a cardiovascular risk factor: the dangers of chronic fight or flight. Mayo Clin Proc. 2002;77:45–54.
53. Tan AY, Verrier RL. The role of the autonomic nervous system in cardiac arrhythmias. Handb Clin Neurol. 2013;117:135–45.
54. Alfano KM, Cimino CR. Alteration of expected hemispheric asymmetries: valence and arousal effects in neuropsychological models of emotion. Brain Cogn. 2008;66:213–20.
55. Hagemann D, Waldstein SR, Thayer JF. Central and autonomic nervous system integration in emotion. Brain Cogn. 2003;52:79–87.

56. Taggart P, Boyett MR, Logantha S, Lambiase PD. Anger, emotion, and arrhythmias: from brain to heart. Front Physiol. 2011;2:67.
57. Steptoe A, Kivimäki M. Stress and cardiovascular disease: an update on current knowledge. Annu Rev Public Health. 2013;34:337–54.
58. von Känel R, Mills PJ, Fainman C, Dimsdale JE. Effects of psychological stress and psychiatric disorders on blood coagulation and fibrinolysis: a biobehavioral pathway to coronary artery disease? Psychosom Med. 2001;63:531–44.
59. Wirtz PH, Ehlert U, Emini L, Rüdisüli K, Groessbauer S, Gaab J, Elsenbruch S, von Känel R. Anticipatory cognitive stress appraisal and the acute procoagulant stress response in men. Psychosom Med. 2006;68:851–8.
60. Shimbo D, Child J, Davidson K, Geer E, Osende JI, Reddy S, Dronge A, Fuster V, Badimon JJ. Exaggerated serotonin-mediated platelet reactivity as a possible link in depression and acute coronary syndromes. Am J Cardiol. 2002;89:331–3.
61. Zafar MU, Paz-Yepes M, Shimbo D, Vilahur G, Burg MM, Chaplin W, Fuster V, Davidson KW, Badimon JJ. Anxiety is a better predictor of platelet reactivity in coronary artery disease patients than depression. Eur Heart J. 2010;31:1573–82.
62. Lesch KP, Wolozin BL, Murphy DL, Reiderer P. Primary structure of the human platelet serotonin uptake site: identity with the brain serotonin transporter. J Neurochem. 1993;60:2319–22.
63. Becker RC. Editor's page: fundamentals in neurocardiology: the brain-platelet-coronary artery interface. J Thromb Thrombolysis. 2008;26:74–7.
64. Wirtz PH, Redwine LS, Baertschi C, Spillmann M, Ehlert U, von Känel R. Coagulation activity before and after acute psychosocial stress increases with age. Psychosom Med. 2008;70:476–81.
65. Jern C, Eriksson E, Tengborn L, Risberg B, Wadenvik H, Jern S. Changes of plasma coagulation and fibrinolysis in response to mental stress. Thromb Haemost. 1989;62:767–71.
66. von Känel R, Bellingrath S, Kudielka BM. Association between burnout and circulating levels of pro- and anti-inflammatory cytokines in schoolteachers. J Psychosom Res. 2008;65:51–9.
67. von Känel R, Dimsdale JE, Ziegler MG, Mills PJ, Patterson TL, Lee SK, Grant I. Effect of acute psychological stress on the hypercoagulable state in subjects (spousal caregivers of patients with Alzheimer's disease) with coronary or cerebrovascular disease and/or systemic hypertension. Am J Cardiol. 2001;87:1405–8.
68. Steptoe A, Wardle J, Marmot M. Positive affect and health-related neuroendocrine, cardiovascular, and inflammatory processes. Proc Natl Acad Sci U S A. 2005;102:6508–12.
69. Preckel D, von Känel R. Regulation of hemostasis by the sympathetic nervous system: any contribution to coronary artery disease? Heart. 2004;4:123–30.
70. von Känel R, Dimsdale JE. Effects of sympathetic activation by adrenergic infusions on hemostasis in vivo. Eur J Haematol. 2000;65:357–69.
71. von Känel R, Mills PJ, Ziegler MG, Dimsdale JE. Effect of beta2-adrenergic receptor functioning and increased norepinephrine on the hypercoagulable state with mental stress. Am Heart J. 2002;144:68–72.
72. Stämpfli SF, Camici GG, Keller S, Rozenberg I, Arras M, Schuler B, Gassmann M, Garcia I, Lüscher TF, Tanner FC. Restraint stress enhances arterial thrombosis in vivo – role of the sympathetic nervous system. Stress. 2014;17:126–32.
73. Allen MT, Patterson SM. Hemoconcentration and stress: a review of physiological mechanisms and relevance for cardiovascular disease risk. Biol Psychol. 1995;41:1–27.
74. Austin AW, Patterson SM, von Känel R. Hemoconcentration and hemostasis during acute stress: interacting and independent effects. Ann Behav Med. 2011;42:153–73.
75. Nater UM, Skoluda N, Strahler J. Biomarkers of stress in behavioural medicine. Curr Opin Psychiatry. 2013;26:440–5.
76. Sojka P, Stålnacke BM, Björnstig U, Karlsson K. One-year follow-up of patients with mild traumatic brain injury: occurrence of post-traumatic stress-related symptoms at follow-up and serum levels of cortisol, S-100B and neuron-specific enolase in acute phase. Brain Inj. 2006;20:613–20.
77. Michaud K, Matheson K, Kelly O, Anisman H. Impact of stressors in a natural context on release of cortisol in healthy adult humans: a meta-analysis. Stress. 2008;11:177–97.
78. Poll EM, Kreitschmann-Andermahr I, Langejuergen Y, Stanzel S, Gilsbach JM, Gressner A, Yagmur E. Saliva collection method affects predictability of serum cortisol. Clin Chim Acta. 2007;382:15–9.
79. Bozovic D, Racic M, Ivkovic N. Salivary cortisol levels as a biological marker of stress reaction. Med Arh. 2013;67:374–7.
80. Elenkov IJ, Chrousos GP. Stress hormones, Th1/Th2 patterns, pro/anti-inflammatory cytokines and susceptibility to disease. Trends Endocrinol Metab. 1999;10:359–68.
81. Moretti M, Colla A, de Oliveira BG, dos Santos DB, Budni J, de Freitas AE, Farina M, Severo Rodrigues AL. Ascorbic acid treatment, similarly to fluoxetine, reverses depressive-like behavior and brain oxidative damage induced by chronic unpredictable stress. J Psychiatr Res. 2012;46:331–40.
82. Bertone-Johnson ER, Whitcomb BW, Missmer SA, Karlson EW, Rich-Edwards JW. Inflammation and early-life abuse in women. Am J Prev Med. 2012;43:611–20.
83. Chavda N, Kantharia ND, Jaykaran. Effects of fluoxetine and escitalopram on C-reactive protein in patients of depression. J Pharmacol Pharmacother. 2011;2:11–6.

84. Antoni MH, Lutgendorf SK, Blomberg B, Carver CS, Lechner S, Diaz A, Stagl J, Arevalo JM, Cole SW. Cognitive-behavioral stress management reverses anxiety-related leukocyte transcriptional dynamics. Biol Psychiatry. 2012;71:366–72.
85. Lu XT, Zhao YX, Zhang Y, Jiang F. Psychological stress, vascular inflammation, and atherogenesis: potential roles of circulating cytokines. J Cardiovasc Pharmacol. 2013;62:6–12.
86. Skurk T, van Harmelen V, Hauner H. Angiotensin II stimulates the release of interleukin-6 and interleukin-8 from cultured human adipocytes by activation of NF-kappaB. Arterioscler Thromb Vasc Biol. 2004;24:1199–203.
87. Tsuchiya K, Yoshimoto T, Hirono Y, Tateno T, Sugiyama T, Hirata Y. Angiotensin II induces monocyte chemoattractant protein-1 expression via a nuclear factor kappaB- dependent pathway in rat preadipocytes. Am J Physiol Endocrinol Metab. 2006;291:E771–8.
88. Lu XT, Zhao YX, Zhang Y, Jiang F. Psychological stress, vascular inflammation, and atherogenesis: potential roles of circulating cytokines. J Cardiovasc Pharmacol. 2013;62:6–12.
89. Hapuarachchi JR, Chalmers AH, Winefield AH, Blake-Mortimer JS. Changes in clinically relevant metabolites with psychological stress parameters. Behav Med. 2003;29:52–9.
90. Tyagi N, Sedoris KC, Steed M, Ovechkin AV, Moshal KS, Tyagi SC. Mechanisms of homocysteine-induced oxidative stress. Am J Physiol Heart Circ Physiol. 2005;289:H2649–56.
91. Hiroki J, Shimokawa H, Higashi M, Morikawa K, Kandabashi T, Kawamura N, Kubota T, Ichiki T, Amano M, Kaibuchi K, Takeshita A. Inflammatory stimuli upregulate Rho-kinase in human coronary vascular smooth muscle cells. J Mol Cell Cardiol. 2004;37:537–46.
92. Bierhaus A, Wolf J, Andrassy M, Rohleder N, Humpert PM, Petrov D, Ferstl R, von Eynatten M, Wendt T, Rudofsky G, Joswig M, Morcos M, Schwaninger M, McEwen B, Kirschbaum C, Nawroth PP. A mechanism converting psychosocial stress into mononuclear cell activation. Proc Natl Acad Sci U S A. 2003;100:1920–5.
93. Sivonová M, Zitnanová I, Hlincíková L, Skodácek I, Trebaticlá J, Duracková Z. Oxidative stress in university students during examinations. Stress. 2004;7:183–8.
94. Mauck HP, Hockman CH. Central nervous system mechanisms mediating cardiac rate and rhythm. Am Heart J. 1967;74:106–9.
95. Engel GL. Sudden and rapid death during psychological stress. Ann Intern Med. 1971;74:771–82.
96. Trichopoulos D, Katsoutanni K, Zavitsanos X, Tronou A, Dalla-Vorgia P. Psychological stress and fatal heart attack: the Athens earthquake natural experiment. Lancet. 1983;1:441–3.
97. Meisel SR, Kutz I, Dayan KI, Pauzner H, Chetbourg I, Arbel Y, David D. Effect of Iraqi missile war on incidence of acute myocardial infarction and sudden death in Israeli civilians. Lancet. 1991;338:660–1.
98. Leor J, Poole WK, Kloner RA. Sudden cardiac death triggered by an earthquake. N Engl J Med. 1996;334:413–9.
99. Steinberg JS, Arshad A, Kowalski M, Kukar A, Suma V, Vloka M, Eklert F, Herweg B, Donelly J, Phillip J, Reed G, Rozanski A. Increased incidence of life threatening arrhythmias in implantable defibrillator patients after the World Trade Centre attack. J Am Coll Cardiol. 2004;44:1261–4.
100. Lampert R, Jain D, Burg MM, Batsford WP, McPherson CA. Destabilising effects of mental stress on ventricular arrhythmias in patients with implantable cardio-verter defibrillators. Circulation. 2000;101:158–64.
101. Toivonen L, Helenius K, Vitasalo M. Electrocardiographic repolarization during stress from awakening on alarm call. J Am Coll Cardiol. 1997;30:774–7.
102. James PR, Taggart P, McNally ST, Newman SP, Sporton SC, Hardman SMC. Acute psychological stress and the propensity to ventricular arrhythmias. Eur Heart J. 2000;21:1023–8.
103. Kop WJ, Krantz DS, Nearing BD, Gottdiener JS, Quigley JF, O'Callahan M, DelNegro AA, Friehling TD, Karasik P, Suchday S, Levine J, Verrier RL. Effects of acute mental stress and exercise on T-wave alternans in patients with implantable cardioverter defibrillators and controls. Circulation. 2004;109:1864–9.
104. Taggart P, Sutton P, Redfern C, Batchvarov VN, Hnatkova K, Malik M, James U, Joseph A. The effect of mental stress on the non-dipolar components of the T wave: modulation by hypnosis. Psychosom Med. 2005;67:376–83.
105. Lampert R, Shusterman V, Burg M, McPherson C, Batsford W, Goldberg A, Soufer R. Anger induced T wave alternans predicts future ventricular arrhythmias in patients with implantable cardioverter defibrillators. J Am Coll Cardiol. 2009;53:774–8.
106. Zipes DP, Rubart M. Neural modulation of cardiac arrhythmias and sudden cardiac death. Heart Rhythm. 2006;3:108–13.
107. Coote JH. Landmarks in understanding the central nervous control of the cardiovascular system. Exp Physiol. 2007;92:3–18.
108. Sengupta P. Health impacts of yoga and pranayama: a state-of-the-art review. Int J Prev Med. 2012;3(7):444–58.
109. Schwartz PJ. The rationale and the role of left stellectomy for the prevention of malignant arrhythmias. Ann N Y Acad Sci. 1984;427:199–221.
110. Schwartz PJ, Zipes DP. Autonomic modulation of cardiac arrhythmias. In: Zipes DP, Jalife J, editors. Cardiac electrophysiology. From cell to bedside. 4th ed. Philadelphia: W. B. Saunders; 2004. p. 300–14.
111. Umetani K, Singer DH, McCraty R, Atkinson M. Twenty-four hour time domain heart rate variability and heart rate: relations to age and

gender over nine decades. J Am Coll Cardiol. 1998;31(3):593–601.
112. Leenen FHH. Brain mechanisms contributing to sympathetic hyperactivity & heart failure. Circ Res. 2007;101:221–3.
113. Ajijola OA, Lux RL, Khahera A, Kwon O, Aliotta E, Ennis DB, Fishbein MC, Ardell JL, Shivkumar K. Sympathetic modulation of electrical activation in normal and infarcted myocardium: implications for arrhythmogenesis. Am J Physiol Heart Circ Physiol. 2017;312(3):H608–21. https://doi.org/10.1152/ajpheart.00575.2016. Epub 2017 Jan 13
114. Vinik A, Ziegler D. Diabetic cardiovascular autonomic neuropathy. Circulation. 2007;115:387–97.
115. La Rovere MT, Bigger JT, Marcus FI, Mortara A, Schwartz PJ. Baroreflex sensitivity and heart rate variability in prediction of total cardiac mortality after myocardial infarction. Lancet. 1998;351:478–84.
116. Gottlieb SS, McCarter RJ, Vogel RA. Effect of beta blockade on mortality among high-risk and low risk patients after myocardial infarction. N Engl J Med. 1998;339:489–97.
117. Schwartz PJ, De Ferrari GM. Sympathetic-parasympathetic interaction in health and disease:abnormalities and relevance in heart failure. Heart Fail Rev. 2011;16:101–7.
118. Koizumi K, Kollai M. Control of reciprocal and non reciprocal action of vagal and sympathetic efferents: study of centrally induced reactions. J Auton Nerv Syst. 1981;3:483–501.
119. Zipes DP, Miyazaki T. The autonomic nervous system and the heart: basis for understanding interactions and effects on arrhythmia development. In: Zipes DP, Jalife J, editors. Cardiac electrophysiology: from cell to bedside. Philadelphia: W. B. Saunders; 1990. p. 312–30.
120. Paton JFR, Boscan P, Pickering AE, Nalivaiko E. The yin and yang of cardiac autonomic control: vago-sympathetic interactions revisited. Brain Res Rev. 2005;49:555–65.
121. Porges SW. The polyvagal theory: neurophysiological foundations of emotions, attachment, communication, and self-regulation. New York: WW Norton & Co., Inc; 2011.
122. Randall WC, Szentivanyi M, Pace JB, Wechsler JS, Kaye MP. Patterns of sympathetic nerve projections onto the canine heart. Circ Res. 1968;22(3):315–23.
123. Katritsis DG, Pokushalov E, Romanov A, et al. Autonomic denervation added to pulmonary vein isolation for paroxysmal atrial fibrillation: a randomized clinical trial. J Am Coll Cardiol. 2013;62:2318–25.
124. Wu J, Wu J, Zipes DP. Mechanisms of initiation of ventricular tachyarrhythmias. In: Zipes DP, Jalife J, editors. Cardiac electrophysiology; from cell to bedside. 4th ed. Philadelphia: Saunders; 2004. p. 380–9.
125. Levy MN, Ng ML, Zieske H. Functional distribution of the peripheral sympathetic pathways. Circ Res. 1966;14:650–61.
126. Yanowitz F, Preston JB, Abildskov JA. Functional distribution of right and left stellate innervation to the ventricles: production of neurogenic electrocardiographic changes by unilateral alteration of sympathetic tone. Circ Res. 1966;28:416–28.
127. Randall WC, Ardell JL. Nervous control of the heart: anatomy and pathophysiology. In: Zipes DP, Jalife J, editors. Cardiac electrophysiology: from cell to bedside. Philadelphia: W. B. Saunders; 1990. p. 291–9.
128. Kralios FA, Martin L, Burgess MJ, Millar K. Local ventricular repolarization changes due to sympathetic nerve-branch stimulation. Am J Phys. 1975;228:1621–6.
129. Chen PS, Chen LS, Cao JM, Sharifi B, Karagueuzian HS, Fishbein MS. Sympathetic nerve sprouting, electrical remodeling and the mechanisms of sudden death. Cardiovasc Res. 2001;50:409–16.
130. Chen LS, Chen PS. Nerve sprouting and cardiac arrhythmias. In: Zipes DP, Jalife J, editors. Cardiac electrophysiology: from cell to bedside. Philadelphia: W. B. Saunders; 2004. p. 299–305.
131. Schwartz PJ. The rationale and the role of left stellectomy for the prevention of malignant arrhythmias. Ann N Y Acad Sci. 1984;427:199–221.
132. Umetani K, Singer DH, McCraty R, Atkinson M. Twenty-four hour time domain heart rate variability and heart rate: relations to age and gender over nine decades. J Am Coll Cardiol. 1998;31(3):593–601.
133. McNeill EM, Roos KP, Moechars D, Clagett-Dame M. Nav2 is necessary for cranial nerve development and blood pressure regulation. Neural Dev. 2010;5:6. https://doi.org/10.1186/1749-8104-5-6.
134. Malpas SC. The rhythmicity of sympathetic nerve activity. Prog Neurobiol. 1998;56:65–96.
135. Hainsworth R. Reflexes from the heart. Am J Physiol. 1991;71:617–58.
136. Longhurst JC, Tjen-A-Looi S, Fu L-W. Cardiac sympathetic afferent activation provoked by myocardial ischemia and reperfusion: mechanisms and reflexes. Ann N Y Acad Sci. 2001;940:74–95.
137. Critchley HD. Psychophysiology of neural, cognitive and affective integration: fMRI and autonomic indicants Int. J Psychophysiol. 2009;73:88–94.
138. Patterson E, Po SS, Scherlag BJ, Lazzara R. Triggered firing in pulmonary veins initiated by in vitro autonomic nerve stimulation. Heart Rhythm. 2005;2:624–31.
139. Pope ML, Smith TW. Cortisol excretion in high and low cynically hostile men. Psychosom Med. 1991;53:386–92.
140. Suarez EC, Shiller AD, Kuhn CM, Schanberg SM, Williams RB Jr, Zimmerman EA. The relationship between hostility and beta adrenergic receptor physiology in healthy males. Psychosom Med. 1997;59:481–7.
141. Mattioli AV, Bonatti S, Zennaro M, Melotti R, Mattioli G. Effect of coffee consumption, lifestyle and acute life stress in the development of acute lone

atrial fibrillation. J Cardiovasc Med. (Hagerstown). 2008;9:794–8.
142. James W. What is an emotion? Mind. 1884;9:188–205.
143. Cannon WB. The James-Lange theory of emotions: a critical examination and an alternative theory. Am J Psychol. 1927;39:106–24.
144. Lampert R, Joska T, Burg MM, Batsford WP, McPherson CA, Jain D. Emotional and physical precipitants of ventricular arrhythmias. Circulation. 2002;106:1800–5.
145. Narayan SM. T-wave alternans and the susceptibility to ventricular arrhythmias. J Am Coll Cardiol. 2006;47(2):269–81. Epub 2006 Jan 4. Review.
146. Ekman P, Levenson RW, Friesen WV. Autonomic nervous system activity distinguishes among emotions. Science. 1983;221:1208–10.
147. Levenson RW, Ekman P, Friesen WV. Voluntary facial action generates emotion-specific autonomic nervous system activity. Psychophysiology. 1990;27:363–84.
148. Christie IC, Friedman BH. Autonomic specificity of discrete emotion and dimensions of affective space: a multivariate approach. Int J Psychophysiol. 2004;51:143–53.
149. Rainville P, Bechara A, Naqvi N, Damasio AR. Basic emotions are associated with distinct patterns of cardiorespiratory activity. Int J Psychophysiol. 2006;61:5–18.
150. McCraty R, Atkinson M, Tiller WA, Rein G, Watkins AD. The effects of emotions on short-term power spectrum analysis of heart rate variability. Am J Cardiol. 1995;76:1089–93.
151. Lampert R, Shusterman V, Burg MM, Jee FA, Earley C, Goldberg A, McPherson CA, Batsford WP, Soufer R. Effects of psychological stress on repolarization and relationship to autonomic and haemodynamic factors. J Cardiovasc Electrophysiol. 2005;16:372–7.
152. Bernardi L, Wdowczyk-Szulc J, Valenti C, Castoldi S, Passino C, Spadacine G, Sleight P. Effects of controlled breathing, mental activity, and mental stress with or without verbalisation on heart rate variability. J Am Coll Cardiol. 2000;35:1462–9.
153. Stopper M, Joska T, Burg MM, Batsford WP, McPherson CA, Jain D, Lampert R. Electrophysiologic characteristics of anger–triggered arrhythmias. Heart Rhythm. 2007;4:268–73.
154. Friedman BH, Thayer JF. Autonomic balance revisited: panic anxiety and heart rate variability. J Psychosom Res. 1998;44:133–51.
155. Taggart P, Carruthers M, Somerville W. Some effects of emotion on the normal and abnormal heart. Curr Probl Cardiol. 1983;12:1–29.
156. Golbidi S, Frisbee JC, Laher I. Chronic stress impacts the cardiovascular system: animal models and clinical outcomes. Am J Physiol Heart Circ Physiol. 2015;308:H1476–98.
157. Thayera JF, Sternberg EM. Neural aspects of immunomodulation: focus on the vagus nerve. Brain Behav Immun. 2010;24(8):1223–8.
158. Miller AH, Maletic V, Raison CL. Inflammation and its discontents: the role of cytokines in the pathophysiology of major depression. Biol Psychiatry. 2009;65:732–41. https://doi.org/10.1016/j.biopsych.2008.11.029. (p737).
159. Huston M, Tracey KJ. The pulse of inflammation: heart rate variability, the cholinergic anti-inflammatory pathway and implications for therapy. J Intern Med. 2011;269(1):45–53.
160. Cohen S, Janicki-Deverts D, Doyle WJ, Miller GE, Frank E, Rabin BS, Turner RB. Chronic stress, glucocorticoid receptor resistance, inflammation, and disease risk. Proc Natl Acad Sci U S A. 2012;109(16):5995–9. https://doi.org/10.1073/pnas.1118355109. Epub 2012 Apr 2.
161. Critchley HD, Corfield DR, Chandler MP. Cerebral correlates of autonomic cardiovascular arousal: a functional neuroimaging investigation. J Physiol (Lond). 2000;523:259–70.
162. Napadow V, Dhond R, Conti G, Makris N, Brown EN, Barberi R. Brain correlates of autonomic modulation: combining heart rate variability with fmri. NeuroImage. 2008;42:169–77.
163. Xavier CH, Nalivaiko E, Beig MI, Menezes GB, Cara DC, Campagnole-Santos MJ, Fontes MAP. Functional asymmetry in the descending cardiovascular pathways from dorsomedial hypothalamic nucleus. Neuroscience. 2009;164:1360–8.
164. Mujica-Parodi LR, Korgaonkar M, Ravindranath B, Greenberg T, Tomasi D, Wagshul M, Ardekani B, Guilfoyle D, Khan S, Zhong Y, Chon K, Malaspina D. Limbic dysregulation is associated with lowered heart rate variability and increased trait anxiety in healthy adults. Hum Brain Mapp. 2009;30:47–58.
165. Oppenheimer SM, Gelb AW, Girvin JP, Hachinski VC. Cardiovascular effects of human insular cortex stimulation. Neurology. 1992;42:1727–32.
166. Wittling W. Brain asymmetry in the control of autonomic-physiologic activity. In: Davidson RJ, Hugdahl KJ, editors. Brain asymmetry. Cambridge, MA: The MIT Press; 1995. p. 305–57.
167. Rozanski A, Bairey CN, Krantz DS, Friedman J, Ressler KJ, Morell M, Hilton-Chalfen S, Hestrin L, Bietendorf J, Berman DS. Mental stress and the induction of silent myocardial ischemia in patients with coronary artery disease. N Engl J Med. 1988;318:1005–12.
168. Burg MM, Soufer JD, Kerns RD, Zaret BL. Role of behavioural and psychological factors in mental stress induced silent left ventricular dysfunction in coronary artery disease. J Am Coll Cardiol. 1993;22:440–8.
169. Gottdiener JS, Krantz DS, Howell RH, Hecht GM, Klein J, Falconer JJ, Rozanski A. Induction of silent myocardial ischemia with mental stress testing: relation to the triggers of ischemia during daily life activities and to ischemia functional severity. J Am Coll Cardiol. 1994;24:1645–51.
170. Goldberg AD, Becker LC, Bonsall R, Cohen JD, Ketterer MW, Kaufman PG, Krantz DS, Light KC,

McMahon RP, Noreuil T, Pepine CJ, Raczynski J, Stone PH, Strother D, Taylor H, Sheps DS. Ischemic, haemodynamic and neurohumoral responses to mental and exercise stress. Circulation. 1996;94:2402–9.
171. Raadsheer FC, Hoogendijk WJ, Stam FC, Tilders FJ, Swaab DF. Increased numbers of corticotropin-releasing hormone expressing neurons in the hypothalamic paraventricular nucleus of depressed patients. Neuroendocrinology. 1994;6:436–44.
172. Purba JS, Raadsheer FC, Hofman MA, Ravid R, Polman CH, Kamphorst W, Swaab DF. Increased number of corticotropin-releasing hormone expressing neurons in the hypothalamic paraventricular nucleus of patients with multiple sclerosis. Neuroendocrinology. 1995;62:62–70.
173. Frasure-Smith N, Lespérance F, Gravel G, Masson A, Juneau M, Talajic M, Bourassa MG. Depression and health-care costs during the first year following myocardial infarction. J Psychosom Res. 2000;48(4–5):471–8.
174. Sternberg EM. Neural regulation of innate immunity: a coordinated nonspecific host response to pathogens. Nat Rev Immunol. 2006;6(4):318–28. Review.
175. Hintsa T, Puttonen S, Toivonen L, Kontula K, Swan H, Keltikangas-Jarvinen L. A history of stressful life events, prolonged mental stress and arrhythmic events in inherited long QT syndrome. Heart. 2010;96:1281–6.
176. Dyson KS, Shoemaker JK, Hughson RL. Effect of acute sympathetic nervous system activation on flow-mediated dilation of brachial artery. Am J Physiol Heart Circ Physiol. 2006;290:H1446–53.
177. Poitras VJ, Pyke KE. The impact of acute mental stress on vascular endothelial function: evidence, mechanisms and importance. Int J Psychophysiol. 2013;88:124–35.
178. Hijmering ML, Stroes ES, Olijhoek J, Hutten BA, Blankestijn PJ, Rabelink TJ. Sympathetic activation markedly reduces endothelium-dependent, flow-mediated vasodilation. J Am Coll Cardiol. 2002;39:683–8.
179. Eriksson M, Johansson K, Sarabi M, Lind L. Mental stress impairs endothelial vasodilatory function by a beta-adrenergic mechanism. Endothelium. 2007;14:151–6.
180. Black PH, Garbutt LD. Stress, inflammation and cardiovascular disease. J Psychosom Res. 2002;52:1–23.
181. Kaplan JR, Manuck SB, Clarkson TB, Lusso FM, Taub DM. Social stress and atherosclerosis in normocholesterolemic monkeys. Science. 1983;220:733–5.
182. Manuck SB, Adams MR, McCaffery JM, Kaplan JR. Behaviorally elicited heart rate reactivity and atherosclerosis in ovariectomized cynomolgus monkeys (Macaca fascicularis). Arterioscler Thromb Vasc Biol. 2000;17:1774–9.
183. Groeschel M, Braam B. Connecting chronic and recurrent stress to vascular dysfunction: no relaxed role for the renin-angiotensin system. Am J Physiol Renal Physiol. 2011;300:F1–F10.
184. Spieker LE, Hürlimann D, Ruschitzka F, Corti R, Enseleit F, Shaw S, Hayoz D, Deanfield JE, Lüscher TF, Noll G. Mental stress induces prolonged endothelial dysfunction via endothelin-A receptors. Circulation. 2002;105:2817–20.
185. Seya Y, Fukuda T, Isobe K, Kawakami Y, Takekoshi K. Effect of norepinephrine on RhoA, MAP kinase, proliferation and VEGF expression in human umbilical vein endothelial cells. Eur J Pharmacol. 2006;553:54–60.
186. Ghiadoni L, Donald AE, Cropley M, Mullen MJ, Oakley G, Taylor M, O'Connor G, Betteridge J, Klein N, Steptoe A, Deanfield JE. Mental stress induces transient endothelial dysfunction in humans. Circulation. 2000;102:2473–8.
187. Uji M, Yoshida K, Shitani-Ishida K, Morimoto K. Sex difference in norepinephrine surge in response to psychological stress through nitric oxide in rats. Life Sci. 2007;80:860–6.
188. Toda N, Nakanishi-Toda M. How mental stress affects endothelial function. Pflügers Arch. 2011;462:779–94.
189. Aberg G, Ferrer P. Effects of captopril on atherosclerosis in cynomolgus monkeys. J Cardiovasc Pharmacol. 1990;15:s65–72.
190. Keidar S, Kaplan M, Hoffman A, Aviram M. Angiotensin II stimulates macrophage-mediated oxidation of low density lipoproteins. Atherosclerosis. 1995;115:201–15.
191. Kaplan M, Aviram M, Knopf C, Keidar S. Angiotensin II reduces macrophage cholesterol efflux: a role for the AT-1 receptor but not for the ABC1 transporter. Biochem Biophys Res Commun. 2002;290:1529–34.
192. Keidar S, Heinrich R, Kaplan M, Hayek T, Aviram M. Angiotensin II administration to atherosclerotic mice increases macrophage uptake of oxidized LDL: a possible role for interleukin-6. Arterioscler Thromb Vasc Biol. 2001;21:1464–9.
193. Mateo T, Abu Nabah YN, Abu Taha M, Mata M, Cerda-Nicolas M, Proudfoot AE, Stahl RA, Issekutz AC, Cortijo J, Morcillo EJ, Jose PJ, Sanz MJ. Angiotensin II-induced mononuclear leukocyte interactions with arteriolar and venular endothelium are mediated by the release of different CC chemokines. J Immunol. 2006;176:5577–86.
194. Mateo T, Naim Abu Nabah Y, Losada M, Estelles R, Company C, Bedrina B, Cerda-Nicolas JM, Poole S, Jose PJ, Cortijo J, Morcillo EJ, Sanz MJ. A critical role for TNFalpha in the selective attachment of mononuclear leukocytes to angiotensin-II-stimulated arterioles. Blood. 2007;110:1895–902.
195. Piqueras L, Kubes P, Alvarez A, O'Connor E, Issekutz AC, Esplugues JV, Sanz MJ. Angiotensin II induces leukocyte-endothelial cell interactions in vivo via AT1 and AT2 receptor-mediated P-selectin upregulation. Circulation. 2000;102:2118–23.
196. Zhao Q, Ishibashi M, Hiasa K, Tan C, Takeshita A, Egashira K. Essential role of vascular endothelial growth factor in angiotensin II induced vascular

inflammation and remodeling. Hypertension. 2004;44:264–470.
197. Chan YC, Leung PS. Angiotensin II type 1 receptor-dependent nuclear factor-kappaB activation-mediated proinflammatory actions in a rat model of obstructive acute pancreatitis. J Pharmacol Exp Ther. 2007;323:10–8.
198. Hsu YH, Chen JJ, Chang NC, Chen CH, Liu JC, Chen TH, Jeng CJ, Chao HH, Cheng TH. Role of reactive oxygen species-sensitive extracellular signal-regulated kinase pathway in angiotensin II-induced endothelin-1 gene expression in vascular endothelial cells. J Vasc Res. 2004;41:64–74.
199. Liu HQ, Wei XB, Sun R, Cai YW, Lou HY, Wang JW, Chen AF, Zhang XM. Angiotensin II stimulates intercellular adhesion molecule-1 via an AT1 receptor/nuclear factor-kappaB pathway in brain microvascular endothelial cells. Life Sci. 2006;78:1293–8.
200. Pueyo ME, Gonzalez W, Nicoletti A, Savoie F, Arnal JF, Michel JB. Angiotensin II stimulates endothelial vascular cell adhesion molecule-1 via nuclear factor-kappaB activation induced by intracellular oxidative stress. Arterioscler Thromb Vasc Biol. 2000;20:645–51.
201. Ruiz-Ortega M, Lorenzo O, Ruperez M, Suzuki Y, Egido J. Angiotensin II activates nuclear transcription factor-kappaB in aorta of normal rats and in vascular smooth muscle cells of AT1 knockout mice. Nephrol Dial Transplant. 2001;16:S27–33.
202. Suzuki Y, Ruiz-Ortega M, Lorenzo O, Ruperez M, Esteban V, Egido J. Inflammation and angiotensin II. Int J Biochem Cell Biol. 2003;35:881–900.
203. Kaplan JR, Adams MR, Clarkson TB, Manuck SB, Shively CA, Williams JK. Psychosocial factors, sex differences, and atherosclerosis: lessons from animal models. Psychosom Med. 1996;58:598–611.
204. Wassmann S, Czech T, van Eickels M, Fleming I, Bohm M, Nickenig G. Inhibition of diet-induced atherosclerosis and endothelial dysfunction in apolipoprotein E/angiotensin II type 1A receptor double-knockout mice. Circulation. 2004;110:3062–7.
205. Fukuda D, Sata M, Ishizaka N, Nagai R. Critical role of bone marrow angiotensin II type 1 receptor in the pathogenesis of atherosclerosis in apolipoprotein E deficient mice. Arterioscler Thromb Vasc Biol. 2008;28:90–6.
206. Pavel J, Benicky J, Murakami Y, Sanchez-Lemus E, Saavedra JM. Peripherally administered angiotensin II AT1 receptor antagonists are anti-stress compounds in vivo. Ann N Y Acad Sci. 2008;1148:360–6.
207. Schiavone MT, Santos RA, Brosnihan KB, Khosla MC, Ferrario CM. Release of vasopressin from the rat hypothalamo-neurohypophysial system by angiotensin (1–7) heptapeptide. Proc Natl Acad Sci U S A. 1988;85:4095–8.
208. Benter IF, Yousif MH, Anim JT, Cojocel C, Diz DI. Angiotensin-(1–7) prevents development of severe hypertension and end-organ damage in spontaneously hypertensive rats treated with l-NAME. Am J Physiol Heart Circ Physiol. 2006;290:H684–91.
209. Grobe JL, Mecca AP, Lingis M, Shenoy V, Bolton TA, Machado JM, Speth RC, Raizada MK, Katovich MJ. Prevention of angiotensin II-induced cardiac remodeling by angiotensin-(1–7). Am J Physiol Heart Circ Physiol. 2007;292:H736–42.
210. Saladin K. Chapter 15: the autonomic nervous and visceral reflexes. In: Anatomy. New York: The McGraw-Hill; 2004.
211. Gilsanz P, Mayeda ER, Glymour MM, Quesenberry CP, Mungas DM, DeCarli C, Dean A, Whitmer RA. Female sex, early-onset hypertension, and risk of dementia. Neurology. 2017;89(18):1886–93.
212. Otite FO, Liaw N, Khandelwal P, Malik AM, Romano JG, Rundek T, Sacco RL, Chaturvedi S. Increasing prevalence of vascular risk factors in patients with stroke: a call to action. Neurology. 2017;89(19):1985–94.
213. Otite FO, Liaw N, Khandelwal P, Malik AM, Romano JG, Rundek T, Sacco RL, Chaturvedi S. Increasing prevalence of vascular risk factors in patients with stroke: a call to action. Neurology. 2017;89(19):1985–94.
214. Andersson U, Tracey KJ. Neural reflexes in inflammation and immunity. J Exp Med. 2012;209(6):1057–68. https://doi.org/10.1084/jem.20120571.
215. Pavlov VA, Tracey KJ. The vagus nerve and the inflammatory reflex – linking immunity and metabolism. Nat Rev Endocrinol. 2012;8(12):743–54. https://doi.org/10.1038/nrendo.2012.189.
216. Borovikova LV, et al. Vagus nerve stimulation attenuates the systemic inflammatory response to endotoxin. Nature. 2000;405:458. https://doi.org/10.1038/35013070.
217. Clancy JA, Mary DA, Witte KK, Greenwood JP, Deuchars SA, Deuchars J. Non-invasive vagus nerve stimulation in healthy humans reduces sympathetic nerve activity. Brain Stimul. 2014;7(6):871–7. https://doi.org/10.1016/j.brs.2014.07.031. Epub 2014 Jul 16.
218. Sundman E, Olofsson PS. Neural control of the immune system. Adv Physiol Educ. 2014;38:135–9. https://doi.org/10.1152/advan.00094.2013.
219. Gold MR, Van Veldhuisen DJ, Hauptman PJ, Borggrefe M, Kubo SH, Lieberman RA, Milasinovic G, Berman BJ, Djordjevic S, Neelagaru S, Schwartz PJ, Starling RC, Mann DL. Vagus nerve stimulation for the treatment of heart failure: the INOVATE-HF trial. J Am Coll Cardiol. 2016;68(2):149–58. https://doi.org/10.1016/j.jacc.2016.03.525. Epub 2016 Apr 4.
220. Hauptman PJ, Schwartz PJ, Gold MR, Borggrefe M, Van Veldhuisen DJ, Starling RC, Mann DL. Rationale and study design of the increase of vagal tone in heart failure study: INOVATE-HF. Am Heart J. 2012;163(6):954–962.e1. https://doi.org/10.1016/j.ahj.2012.03.021.
221. Van Wagoner DR. Chronic vagal nerve stimulation for the treatment of human heart failure: progress in translating a vision into reality. Eur Heart J. 2011;32(7):788–90. https://doi.org/10.1093/eurheartj/ehq424. Epub 2010 Nov 18.

222. De Ferrari GM, Crijns HJ, Borggrefe M, Milasinovic G, Smid J, Zabel M, Gavazzi A, Sanzo A, Dennert R, Kuschyk J, Raspopovic S, Klein H, Swedberg K, Schwartz PJ, CardioFit Multicenter Trial Investigators. Chronic vagus nerve stimulation: a new and promising therapeutic approach for chronic heart failure. Eur Heart J. 2011;32(7):847–55. https://doi.org/10.1093/eurheartj/ehq391. Epub 2010 Oct 28.
223. Premchand RK, Sharma K, Mittal S, Monteiro R, Dixit S, Libbus I, DiCarlo LA, Ardell JL, Rector TS, Amurthur B, KenKnight BH, Anand IS. Autonomic regulation therapy via left or right cervical vagus nerve stimulation in patients with chronic heart failure: results of the ANTHEM-HF trial. J Card Fail. 2014;20(11):808–16. https://doi.org/10.1016/j.cardfail.2014.08.009. Epub 2014 Sept 1.
224. Zannad F, De Ferrari GM, Tuinenburg AE, Wright D, Brugada J, Butter C, Klein H, Stolen C, Meyer S, Stein KM, Ramuzat A, Schubert B, Daum D, Neuzil P, Botman C, Castel MA, D'Onofrio A, Solomon SD, Wold N, Ruble SB. Chronic vagal stimulation for the treatment of low ejection fraction heart failure: results of the Neural Cardiac Therapy for Heart Failure (NECTAR-HF) randomized controlled trial. Eur Heart J. 2015;36(7):425–33. https://doi.org/10.1093/eurheartj/ehu345. Epub 2014 Aug 31.
225. De Ferrari G, et al. Chronic vagus nerve stimulation: a new and promising therapeutic approach for chronic heart failure. Eur Heart J. 2011;32:847. https://doi.org/10.1093/eurheartj/ehq391.
226. Stavrakis S, et al. Low-level transcutaneous electrical vagus nerve stimulation suppresses atrial fibrillation. J Am Coll Cardiol. 2015;65:867. https://doi.org/10.1016/j/jack.2014.12.026.
227. Galbarriatu L, et al. Vagus nerve stimulation therapy for treatment-resistant epilepsy: a 15-year experience at a single institution. Clin Neurol Neurosurg. 2015;137:89. https://doi.org/10.1016/j.clineuro.2015.06.023.
228. Bonaz B, et al. Vagus nerve stimulation: from epilepsy to the cholinergic anti-inflammatory pathway. Neurogastroenterol Motil. 2013. https://doi.org/10.1111/nmo.12076.
229. Grimonprez A, et al. The antidepressant-like effect of vagus nerve stimulation is mediated through the locus coeruleus. J Psychiatr Res. 2015;68:1. https://doi.org/10.1016/j.psychires.2015.05.002.
230. Premchand R, et al. Autonomic regulation therapy via left or right cervical vagus nerve stimulation in patients with chronic heart failure: results of the ANTHEM-HF trial. J Card Fail. 2014;20:808. https://doi.org/10.1016/j.cardfail.2014.08.009.
231. Jacobs H, et al. Transcutaneous vagus nerve stimulation boosts associative memory in older individuals. Neurobiol Aging. 2015;36:1860. https://doi.org/10.1016/j.neurobiolaging.2015.02.023.
232. Gaul C, et al. Non-invasive vagus nerve stimulation for PREVention and Acute treatment of chronic cluster headache (PREVA): a randomised controlled study. Cephalalgia. Published online September 21, 2015. https://doi.org/10.1177/0333102415607070.
233. Wang S, et al. Transcutaneous vagus nerve stimulation induces tidal melatonin secretion and has an antidiabetic effect in Zucker fatty rats. PLOS One. Published online April 16, 2015. https://doi.org/10.1371/journal.pone.0124195.
234. Groves DA, Brown VJ. Vagal nerve stimulation: a review of its applications and potential mechanisms that mediate its clinical effects. Neurosci Biobehav Rev. 2005;29:493. https://doi.org/10.1016/j.neubiorev.2005.01.004.
235. Jacobs HI, Riphagen JM, Razat CM, Wiese S, Sack AT. Transcutaneous vagus nerve stimulation boosts associative memory in older individuals. Neurobiol Aging. 2015;36(5):1860–7. https://doi.org/10.1016/j.neurobiolaging.2015.02.023. Epub 2015 Feb 28.
236. Yuan H, Silberstein SD. Vagus nerve and vagus nerve stimulation, a comprehensive review: part III. Headache. 2016;56(3):479–90. https://doi.org/10.1111/head.12649. Epub 2015 Sept 14. Review.
237. Ben-Menachem E, Revesz D, Simon BJ, Silberstein S. Surgically implanted and non-invasive vagus nerve stimulation: a review of efficacy, safety and tolerability. Eur J Neurol. 2015;22(9):1260–8. https://doi.org/10.1111/ene.12629.
238. Grazzi L, Egeo G, Liebler E, Padovan AM, Barbanti P. Non-invasive vagus nerve stimulation (nVNS) as symptomatic treatment of migraine in young patients: a preliminary safety study. Neurol Sci. 2017;38(Suppl 1):197–9. https://doi.org/10.1007/s10072-017-2942-5.
239. Larkum ME, Launey T, Dityatev A, Lüscher H-R. Integration of excitatory postsynaptic potentials in dendrites of motoneurons of rat spinal cord slice cultures. J Neurophysiol. 1998;80(2):924–35.
240. Myers B, Greenwood-Van MB. Role of anxiety in the pathophysiology of irritable bowel syndrome: importance of the amygdala. Front Neurosci. 2009;3:47. https://doi.org/10.3389/neuro.21.002.2009. eCollection 2009.
241. Jezova D, Makatsori A, Smriga M, Morinaga Y, Duncko R. Subchronic treatment with amino acid mixture of L-lysine and L-arginine modifies neuroendocrine activation during psychosocial stress in subjects with high trait anxiety. Nutr Neurosci. 2005;8(3):155–60.
242. Sherwood A, Hinderliter AL, Watkins LL, Waugh RA, Blumenthal JA. Impaired endothelial function in coronary heart disease patients with depressive symptomatology. J Am Coll Cardiol. 2005;46(4):656–9.
243. Hatcher S, Arroll B. Newer antidepressants for the treatment of depression in adults. BMJ. 2012;344:d8300. https://doi.org/10.1136/bmj.d8300.
244. Jolly K, Langman MJS. Psychotropic medication: curing illness or creating problems? Heart. 2009;95:1893–4. https://doi.org/10.1136/hrt.2009.179127.

245. Olfson M, Marcus SC. National patterns in antidepressant medication treatment. Arch Gen Psychiatry. 2009;66:848–56. https://doi.org/10.1001/archgenpsychiatry.2009.81.
246. Lockhart P, Guthrie B. Trends in primary care antidepressant prescribing 1995–2007: a longitudinal population database analysis. Br J Gen Pract. 2011;61:e565–72. https://doi.org/10.3399/bjgp11X593848.
247. Stephenson CP, Karanges E, McGregor IS. Trends in the utilisation of psychotropic medications in Australia from 2000 to 2011. Aust N Z J Psychiatry. 2013;47:74–87. https://doi.org/10.1177/0004867412466595.
248. Cohn JN, Tognoni G, for the Valsartan Heart Failure Trial Investigators. A randomized trial of the angiotensin-receptor blocker valsartan in chronic heart failure. N Engl J Med. 2001;345:1667–75.
249. Lachmann J, Banerjee A, Davoudi M, Aragon D, Talerja A, Sonnenblick EH, Shirani J, LeJemtel TH. Withdrawal of angiotensin receptor blocker (ARB) from triple neurohormonal therapy partially restores sympathetic activity in patients with chronic congestive heart failure. Am Heart Assoc. Scientific Sessions, 2001. Circulation. 2001;104:e9051–e9052.
250. US Food and Drug Administration. FDA Drug Safety Communication. FDA Drug Safety Communication: abnormal heart rhythms associated with high doses of Celexa (citalopram hydrobromide). 2011. www.fda.gov/Drugs/DrugSafety/ucm269086.htm
251. Castro VM, Clements CC, Murphy SN, et al. QT interval and antidepressant use: a cross sectional study of electronic health records. BMJ. 2013;346:f288. https://doi.org/10.1136/bmj.f288.
252. Girardin FR, Gex-Fabry M, Berney P, Shah D, Gaspoz JM, Dayer P. Drug-induced long QT in adult psychiatric inpatients: the 5-year cross-sectional ECG screening outcome in psychiatry study. Am J Psychiatry. 2013;170:1468–76. https://doi.org/10.1176/appi.ajp.2013.12060860.
253. El-Sherif N, Turitto G. Torsade de pointes. Curr Opin Cardiol. 2003;18:6–13. https://doi.org/10.1097/00001573-200301000-00002.
254. Coupland C, Hill T, Morriss R, Moore M, Arthur A, Hippisley-Cox J. Antidepressant use and risk of cardiovascular outcomes in people aged 20 to 64: cohort study using primary care database. BMJ. 2016;352:i1350. https://doi.org/10.1136/bmj.i1350.
255. Cadegiani FA, Kater CE. Adrenal fatigue does not exist: a systematic review. BMC Endocr Disord. 2016;16(1):48. https://doi.org/10.1186/s12902-016-0128-4.
256. Rosengren A, Hawken S, Ounpuu S, Sliwa K, Zubaid M, Almahmeed WA, Blackett KN, Sitthi-amorn C, Sato H, Yusuf S, INTERHEART investigators. Association of psychosocial risk factors with risk of acute myocardial infarction in 11119 cases and 13648 controls from 52 countries (the INTERHEART study): case-control study. Lancet. 2004;364(9438):953–62.
257. Landsbergis PA, Schnall PL, Pickering TG, et al. Life-course exposure to job strain and ambulatory blood pressure in men. Am J Epidemiol. 2003;157:998–1006.
258. Vrijkotte TG, van Doornen LJ, de Geus EJ. Effects of work stress on ambulatory blood pressure, heart rate, and heart rate variability. Hypertension. 2000;35:880–6.
259. Herd JA. Cardiovascular response to stress. Physiol Rev. 1991;71:305–30.
260. Malik M, The Task Force of the European Society of Cardiology and the North American Society of Pacing and Electrophysiology. Heart rate variability, standards of measurement, physiological interpretation, and clinical use. Circulation. 1996;93:1043–65.
261. Malik M, The Task Force of the European Society of Cardiology and the North American Society of Pacing and Electrophysiology. Heart rate variability, standards of measurement, physiological interpretation, and clinical use. Eur Heart J. 1996;17:354–81.
262. Gawaz M, Langer H, May AE. Platelets in inflammation atherogenesis. J Clin Invest. 2005;115:3378–84.
263. von Känel R, Mills PJ, Fainman C, Dimsdale JE. Effects of psychological stress and psychiatric disorders on blood coagulation and fibrinolysis: a biobehavioral pathway to coronary artery disease? Psychosom Med. 2001;63(4):531–44.
264. Kessler R, et al. Posttraumatic stress disorders in a national comorbidity survey. Arch Gen Psychiatry. 1995;52:1048–60.
265. Kubzanski LD, et al. Prospective study of the posttraumatic stress disorder symptom in coronary artery disease and normative aging study. Arch Gen Psychiatry. 2007;64:109–16.
266. Mewisse ML, et al. Cortisol and posttraumatic stress disorder in adults: systemic review of metaanalysis. Br J Psychiatry. 2007;191:387–92.
267. Sack M, et al. Low respiratory sinus arrhythmia and prolonged psychophysiological arousal in posttraumatic disorder: heart rate dynamics and individual differences in arousal regulation. Biol Psychiatry. 2004:55, 284–290.
268. Tracy KD. Physiology and immunology of the cholinergic antiinflammatory pathway. J Clin Invest. 2007;117:289–96.
269. Bhaskar L, Kharya C, Deepak KK, Kochupillai V. Assessment of cardiac autonomic tone following Long Sudarshan Kriya yoga in art of living practitioners. J Altern Complement Med. 2017;23(9):705–12. https://doi.org/10.1089/acm.2016.0391. Epub 2017 Jul 10.
270. Gothe NP, Keswani RK, McAuley E. Yoga practice improves executive function by attenuating stress levels. Biol Psychol. 2016;121(Pt A):109–16. https://doi.org/10.1016/j.biopsycho.2016.10.010. Epub 2016 Oct 26.

271. Jones SM, Guthrie KA, Reed SD, Landis CA, Sternfeld B, LaCroix AZ, Dunn A, Burr RL, Newton KM. A yoga & exercise randomized controlled trial for vasomotor symptoms: effects on heart rate variability. Complement Ther Med. 2016;26:66–71. https://doi.org/10.1016/j.ctim.2016.03.001. Epub 2016 Mar 4.

272. Doufesh H, Ibrahim F, Ismail NA, Wan Ahmad WA. Effect of Muslim prayer (Salat) on α electroencephalography and its relationship with autonomic nervous system activity. J Altern Complement Med. 2014;20(7):558–62. https://doi.org/10.1089/acm.2013.0426. Epub 2014 May 14.

273. Tyagi A, Cohen M. Yoga and hypertension: a systematic review. Altern Ther Health Med. 2014;20(2):32–59.

274. Berntson GG, Norman GJ, Hawkley LC, Cacioppo JT. Spirituality and autonomic cardiac control. Ann Behav Med. 2008;35(2):198–208. https://doi.org/10.1007/s12160-008-9027-x. Epub 2008 Mar 21.

# Mind-Body Wellness Program Benefits

# 9

In this chapter, examples of the benefits of the Mind-Body Wellness Program (see Insert below[1]) are presented. The Mind-Body Wellness Program cocktail for autonomic and mitochondrial dysfunction along with exercise, stress reduction, and Mediterranean diet consists of the following:

1. Alpha-lipoic acid 400–1800 mg a day
2. Coenzyme Q10 200–300 mg a day
3. L-Carnitine 1 g a day
4. L-Arginine 2–3 g a day
5. L-Citrulline 1 g a day
6. Beetroot extract 500 mg a day (important source of inorganic nitrates)
7. Lysine 1–3 g a day
8. Folic acid, B vitamins, magnesium, and vitamin D at recommended daily allowances[2]
9. Omega-3 fatty acid 1200 mg a day
10. (Optional) N-acetylcysteine (NAC) 600–1800 mg a day

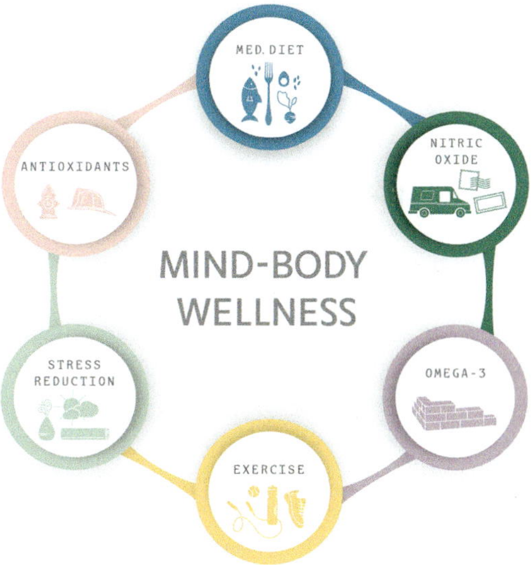


## Contraindications or Interactions[3]

As always, all medications should be closely supervised by an individual's personal physician, whether it may be pharmaceutical, nutraceutical, or supplemental.

[1]Illustration by Elysian Creative Studio, www.elysiancreativestudio.com, Lizzy Colombo.

[2]First consult your physician. Adult RDAs: folic acid ($B_9$) = 400 to 800 µg, thiamin ($B_1$) = 1.1 to 1.6 mg, riboflavin ($B_2$) = 1.1 to 1.6 mg, niacin ($B_3$) = 14 to 18 mg, pantothenic acid ($B_5$) = 5 to 7 mg, vitamin $B_6$ = 1.3 to 2.0 mg, vitamin $B_{12}$ = 2.4 to 2.8 µg (sublingual preferred), magnesium = 300 to 400 mg, vitamin D = 600 to 800 IU, and calcium = 1000 to 1200 mg.

[3]Unless otherwise stated, the contraindications or indications are published on WebMD.


N. L. DePace, J. Colombo, *Clinical Autonomic and Mitochondrial Disorders*,
https://doi.org/10.1007/978-3-030-17016-5_9

## Alpha-Lipoic Acid Interactions

Alpha-Lipoic acid (ALA) may cause stomach awareness. If so, recommend taking ALA with food or lower dose until tolerance is built. ALA may also lower BP and maybe contraindicated for antihypertensive therapy or for patients who are hypotensive.

*Medications for cancer (Chemotherapy)* – (Possible moderate interaction) Interacts with alpha-lipoic acid (ALA). ALA is an antioxidant. There is some concern that antioxidants might decrease the effectiveness of some medications used for cancers. But it is too soon to know if this interaction occurs.

*Medications for diabetes (Anti-diabetes drugs)* – (Possible minor interaction) Interacts with ALA. ALA might decrease blood sugar. Diabetes medications are also used to lower blood sugar. Taking ALA along with diabetes medications might cause low blood sugar. But more evidence is needed to know if this interaction is a big concern. Monitor blood sugar closely. Some medications used for diabetes include glimepiride (Amaryl), glyburide (DiaBeta, Glynase PresTab, Micronase), insulin, pioglitazone (Actos), rosiglitazone (Avandia), chlorpropamide (Diabinese), glipizide (Glucotrol), tolbutamide (Orinase), and others.

## Coenzyme Q-10 Interactions

*Medications for cancer (Chemotherapy)* – (Possible moderate interaction) Interacts with coenzyme Q-10 (CoQ-10). CoQ-10 is an antioxidant. There is some concern that antioxidants might decrease the effectiveness of some medications used for cancers. But it is too soon to know if the interaction occurs.

*Antihypertensive drugs* – (Possible moderate interaction) Medications for high BP interact with CoQ-10. CoQ-10 seems to decrease BP. Taking CoQ-10 along with medications for high BP might cause BP to go too low. Some medications for high BP include captopril (Capoten), enalapril (Vasotec), losartan (Cozaar), valsartan (Diovan), diltiazem (Cardizem), amlodipine (Norvasc), hydrochlorothiazide (HydroDiuril), furosemide (Lasix), and many others.

*Warfarin (Coumadin)* – (Possible moderate interaction) Interacts with CoQ-10. Warfarin (Coumadin) is used to slow blood clotting. CoQ-10 might help the blood clot. By helping the blood clot, CoQ-10 might decrease the effectiveness of Warfarin. Decreasing the effectiveness of warfarin might increase the risk of clotting. Be sure to check blood regularly. The dose of warfarin might need to be changed.

## L-Arginine Interactions

*Antihypertensive drugs* – (Possible moderate interaction) Medications for high BP interact with L-arginine. L-Arginine may decrease BP. Taking L-arginine along with medications for high BP might cause BP to go too low. Some medications for high BP include captopril (Capoten), enalapril (Vasotec), losartan (Cozaar), valsartan (Diovan), diltiazem (Cardizem), amlodipine (Norvasc), hydrochlorothiazide (HydroDiuril), furosemide (Lasix), and many others.

*Nitrates* – (Possible moderate interaction) Medications that increase blood flow to the heart interact with L-arginine. L-Arginine increases blood flow. Taking L-arginine with medications that increase blood flow to the heart might increase the chance of dizziness and lightheadedness. Some of these medications that increase blood flow to the heart include nitroglycerin (Nitro-Bid, Nitro-Dur, Nitrostat) and isosorbide (Imdur, Isordil, Sorbitrate).

*Sildenafil (Viagra)* – (Possible moderate interaction) Interacts with L-arginine. Sildenafil may lower BP. L-Arginine can also lower blood pressure. Taking sildenafil and L-arginine together might cause the BP to go too low. BP that is too low can cause lightheadedness and other side effects.

## L-Carnitine Interactions

*Acenocoumarol (Sintrom)* – (Possible moderate interaction) Interacts with L-carnitine.

Acenocoumarol is used to slow blood clotting. L-Carnitine might increase the effectiveness of acenocoumarol. Increasing the effectiveness of acenocoumarol might slow blood clotting too much. The dose of acenocoumarol might need to be changed.

*Thyroid hormone* – (Possible moderate interaction) Interacts with L-carnitine. L-Carnitine seems to decrease how well thyroid hormone works in the body. Taking L-carnitine with thyroid hormone might decrease the effectiveness of the thyroid hormone.

*Warfarin (Coumadin)* – (Possible moderate interaction) Interacts with L-carnitine. Warfarin is used to slow blood clotting. L-Carnitine might increase the effects of warfarin and increase the chances of bruising and bleeding. Be sure to check blood regularly. The dose of warfarin might need to be changed.

## L-Citrulline Interactions

No known interactions listed.

## Beetroot Extract (Nitric Oxide Supplement) Interactions

See section "L-Arginine Interactions"

## Lysine Interactions

*Calcium supplements* – (Possible moderate interaction) Interact with lysine. Lysine can increase how much calcium the body absorbs. Taking calcium along with lysine can increase the amount of calcium in the body. Avoid taking large amounts of calcium and lysine at the same time.

## Folic Acid Interactions

*Anti-seizure medications* – (Possible moderate interaction) Interact with folic acid. Medications such as fosphenytoin (Cerebyx), primidone (Mysoline), phenytoin (Dilantin), and phenobarbital (Luminal) interact with folic acid. Fosphenytoin, primidone, phenytoin, and phenobarbital are used for seizures. The body breaks down fosphenytoin to get rid of it. Folic acid can increase how quickly the body breaks down fosphenytoin. Taking folic acid along with fosphenytoin might decrease the effectiveness of fosphenytoin, primidone, phenytoin, or phenobarbital for preventing seizures.

*Medications for cancer (Chemotherapy)* – (Possible moderate interaction) Interact with folic acid. Medications such as methotrexate (MTX, Rheumatrex) interact with folic acid. Methotrexate works by decreasing the effects of folic acid in the body's cells. Taking folic acid pills along with methotrexate might decrease the effectiveness of methotrexate.

*Pyrimethamine (Daraprim)* – (Possible moderate interaction) Interacts with folic acid. Pyrimethamine (Daraprim) is used to treat parasite infections. Folic acid might decrease the effectiveness of pyrimethamine (Daraprim) for treating parasite infections.

## Omega-3, Fish Oil Interactions

Fish oil may cause stomach awareness or a bad taste. Consider taking fish oil with food.

*Birth control pills (Contraceptive drugs)* – (Possible moderate interaction) Interacts with fish oil. Fish oils seem to help reduce some fat levels in the blood. These fats are called triglycerides. Birth control pills might decrease the effectiveness of fish oils by reducing these fat levels in the blood. Some birth control pills include ethinyl estradiol and levonorgestrel (Triphasil), ethinyl estradiol and norethindrone (Ortho-Novum 1/35, Ortho-Novum 7/7/7), and others.

*Medications for high blood pressure (antihypertensive drugs)* – (Possible moderate interaction) Interacts with fish oil. Fish oils seem to decrease BP. Taking fish oils along with medications for BP pressure might cause BP to go too low. Some medications for high BP include captopril (Capoten), enalapril (Vasotec), losartan (Cozaar), valsartan (Diovan), diltiazem (Cardizem), amlodipine (Norvasc), hydrochlorothiazide (HydroDiuril), furosemide (Lasix), and many others.

*Orlistat (Xenical, Alli)* – (Possible moderate interaction) Interacts with fish oil. Orlistat (Xenical, Alli) is used for weight loss. It prevents dietary fats from being absorbed from the gut. There is some concern that orlistat (Xenical, Alli) might also decrease absorption of fish oil when they are taken together. To avoid this potential interaction, take orlistat (Xenical, Alli) and fish oil at least 2 hours apart.

*Medications that slow blood clotting (anticoagulant and antiplatelet drugs)* – (Possible minor interaction) Interacts with fish oil. Fish oils might slow blood clotting. Taking fish oils along with medications that also slow clotting might increase the chances of bruising and bleeding. Some medications that slow blood clotting include aspirin, clopidogrel (Plavix), diclofenac (Voltaren, Cataflam, others), ibuprofen (Advil, Motrin, others), naproxen (Anaprox, Naprosyn, others), dalteparin (Fragmin), enoxaparin (Lovenox), heparin, warfarin (Coumadin), and others.

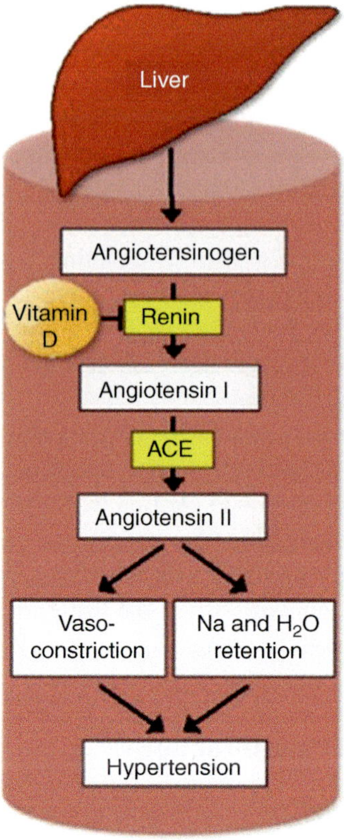


**Fig. 9.1** The effects of vitamin D on the renin-angiotensin system. 1,25-Dihydroxyvitamin D suppresses renin gene expression, thereby inhibiting the renin-angiotensin system. ACE, angiotensin-converting enzyme; $H_2O$, water; Na, sodium [1] (Open Access, Society of Diabetic Nephropathy Prevention)

## Pharmacology and "Functional Medicine" Are Complimentary

As the title of this section states, pharmacology and "functional medicine" are complimentary. The body's systems are very intricate and involved. Every process has many steps that either lead to wellness (if healthy), or illness (if not healthy). While one small step is all it takes to lead to illness, a similarly small step leads to wellness, just as easily. For example, the renin-angiotensin-aldosterone system (RAAS) is critical in maintaining blood volume and thereby BP. While renin, an enzyme, leads to thirst, an increase in blood volume, and eventually increased blood pressure, all to restore proper perfusion pressure in the kidneys, excessive renin expression may lead to excessive blood volume, high BP (and ultimately hypertension), and possible renal damage and disease. As mentioned earlier, half the hypertension patients prescribed up to three antihypertensives are still hypertensive. Vitamin D (either from the diet or as a supplement), among the other functions discussed in this volume, also blocks Renin expression in patients with high BP due to high blood volume (including those with renal disease) helping to reduce blood volume, and in turn BP, which may then help to reverse hypertension and kidney disease (see Fig. 9.1) [1].

However, "bad" habits, which seem easier because they are habits already, often lead to illness. Unfortunately this happens very slowly, so that by the time they are recognized, they are hard to break and illness is just waiting to appear (if not already) because the process has already begun. It is just that the results have yet to surface. The complexity of the human body may both help and hurt. It provides many opportunities for repair and prevention, but it also takes multiple approaches (prongs) to affect repair and prevention in order to maintain health and wellness.

As another example, vitamin E by itself does not prevent the formation of oxidized lipids, and more than just vitamin E alone is required. Also, just lowering the LDL cholesterol particle count with statins, pharmacology, or other dietary measures will not prevent atherosclerosis since the oxidation of these lipids also needs to be prevented even though they are in lower quantity. One of the disadvantages of oxidative stress is that when LDL and lipoprotein particles become oxidized and enter the vascular system in the form of foam cells (see Fig. 3.5), atherosclerosis has already begun. Foam cells increase platelet aggregation and cause them to clump together, forming clots, decreasing nitric oxide and PGI2 (which are vasodilating substances), and causing endothelial cell dysfunction. Foam cells damage endothelial cells and promote inflammation. Therefore, oxidized LDL particles promote heart disease and need to be prevented. It has been shown that statins have the ability to remove oxidized LDL cholesterol from plaques. This may be measured in very sophisticated scientific experiments. However, preventing the plaque from forming in the first place, or limiting its formation, is a goal of wellness.

Since the first mitochondrial dysfunction was described in the 1960s, medicine has advanced in its understanding the role mitochondria play in health, disease, and aging. A wide range of seemingly unrelated disorders, such as schizophrenia, bipolar disease, dementia, Alzheimer's disease, epilepsy, migraine headaches, strokes, neuropathic pain, Parkinson's disease, ataxia, transient ischemic attack, cardiomyopathy, coronary artery disease, chronic fatigue syndrome, fibromyalgia, retinitis pigmentosa, diabetes, hepatitis C, and primary biliary cirrhosis, have underlying pathophysiological mechanisms in common, namely, reactive oxygen species (ROS) production. Healthy mitochondria generate small amounts of ROS and other oxidative agents, but these are healthy levels and used by the body, including the immune system to defeat the body's invaders.

However, in unhealthy situations, the accumulation of mitochondrial DNA (mtDNA) damage from ROS production results in mitochondrial dysfunction. Antioxidant therapies hold promise for improving mitochondrial performance. Physicians seeking systematic treatments for their patients might consider testing urinary organic acids to determine how best to treat them [2]. In general, developing as much of an antioxidant buffer mitigates the effect of ROS and other oxidative agents, helping to maintain healthy mitochondrial function (see Fig. 9.2), and prevent or slow the progression of oxidative disease and aging effects. Developing and maintaining an antioxidant buffer (with exercise, Mediterranean diet, reduced oxidative stress, and reduced psychosocial stress) is another goal of wellness.

## Cannabidiol (Marijuana)

Marijuana, also known as cannabis, is considered the most commonly used illegal psychoactive drug worldwide [4]. Medical marijuana has long been used to help relieve or control pain, mood disorders (e.g., anxiety, depression, and related disorders), inflammatory disorders, posttraumatic stress, possibly seizure disorders, and much more. Some even believe that it has helped to control some forms of cancer. Whether this is perceived (as a result of the psychotropic nature of marijuana) or real is still contentious. With its recent legalization in many states within the United States, marijuana research into its purported benefits has significantly increased. The primary argument for its legalization is that it is believed by some to possibly limit the use of alcohol and opiates by individuals.

There are two active components to marijuana: cannabidiol (CBD) and tetrahydrocannabinol (specifically, delta 9 tetrahydrocannabinol; aka, THC). THC is one of potentially many psychotropic and addictive factors of marijuana. THC is the primary psychoactive and addictive component, whereas CBD has little, if any, known toxic effects on humans. It is CBD that seems to hold the key to the wide variety of medicinal and therapeutic effects that marijuana

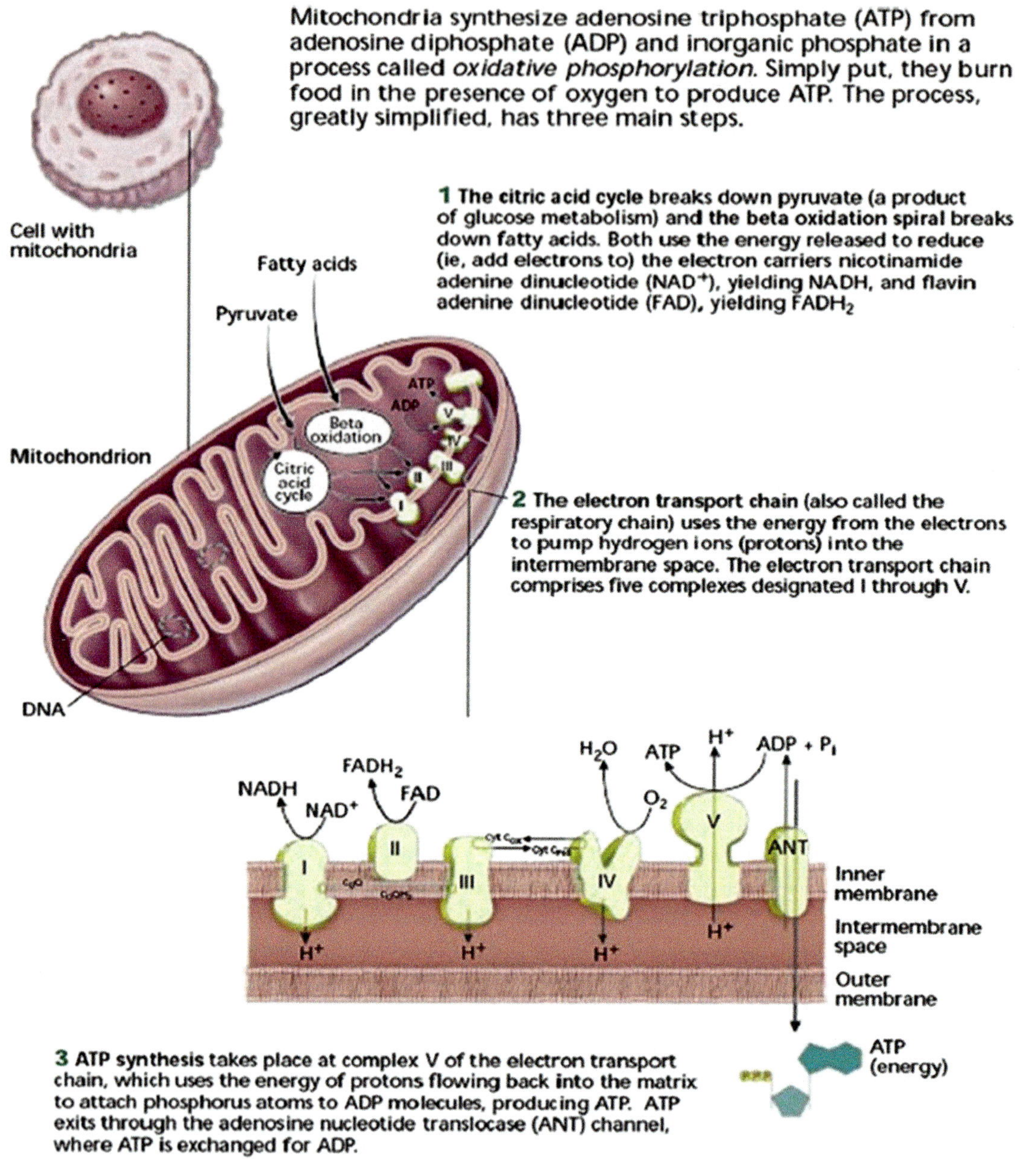


**Fig. 9.2** Healthy mitochondrial function [3]. (Republished with permission from Cleveland Clinic J. of Med)

seems to offer. As with any supplement or nutraceutical, it does not necessarily work for everyone. If after a month of CBD, or even medical marijuana therapy, there is no relief, then it is not the right choice of therapy.

For all its perceived benefit, there are significant concerns regarding widespread use of marijuana, even under physician supervision. There has long been noted an association between marijuana and cardiovascular diseases in some individuals. An article published in August 2017 [5] found that marijuana use increased the risk of hypertensive mortality. A follow-up study of 19,569 person years demonstrated that adjusted hazard ratio for death from hypertension among marijuana users compared to non-marijuana users was 3.42 and for each year of marijuana use was 1.04. The study controlled for cigarette smoking and other relevant variables.

It is known that cannabis intake can acutely increase sympathetic activity and decrease parasympathetic activity. This results in release of catecholamines and can produce tachycardia, vasodilatation, increase in cardiac output, and an increase in myocardial oxygen demand with little or no increase in BP [6, 7]. Orthostatic hypotension has also been associated with cannabis use [8]. The cannabinoid CB1 receptor antagonist rimonabant attenuates the hypotensive effect of smoked marijuana in male smokers. It has been shown that cannabis smoking causes a short-term increase in risk of acute myocardial infarction even in individuals that have history of coronary disease, angina, or high BP. This was shown in a prospective study of 3886 adult patients with acute myocardial infarction, 3.2% of whom smoked cannabis within the prior year [9]. Another study of 1913 subjects showed that after medium 3.8 years, weekly cannabis users have a hazard ratio of 4.2 [10]. Lung cancer also has been investigated. A 2006 systemic review of 19 studies showed associated cannabis smoking lung cancer with alveolar macrophage dysfunction, oxidative stress, and bronchial mucosa abnormalities, but no association with lung cancer after adjusting for tobacco use [11]. This was somewhat comforting. Cannabis has been also been associated with:

- Atrial fibrillation in a growing a number of case reports, although the risk also appears to be small [12, 13]
- Stroke, although the absolute risk also appears to be small [14]
- Arthritis of the limbs [15]

While cannabis is used for medical use in many entities, the risk of cardiovascular harm has been of some concern. It is potentially possible that there are long-lasting P&S dysfunction effects produced by cannabis. P&S function tests were conducted on patients who had never been exposed to medical marijuana, who subsequently took medical marijuana for 3 months. There seem to be two marijuana-naïve subpopulations identified by P&S monitoring, those with baseline, primary sympathetic excess (SE) and those with baseline, secondary SE to a primary parasympathetic excess (PE). For those with a history of marijuana use, whether PE is a result of marijuana use or exacerbated by marijuana use is still in question.

## B Vitamins

Limiting both defects and prolonging life expectancy are the goals of all physicians. It has been shown, including throughout this text, that B vitamins (primarily from dark green leafy vegetables in the diet) are essential to wellness. In this example, the focus is on vitamin $B_3$ (Niacin) and vitamin $B_9$ (folic acid). Folic acid and nicotinamide adenine dinucleotide (NAD) are important cofactors in various biochemical systems in the body. The importance of folic acid in nitric oxide production and nitric oxide synthases has been described earlier. The NAD de novo synthesis pathway involves the essential amino acid L-tryptophan. This is also known as the kynurenine pathway, as described earlier. Niacin, among its other functions, is involved in the production of NAD. There is an NAD salvage pathway where NAD becomes nicotinamide, which becomes nicotinamide mononucleotide, which then gets turned back into NAD. Tryptophan and niacin, which is supplied as nicotinic acid and nicotinamide, represent dietary inputs.

Disruption of NAD synthesis causes a deficiency in NAD and congenital malformations [16]. Niacin supplementation during gestation helps to prevent, specifically, neural tube[4] malformation. Severe niacin deficiency in adults

[4]The neural tube is the foundation of the nervous system occurring in utero by the fourth week of pregnancy. As the neural plate folds and forms the neural tube, separating from the epidermis, the central nervous system begins development from the neural tube, and, among other structures, the peripheral nervous system is formed from the epidermis.

causes pellagra characterized by dermatitis, diarrhea, dementia, and death. Severe niacin deficiency in utero causes deficiencies of the GI and neurological systems and possibly defects predominantly affecting the thoracic and lumbar spine, cleft palate, bifid uvula, and laryngeal webs and laryngeal tracheomalacia, cognitive defects, and postnatal growth abnormalities. Therefore, NAD deficiency in utero due to maternal niacin deficiency can cause significant congenital defects.

NAD is essential to energy metabolism; it is an essential coenzyme in glycolysis, the tricarboxylic acid cycle (Krebs cycle) in the mitochondria electron transport chain, and is also essential to production of macromolecules, including nucleotides (see Energy Production). Also, NAD regulates sirtuin-mediated deacetylation, which modulates transcription factors and metabolic enzymes that promote mitochondrial oxidative function and enhance cell survival under stress conditions [17, 18, 19]. Thirdly, DNA repair is active during embryogenesis and is required for normal development. There is evidence that NAD deficiency impairs DNA repair and that a DNA fragmentation disorder in humans, Fanconi's anemia, can result in multiple congenital abnormalities, which define the VACTERL association [7]. Patients are considered to have VACTERL associations if they have any three of the following defects in the absence of a genetic cause: malformations and vertebral defects, anal atresia, cardiac defects, transesophageal fistula, renal anomalies, and limb abnormalities.

The article in *The New England Journal of Medicine* [16] nicely shows the NAD de novo synthesis pathway and how nicotine and nicotinic acid are important participants. There also is a perspective written by Dr. Vander Heiden. He states that it is well known that metabolism needs to be tightly controlled to support the needs of individual cells in tissues [20]. Nutrient oxidation is necessary for the production of ATP. It supports energetically unfavorable processes in cells. It is also necessary for the metabolic conversion of nutrients to build biomass to support cell proliferation. The perspective gives the example of folic acid deficit delaying neural tube closure, resulting in ANS anencephaly or spina bifida. It continues in that cereal foods need to be fortified to prevent this. Therefore, this is one area where a cofactor, namely, folic acid, prevents defects at birth. Now, NAD is well known to be an important cofactor that is needed in utero to prevent genetic defects.

As described in the perspective and elsewhere (see Fig. 5.48), NAD is synthesized from tryptophan in the diet. Through the kynurenine pathway, it is metabolized to produce NAD. $NAD^+$ can accept electrons and become NADH. NADH is cycled back to $NAD^+$ when pyruvate through oxygen makes water through lactate. NAD has an essential role in cell metabolism as an electron carrier for the reduction action in cells. Oxidized NAD or $NAD^+$ can accept an electron and pair as a cofactor in oxidation reactions, including those involving glycolysis and tricarboxylic acid that are important in ATP production. $NAD^+$ is also an electronic acceptor in biosynthetic pathways, including pathways which consist of purine and pyrimidine nucleotides, which are fundamental building blocks of RNA and DNA. When $NAD^+$ accepts electrons, it is reduced to NADH. Because the pool of $NAD^+$ is relatively small due to metabolic pathways involving oxidative reactions, NAD must be continually regenerated by transferring the electron from NADH to another substrate such as terminal electron acceptors, oxygen or pyruvate. Thus, the continued shuttling of electrons between NADH and $NAD^+$ is crucial to many cellular processes including generations of ATP and the synthesis of nucleotides. $NAD^+$ is also a substrate for enzymes that signal the presence of DNA damage and other types of cell stress. It is now known that NAD deficiency causes congenital malformations. Folic acid and NAD, not only in utero, but throughout life, are important in maintaining normal DNA, DNA repair, and appropriate mitochondrial function to produce the ATP. This is why B vitamins such as $B_3$ (niacin) and $B_9$ (folic acid) are strongly recommended as part of the necessary cofactors in this six-pronged approach.

## Questionnaires

Having patients complete questionnaires and participate in extensive interviews helps to better understand patients' histories so that all the systems of the body and the whole person may be considered. This helps to individualize therapy (pharmaceutical, nutraceutical, lifestyle, and supplemental therapies). This is the primary reason for questionnaires, including a few different autonomic questionnaires (for diabetics and nondiabetics) and an Ehlers-Danlos[5] questionnaire [21].

## Compass 31 Questionnaire

The Composite Autonomic Symptom Score (COMPASS) questionnaire is a concise and statistically robust instrument to assess autonomic symptoms that provide clinically relevant scores of autonomic symptom severity based on the well-established 169-item Autonomic Symptom Profile (ASP) and its validated 84-question scoring instrument, COMPASS. COMPASS 31 is a refined (31-question), internally consistent, and markedly abbreviated quantitative measure of autonomic symptoms. It is based on the original ASP and COMPASS (84-question), applies a much simplified scoring algorithm, and is suitable for widespread use in autonomic research and practice [22]. The COMPASS 31 questionnaire assesses symptoms of dysautonomia. It has good psychometric properties and is useful as an initial screening tool [23].

### Compass 31 Questionnaire

1. In the past year, have you ever felt faint, dizzy, "goofy," or had difficulty thinking soon after standing up from a sitting or lying position?
   a. Yes
   b. No (if you marked No, please skip to question 5)
2. When standing up, how frequently do you get these feelings or symptoms?
   a. Rarely
   b. Occasionally
   c. Frequently
   d. Almost always
3. How would you rate the severity of these feelings or symptoms?
   a. Mild
   b. Moderate
   c. Severe
4. In the past year, have these feelings or symptoms that you have experienced:
   a. Gotten much worse
   b. Gotten somewhat worse
   c. Stayed about the same
   d. Gotten somewhat better
   e. Gotten much better
   f. Completely gone
5. In the past year, have you ever noticed color changes in your skin, such as red, white, or purple?
   a. Yes
   b. No (if you marked No, please skip to question 8)
6. What parts of your body are affected by these color changes? (Check all that apply)
   a. Hands
   b. Feet
7. Are these changes in your skin color:
   a. Getting much worse
   b. Getting somewhat worse
   c. Staying about the same
   d. Getting somewhat better
   e. Getting much better
   f. Completely gone
8. In the past 5 years, what changes, if any, have occurred in your general body sweating?
   a. I sweat much more than I used to.
   b. I sweat somewhat more than I used to.
   c. I haven't noticed any changes in my sweating.
   d. I sweat somewhat less than I used to.
9. Do your eyes feel excessively dry?
   a. Yes
   b. No

[5]Ehlers-Danlos is a connective tissue disorder marked by hyper-flexibility and "elastic skin" which bruises easily due to "weak" blood vessels and is well known to involve the P&S nervous systems. It is considered a hereditary disease.

10. Does your mouth feel excessively dry?
    a. Yes
    b. No
11. For the symptom of dry eyes or dry mouth that you have had for the longest period of time, is this symptom:
    a. I have not had any of these symptoms.
    b. Getting much worse.
    c. Getting somewhat worse.
    d. Staying about the same.
    e. Getting somewhat better.
    f. Getting much better.
    g. Completely gone.
12. In the past year, have you noticed any changes in how quickly you get full when eating a meal?
    a. I get full a lot more quickly now than I used to.
    b. I get full more quickly now than I used to.
    c. I haven't noticed any change.
    d. I get full less quickly now than I used to.
    e. I get full a lot less quickly now than I used to.
13. In the past year, have you felt excessively full or persistently full (bloated feeling) after a meal?
    a. Never
    b. Sometimes
    c. A lot of the time
14. In the past year, have you vomited after a meal?
    a. Never
    b. Sometimes
    c. A lot of the time
15. In the past year, have you had a cramping or colicky abdominal pain?
    a. Never
    b. Sometimes
    c. A lot of the time
16. In the past year, have you had any bouts of diarrhea?
    a. Yes
    b. No (if you marked No, please skip to question 20)
17. How frequently does this occur?
    a. Rarely
    b. Occasionally
    c. Frequently _________ times per month
    d. Constantly
18. How severe are these bouts of diarrhea?
    a. Mild
    b. Moderate
    c. Severe
19. Are your bouts of diarrhea getting:
    a. Much worse
    b. Somewhat worse
    c. Staying the same
    d. Somewhat better
    e. Much better
    f. Completely gone
20. In the past year, have you been constipated?
    a. Yes
    b. No (if you marked No, please skip to question 24)
21. How frequently are you constipated?
    a. Rarely
    b. Occasionally
    c. Frequently _________ times per month
    d. Constantly
22. How severe are these episodes of constipation?
    a. Mild
    b. Moderate
    c. Severe
23. Is your constipation getting:
    a. Much worse
    b. Somewhat worse
    c. Staying the same
    d. Somewhat better
    e. Much better
    f. Completely gone
24. In the past year, have you ever lost control of your bladder function?
    a. Never
    b. Occasionally
    c. Frequently _________ times per month
    d. Constantly
25. In the past year, have you had difficulty passing urine?
    a. Never
    b. Occasionally
    c. Frequently _________ times per month
    d. Constantly
26. In the past year, have you had trouble completely emptying your bladder?
    a. Never
    b. Occasionally
    c. Frequently _________ times per month
    d. Constantly

27. In the past year, without sunglasses or tinted glasses, has bright light bothered your eyes?
    a. Never (if you marked Never, please skip to question 29)
    b. Occasionally
    c. Frequently
    d. Constantly
28. How severe is this sensitivity to bright light?
    a. Mild
    b. Moderate
    c. Severe
29. In the past year, have you had trouble focusing your eyes?
    a. Never (if you marked Never, please skip to question 31)
    b. Occasionally
    c. Frequently
    d. Constantly
30. How severe is this focusing problem?
    a. Mild
    b. Moderate
    c. Severe
31. Is the most troublesome symptom with your eyes (i.e., sensitivity to bright light or trouble focusing) getting:
    a. I have not had any of these symptoms.
    b. Much worse.
    c. Somewhat worse.
    d. Staying about the same.
    e. Somewhat better.
    f. Much better.
    g. Completely gone.

## SF-36 Questionnaire

The Short Form-36 (SF-36) is a 36-item questionnaire which measures quality of life (QoL) across eight domains, which are both physically and emotionally based, including physical functioning, role limitations due to physical health, role limitations due to emotional problems, level of energy or fatigue, emotional well-being, social functioning, pain, and general health. A single item is also included that identifies perceived change in health, making the SF-36 a useful indicator for change in QoL over time and treatment. The SF-36 has been widely validated (over 5000 published studies) for numerous professions and patient groups and can be administered by clinicians or by the patient at home. An aggregate percentage score is produced for each of the eight domains that the SF-36 measures. The percentage scores range from 0% (lowest or worst possible level of functioning) to 100% (highest or best possible level of functioning).

Scores are calculated through a two-step system. Each of the question responses relates to a different pre-coded numeric value. The raw scores are translated into one from 0 to 100, with 0 representing a very low level of QoL in that item and 100 representing a very positive response to that item. In the second step, work out the mean average for each of the eight scales from the translated scores. Add up the translated scores for each of the scale items to calculate the average. For example, add up the scores for questions 21 and 22 and divide by two to assess the scale "pain"; add up the scores for items 17, 18, and 19 and divide by three to assess the scale "role limitations due to emotional problems"; continue to do this for all eight scales. A summary of physical QoL (Physical Component Summary; PCS) and emotional QoL (Mental Component summary; MCS) is computed by taking the mean of all of the physically relevant questions and of all of the emotionally relevant items.

The SF-36 QoL measures are quite individual. Two patients who have the same scores on the SF-36 may actually feel very different about their QoL. Therefore, it makes little sense to present normative values. No normative values or cutoff scores are therefore presented. However, the scoring of the SF-36 indicates that 0% in a domain represents the poorest possible QoL and 100% indicates full QoL (the best possible result). Taking this into account, it is easy to see that the higher the scores on the SF-36 indicate, the better QoL. Upon repeat of SF-36 QoL measures (either for a group of patients or a single patient), an increase in the score marks an improvement in QoL.

### SF-36 Questionnaire

1. In general, would you say your health is:
   - □ 0. Excellent
   - □ 1. Very good
   - □ 2. Good
   - □ 3. Fair
   - □ 4. Poor

2. Compared to 1 year ago, how would you rate your health in general now?
   - □ 0. Much better than 1 year ago
   - □ 1. Somewhat better now than 1 year ago
   - □ 2. About the same as 1 year ago
   - □ 3. Somewhat worse than 1 year ago
   - □ 4. Much worse than 1 year ago

The following items are about activities you might do during a typical day. Does your health now limit you in these activities? If so, how much?

| | Activities | No, not limited at all (0) | Yes, limited a little (2) | Yes, limited a lot (4) |
|---|---|---|---|---|
| 3. | *Vigorous activities* such as running, lifting heavy objects, or participating in strenuous sports | | | |
| 4. | *Moderate activities* such as moving a table, pushing a vacuum cleaner, bowling, or playing golf | | | |
| 5. | Lifting or carrying groceries | | | |
| 6. | Climbing *several flights* of stairs | | | |
| 7. | Climbing *one flight* of stairs | | | |
| 8. | Bending, kneeling, or stooping | | | |
| 9. | Walking *more than a mile* | | | |
| 10. | Walking *several blocks* | | | |
| 11. | Walking *one block* | | | |
| 12. | Bathing or dressing yourself | | | |

During the past 4 weeks, have you had any of the following problems with your work or other regular daily activities as a result of your physical health?

| | Activities | Yes (1) | No (0) |
|---|---|---|---|
| 13. | Cut down the amount of time you spent on work or other activities | | |
| 14. | Accomplished less than you would like | | |
| 15. | Were limited in the kind of work or other activities | | |
| 16. | Had difficulty performing the work or other activities | | |

During the past 4 weeks, have you had any of the following problems with your work or other regular daily activities as a result of any emotional problems (such as feeling depressed or anxious)?

| | Activities | Yes (1) | No (0) |
|---|---|---|---|
| 17. | Cut down the *amount of time* you spent on work or other activities | | |
| 18. | *Accomplished less* than you would like | | |
| 19. | Didn't do work or other activities as *carefully* as usual | | |

20. During the past 4 weeks, to what extent has your physical health or emotional problems interfered with your normal social activities with family, friends, neighbors, or groups?
    - □ 0. Not at all
    - □ 1. A little bit
    - □ 2. Moderate
    - □ 3. Quite a bit
    - □ 4. Extremely
21. How significant has your *bodily* pain been during the *past 4 weeks*?
    - □ 0. None
    - □ 1. Very mild
    - □ 2. Mild
    - □ 3. Moderate
    - □ 4. Severe
    - □ 5. Very severe
22. During the past 4 weeks, how much did pain interfere with your normal work (including both work outside the home and housework)?
    - □ 0. Not at all
    - □ 1. A little bit
    - □ 2. Moderate
    - □ 3. Quite a bit
    - □ 4. Extremely

The next sets of questions are about how you have felt the past 4 weeks.

23. Did you feel full of pep?
   - □ 0. All the time
   - □ 1. Most of the time
   - □ 2. Some of the time
   - □ 3. A Little of the time
   - □ 4. None of the time
24. Have you been very nervous person?
   - □ 0. None of the time
   - □ 1. A little of the time
   - □ 2. Some of the time
   - □ 3. Most of the time
   - □ 4. All the time
25. Have you felt so down in the in the dumps that nothing could cheer you up?
   - □ 0. None of the time
   - □ 1. A little of the time
   - □ 2. Some of the time
   - □ 3. Most of the time
   - □ 4. All the time
26. Have you felt calm and peaceful?
   - □ 0. All the time
   - □ 1. Most of the time
   - □ 2. Some of the time
   - □ 3. A little of the time
   - □ 4. None of the time
27. Did you have a lot of energy?
   - □ 0. All the time
   - □ 1. Most of the time
   - □ 2. Some of the time
   - □ 3. A little of the time
   - □ 4. None of the time
28. Have you felt downhearted and blue?
   - □ 0. None of the time
   - □ 1. A little of the time
   - □ 2. Some of the time
   - □ 3. Most of the time
   - □ 4. All the time
29. Did you feel worn out?
   - □ 0. None of the time
   - □ 1. A little of the time
   - □ 2. Some of the time
   - □ 3. Most of the time
   - □ 4. All the time
30. Have you been a happy person?
   - □ 0. None of the time
   - □ 1. A little of the time
   - □ 2. Some of the time
   - □ 3. Most of the time
   - □ 4. All the time
31. Did you feel tired?
   - □ 0. None of the time
   - □ 1. A little of the time
   - □ 2. Some of the time
   - □ 3. Most of the time
   - □ 4. All the time
32. During the past 4 weeks, how much of the time has your physical health or emotional problems interfered with your social activities?
   - □ 0. None of the time
   - □ 1. A little of the time
   - □ 2. Some of the time
   - □ 3. Most of the time
   - □ 4. All the time
33. I seem to get sick a little easier than other people.
   - □ 0. Definitely false
   - □ 1. Mostly false
   - □ 2. Don't know
   - □ 3. Mostly true
   - □ 4. Definitely true
34. I am as healthy as anyone I know.
   - □ 0. Definitely true
   - □ 1. Mostly true
   - □ 2. Don't know
   - □ 3. Mostly false
   - □ 4. Definitely false
35. I expect my health to get worse.
   - □ 0. Definitely false
   - □ 1. Mostly false
   - □ 2. Don't know
   - □ 3. Mostly true
   - □ 4. Definitely true
36. My health is excellent.
   - □ 0. Definitely true
   - □ 1. Mostly true
   - □ 2. Don't know
   - □ 3. Mostly false
   - □ 4. Definitely false

TOTAL: 124 - _ _ _ = _ _ _

Table 9.1 (in two parts) offers examples of SF-36 QoL responses for individuals who are considered normal. These values are offered for comparative purposes. They are not proposed as normal values. As with the P&S nervous systems, the QoL declines with age in the overall score or in the eight individual domains, parallel to the P&S decline (*c.f.*, Fig. 7.6).

**Table 9.1** Mean (SD) scores for the SF-36 dimensions by age and gender, social class, and health variables [24]

| | Physical functioning | | | Role limitations (physical) | | | Bodily pain | | | General health perceptions | | |
|---|---|---|---|---|---|---|---|---|---|---|---|---|
| Total score | Mean | (SD) | (*n*) | Mean | (SD) | (*n*) | Mean | (SD) | (*n*) | Mean | (SD) | (*n*) |
| *Age* | | | | | | | | | | | | |
| 16–24 | 95.5 | (12.1) | (204) | 90.7 | (24.5) | (202) | 86.0 | (22.6) | (203) | 78.6 | (17.7) | (204) |
| 25–34 | 94.5 | (13.5) | (415) | 87.5 | (29.8) | (414) | 86.7 | (22.6) | (414) | 79.4 | (17.9) | (416) |
| 35–44 | 93.3 | (13.4) | (319) | 88.2 | (28.0) | (318) | 84.9 | (21.8) | (318) | 75.5 | (19.5) | (319) |
| 45–54 | 87.2 | (20.9) | (297) | 83.5 | (33.8) | (296) | 80.7 | (25.5) | (298) | 71.3 | (23.4) | (297) |
| 55–64 | 78.0 | (26.3) | (297) | 72.7 | (40.6) | (295) | 74.4 | (28.6) | (296) | 65.3 | (26.5) | (295) |
| 65–74 | 72.7 | (26.7) | (281) | 72.6 | (39.5) | (279) | 75.5 | (27.2) | (279) | 65.0 | (24.1) | (279) |
| 75–84 | 57.9 | (28.6) | (296) | 62.2 | (42.1) | (176) | 70.3 | (29.5) | (178) | 58.7 | (24.5) | (175) |
| 85+ | 39.3 | (31.5) | (36) | 65.0 | (42.5) | (35) | 65.7 | (30.5) | (35) | 60.3 | (22.2) | (34) |
| *Sex* | | | | | | | | | | | | |
| Male | 86.3 | (22.5) | (925) | 82.7 | (33.7) | (921) | 83.2 | (24.4) | (922) | 71.9 | (23.0) | (921) |
| Female | 81.8 | (25.7) | (1117) | 79.0 | (36.5) | (1109) | 78.1 | (26.8) | (1114) | 71.3 | (22.8) | (1113) |
| *Social class* | | | | | | | | | | | | |
| I Prof | 89.9 | (18.0) | (73) | 83.5 | (33.3) | (71) | 83.7 | (21.0) | (73) | 76.7 | (18.9) | (72) |
| II Semi-prof | 85.5 | (19.2) | (481) | 86.4 | (30.1) | (480) | 85.2 | (22.1) | (481) | 75.5 | (19.4) | (479) |
| IIInm | 85.8 | (22.6) | (474) | 82.2 | (33.8) | (473) | 80.4 | (24.5) | (474) | 72.9 | (22.0) | (473) |
| IIIm | 82.0 | (26.0) | (447) | 77.1 | (38.2) | (443) | 79.0 | (27.2) | (444) | 69.7 | (23.9) | (446) |
| IV | 79.9 | (27.3) | (339) | 77.2 | (36.8) | (337) | 75.5 | (28.7) | (337) | 68.4 | (25.2) | (338) |
| V | 75.7 | (29.5) | (151) | 75.7 | (40.1) | (149) | 75.6 | (28.7) | (151) | 65.6 | (25.2) | (150) |
| *Cut down activities because of illness (in last 2 weeks)* | | | | | | | | | | | | |
| Yes | 63.0 | (33.4) | (319) | 27.7 | (37.4) | (316) | 49.8 | (29.8) | (318) | 51.5 | (27.5) | (316) |
| No | 87.7 | (20.2) | (1722) | 90.4 | (24.7) | (1713) | 86.1 | (20.6) | (1717) | 75.3 | (19.9) | (1717) |
| *Long-term health problem* | | | | | | | | | | | | |
| Yes | 52.3 | (28.9) | (449) | 44.1 | (42.5) | (444) | 56.0 | (30.2) | (447) | 44.8 | (23.5) | (444) |
| No | 92.7 | (13.1) | (1590) | 90.9 | (24.7) | (1583) | 87.4 | (19.6) | (1586) | 79.0 | (16.1) | (1587) |
| *Attended A&E or hospital out-patient (in past 3 months)* | | | | | | | | | | | | |
| Yes | 71.5 | (30.8) | (353) | 60.4 | (43.0) | (353) | 65.3 | (30.9) | (353) | 60.4 | (27.0) | (351) |
| No | 86.4 | (22.1) | (1689) | 84.9 | (31.9) | (1677) | 83.6 | (23.5) | (1683) | 73.9 | (21.2) | (1683) |
| *Been hospital in-patient (in past 12 months)* | | | | | | | | | | | | |
| Yes | 70.2 | (31.3) | (256) | 58.2 | (44.0) | (255) | 67.6 | (31.8) | (256) | 59.7 | (27.4) | (256) |
| No | 85.8 | (22.7) | (1786) | 83.9 | (32.7) | (1775) | 82.3 | (24.4) | (1780) | 73.2 | (21.7) | (1778) |

| | Energy/vitality | | | Social functioning | | | Role limitations (emotional) | | | Mental health | | |
|---|---|---|---|---|---|---|---|---|---|---|---|---|
| Total score | Mean | (SD) | (*n*) | Mean | (SD) | (*n*) | Mean | (SD) | (*n*) | Mean | (SD) | (*n*) |
| *Age* | | | | | | | | | | | | |
| 16–24 | 68.3 | (19.0) | (203) | 91.5 | (17.2) | (203) | 91.1 | (24.6) | (203) | 79.6 | (15.2) | (203) |
| 25–34 | 66.8 | (18.4) | (415) | 91.1 | (16.9) | (413) | 90.3 | (26.2) | (414) | 77.2 | (16.2) | (415) |
| 35–44 | 64.9 | (18.2) | (319) | 90.5 | (19.4) | (317) | 88.2 | (28.7) | (317) | 76.0 | (18.3) | (319) |
| 45–54 | 63.0 | (23.1) | (296) | 87.7 | (22.8) | (297) | 88.4 | (28.6) | (297) | 75.6 | (20.2) | (297) |
| 55–64 | 61.8 | (24.6) | (297) | 84.7 | (25.6) | (297) | 81.8 | (35.8) | (296) | 76.0 | (20.2) | (297) |
| 65–74 | 63.0 | (24.1) | (279) | 85.8 | (25.6) | (279) | 88.1 | (29.8) | (280) | 80.0 | (18.3) | (279) |
| 75–84 | 54.2 | (24.9) | (176) | 75.9 | (29.1) | (176) | 82.8 | (34.7) | (174) | 75.6 | (19.5) | (176) |
| 85+ | 52.1 | (20.8) | (35) | 73.7 | (24.7) | (35) | 87.6 | (32.4) | (35) | 73.9 | (17.8) | (34) |
| *Sex* | | | | | | | | | | | | |
| Male | 67.2 | (21.7) | (923) | 88.8 | (21.4) | (920) | 90.4 | (26.6) | (912) | 79.5 | (17.7) | (920) |
| Female | 60.6 | (21.6) | (1112) | 86.2 | (23.4) | (1112) | 85.3 | (32.0) | (1110) | 75.1 | (18.6) | (1115) |
| *Social class* | | | | | | | | | | | | |
| I Prof | 69.0 | (18.5) | (73) | 90.7 | (17.8) | (73) | 93.4 | (17.5) | (73) | 81.2 | (15.3) | (73) |

**Table 9.1** (continued)

| | Energy/vitality | | | Social functioning | | | Role limitations (emotional) | | | Mental health | | |
|---|---|---|---|---|---|---|---|---|---|---|---|---|
| Total score | Mean | (SD) | (*n*) | Mean | (SD) | (*n*) | Mean | (SD) | (*n*) | Mean | (SD) | (*n*) |
| II Semi-prof | 65.9 | (19.3) | (480) | 91.4 | (18.3) | (479) | 89.7 | (26.2) | (481) | 79.0 | (16.7) | (481) |
| IIInm | 62.8 | (19.7) | (474) | 88.0 | (21.1) | (473) | 88.7 | (28.2) | (472) | 76.6 | (16.6) | (475) |
| IIIm | 64.3 | (23.1) | (445) | 86.2 | (23.0) | (445) | 88.2 | (29.5) | (443) | 78.7 | (18.6) | (444) |
| IV | 60.5 | (24.8) | (338) | 84.3 | (26.0) | (337) | 83.1 | (34.3) | (338) | 74.1 | (20.7) | (338) |
| V | 60.7 | (25.2) | (149) | 81.9 | (27.7) | (149) | 82.8 | (36.5) | (149) | 73.8 | (21.1) | (149) |
| *Cut down activities because of illness (in last 2 weeks)* | | | | | | | | | | | | |
| Yes | 44.0 | (24.8) | (315) | 60.8 | (30.9) | (316) | 66.4 | (45.1) | (316) | 66.3 | (21.8) | (316) |
| No | 67.1 | (19.3) | (1719) | 92.3 | (16.6) | (1715) | 91.6 | (23.9) | (1714) | 79.1 | (16.9) | (1718) |
| *Long-term health problem* | | | | | | | | | | | | |
| Yes | 44.1 | (23.9) | (446) | 65.3 | (30.5) | (445) | 71.6 | (41.7) | (444) | 67.5 | (22.1) | (446) |
| No | 69.0 | (17.9) | (1586) | 93.5 | (14.9) | (1584) | 92.1 | (23.5) | (1584) | 79.8 | (16.1) | (1586) |
| *Attended A&E or hospital out-patient (in past 3 months)* | | | | | | | | | | | | |
| Yes | 54.2 | (25.0) | (351) | 74.7 | (30.2) | (352) | 79.5 | (37.7) | (352) | 72.5 | (20.3) | (351) |
| No | 65.5 | (20.7) | (1684) | 90.0 | (19.7) | (1680) | 89.3 | (27.5) | (1679) | 78.1 | (77.7) | (1684) |
| *Been hospital in-patient (in past 12 months)* | | | | | | | | | | | | |
| Yes | 50.9 | (26.1) | (254) | 72.1 | (31.9) | (255) | 79.9 | (37.2) | (255) | 71.3 | (21.5) | (255) |
| No | 65.4 | (20.6) | (1781) | 89.5 | (20.1) | (1777) | 88.7 | (28.4) | (1777) | 77.9 | (17.7) | (1780) |

## Nottingham Health Profile

The Nottingham Health Profile measures perceived health status as a predictor of, need for, and utilization of health services. It is a health-related QoL measure with 38 questions grouped into 6 domains: physical mobility (8 items), social isolation (5 items), emotional reactions (9 items), pain (8 items), sleep (5 items), and energy (3 items). The items include frequency of health-related problems pertaining to paid employment, housework, hobbies, family life, social life, sex life, and holidays. Each question is answered "yes" or "no" according to whether the symptom is present or absent "in general." It is well documented with regard to reliability and validity and is useful in describing the impact of chronic disease. It is also a useful tool to evaluate patients with more pronounced disability [25].

Items in each domain are assigned a weight; the total score for each domain is 100 where a score of 0 indicates good subjective health status and 100 indicates poor subjective health status. The total score is obtained by averaging the six domain scores. Results showed that the profile was capable of discriminating between groups differing in terms of diagnosed chronic illness, number of consultations at primary care level, and physiological fitness. Age, sex, and marital status were not significant overall in affecting scores. In elderly subjects, perceived health status accorded well with objective health status.

## Nottingham Health Profile

Please check the Yes or No box for the following questions.

Part I. Total: 100 - _ _ _ = _

| | Question | Yes | No | Section | Weight |
|---|---|---|---|---|---|
| 1 | I'm tired all the time | | | EL | 39.20 |
| 2 | I have pain at night | | | P | 12.91 |
| 3 | Things are getting me down | | | ER | 10.47 |
| 4 | I have unbearable pain | | | P | 19.74 |
| 5 | I take pills to help me sleep | | | S | 22.37 |
| 6 | I've forgotten what it's like to enjoy myself | | | ER | 9.31 |
| 7 | I'm feeling on edge | | | ER | 7.22 |
| 8 | I find it painful to change position | | | P | 9.99 |

| | Question | Yes | No | Section | Weight |
|---|---|---|---|---|---|
| 9 | I feel lonely | | | SI | 22.01 |
| 10 | I can walk about but only indoors | | | PA | 11.54 |
| 11 | I find it hard to bend | | | PA | 10.57 |
| 12 | Everything is an effort | | | EL | 36.80 |
| 13 | I'm waking up in the early hours of the morning | | | S | 12.57 |
| 14 | I'm unable to walk at all | | | PA | 21.30 |
| 15 | I'm finding it hard to make contact with people | | | SI | 19.36 |
| 16 | The days seem to drag | | | ER | 7.08 |
| 17 | I have trouble getting up and down stairs and steps | | | PA | 10.79 |
| 18 | I find it hard to reach things | | | PA | 9.30 |
| 19 | I'm in pain when I walk | | | P | 11.22 |
| 20 | I lose my temper easily these days | | | ER | 9.76 |
| 21 | I feel there is nobody I am close to | | | SI | 20.13 |
| 22 | I lie awake for most of the night | | | S | 27.26 |
| 23 | I feel as if I'm losing control | | | ER | 13.99 |
| 24 | I'm in pain when I'm standing | | | P | 8.96 |
| 25 | I find it hard to get dressed by myself | | | PA | 12.61 |
| 26 | I run out of energy | | | EL | 24.00 |
| 27 | I find it hard to stand for long (e.g., at the kitchen sink, waiting in line) | | | PA | 11.20 |
| 28 | I'm in constant pain | | | P | 20.86 |
| 29 | It takes me a long time to get to sleep | | | S | 16.10 |
| 30 | I feel I am a burden to people | | | SI | 22.53 |
| 31 | Worry is keeping me awake at night | | | ER | 13.95 |
| 32 | I feel as though life is not worth living | | | ER | 16.21 |
| 33 | I sleep badly at night | | | S | 21.70 |
| 34 | I'm finding it hard to get along with people | | | SI | 15.97 |
| 35 | I need help to walk outside (e.g., a walking aid or someone to support me) | | | PA | 12.69 |
| 36 | I'm in pain when going up or down stairs | | | P | 5.83 |
| 37 | I wake up feeling depressed | | | ER | 12.01 |
| 38 | I'm in pain when I'm sitting | | | P | 10.49 |

Total: 100- _ _ _ = _ _ _

| | | Yes | No |
|---|---|---|---|
| 39 | Is your present state of health causing problems with your: | | |
| 40 | Work? (i.e., paid employment) | | |
| 41 | Looking after the home? (Cleaning and cooking, repairs, odd jobs around the home, etc.) | | |
| 42 | Social life? (Going out, seeing friends, going to the movies, etc.) | | |
| 43 | Home life? (i.e., relationships with other people in your home) | | |
| 44 | Sex life? | | |
| 45 | Interests and hobbies? (Sports, arts and crafts, do-it-yourself, etc.) | | |
| 46 | Vacations? (Summer or winter vacations, weekends away, etc.) | | |

## Simplified Autonomic Questionnaire

Based on the previous two questionnaires and clinic experiences, the following questionnaire was developed. This is less a measure of QoL and more a measure of clinical necessity. It is used to identify the need for autonomic and other tests and to begin to build a therapy plan.

Circle which symptoms you have:

1. Light-headed
2. Fainting and near fainting
3. Fatigue
4. Brain fog or mental cloudiness
5. Difficulty finding words
6. Short-term memory loss
7. Sensory: hypersensitive to light, sound, motion, touch
8. Pins and needs in arms/legs
9. Numbness in hands and feet
10. Coat hanger pain (in neck and shoulders)
11. Migraine or headache
12. Tension headaches

13. Nausea, vomiting
14. Difficulty standing
15. Chest pain, palpitations
16. Short of breath
17. Hypermobility joints or joints pop out
18. Depression or anxiety
19. Sweat too much
20. Sweat too little
21. Salivate too little, or have dry mouth
22. Cold hands or feet
23. Dimmed vision
24. Dimmed hearing or ringing in ears
25. Does hot or cold weather bother you

## Questionnaire on Hypermobility Syndromes (EDS and Related Disorders)

This is a simple and reproducible self-reporting questionnaire that identifies individuals with hypermobility. The Ehlers-Danlos Society promotes the Beighton score [26].

### How To Assess Joint Hypermobility

- A numerical mobility score of 0–9, 1 point allocated for the ability to perform each of the following tests:

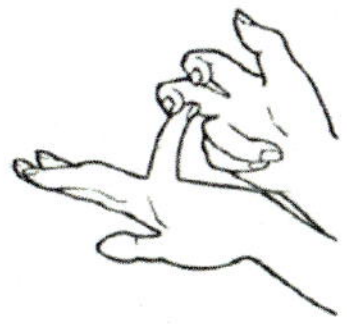

Pull little finger back beyond 90°
*(one point for each side)*

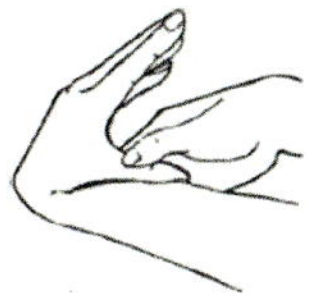

Pull thumb back to touch forearm
*(one point for each side)*

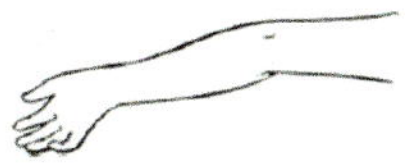

Bend elbow backwards beyond 10°
*(one point for each side)*

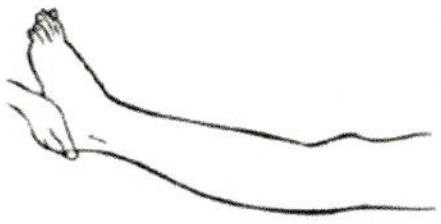

Bend knee backwards beyond 10°
*(one point for each side)*

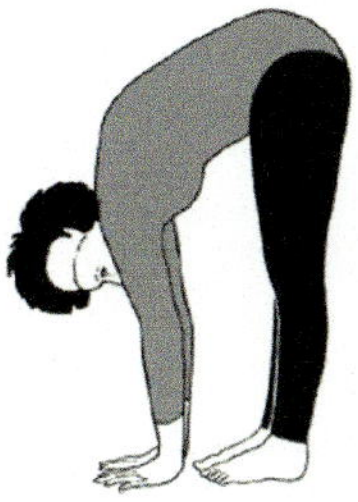

Lie hands flat on floor while keeping knees straight and bending forward at waist

- A positive Beighton score for adults [27] is 5 out of the 9 possible points; for children [28], a positive score is at least 6 out of 9 possible points.
- As joint mobility is known to decrease by age for adults, include historical information by asking, "Can you now or have you previously been able to …."

The Soloway-DePace mobility scale developed with Dr. Stephen Soloway is also used. Of note, while postural orthostatic tachycardia syndrome (POTS) is one of many symptoms of Ehlers-Danlos syndrome (EDS), and it is considered a hallmark of EDS, parasympathetic excess (with sympathetic challenge [29]) is the primary finding. The Soloway-DePace scoring system (Copyright 2018) is:

**Soloway-DePace Hypermobility Questionnaire**
**Questionnaire on Hypermobility Syndromes (EDS and Related Disorders)**
**Please circle Yes or No:**

| | | |
|---|---|---|
| 1. Do you develop pain in joints that is continuous or intermittent that is difficult to relieve and causes discomfort, and also possible abdominal discomfort or migraines? | Yes | No |
| 2. Do you have significant fatigue during the day or on awakening? | Yes | No |
| 3. Do your limbs feel like lead and become heavy at times? | Yes | No |
| 4. Do you get bouts of drowsiness or sleepiness? | Yes | No |
| 5. Do you have difficulty standing up for long periods of time? | Yes | No |
| 6. Do you have profuse sweating? | Yes | No |
| 7. Do you get chills or cold extremities? | Yes | No |

| | | |
|---|---|---|
| 8. Do you believe that you have a drop in blood pressure periodically? | Yes | No |
| 9. Do you bruise easy, do you have bleeding from your gums, mouth, nose, or heavy periods? | Yes | No |
| 10. Are you hypersensitive to sound, smells, sudden positional changes, flickering lights, or any cutaneous stimulation? | Yes | No |
| 11. Do you have problems with blurred vision or does the image ever split? Does your vision at times feel as though it gets tired? | Yes | No |
| 12. Do you get shortness of breath on minimal exertion? | Yes | No |
| 13. Do you have memory deficits? | Yes | No |
| 14. Do you get brain fog, orientation difficulties, difficulty concentrating, or have attention-deficit problems? | Yes | No |
| 15. Do you have clumsiness when you walk? Do you fall? | Yes | No |
| 16. Do you get frequent sprains, dislocate, or sublux your joints, such as your ankles, knees, jaw, or any other joints? Please list joints that are affected. | Yes | No |
| 17. Have you suffered numerous miscarriages (if female)? | Yes | No |
| 18. Do you have urological problems such as losing urine or retaining urine? | Yes | No |
| 19. Do you get sleep disturbances? | Yes | No |
| 20. Do you get pneumothoraces? | Yes | No |
| 21. Have you ever had swelling of the legs or lymphedema? | Yes | No |
| 22. Have you ever had a history of arterial aneurysms? | Yes | No |
| 23. Do you have excessive elasticity or stretchability of your skin? | Yes | No |
| 24. Do you have easy bruisability? | Yes | No |
| 25. Do you have scars that formed oftentimes on your skin? | Yes | No |
| 26. Do you have stretch marks before pregnancy or do you get stretch marks easily? | Yes | No |
| 27. Do you have delayed healing? | Yes | No |
| 28. Do you have thin skin? | Yes | No |
| 29. Do you have transparent skin? | Yes | No |
| 30. As a child did you participate or excel in gymnastics, swimming, or cheerleading? | Yes | No |
| 31. Do you get fractures often? If so how many fractures______ | Yes | No |
| 32. Do you or a family member have diverticulitis or diverticulosis? | Yes | No |
| 33. Do you have a cleft lip or cleft palate? | Yes | No |
| 34. Is the white of your eyes discolored either blue gray or off-white? | Yes | No |
| 35. Do you have hernias? | Yes | No |
| 36. Do you have scoliosis? | Yes | No |
| 37. Do you have herniated discs, ruptured disc, or bulging disc? | Yes | No |
| 38. Do you have mitral valve prolapse? | Yes | No |
| 39. Do you have family history of Ehlers-Danlos, Marfan's osteogenesis imperfecta, sickle cell syndrome, and pseudoxanthoma elasticum? | Yes | No |
| 40. Do you develop cigarette paper skin after a cut, stitches, or when you form a scar? | Yes | No |
| 41. Are you double jointed such as touch your thumb on your wrist or put palms on the floor when bending waist without bending knee? | Yes | No |
| 42. Can you put your thumb through your closed fist and have it come out the other side? | Yes | No |
| 43. Can you pull the skin from your elbow more than 2 inches? | Yes | No |
| 44. Is your hair very thick? | Yes | No |
| 45. Is your hair very thin? | Yes | No |
| 46. Are your nails weak and fragile? | Yes | No |
| 47. Are your nails strong and grow back fast? | Yes | No |
| 48. Does your chest cave in or does it appear to cave in or have you had any family members who had to have their chest bone or sternum removed because it was pushing on your heart? | Yes | No |

## Dysautonomia Drugs Taken in the Past or Present

Many autonomic disordered patients have sensitivities to many medications or have been prescribed medications (typically) in relatively, very high dosages and were not responsive. As discussed with patients, the P&S nervous systems are like pendulums; they require gentle nudges (very small dosing) and time to correct. Knowing what the patient has been prescribed in the past helps to further diagnose the patient and develop the therapy plan.

| **Dysautonomia drugs taken in the past or present** Indicate all that apply: | *Currently on* | *Past use* | *Has side effects* |
|---|---|---|---|
| 1. Florinef (fludrocortisone) | □ | □ | □ |
| 2. Midodrine (Proamatine) | □ | □ | □ |
| 3. Beta-blocker (carvedilol, propranolol, atenolol, metoprolol, nadolol) | □ | □ | □ |

| | | | |
|---|---|---|---|
| 4. Pyridostigmine (Mestinon) | □ | □ | □ |
| 5. Clonidine (Catapres) | □ | □ | □ |
| 6. Tenex | □ | □ | □ |
| 7. Aldomet | □ | □ | □ |
| 8. Amphetamine (Adderall) | □ | □ | □ |
| 9. Methylphenidate (Ritalin, Concerta) | □ | □ | □ |
| 10. Northera (droxidopa) | □ | □ | □ |
| 11. Yohimbe | □ | □ | □ |
| 12. Tricyclic (nortriptyline, amitriptyline) | □ | □ | □ |
| 13. SSRI (Zoloft, Celexa, Prozac, Paxil) | □ | □ | □ |
| 14. SNRI (Cymbalta, Wellbutrin, Effexor) | □ | □ | □ |
| 15. Desmopressin (DDAVP) | □ | □ | □ |
| 16. Bethanechol (Urecholine) | □ | □ | □ |
| 17. Levsin | □ | □ | □ |
| 18. Antihistamines (Zantac, Pepcid, Claritin, Benadryl, Zyrtec) | □ | □ | □ |
| 19. Spiriva inhaler (Incruse inhaler) | □ | □ | □ |
| 20. Scopolamine patch | □ | □ | □ |
| 21. Sandostatin (octreotide) | □ | □ | □ |
| 22. Ivabradine (Corlanor) | □ | □ | □ |
| 23. Procrit (erythropoietin) | □ | □ | □ |

## Composite Autonomic Scoring Scale (CASS)

This is a generalized autonomic scoring scale applicable to all autonomic disorders, whether the etiology is genetic, lifestyle, chronic disease, injury, or acute condition. An autonomic reflex screen, consisting of a (1) quantitative sudomotor axon reflex test (QSART), (2) orthostatic blood pressure and heart rate response to positive head-up postural change (PC: tilt or stand), (3) heart rate response to deep breathing, (4) the Valsalva ratio, and (5) beat-to-beat blood pressure measurements during deep breathing, phases II and IV of the Valsalva maneuver, and PC was used to develop a 10-point composite autonomic scoring scale of autonomic function. The scheme allots 4 points for adrenergic dysfunction (Valsalva and PC, including orthostatic dysfunction) and 3 points each for sudomotor and cardio-vagal (deep breathing) dysfunction. Each score is normalized for the compounding effects of age and gender. Patients with a score of 3 or less on the composite autonomic scoring scale have only mild autonomic failure, those with scores of 7–10 have severe failure, and those with scores between these two ranges have moderate autonomic failure. The sensitivity and specificity of the method is high. Thus, autonomic laboratory tests should be useful in grading the degree of autonomic failure.

The main findings are that patients with central (multisystem atrophy) or peripheral neuropathy and symptomatic autonomic failure will be identifiable with CASS with sensitivity and specificity and that patients without clinical autonomic failure, whether neurologic involvement is peripheral (peripheral neuropathy but no autonomic symptoms) or central (Parkinson's disease), will be easily separable from them without overlap. If a score of 7 or more is used as an index of severe autonomic failure, the test has a sensitivity of 94% and a specificity of 100% [30].

## Elements of the Autonomic Reflex Screen

- 1 = Quantitative sudomotor axon reflex test – one upper and three lower limb sites
- 2 = Orthostatic blood pressure and heart rate response to tilt
- 3 = Heart rate response to deep breathing
- 4 = The Valsalva ratio
- 5 = Beat-to-beat blood pressure measurements during the Valsalva maneuver, tilt, and deep breathing

## Laboratory Grading of Autonomic Failure[6]

*Sudomotor Index*

- 1 = Single site abnormal on quantitative sudomotor axon reflex test *or* length-dependent pattern (distal sweat volume < $\frac{1}{3}$ of

[6] BP = blood pressure; HRDB = heart rate response to deep breathing; VR = Valsalva ratio

proximal value) *or* persistent sweat activity at foot [on thermoregulatory sweat test, anhydrosis present but <25%][7]
- 2 = Single site <50% of lower limit on quantitative sudomotor axon reflex test [on thermoregulatory sweat test, anhydrosis 25–50%][5]
- 3 = Two or more sites <50% of lower limit on quantitative sudomotor axon reflex test [on thermoregulatory sweat test, anhydrosis >50%][5]

*Adrenergic Index*[8]
- 1 = Phase $II_e$ decrease of <40 but >20 mmHg mean BP *or*
- phase III does not return to baseline *or*
- decrease in pulse pressure to ≤50% of baseline
- 2 = Phase $II_e$ decrease of <40 but >20 mmHg mean BP + phase $II_l$ or phase IV absent
- 3 = Phase $II_e$ decrease of >40 mmHg + absent phases III and IV
- 4 = Criteria for 3 + orthostatic hypotension (systolic BP decrease of ≥30 mmHg; mean decrease of ≥20 mm Hg)

*Cardiovascular Heart Rate Index*
- 1 = $HR_{DB}$ or VR mildly decreased (above 50% of minimum)
- 2 = $HR_{DB}$ or VR decreased to <50% of minimum
- 3 = Both $HR_{DB}$ and VR decreased to <50% of minimum

## Suggested Laboratory Grading of Autonomic Failure

| Composite autonomic scoring scale | Degree of autonomic failure |
|---|---|
| 1–3 | Mild |
| 4–6 | Moderate |
| 7–10 | Severe |

[7]Could be substituted for results of quantitative sudomotor axon reflex test.

[8]Phases refer to components of the Valsalva maneuver: $II_e$ and $II_l$ = early and late portions, respectively, of phase II.

## Autonomic Neuropathy Scoring

This is a simplified version of CASS originally developed for patients diagnosed with diabetes as an attempt to document earlier onset of cardiovascular autonomic neuropathy (CAN). The indication of diabetic autonomic neuropathy (DAN) provided earlier documentation of the onset of CAN which enabled physicians to be more aggressive with the patient's diabetes to reduce symptoms, delay the onset of debilitating symptoms, and help maintain and prolong QoL. Since its inception, diabetes has become a model of chronic disease. As a result, DAN is equivalent to advanced autonomic dysfunction (AAD), but without issues related to diabetes. This scoring is based on the time-domain ratios (TDRs) computed from Ewing challenges as developed by Vinik et al. The three TDRs, E/I ratio from deep breathing, Valsalva ratio, and 30:15 ratio from PC, are compared with normal, age-matched thresholds.

- If less than two of the three (any one or no) TDRs are low, then no autonomic neuropathy is possible.
  - In these cases, central autonomic dysfunction is being considered.
  - Only one TDR low may be associated with possible peripheral autonomic dysfunction (neuropathy).
- If any two of the three are low, then DAN or AAD (similar to DAN, but without the diabetes issues) is possible.
- If all three are low, then CAN is possible.

AAD or DAN is associated with increased morbidity risk, and CAN is associated with increased mortality risk. Everyone who dies of "natural causes" will die as a result, in part, due to the progression of autonomic neuropathy. With CAN, there is not enough parasympathetic activity to prevent a heart attack or mobilize the immune system to prevent pneumonia, as examples. With both AAD (DAN) and CAN, risks are stratified by sympathovagal balance (SB; the resting S/P ratio). Once CAN is documented, patients should have a full cardiac work-up to establish a baseline and then work to normalize SB. CAN with high SB indicates high risk of major cardiac events (MACE risk). CAN with low SB indicates high risk of "Broken Heart syndrome" and the like. CAN with low-normal SB ($0.4 < SB < 1.0$) indicates minimal risk; at this level, CAN simply means that an older person has a greater chance of dying (naturally) than a younger person.

## Supplements and Nutraceuticals Help to Improve Pharmacology

Major depression and anxiety disorders have high prevalence rates and are frequently comorbid. Depression is one of the most common psychiatric disorders and the fourth leading cause of long-term disability throughout the world. This in part contributes to anxiety, which is the most diagnosed disorder in the world. Despite the availability of different classes of antidepressant and anxiolytic (generally anticholinergic) drugs, most of them are not completely effective and above all are associated with many serious adverse effects. Recently, accumulating evidence suggests that dietary supplements rich in important phytochemicals possess beneficial therapeutic roles in depression. Green tea catechins have been shown to decrease depressive symptoms, possibly in part through the inhibition of monoamine oxidase (MAO). Anthocyanins and their glycols, responsible for the typical color of berries, inhibit MAO. Other studies suggest that cocoa extracts, whose main components are procyanidins, attenuate depressive symptoms. Resveratrol (Fig. 6.13), one of the most important natural stilbenoids, inhibits noradrenaline and serotonin reuptake and significantly decreases anxiety-depressive behaviors while increasing hippocampal serotonin and noradrenaline levels. Trans-resveratrol possesses MAO-A inhibitory effects in different brain areas, particularly in the frontal cortex and hippocampus, as already reported for tea catechins. There is correlative evidence between certain nutrients, such as omega-3 polyunsaturated fatty acids, B vitamins, and resveratrol, and depression-anxiety in human population studies. Growing evidence suggests that consumption of these compounds may represent an alternative strategy to delay the onset and progression of depression and depressive-like symptoms [31].

Over the past decade, there has been growing evidence for the use of N-acetylcysteine (NAC) in treating psychiatric and neurological disorders, considering its role in attenuating pathophysiological processes associated with these disorders, including oxidative stress, apoptosis, mitochondrial dysfunction, neuro-inflammation, and glutamate and dopamine dysregulation. Favorable evidence from a systematic review was found for the use of NAC in several psychiatric and neurological disorders, particularly autism, Alzheimer's disease, cocaine and cannabis addiction, bipolar disorder, depression, trichotillomania, nail-biting, skin picking, obsessive-compulsive disorder, schizophrenia, drug-induced neuropathy, and progressive myoclonic epilepsy [32].

Low folate levels are linked to a poor response to antidepressants, and treatment with folic acid is shown to improve response to antidepressants. It has also been suggested that high vitamin $B_{12}$ status may be associated with better treatment outcome. On the basis of current data, oral doses of both folic acid (800 μg daily) and vitamin $B_{12}$ (1 mg daily) should be tried to improve treatment outcome in depression-anxiety syndromes [33].

Exposure to stressful stimuli has been found to be associated with activation of nitric oxide synthase (NOS) and generation of nitric oxide, which reacts with spontaneous oxygen species to aid formation of active nitrogen radicals. High concentrations of reactive nitrogen radicals may cause damage to intracellular proteins, in addition to causing impairment to components of the mitochondrial transport chain, leading to cellular energy deficiency. This may further serve as an etiological link to the development of secondary neurological diseases associated with chronic stress. Also, during stress exposure, pharmacological inhibition of nitric oxide production displays reduction in indicators of anxiety- and depressive-like behavior [34].

mechanism(s) linking larger lean body mass to AFib are not established. However, a critical mass of tissue is suggested as necessary to maintain AFib [45], and atrial size is a key determinant of sustained AFib [46]. Studies suggest that larger atria may make AFib more stable [47]. Thus, the simplest explanation of the relationship between lean body mass and AFib is that the larger the person, the larger their atria, and the more likely it is that AFib will occur and be sustained [43].

An alternate explanation [48] suggests that obesity is not an independent determinant of AFib. This does not invalidate obesity as an AFib risk factor. It implies that, while obesity is well-established as a significant risk factor for AFib, it may not be independent and due to adiposity per se. Rather, the effect may be mediated by the increase in lean body mass caused by obesity. As body weight increases, so does the skeletal muscle mass needed to carry it and the mass of cardiac tissue needed to perfuse the skeletal muscle and adipose tissue beds. Obesity typically causes left ventricular hypertrophy and dilation as well as left atrial enlargement [48].

Whether one or the other is correct, or some combination of the two, or something more complex, does not diminish the importance of weight loss and associated lifestyle modifications. Furthermore, these two modifications include stress reduction, moderate exercise, and diet modifications, all of which tend to increase nitrate, omega-3 fatty acid, and antioxidant levels. The combined total effect is to naturally reduce AFib risk or enable a reduction in AFib load [48].

## Anxiety

Anxiety is a complex disorder that may not always be only psychological. Anxiety disorders include generalized anxiety disorder (GAD), social anxiety disorder (also known as social phobia), specific phobia, panic disorder with and without agoraphobia,[9] posttraumatic stress disorder (PTSD), anxiety secondary to medical condition, acute stress disorder (ASD), and substance-induced anxiety disorder [49]. Therefore, by definition, persistent psychosocial stress is anxiety. PTSD will be addressed separately below. The DSM-V no longer includes obsessive-compulsive disorders as anxiety. Through (physiological) work in the P&S nervous system, additional forms of "anxiety" have been documented [29, 44]. The only "anxiety" that is officially recognized is (primary) anxiety which qualifies under the DSM-V definition (e.g., generalized anxiety disorder. 300.02 (F41.1) A, and its related forms, as listed above). In general, anxiety is clinically defined as excessive anxiety and worry (apprehensive expectation), occurring more days than not for at least 6 months, about a number of events or activities (such as work or school performance) [49]. However, recognizing that patients call many things "anxiety," P&S monitoring helps to differentiate four pathophysiologic states that present with anxiety-like symptoms.[10] The four additional forms of anxiety are based on P&S dysfunction that often involves poor brain perfusion. They include:

- Sympathetic withdrawal (SW) documented with standing (positive head-up tilt), associated with possible (preclinical) orthostatic dysfunction that may, indirectly, compromise brain perfusion, possibly leading to "adrenaline storms" that may cycle "anxiety."
  - This is therefore, by definition, a vascular or blood volume issue, able to be further differentiated by P&S testing, and may be treated, thereby treating "anxiety."
- Sympathetic excess (SE) upon standing, associated with possible (preclinical) syncope that may, indirectly or directly, compromise brain perfusion, possibly leading to "adrenaline storms" that may cycle "anxiety."
  - This is therefore, by definition, a syncope issue, able to be further differentiated by P&S testing, and may be treated, thereby treating "anxiety."
- Arrhythmia, causing inefficient blood pumping that may compromise brain perfusion,

[9] Extreme or irrational fear of crowded spaces or enclosed public places.

[10] Patients with anxiety-like symptoms have conditions that include the same symptoms as anxiety, but they are either not fully relieved by anxiety therapy or have documented additional dysfunction (i.e., P&S dysfunction that causes poor brain perfusion) that may lead to similar or the same symptoms.

possibly leading to "adrenaline storms" that may cycle "anxiety."
  - P&S testing elucidates the involvement of the P&S systems, helping to provide more information when developing treatment plans to relieve arrhythmia, including autonomically induced arrhythmia, and thereby treat "anxiety."
- Parasympathetic excess (PE), regardless of when it is demonstrated by P&S testing (at rest or in response to challenge), may indirectly or directly compromise brain perfusion, possibly leading to "adrenaline storms" that may cycle "anxiety."
  - This is an autonomic issue, further differentiated by P&S testing, and may be treated, thereby treating "anxiety."

The hallmark of the P&S forms of anxiety is poor brain perfusion. Poor brain perfusion causes the brain or portions of the brain to function slower or "go to sleep." This makes them all primary depression-based syndromes. Again, poor brain perfusion reduces brain function, resulting in (typically) pre-clinical depression, and any further drop in BP (e.g., due to emotions, large meals, bed-time, meditation, medications, etc.) may trigger an "adrenaline storm" that cycles the anxiety, until proper (or nominal) brain perfusion is restored. Any or all of these, together with primary anxiety itself, may all be comorbid. In general, all may be treated simultaneously as well, history dependent.

Anxiety is a natural response and a necessary warning adaptation in humans. Anxiety can become a pathologic disorder when it is excessive and uncontrollable, requires no specific external stimulus, and manifests with a wide range of physical and affective symptoms as well as changes in behavior and cognition. Patients often present with complaints of poor physical health as their primary concern. If only symptoms are considered, this can be misleading. Poor health is particularly common in panic attacks, which are characterized by a short period of intense fear and a sense of impending doom, with accompanying physical symptoms, such as chest pain, dizziness, and shortness of breath. Very often, these patients first present to an emergency department. When panic disorder is complicated by agoraphobia, the person fears having a panic attack in a place from which escape is perceived to be difficult. The patient then avoids such situations, with subsequent disturbances in functioning. When the emergency department tries to send them home after negative tests for heart attack or stroke, the patients do not believe it and refuse. Often, patients are then sent for psychiatric evaluation because physicians, without P&S Monitoring, find nothing physiological. This is how patients come to feel disenfranchised and begin the merry-go-round of multiple doctors and therapies, including psychiatry, psychology, and physiology; all to no avail without P&S Monitoring.

Anxiety is one of the most prevalent of all psychiatric disorders in the general population. Simple phobia is the most common anxiety disorder, with up to 49% of people reporting an unreasonably strong fear and 25% of those people meeting criteria for simple phobia. Social anxiety disorder is the next most common disorder of anxiety, with roughly 13% of people reporting symptoms that meet the DSM criteria. PTSD, which is often unrecognized, afflicts approximately 7.8% of the overall population and 12% of women, in whom it is significantly more common. In victims of war trauma, PTSD prevalence reaches 20% [50]. A subjective experience of distress with accompanying disturbances of sleep, concentration, and social or occupational functioning are common symptoms in many of the anxiety disorders. Despite their similarities, these disorders often differ in presentation, course, and treatment. Diagnosis is often complicated by other psychiatric disorders. Many of anxiety disorders have overlapping signs and symptoms, requiring the clinician to explore several lines of questioning to clarify the primary diagnosis. Anxiety disorders that are more commonly recognized have lower lifetime prevalence rates. GAD and panic disorder, for example, have lifetime prevalence rates of roughly 5% and 3.5%, respectively. Of the panic sufferers, up to 40% also meet criteria for agoraphobia.

Clinically important risk factors include comorbid substance abuse and family history (including possible genetic predisposition[11]). One 20-year study of the offspring of depressed

[11]There is also a possible genetic predisposition to autonomic dysfunction, including PE, which may underlie anxiety.

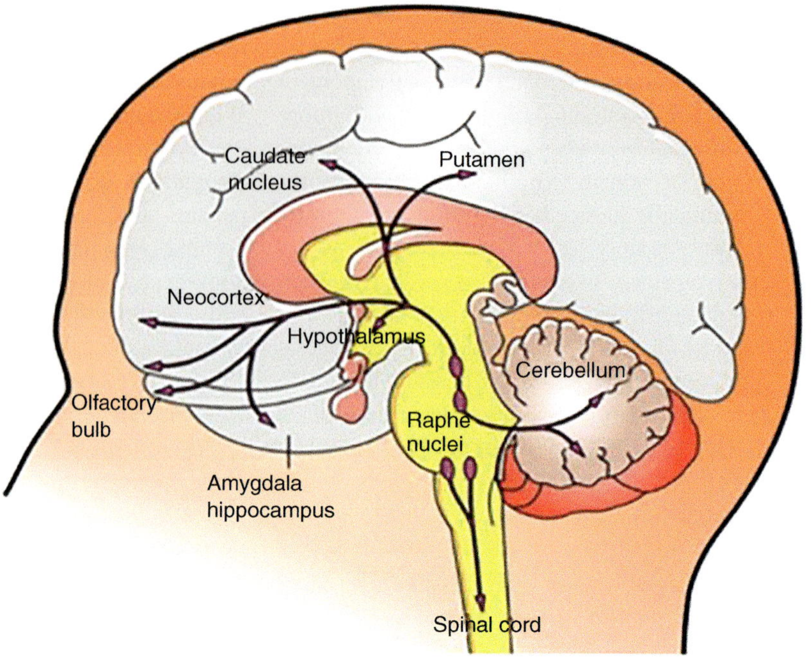


**Fig. 9.4** Principal serotonergic projections from the reticular formation [52, Fig. 4.8]. (Republished with permission from Springer International Publishing AG)

parents found a threefold increase in anxiety disorders, including greater substance abuse, younger onset, and more significant physical health concerns [51]. Otherwise, definitive pathophysiologic mechanisms have not yet been determined for primary anxiety. However, anxiety symptoms and the resulting disorders are believed to be due to disrupted modulation within the central nervous system, including hormonal and neurotransmitter imbalances; trauma, stroke, and other brain injuries (including concussion); and poor brain perfusion. Environmental stressors clearly play a role to varying degrees. All primary anxiety disorders are affected in some way by external cues. Abnormal processing of and responses to these cues often underlie primary anxiety. Physical and emotional manifestations of this dysregulation are the result of heightened sympathetic arousal of varying degrees, including sympathetic excess secondary to parasympathetic excess. The anxiety, worry, or physical symptoms cause clinically significant distress or impairment in social or occupational functioning. Several neurotransmitter systems have been implicated in one or several of the modulatory steps involved.

In primary anxiety, the most commonly considered neurotransmitter systems are the serotoninergic (Fig. 9.4) and noradrenergic (Fig. 9.5) systems. In very general terms, it is believed that an under-activation of the serotoninergic system and an over-activation of the noradrenergic system are involved. These systems regulate and are regulated by other pathways and neuronal circuits in various regions of the brain, including the locus coeruleus and limbic structures, resulting in dysregulation of physiologic arousal and the emotional experience of this arousal.

In some forms of primary anxiety, a disruption of the gamma-aminobutyric acid (GABA) system has also been implicated because of the response of many of the anxiety-spectrum disorders to treatment with benzodiazepines. There has also been some interest in the role of corticosteroid regulation and its relation to symptoms of fear and anxiety. Corticosteroids might increase or decrease the activity of certain neural pathways, affecting not only behavior under stress but also the brain's processing of fear-inducing stimuli.

An important part of any intervention with a patient with an anxiety disorder is education. The practice guidelines for panic disorder recommend

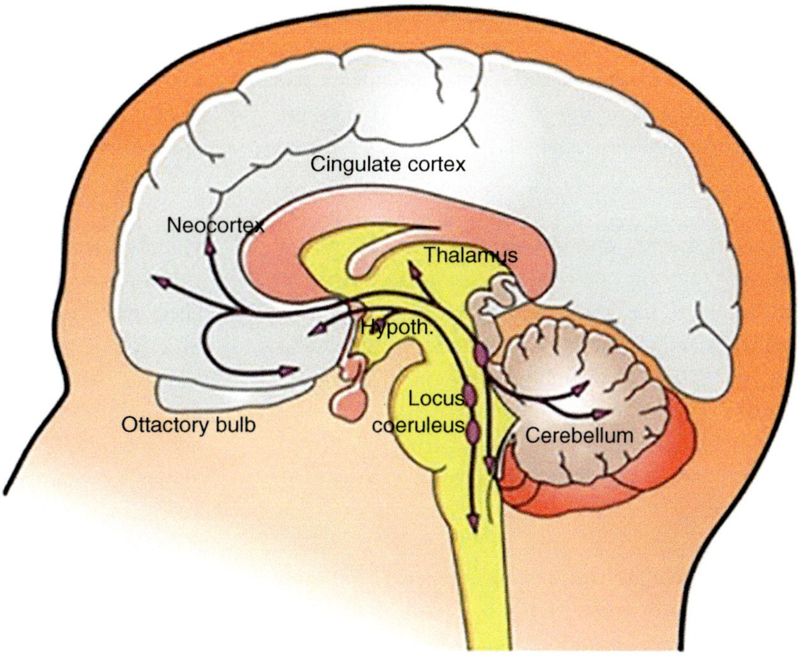


**Fig. 9.5** Principal noradrenergic projections from the reticular formation [52, Fig. 4.6]. (Republished with permission from Springer International Publishing AG)

education of the family as well. Many people are confused by the symptoms and behavior and are reassured to know they are not alone and that there are effective interventions. The patient should receive an appropriate medical work-up, such as a physical examination, and studies (e.g., electrocardiogram, thyroid-stimulating hormone) when indicated. After ruling out a medical condition, developing a working alliance with the patient provides a basis for ongoing management and prevents further inappropriate use of the medical system.

Selective serotonin reuptake inhibitors (SSRIs, an antidepressant and, in low doses, an indirect anticholinergic) and cognitive behavioral therapy (CBT) are considered first-line defense for primary anxiety. SSRIs have been shown to be the best-tolerated medications, and response rates are significantly higher than placebo for panic disorder, OCD, PTSD, social anxiety disorder, and GAD. SSRIs are preferred by cardiologists due to their minimal effect on blood pressure. SSRIs and CBT also have the least potential for addiction, which is especially helpful given the prevalence of addictive behaviors noted in anxiety patients. However, SSRIs have a minimal effect on the P&S nervous system, as measured by P&S monitoring. In cases of anxiety with P&S dysfunction or anxiety-like symptoms, SSRIs are often discontinued and patients titrated on very low-dose tricyclic or SNRI to relieve the P&S dysfunction and treat the anxiety-like symptoms. In all of the anxiety disorders, SSRIs should be started at low doses and gradually titrated up to therapeutic levels to avoid an initial exacerbation of anxiety.

The choice of medications is well defined both by the tests listed above and P&S monitoring. Often however, these medications do not completely relieve the symptoms, and the psychology therapies (e.g., CBD) are long term and drawn out and serve to create dependence between patient and therapist. As with the "Statin Gap" and other shortcomings of typical therapy plans for other diseases, the Mind-Body Wellness Program helps to fill the "gaps." Unlike the commercial that says to take another medication if the primary depression medication is not working, stop simply treating symptoms and re-establish a firm foundation and then rebuild or remodel the house. In other words, establish health and wellness in the nervous and cardiovascular systems (the brain and heart connected by the P&S nervous systems and the vascular system). If the nervous system (including the brain) and the heart are not receiving the proper amount of energy, and if they are constantly fighting against the effects of stress and disease by not having enough antioxidants to deal with free radicals and reactive oxygen and nitrogen species, and if nitric oxide levels are low causing (among other things) poor blood flow to all areas of the body and not delivering these nutrients and removing waste products, then anxiety is a result. No wonder it is the most diagnosed disease or disorder *in the world!*

All six prongs of the Mind-Body Wellness Program work together to help relieve anxiety in any form.

1. Antioxidants, vitamins, amino acids, and minerals are shown to improve, in part, depression and depression-related disorders (including anxiety, psychosocial stress, and obsessive-compulsive disorders) [53]. Antioxidants known to help relieve anxiety include alpha-lipoic acid [54], N-acetylcysteine (NAC, see Fig. 5.66 and the "Homocysteine" section of Chap. 5) [32, 55], resveratrol [31], folate[12] (vitamin $B_9$) [56], and L-arginine [57]. Antioxidants, with these other supplements, and of course directly reducing oxidative stress [58], all help relieve oxidative stress which can be caused by anxiety, thereby helping to reduce the effects of anxiety and thereby helping to maintain health and wellness.
2. Omega-3 fatty acids including eicosapentaenoic acid (EPA) and docosahexaenoic acid (DHA) [31, 35–38] help relieve anxiety by helping to repair what chronic psychosocial and oxidative stress damages through free radical and reactive oxygen and nitrogen species. Fish oil supplementation is safe and well tolerated and, in part, has adjunctive therapeutic benefits in anxiety and anxiety-like syndromes without notable side effects and with enduring benefit, including in children.
3. That unique neuromodulator, nitric oxide, influences and modulates several other conventional messengers which play an important role in anxiety, thereby helping to reduce anxiety [32, 59].
4. Exercise is arguably the single most powerful antioxidant. Given that Parasympathetic Excess (PE, see "Dynamic Parasympathetic Excess" section of Chap. 8) is common in anxiety patients, "low and slow" exercise programs are recommended until P&S balance is restored. Then any remaining anxiety may be more directly and reliably treated. "Low and slow" exercise: Moderate to strenuous exercise has become a stress for the patient with PE and will only exacerbate PE. As an alternative to pharmaceutical therapy for PE, consider a lifestyle change to include mild, intensive cardiovascular exercise. For the first six weeks, only zero impact, pure cardiac workouts (e.g., long easy walks at about 2 miles per hour, or very easy bike rides, or walking in a pool with the water level above the belly-button) to avoid any tissue breakdown or stress that will stimulate Parasympathetic activity, and to avoid (at first) any significant increases in HR or BP that may be interpreted by the nervous system as a stress and exacerbate PE. Although very easy elliptical machine workouts, or swimming, etc., are also zero impact these modalities tend to elevate HR & BP too fast, causing additional stress in these patients. The goal is to only stimulate, gently, sympathetic activity and retrain the autonomic nervous system to react normally to stresses. This exercise must be for 40 contiguous minutes per day (you may need to work up to this) for 6 days per week. Remember, a habit has been formed which must now be broken and a new habit formed to replace it. Target HR or BP is not the goal. For example, after 40 minutes of walking the patient should be able to carry on a normal conversation without being winded. They will still have increased HR and BP and sweated, but perhaps not within the first 15 to 20 minutes. Skipping a week, starts the 6 weeks over again. Then for the remainder of the first six months, the exercise may be decreased to 4 days per week, maintaining a contiguous 40 minutes per event. After the six months and a normalization of Parasympathetic activity, activities that might damage tissue may be

[12] Folate deficiency is associated with problems in cognition, mood, psychosis, and anxiety.

returned (e.g., more strenuous exercise, including weight lifting and contact sports). In this way the parasympathetics are (re-) trained to not over-react to stressful stimuli, making for a more normal autonomic response.

5. The Mediterranean diet provides the nutrients, including antioxidants, vitamins, minerals, amino acids, omega-3 fatty acids, nitric oxide, and their building blocks, and the energy need to power all of these activities.
6. Lastly, but by no means less important, by reducing psychosocial stress itself, you relieve the many effects of anxiety and perhaps anxiety itself.

## Anxiety and Depression

According to a recent *Journal of the American Medical Association* study, more than one-third of American adults may be using prescription medications that can potentially cause depression or increase the risk of suicide [60]. These prescription medications include hormonal birth control pills, heart and blood pressure medications, proton pump inhibitors, antacids, and painkillers. There are over 200 commonly used prescription drugs that have depression or suicide listed as a potential side effect. Researchers from the University of Illinois at Chicago studied more than 26,000 people from 2005 to 2014 who used these medications. Because of the wide use of these medications, doctors and healthcare providers may not be aware of any increased risk of depression or suicide, even though they are known side effects. Note, P&S monitoring referenced throughout this book is able to differentiate those who are at risk from those who are not. Approximately 15% of adults who used three or more of these medications at the same time may be at risk for depression. For those using one of these medications, 7% are at risk, and for those taking two of these drugs simultaneously, 9% are at risk for depression.

The study highlights the fact that polypharmacy[13] can lead to depressive symptoms and that patients and healthcare providers need to be aware of the risk of depression that comes with all kinds of common prescription drugs. Further, many of these drugs, albeit in reduced dosages, are also available over the counter. Due to their nature of suppressing systems of the body, they may limit blood flow to the brain or limit brain function itself, thereby inducing depression. Examples include (1) medications to suppress blood pressure or heart rate to treat hypertension or arrhythmia, (2) diuretics which reduce blood volume and reduce blood flow to the brain, (3) anxiolytics or medications to treat ADD or ADHD which reduce or limit brain function, or (4) pain medications to limit pain. Underlying the clinical effects of these medications is the fact that these medications suppress or limit sympathetic activity. While a little limitation may be beneficial to prevent the diseases for which these medications are prescribed, too much sympathetic suppression leads to parasympathetic excess which is a hallmark of depression. Further, sympathetic insufficiency is associated with light-headedness, exercise intolerance, sex dysfunction, "brain fog," cognitive dysfunction, poor circulation, and more. As a result, many may be surprised to learn that these medications may increase their risk of depression, even though they may have nothing to do with mood, depression, or anxiety.

For example, consider over-the-counter antihistamines. It is well known that temporary or transient histaminergic-induced inflammation aids in healing. It is well known that inflammation is mediated by the sympathetic nervous system, and it is well known that too much inflammation and too much sympathetic activity are detrimental. In the brain, histaminergic projections arise from the tuberomammillary nucleus (TMN) in the hypothalamus (see Fig. 9.6). The histaminergic system in the brain is a phylogenetically old group of neurons that project to most of the central nervous system. It holds a key position in the regulation of basic body functions, including the sleep-wake cycle, energy and endocrine homeostasis, synaptic plasticity and learning, consciousness, thermoregulation, metabolism, and other life-sustaining functions [61]. Histaminergic neurons from the TMN are pacemakers that fire at slow regular rates. Their rates vary based on

[13] Polypharmacy is defined as more than one drug prescribed at the same.

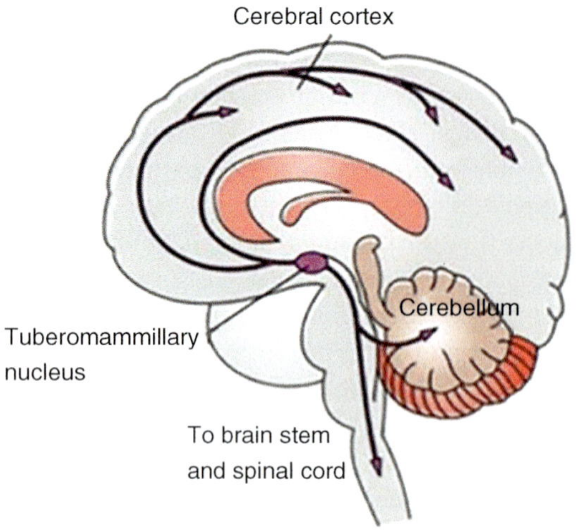


**Fig. 9.6** Histaminergic projections originating in the tuberomammillary nucleus (TMN) of the hypothalamus [52, Fig. 4.10a]. (Republished with permission from Springer International Publishing AG)

metabolic state. Their activity is high during waking and attentive states and low or absent during sleep. These neurons have been shown to protect against convulsions. Malfunctions in this system are associated with neurological diseases, including Alzheimer's and Parkinson's, as well as headaches and migraines, difficulty falling asleep, easy arousal, hypertension, vertigo or dizziness, arrhythmia, accelerated heart rate, difficulty regulating body temperature, anxiety, nausea, vomiting, abdominal cramps, flushing, nasal congestion, sneezing, difficulty breathing, abnormal menstrual cycle, hives, fatigue, and tissue swelling. Blocking histaminergic activity in the brain may cause low or absent pacemaker activity. Antihistamines are known to have a sedative side effect by, among other things, reducing the energy and wakefulness functions of the histaminergic system. Prolonged antihistamine therapy, by reducing histamine neuron activity, therefore can lead to the depression-like symptoms of low energy, cognitive difficulty, disrupted endocrine and hormonal function, reduced metabolic states, and excessive desire for sleep.

With the national suicide rate increasing, depression has become a public health issue. As a result, the use of these medications should be reconsidered to reduce or minimize the risk of depression. To this end, "Psychopharmacology and Cardiovascular Disease" is arguably the most important *Journal of the American College of Cardiology* review ever published in this area [62]. The review's epidemiology shows there are many physiologic and lifestyle risk factors for the development of atherosclerosis. These include high lipid levels, hypertension, diabetes, abdominal obesity, physical inactivity, low daily fruit and vegetable consumption, alcohol over consumption, and psychological factors [63]. There are several psychological factors as well, such as depression, anxiety, hostility, and type A personality. These psychological factors have not only been shown to be risk factors for cardiovascular disease but have also been shown to affect clinical outcomes. It is believed that hypercortisolism can cause a lower than expected response to corticotropin-releasing factor administration [64, 65]. Platelet function is also abnormal with high reactivity and release of factor 4 and beta-thyroglobulin [66]. Both of these factors are atherogenic. Furthermore, patients with these psychological problems have abnormal heart rate variability, which can lead to arrhythmias [67].

Acute stress has been well studied. Acute stress activates the sympathetic nervous system, resulting in arrhythmias, endothelial dysfunction, inflammation, and platelet activation [68]. Also, acute stress may affect coronary blood flow, which is mediated by the neuronal nitric oxide synthase (nNOS) pathway [69]. Inflammation is implicated in coronary plaques and patients who are depressed with multiple cytokines such as C-reactive protein, tumor necrosis factor, and interleukin-6, among others [70]. Excessive sympathetic activation amplifies and exaggerates the acute stress responses. Sympathetic excess (SE) is an autonomic dysfunction (imbalance) and may be a primary dysfunction (e.g., high sympathovagal balance) or a secondary dysfunction, secondary to an abnormal parasympathetic excess (PE) in response to the stress itself [29].

Subjects with depression have an 80% increase in risk for development of new worsening cardiovascular disease and death from cardiovascular disease [71]. Depression increases the risk of developing cardiovascular disease, and cardiovascular disease can increase the risk of developing depression. Depression is associated with PE, which may lead to secondary SE, thereby accelerating the stress effects (i.e., endothelial dysfunction, inflammation, and platelet activation) leading to the risk increase. PE may also suppress the immune system effecting cell senescence and apoptosis. Meta-analyses have shown from perspective studies that depression significantly increases the risk of cardiovascular disease. Furthermore, treatment of depression has been shown to be effective in some studies. It has also been shown that reductions in depression are associated with modestly reduced coronary heart disease (CHD) risks, but only among patients with mild depression at baseline [72]. A 10-year-follow-up study shows that anxiety was found to be associated with a 77% increased mortality risk and nearly threefold increased risk for CHD. However, in this study, depression was not shown to be associated with these risks [73].

Exercise training (the HF-ACTION study [74]) of patients with heart failure with reduced ejection fraction to exercise training demonstrated a moderate decline in depression symptoms at 3 months. The decline was measured as an improvement in the Beck Depression Inventory (BDI) scoring system. The relationship between anxiety disorders and increasing symptoms of anxiety and CHD events has been evaluated in several studies. In a study of over 49,000 Swedish men, the presence of anxiety was associated with more than twice the risk of CHD and acute MI [75]. Meta-analyses of 20 studies of more than 11-year duration demonstrate that anxiety is correlated with an increased risk for CHD and sudden cardiac death [5198]. In addition, it has been shown that patients with generalized anxiety disorder and depression were at greater risk of CHD than patients with either condition alone [76, 77]. Associations between anger, hostility, and CHD have been studied. Meta-analysis has shown that higher levels of anger and hostility are associated with poor clinical outcomes in both healthy and cardiac patients [78]. For example, anger is associated with increase incidences of implantable cardiac defibrillator discharge among cardiac patients [79].

In landmark studies, acute mental stress has shown adverse cardiac events. Acute mental stress from intense activities such as (1) intense sporting events, (2) catastrophe such as earthquakes and blizzards, and (3) acute physical activity may increase risk for arrhythmias, myocardial infarction, and sudden cardiac death [79–81].

Chronic factors such as work-related stress and marital dissatisfaction increases the risk for CHD through elevated blood pressure and abnormalities of the coagulation system [79, 82–85]. Similarly, family stress and psychosocial stresses in general increase risk of adverse cardiac events.

Chronic work stress (low decision latitude and heavy job demands) has been studied extensively. From the field of neuroimmunology, it is well known that subordinates are more likely to be ill than are superiors [86]. In meta-analysis, the men show that high psychological demands, lack of social support, and strain were associated with increased risk for ischemic heart disease, whereas effort, reward and balance, job sensitivity, and long working hours were not related [84]. The landmark article INTERHEART from 52 countries showed that patients who had their first MI had greater work stress, stress at home, general stress, and impairment stress in comparison with age-matched controls [87]. Stress has been associated with a threefold increase in risk for recurrence of CHD during a 5-year follow-up, adjusting for background- and health-related factors [88].

All in all, chronic stress is an extreme risk factor for coronary heart disease events. In addition to the various psychological stresses, strenuous physical activity and stressful mental activities were predictive of myocardial ischemia [89]. Another study showed that the level of risk of ischemia increased twofold among cardiac patients during appearance when they reported feeling tension, sadness, or frustration [90]. The presence of mental stress-induced ischemia is predictive of clinical events in patients with CHD. This is a threefold increase risk for recurrent cardiac events among patients with CAD and that the change in ejection fraction during mental stress was an important predictor of event-free survival [91]. Type A personality demonstrates controversial results [92]. A meta-analysis that included trials that performed psychological or behavioral interventions demonstrated that psychotherapy was associated with a 28% reduction in mortality in comparison with controls from a 2-year follow-up. Cardiac patients had significant benefit [76].

ENRICHD (Enhancing Recovery in Coronary Heart Disease Patients) studied post-MI patients who were depressed or had low levels of social support. Cognitive behavioral therapy was initiated within several weeks following an MI. The trial demonstrated greater improvement in psychological outcome such as reduced depression and increased social support, but this was not associated with reduction in event-free survival [79, 93]. SSRIs were also prescribed in this study. Other studies have shown that stress management and aerobic exercise in patients with cardiovascular disease and evidence of stress-induced myocardial ischemia demonstrate reductions in myocardial ischemia during mental stress and decreasing cardiac events [78, 94]. They had improvements in quality of life, lower reductions in ejection fraction during mental stress, fewer wall motion abnormalities, and improvement in flow-mediated dilation [78].

Antidepressants such as tricyclics, serotonin, norepinephrine, serotonin antagonists and reuptake inhibitors, and noradrenergic and specific serotonergic antidepressants may be less desirable in patients with coronary artery disease (CAD) with depression because of the potential for QT interval prolongation. In the case of tricyclic antidepressants, an increase in serotonin-norepinephrine with serotonin-norepinephrine reuptake inhibitors (SNRIs) may lead to worsening hypertension. However, all of these issues are at clinical doses which are often required in the absence of P&S assessment. Frequently, these agents are required at significantly less doses (as little as a one-fourth to one-tenth the standard clinical dose) once properly paired with any underlying P&S dysfunction. While selective serotonin reuptake inhibitors (SSRIs) have the least effect on BP and have an antiplatelet effect that may be beneficial in coronary artery disease, they have the least effect on any PE that may underlie the depression. SSRIs (i.e., citalopram, fluoxetine, fluvoxamine, paroxetine, sertraline (Zoloft), and venlafaxine) prescribed with antiplatelet agents may inhibit platelets, but failed to link bleeding to these agents. Benzodiazepines are the most commonly used antianxiety agents. Since coronary patients receive statins and since benzodiazepines and statins are both metabolized through the P450 CYP3A4 enzyme system, an interaction between the two is possible. Further studies into this enzyme pathway are needed.

SSRIs include escitalopram, sertraline, citalopram, fluoxetine, fluvoxamine, and paroxetine and are important in treating depression. The American Heart Association has shown that depression is now an independent risk factor for poor outcomes in acute coronary syndrome. SSRIs have been the preferred therapy for depression in patients with cardiovascular disease because of their overall safety profile and effectiveness. They will mildly prolong the corrected QT interval at reasonable therapeutic levels, but the risk increases at ranges higher than the recommended doses. Sertraline, in the SADHART study, is a study of patients with post-MI and unstable angina [95]. It did not alter ejection fraction or ventricular ectopic beats. It did not significantly increase QT interval or other cardiovascular outcomes. It was effective on depressive symptoms.

In the ENRICHD trial, which included behavioral therapy with an SSRI started 50 weeks after behavioral therapy, patients on sertraline or Zoloft had a significant reduction in death or a nonfatal MI compared with no drug therapy. This benefit was seen only with SSRIs (at clinical doses) and not with other antidepressant categories (at clinical doses). A meta-analysis in 2011 showed reduction in readmissions with SSRIs [96]. The older SSRIs have little effect on the QTc interval as compared with citalopram [97]. Higher doses of citalopram (over 40 mg) increase the QTc sometimes significantly. SSRIs have some important effects on heart rate variability, and they have moderate vagolytic effects, especially with paroxetine. Also, sertraline may have anti-inflammatory effects with reduction levels of C-reactive protein and interleukin-6 [98].

The SNRI class includes venlafaxine, duloxetine, desvenlafaxine, and levomilnacipran. They inhibit the reuptake of both neurotransmitters, serotonin and norepinephrine, from the synaptic cleft. With higher levels of both neurotransmitters, cardiac sympathetic activities are elevated. This may lead to tachycardia, hypertension, and arrhythmias. At clinical doses, SNRIs have more side effects than SSRIs, including hypertension, especially at high doses; therefore, people on antidepressant therapy should be monitored closely. However, a comparison study of venlafaxine with sertraline showed no difference in risk adverse cardiac outcomes and actually lower heart failure risk with venlafaxine [99].

Tricyclic antidepressants are among the oldest agents for depression therapy and include amitriptyline, desipramine, doxepin, imipramine, clomipramine, and nortriptyline [100]. At clinical doses, they cause a significant QRS interval prolongation, and corrected QTc interval is increased. These have anticholinergic effects and at clinical doses include the possibility of associated arrhythmias, including ventricular tachycardia and atrial fibrillation [101, 102]. Therefore, patients with cardiac disease and ventricular arrhythmias should be carefully treated with these agents or not treated at all. In non-depressed patients, both nortriptyline and imipramine failed to alter ventricular function. However, although there is no evidence of worsening ventricular arrhythmia, the risk of ventricular arrhythmia makes the use of tricyclics at times less desirable [103].

Atypical agents such as dopamine or epinephrine and serotonin reuptake inhibitors such as bupropion, trazodone, nefazodone, vortioxetine, vilazodone, buspirone, and mirtazapine had been studied. The FDA has approved buspirone for smoking cessation, although the mechanism is not well understood [104, 105]. Trazodone is second generation of selective serotonin receptor antagonist and reuptake inhibitor, and it is the best studied. It is used as a hypnotic agent and has been preferred because of better cardiovascular profile and less anticholinergic effects in animal studies. It causes less myocardial depression than imipramine without alterations in chronotropy or inotropy and with an increase in coronary flow. However, there are some patients with increased QTc interval with overdose that could lead to lethal arrhythmia [106]. One must be careful with this drug on amiodarone [107, 108].

Benzodiazepines include alprazolam, clonazepam, diazepam, lorazepam, triazolam, oxazepam, and midazolam which are used for anxiety. Increase in heart rate has been observed with triazolam [109]. There is a 30% excess risk for ischemic disease associated with benzodiazepines, and users of benzodiazepines were twice as likely to have events compared with nonusers [110]. This was in a community study of 7000 subjects. This study was confounded by risk factors and small number events. On meta-analysis of eight single studies reported overall, the use of hypnotic agents was associated with lower CVD risk mortality. However, the type of hypnotic agent did not make a difference; rather it did affect the difference with zolpidem and had a decrease risk for heart disease [111]. Long-acting agents such as clonazepam, lorazepam, and alprazolam are preferred anxiolytics within this class, but should be prescribed with caution, as prolonged use may require dose escalation due to resistance or difficulty achieving a similar therapeutic effect.

Beta-blockers are useful for situational episodes taken 1 hour before activities that cause anxiety-like symptoms [112]. An advantage of beta-blockers is that they generally decrease the QT interval. Questionnaires failed to show that beta-blockers increase depression or anxiety symptoms [113]. Given that many of these drugs are co-prescribed, drug-drug interactions are very important to consider and follow closely.

## Neurofeedback

The electroencephalogram (EEG) is a recording of the electrical activity of the brain. A study of the EEG demonstrates certain waveforms at certain frequencies that have been associated with certain (normal) and essential daily activities, such as sleep, relaxed attention, and hyperattention. The different types of brain waves that have been identified and correlated are [114]:

- *Alpha* – waveforms associated generally with a state of relaxation (8–12 Hz)
- *Beta* – the fastest of the waveforms correlated, which represent a state of mental, intellectual activity and outward focused attention (12–35 Hz)
  - The lower end of this frequency band (e.g., sensorimotor rhythm or SMR) corresponds to a state of relaxed attentiveness (12–15 Hz).
  - The hyper-state of high-frequency beta brain waves is as high as 35 Hz.
- *Delta* – the slowest of the waveforms correlated, which are associated with deep restorative sleep (0.5–3.5 Hz).
- *Theta* – waveforms represent a deeply relaxed, daydreaming state (4–8 Hz)

It should be noted that each of these brain wave frequencies is always present to some degree in different parts of the brain. For example, if someone is experiencing acute anxiety, an excess of high-frequency beta brain waves may be present in a certain brain region, or it may be a result of an excessive amount of alpha brain waves in the frontal regions of the brain that are associated with the control of emotions.

Neurofeedback, a type of biofeedback, is an operant conditioning technique used to reinforce or inhibit specific forms of EEG activity [115, 116]. It is a therapeutic method designed to train the mind and body to act in a more optimal way in order to improve emotional, cognitive, physical, and behavioral experiences [117]. By challenging the brain, much as the body is challenged in physical exercise, the brain may be helped to learn to function better. Based on the research in neuropathology, this method has shown evidence of turning abnormal rhythms and frequencies (based on Quantitative-EEG[14]) into normal (or relatively normal) rhythms and frequencies, thereby turning abnormal psychological states into normal ones [118].

Neurofeedback, for example, has been used to treat ADHD [119–122], epilepsy [123], depression [124], anxiety and affective disorders [125, 126], fibromyalgia [127], and obsessive-compulsive disorder [128] and also to enhance attention and memory performance in healthy subjects [129–132]. This technique also has been used as a therapeutic method for substance- or alcohol-dependent patients, and results have corroborated the efficiency of neurofeedback treatment on negative neuropsychological consequences of these disorders [126, 133, 134–138]. Heterogeneity in the EEG brain wave patterns is often the case and is associated with different conditions, such as anxiety and ADD/ADHD [139]. The diagnostic considerations become even more complex when comorbid problems are present. It is critical, therefore, that accurate assessment is made prior to neurofeedback treatment in order to determine excesses and deficiencies of given brain wave frequencies and where these abnormalities may occur in the brain, taking into consideration comorbidities to ensure individualized patient treatment [140].

Alpha neurofeedback training (30 50-minute SMR training sessions in the central brain cortex area over 2 months) has been demonstrated to reduce anxiety, improving aspects of personality, and decrease stress-related and blood-based beta-endorphins. Alpha-theta training (30 20-minute SMR training sessions in the parietal brain cortex area over 2 months) showed improvement in mood, personality inventory scales, ability to focus, and ability to processes information. Preliminary research suggests that neurofeedback could be effective in helping adolescents. Despite all these promising results, neurofeedback treatment has not yet been well accepted [141].

In alpha training (visual, relaxed attention), the reinforcement band was 12–15 Hz (SMR) frequency band, and the suppressed frequencies were delta (2–5 Hz), theta (5–8 Hz), and high beta (18–30 Hz). Thresholds were adjusted in a way that if the participant maintained the reinforcement band above the threshold for 80% of the time during at least 0.5 seconds, and the suppressed band under the threshold for 20% of the time, feedback was received. Whenever participants could maintain the reinforcement band's above the threshold for 90% of the time during two continuous trials, the threshold was changed automatically so that it was closer to the optimal threshold.

In the alpha-theta training (audio, eyes closed, relaxed attention), the reinforcement band was 5–8 Hz (theta) and 8–12 Hz (alpha). The initial sessions were used to train patients to decrease alpha levels that were above 12 mV (peak to peak) while augmenting theta, until the alpha amplitude dropped below that of theta. Next, both alpha and theta frequencies were augmented, and the delta (2–5 Hz) range was inhibited. This seems to discourage the sleep transition during low-arousal states.

Research indicates that after 15 sessions of neurofeedback, patients experienced long-term benefits (positive changes) in personality variables. Although there is no general consensus as to the exact mechanism of alpha-theta neurofeed-

[14]As a comprehensive assessment tool endorsed by both the American Psychological Association and the International Society for Neurofeedback and Research, QEEG is used by qualified healthcare professionals to objectively and scientifically evaluate a patient's brain wave function to determine whether brain wave patterns are abnormal and, if so, where and why these abnormalities occur.

back, it is believed to increase beta-endorphin levels related to the stress [142–145]. Neurofeedback can help to:

- Improve sleep patterns. More efficient sleep is associated with being more alert during the day, reduced anxiety and depression, and reduced migraine or chronic pain.
- Improve focus and enable more attention, as measured by how well one persists even at an unwanted task.
- Improve the management of emotions. Emotions, like perceptions, are real to the individual, but the brain has a lot to say about how the individual will respond to emotions and how the individual will feel and react. Out-of-control emotions are not good, but one can be trained. No emotions (i.e., a lack of empathy) are not good, but one can be trained.
- Reduce some forms of seizures by reorganizing the brain to bypass the circuits that generate seizure.
- Normalize traumatic brain injury, including concussion and stroke, by reorganizing the brain to bypass injured circuits.
- Train (retrain) the brain in autism to function better and possibly engage the circuits that are being bypassed.

Before the training begins, specific objectives are established by the patient or in cooperation with the patient's loved ones. In order to reach a specific objective, the training usually continues for a specific number of sessions. If there is a loss of optimal training effect after completion, due to stresses in life, a few booster sessions may be recommended. However, just as concert pianists practice more than the rest, rather than less, neurofeedback training can be used without limit to enhance performance. This "peak performance training" may be of interest to many, including professional athletes, corporate executives, and performing artists.

## Atherosclerosis

For details on atherosclerosis, please see earlier sections of the book including, "Details of Oxidized LDL and Atherosclerosis Production." All six prongs of the Mind-Body Wellness Program work to reverse and prevent atherosclerosis. The program provides the supplements (antioxidants such as alpha-lipoic acid, Co-Q10, and vitamins to prevent oxidation of LDLs; omega-3 fatty acids to establish and maintain a proper HDL-LDL balance; a nitric oxide compound, to provide the anti-atherosclerotic molecule) and lifestyle routines (exercise, the most powerful antioxidant, to prevent LDL oxidation; Mediterranean diet to provide more omega-3s, antioxidants, and nitric oxide; and stress reduction to reduce oxidants).

## Autonomic Dysfunction and Small Fiber Neuropathy and Their Measurements

Peripheral nerves contain myelinated and unmyelinated fibers. Both serve somatic and autonomic functions. Peripheral nerve fibers are classified according to size, which correlates with the degree of myelination. Large nerve fibers (e.g., A fibers[15]) are heavily myelinated, and they control motor strength and vibratory and touch sensation. Medium-sized fibers (e.g., B fibers[16]) are myelinated and carry information to muscle spindles. Small fibers (e.g., C fibers[17]) include lightly myelinated and unmyelinated fibers. They

[15]Type A fibers are the thickest and fastest conducting. They are myelinated, with diameters of 1.5–20 microns and conduction speeds of 4–120 m/sec. They are the sensory or motor fibers found in the somatic nerves; examples include skeletomotor fibers, fusimotor fibers, and afferent fibers to the skin. They comprise four subgroups, from highest to lowest speed: $\alpha$, $\beta$, $\gamma$, and $\delta$. The A fibers found in the ANS are A$\delta$.

[16]Type B fibers are medium in size, i.e., they are smaller than type A fibers but larger than type C fibers. Type B fibers are myelinated, with diameters of 1.0–3.5 microns and conduction speeds of 3–15 m/sec; examples include preganglionic autonomic efferents. In the ANS, they constitute the white communicating branches (preganglionic afferents) of the sympathetic chain.

[17]Type C fibers are the smallest and thinnest of the nerve fibers. They are nonmyelinated, with diameters of 0.1–2 microns and conduction speeds 0.5–4 m/sec; examples include postganglionic autonomic efferents and afferent fibers to the skin. In fact, these constitute the majority of the ANS fibers in the body, e.g., the afferent amyelinated fibers of the visceral nerves and the sympathetic postganglionic nerves.

mediate pain, thermal sensation, and autonomic function. Small fiber neuropathy occurs when only these small fibers are selectively impaired. Small fiber neuropathy may affect small somatic fibers, autonomic fibers, or both. Small fiber neuropathy as it transmits thermal and pain sensation may present with autonomic dysfunction or lack of thermal and pain sensation, neuropathic pain, dysesthesias, or combination of the above symptoms. Small fiber neuropathy can present with both positive and negative symptoms of pain and temperature fibers. EMGs are normal in patients with isolated small fiber disease. Small fiber neuropathy and autonomic neuropathy are often concurrent, for two reasons: (1) autonomic fibers are small fibers, and (2) given that they are unmyelinated, they are more susceptible to hypoxia from poor peripheral circulation resulting from autonomic dysfunction (i.e., peripheral autonomic neuropathy). In addition to hypoxia, autonomic dysfunction leading to poor peripheral circulation may also be due to sugar acidosis (i.e., from diabetes), or uremia toxicity (i.e., from kidney disease). Small fiber neuropathy almost always indicates the presence of early autonomic dysfunction.

Small fiber neuropathy manifests in a variety of different illnesses and often results in symptoms of burning pain, shooting pain, allodynia, and hyperesthesia and also autonomic dysfunction since it can affect the autonomic and enteric function. Usually a sensory function includes fibers or the thermal perception and nociception. These are usually peripheral nerves that are either small myelinated A fibers or unmyelinated C fibers. Most small fiber neuropathies occur in length-dependent fashion, resulting in loss of function in a stocking distribution in the lower extremities. When the condition is advanced, glove-like loss in the upper extremities may occur. Burning pain is often a symptom first noted. Also, cold-like pain, tingling, or pins and needle sensation may be found. Some patients report a transient electric shock-like pain that last seconds, but it can be quite severe. Also, allodynia and hyperesthesia may be noted. Many people wear socks to bed because bedsheets can precipitate pain in the feet.

It is well known that small fiber neuropathies can result in autonomic and enteric dysfunction. Patients may report dry eyes, dry mouth, and skin changes such as atrophic dry skin, postural light-headedness, pre-syncope, syncope, orthostatic hypotension, orthostatic dizziness, abnormal sweating, sexual dysfunction (both erectile dysfunction and vaginal dryness), nausea, vomiting, constipation, early satiety, difficulty with urinary frequency, nocturia, and voiding [146, 147]. Sometimes the skin is mildly swollen or edematous. Biopsies were taken 10 centimeters above the lateral malleolus, and 5-micrometer sections were stained with H&E [147]. Autonomic involvement occurs in patients with sensory small fiber neuropathy, and punch skin biopsies used in sections in simple and conventional methods to detect dermal autonomic small fiber abnormalities have been used. There are many causes of small fiber neuropathy. These include diabetes, dyslipidemia, familial amyloid polyneuropathy, Tangier disease, hereditary sensory autonomic neuropathy (HSAN), Fabry's disease, vasculitis, hepatitis C, HIV post-viral, Sjögren's syndrome, alcohol, drugs, nutritional disease, liver disease, and so forth. Oftentimes, people believe they are not diabetics but have impaired glucose tolerance, and this is usually the cause of their small fiber neuropathy.

Fabry's disease is a rare X-linked disorder. It is hereditary due to a deficiency of alpha-galactosidase A. It affects the heart, central nervous system, GI tract and metabolism. Patients have severe burning in extremities, usually males. They can have paresthesias, do not sweat, and have heat intolerance and reduced tear and saliva production. Tangier disease, hereditary high-density lipoprotein deficiency, is autosomal recessive, and it can manifest as extensive loss of pain and temperature sensation. They often have orange-colored tonsils.

Skin biopsy is probably the most accurate way to diagnose small fiber disease. As a result, it has become the most widely accepted technique to investigate structural integrity of small nerve fibers [148]. Biopsy specimens are immunostained using an antibiotic against protein gene product 9.5, which is a pan-axonal marker. Quantitative sudomotor axon reflex test or QSART measures sweat output. Reflexive function of certain population of small fiber nerves. In this test, electrodes are produced on the arms and legs to record the volume of sweat produced. The output is compared with normal people. One study showed that 73% of patients with painful feet had abnormal results on QSART [149, 150]. Celiac sprue has also been associated with small fiber disease [151]. A lip biopsy should be considered if there is suspicion of Sjögren's disease or amyloid or sicca syndrome. If sarcoid is suspected clinically, one may even have to do additional tests.

Multiple medications have been used to treat symptoms of small fiber neuropathy. Tricyclic antidepressants are usually first tier in guidelines. The mechanism of action is inhibition of serotonin and norepinephrine uptake. However, they also have anticholinergic effects that may cause significant side effects in some patients. They are contraindicated in patients with significant cardiac history or glaucoma or recent monoamine oxidase inhibitor use. SNRIs or other classes of antidepressants are used to treat neuropathic pain. Both duloxetine and venlafaxine have been recommended. One should be careful when using these medicines for uncontrolled narrow angle glaucoma or being treated with MAO inhibitors. Venlafaxine may be useful in treating painful diabetic neuropathy or mixed neuropathy. Anticonvulsants have been used such as gabapentin and pregabalin for treatment of neuropathic pain. Topical lidocaine may be used. Opiates and tramadol are also frequently used. However, dependence for these medications, including tramadol, can occur. In published studies, specifically examining small fiber neuropathy, both gabapentin and tramadol were found to be effective [152].

In regard to autonomic neuropathy, with the exception of SNRIs and tricyclics, many of these medications have not been effective in improving autonomic nervous system function [personal communication, Drs. DePace and Colombo]. However, alpha-lipoic acid and other antioxidants have been found to be effective in empiric observations. While most of the medications discussed improve symptoms in small fiber disease, none of them have shown to increase the density of small fibers. However, antioxidants may have that capability. Specifically, supplemental antioxidants may be the best way to protect nerves. Many of the nutrients that support energy production in mitochondria include alpha-lipoic acid, carnitine, and coenzyme Q10. Alpha-Lipoic acid, in particular, has been well studied and proven to minimize nerve damage and painful symptoms in diabetics [153–155].

There is a medication, Metanx, which is a prescription medical food made by Pamlab that contains L-methylfolate. It is a vitamin B supplement. It is indicated in the management of peripheral neuropathy. It contains folate, L-methylfolate, pyridoxal 5, phosphate, and methylcobalamin. It has been suggested that the use of this medicine has increased small nerve fiber density on biopsies. After 6 months of treatment with Metanx, 80% of patients with diabetic neuropathy reported reduced pain and numbness [156]. The study found that Metanx actually increased the number of nerve fibers, possibly reversing the damage done by diabetes. It is generally well tolerated. It can cause an upset stomach, and it should be taken with meals.

Metanx treatment seems to counteract endothelial NOS uncoupling, inducible NOS upregulation, and methylglyoxal-derived advanced glycation end product, nitrotyrosine, and nitrite/nitrate accumulation in the peripheral nerve. In other words, Metanx maintains blood flow in vessels that supply peripheral nerves and facilitates peripheral nerve repair. Unlike commonly used agents such as pregabalin, which are palliative in action, preparations such as Metanx may have both analgesic and a neurotrophic effect on peripheral nerve health and function [157, 158].

In the autonomic lab, various techniques are used to diagnose and treat the autonomic nervous systems (ANS), including the parasympathetic (P) and sympathetic (S) nervous systems (P&S). Traditionally, autonomic dysfunctions are classified based on their primary or secondary nature. The pathophysiological classifications are [52]:

- Primary
  - Pure autonomic failure
  - Multisystem atrophy (Shy-Drager syndrome)
  - Parkinson's disease
  - Pan-dysautonomic neuropathy
  - Paraneoplastic autonomic neuropathy
- Secondary
  - General diseases: diabetes, alcoholism, renal failure, amyloidosis, neoplasms, dysautonomia of aging

- Autoimmune diseases: acute and chronic inflammatory polyneuropathy, Lambert-Eaton syndrome, rheumatoid arthritis, lupus erythematosus
- Metabolic diseases: porphyria, Tangier disease, Fabry's disease, pernicious anemia
- Hereditary disorders: familial dysautonomia, hereditary motor and sensory neuropathies, sensorial and autonomic congenital neuropathy, Friedreich's ataxia
- Infections: Chagas disease, AIDS, botulism, leprosy, syphilis
- Diseases of the central nervous system: medullary lesions, strokes, tumors, multiple sclerosis, amyotrophic lateral sclerosis, Adie syndrome
- Intoxications: by acrylamide, heavy metals, organic solvents
- Pharmacological: by antineoplastics, antidepressants, sedatives, hypotensives, adrenergic blockers, cholinergic blockers

Autonomic dysfunctions are also classified clinically in four organizational levels. It is also possible that multiple dysfunctional levels may occur simultaneously. The clinical classifications are [52]:

- Level 1 disorders (spinal cord)
  - Autonomic disorders with spinal cord involvement
    - Traumatic quadriplegia
    - Syringomyelia
    - Multiple sclerosis and neuromyelitis optica
    - Amyotrophic lateral sclerosis
    - Tetanus
    - Spinal cord tumors
  - Autonomic neuropathies
    - Acute/subacute autonomic neuropathies
      - Subacute autoimmune autonomic ganglionopathy
        - Subacute paraneoplastic autonomic neuropathy
        - Guillain-Barré syndrome
        - Lambert-Eaton syndrome
        - Botulism
        - Porphyria
        - Drug-induced autonomic neuropathies
        - Toxin-induced autonomic neuropathies
    - Chronic peripheral autonomic neuropathies
      - Distal small fiber neuropathy
      - Combined sympathetic and parasympathetic failure
        - Amyloid
        - Diabetic autonomic neuropathy
        - Autoimmune autonomic ganglionopathy (paraneoplastic and idiopathic)
        - Sensory neuronopathy with autonomic failure
        - Familial dysautonomia (Riley-Day syndrome)
        - Uremic or nutritional deficiency
        - Dysautonomia of old age
      - Disorders of reduced orthostatic intolerance: idiopathic orthostatic hypotension, reflex syncope, postural orthostatic tachycardia syndrome, associated with prolonged bedrest, associated with space flight, chronic fatigue
- Level 2 disorders (brain stem and cerebellum)
  - Vertebrobasilar and lateral medullary (Wallenberg) syndromes
  - Posterior fossa tumors
  - Syringobulbia and Arnold-Chiari malformation
  - Horner's syndrome
  - Disorders of blood pressure control (hypertension, hypotension)
  - Cardiac arrhythmias
  - Baroreflex failure
  - Central sleep apnea
  - Brain stem encephalitis
- Level 3 disorders (hypothalamus)
  - Thiamine deficiency (Wernicke-Korsakoff syndrome)
  - Diencephalic syndrome
  - Neuroleptic malignant syndrome
  - Serotonin syndrome
  - Fatal familial insomnia

  - Arginine vasopressin syndromes (diabetes insipidus, inappropriate arginine vasopressin secretion)
  - Disturbances of temperature regulation (hyperthermia, hypothermia)
  - Disturbances of sexual function
  - Disturbances of appetite
- Level 4 disorders (focal central nervous system disorders)
  - Frontal cortex lesions causing urinary/bowel incontinence
  - Focal seizures (temporal lobe or anterior cingulate)
  - Cerebral infarction of the insula
  - Shapiro syndrome (agenesis of the corpus callosum, hyperhidrosis, hypothermia)
  - Autonomic seizures
  - Limbic encephalitis
- Multilevel disorders (focal central nervous system disorders)
  - Multilevel autonomic nervous system disorders
  - Multisystem degeneration: autonomic failure clinically prominent
    - Multiple system atrophy (Shy-Drager syndrome)
    - Parkinson's disease with autonomic failure
    - Diffuse Lewy body disease (some cases)
  - Multisystem degeneration: autonomic failure clinically not usually prominent
    - Parkinson's disease
    - Other extrapyramidal disorders (inherited spinocerebellar atrophies, progressive supranuclear palsy, corticobasal degeneration, Machado-Joseph disease, fragile X syndrome)

All of these classifications notwithstanding, the traditional signs of autonomic dysfunction include, as grouped by organ or organ system:

| | | |
|---|---|---|
| Cardiovascular | Sudomotor | Genitourinary tract |
| Tachycardia at rest | Hypohidrosis, anhydrosis | Bladder dysfunction |
| Orthostatic hypotension | Hyperhidrosis | Urinary retention |
| Arterial hypertension | Gustatory sweating | Incontinence |
| Arrhythmias | Eye | Impotence |
| Syncope | Anisocoria | Central nervous system |
| Gastrointestinal tract | Nyctalopia | Anxiety |
| Dysphagia, regurgitation | Close blurred vision | Insomnia |
| Gastroparesis, vomiting | Tunnel vision | Chronic fatigue |
| Constipation | Double vision | Brain fog |
| Episodes of diarrhea | | Vertigo |
| | | Dizziness |
| | | Weakness |

While all of this is useful clinically, the primary focus is to maintain wellness by detecting and treating P&S dysfunction before symptoms present, before quality of life, let alone life itself, is threatened. The focus is on maintaining wellness by asking "are you truly healthy or merely symptom-free." Since the P&S nervous systems control the organs and organ systems, they will typically become dysfunctional before symptoms. However, symptoms typically present only after the organs become dysfunctional. The main purpose of the P&S systems is to maintain normal organ function even if they themselves are dysfunctional. P&S monitoring enables physicians to detect and treat P&S dysfunction prior to symptoms, thereby maintaining wellness. Yet, patients do become ill and P&S monitoring helps physicians to gain more information about the individual patient, thereby tailoring the therapy plan to the individual patient rather than simply classifying the patient and treating them like everyone else. This may also help to minimize the amount of medication deemed necessary and help to minimize the duration that a patient will need to take the medication. By not waiting until the organs or organ systems are dysfunctional, the purpose of the medication will be to retrain the nervous system to maintain proper function and proper balance. Once the organs are dysfunctional, then the purpose of the medication turns to supporting or even replacing the function of the organs as opposed to normalizing their control. When medication is needed to support or replace function, then they may become lifelong. The goal is to delay this eventuality as long as possible. A brief summary of the relationship between the P&S nervous systems and the organs or organ systems is listed in Table 9.2.

**Table 9.2** Autonomic nervous system effects on effector organs [52]

| Organ, tissue | Parasympathetic stimulation | Sympathetic stimulation |
|---|---|---|
| *Pupils* | | |
| Radial muscle of the iris | – | Contraction, α1 adrenoceptor mediated |
| Sphincter muscle of the iris | Contraction, M3, M2-receptor mediated | – |
| Ciliary muscle | Contraction, M3, M2-receptor mediated | Weak relaxation, β2 receptor mediated |
| Tracheobronchial muscle | Contraction, M2,M3-receptor mediated | Relaxation, β2 adrenoceptor mediated |
| Heart | Bradycardia, negative inotropism, M2 receptor mediated | Tachycardia, positive inotropism, β1 adrenoceptor mediated |
| *Arteries* | | |
| Skin, mucosas | – | Constriction, α1 adrenoceptor mediated |
| Abdomen | – | Constriction, α1 adrenoceptor-mediated dilatation (blood epinephrine), β2 adrenoceptor mediated |
| Skeletal muscle | – | Dilation, M2 receptor mediated |
| Dilatation (blood epinephrine), β2 adrenoceptor mediated | | |
| Coronary arteries | – | Constriction, α1 adrenoceptor-mediated dilation, β2 adrenoceptor mediated |
| CNS arteries | Dilation (?) | Constriction, α1 adrenoceptor mediated |
| Penis | Dilation, M2 receptor mediated | – |
| Kidney | – | Constriction, α1 adrenoceptor mediated |
| Veins | – | Constriction, α1 adrenoceptor mediated |
| Endothelium | Stimulation of NO synthase, M3 receptor mediated | |
| *Bladder* | | |
| Detrusor muscle | Contraction, M3 receptor mediated | Relaxation, β2 adrenoceptor mediated |
| Internal sphincter | Relaxation, M2 receptor mediated | Constriction, α1 adrenoceptor mediated |
| *Genital tract* | | |
| Seminal vesicles | – | Constriction, α1 adrenoceptor mediated |
| Vas deferens | – | Constriction, α1 adrenoceptor mediated |
| Intercourse | Erection, M3 receptor mediated | Ejaculation, α1 adrenoceptor mediated |
| Uterus | – | Constriction, α1 adrenoceptor-mediated relaxation, β2 adrenoceptor mediated |
| *Gastrointestinal tract* | | |
| Circular and longitudinal muscle | Contraction, M3 receptor mediated | Relaxation (direct) β adrenoceptor-mediated parasympathetic inhibition, α1 adrenoceptor mediated |
| Sphincters | Relaxation | Constriction, α adrenoceptor mediated |

**Table 9.2** (continued)

| Organ, tissue | Parasympathetic stimulation | Sympathetic stimulation |
|---|---|---|
| *Exocrine glands* | | |
| Salivary | Secretion, M3 receptor mediated | |
| Lacrimal | Secretion, M3 receptor mediated | – |
| Digestive | Secretion, M3 receptor mediated | Inhibition, α adrenoceptor mediated |
| Nasopharyngeal | Secretion, M3 receptor mediated | – |
| Sweat | – | Secretion, M3 receptor mediated |
| Bronchial | Secretion, M3 receptor mediated | Weak inhibition, α1 adrenoceptor mediated. Weak stimulation, β adrenoceptor mediated |
| Adipose tissue | – | Lipolysis, β1 adrenoceptor mediated |
| *Immune system* | | |
| Lymph nodes, spleen | Stimulation | Inhibition, α1 adrenoceptor mediated |
| Splenic capsule | – | Constriction, α1 adrenoceptor mediated |
| *Endocrine system* | | |
| Juxtaglomerular apparatus | – | Renin secretion, β1 adrenoceptor mediated |
| Thyroid follicles | Thyroid growth, secretion of T4, M receptor mediated | Inhibition of T4 secretion, α1 mediated. Weak stimulus of T4 secretion, β adrenoceptor mediated |
| Thyroid C cells | Inhibition of CT secretion | Inhibition of CT secretion, α1 mediated. Weak stimulus of CT secretion, β adrenoceptor mediated |
| Parathyroid glands | Inhibition of PTH secretion | Inhibition of PTH secretion |
| Pineal gland | – | Melatonin release, β2 adrenoceptor mediated. Weak stimulus of melatonin release, α1 adrenoceptor mediated |
| Adrenal medulla | | Preganglionic stimulation, M1 receptor mediated |
| Anterior pituitary | | Postganglionic SCG sympathetic neurons inhibit FSH, LH, GH, PRL, and TSH secretion and augments ACTH secretion |
| Posterior hypophysis | – | Postganglionic SCG sympathetic neurons inhibit ADH secretion, β adrenoceptor mediated |
| Exocrine pancreatic glands | Secretion, M1 receptor mediated | Inhibition, α adrenoceptor mediated |
| Pancreatic islets, α-cells | Secretion, M1 receptor mediated | Inhibition of glucagon secretion, α2 adrenoceptor mediated. Weak stimulation of glucagon secretion, β2 adrenoceptor mediated |
| Pancreatic islets, β-cells | Secretion, M1 receptor mediated | Inhibition of insulin secretion, α2 adrenoceptor mediated. Weak stimulation of insulin secretion, β2 adrenoceptor mediated |
| Liver | Glycogen synthesis (?) | Glycogenolysis, α1 adrenoceptor-mediated gluconeogenesis, β2 adrenoceptor-mediated lipolysis, β1 adrenoceptor mediated |

*NO* nitric oxide, *CT* calcitonin, *PTH* parathyroid hormone, *SCG* superior cervical ganglion, *FSH* follicle-stimulating hormone, *LH* luteinizing hormone, *GH* growth hormone, *PRL* prolactin, *TSH* thyroid-stimulating hormone, *ACTH* adrenocorticotropic hormone, *ADH* antidiuretic hormone

Whether on a tilt table or not, there are several other autonomic challenges designed to help diagnose autonomic dysfunction. Note that the autonomic nervous system is a dynamic system designed to change and mediate change. The difficulty most have and the reason why most autonomic dysfunctions go undiagnosed by many doctors over many visits is that most often when a doctor assesses a patient the patient is at rest, sitting or lying down. Most autonomic dysfunctions do not present at rest, until very late in the progression of autonomic neuropathy.

As discussed above, like a thermostat, the P&S systems are designed to maintain normal organ function, even if they themselves are abnormal. So the resting state is the baseline and enables the patient to be their own control, so that the results of the test may be assessed and prescribed the same day.

Therefore, typical ANS challenges are dynamic in nature. Currently, the three most common are deep breathing, Valsalva, and postural change (either tilt table or stand). Others have included isometric handgrip, cold water, and counting backward from 100 by sevens. All but the deep breathing challenge are (net) sympathetic challenges. The three most common are also known as the Ewing challenges after David J. Ewing, MD, who first proposed a standard for them in the 1980s. The three Ewing ratios, or time-domain ratios, that are used to assess the Ewing challenges are the exhalation/inhalation (E/I) ratio, Valsalva ratio, and 30:15 ratio [44]. These are thresholded measures of more or less heart rate variability (HRV), which makes them qualitative measures of parasympathetic activity (including the Valsalva ratio). There is no known maximum for normal, which has led to the impression that more parasympathetic activity is always best. Yet it is well known that too much parasympathetic activity leads to depression, hypotension, fatigue, suppressed immune function, and even "Broken Heart" syndrome which may lead to sudden cardiac death.

Postural change is considered a net, sympathetic challenge, because first the parasympathetics are expected to decrease and then the sympathetic increase to cause the orthostatic response. The other traditional parameters to measure ANS responses are either time-domain or frequency-domain HRV measures. In the frequency domain, there are low-frequency (LF) and high-frequency (HF) measures. LF is a mix of both S- and P-activity (S-responses are limited to 0.15 Hz; P-responses can go up to 0.40 Hz). HF is a broadband measure of P-activity but usually includes harmonics and other noise, corrupting the P-measure, assuming the P-activity is even to be found in the HF region. The sum of LF and HF is known as total spectral power, another mixed measure. The ratio of LF/HF is intended to be a ratio of the two autonomic branches; however, the two measures are mixed which makes their ratio mixed and of little help.

In the time domain, the standard deviation of beat-to-beat intervals (sdNN) is a mixed measure of both P&S activity. The root-mean-square of the standard deviation (rmsSD) or the percent of the beat-to-beat intervals greater than 50 msec (pNN50) are relative measures of more or less parasympathetic activity. Because P-activity is able to reach higher frequencies, the rmsSD and pNN50 measure only measures of P-activity. However, sdNN, rmsSD, and pNN50 are only valid with a minimum of 5 minutes of stationary data, which is too long to measure in response to deep breathing or Valsalva and cannot be used in response to postural change because of its dynamic nature.

Beat-to-beat BP (btbBP) and pulse wave velocity are other types of heartbeat interval monitoring, but require waveform analyses, which leaves much to the imagination and is limiting once autonomic responses are too low to visualize. BTBBP is often pared with tilt table testing as an attempt to better differentiate P-from S-responses, more on this later. From the btbBP recordings in response to stand, the baroreceptor reflex may be measured and quantified [159]. A summary of the tests used by organ system is summarized in Table 9.3.

Often considered the so-called gold standard in diagnosing autonomic testing, the tilt test has had many problems. First of all, it is long and cumbersome and uncomfortable for the patient. It is also stressful. By increasing sympathetic drive, for example, as in white coat syndrome, it may blunt many of the testing effects needed to be observed to accurately diagnose. These effects are often overshadowed by the initial high sympathetic activity caused by preparing the patient for the test. Tilt testing with a prolonged protocol and with drug infusions may be useful at times in confirming reflux or vagal-type syncope from orthostatic hypotension-type symptoms. However in these instances, it is usually a vasovagal reflex syncope that is declared and not orthostatic hypotension (OH). With P&S monitoring,

**Table 9.3** Some tests of ANS function

| Test | Parameter | Main part of the reflex arc tested |
|---|---|---|
| *Cardiovascular system* | | |
| RR interval during respiration | HR | Vagal afferent and efferent limbs |
| Heart rate variability | HR | Vagal afferent and efferent limbs |
| Valsalva maneuver | HR, BP | Afferent and efferent limbs |
| Mueller maneuver | HR, BP | Afferent and efferent limbs |
| BP response to standing or vertical tilt | BP | Afferent and sympathetic efferent limbs |
| Heart rate response to standing | HR | Vagal afferent and efferent limbs |
| Handgrip | HR, BP | Sympathetic efferent limb |
| Cold pressor test | HR, BP | Sympathetic efferent limb |
| Radiant heating of the trunk | Hand blood flow | Sympathetic efferent limb |
| Immersion of the hand in hot water | Blood flow of the opposite hand | Sympathetic efferent limb |
| Emotional stress | HR, BP | Sympathetic efferent limb |
| Baroreflex sensitivity | HR, BP | Vagal afferent and efferent limbs |
| Doppler | Blood flow | Sympathetic efferent limb |
| Plasma norepinephrine levels | Rises on tilting from horizontal to vertical | Sympathetic efferent limb |
| Plasma arginine vasopressin levels | Rise with induced hypotension | Afferent limb |
| *Sudomotor system* | | |
| Sweat tests | Sweat | Sympathetic efferent limb |
| Quantitative sudomotor axon reflex test | Evaporation rate | Sympathetic efferent limb |
| Sympathetic skin response | Potentials | Sympathetic efferent limb |
| *Pupil* | | |
| Pharmacological tests of pupillary innervation | Pupil diameter | Afferent and efferent limbs |
| Pupil cycle time | Pupil diameter | Afferent and efferent limbs |
| Pupillometry | Pupil diameter and latency | Afferent and efferent limbs |
| *Others* | | |
| Microneurography | Potentials | Sympathetic efferent limb |
| Sympathetic neuroimaging | 123I-Metaiodobenzylguanidine uptake by NE vesicles in cardiac sympathetic nerves | Sympathetic efferent limb |
| Skin biopsy | Peripheral adrenergic and cholinergic fibers innervating sweat glands and arrector pili muscles | Sympathetic efferent limb |

rarely is tilt testing needed to diagnose autonomic dysfunction or the type.

Beat-to-beat blood pressure, even in abbreviated algorithms using short-term tilt testing, provides only some information on sympathetic reflux in recovery with Valsalva and stand responses, but does not provide much detail, especially given that it forces waveform reading which can be highly subjective or obscured by noise. Heart rate variability (HRV) testing oftentimes does not provide an idea of what agent is most efficient or what part of the ANS is more excessive or deficient and needs to be targeted with therapy. P&S monitoring has shown the ability to differentiate P&S activity. When testing patients not only does P&S monitoring provide significant information on the type of autonomic (P&S) dysfunction but also what type of treatment could be started initially. This is beneficial for the patient and is a cost saving when the patient responds quickly to therapy. The quicker response is because the therapy is not just empirically started in a trial by error basis, but with some scientific basis. Ultimately, the patient is better quicker and is more confident which reinforces the treatment plan. Also, on following patients serially, P&S monitoring is invaluable in showing improvements in various branches of the ANS and therefore diagnosing how to titrate therapy or add additional agents. Not only pharmacology but lifestyle changes and supplements are important to institute during various stages (e.g., fish oils to help close the Statin Gap or alpha-lipoic acid (ALA) to help reduce hypertension secondary to OH).

Sudomotor testing is valuable in showing inflammation of sweat fibers or deficiency of sweat fibers. With inflammation, antioxidants, such as ALA, have been found to be very effective when titrated to high doses. With deficiency, ALA has also been shown to be important. With low sudomotor testing responses, this obviates the need for skin biopsies for small fiber density or disease, which is an invasive procedure and can be hit or miss. Sudomotor testing may involve quantitative sudomotor axon reflex test (QSART), quantitative direct and indirect axon reflex test (QDIRT), quantitative sensory test, thermoregulatory sweat test, silastic sweat imprint, sympathetic skin response, or electrochemical sweat conductance (QSweat). The most frequent utilized is the QSART, quantitative sudomotor axon reflex test, a measure of postganglionic sympathetic cholinergic function. Local sweating is produced through iontophoresis of acetylcholine; this method uses a mild electrical current to draw acetylcholine, a charged substance, into the skin, causing activation of local sweat glands. This triggers an axon reflex, resulting in neighboring sweat glands, not stimulated by acetylcholine to produce sweat. Dry gas is passed over a non-stimulated region and quantifying a change in humidity of the gas. Sudomotor dysfunction may be the earliest manifestation of distal small fiber neuropathy. Other tests including sweat imprint test, thermoregulatory sweat testing, and quantitative direct and indirect sudomotor testing also detect abnormalities and small fiber neuropathy.

P&S monitoring provides more information, including valuable baseline information in terms of sympathovagal balance (SB). It can demonstrate vagal dominance at rest (resting P-excess measured as low SB, as associated with depression and hypotension). Also, P&S monitoring is the only measurement that is able to measure

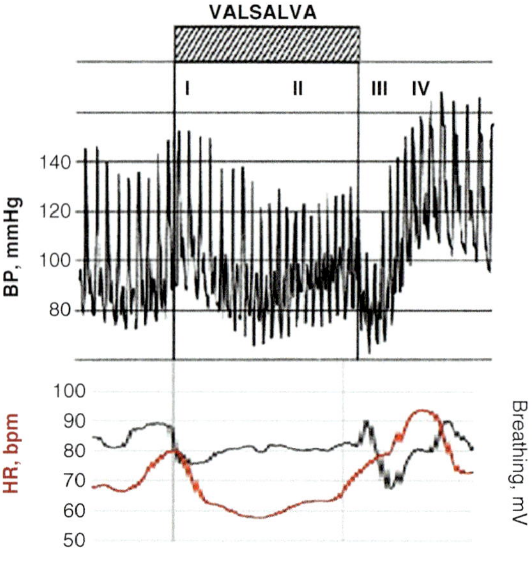


**Fig. 9.7** Simultaneous beat-to-beat BP (btb-BP), instantaneous HR, and respiratory activity recordings from a young healthy subject in response to a 15-second Valsalva maneuver at 40 mmHg pressure. From the BTB-BP waveform, the four phases of a Valsalva response are indicated in roman numerals. They are also reflected in the HR (red) curve. The subject's average BP in response to the Valsalva maneuver is 136/62 mmHg, an increase of 25 mmHg systolic. The Valsalva ratio is 1.60. The HRV measure is 43 bpm. The P&S measures are 14.19 $bpm^2$ and 48.26 $bpm^2$, respectively.

P-activity, independent of but simultaneously with S-activity, especially during dynamic maneuvers such as Valsalva or postural change (e.g., stand or tilt). For example, simultaneous beat-to-beat BP (btbBP), instantaneous HR, and respiratory activity recordings from a young healthy subject in response to a 15-second Valsalva maneuver at 40 mmHg pressure are presented in Fig. 9.7.

Other ANS tests include:

- Pulse wave velocity testing
  - A simplified form of btbBP; requires waveform reading and is difficult to differentiate P from S-activity.
- Norepinephrine spillover
  - A measure of the amount of norepinephrine that is not taken back into the sympathetic nerve endings near the heart. It is a sympathetic measure only. It is a qualita-

tive measure of the dysfunction of the sympathetic nerves that innervate the heart (the more spillover, the less uptake, the more dysfunctional). This is confounded by age and duration of chronic illness ("physiologic age," not chronologic age).

- Baroreflex assessment
  - A measure of sympathetic nerve function, only.
- Microneurography
  - Nerve activity recorded directly from intraneural microelectrodes inserted percutaneously into a peripheral nerve in awake human subjects. It is not a quantitative test, nor is it intended to be diagnostic. Two forms of microneurography include muscle sympathetic nerve activity (MSNA) recordings and skin sympathetic nerve activity (SSNA).
- Nerve conduction velocity
  - An electrical test that is used to determine the adequacy of the conduction of the nerve impulse as it courses down a nerve. This test is used to detect signs of nerve injury, including autonomic neuropathy. However, it is primarily a measure of the larger diameter sensory and motor nerve fibers (A- and B-nerve fibers), rather than the smaller C fibers that include the autonomic and pain fibers.
- $^{123}$I-meta-iodobenzylguanidine ($^{123}$I-MIBG)
  - An anatomical label measure of sympathetic nerve function, only. It does not measure activity level, only nerves that are active or not. It cannot quantitate activity level.

All of these other ANS tests require assumption or approximation to hypothesize P&S activity. They are either mixed measures of P&S activity or of only sympathetic activity. If P&S levels cannot be differentiated properly, it is very difficult to know where to start with therapy and to know how to titrate therapy. Furthermore, follow-up testing is not possible, because the assumptions and approximations are invalidated by the therapy. Further, it is not possible to fully document patient response to therapy or disease. Nor is it possible to fully know morbidity or mortality risks or to document patient outcomes.

Autonomic dysfunction is known to precede autonomic neuropathy (see Fig. 7.4). Autonomic neuropathy is often asymptomatic. The preceding autonomic dysfunction, therefore, is asymptomatic. Autonomic dysfunction and neuropathy are mostly asymptomatic due to the simple fact that symptoms are mostly a function of end-organ dysfunction. The P&S controls the organs. Between the two branches, even when they are dysfunctional, the ANS will find a strategy to maintain homeostasis for up to decades prior to end-organ failure and symptom presentation. Autonomic dysfunction and neuropathy are characterized by autonomic imbalance. Autonomic imbalance (autonomic dysfunction or neuropathy as measured by abnormal sympathovagal balance, SB: $0.4 < SB < 3.0$) accelerates the onset of end-organ failure and the presentation of symptoms. Chronic disease is known to lead to autonomic neuropathy [44, 160, 161, 162–165]. Therefore, chronic disease, which causes autonomic imbalance, causes autonomic dysfunction. The asymptomatic nature of autonomic dysfunction and neuropathy leaves only the chronic disease itself as the indicator for autonomic dysfunction and therefore P&S monitoring.

By way of an example, consider the thermostat on the wall of your house. Assume that you have no knowledge of and cannot access or hear the heating and cooling systems of your house. Further, assume that you like your house temperature to be 70 °F (like heart rate at 70 bpm), and that is what your thermostat is set to. As long as the thermostat reads "70," everyone is happy. Now pretend it is a hot, humid, August day in the city, the cooling system is working well, and a $5 heater switch fails and the heater comes on full. What happens to the temperature in the house as read on the thermostat? … *Nothing!* … The cooling system is working well, so it "amps up" and compensates, not only for the ambient but also for the dysfunctional heating system (heart rate does not change; 70 is still the reading). The question becomes, how long will the dysfunctional situation last until there is a catastrophic failure (costing $5000, or more) in one or both of the cooling and heating systems? Meanwhile you are totally unaware (like your heart rate is still normal, 70) until the catastrophic failure (like a heart attack), when it is too late. P&S monitoring detects when the $5 switch fails (all other noninvasive, autonomic measures only measure the thermostat), and the lifestyle and supplement recommendations herein help keep the systems functioning normally (healthy) and a proper balance between the cooling (parasympathetic) and heating (sympathetic) systems to help keep the "$5 switches" functioning normally (healthy and well).

Autonomic neuropathy (the catastrophic failure) places patients at risk for increased morbidity and mortality. With P&S monitoring, autonomic dysfunction (the $5 switch failure) may now be detected early and clinically followed, before the onset of autonomic neuropathy (the $5000 failure). When P&S balance is restored, by normalizing SB, the onset of autonomic neuropathy is slowed or stayed. Normal aging, as dictated by an individual's history, lifestyle, and genetic makeup, causes autonomic decline, ultimately leading to autonomic neuropathy; this is the target rate of autonomic decline (see Figs. 7.6 and 7.7), and each individual is different. Even after the onset of autonomic neuropathy, normalizing SB slows the progression of autonomic neuropathy by limiting the morbidity [166] and mortality [167] risk, optimizing quality of life, and promoting normal longevity for the individual. Establishing and maintaining normal SB, appropriate for the individual, also reduces secondary symptoms which reduces medication load, prevents hospitalizations, and thereby lowers healthcare costs [29, 168, 169–176].

Studies [177, 178] have demonstrated a progression of autonomic dysfunction that is finer than previously thought. Using the effects of diabetes as a model of the effects of chronic disease [168, 169, 171, 172] on the ANS, the progression (Fig. 7.4) starts with peripheral autonomic neuropathy (PAN), followed by advanced autonomic dysfunction (AAD) or diabetic autonomic neuropathy (DAN, which is AAD with blood glucose and insulin issues), and ends with cardiovascular autonomic neuropathy (CAN) [179]. CAN defines the risk for sudden cardiac death due to damage to the autonomic nerves that innervate the heart and blood vessels, characterized by very low, resting parasympathetic activity ($P < 0.1$ bpm$^2$, as measured by P&S monitoring). This is like having very worn brakes on the car. Regardless of how strong the accelerator, eventually the car will roll down a hill and cannot be stopped. The accident at the bottom of the hill is a heart attack or stroke. While the "brakes" will eventually wear out (and the ones inside the body, the parasympathetics, cannot be replaced), balancing the brakes and accelerator will keep the brakes functioning longer and help prevent crashes.

CAN results in dysfunction in HR and BP control and vascular dynamics [166, 167] (e.g., Fig. 9.8). AAD or DAN defines a set of early symptoms, which, if detected and treated early enough, reduces the risk of CAN and associated morbidity and mortality risks [180]. These symptoms include resting tachycardia, exercise intolerance, orthostatic hypotension, constipation, gastroparesis, erectile dysfunction, sudomotor dysfunction, impaired neurovascular function, and, in the case of diabetics, "brittle diabetes," or hypoglycemic autonomic failure [166]. PAN is characterized by (1) vasomotor changes including poor peripheral circulation leading to poor wound healing, pallor sometimes alternating with rubor, dry and brittle skin, cyanosis, and mottling and (2) sudomotor dysfunction including excessive sweating or anhydrosis of the extremities.

Recent studies have shown a finer gradation with earlier phases [177, 178]. These studies are based on the accepted and American Diabetes Association-approved and American College of Clinical Endocrinology and American College Of Endocrinology-recommended methodology for P&S assessment [146, 147, 181]. These studies include (A) 5 minutes of resting baseline; (B) 1 minute of slow, paced breathing (*aka* deep breathing); (C) a 1-minute return to baseline; (D) a series of (up to five) short Valsalva maneuvers (of 15 seconds or less duration); (E) a 2-minute return to baseline; and (F) a quick, head-up, postural change (e.g., quick standing or tilt) followed by 5 minutes of quiet head-up posture (e.g., standing or tilt). The resting baseline challenge assesses the absolute and relative measures of P&S activity, including SB (= S/P). Abnormal resting baseline results are associated with mortality risk

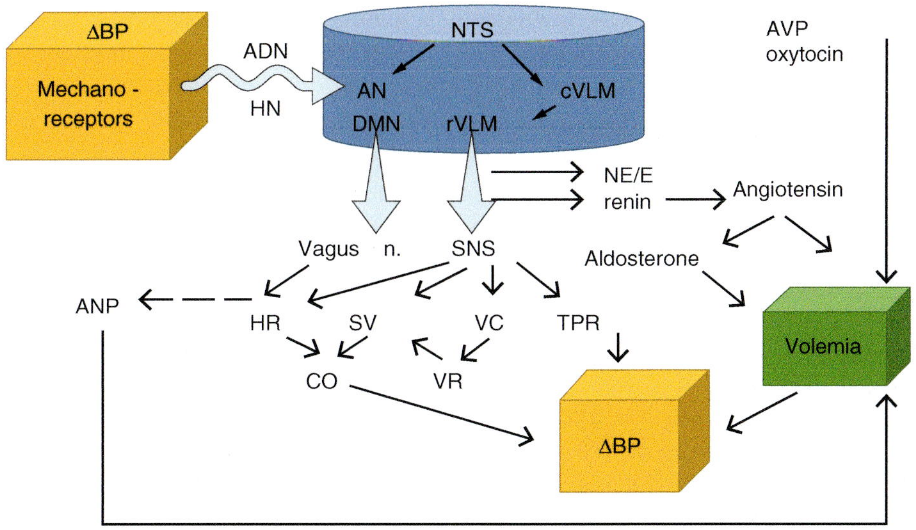


**Fig. 9.8** Schematic representation of neurohormonal responses triggered by the stimulation of vascular mechanoreceptors by changes in BP. Abbreviations: ADN aortic depressor nerve, AN ambiguous nucleus, ANP atrial natriuretic peptide, CO cardiac output, cVLM caudal ventrolateral medulla, DMN dorsomedial nucleus of the vagus, HN Hering's nerve, HR heart rate, rVLM rostral ventrolateral medulla, SNS sympathetic nervous system, SV systolic volume, TPR total peripheral resistance, VC venous capacity, and VR venous return [52, Fig. 4.12]. (Republished with permission from Springer International Publishing AG)

[182], including risk of sudden cardiac death or other MACE events. Morbidity risk is defined as very low, resting, parasympathetic activity. Very low, resting, parasympathetic activity (RFa[18] < 0.1 bpm$^2$) is the definition of CAN. Deep breathing is a P-challenge where the patient's breathing is paced at six breaths per minute, slowly and relaxed. The Valsalva challenge is a S-challenge, where the parasympathetics are expected to decline or at least not increase significantly. DB and Valsalva challenges are early indicators of autonomic decline or autonomic dysfunction, as well as small fiber disease.

The postural challenge (PC) is also a (net) S-challenge in the sense that sympathetics are expected to increase in a bounded manner. Preceding the bounded S-increase, the parasympathetics are expected to decrease. It is often better to regard the postural change challenge as a challenge to the coordination between P&S. Abnormal postural change challenge results are associated with morbidity risk, including dizziness or light-headedness [166]. A lack of coordination between the P&S nervous systems, including during the Valsalva challenge, as well as the postural change challenge, leads to secondary symptoms that may also include hypertension secondary to autonomic dysfunction, orthostasis, sleep disturbances, depression, fatigue, exercise intolerance, GI upset, or frequent headache or migraine.

Examples of autonomic diseases include fibromyalgia, Ehlers-Danlos syndrome, Sjögren's syndrome, bipolar disorder, chronic regional pain syndrome, PTSD, abnormal sweating, and central (non-obstructive) sleep apnea. Autonomic diseases are correlated with mitochondrial diseases. Regardless, *balance is key* to proper autonomic function and therefore health and wellness. Consider the following:

- Oxygen – Too little oxygen leads to suffocation. Too much oxygen, tissues burn (fire is the oxidation of carbon: wood, paper, etc.). A proper amount (read that "a balance") of oxygen (antioxidants and oxidants, including a level of reactive oxygen species (ROS) and free

[18] Respiratory Frequency area (RFa) is the measured parameter that is the measure of parasympathetic activity.

radicals to help the immune system) is required for health and wellness. Oxygen is needed for proper metabolic function, especially in energy production. However, too many oxidants "burn" (oxidize) DNA, cell membranes, LDLs, and more. Supplements (antioxidants such as alpha-lipoic acid, Co-Q10, and vitamins) and lifestyle routines (exercise, Mediterranean diet, and stress reduction) help to preserve a proper antioxidant-oxidant balance, by establishing and maintaining an antioxidant buffer that the body may draw on in times of stress.

- Water – Too little water leads to dehydration. Too much water causes people to drown in their own tissues. Proper hydration for all cells of the body is crucial. Remember, the body is made mostly of water. Water keeps the skin and hair supple (among other things) and helps to rid the body of wastes and toxins through sweat and exhaled water vapor. The supplements mentioned above and lifestyle routines (exercise and Mediterranean diet) that help to preserve a proper hydration-dehydration (water) balance prevent many disorders and symptoms.
- Nitric oxide – Too little nitric oxide, blood flow, and cellular communications are significantly disrupted. Too much nitric oxide, and the oxidant (reactive nitrogen species)-antioxidant balance is compromised. Compromised blood flow is caused by atherosclerosis caused by too little nitric oxide enabling the LDLs to burn and the walls of blood vessels to become "sticky," enabling plaque to form, causing turbulent blood flow which exacerbates and accelerates the progression of atherosclerosis, leading to heart attack, stroke, or aneurysm. Supplements (a nitric oxide compound) and lifestyle routines (exercise and Mediterranean diet) help to preserve a proper nitric oxide balance.
- LDLs – Too few LDLs, nerves stop working properly and cell membranes become rigid and inefficient in passing things in and out of cells. Too much LDL, and the risk of atherosclerosis and atherosclerotic cardiovascular disease is high. The nerves stop working because the myelin sheath (like the plastic coating on wires) that helps with the transduction of electricity becomes too thin, and patients experience cognitive difficulties, muscle weakness, and coordination issues. Supplements (omega-3 fatty acids in the form of fish oils) and lifestyle routines (exercise and Mediterranean diet) help to preserve a proper LDL-HDL-triglyceride balance.
- P&S activity – Too much P-activity, and the risk of depression, fatigue, exercise intolerance, GI upset (GERD), light-headedness, and sex dysfunction is high. Too little P-activity, and the risk of heart attack and stroke, as well as GI upset (Gastroparesis), and sex dysfunction is high. Too much S-activity, and the risk of anxiety, pain, sleep difficulties, high blood pressure (hypertension), diabetes, light-headedness, and sex dysfunction is high. Too little S-activity, and the risk of sex dysfunction (impotence or lack of orgasm), malaise, exercise intolerance, low blood pressure (hypotension), and light-headedness is high. Balance minimizes morbidity and mortality risk. Supplements and lifestyle routines help to preserve P&S balance, both at rest and dynamically.

A common example of the effects of an imbalance between the P&S nervous systems is metabolic syndrome (Fig. 9.9). In this case, the P&S balance involves sympathetic excess (SE). The SE is often secondary to parasympathetic excess, with both occurring simultaneously. These are not typically resting responses, which is why they are difficult to document[19] without P&S monitoring. They typically occur in response to challenges [29]. Both ANS branches excessively activated explain the symptoms of metabolic syndrome, including difficulty to manage symptoms. Since the parasympathetics set the threshold around which the sympathetics react, the typical protocol (for all such P&S imbalances, not just metabolic syndrome) for treating the ANS is to first treat the PE and then any remaining SE symptoms. This is in parallel with typical metabolic syndrome (or other disease) therapy. As PE and then SE are normalized, typically symptoms are relieved (unless a history of end-organ dys-

[19] Dynamic autonomic responses are difficult to document, because most medical tests are performed with the patient at rest (sitting or supine). However, most autonomic dysfunctions are dynamic and require dynamic tests to document them.

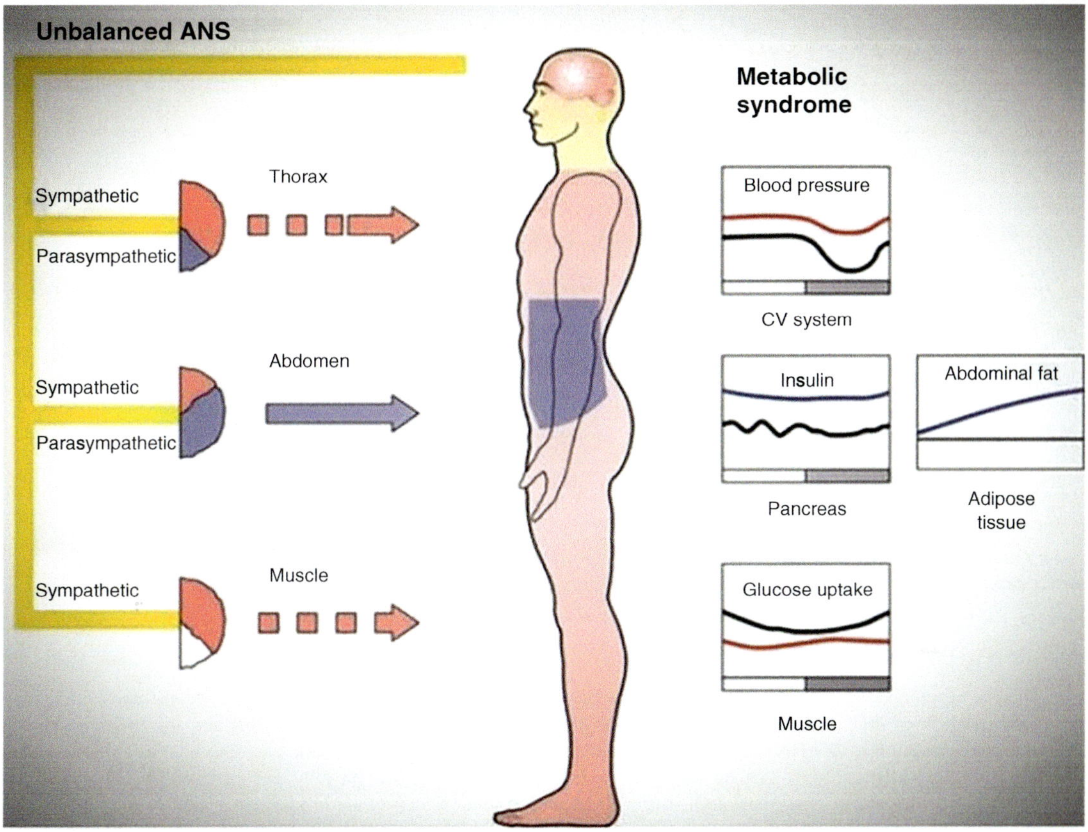


**Fig. 9.9** Parasympathetic and sympathetic (P&S) nervous system (or autonomic nervous system, ANS) imbalances, including in the abdominal and thoraco-muscular regions, are known to underlie metabolic syndrome. The result includes hypertension, increased insulin resistance, and abdominal obesity [52, Fig. 5.35]. (Republished with permission from Springer International Publishing AG)

function). As symptoms are relieved, consider weaning from therapy (if the patient does not wean themselves), both P&S therapy and the primary disease therapy. With the P&S nervous systems "re-trained" (like the rest of the nervous system they are able to learn, either chemically through pharmaceuticals or nutraceuticals or through lifestyle modifications such as exercise and diet), the nervous systems and their control of the organs may carry forward without chemical therapy to help maintain their proper balance.

## Breast Cancer, Oxidative Stress, and Cardiovascular Disease

Breast cancer therapy, while very effective, carries a significant risk of therapy-induced cardiovascular disease [183–185], a dose-dependent risk of heart failure and cardiomyopathy, and an increased incidence of cardiotoxicity. Oxidative and nitrosative stress (reactive oxygen and nitrogen species, RONS) and endothelial dysfunction may be central to cancer therapy-induced cardiovascular disease. Oxidants (e.g., superoxide) react with several molecules, suggesting that the pathways involved are likely to be multiple and complex. One molecule is nitric oxide. These reactions result in the production of RONS, disrupting cellular redox balance, thereby, further increasing oxidative or nitrosative stress [186–188]. Higher circulating levels of oxidative stress are associated with increased cardiovascular risk in breast cancer patients [189, 190]. Endothelial dysfunction further promotes cardiovascular disease by disrupting normal interactions between endothelial cells and cardiomyocytes through signaling factors such as nitric oxide, vascular

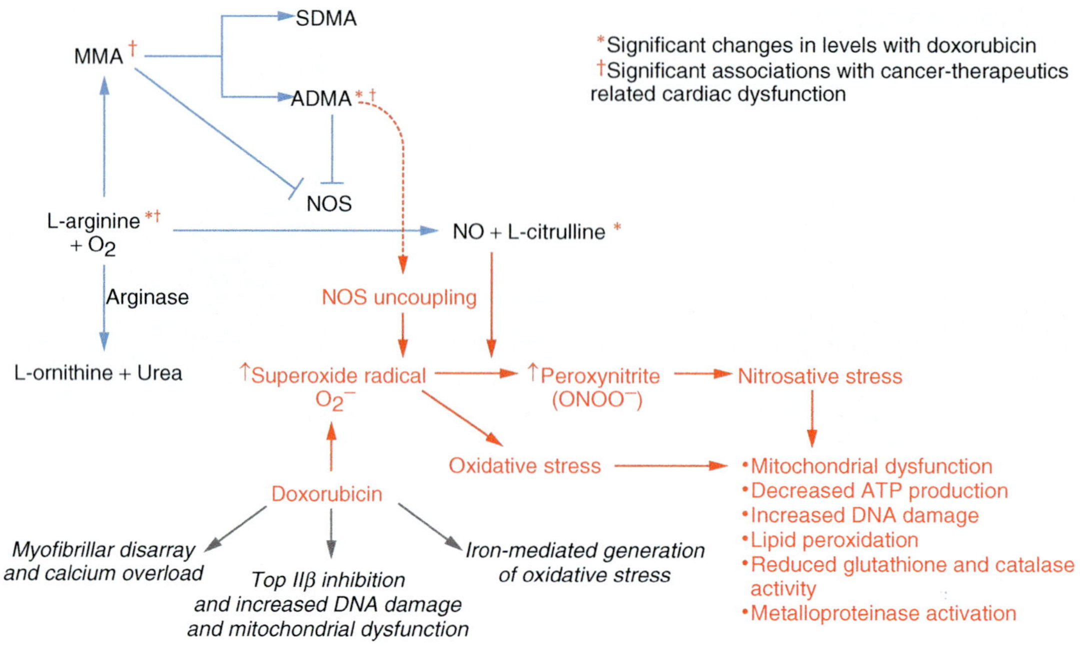


**Fig. 9.10** Pathophysiology of nitric oxide production, arginine metabolism, and anthracycline-induced cardiotoxicity. Anthracycline is an effective breast cancer therapy. L-Arginine (substrate) is oxidized by nitric oxide synthase (NOS) to form citrulline and nitric oxide. Alternatively, L-arginine can be catabolized by arginase to form ornithine or shunted to the methylation pathway to form N-monomethylarginine (MMA), symmetric dimethylarginine (SDMA), and asymmetric dimethylarginine (ADMA). Both MMA and ADMA inhibit NOS. Anthracycline-induced cardiotoxicity occurs through formation of superoxide radical, a potent cause of oxidative stress. The superoxide interacts with a variety of molecules, including nitric oxide, to produce toxic peroxynitrites that lead to further nitrosative stress. Reductions in nitric oxide can also lead to anthracycline-induced cardiotoxicity by disrupting the beneficial physiological effects of nitric oxide on normal, well-functioning endothelium. Doxorubicin also results in calcium overload and myofibrillar disarray, topoisomerase (Top)-IIb inhibition, which may further exacerbate oxidative stress via alterations in the transcriptome and iron-mediated generation of oxidative stress. Abbreviations: ATP adenosine triphosphate; DNA deoxyribonucleic acid [197]. (Republished with permission from Elsevier)

endothelial growth factor (VEGF), and neuregulin-1 [191, 192] and by leading to increases in BP and afterload [193]. These increases exacerbate cardiovascular diseases, resulting in worse oxidative stress and cardiomyocyte and endothelial cell dysfunction [192, 194, 195].

The arginine-nitric oxide metabolic pathway (see Fig. 4.33), which has been implicated in a variety of cardiovascular disease states [196], plays a central role in both cellular oxidative and nitrosative stress and endothelial dysfunction (Fig. 9.10). Nitric oxide is an essential molecular mediator of normally functioning endothelium. Reductions in nitric oxide bioavailability lead to DNA damage, lipid peroxidation, cardiomyocyte apoptosis, endothelial cell dysfunction, and reduced cardiac contractility [198, 199]. L-Arginine, a key substrate in nitric oxide production, can be alternatively catabolized to urea or converted to N-monomethylarginine (MMA), which results in nitric oxide synthase (NOS) inhibition and less nitric oxide bioavailability. MMA is a precursor to two amino acid derivatives: asymmetric dimethylarginine (ADMA), which potently inhibits NOS, and symmetrical dimethylarginine (SDMA), which is inactive against NOS. Increased level of ADMA, as an inhibitor of endothelial NOS, is a predictor of cardiovascular mortality in individuals with coronary artery disease [200], myocardial infarction [201], and heart failure [202] and is an independent risk factor for heart failure, hypertension, coronary artery disease, diabetes, and renal dysfunction [203].

Today, with breast cancer (like many cancers), the good news is that cancer has a much higher chance of being relieved than even a generation ago. However, the cancer therapy is likely to also significantly affect quality of life, including the effects of cardiovascular disease (e.g., lightheadedness, GI upset, sleep and sex dysfunction, hypertension). It is likely that cancer therapy causes these quality of life deficits through changes in arginine-nitric oxide metabolism, specifically in the balance between arginine, ADMA, and MMA. These imbalances manifest as P&S imbalances. Establishing and maintaining a proper antioxidant-oxidant balance, or better, a significant antioxidant reserve, and a nitric oxide reserve to be available buffers the effects of cancer therapy. Supplements (antioxidants such as alpha-lipoic acid, Co-Q10, vitamins, and nitric oxide) and lifestyle routines (exercise as the most powerful of antioxidants, Mediterranean diet providing antioxidants and nitric oxide, and stress reduction which is also an antioxidant) help to preserve a proper antioxidant-oxidant balance, by establishing and maintaining an antioxidant and nitric oxide buffer that the body may draw on in times of stress, including with both the cancer and the cancer therapy. As always, consult with your physician before starting anything new. For example, antioxidants may interfere with the oxidative agents used to kill (burn) the cancer cells.

## Chronic Fatigue Syndrome

Chronic fatigue syndrome (CFS) is also known as systemic exertion intolerance disease, or myalgic encephalomyelitis. CFS, which has a very specific set of criteria upon which it is diagnosed, is differentiated from "persistent" fatigue (see the later section of this chapter), which applies to everyone else who is *persistently* fatigued. CFS is a complex of symptoms characterized by fatigue for a long period of time, usually more than 6 months, in which a person's daily activities are significantly curtailed. A great majority of patients become disabled or are unable to maintain gainful employment. Also, quality of life is severely affected. There are many definitions for the term "chronic fatigue syndrome" or the alternates. These definitions have changed over time. Significant problems with post-exertional fatigue are a hallmark of this syndrome. Also, sleep problems, autonomic dysfunction with orthostatic-related symptoms, cognitive impairment, and memory impairments are part of the disorder.

It is estimated that over 880,000 and possibly over 2.5 million Americans are affected with CFS [204]. In 2003, the Canadian consensus definition was written to aid and diagnose on the basis of symptoms of chronic fatigue. These criteria were further developed into the 2011 International Consensus Criteria [205, 206]. The cause of CFS is not known. Dysregulation of the autonomic nervous system has been implicated. Infection, immune system abnormalities, mitochondrial dysfunction, and genetics may also contribute to the etiology (and autonomic dysfunction). However, CFS is correlated with autonomic disease [207–211] and mitochondrial disease [212–214] and may be a result of both. Studies on genetics have shown a familial predisposition of CFS, although the studies have been small. Because CFS may cause sore throat, lymphadenopathy, arthralgias, and muscle pain, it has been linked to the immune system and inflammatory process. Most of the studies have been inclusive regarding characteristic immune features of chronic fatigue syndrome.

CFS is classified by the WHO as a chronic neurological condition [215]. CFS symptoms including palpitations, bowel and bladder dysfunction, dizziness, and temperature dysregulation are commonly seen and are regulated by the autonomic (P&S) nervous system. This strongly suggests that P&S nervous system dysfunction is key in CFS. In fact, there is overlap between orthostatic intolerance and postural BP drops (postural hypotension) and multiple sclerosis and CFS [216]. The strongest relationship between CFS and the P&S nervous systems is shown between the association of CFS and postural orthostatic tachycardia syndrome (POTS). In POTS, the HR responses are abnormal to standing position. A similar cause of mechanism with POTS and CFS has been postulated by many investigators [211, 217]. However, P&S monitoring often finds challenge parasympathetic excess [29] more often than POTS; both produce similar symptoms. The hypothalamic-pituitary axis

(HPA, see Fig. 8.3) has also been implicated in the cause of CFS with dysregulation of this axis being seen in many patients. Reduced cortisol levels and decreased variability of the HPA axis have been found [218, 219], but some of these results have also been inconsistent [219, 220].

Inflammation has been implicated. Inflammation is one of many sympathetic functions. Cytokines and proteins have been shown to be abnormal in CFS, including various interleukins and tumor necrosis factors. However, again, studies have been inconsistent in these findings. The role of the immune system has been conflicting. Prognoses of CFS have had variable numbers. Studies point to patterns of recovery: 0–20% a full recovery, 8–63% some improvement in symptoms, 5–20% have worsening symptoms, 24–57% report no change [221]. Cost and expenditure of money has been very significant. The P&S nervous systems are invariably affected in this disorder. Whether this is a cause and effect relationship needs to be discerned. As a result of P&S dysfunction, baroreceptor reflex may be impaired. Many studies show a relationship between CFS and P&S dysfunction. The findings are not always reproducible, however. A cross-sectional study using the COMPASS questionnaire showed that almost 90% of CFS patients experienced symptoms related to P&S dysfunction [222].

There has been some literature that suggests that controlling P&S symptoms can improve function in CFS, and effective trials of medications to treat P&S symptoms should be pursued. Studies have shown that functional ability or disability in CFS has been better predicted by P&S dysfunction [223, 224]. Orthostatic hypotension is a common P&S symptom and, as a result, a common feature of many chronic diseases, including CFS [225]. As mentioned above, POTS is another orthostatic dysfunction. POTS is a disorder of orthostatic intolerance involving increase in HR of greater than 30 bpm above the baseline without a drop in BP (without orthostatic hypotension). In POTS, growing evidence suggests an association between it and CFS. In one small study, nearly one-third of the participants within a CFS cohort presented with a diagnosis of POTS, based on hemodynamic testing [226]. Another small study found that 93% of the group had symptoms of severe fatigue and fulfilled CES criteria for CFS when assessing patients with POTS [227].

Studies need to be done with pharmaceutical agents for CFS. Midodrine has not been subject to a large randomized trial, although preliminary studies have shown that six out of ten patients with CFS had improvement in subjective or objective symptoms during 10 months of treatment with Midodrine, suggesting a potential role [228, 229]. There is no specific treatment of CFS that has been shown to be universally effective. Some studies suggest that cognitive behavioral (psychiatric) therapy may be effective. The rate of exercise therapy, going very slowly ("low and slow"), has also been shown to be effective in some instances (suggestive of parasympathetic excess as a potential etiology [29]). A number of medicines may be effective; however, there is an associated trial-and-error basis to determine to which agent a given patient may respond best. No anti-infectious agents have been shown to be universally effective. Medications used in a supportive approach are very important.

Patients must know that there is no diagnostic test that is accurate enough to prove that a person has CFS. One has to avoid the controversy of whether this is psychogenic or an organic symptom and whether it is caused by infection. Medications used to treat CFS have included centrally acting acetylcholinesterase inhibitors such as galantamine. However, studies have been negative with this agent. Intravascular immunoglobulin was beneficial in one small study, but had high adverse effects [230]. Rituximab, an anti-CD20 monoclonal antibody which depletes B cells, was shown to be effective in one small double-blind study [231, 232]. Antidepressants have been used and may be effective in depression, insomnia, and muscle aches that accompany this disorder. Most studies do not show any significant beneficial effect of antidepressants.

Double-blind studies with methylphenidate may have potential benefits; mixed effects were seen in a small study. Glucocorticoids have been useful in some studies and others not. A randomized glucocorticoid trial showed clinical improvement was reserved in response to 10 mg a day of hydrocortisone in of 1 of 32 people with CFS [233]. Other studies have been done with cytokine inhibitors, still in their infancy. Since neurally mediated hypotension has been linked to CFS, studies have been done with fludrocortisone with no significant improvement. As mentioned above, midodrine may have some beneficial effects, at least as far as it will target the orthostatic dysfunction (POTS, orthostatic intolerance, or orthostatic hypotension) associated with CFS. With cardiorespiratory (P&S) testing, abnormalities in P&S function are documented, and medications are adjusted in an attempt to get better autonomic balance, both at rest (e.g., anticholinergic or sympatholytic therapy), and dynamically (e.g., midodrine). The six-prong supplement and lifestyle routines are recommended, including (1) antioxidants such as alpha-lipoic acid, Co-Q10, and vitamins to ensure mitochondrial health to provide more energy, (2) omega-3 fatty acids to reduce inflammation and help repair P&S nerve damage, (3) nitric oxide to ensure abundant blood flow and cardiovascular health, (4) exercise as the most powerful of antioxidants, (5) Mediterranean diet to provide fuel and additional antioxidants and nitric oxide, and (6) stress reduction which is also an antioxidant. All six prongs address areas of research that have been shown to help relieve the symptoms of CFS.

## Persistent Fatigue

Chronic fatigue syndrome (CFS) addressed in the previous section of this chapter is a specific diagnosis into which the majority of fatigue patients do not fit. "Persistent" fatigue is differentiated from CFS to be able to better address the symptoms of fatigue [234]. Mitochondrial dysfunction and P&S dysfunction are considered to be biological mechanisms of fatigue. Fatigue is described as a lack of energy and mental or physical tiredness, diminished endurance, and prolonged recovery after physical activity. Mitochondrial dysfunction, including deficits in mitochondrial enzymes and excesses in oxidative or nitrosative stress, has been implicated as causes of deficits in mitochondrial energy metabolism and ATP production from fatty acid metabolism. Coenzyme Q10 was the most commonly investigated mitochondrial enzyme. Low levels of Co-Q10 were consistently associated with fatigue. Mitochondria have an essential role in energy production from oxidative phosphorylation of electrons into ATP which powers the activities of most cells. Mitochondria have been implicated in various physiologic processes including the production of reactive oxygen species (ROS[20]).

Fatigue is the hallmark of mitochondrial dysfunction. Many of these studies use cross-sectional designs that were published in the last 25 years. Eighteen of these studies investigated patients with CFS. Alternations in energy and metabolism may contribute to fatigue. As noted, many of these studies were cross-sectional and only studied patients with CFS, and the findings were inconsistent between mitochondrial biomarkers and fatigue. Reduced levels of Co-Q10 have been found in some studies and reduced levels of succinate reductase. Increased levels of ROS and decreased levels of antioxidants have been found. Fatty acid metabolism has also been impaired by evidence of abnormal carnitine levels.

Alterations in intramuscular ATP and phosphocreatine (PCR) were found in fibromyalgia patients and probably reflect a combination of an activity related to pain and dysfunction of muscle mitochondria [235]. Could mitochondrial dysfunction be a differentiating marker between CFS and fibromyalgia [236]? Mitochondrial citrates and PCR activity are significantly lower in fibromyalgia patients but not in CFS patients. Also, mitochondrial DNA content was normal with CFS patients and reduced in fibromyalgia patients. Both CFS and fibromyalgia patients had significantly increased levels of lipid peroxidation, which indicates oxidative stress-induced damage. Also, peripheral blood mononuclear

[20]In small amounts, these ROS are beneficial in "burning the trash" (waste products and worn membranes) and helping the immune systems to "burn out" invaders attempting to make one sick.

cells showed decreased levels of Co-Q10 from both CFS and fibromyalgia patients.

Another study concludes that deficiencies of various B vitamins, vitamin C, magnesium, sodium, zinc, L-tryptophan, L-carnitine, alpha-lipoic acid, Co-Q10, and essential fatty acids may have etiological relevance [237]. Deficiencies in L-creatinine, NADH, and membrane phospholipids did not demonstrate statistical relevance. Other clinical trials have shown the utility of using oral replacement supplements, such as L-carnitine, alpha-lipoic acid, Co-Q10, NADH, membrane phospholipids, and other supplements. One drawback to these studies is that the agents referenced are studied in isolation. Combinations of these agents may have significantly greater effects that they do alone. Clinical experience has been that in many cases the combination of these supplements significantly reduces the fatigue and other symptoms associated with chronic disease. Long-term use of these combinations often restores mitochondrial function, even for long-term patients with intractable fatigue.

Co-Q10 is an important component in the mitochondrial oxidative phosphorylation system. In this regard, it is an important supplement, and individuals with reduced levels, when supplemented, demonstrate increased energy production and reduced fatigue. L-carnitine is a fatty acid transporter found in all species of mammals. It plays a critical role in the process of mitochondrial beta-oxidation of fatty acids. L-carnitine supplementation has been successfully used in clinical disorders that are characterized by low concentrations of L-carnitine. In fatty acid oxidation, such as diabetes, sepsis, renal disease, and cardiomyopathy, supplemental L-carnitine restores proper fatty acid oxidation. Diet is the source of 75% of carnitine, and 25% of it is synthesized in the body, predominately within the muscle, liver, and kidneys. Creatinine in the presence of cells combines a phosphate and a mitochondrial deformed PCR. This serves as a source of high-energy phosphate released during anaerobic metabolism. Tissues with high-energy demands have high concentrations of this substance, such as the skeletal muscle and brain. Alpha-Lipoic acid as a super-antioxidant is important in mitochondrial oxidative decarboxylation reactions and is used as a treatment in complications associated with type 2 diabetes. It is also used in conditions where ceramide accumulation of mitochondria is damaging to cardiac tissues. In certain chronic conditions, these sphingolipids, especially ceramide, accumulate in mitochondria and are damaging.

Fatigue may also be induced by P&S imbalance. P&S imbalance may be induced by mitochondrial dysfunction. Parasympathetic excess (PE) is associated with low HR and low BP. Either condition causes hypoperfusion of the brain, the heart, muscles, etc. As a result, patients demonstrate subclinical depression and low energy. PE is also associated with sleep dysfunction, either non-restorative sleep, such as associated with subclinical depression typically from resting PE (low sympathovagal balance), or difficulty falling asleep[21] or frequent waking during the night, such as associated with dynamic PE (as measured during sympathetic challenge). Either condition is often relieved by low-dose anticholinergic (very low-dose antidepressant[22]).

The stresses of the typical American lifestyle significantly disrupt normal sleep patterns which both affect and are effected by mitochondrial dysfunction or P&S dysfunction causing circadian misalignment which initiates a cascade of dysfunctions that lead to disease (Fig. 9.11). Sleep dysfunction is exacerbated by aging and accelerates the aging process (Fig. 9.12). Balancing the P&S nervous system, including melatonin function, can restore proper sleep habits and provide restorative sleep (Fig. 9.13).

[21] The reason why people who faint fall down is that once horizontal, the brain and the heart are at the same level; therefore, the brain is fully perfused. If while upright all day long the brain is only marginally perfused, the brain is not fully awake. Once supine, ready for sleep, the brain is finally fully perfused and is now fully awake, even though the rest of the body is ready for sleep. If based on subclinical or clinical forms of orthostatic dysfunction, syncope, or PE, falling asleep is a problem, then lying down for 15–20 minutes about 2 hours before bedtime may help to shorten the time it takes to fall asleep, because once fully perfused the brain is able to process the day and prepare for sleep normally.

[22] Clinical doses of antidepressants, used for anticholinergic purposes, often induce additional (secondary) symptoms associated with too much anticholinergic. Remember, the P&S systems are like a pendulum; they cannot be altered with force, only gentle nudges.

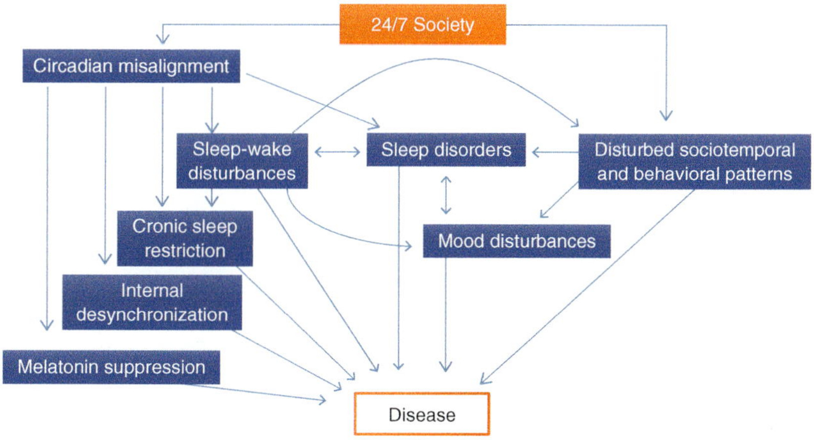


**Fig. 9.11** The impact of a 24/7 Society [52, Fig. 8.1]. (Republished with permission from Springer International Publishing AG)

Whether mitochondrial dysfunction or P&S dysfunction, all six prongs of the Mind-Body Wellness Program work to relieve and prevent fatigue.

The program provides supplements including:

- Antioxidants such as alpha-lipoic acid, Co-Q10, and vitamins to prevent oxidation of mitochondria and to energize the heart.
- Omega-3 fatty acids to establish and maintain a proper HDL-LDL balance to help keep blood flowing properly and to provide the building blocks for repair work (especially brain, nervous system, and heart) mediated by nitric oxide.
- A nitric oxide compound to maintain smooth blood vessel walls for free and abundant circulation of oxygen and nutrients throughout the body, especially to the heart and brain.

The program provides the lifestyle routines including:

- Exercise, the most powerful antioxidant to further reduce oxidation and improve cardiovascular function (*under close physician supervision*);
- Mediterranean diet to provide more omega-3s, antioxidants, and nitric oxides; and
- Stress reduction to further reduce oxidation, including from free radicals and reactive oxygen and nitrogen species.

Also, nitric oxide and antioxidant compounds provide supplements that are known to reduce depression, anxiety, and brain fog, improve restorative sleep, and more.

## Congestive Heart Failure

Approximately 6.5 million American adults are estimated to have heart failure, and the number of persons is projected to increase by 46% by 2030 [238]. Approximately half of these patients have heart failure with preserved left ventricular ejection fraction[23] [239]. There is no single disease that can be defined by a phenotype of a constellation of symptoms, blood tests, or symptoms to define heart failure, although left ventricular diastolic dysfunction, which represents stiffness of the heart or high filling pressures on the left side of the heart, seems to be a common denominator. Also associated are abnormalities occasionally with the squeezing function of the heart, stiffness in the vessels, stiffness of conduit vessels, stiffening of pulmonary vessels, and abnormal function of the right side of the heart. In addition, microvascular function, that is, the small blood vessels, is often abnormal in diastolic heart failure, as is skeletal muscle function and body composition with fat, specifically fat around the pericardium, epicardium, in between skeletal muscles in the viscera, and subcutaneously. Of interest to date, no randomized trials have really shown any

[23] An ejection fraction greater than 45% or 50%.

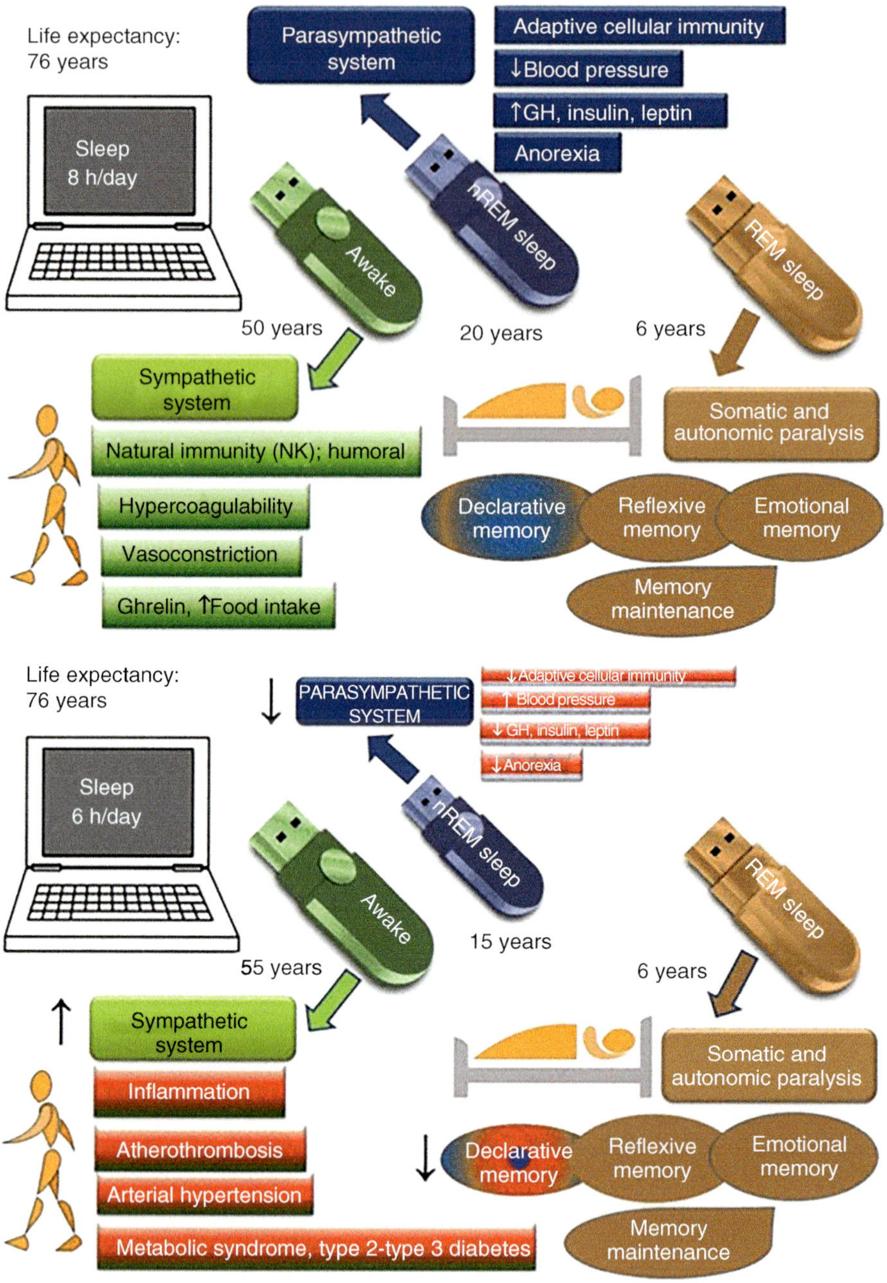


**Fig. 9.12** Three different wakefulness states (awake, slow-wave or nREM sleep, and REM sleep) must necessarily follow each other for normal health and wellness. (Upper panel) A 76 y/o sleeping 8 hrs/day will live 50 years in the physiological state or wakefulness, 20 years in nREM sleep, and 6 years in REM sleep. (Lower panel) A 25% reduction in sleep duration over the last 40 years of life leads to predominance of the wakefulness state and a reduction in nREM sleep. The effects of this reduction are associated with cardiovascular disease, metabolic syndrome, obesity, and type 2 diabetes [52, Fig. 8.2]. (Republished with permission from Springer International Publishing AG)

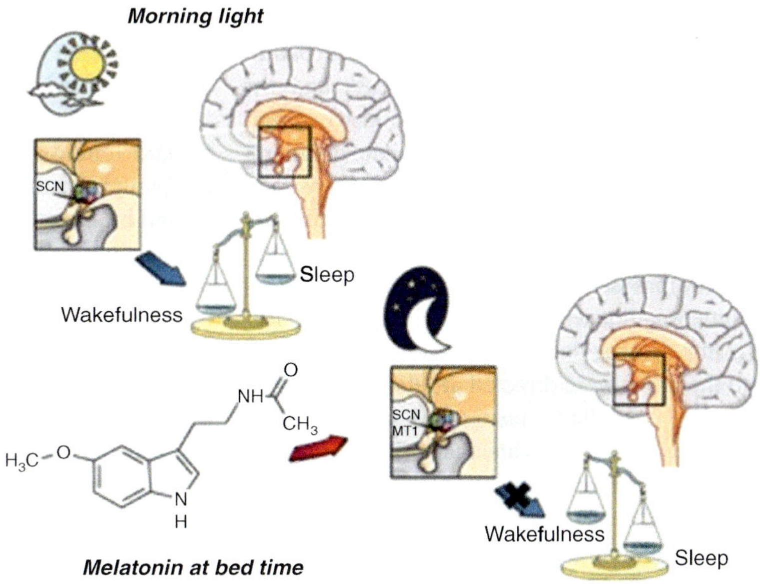


**Fig. 9.13** Parasympathetic and sympathetic (P&S) nervous system (or autonomic nervous system, ANS) imbalances, including in the abdominal and thoraco-muscular regions, are known to underlie metabolic syndrome. The result includes hypertension, increased insulin resistance, and abdominal obesity [52, Fig. 8.8]. (Republished with permission from Springer International Publishing AG)

excellent interventions to be able to treat diastolic heart failure patients.

As the population ages and as the population becomes more obese, heart failure with preserved ejection fraction is becoming to be more prevalent as the common cause of hospital admissions. The vast majority of individuals are indeed overweight with heart failure with preserved ejection fraction (HFpEF) [240]. Diabetes often accompanies obese patients with heart failure with preserved ejection fraction (HFpEF). It appears that two central abnormalities in obesity-related HFpEF exist: (1) sodium retention and (2) systemic inflammation. It appears obese people reabsorb a significant amount of sodium into the plasma volume and cause expansion, and this is related to their body mass [241].

Over time obese people's adipose tissue undergoes a biological transformation to an inflammatory state, which adversely affects the structural and function of vasculature and most visceral organs. Vascular inflammation contributes to stiffness of large arteries and great vessels and a marked reduction in capillary density, which leads to microcirculatory rarefaction [242]. Inflammation may cause microvascular abnormalities with fibrosis in the heart, kidneys, lungs, and other organs and leads to many of the comorbidities associated with HFpEF. Inflammation in epicardial tissue has recently been emphasized.

Adipose tissue inflammation has adverse effects on coronary and systemic arteries and also the microvascular endothelial system and capillaries and also has effects on impaired skeletal muscle mitochondrial function with protein synthesis that results in reduced skeletal muscle oxygen delivery and extraction [243].

Obese patients with HFpEF have large fat in abdominal and thigh adipose tissue and smaller amounts of epicardial fat (recently recognized). They also had intramuscular fluid and fat deposits. This could be measured in the thigh. The increased thigh intramuscular fat (IMF) is associated with increased anaerobic metabolism during submaximal exercise and may be related to the abnormal effects of skeletal muscle mitochondrial function. Fat volume from thigh IMF measurements is negatively associated with skeletal muscle citrate synthesis activity in sedentary older individuals. Obese people with HFpEF with obesity have decreased skeletal muscle oxidative fibers, enzyme capillaries, and mitochondrial function that result in decreased diffusion oxygen transport and impaired peak and reserve oxygen use by active muscles [244, 245].

Antidepressants such as nortriptyline have been the initial therapies. Also, using anti-seizure medicines in more advanced forms such as gabapentin and pregabalin has been used along with SNRIs, such as Cymbalta. Cognitive behavioral therapy may have small effects. Exercise can improve fitness and sleep. There is some evidence that cardiovascular exercise is effective for some people [257]. P&S dysfunction has strongly been linked with fibromyalgia. Increased levels of pro-inflammatory cytokines in fibromyalgia have been shown in one study which may increase sensitivity to pain and contribute to mood problems [258].

With implications of oxidation, inflammation, P&S dysfunction, and nitric oxide dysfunction, and no known specific therapy for fibromyalgia, antioxidants, and nitric oxide supplements are well recommended. Perhaps the combinations of therapies (anticholinergics, antioxidants, nitric oxide supplements, etc.) merely "trample" the problem, as opposed to specifically addressing the problem; however, relieving it is the goal. The fact that fibromyalgia is a multifaceted disease and that each patient seems to have an individualistic response suggests a multipronged approach and further indicates it as a P&S disorder. All six prongs of the program work to relieve fibromyalgia:

- Antioxidants such as alpha-lipoic acid, Co-Q10, and vitamins to prevent oxidation
- Omega-3 fatty acids to provide the building blocks for repair work (especially brain and nervous system)
- A nitric oxide compound to restore normal nitric oxide function
- Exercise as the most powerful antioxidant to further reduce oxidation (*under close physician supervision*)
- Mediterranean diet to provide more omega-3s, antioxidants, and nitric oxide
- Stress reduction to further reduce oxidation, including from free radicals and reactive oxygen and nitrogen species

Also, nitric oxide and antioxidant compounds provide supplements that are known to reduce depression and anxiety and brain fog and improve restorative sleep, and many of the other symptoms associated with fibromyalgia.

## Hypertension

Hypertension is usually defined by the presence of chronic elevated systemic arterial blood pressure (BP) above a certain threshold value. The threshold associated with cardiovascular risk is above approximately 115/75 mm Hg. Strictly speaking, hypertension is a progressive cardiovascular syndrome arising from complex and interrelated etiologies. Early markers of the syndrome are often present before BP elevation is sustained; therefore, hypertension cannot be classified solely by discrete BP thresholds. Progression is strongly associated with functional and structural cardiac and vascular abnormalities that damage the heart, kidneys, brain, vasculature, and other organs and lead to premature morbidity and death. Reduction of BP when target organ damage is demonstrable or the functional precursor of target organ damage is present and still reversible generally reduces the risk for CV events. Elevated BP (one manifestation of the disease) is typically separated from hypertension (the disease). This defines primary hypertension [259].

P&S monitoring helps to improve outcomes in primary hypertensives by enabling therapy to be titrated to the individual patient's specific (excessive) levels of S-activity. If after therapy, even with a decrease in resting BP, SE (albeit reduced) persists, then additional antihypertensive therapy may be safely administered without causing exercise intolerance and other side effects of low, resting S-activity. If after therapy, with a decrease in BP, the resting S-response is now too low, then the patient will become light-headed and more (other symptoms associated with hypotension) and probably not comply with the therapy, thereby remaining at risk for MACE. If after therapy resting SE is also relieved, then the patient is responding to therapy as planned. However, retesting is recommended after 6 months to ensure the patient remains normalized, for as the nervous system adapts to the therapy, it may arrive at a new set point that may lead to further symptoms that may be prevented.

## Hypertension Secondary to Parasympathetic Excess

P&S monitoring has identified some autonomic or secondary forms of hypertension. The symptoms of these secondary forms of hypertension are considered by some to be "labile" or "difficult to manage" forms of hypertension. The secondary forms presented here are secondary to autonomic or P&S dysfunction. Given that the sympathetics (including the angiotensin-renin system, a part of the sympathetic nervous system) control baroreceptor reflex which controls BP, high BP that leads to hypertension is associated with sympathetic excess (SE). Of course, high BP may also be caused by atherosclerosis, inflammation, hardening of the arteries, stress, and more, which are all associated with SE. It is known that the sympathetic nervous system is the reactionary nervous system, reacting to the threshold established by the parasympathetic nervous system. P&S monitoring has demonstrated where parasympathetic excess responses to stress induce (secondary) SEs [29], which raise BP and involve hypertension. This is a form of hypertension that often involves depression or depression and anxiety syndromes. Also vasovagal syncope involves PE (the vagal component) and may be associated with the more labile forms of hypertension with the PE causing periods of low BP and the reactionary SE causing periods of high BP.

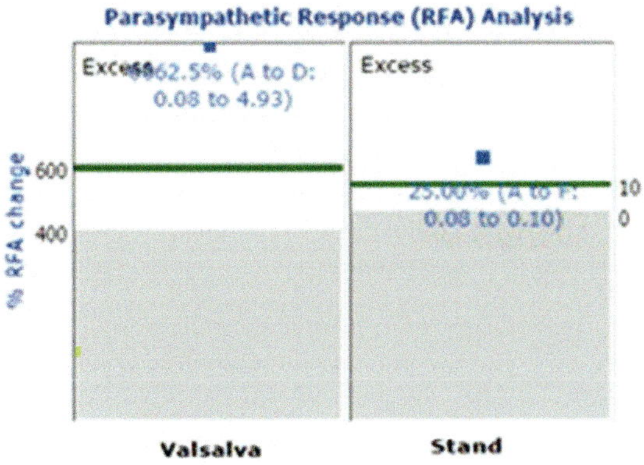


In these cases, the dynamic PE (see insert above) must be treated as the primary autonomic condition: (1) if no cardiovascular disease, consider very low-dose anticholinergic therapy, history dependent; or (2) if cardiovascular disease (CVD), switch to or titrate low-dose carvedilol to treat both PE and CVD (SE). If PE is not treated as the primary autonomic condition, SE therapy (including beta-blockers and antihypertensives) may exacerbate the PE. The SE therapy will block some of the extant sympathetic activity, enabling greater parasympathetic activity, increasing the PE. Typically, treating PE (assuming no adverse end-organ effects), thereby reducing P-activity, will organically reduce S-activity (after a month or so), which will then reduce baroreceptor reflex, which will then reduce BP and relieve the hypertension.

Note, in cases of long-standing PE, even light exercise may be perceived as a stress. Remember the parasympathetics are the "protective" branch, as well. They are also the branch that is involved in healing. Many forms of exercise break down tissue to strengthen. Even the micro-tears in cartilage during jogging will involve P-activity to heal. Alternative exercise therapy for PE must avoid as much of this as possible, as well as avoiding increasing HR and BP too fast during exercise. The goal cannot be "target HRs and BPs" as recommended in most cases.

As an alternative to pharmaceutical therapy for PE, consider a lifestyle change to include mild, intensive cardiovascular exercise, e.g., for the first 6 weeks, only zero or minimum impact or pure cardiac workouts (e.g., long easy walks[24]) to avoid any tissue breakdown that will stimulate P-activity and to avoid (at first) any significant increases in HR or BP that may be interpreted by the patient's system as a stress and exacerbate PE. The goal is to only stimulate, gently, S-activity and, thereby, retrain the autonomic nervous system to react normally to stresses. This exercise must be for 40 contiguous minutes per day (you may need to work up to this) for 6 days per week. Again, target HR or BP is not the goal. For example, after 40 minutes of walking, the patient should be able to carry on a normal conversation without being

[24]Although very easy elliptical machine workouts, swimming, etc., are also zero impact, they tend to elevate HR and BP too fast and may be perceived as stresses.

winded. They will still have increased HR and BP and sweated, but perhaps not within the first 15–20 minutes. Skipping a week starts the 6 weeks over again. Then for the remainder of the first 6 months, the exercise may be decreased to 4 days per week, maintaining a contiguous 40 minutes per event. After the 6 months and a normalization of P-activity, activities that might damage tissue may be returned. In this way the parasympathetics are (re-)trained to not overreact to stressful stimuli, making for a more normal autonomic response.

Since the first 3 of the 6 months the patient typically does not feel any different, an interim 3-month P&S test is recommended to encourage the patient. The patient is reminded that the P&S systems are foundational and must be normalized first before organ function will change and thereby symptoms will change. After PE and SE are normalized, any remaining symptoms are then treated, perhaps lifelong, depending on end-organ damage, if any.

PE may be a factor in renal ablation candidates. The findings of the SYMPLICITY HTN-3 were not as compelling as the previous two studies by the same name, primarily due, in part, to the fact that the first two were high selective of patients, and the third generalized the study population [260]. It is hypothesized that the portion of the renal ablation candidates who do not respond, in fact that their BP further increases post-ablation, is suffering from PE. The renal ablation procedure reduces SE by ablating the sympathetic innervation to the kidneys. This seems to exacerbate the (primary) PE, which in turn further increases the SE it was designed to reduce. In other words, the body, via the other sympathetic pathways, found a way to defeat the ablation therapy and, in response to the abnormal PE, maintains an abnormal SE, perpetuating or even exacerbating the hypertension.

## Hypertension Secondary to Orthostatic Dysfunction

Normally, the orthostatic response starts with a decrease in vagal or P-activity followed by an increase in S-activity, specifically alpha-S-activity (αS-activity). The increase in αS-activity (see top panel of insert below) causes the vasoconstriction of the lower-peripheral vasculature to move the blood to the abdomen to aid the heart in delivering the blood to the brain upon standing. S-withdrawal (SW, see bottom panel of insert below) is an abnormal S-response to standing (upright posture) and underlies orthostatic dysfunction, including orthostatic hypotension (OH, where SW underlies the characteristic drop in BP upon standing), orthostatic intolerance (OI, where BP and HR responses are within normal limits), and postural orthostatic tachycardia syndrome (POTS; where SW underlies the characteristic excessive HR response or tachycardia). Of course, vascular dysfunction ("lazy walls" and venous valve dysfunction) may also cause orthostatic dysfunction, as well.

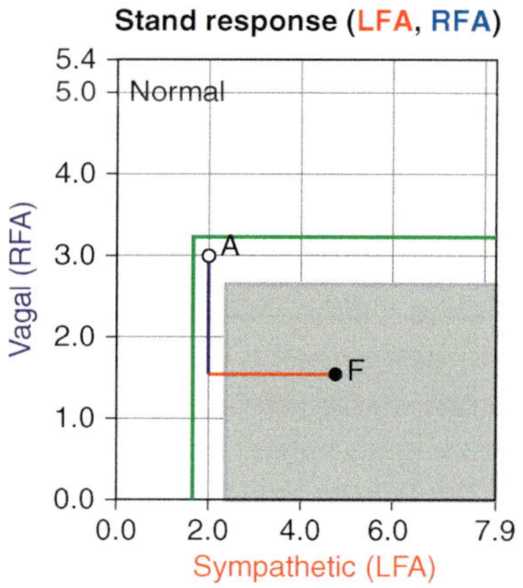


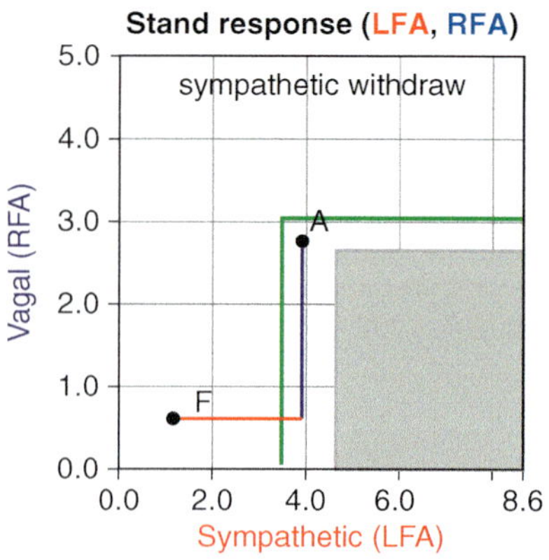

Note, the stand test helps to improve the differential diagnosis between orthostatic dysfunction (an αS-dysfunction) and syncope (a βS-dysfunction). Stand SW underlies orthostatic dysfunction. Stand S-excess (SE) underlies syncope. BP and HR responses to stand as compared with rest differentiate the subforms of syncope: vasovagal and neurogenic; cardiogenic syncope is a diagnosis by omission. In this way neurocardiogenic syncope is an actual measurement [261]. This also enables the combined diagnosis of orthostatic dysfunction and syncope concurrently, a foreign concept to most. With improved differential diagnoses, alternate therapy plans are available such as those discussed herein.

Often high BP or hypertension is found to accompany SW or orthostatic dysfunction. Note, the coexistence of SW with SE is possibly given that SW is an αS-response and SE is a βS-response. SE or high BP or hypertension seems to be compensatory for SW or orthostatic dysfunction, whether OH, OI, or POTS. Take, for example, OH. In the presence of a drop in BP, the brain becomes hypoperfused and may initiate an "adrenaline storm" to ensure proper perfusion upon standing. If this occurs often enough the frequent adrenaline surges, lead to SE. SE leads to increased (resting) BP. This may be similar to "priming the pump." If, for example, there is a 10 mmHg drop in pressure upon standing and the brain requires a 5 mmHg increase in pressure, the brain may reset the resting pressure to be 15–20 mmHg higher, so that now a 10 mmHg drop is still above the 5 mmHg increases needed in order to ensure proper perfusion with the abnormal orthostatic changes.

In these cases if the high BP or SE or hypertension were treated as the primary dysfunction, the patient would become light-headed upon standing and present with the other symptoms typical of orthostatic dysfunction. As a result, they may become non-compliant, and since high BP is asymptomatic, they feel better off the medication. Of course that leaves them at higher risk. Whereas if the SW or orthostatic dysfunction were treated as the primary disorder, as the SW is relieved, the compensatory SE may then be relieved as well, assuming no other reasons for SE [168]. In fact, in the referenced study [168], patients whose SW was relieved with the α-adrenergic agonist midodrine (2.5 mg QD, dinner), who remained on the midodrine, demonstrated an average 8 mmHg decrease in BP while still on the midodrine. Perhaps this indicates the reduction in cardiac workload as a result of the reintegration of the vasculature with the heart. For patients that do not respond to midodrine, consider reducing diuretics or increasing oral fluid and salt intake to increase plasma volume or titrating fludrocortisone or droxidopa, history dependent.

Dr. Gary Murray has recently completed a preliminary study documenting the positive effects of alpha-lipoic acid (ALA[25]) on OH and OI, including SW [262]. He finds ALA safely improved OH and OI by increasing standing αS-activity, as measured by LFa. ALA is already known to decrease resting BP (a βS-activity). Specifically, he writes, although previous human studies of the effect of ALA upon high BP have been mixed [263], it can reduce high BP, increase baroreceptor reflex afferent limb sensitivity, improve endothelial dysfunction, increase nitric oxide, and improve diabetic dysautonomia [264–270]. In the OH responders to ALA (approximately 700 mg to 1000 mg per day), mean changes in BP to standing from pre- to posttreatment were −28/−6 mmHg (sitting to standing, pretreatment) to 0/+2 mmHg (sitting to standing, posttreatment). The concurrent change in mean, resting BP was 145/73 mmHg to 126/66 mmHg. To date, there are no known other pharmacologic treatments that both decrease resting hypertension and OH. Such treatment has the potential to reduce substantially major cardiovascular events such as stroke, congestive heart failure, myocardial infarction, and cardiovascular death (MACE), as well as therapeutic costs and side effects. Nausea, rare flushing, and biotin depletion are the only known side effects of ALA and are harmless and easily treatable. The fact that ALA may also increase standing αS-activity is very positive.

[25]ALA exists as two enantiomers: r- or s-. (R)ALA is much more active than (s)ALA, and neither requires a prescription. The (r + s)ALA is the less expensive and less effective form.

## Migraine Headaches

Migraine is a disorder which occurs episodically. It is a severe headache with nausea, usually pulsation, and sensitivity to light or sound. It is extremely common in clinical practice. At one time, it was thought that vasodilation and vasoconstriction were etiological events in migraine. It is now believed that there is a relationship between migraine aura and headache that is linked to a cortical spreading phenomena where there is an actual self-propagating wave of neurological depolarization that spreads across the cortex of the brain [271, 272].

Disease classification of migraines is defined in the *International Classification of Headache Disorder*, Third Edition, ICHD-3 [273]. These classifications require at least five attacks filling the following criteria: headaches lasting 4–72 hours have at least two of the four following characteristics: (1) unilateral location, (2) pulsating quality, (3) moderate to severe pain intensity, and (4) aggravation by causing avoidance of routine physical activity, for example, walking or climbing stairs. During headache, at least one of the following should be noted: (1) nausea and vomiting and (2) photophobia and phonophobia. Also, headaches should not be better accounted for by another ICHD-3 diagnosis. Migraine validation should also include headaches with at least two of the following during the past 3 months: nausea or sickness to stomach, sensitivity to light or sound, and limited ability to work, study, or do what is needed for at least 1 day.

On the cellular level, it is believed that there is a possible role for mitochondrial dysfunction in migraine. Abnormal myocardial function translates into high intracellular penetration of calcium, excessive production of free radicals, and deficient oxidative phosphorylation which causes energy failure in neurons and astrocytes. This can trigger the migraine mechanism including the spreading depression, which is thought to be the most common mechanism [274], possibly compounded by poor brain perfusion. This is supported by the fact that there are markers of low activity of the protective superoxide dismutase enzyme which sequesters free radical and high levels of lactate and pyruvate, which are markers of increasing mitochondrial dysfunction. Migraine sufferers have also been found to have ragged red[26] in cytochrome C oxidase-negative fibers in biopsies of muscles with so-called paracrystalline inclusions. This supports the contention that mitochondrial dysfunction is associated with migraines [275].

As further data supports oxidative stress and mitochondrial dysfunction contributing to migraine phenomenon, attention has also been toward migraine and P&S nervous system dysfunction [276]. HR variability (HRV, measured at rest by the standard deviation of the beat-to-beat interval; sdNN) during deep breathing and the Valsalva maneuver (as measured by Ewing ratios) were significantly lower in disabled migraineurs compared to disabled and controls. Lower deep breathing and Valsalva ratios (Ewing ratios) indicate more advanced autonomic dysfunction. The reduction in HRV was significantly greater in females (two to three times more common in women as in men [277]) and in chronic migraine patterns when compared to new-onset cases. It appears migraineurs with disabling headaches were more susceptible to impaired P&S activity. It was postulated that the dysfunction of the P&S nervous systems may increase the tendency to headaches by lowering the threshold to migraine triggers. The fact that symptoms include nausea, vomiting, diarrhea, pallor, flushing, and diaphoresis further supports P&S dysfunction is associated [276]. Previous studies corroborate P&S imbalance in migraine [278]. It was also noted that in children with migraine, equivalents occur in abdominal pain and cyclical vomiting, which are symptoms of P&S nervous system dysfunction [279–281].

There are many triggers for migraine that could be identified: food, light, sound, odors, and so forth. Aura symptoms may often precede migraines. Usually they can include visual distur-

[26]Ragged-red fibers – clumps of diseased mitochondria accumulate in the subsarcolemmal regions' muscle fibers and appear as "ragged-red fibers" when the muscle is stained with modified Gömöri trichrome stain. It is a symptom of progressive myoclonic epilepsy. In fact, some believe that migraine with spreading depression and epilepsy are two ends of the same spectrum.

bances such as wavy lines, bright or dark spots, or sensory changes such as numbness or tingling. They also sometimes include language dysfunction, vertigo, and cutaneous allodynia, which is an exaggerated response to normal touch. Although migraines are severe, unilateral, and throbbing, it may be moderate, bilateral, and constant in quality [280]. Migraines often interfere with the ability of people to function.

Migraine is associated with other disorders including asthma, stroke, anxiety, depression, and other pain disorders [282]. Lifestyle factors may precipitate migraines or make the occurrences more frequent, such as skipping meals, irregular sleep, stress, irregular caffeine intake, and so forth. Medicines can exaggerate migraine. Postmenopausal hormone therapy, nasal decongestants, oral contraceptives, selective serotonin reuptake inhibitors, antidepressants, and proton pump inhibitors have been identified. Regular use of analgesic medicines including opiates and barbiturates and caffeine analgesics may also increase migraines [283].

There are preventative therapies for migraine. These include antihypertensive drugs, such as beta-adrenergic blockers and angiotensin receptor blockers such as candesartan; anticonvulsant agents, such as topiramate and divalproex sodium; and tricyclic antidepressants (amitriptyline and nortriptyline) as standard preventative therapies. For chronic migraine defined as more than 15 migraines per month, onabotulinumtoxin A is approved by the Food and Drug Administration. Treatment for acute migraine often employs nonsteroidal anti-inflammatory agents, multiple ergotamine preparations, and anti-emetics, particularly in patients with substantial nausea. Acetaminophen has also been used in combinations with aspirin, caffeine, and nonsteroidals with sumatriptan.

As noted, mitochondrial dysfunction has been implicated in many neurodegenerative diseases: migraine, chronic fatigue, and fibromyalgia. Antioxidants hold promise for treatment in all of these disorders. Diets rich in antioxidants are known to increase glutathione [284], such as those composed of protein with vitamins C and E, L-carnitine, alpha-lipoic acid, glutathione, broccoli, marine (fish or Krill) oil, curcumin, selenium, yeast, flavonoid, polyphenols, and carotenoid. A role for coenzyme NADH and FADH, the pyruvate dehydrogenase pathway and substrates for the PDH complex coenzyme-QA, which is derived from pantothenic acid, is suggested. B vitamins, FAD, and alpha-lipoic acid may also be helpful. There are nine intermediates in the TCA, or Krebs, cycle that require cofactor (see Fig. 2.16): cysteine, iron, niacin, magnesium, manganese, thiamin, riboflavin, pantothenic acid, and alpha-lipoic acid.

Hyperglycemia may trigger migraine, and it induces mitochondrial superoxide production by endothelial cells which is an important mediator of diabetic complications such as cardiovascular disease. Endothelial superoxide production also contributes to atherosclerosis, hypertension, heart failure, aging, sepsis, ischemia perfusion injury, and hypercholesterolemia. The antioxidants listed above are useful in combating oxidative stress.

Other points of interest in migraines include the following: (1) serotonin and activation of serotonin receptors may be involved in migraine, (2) calcitonin gene-related peptides may be involved, (3) genetics may be involved in common forms of migraines, and migraines are also associated with (4) right to left shunt, (5) emotional stress, (6) hormones in women, (7) not eating, (8) weather, (9) sleep disturbances, (10) odors, (11) neck pain, (12) lights, (13) alcohol, (14) smoke, (15) sleeping late, (16) heat, (17) food, (18) exercise, and (19) sexual activity, and (20) cutaneous allodynia such as brushing hair or touching the scalp, shaving, or wearing contact lenses may trigger allodynic symptoms during migraine [285].

With all of the different triggers, most P&S imbalances are implicated. Resting parasympathetic excess (PE) can cause poor brain perfusion leading to insufficient oxygenation or temporary drops in electrolyte levels which can trigger migraine. Parasympathetic hypofunction in migraineurs was present and a mark of poor prognosis [286]. It is also known to lead to activation and sensitization of the trigeminal system with a trigeminal parasympathetic-type reflex activation causing autonomic symptoms and signs observed in migraine attacks. Dynamic PE causing a secondary sympathetic excess (SE) can lead to overstimulation of brain centers that may trigger migraine. A similar result may be caused by (primary) resting or dynamic SE in response to even common stimuli (e.g., stress-related amplification of a normal stressor, including Valsalva-like stressors) or parasympathetic insufficiency causing a (secondary) relative SE. While the cause is important to determine etiology, it is more important in the selection and titration of therapy. In this way, P&S monitoring helps to individualize therapy, thereby improving patient outcomes.

Agents such as riboflavin, niacin, and the other B vitamins, alpha-lipoic acid, Co-Q10, magnesium, niacin, creatine, melatonin, and topiramate are agents which have a positive effect on P&S function and mitochondrial metabolites and have been shown to be effective in treatment of migraines, including decreasing frequency and pain intensity ($p = 0.03$) and improving scoring on the HIT-6 questionnaire (a headache version of the SF-36 questionnaire, see the corresponding section earlier in this chapter; $p = 0.01$) [274, 287]. Many of these treatments are included in the antioxidant, nitric oxide, and fish oil supplements recommended herein and are amplified and potentiated by the lifestyle modifications:

- Antioxidants such as alpha-lipoic acid, Co-Q10, vitamins, minerals, and amino acids to prevent oxidation and inflammation
- Omega-3 fatty acids to help prevent inflammation
- A nitric oxide compound to restore normal nitric oxide function in the brain and in the vasculature to help improve circulation
- Exercise as the most powerful antioxidant to further reduce oxidation (*under close physician supervision*)
- Mediterranean diet to provide more omega-3s, antioxidants, and nitric oxide, as well as vitamins, minerals, nutrients, amino acids, and fuel
- Stress reduction to further reduce oxidation, including from free radicals and reactive oxygen and nitrogen species

Also, nitric oxide and antioxidant compounds provide supplements that are known to reduce depression and anxiety and brain fog and improve restorative sleep and many of the other symptoms associated with migraine.

## Mitochondrial Dysfunction and Neurodegenerative Disorders

Recent data has shown that the role of mitochondria is not limited to cellular, and thereby systemic, energy production [288]. They are not only isolated power plants (Fig. 9.14) [289]. As already shown, mitochondria play a role in ROS and free radical production and the antioxidant-oxidant balance, which affects inflammatory processes and immune function and alters gene expression and protein function, which effects macromolecule biosynthesis (including hormones and others that enable cell growth and replication) [290–292]. In fact, mitochondria are not "simple" (as compared to the cell as a whole) organelles but rather should be considered "symbiotic microorganisms," with DNA of their own, and able to act and interact with each other and their surroundings, similar to the beneficial, symbiotic bacteria that exist in the gut (Fig. 9.15):

- Mitochondrial exchange information with each other via inter-organelle fusion, the release of soluble mediators, and inter-mitochondrial junctions
- Mitochondrial redox signaling shifts signal transduction pathways in the cytoplasm by modifying redox-sensitive amino acids and altering the activity of kinases, phosphatases, and proteases
- Mitochondrial metabolic intermediates and ROS travel to the nucleus where they impact epigenetic and transcriptional processes that alter gene expression profiles
- Mitochondria release signals that travel to the systemic circulation, influencing the behavior of surrounding cells and tissues, and the physiological function of neuroendocrine, cardiovascular, and nervous systems that indirectly feedback onto the brain to impact neuronal

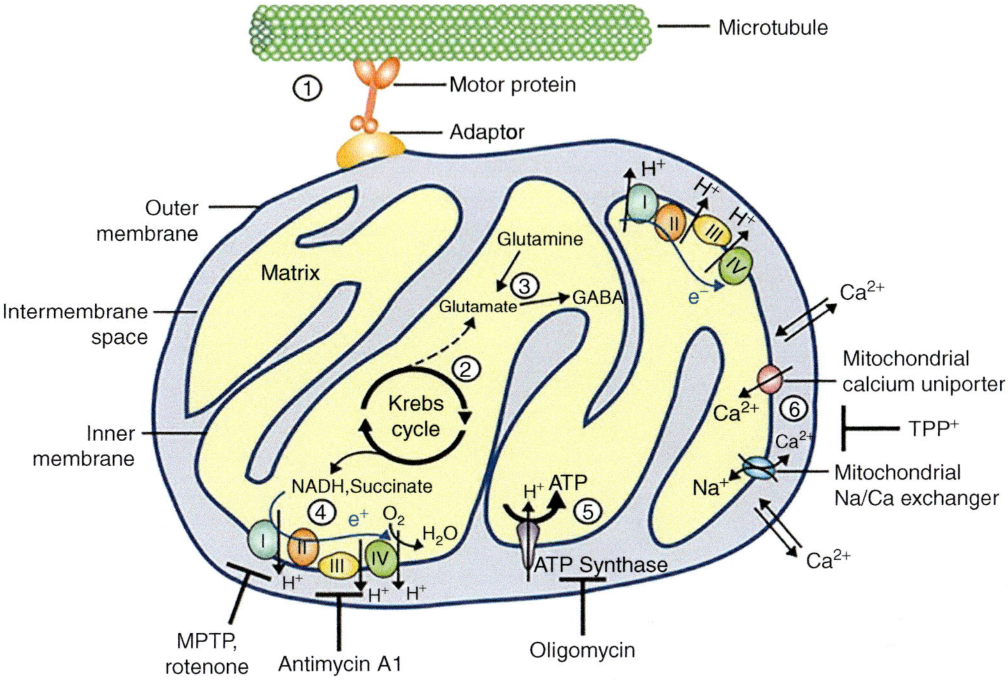


**Fig. 9.14** Mitochondrial functions which may affect neurotransmission are presented in a schematic representation of a mitochondrion illustrating mitochondrial functions. (1) Mitochondria are dynamic organelles, able to move bidirectionally along microtubule tracts with the help of motor proteins (kinesin for anterograde and dynein for retrograde axonal transport, respectively) and adaptor proteins (e.g., Milton and the associated Rho-GTPase Miro or syntabulin). Short-distance transport along actin filaments is mediated by myosin motors (not shown). (2) The Krebs cycle takes place in the mitochondrial matrix, generating α-ketoglutarate and electron donors (NADH and succinate). (3) Transamination of α-ketoglutarate yields the neurotransmitter glutamate, which can also be formed by glutamine hydrolysis. Glutamate can be further decarboxylated to yield GABA, another neurotransmitter. (4) The electron transport chain (ETC), consisting of four multiprotein complexes, mediates electron transfer (blue arrow) from NADH and succinate to the electron acceptor $O_2$. Numerous drugs target components of the ETC, for example, MPTP (1-methyl-4-phenyl-1,2,3,6-tetrahydropyridine) and rotenone affect complex I, while antimycin A1 inhibits complex III. Electron transfer is coupled with proton extrusion out of the matrix toward the intermembrane space, producing an electrochemical gradient across the inner membrane (about – 200 mV). (5) Protons ultimately return to the matrix through the ATP synthase, using the free energy produced by the ETC to drive ATP synthesis. Oligomycin is an inhibitor of the ATP synthase. (6) Mitochondria are also involved in calcium homeostasis, and $Ca^{2+}$ ions can be sequestered in the matrix under the form of a reversible phosphate complex. While the outer mitochondrial membrane is rather permeable to $Ca^{2+}$, $Ca^{2+}$ entry across the inner mitochondrial membrane is mediated by a uniporter, and its extrusion largely relies on a sodium/calcium exchanger. Mitochondrial $Ca^{2+}$ transport can be inhibited by $TPP^+$ (tetraphenylphosphonium). Close interactions between the endoplasmic reticulum (ER) and mitochondria are essential for rapid and sustained $Ca^{2+}$ uptake by mitochondria. $Ca^{2+}$ buffering by mitochondria regulates $Ca^{2+}$ release from the ER. Among other functions, $Ca^{2+}$ buffering modulates cellular (electrical) polarity. For example, in neurons mitochondria localized near $Ca^{2+}$ channels, such as N-methyl-d-aspartate receptors, accumulate $Ca^{2+}$ locally to assist in synaptic vesical transport, fusion with the cell membrane, and neurotransmitter release [289] (Open Access, Frontiers in Neuroscience)

structure (including memory) and function (i.e., cognitive behavior) and contribute to neurodegeneration

At the biochemical level, in addition to ATP synthesis, mitochondria help to regulate calcium ($Ca^{2+}$) uptake and release impacting (1) energy production regulation itself (Fig. 9.16) [293], (2) intracellular signaling and vesicular endocytosis (Fig. 9.17) [295], and (3) mitochondria and cell death (autophagy (Fig. 9.18) and apoptosis (Fig. 9.19), respectively) [296, 297].

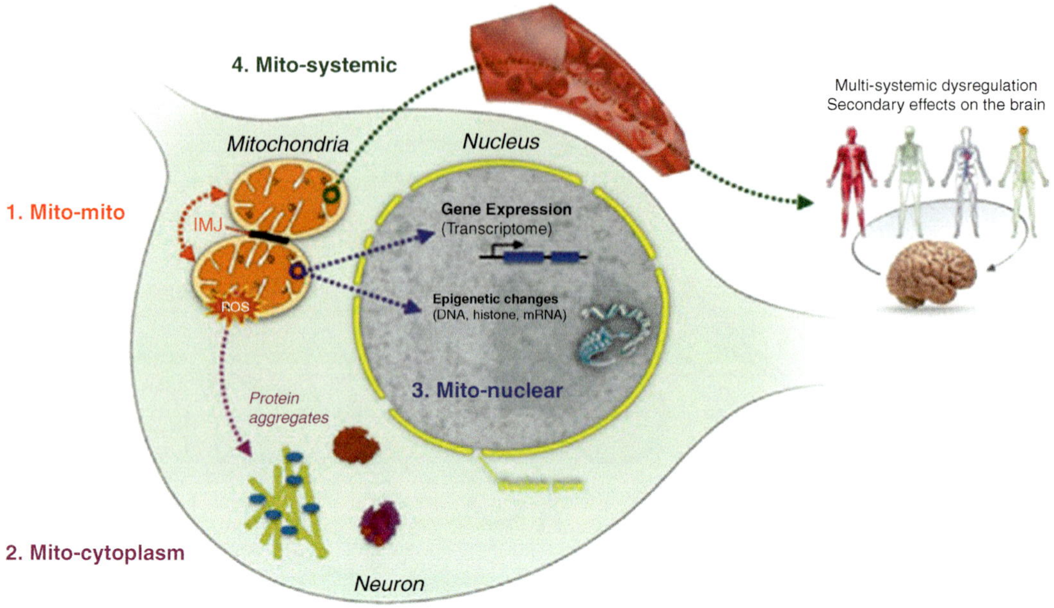


**Fig. 9.15** Overview of mitochondrial signaling. (1) Mitochondrial exchange information with each other via inter-organelle fusion, the release of soluble mediators, and inter-mitochondrial junctions (IMJ). (2) Mitochondrial redox signaling shifts signal transduction pathways in the cytoplasm by modifying redox-sensitive amino acids and altering the activity of kinases, phosphatases, and proteases. (3) Mitochondrial metabolic intermediates and ROS travel to the nucleus where they impact epigenetic and transcriptional processes that alter gene expression profiles. (4) Mitochondria release signals that travel to the systemic circulation, influencing the behavior of surrounding cells and tissues and the physiological function of neuroendocrine, cardiovascular, and nervous systems that indirectly feedback onto the brain to impact neuronal structure (including memory) and function (i.e., cognitive behavior) and contribute to neurodegeneration [288, Fig. 5.1]. (Republished with permission from Springer International Publishing AG. Source: [184])

As an example of mitochondrial signaling at the cellular level, in the neuron, presynaptic $Ca^{2+}$ influx triggers synaptic vesicle (SV) exocytosis and modulates subsequent SV endocytosis. A number of $Ca^{2+}$ clearance mechanisms are present in central nerve terminals that regulate intracellular free $Ca^{2+}$ levels both during and after stimulation. During action potential stimulation, mitochondria rapidly accumulate presynaptic $Ca^{2+}$ via the mitochondrial $Ca^{2+}$ uniporter (MCU, Fig. 9.20 [298]). The accumulated $Ca^{2+}$ is a local phenomenon, helping to maintain depolarization near the end of the presynaptic neuron, assisting in, and providing the energy for, SV transport, SV fusion with the cell membrane, and neurotransmitter release (SV exocytosis), and reuptake (SV endocytosis) [288].

As an example of mitochondrial signaling at the system level, mitochondrial ("bioenergetic") control of substantia nigra pars compacta (SNc) dopaminergic (DA) neurons appears to have both feedback and feed-forward mechanisms (Fig. 9.21). In general, feedback mechanisms control static levels of DA and feed-forward mechanisms to regulate (up or down) "spike-driven" DA levels under excessive (both high and low) conditions.[27] $Ca^{2+}$ entry drives oxidative phosphorylation in anticipation of need (feed-forward mode), rather than in response to a drop in ATP levels (feedback mode). Feed-forward

[27] In the brain, DA affects emotions, movements, and your sensations of pleasure and pain. Too little DA in the brain may cause muscle cramps, spasms, or tremors. Aches and pains and in the extreme Parkinson's disease. Too much DA in the brain is linked to suspicious personality, paranoia, and withdrawal from social situations. Drugs, such as amphetamines and cocaine, cause buildup of DA, which leads to drug-induced psychosis or schizophrenia.

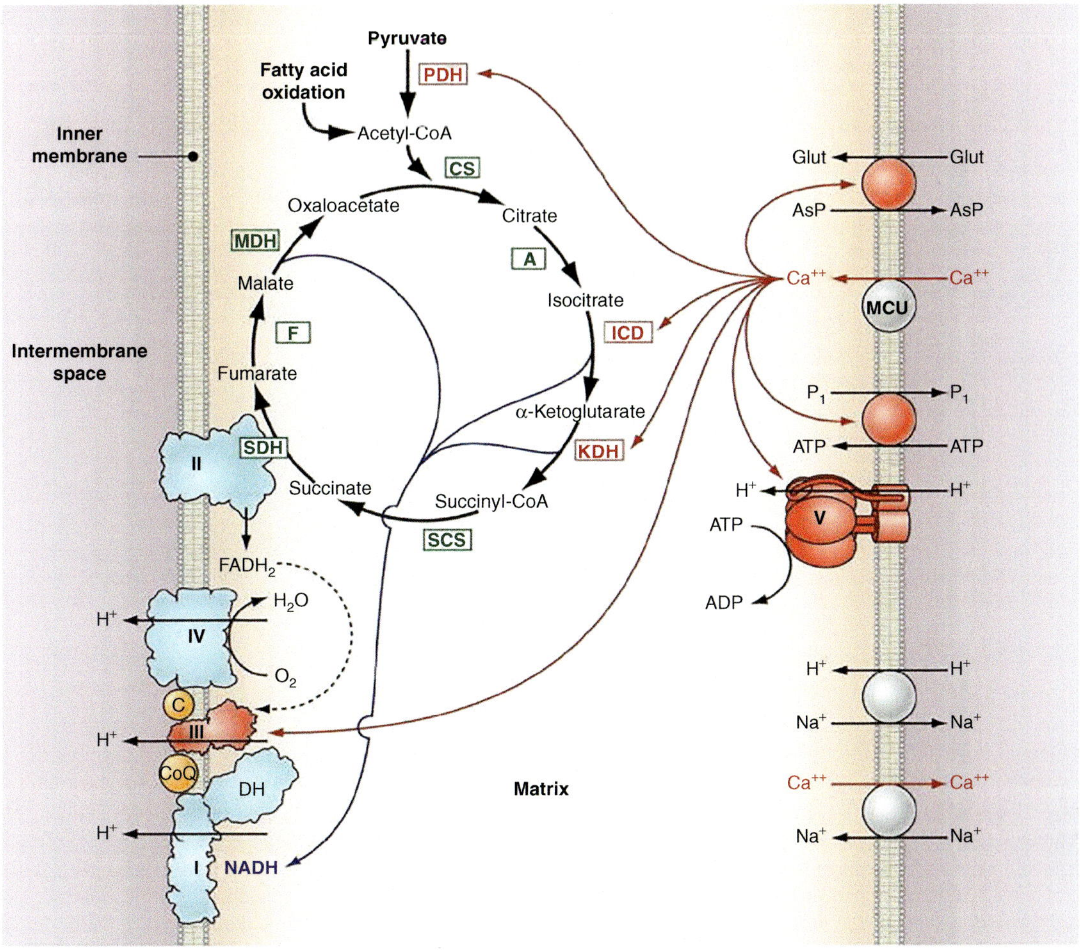


**Fig. 9.16** Schematic diagram of the interaction of matrix $Ca^{2+}$ with processes involved in oxidative phosphorylation. $Ca^{2+}$ is a primary candidate as the molecular signal in the maintenance of the cellular metabolic homeostasis. The activation of metabolism by $Ca^{2+}$ in cells is apparently distributed over many elements of oxidative phosphorylation. The best evidence for $Ca^{2+}$ activation downstream of the dehydrogenases is a $V_{max}$ activation of complex V, but the specific mechanisms remain elusive. Thus, it is evident that $Ca^{2+}$ is playing a much more integrative role in the regulation of mitochondrial energy metabolism that exceeds a simple activation of dehydrogenases and may include a systemic activation of the metabolic network contributing to the overall metabolic homeostasis of the cell. Enzyme abbreviations: PDH pyruvate dehydrogenase, CS citrate synthase, A aconitase, ICD isocitrate dehydrogenase, KDH α-ketoglutarate dehydrogenase, SCS succinyl-CoA synthetase, SDH succinate dehydrogenase (also complex II), F fumarase, MDH malate dehydrogenase, MCU mitochondrial calcium uniporter. The complexes of oxidative phosphorylation are labeled as roman numerals from I to V. The DH on complex I refers to the intrinsic and possibly associated NADH dehydrogenase activity. The red arrows from $Ca^{2+}$ to the different interaction sites imply either a direct or indirect modulation of the transport or enzymatic activity [293, Fig. 4]. (Republished with permission from American Chemical Society. Source: [292])

control, associated with pacemaking, is well-established in cardiac cells and is emerging in the regulation of SNc DA cells. SNc pacemaking is thought to be associated with motor learning, reward motivation, memory, and cognition. Dysfunction in SNc pacemaking, including as a result of acquired mitochondrial dysfunction may lead to schizophrenia, addiction, obsessive-compulsive disorder, depression, Parkinson's disease, and attention-deficit and hyperactivity disorder. The feed-forward mechanism is critical in preventing energy depletion in

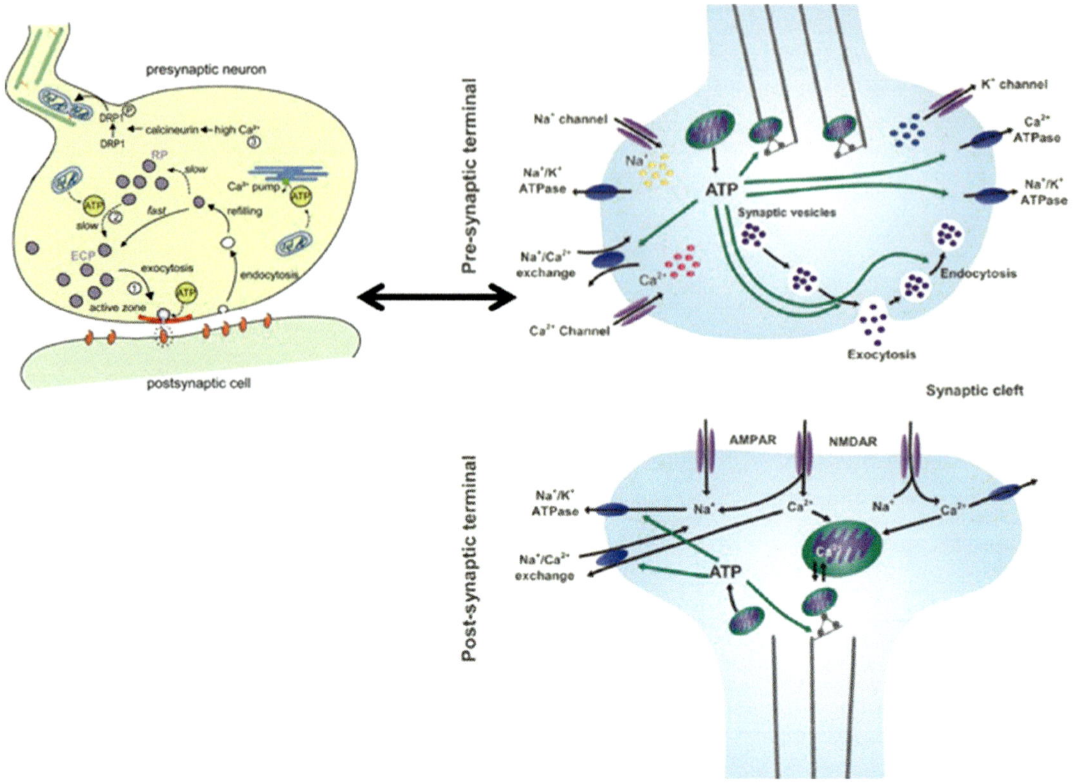


**Fig. 9.17** Synaptic mitochondrial functions. Mitochondria are enriched at synaptic sites (axonal terminals and neuronal dendrites), where their function is crucial for synaptic transmission. Left: schematic representation of a mitochondrial involvement in the organization of presynaptic vesicle pools. (1) Synaptic vesicles (SVs) from the exo- and endocycling pool (ECP) participate in neurotransmitter release at active zones (in red). Upon arrival of an action potential at the nerve terminal, these vesicles fuse with the presynaptic membrane and discharge neurotransmitters in the synaptic cleft. (2) In contrast, SVs from the reserve pool (RP), which contains the majority of vesicles in most synapses, are tethered to cytoskeletal elements and are only recruited to the active zone during intense stimulation. This recruitment of the RP depends on ATP produced by the mitochondria. (3) The ATP produced by the mitochondria also plays an important role for presynaptic $Ca^{2+}$ buffering in the endoplasmic reticulum (ER). High $Ca^{2+}$ induced by exo- and endocytosis activates calcineurin that in turn activates and dephosphorylates DRP1, resulting in mitochondrial fission and transport. Right: in addition to the above, at the presynaptic terminal, mitochondrion-generated ATP is used to also regulate ionic fluxes necessary for action potential propagation (via fueling ATPases) and motor-protein-assisted organelle transport to/from the synapse. Postsynaptic mitochondria are essential for synaptic transmission preservation since mitochondrial ATP production and $Ca^{2+}$ buffering capacities are key for reversing ionic gradients generated following transmitter release and uptake. Left: [289, Fig. 2] (Open Access, Frontiers in Neuroscience). Right: [294, Fig. 9.1], republished with permission from Springer International Publishing AG.(Sources: left: [279], right [295])

acute high-stress conditions (e.g., normal, sympathetically mediated fight or flight situations). Similar to over-activation of feed-forward control of pacemaking in cardiac cells (which paradoxically may lead to arrhythmia, including ventricular tachyarrhythmia which may lead to sudden death), over-activation of mitochondria driven $Ca^{2+}$ drive feed-forward control in SNc cells may paradoxically lead to depression, depression-based anxiety, attention-deficit hyperactivity, addiction, obsessive-compulsive disorder, as well as schizophrenia and Parkinson's diseases.

Mitochondria-cellular signaling are from mitochondria-generated diffusible signals that are communicated to both the cytoplasm and cell nucleus. Many of these signals ultimately alter signal transduction pathways and protein processing. Mitochondrial signals, including metabolic intermediates, are also the epigenetic language that directs chromatin accessibility.

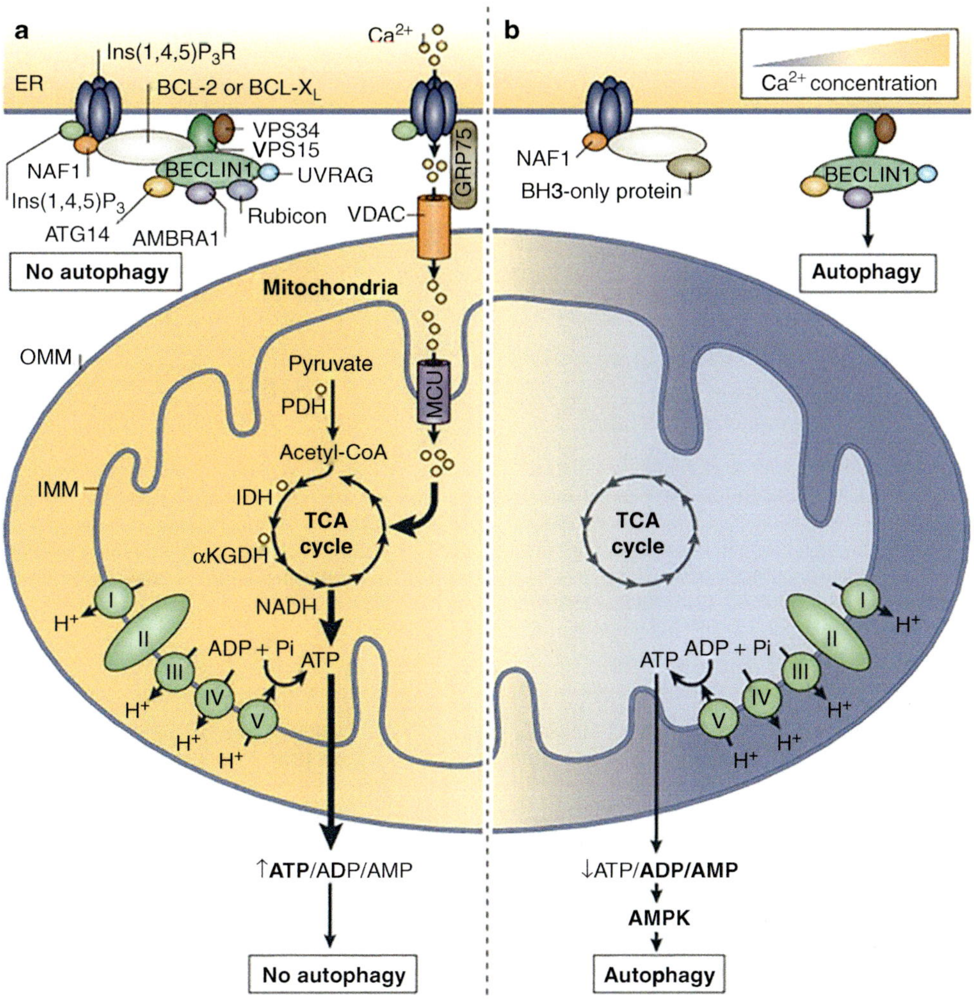


**Fig. 9.18** The regulation of aerobic metabolism and mitochondrial autophagy. (a) Conditions that inhibit autophagy. (b) Conditions that promote autophagy. A reduction in ATP synthesis, with a buildup of ADP and AMP leads to mitochondrial autophagy. One mechanism that may cause mitochondrial autophagy is the buildup of oxidants, including ROS and free radicals generated by the mitochondria themselves. TCA cycle – tricarboxylic acid cycle, aka, Krebs cycle [296, Fig. 4]. (Republished with permission from Springer Nature.Source: [295])

Mitochondria-cellular signaling helps to mediate responses to stress and inflammation, including neurodegenerative pathogenesis (Fig. 9.22).

In neurodegenerative diseases, microglia become "primed" and contribute to inflammatory changes within the brain. Under acute conditions, this is normal and helpful. Under chronic conditions, this may actually perpetuate the damage, for once the microglia consume the dead and dying matter, they may turn on the developing, regenerating, or non-mature structures, preventing the damaged structure from fully healing. Parasympathetic activity aids in the activation of microglia. Empirically, it has been noted that chronic parasympathetic excess is also involved in chronic microglia activation.

Figure 9.23 depicts a current hypothesis linking neuronal mitochondrial dysfunction and the initiation of microglial activation through the release of immunogenic signals of stress (SOS). Mitochondrial SOS include ROSs and damage-associated molecular patterns or DAMPs; mtDNA, RNA, and N-formyl peptides that activate toll-like receptors 4 and 9 (TLR4, TLR9), thereby inducing the innate immune response from microglia and systemic macrophages. In the aging brain, chronic

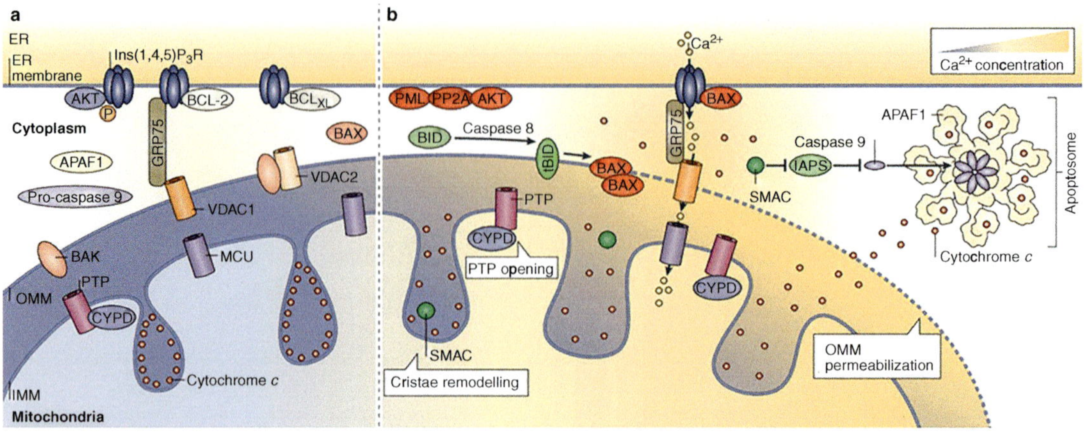


**Fig. 9.19** Mitochondrial $Ca^{2+}$ signals in the regulation of cell death pathways. (a) Conditions that prevent massive $Ca^{2+}$ transfer from the endoplasmic reticulum (ER) to mitochondria through proper regulation of the $Ca^{2+}$ channels, including (1) inositol-1,4,5-trisphosphate (Ins(1,4,5) P3) receptor (Ins(1,4,5)P3R)), (2) voltage-dependent anion channel (VDAC), and (3) the mitochondrial $Ca^{2+}$ uniporter (MCU), generally protect cells from cell death by necrosis (not shown) and apoptosis. (b) Excessive opening of the $Ca^{2+}$ channels enables the massive transfer of $Ca^{2+}$, leading to apoptosis and possibly necrosis [296, Fig. 5]. (Republished with permission from Springer Nature. Source: [295])

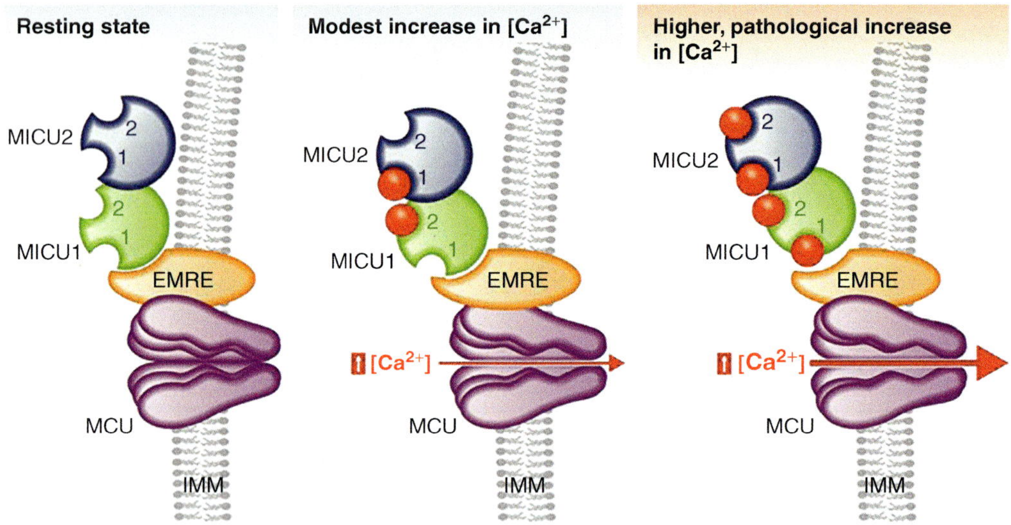


**Fig. 9.20** The uniporter complex is composed of the pore-forming mitochondrial $Ca^{2+}$ uniporters (MCU), MICU1 and MICU2, which are connected by essential MCU regulator (EMRE). In the resting state, EMRE recruits MICU1 and MICU2 to MCU to keep MCU in the closed state. Modest increase in $Ca^{2+}$ concentration ($[Ca^{2+}]$) above about 2–3 μM results in binding of $Ca^{2+}$ to site #2 of MICU1 and site #1 of MICU2 to increase MCU open probability without disrupting the complex. Higher, pathological increase in $[Ca^{2+}]$ results in $Ca^{2+}$ binding to all MICU sites locking MCU in the open state resulting in large mitochondrial $Ca^{2+}$ accumulation. Binding of $Ca^{2+}$ to all sites may partially dissociate the MCU complex, releasing MICU1 and MICU2 [298]. (Source: [297])

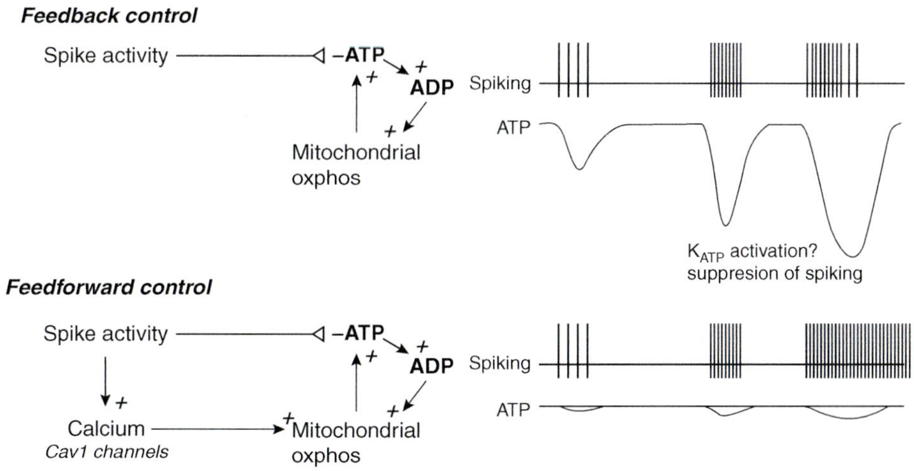


**Fig. 9.21** Schematic representation of feedback (top) and feed-forward (bottom) metabolic control of mitochondrial respiration. Hypothetical changes in cytosolic ATP levels are also shown, $Ca^{2+}$ influx through Cav 1 channels during pacemaking triggers $Ca^{2+}$-induced $Ca^{2+}$ release from endoplasmic reticulum stores, which prolongs oxidative phosphorylation ("oxphos") which ultimately increases ATP synthesis to enable prolonged action potentials and the neuronal depolarization needed for pacemaking [288, Fig. 6.2]. (Republished with permission from Springer International Publishing AG. Source: [287, Fig. 6.2])

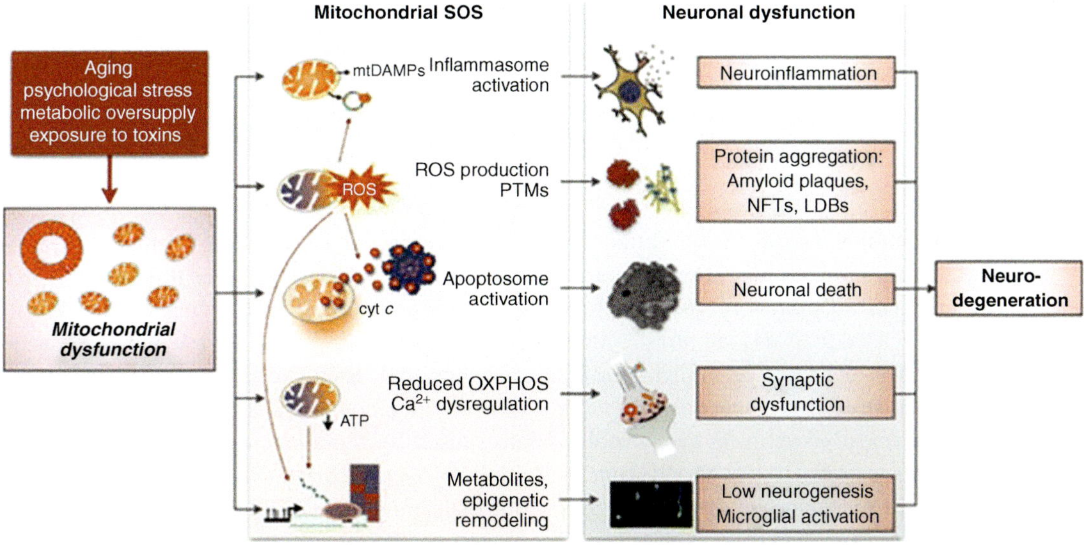


**Fig. 9.22** Mitochondrial signals of stress: from mitochondrial dysfunction to neurodegenerative disease. Common stressors such as aging, psychological and metabolic stress, and exposure to toxins cause mitochondrial dysfunction and aberrant morphology, including donut-shaped mitochondria. Mitochondria respond by sending signals of stress (SOS), which induces molecular changes within the cytoplasm and nucleus that directly contribute to the established hallmarks of neurodegenerative diseases, including protein aggregates and transcriptional dysregulation. Abbreviations: OXPHOS oxidative phosphorylation, "Cyt c" cytochrome C, PTMs posttranslational modifications, NFTs neurofibrillary tangles, LBs Lewy bodies [288, Fig. 5.2]. (Republished with permission from Springer International Publishing AG. Source: [287, Fig. 5.2])

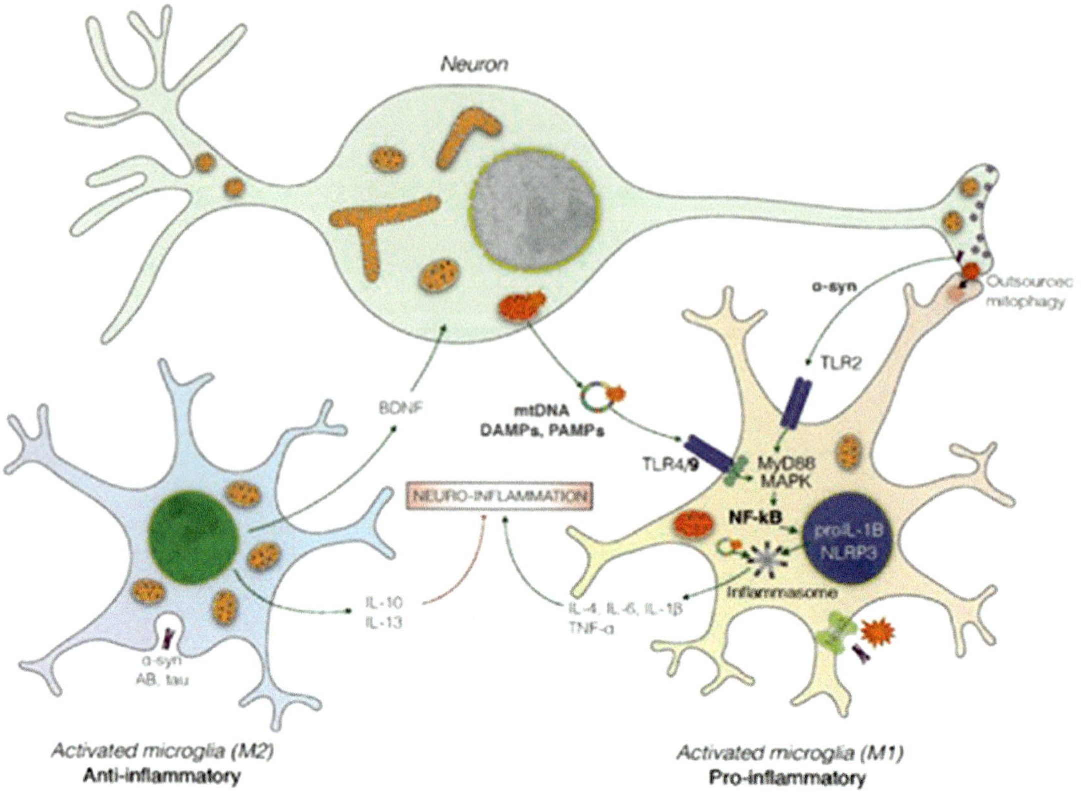


**Fig. 9.23** Mitochondrial signals of stress and neuro-inflammation. See text for details [288, Fig. 5.3]. (Republished with permission from Springer International Publishing AG. Source: [287, Fig. 5.3])

stimulation by mitochondrial SOS shifts the response of "primed" microglia from primarily phagocytic and anti-inflammatory (M2) to pro-inflammatory (M1) and induces their proliferation. TLR4/9 stimulation activates M1 microglia by MyD88 or mitogen-activated protein kinases (MAPK), which sends NF-κB from the cytosol to the nucleus to induce proIL-1β and NLRP3 (nucleotide-binding domain, leucine-rich-repeat containing family, pyrin domain-containing 3) transcription. When activated oxidized mtDNA, the NLRP3-inflammasome cleaves pro-capase-1 and induces the release of cytokines (IL-4, IL-8, IL-1B, and TNF-α) that promote neuro-inflammation, gliosis, and neuronal damage. Secondary insult from protein aggregates or glucocorticoids may exaggerate this response in sensitive brain regions, contributing to the mood disorders, cognitive decline, and cell death associated with neurodegenerative disease. Microglia may also contribute to elimination of dysfunctional mitochondria within the axon terminal, in a process whereby neurons outsource mitophagy [288].

There are two general categories of mitochondrial dysfunction: genetic and acquired. Genetic mitochondrial diseases are not addressed herein. Genetic mitochondrial dysfunctions are those that are caused by mutations in either the mitochondrial DNA or nuclear DNA that lead to dysfunction of the mitochondria and inadequate production of energy. Those caused by mutations in mitochondrial DNA are transmitted by maternal inheritance. Those caused by mutations in nuclear DNA may follow an autosomal dominant, autosomal recessive, or X-linked pattern of inheritance. Acquired mitochondrial dysfunctions are addressed herein. Acquired mitochondrial dysfunctions are those that may be slowed or reverse with a proper antioxidant-oxidant balance, a proper autonomic balance, a proper nitric oxide environment to promote proper oxygenation through proper blood flow, and proper glucose

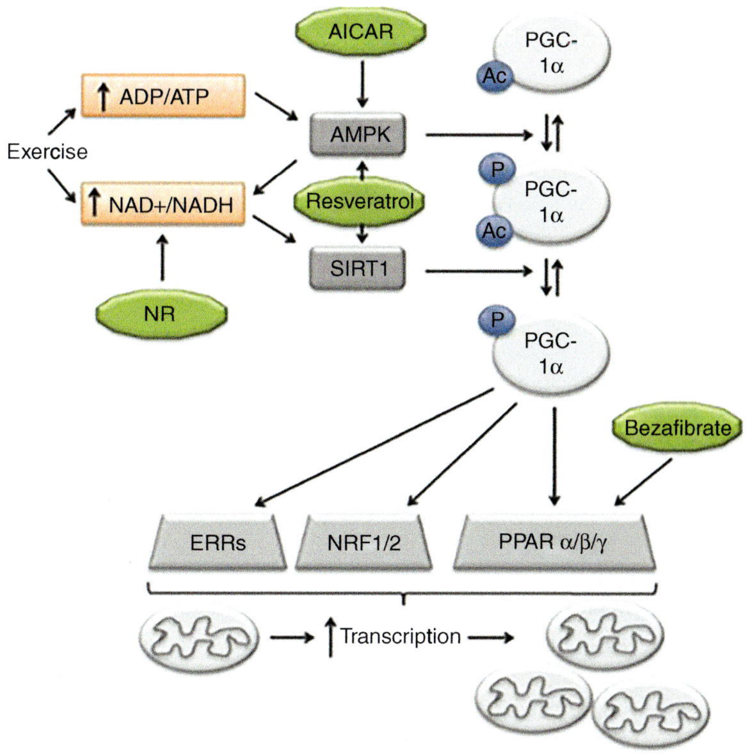


**Fig. 9.24** Compounds that stimulate mitochondrial biogenesis. See text for details. Abbreviations: ERR estrogen-related receptor, NRF nuclear respiratory factor, and PPAR peroxisome proliferator-activating receptor; see text for additional abbreviations [288, Fig. 15.1]. (Republished with permission from Springer International Publishing AG.Source: [287, Fig. 15.1]

metabolism through treating metabolic syndrome, diabetes, cardiovascular diseases, hypertension, chronic kidney disease, autonomic dysfunctions, and other related diseases.

Mitochondria biogenesis is a current leading research field in relieving or reversing mitochondrial dysfunction. Resveratrol has been shown to increase mitochondrial biogenesis and oxidative respiration [299, 300]. As depicted in Fig. 9.24, resveratrol,[28] AICAR (5-amino-4-imidazolecarboxamide 1-β-d-ribofuranoside),[29] bezafibrate,[30] and NR[31] (nicotinamide riboside) are different compounds that stimulate mitochondrial biogenesis in different ways. Mitochondria biogenesis starts with ATP and NADH depletion during energy expenditure, such as exercise. The subsequent increase in the ADP/ATP ratio is sensed by AMP-activated protein kinase (5′ adenosine monophosphate-activated protein kinase or AMPK) that activates peroxisome proliferator-activated receptor gamma coactivator 1-alpha (PGC-1α). AMPK is also known to effect NAD+/NADH ratio via nicotinamide phosphoribosyltransferase (NAMPT, aka, pre-B-cell colony-enhancing factor 1 (PBEF1) or visfatin). The NAD+/NADH ratio regulates the deacetylase NAD-dependent deacetylase sirtuin-1 (SIRT1) that fully activates PGC-1α. PGC-1α interacts with groups of transcription factors to increase the transcription of nuclear-encoded and subsequently mitochondrial-encoded mitochondrial genes. The resulting increase in mitochondrial gene transcription leads to an increase in mitochondrial biogenesis [288].

[28] Resveratrol (3,5,4′-trihydroxy-trans-stilbene) is a stilbenoid, a type of natural phenol, and a phytoalexin produced by several plants in response to injury or when the plant is under attack by pathogens such as bacteria or fungi. Sources of resveratrol in food include the skin of grapes, blueberries, raspberries, mulberries.

[29] AICARA is an analog of adenosine monophosphate (AMP) that is capable of stimulating AMP-dependent protein kinase (AMPK) activity.

[30] Bezafibrate is a fibrate drug that is an agonist of PPARα. It is primarily used as a lipid-lowering agent to treat hyperlipidemia. It helps to lower LDL cholesterol and triglyceride in the blood and increase HDL.

[31] Nicotinamide riboside is a pyridine-nucleoside form of vitamin $B_3$ that functions as a precursor to nicotinamide adenine dinucleotide or NAD+.

## Posttraumatic Stress Disorder

Posttraumatic stress disorder (PTSD) is characterized by the persistence of intense reactions to reminders of a traumatic event. The event may include exposure to actual or threatened death, serious injury, or sexual violence. The event must be (1) directly experienced; (2) witnessed as it occurred to others; (3) learned of as the traumatic event occurred to a close family member or friend; or (4) experienced as an extreme exposure, or repeated exposure, to aversive details of the event, but not applied in the case of media, television, movies, or pictures. PTSD is further characterized by (1) altered mood, a (2) sense of imminent threat, (3) disturbed sleep, and (4) hypervigilance. Cognitive behavioral therapy and anxiolytic or antidepressant agents can ameliorate some symptoms [301]. Through the DSM-5, the American Psychiatric Association has outlined four distinct diagnostic symptom clusters of PTSD which must persist for at least a month [302]:

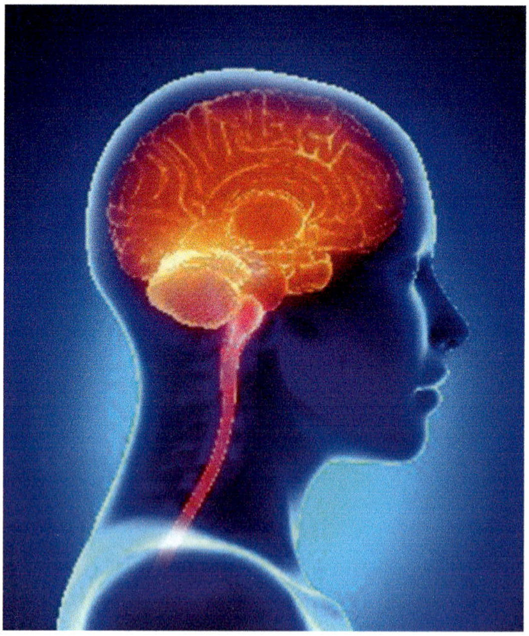

Insert: From Shutterstock: Royalty-free stock illustration ID: 511446631, brain power concept with 3D rendering human brain, by Phonlamai Photo).

1. Re-experiencing – involves the persistent re-experiencing the experience through thoughts or perceptions, images, dreams, illusions or hallucinations, dissociative flashback episodes or intense psychological distress, or reactivity to cues that symbolize some aspects of the original traumatic event. The traumatic event is persistently re-experienced in at least one of the following ways:
   - Recurrent and intrusive distressing recollections of the original traumatic event, including images, thoughts, or perceptions
   - Recurrent vivid, distressing memories or recurring dreams of the event
   - Acting or feeling as if the traumatic event were recurring, including a sense of reliving the experience, illusions, hallucinations, and intrusive flashback episodes
   - Intense psychological distress at exposure to cues that symbolize an aspect of the traumatic event
   - Physiologic reactivity on exposure to cues that symbolize or resemble an aspect of the traumatic event
2. Avoidance – involves avoidance of stimuli that are associated with the original trauma and numbing of general responsiveness. The person persistently avoids stimuli associated with the trauma and has numbing of general responsiveness including at least one of the following:
   - Efforts to avoid distressing memories, thoughts, feelings, or conversations associated with the original trauma
   - Efforts to avoid activities, places, people, or other external reminders that arouse recollections of the trauma
   - Inability to recall an important aspect of the trauma
   - Markedly diminished interest or participation in significant activities
   - Feelings of detachment or estrangement from others
   - Restricted range of affect
     - PTSD is specified as "with prominent dissociative symptoms" if the patient reports being detached from one's mind or body or has experiences in which the world seems unreal, dreamlike, or distorted.

3. Negative cognitions and moods – involves negative alterations in thought and mood as characterized by symptoms like:
   - Inability to remember an important aspect of the original traumatic event(s)
   - Persistent and exaggerated negative beliefs or expectations about oneself, others, or the world
   - Persistent, distorted cognitions about the cause or consequences of the traumatic event that lead the individual to blame her or himself or others
   - Persistent negative emotional state
   - Persistent inability to experience positive emotions
4. Arousal – involves alteration in arousal and reactivity. Persistent symptoms of increased arousal are indicated by at least two of the following:
   - Difficulty falling or staying asleep
   - Irritability or outbursts of anger or aggression
   - Reckless or self-destructive behavior
   - Difficulty concentrating
   - Hypervigilance
   - Exaggerated startle response

The disturbance causes clinically significant distress or impairment in social, occupational, or other important areas of functioning. PTSD is developmentally sensitive in that lower diagnostic thresholds have been established for children and adolescents, and separate criteria are included for children age 6 years or younger. For children 6 years of age or younger, PTSD is specified as the "Preschool Type." The acute phase of PTSD is defined as during the first 3 months of the onset of symptoms. From the third month on, PTSD is defined as chronic. However, the goal is to discover PTSD long before symptoms. If possible, PTSD is documented immediately after trauma. As such it is considered as preclinical and as soon as P&S imbalance(s) present, even before symptoms, it may be treated to prevent, or minimize, symptoms. PTSD is specified as "with delayed onset" if symptom onset is at least 6 months after the original traumatic event.

Important in the diagnosis of PTSD is identifying a history of trauma and being sure, in the face of the triggering stimuli, to ask questions related to the four symptom clusters listed above. The most common nonmilitary trauma associated with PTSD is rape (or sexual abuse; although, unfortunately, many in the military also report rape as the original trauma as well). The symptoms of PTSD may be mistaken for depression, other anxiety disorders, or dysfunctional personality traits. Patients might not be able to identify a connection between the symptoms and the trauma history, especially in the delayed onset mode when there may be up to 3 years between the initiating trauma and symptoms. PTSD requires the clinician be sensitive to the possibility that a trauma history exists. This is especially true since PTSD has a delayed onset that is often several years long or more. If the patient presents with complaints within 4 weeks of the trauma (with resolution within 4 weeks of symptom onset), then PTSD may not be the diagnosis; rather, a diagnosis of acute stress disorder is likely [50], although both are possible.

To qualify as having been exposed to a traumatic event, both of the following must be present:

1. The patient experienced, witnessed, or was confronted with an event that involved actual or threatened death or serious injury or a threat to the physical integrity of others.
2. The patient's response involved intense fear, helplessness, or horror.

The P&S monitoring findings from PTSD patients are parasympathetic excess (PE), definitely in response to stress (sympathetic challenge [29]), but also at rest. Either way, the psychology model of "Undischarged Traumatic Stress" (Fig. 9.25) is explained by PE. The P-nervous system sets the metabolic baseline around which the S-nervous system reacts. Therefore, any S-response is exaggerated or overly amplified by this abnormal and untimely P-response. As it is taught in medical school, the normal P&S response is the "seesaw" affect. In normal responses to a S-stimulus, or stress, the P-nervous system responds first, by decreasing, and then the S-nervous system responds in a minimalistic fashion. In fact, the initial P-response potentiates and facilitates the reactionary S-response, thereby, minimizing the S-responses. In cases with underlying (abnormal) PE, the P-nervous system also responds (increases), forcing an excessive S-response (SE), thereby, amplifying or overly exaggerating what would otherwise be a normal S-response. The result is the "stuck 'on'" feeling. Note, given that the S-response is the reactionary response, SE is therefore the secondary effect and must be treated as such; otherwise, the patients are found unresponsive or perhaps even considered non-compliant (Fig. 9.25).

PE with secondary SE fully explains confounding symptoms such as depression with anxiety or hypertension, or low HR with excessive pain or hyperactivity. Both P&S branches are high. The seesaw is broken (*both ends are high at the same time*[32]). This abnormal response cannot be not measured with HRV or beat-to-beat blood pressure, or any other form of heartbeat interval alone measurement. These heartbeat interval alone measurements are only of total autonomic function and force assumption and approximation that precludes discovery of dynamic PE.

PE, even without an S-stimulus, still persists and also amplifies or exaggerates the relaxation phases (see Fig. 9.25). The normal P-responses are exaggerated and cause even lower HRs and BPs, causing brain hypoperfusion, possibly leading to or exacerbating depression, fatigue, exhaustion, non-restorative sleep, malaise, etc. The depression then worsens into disorientation, disconnection, disassociation, etc., as the downward spiral persists. The result is the "stuck 'off'" feeling.

The cure begins with relief of this (dynamic) PE, and then further testing and therapy may be indicated as the dominoes effect progresses: (1) relieving PE helps to relieve the depression and sleep issues while (2) reducing the secondary SE; (3) relieving the secondary SE then reduces the amplified pain responses (such as in fibromyalgia-like symptoms associated with PTSD), and relieving (4) the anxiety and panic attacks, etc.; (5) GI and sex dysfunction and other associated dysfunction often follow as the nervous system is normalized. In all, quality of life is restored, helping the patients to feel better about themselves. While relieving PE does not deal with the trigger that is at the root of PTSD, it helps the person to an improved self-image and self-esteem, thereby, enabling them to better manage their trigger. This also facilitates the psychiatrists work in helping the patient cope with the trigger.

Ultimately, the findings are that PTSD is not "all in your head." The symptoms of trauma are the result of a dysregulation of the P&S nervous systems that then manifests as organ dysfunctions, including higher resting HRs and BPs, decreased HRV, and increased plasma and urine catecholamine levels typical with PTSD. Some of these symptoms implicate the renin-angiotensin system [303] which is part of the sympathetic nervous system. P&S systems have an inherent capacity to self-regulate that is undermined by trauma. This can include the failure of BP to decrease by $\geq 10\%$ nocturnally (non-dipping), which is thought to be mediated by SE. SE, often associated with parasympathetic insufficiency (aka, cardiovascular autonomic neuropathy, or CAN), is associated with increased cardiovascular risk, which is a result of long-term PTSD. In fact, PTSD typically accelerates the onset of CAN.

Humans (as with other mammals) automatically regulate survival responses from parts of the brain (primarily the limbic system with the amygdala, hypothalamus, and hippocampus, and the brain stem) associated with the autonomic nervous system. In the wild, animals spontaneously "discharge" this excess energy once safe. Involuntary movements such as shaking, trembling, and deep spontaneous breaths reset the P&S and restore balance. Humans disrupt this discharge as a result of conforming to the culture through rational thinking, shame, judgments, and fear of bodily sensations. Humans compound these problems by adding psychosocial stresses that are associated with feelings of inadequacy, low self-confidence, and low self-esteem. Expectations are set on others, others that will ultimately disappoint. A goal is to restore both

[32]To use the car analogy the person is "riding the brakes" (PE) and must "over-rev the engine" (SE) to get to speed or go anywhere.

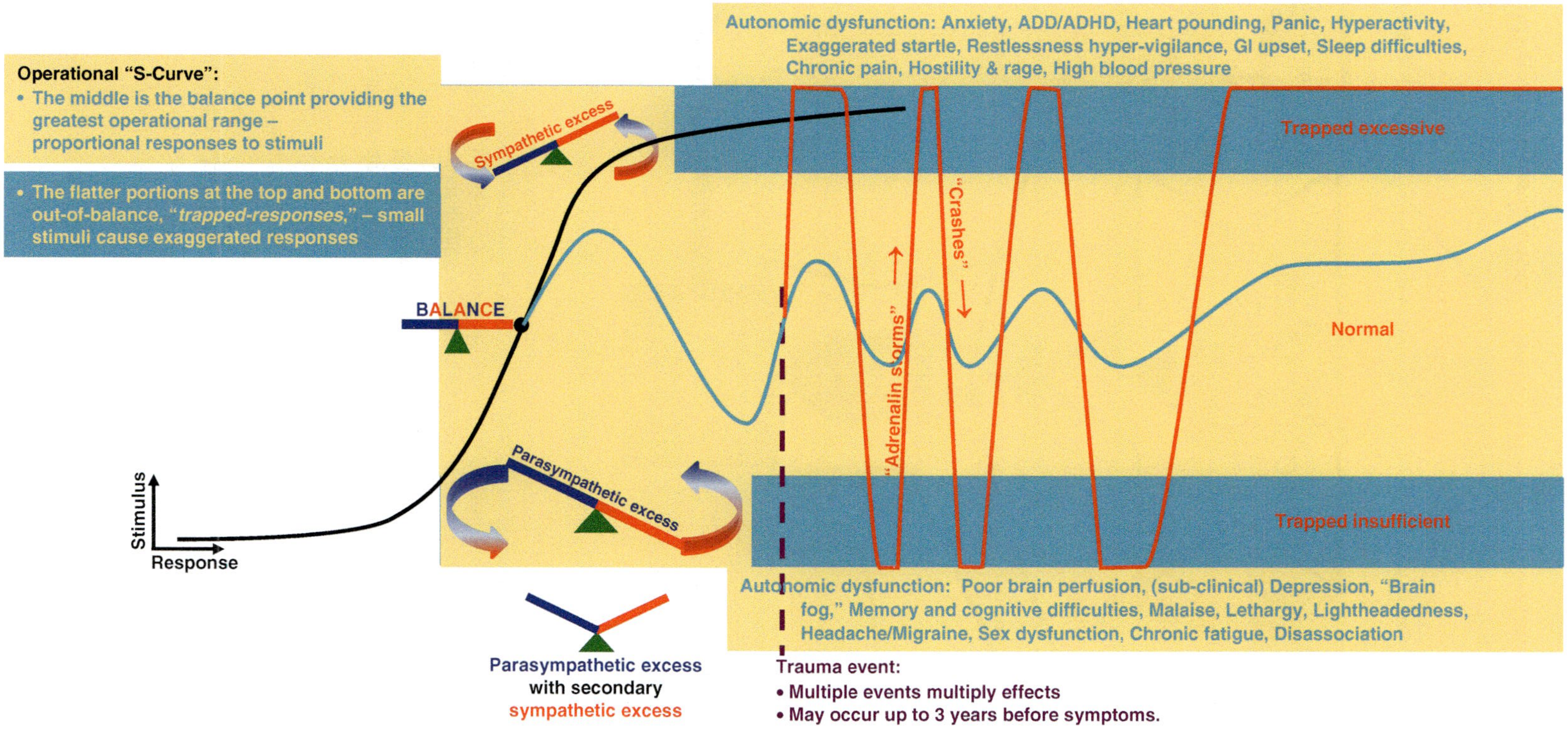


**Fig. 9.25** Undischarged traumatic stress model. Traumatic events may significantly or excessively amplify the normal mood changes that normally occur over time. When the active phases of life (upward swings in the blue curve in the figure) are amplified, the results may be some or all of anxiety, panic, hyperactivity, exaggerated startle, inability to relax, restlessness, hypervigilance, digestive problems, emotional flooding, chronic pain, sleeplessness, or hostility or rage. Some describe the feel of being "stuck 'on'." When the relaxation phases of life (downward swings in the blue curve in the figure) are amplified, the results (red curve) may be some or all of depression, flat effect, lethargy, deadness, exhaustion, chronic fatigue, disorientation, disconnection, disassociation complex syndrome, pain, low blood pressure, or poor digestion. Some describe the feel of being "stuck 'off'" [44]. (Source: Reed SB, Ross M, Mcmannemin F. Results from Treating Trauma (PTSD) Survivors and Measuring Treatment Effect with Heart Rate Variability Analysis. 2006. from Somatic Experiencing – http://hesed.info/blog/somatic-experiencing.abp)

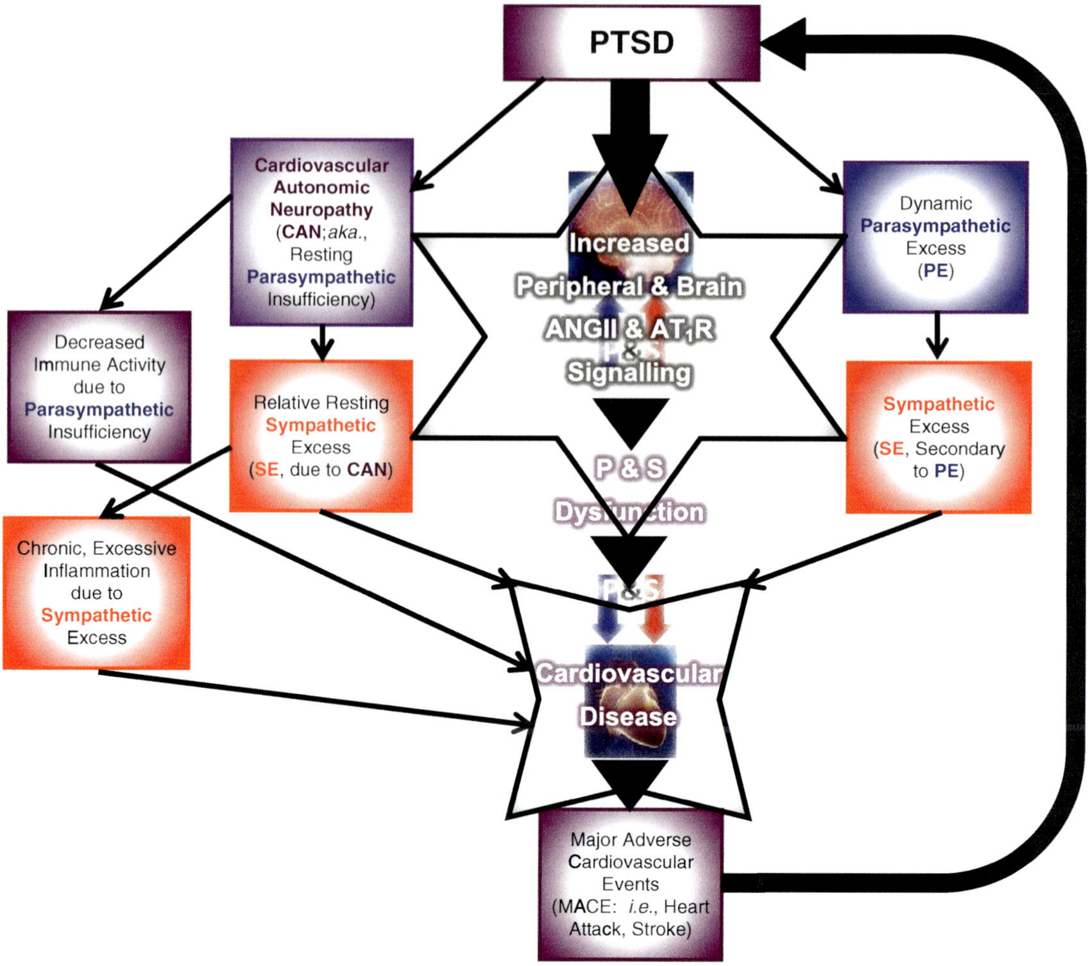


**Fig. 9.26** Pathways involved in PTSD-associated cardiovascular disease development and PTSD induced from cardiovascular related events. Consequences of PTSD can lead to increased immune cell dysfunction and inflammation, heightened sympathetic nerve activity (hyperarousal, typically a result of parasympathetic insufficiency), and activation of the renin-angiotensin system (star). It is proposed that renin-angiotensin system activation further promotes autonomic and immune disturbances in the setting of PTSD, and these changes ultimately contribute to the culmination of increased cardiovascular disease risk. PTSD symptoms can also be induced thick arrow, right by a single cardiovascular related event such as a stroke or heart attack, thus putting these individuals at greater risk for future adverse cardiovascular events (a function of sympathetic excess, that in the face of PTSD is typically secondary to a dynamic parasympathetic excess – a parasympathetic excess during a sympathetic (stress) stimulus [29]). Abbreviations: ANGII angiotensin 2, $AT_1R$ angiotensin type 1 receptor [303].

physiologic health and psychologic health by restoring the health and wellness of the connection between the two, the Mind-Body connection: the P&S nervous systems.

The P&S nervous systems have extensive communications with the immune system (see Fig. 9.26) [304]. P&S imbalance may induce immune dysregulation, leading to inflammation. The P&S imbalance is a consequence of the trauma that underlies PTSD. Chronic elevations in catecholamines increase cytokine production via stimulation of beta-2 adrenergic receptors on immune cells [304], which may contribute to the increased levels of inflammatory markers (i.e.,

C-reactive protein, CRP) and increased inflammation in PTSD [305]. CRP is predictive of cardiovascular disease [306] and is also increased and frequently associated with PTSD.

When considering inflammation as a contributing factor or consequence of PTSD, it is important to keep in mind that inflammation and cytokines may have secondary effects on neurotransmitters, which could contribute to the impairments in fear memory and extinction processes found in PTSD and other psychiatric diseases [307]. For example, under stress, microglia, endothelial cells, and macrophages release IL-1β, and many IL-1β receptors are concentrated near the hippocampus and amygdala. These may alter fear memory [308, 309] by influencing synaptic strength and signaling between neurons. Both IL-1β and nitric oxide are thought to play a role in long-term potentiation (increased postsynaptic response to a fixed stimulus), which can serve to enhance learning and memory [308, 310]. Interestingly, IL-1β has been found to promote fear memory and the conditioned fear response.

Often with PTSD, especially by the time symptoms present, pharmaceuticals are needed to chemically retrain the P&S nervous systems to re-establish balance. However, there are few medications that are specifically designed to address P&S imbalance, especially when a relatively healthy (just imbalanced) P&S nervous system still exists. Just like with the "Statin Gap" discussed with atherosclerosis, pharmaceuticals do not always complete the therapy needed by patients with PTSD. Again, as with the "Statin Gap," antioxidants, nitric oxide, and fish oil supplements help to "close the gap":

- Antioxidants such as alpha-lipoic acid, Co-Q10, vitamins, minerals, and amino acids to prevent oxidation and inflammation, and boost immune responses
- Omega-3 fatty acids to help prevent inflammation and repair nerve and vascular tissue, and more
- A nitric oxide compound to restore normal nitric oxide function (communications) in the brain and in the vasculature to help improve cognition and circulation
- Exercise as the most powerful antioxidant to further reduce oxidation and increase blood flow to the brain and heart (*under close physician supervision*)
- Mediterranean diet to provide more Omega-3s, antioxidants, and nitric oxide, as well as vitamins, minerals, nutrients, amino acids, and fuel
- Stress reduction to further reduce oxidation, including from free radicals and reactive oxygen and nitrogen species

Also, nitric oxide and antioxidant compounds provide supplements that are known to reduce depression and anxiety and brain fog and improve restorative sleep and many of the other symptoms associated with PTSD.

## Telomere Length, Longevity, Fish Oils, and Antioxidants

A telomere is a region of repetitive nucleotide sequences (in humans: the sequence TTAGGG bound by a set of specialized proteins [311]) at each end of eukaryotic chromosomes. Like the plastic tips at the end of shoelaces, telomeres are the caps at the end of each strand of DNA that protect chromosomes from deterioration or from fusion with neighboring chromosomes. Without the cap, shoelaces become frayed until they can no longer do their job, just as without telomeres, DNA strands become damaged, and cells can't do their job.

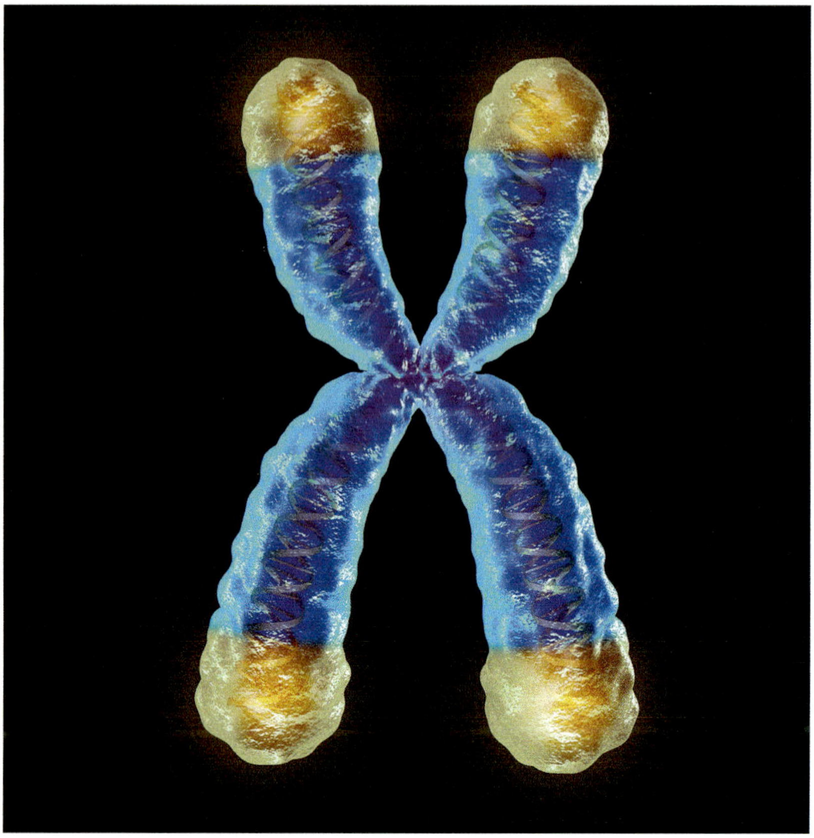

(Insert: From Shutterstock: Royalty-free stock illustration ID: 609519446, telomere length medical concept and telomeres located on the end caps of a chromosome resulting in aging by damaging DNA or protection resulting in living longer or longevity as a 3D illustration, by Lightspring)

The length of telomeres, and in particular the abundance of short telomeres, may be a biomarker of aging and of general health status. A wide variety of studies show the association of short telomeres with age-related pathologies and cancer, as well as with life span and mortality (Fig. 9.27) [311, 313]. In the absence of a compensatory elongating mechanism, telomeres get shorter with each cell division [314]. Telomerase is a reverse transcriptase that can elongate telomeres [315, 316]. After birth, telomerase is silenced in most somatic cells. As a result, telomeres progressively shorten with aging (aging, as measured by the number of cell divisions) [314, 317]. Certain cell types, such as all blood cells, stem cells, and germ cells, have the ability to activate telomerase, but this is not sufficient to prevent telomere shortening with aging [318, 319]. Critically short telomeres cannot be repaired by any of the known DNA repair mechanisms and consequently trigger a persistent DNA damage response, which leads to cellular senescence or apoptosis [320, 321], eventually compromising tissue regenerative capacity and function, and contributing to organismal aging [322]. The frequency of short telomeres, rather than the mean telomere length, is proposed to be a better indicator of telomere dysfunction and, consequently, of cell and tissue dysfunction.

Telomere length is influenced by genetic (endogenous or non-modifiable) factors, as well as environmental (modifiable) factors. Non-modifiable factors that shorten both telomere length and aging include genetic factors [323–330], male gender [331–335], cell division [332, 336, 337], age [160, 332–335], oxidative stress [323, 338–341], and inflammation [338, 340–343]. Non-modifiable factors that inhibit shortening of both telomere length and

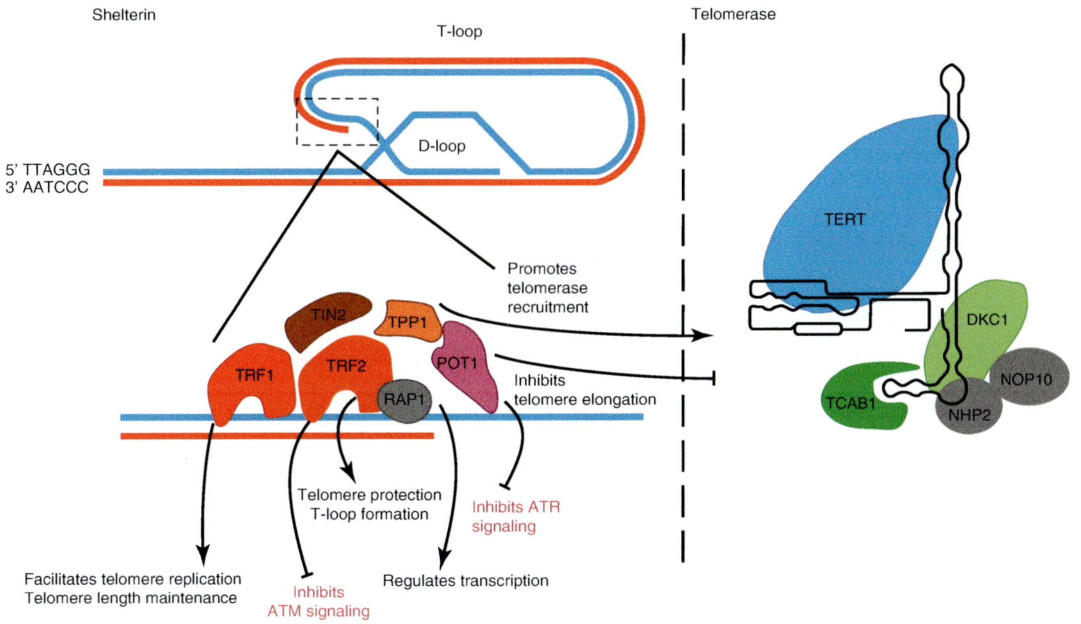


**Fig. 9.27** Shelterin, the telomere-binding complex, protects chromosome ends and controls telomerase function. Telomeric DNA is bound by the double-stranded DNA-binding proteins TRF1 and TRF2 and by the single-stranded DNA-binding protein Pot1. Rap1 binds to TRF2 and functions as a transcriptional regulator. TIN2 nucleates the complex by connecting TRF1 and TRF2 to the Tpp1/Pot1 sub-complex. Each component of sheltering serves a specialized function in telomere maintenance, with TRF2 and Pot1 involved in suppression of DNA damage signaling and TRF1 involved in facilitating replication through difficult to replicate telomeric sequences. Telomerase is recruited to the complex through its interaction with Tpp1; once at the telomere, its action is negatively regulated by Pot1. Telomerase is a ribonucleoprotein composed of a noncoding RNATERC that serves as a scaffold for protein components TERT, TCAB, dyskerin, NOP10, and NHP2. Dyskerin and its associated proteins promote TERC biogenesis and stability, whereas TCAB facilitates trafficking of telomerase to the telomere. TERT is the catalytic subunit, and TERC encodes the template for reverse transcription [312]

aging include telomerase [332, 344–347] and estrogen [348]. Modifiable factors that shorten both telomere length and aging include smoking [349–351], alcohol abuse [352], obesity [349, 350, 353, 354], sedentary lifestyle [323, 355–357], UV irradiation [346], and mental stress [358, 359]. Modifiable factors that inhibit shortening of both telomere length and aging include healthy lifestyle [323, 355–357, 360–365]; vitamins C, D, and E [364, 366–368]; omega-3 fatty acids [369]; healthy diets [370–372]; and statin treatment [373]. As noted, smoking, alcohol abuse, obesity, sedentary lifestyle, UV radiation, and mental stress can cause significant shortening of telomeres and potentially accelerate aging. In contrast, a healthy lifestyle and healthy diets, including antioxidants (vitamins) and omega-3 fatty acids, can significantly inhibit the shortening of telomeres and the acceleration of aging.

Clinical and epidemiological studies listed above have also shown that short telomere length is associated with or is related to cardiovascular risk factors, including atherosclerosis, coronary artery disease, heart failure, and Alzheimer's disease. Short telomere length is also related to diabetes both in type 1 and type 2 and may predict progression of diabetic nephropathy. Whether telomere shortening is causally related to, or is caused by, age-related disease and risk factors remains unclear. Clues to this question are being uncovered through research into (1) tyrosine kinase inhibitors, (2) mitochondrial dysfunction, and (3) oxidative and inflammatory pathways related to chronic diseases.

Kinases are involved in cellular signaling which includes cell growth, differentiation, adhesion, motility, and cell death. Significant research in many and most cancer therapies involves tyrosine kinase inhibitors [337, 345, 347, 348, 363, 374].

Tyrosine kinase inhibitors have also been studied significantly in Alzheimer's disease [323, 337, 356, 362, 375, 376]. Mitochondrial dysfunction and oxidative stress are commonly observed in patients with neurodegenerative diseases with defects in mitochondrial oxidative phosphorylation (see "Reduce Mitochondrial Dysfunction" in Chap. 5).

Two of the factors which are associated with metabolic syndrome are a pro-inflammatory state and an increase in oxidative stress. Both of these have been associated with the aging process. The superoxide which is created in the mitochondria can be converted to hydrogen peroxide by the function of superoxide dismutase. These have antimicrobial action and give rise to more potent antioxidant metabolites that do have significant antimicrobial function and are important in respiratory bursts. Clinical supplements with exogenous antioxidants have not always been shown to be protective against heart disease or cancer [325–328, 377]. For example, vitamin E has been associated with increased heart failure. Fatal heart disease has been associated with men who receive beta-carotene or a combination of beta-carotene and vitamin E [329]. Supplementation with beta-carotene may increase lung cancer in cigarette smokers [330]. Therefore, nonspecific antioxidant therapy may not be necessarily protective against chronic disease but may heighten oxidative stress. Preventing heightened oxidative stress by vitamin-antioxidants is one important reason behind strongly recommending ALA and Co-Q10, because they recycle the more commonly known antioxidants such as vitamins C and E.

The preventing of chromosomal ends from initiating a DNA damage response can be compromised as telomeres erode as a normal part of cellular aging in proliferative tissues. The DNA damage signals and activates the tumor-suppressor protein p53, which then can prompt either cellular senescence or apoptosis. By culling cells with dysfunctional telomeres, p53 plays a critical role in protecting tissues against the effects of critically short telomeres. However, as telomere dysfunction worsens, p53 likely exacerbates short telomere-driven tissue failure diseases, including pulmonary fibrosis, aplastic anemia, and liver cirrhosis. In cells lacking p53, unchecked telomere shortening drives chromosomal end-to-end fusions and cycles of chromosome fusion-bridge-breakage. Precancer cells confronting these telomere barriers must disable p53 signaling to avoid senescence and eventually upregulate telomerase to achieve cellular immortality. The recent findings of highly recurrent activating mutations in the promoter for the telomerase reverse transcriptase gene in diverse human cancers, together with the widespread mutations in p53 in cancer, provide support for the idea that circumvention of a telomere-p53 checkpoint is essential for malignant progression in human cancer [312].

The inability of primary human cells to be cultured indefinitely provided the first suggestion for an inherent limit placed on cell division. This behavior of normal cells directly isolated from tissues contrasted with the indefinite proliferation of cancer cells in culture. The underlying molecular basis for this difference between normal cells and cancer cells is explained by a differential ability to maintain telomeres. The vast majority of human cancer cells express telomerase, the enzyme that elongates telomeres, whereas the primary cell culture models lacked telomerase expression. The roadblocks preventing cell growth in primary cells included two different responses: (1) replicative senescence and (2) crisis. The senescence barrier is enforced by two key tumor-suppressor pathways: p53 and Rb. These barriers are not only relevant in limiting cell proliferation in culture but are critically important in human tissues and in human carcinogenesis [312].

Telomere shortening in cell culture limits the proliferation of primary cells. After a defined number of population doublings in culture, short telomeres in fibroblasts trigger a DNA damage response that acts through p53 to cause cellular senescence and a halt on proliferation. To proceed past senescence, cells must inactivate p53 and Rb, or upregulate telomerase to achieve telomere maintenance. Once cells escape senescence, continued telomere shortening will lead to a period of genomic instability termed crisis, which is characterized by cell death and chromosomal instability. Expression of telomerase will stabilize the genome and allow continued proliferation of the culture [312].

As indicated, telomere length influences diseases of aging and thereby longevity [378]. To that end, factors that influence telomere erosion are of interest and may be intrinsic or environmental. A knowledge of these factors leads to potential solutions to remedy or prevent premature telomere erosion [378]. Aging is a multifactorial process that results in a progressive functional decline at cellular, tissue, and organismal levels. During recent years, a number of molecular pathways have been identified as main molecular causes of aging, including telomere attrition, cellular senescence, genomic instability, stem cell exhaustion, mitochondrial dysfunction, and epigenetic alterations [379]. Interestingly, telomere attrition is considered a primary cause of aging, as it can trigger all the abovementioned hallmarks of aging [379]. Critical telomere shortening elicits the induction of cellular senescence or the permanent inability of cells to further divide, which in turn has been proposed to be at the origin of different disease states [380, 381]. In addition, telomere attrition in the stem cell compartments results in the exhaustion of their tissue- and self-renewal capacity, thus also leading to age-related diseases [382, 383]. When telomere exhaustion occurs prematurely (i.e., telomerase or sheltering gene mutations), a premature loss of the renewal capacity of tissues is triggered leading to aplastic anemia and pulmonary fibrosis, among others [384–387]. Loss of DNA damage checkpoints can also allow the propagation of cells with short or damaged telomeres, thus promoting age-associated diseases like cancer [388, 389]. A link between dysfunctional telomeres and mitochondrial compromise has been also proposed, thus linking dysfunctional telomeres to mitochondrial aging [390].

There are differences in the pace of telomere shortening. The average telomere shortening in human blood cells, for example, occurs at a rate of 31–72 base pairs per year [391, 392]. In addition to the intrinsic end replication problem, there are other factors contributing to telomere attrition [378]. In particular, oxidative damage may severely impact telomere length, whereas antioxidant treatment has the opposite effect [393]. The choice of lifestyle can influence telomere shortening. As an example, smoking, an unhealthy diet (e.g., high cholesterol or high alcohol intake), or obesity might lead to telomere shortening by provoking tissue inflammation and oxidative stress [394–399]. Moreover, accelerated telomere shortening in leukocytes has been associated with psychological stress. In particular, patients with depression disorders have shorter telomeres compared to healthy individuals [400], and this telomere erosion is found in all lymphocyte subpopulations [401]. Stress provoked by physical abuse of children has been also associated with telomere shortening [402]. A number of studies investigating telomere length in major depressive disorder show signs of premature aging [403–405], corresponding to a 10-year increase in biological age [406] compared to healthy subjects. Bipolar disorder patients' shorter telomere cell populations have been described to correspond to a 13-year-older biological age [407]. Shorter telomeres are also associated with cognitive impairment in the elderly [408].

Although cancer and aging have been studied as independent diseases, mounting evidence suggests that cancer is an aging-associated disease and that cancer and aging share many molecular pathways. In particular, recent studies validated telomerase activation as a potential therapeutic target for age-related diseases, and at the same time, abnormal telomerase expression and telomerase mutations have been associated with many different types of human tumors (Fig. 9.28) [409]. Because age is a crucial determinant of cardiovascular diseases [410] and since the attrition of telomeric DNA is a biomarker of aging and health status [411], it is a possibility that telomere attrition might predict cardiovascular risk. Numerous epidemiological studies have investigated the relationship between leukocyte telomere length and cardiovascular ischemic events, but the outcomes are often conflicting or too heterogeneous. One meta-analysis [412] found a significant association between shortened leukocyte telomere length and myocardial infarction, type 2 diabetes,

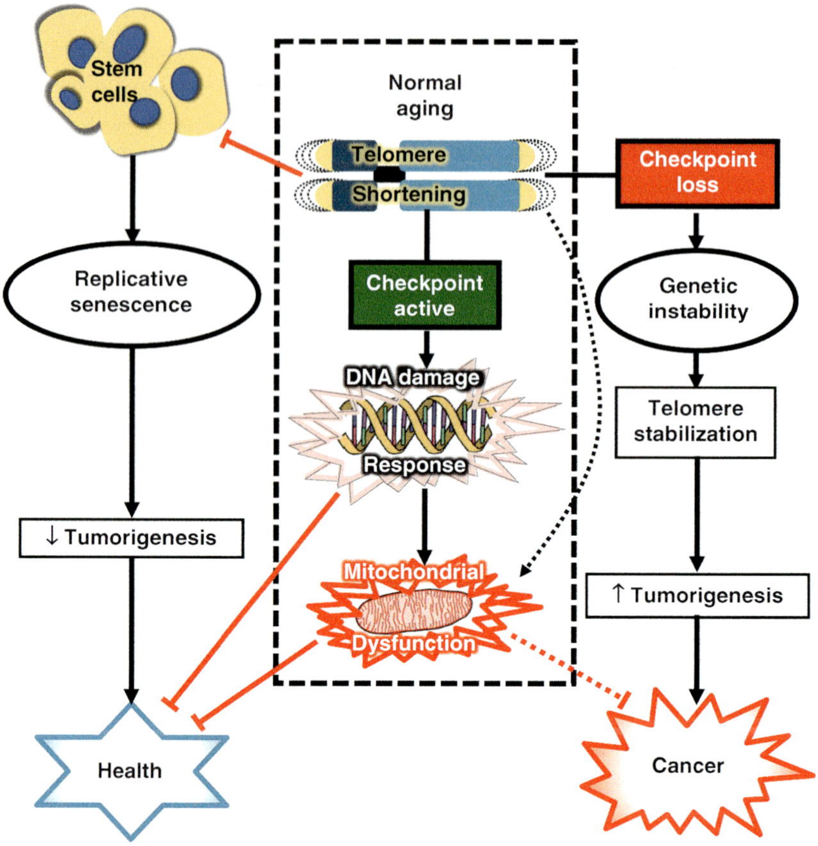


**Fig. 9.28** Major pathways affected by short telomeres and their impact on aging or cancer. DNA damage and tumor-suppressor activity have been shown to impact tissue decline and aging. When DNA damage checkpoints are bypassed, cells with short telomeres could potentially progress to cancer. The role of stem cells with short telomeres in cancer and whether short telomeres could modulate other pathways independently of p53 (such as mitochondrial dysfunction) remains unknown [409]

and stroke. Another meta-analysis [413] also showed a correlation between leukocyte telomere length and myocardial infarction, as well as coronary heart disease death and coronary revascularization, but the association with cerebrovascular disease (stroke) was less certain. The former study [412] did not find a significant association between leukocyte telomere length and coronary artery disease (a secondary outcome defined as angina and nonfatal ischemic heart disease), suggesting that leukocyte telomere length attrition is a marker of plaque rupture and associated ischemic events. This leads to the question of whether shortened leukocyte telomere length is a prognostic biomarker for the early identification of subjects at high risk of developing cardiovascular disease before symptoms appear (e.g., a biomarker for the risk of angiogenesis). However, few epidemiological studies have focused on possible associations between telomere length and subclinical (asymptomatic) atherosclerosis. The results of those few studies of middle-aged men and women free from established cardiovascular disease show that short mean telomere length and the number of short telomeres (<3 kb) in leukocytes are not significant independent determinants of subclinical atherosclerosis burden [414]. Taken together, current evidence suggests that although there is an association between leukocyte telomere length and atherothrombotic cardiovascular events, there is no association with preclinical atherosclerosis [415].

Ultimately, it is in the genes [378]. Telomere length is also dictated by a genetic component [416–419]. Regardless of the method, telomere length shortens with age; length is highly correlated with longevity (the longer the length, the longer the longevity – up to the genetic limit programmed in for total numbers of immune repair cycles), and fish oils (natural anti-inflammatories) and antioxidants are the main agents helping to delay the shortening. While certain lifestyle habits may reduce the detrimental factors causing accelerated telomere shortening, the best that will happen is that the telomere length will be optimized for the individual (if the length is not beyond the critical limit). The lifestyle habits referenced include a diet rich in omega-3 fatty acids [420, 421] (e.g., the Mediterranean diet), physical activity, fitness, and exercise (types of antioxidants), nitric oxide (as anti-inflammatory agents and immune boosters to glean damaged cells) [422–424], and oxidative and psychosocial stress reduction (additional types of antioxidants).

## Summation

P&S monitoring is a means by which to measure patient outcomes. To that end, preliminary data indicates that patient outcomes with the supplement and lifestyle modifications that are recommended herein are significantly improved. The study is a blinded, crossover study, wherein patients are randomly assigned to one of two arms: research or control. All patients, after reading the protocol, initialing each page, and reading and signing a consent form, are assigned. All patients then complete both the SF-36 and the Nottingham Health Profile questionnaires (see respective sections in this chapter above) and are assessed by P&S monitoring. All patients are invited to participate in the research. Exclusion criteria include under 18 y/o; pregnant, nursing, or about to become pregnant; allergies to any of the supplement ingredients; hypotensive patients whose condition may be exacerbated by the blood pressure lowering effects of some supplements; patients who are incapable of the exercise portion of the program; and patients who are not mentally or physically able to follow the program guidelines.

To begin the study, the control arm patients continue their daily activities as before. The research arm patients are educated in the lifestyle modifications and are given the supplements that are the program. After 3 months,[33] all subjects enrolled in the study repeat the questionnaires and P&S monitoring. The research arm cohort continues as before, and the control arm cohort is then educated in the lifestyle modifications and is given the supplements that are the program. After another 3 months (the 6-month mark), all subjects enrolled in the study, again, repeat the questionnaires and P&S monitoring, and the study is concluded. Subjects who report improved outcomes are encouraged to continue the program to maintain the wellness that was established.

Preliminary results demonstrate that all subjects who stayed with both the lifestyle changes and the supplements had statistically significant improvements in both quality of life (QoL) and P&S function, representing the physiology. QoL improvements, as measured by serial questionnaires, included increased restorative sleep, improved upper and lower GI function, improved bladder control, reduced light-headedness (non-vestibular dizziness), normalization in blood pressure, and improved sex function (reduced erectile dysfunction for men and improved vaginal lubrication for women). Physiologic improvements, as measured by serial P&S monitoring, demonstrated normalization of resting sympathovagal balance and normalization of P&S responses to challenge (demonstrating improvements in dynamic P&S balance). Physiologic improvements involve reductions in both mortality and morbidity risks. These are the factors that lead to the reduction in hospitalizations mentioned at the beginning of this section and are quantitative, age-adjusted measures of improved health and wellness.

## References


1. Ajabshir S, Asif A, Nayer A. The effects of vitamin D on the renin-angiotensin system. J Nephropathol. 2014;3(2):41–3. https://doi.org/10.12860/jnp.2014.09.
2. Pieczenik SR, Neustadt J. Mitochondrial dysfunction and molecular pathways of disease. Exp Mol Pathol. 2007;83(1):84–92. Epub 2007 Jan 18.


[33] In general, it takes 2–3 months (depending on physiologic age; the older or sicker, the longer) for the P&S nervous systems to fully adapt to a new condition, including changing or titrating therapy, changing lifestyle, or responding to a new disease or injury (whether physiologic or psychologic).

3. Cohen BH, Gold DR. Mitochondrial cytopathy in adults: what we know so far. Cleve Clin J Med. 2001;68(7):625–42.
4. Vanderplasschen W, et al. Poly substance use and mental health among individuals presenting for substance abuse treatment. Science and society series. Ghent: Academia Press; 2012.
5. Yankey BA, Rothenberg R, Strasser S, Ramsey-White K, Okosun IS. Effect of marijuana use on cardiovascular and cerebrovascular mortality: a study using the National Health and Nutrition Examination Survey linked mortality file. Eur J Prev Cardiol. 2017;24(17):1833–40. https://doi.org/10.1177/2047487317723212. Epub 2017 Aug 8.
6. Desbois AC, Cacoub P. Cannabis-associated arterial disease. Ann Vasc Surg. 2013;27(7):996–1005. https://doi.org/10.1016/j.avsg.2013.01.002. Epub 2013 Jul 10. Review.
7. Thomas G, Kloner RA, Rezkalla S. Adverse cardiovascular, cerebrovascular, and peripheral vascular effects of marijuana inhalation: what cardiologists need to know. Am J Cardiol. 2014;113(1):187–90. https://doi.org/10.1016/j.amjcard.2013.09.042. Epub 2013 Oct 5. Review.
8. Gorelick DA, Heishman SJ, Preston KL, Nelson RA, Moolchan ET, Huestis MA. The cannabinoid CB1 receptor antagonist rimonabant attenuates the hypotensive effect of smoked marijuana in male smokers. Am Heart J. 2006;151(3):754.e1–5.
9. Mittleman MA, Lewis RA, Maclure M, Sherwood JB, Muller JE. Triggering myocardial infarction by marijuana. Circulation. 2001;103(23):2805–9.
10. Mukamal KJ, Maclure M, Muller JE, Mittleman MA. An exploratory prospective study of marijuana use and mortality following acute myocardial infarction. Am Heart J. 2008;155(3):465–70. https://doi.org/10.1016/j.ahj.2007.10.049.
11. Mehra R, Moore BA, Crothers K, Tetrault J, Fiellin DA. The association between marijuana smoking and lung cancer: a systematic review. Arch Intern Med. 2006;166(13):1359–67. Review.
12. Korantzopoulos P, Liu T, Papaioannides D, Li G, Goudevenos JA. Atrial fibrillation and marijuana smoking. Int J Clin Pract. 2008;62(2):308–13. Epub 2007 Nov 21. Review.
13. Korantzopoulos P. Marijuana smoking is associated with atrial fibrillation. Am J Cardiol. 2014;113(6):1085–6. https://doi.org/10.1016/j.amjcard.2014.01.001. Epub 2014 Jan 8.
14. Hackam DG. Cannabis and stroke: systematic appraisal of case reports. Stroke. 2015;46(3):852–6. https://doi.org/10.1161/STROKEAHA.115.008680. Review.
15. Desbois AC, Cacoub P. Cannabis-associated arterial disease. Ann Vasc Surg. 2013;27(7):996–1005. https://doi.org/10.1016/j.avsg.2013.01.002. Epub 2013 Jul 10. Review.
16. Shi H, Enriquez A, Rapadas M, Martin EMMA, Wang R, Moreau J, Lim CK, Szot JO, Ip E, Hughes JN, Sugimoto K, Humphreys DT, McInerney-Leo AM, Leo PJ, Maghzal GJ, Halliday J, Smith J, Colley A, Mark PR, Collins F, Sillence DO, Winlaw DS, Ho JWK, Guillemin GJ, Brown MA, Kikuchi K, Thomas PQ, Stocker R, Giannoulatou E, Chapman G, Duncan EL, Sparrow DB, Dunwoodie SL. NAD deficiency, congenital malformations, and niacin supplementation. N Engl J Med. 2017;377(6):544–52. https://doi.org/10.1056/NEJMoa1616361.
17. Cantó C, Menzies KJ, Auwerx J. NAD(+) metabolism and the control of energy homeostasis: a balancing act between mitochondria and the nucleus. Cell Metab. 2015;22:31–53.
18. Huang J-Y, Hirschey MD, Shimazu T, Ho L, Verdin E. Mitochondrial sirtuins. Biochim Biophys Acta. 2010;1804:1645–51.
19. Cheng H-L, Mostoslavsky R, Saito S, et al. Developmental defects and p53 hyperacetylation in Sir2 homolog (SIRT1)-deficient mice. Proc Natl Acad Sci U S A. 2003;100:10794–9.
20. Vander Heiden MG. Metabolism and congenital malformations – NAD's effects on development. N Engl J Med. 2017;377(6):509–11. https://doi.org/10.1056/NEJMp1707487.
21. Sletten DM, Suarez GA, Low PA, Mandrekar J, Singer W. COMPASS 31: a refined and abbreviated composite autonomic symptom score. Mayo Clin Proc. 2012;87(12):1196–201. https://doi.org/10.1016/j.mayocp.2012.10.013.
22. Sletten DM, Suarez GA, Low PA, Mandrekar J, Singer W. COMPASS 31: a refined and abbreviated composite autonomic symptom score. Mayo Clin Proc. 2012;87(12):1196–201. https://doi.org/10.1016/j.mayocp.2012.10.013.
23. Treister R, O'Neil K, Downs HM, Oaklander AL. Validation of the composite autonomic symptom scale 31 (COMPASS-31) in patients with and without small fiber polyneuropathy. Eur J Neurol. 2015;22(7):1124–30. https://doi.org/10.1111/ene.12717. Epub 2015 Apr 23.
24. Bowling A, Bond M, Jenkinson C, Lamping DL. Short Form 36 (SF-36) health survey questionnaire: which normative data should be used? Comparisons between the norms provided by the Omnibus Survey in Britain, the Health Survey for England and the Oxford Healthy Life Survey. J Public Health Med. 1999;21(3):255–70.
25. Hunt SM, McKenna SP, McEwen J, Backett EM, Williams J, Papp E. A quantitative approach to perceived health status: a validation study. J Epidemiol Community Health. 1980;34(4):281–6.
26. https://www.ehlers-danlos.com/assessing-joint-hypermobility/
27. Naal FD, Hatzung G, Müller A, Impellizzeri F, Leunig M. Validation of a self-reported Beighton score to assess hypermobility in patients with femoroacetabular impingement. Int Orthop. 2014;38(11):2245–50. https://doi.org/10.1007/s00264-014-2424-9. Epub 2014 Jul 5.
28. Smits-Engelsman B, Klerks M, Kirby A. Beighton score: a valid measure for generalized hypermobility

in children. J Pediatr. 2011;158(1):119–23, 123.e1–4. https://doi.org/10.1016/j.jpeds.2010.07.021. Epub 2010 Sep 17.
29. Tobias H, Vinitsky A, Bulgarelli RJ, Ghosh-Dastidar S, Colombo J. Autonomic nervous system monitoring of patients with excess parasympathetic responses to sympathetic challenges – clinical observations. US Neurol. 2010;5(2):62–6.
30. Low PA. Composite autonomic scoring scale for laboratory quantification of generalized autonomic failure. Mayo Clin Proc. 1993;68(8):748–52.
31. Nabavi SM, Daglia M, Braidy N, Nabavi SF. Natural products, micronutrients, and nutraceuticals for the treatment of depression: a short review. Nutr Neurosci. 2017;20(3):180–94. https://doi.org/10.1080/1028415X.2015.1103461. Epub 2015 Nov 27.
32. Deepmala, Slattery J, Kumar N, Delhey L, Berk M, Dean O, Spielholz C, Frye R. Clinical trials of N-acetylcysteine in psychiatry and neurology: a systematic review. Neurosci Biobehav Rev. 2015;55:294–321. https://doi.org/10.1016/j.neubiorev.2015.04.015. Epub 2015 May 6.
33. Mathew SJ. Treatment-resistant depression: recent developments and future directions. Depress Anxiety. 2008;25(12):989–92. https://doi.org/10.1002/da.20540.
34. Kumar A, Chanana P. Role of nitric oxide in stress-induced anxiety: from pathophysiology to therapeutic target. Vitam Horm. 2017;103:147–67. https://doi.org/10.1016/bs.vh.2016.09.004. Epub 2016 Dec 2.
35. Müller CP, Reichel M, Mühle C, Rhein C, Gulbins E, Kornhuber J. Brain membrane lipids in major depression and anxiety disorders. Biochim Biophys Acta. 2015;1851(8):1052–65. https://doi.org/10.1016/j.bbalip.2014.12.014. Epub 2014 Dec 24.
36. Hennebelle M, Champeil-Potokar G, Lavialle M, Vancassel S, Denis I. Omega-3 polyunsaturated fatty acids and chronic stress-induced modulations of glutamatergic neurotransmission in the hippocampus. Nutr Rev. 2014;72(2):99–112. https://doi.org/10.1111/nure.12088. Epub 2014 Jan 13.
37. Appleton KM, Sallis HM, Perry R, Ness AR, Churchill R. ω-3 fatty acids for major depressive disorder in adults: an abridged Cochrane. BMJ Open. 2016;6(3):e010172. https://doi.org/10.1136/bmjopen-2015-010172.
38. Vesco AT, Lehmann J, Gracious BL, Arnold LE, Young AS, Fristad MA. Omega-3 supplementation for psychotic mania and comorbid anxiety in children. J Child Adolesc Psychopharmacol. 2015;25(7):526–34. https://doi.org/10.1089/cap.2013.0141. Epub 2015 Aug 19.
39. Ball J, Carrington MJ, McMurray JJ, Stewart S. Atrial fibrillation: profile and burden of an evolving epidemic in the 21st century. Int J Cardiol. 2013;167:1807–24.
40. Lloyd-Jones DM, Wang TJ, Leip EP, et al. Lifetime risk for development of atrial fibrillation: the Framingham Heart Study. Circulation. 2004;110:1042–6.
41. Fenger-Grøn M, Overvad K, Tjønneland A, Frost L. Lean body mass is the predominant anthropometric risk factor for atrial fibrillation. J Am Coll Cardiol. 2017;69(20):2488–97. https://doi.org/10.1016/j.jacc.2017.03.558.
42. Schnabel RB, Yin X, Gona P, et al. 50 year trends in atrial fibrillation prevalence, incidence, risk factors, and mortality in the Framingham Heart Study: a cohort study. Lancet. 2015;386:154–62.
43. Nattel S. Atrial fibrillation and body composition: is it fat or lean that ultimately determines the risk? J Am Coll Cardiol. 2017;69(20):2498–501. https://doi.org/10.1016/j.jacc.2017.03.566.
44. Colombo J, Arora RR, DePace NL, Vinik AI. Clinical autonomic dysfunction: measurement, indications, therapies, and outcomes. New York: Springer Science + Business Media; 2014.
45. Garrey WE. The nature of fibrillatory contraction of the heart: its relation to tissue mass and form. Am J Phys. 1914;33:397–414.
46. Moore EN, Spear JF. Electrophysiological studies on atrial fibrillation. Heart Vessels Suppl. 1987;2:32–9.
47. Zou R, Kneller J, Leon LJ, Nattel S. Substrate size as a determinant of fibrillatory activity maintenance in a mathematical model of canine atrium. Am J Physiol Heart Circ Physiol. 2005;289:H1002–12.
48. Poirier P, Giles TD, Bray GA, et al. Obesity and cardiovascular disease: pathophysiology, evaluation, and effect of weight loss: an update of the 1997 American Heart Association Scientific Statement on Obesity and Heart Disease from the Obesity Committee of the Council on Nutrition, Physical Activity, and Metabolism. Circulation. 2006;113:898–918.
49. https://www.psychiatry.org/psychiatrists/practice/dsm
50. Rowney J, Hermida T, Malone D. Definition and etiology. 2010. http://www.clevelandclinicmeded.com/medicalpubs/diseasemanagement/psychiatry-psychology/anxiety-disorder/
51. Weissman M, Wickramaratne P, Nomura Y, et al. Offspring of depressed parents: 20 years later. Am J Psychiatry. 2006;163:1001–8.
52. Cardinali DP. Autonomic nervous system: basic and clinical aspects. Cham: Springer International Publishing AG; 2018.
53. Grases G, Colom MA, Fernandez RA, Costa-Bauzá A, Grases F. Evidence of higher oxidative status in depression and anxiety. Oxidative Med Cell Longev. 2014;2014:430216. https://doi.org/10.1155/2014/430216. Epub 2014 Apr 29.
54. McIntyre RS, Soczynska JK, Lewis GF, MacQueen GM, Konarski JZ, Kennedy SH. Managing psychiatric disorders with antidiabetic agents: translational research and treatment opportunities. Expert Opin Pharmacother. 2006;7(10):1305–21.
55. Fernandes BS, Dean OM, Dodd S, Malhi GS, Berk M. N-acetylcysteine in depressive symptoms and functionality: a systematic review and meta-analysis. J Clin Psychiatry. 2016;77(4):e457–66. https://doi.org/10.4088/JCP.15r09984.

56. Kinrys G, Coleman E, Rothstein E. Natural remedies for anxiety disorders: potential use and clinical applications. Depress Anxiety. 2009;26(3):259–65. https://doi.org/10.1002/da.20460.
57. Lakhan SE, Vieira KF. Nutritional and herbal supplements for anxiety and anxiety-related disorders: systematic review. Nutr J. 2010;9:42. https://doi.org/10.1186/1475-2891-9-42.
58. Smaga I, Niedzielska E, Gawlik M, Moniczewski A, Krzek J, Przegaliński E, Pera J, Filip M. Oxidative stress as an etiological factor and a potential treatment target of psychiatric disorders. Part 2. Depression, anxiety, schizophrenia and autism. Pharmacol Rep. 2015;67(3):569–80. https://doi.org/10.1016/j.pharep.2014.12.015. Epub 2015 Jan 5.
59. Gulati K, Rai N, Ray A. Nitric oxide and anxiety. Vitam Horm. 2017;103:169–92. https://doi.org/10.1016/bs.vh.2016.09.001. Epub 2016 Oct 31.
60. Qato DM, Ozenberger K, Olfson M. Prevalence of prescription medications with depression as a potential adverse effect among adults in the United States. JAMA. 2018;319(22):2289. https://doi.org/10.1001/jama.2018.6741.
61. Haas H, Panula P. The role of histamine and the tuberomammillary nucleus in the nervous system. Nat Rev Neurosci. 2003;4:121–30.
62. Piña IL, Di Palo KE, Ventura HO. Psychopharmacology and cardiovascular disease. J Am Coll Cardiol. 2018;71(20):2346–59.
63. American Heart Association Nutrition Committee, Lichtenstein AH, Appel LJ, Brands M, Carnethon M, Daniels S, Franch HA, Franklin B, Kris-Etherton P, Harris WS, Howard B, Karanja N, Lefevre M, Rudel L, Sacks F, Van Horn L, Winston M, Wylie-Rosett J. Diet and lifestyle recommendations revision 2006: a scientific statement from the American Heart Association Nutrition Committee. Circulation. 2006;114(1):82–96. Epub 2006 Jun 19. Erratum in: Circulation. 2006 Dec 5;114(23):e629. Circulation. 2006 Jul 4;114(1):e27.
64. Nemeroff CB, Evans DL. Correlation between the dexamethasone suppression test in depressed patients and clinical response. Am J Psychiatry. 1984;141:247–9.
65. Nemeroff CB, Widerlov E, Bissette G, et al. Elevated concentrations of CSF corticotropin releasing factor-like immunoreactivity in depressed patients. Science. 1984;226:1342–4.
66. Musselman DL, Tomer A, Manatunga AK, et al. Exaggerated platelet reactivity in major depression. Am J Psychiatry. 1996;153:1313–7.
67. Carney RM, Saunders RD, Freedland KE, Stein P, Rich MW, Jaffe AS. Association of depression with reduced heart rate variability in coronary artery disease. Am J Cardiol. 1995;76(8):562–4.
68. Rozanski A, Blumenthal JA, Kaplan J. Impact of psychological factors on the pathogenesis of cardiovascular disease and implications for therapy. Circulation. 1999;99(16):2192–217.
69. Khan SG, Melikian N, Shabeeh H, Cabaco AR, Martin K, Khan F, O'Gallagher K, Chowienczyk PJ, Shah AM. The human coronary vasodilatory response to acute mental stress is mediated by neuronal nitric oxide synthase. Am J Physiol Heart Circ Physiol. 2017;313(3):H578–83. https://doi.org/10.1152/ajpheart.00745.2016. Epub 2017 Jun 23.
70. Preisig M, Waeber G, Mooser V, Vollenweider P. PsyCoLaus: mental disorders and cardiovascular diseases: spurious association? Rev Med Suisse. 2011;7:2127–9.
71. Chaddha A, Robinson EA, Kline-Rogers E, Alexandris-Souphis T, Rubenfire M. Mental health and cardiovascular disease. Am J Med. 2016;129:1145–8.
72. Rugulies R. Depression as a predictor for coronary heart disease: a review and meta-analysis1. Am J Prev Med. 2002;23:51–61.
73. Denollet J, Maas K, Knottnerus A, Keyzer JJ, Pop VJ. Anxiety predicted premature all-cause and cardiovascular death in a 10-year follow-up of middle-aged women. J Clin Epidemiol. 2009;62:452–6.
74. Blumenthal JA, Babyak MA, O'Connor C, Keteyian S, Landzberg J, Howlett J, et al. Effects of exercise training on depressive symptoms inpatients with chronic heart failure: the HF-ACTION randomized trial. JAMA. 2012;308:465–74.
75. Janszky I, Ahnve S, Lundberg I, Hemmingsson T. Early-onset depression, anxiety, and risk of subsequent coronary heart disease: 37- year follow-up of 49,321 young Swedish men. J Am Coll Cardiol. 2010;56:31–7.
76. Phillips AC, Batty GD, Gale CR, et al. Generalized anxiety disorder, major depressive disorder, and their comorbidity as predictors of all-cause and cardiovascular mortality: the Vietnam experience study. Psychosom Med. 2009;71:395–403.
77. Rutledge T, Linke SE, Krantz DS, et al. Comorbid depression and anxiety symptoms as predictors of cardiovascular events: results from the NHLBI-sponsored Women's Ischemia Syndrome Evaluation (WISE) study. Psychosom Med. 2009;71:958–64.
78. Chida Y, Steptoe A. The association of anger and hostility with future coronary heart disease: a meta-analytic review of prospective evidence. J Am Coll Cardiol. 2009;53:936–46.
79. Lampert R, Joska T, Burg MM, Batsford WP, McPherson CA, Jain D. Emotional and physical precipitants of ventricular arrhythmia. Circulation. 2002;106:1800–5.
80. Krantz DS, Kop WJ, Santiago HT, Gottdiener JS. Mental stress as a trigger of myocardial ischemia and infarction. Cardiol Clin. 1996;14(2):271–87.
81. Krantz DS, McCeney MK. Effects of psychological and social factors on organic disease: a critical assessment of research on coronary heart disease. Annu Rev Psychol. 2002;53:341–69.

82. Karasek R, Baker D, Marxer F, Ahlbom A, Theorell T. Job decision latitude, job demands, and cardiovascular disease: a prospective study of Swedish men. Am J Public Health. 1981;71:694–705.
83. Greenlund KJ, Kiefe CI, Giles WH, Liu K. Associations of job strain and occupation with subclinical atherosclerosis: the CARDIA study. Ann Epidemiol. 2010;20:323–31.
84. Eller NH, Netterstrøm B, Gyntelberg F, et al. Work-related psychosocial factors and the development of ischemic heart disease: a systematic review. Cardiol Rev. 2009;17:83–97.
85. Leor J, Poole WK, Kloner RA. Sudden cardiac death triggered by an earthquake. N Engl J Med. 1996;334:413–9.
86. Ader R, Felten DL, Cohen N, editors. Psychoneuroimmunology, vol. 2. Waltham Abbey: Academic Press; 2000. ISBN 978-0-12-0443147.
87. Rosengren A, Hawken S, Ôunpuu S, et al. Association of psychosocial risk factors with risk of acute myocardial infarction in 11 119 cases and 13 648 controls from 52 countries (the INTERHEART study): case-control study. Lancet. 2004;364:953–62.
88. Orth-Gomer K, Wamala SP, Horsten M, Schenck-Gustafsson K, Schneiderman N, Mittleman MA. Marital stress worsens prognosis in women with coronary heart disease: the Stockholm Female Coronary Risk Study. JAMA. 2000;284:3008–14.
89. Gabbay FH, Krantz DS, Kop WJ, et al. Triggers of myocardial ischemia during daily life in patients with coronary artery disease: physical and mental activities, anger and smoking. J Am Coll Cardiol. 1996;27:585–92.
90. Gullette EC, Blumenthal JA, Babyak M, et al. Effects of mental stress on myocardial ischemia during daily life. JAMA. 1997;277:1521–6.
91. Jiang W, Babyak M, Krantz DS, et al. Mental stress–induced myocardial ischemia and cardiac events. JAMA. 1996;275:1651–6.
92. Williams RB, Haney TL, Lee KL, Kong Y-H, Blumenthal JA, Whalen RE. Type A behavior, hostility, and coronary atherosclerosis. Psychosom Med. 1980;42:539–49.
93. Tindle HA, Chang YF, Kuller LH, et al. Optimism, cynical hostility, and incident coronary heart disease and mortality in the Women's Health Initiative. Circulation. 2009;120:656–62.
94. Mc Donnell CG, Shorten G, Van Pelt FN. Effect of atorvastatin and fluvastatin on the metabolism of midazolam by cytochrome P450 in vitro. Anaesthesia. 2005;60:747–53.
95. Jiang W, O'Connor C, Silva SG, et al. Safety and efficacy of sertraline for depression in patients with CHF (SADHART-CHF): a randomized, double-blind, placebo-controlled trial of sertraline for major depression with congestive heart failure. Am Heart J. 2008;156:437–44.
96. Pizzi C, Mancini S, Angeloni L, Fontana F, Manzoli L, Costa G. Effects of selective serotonin reuptake inhibitor therapy on endothelial function and inflammatory markers in patients with coronary heart disease. Clin Pharmacol Ther. 2009;86:527–32.
97. Beach SR, Kostis WJ, Celano CM, et al. Metaanalysis of selective serotonin reuptake inhibitor associated QTc prolongation. J Clin Psychiatry. 2014;75:e441–9.
98. Pizzi C, Rutjes AWS, Costa GM, Fontana F, Mezzetti A, Manzoli L. Meta-analysis of selective serotonin reuptake inhibitors in patients with depression and coronary heart disease. Am J Cardiol. 2011;107:972–9.
99. Ho JM, Gomes T, Straus SE, Austin PC, Mamdani M, Juurlink DN. Adverse cardiac events in older patients receiving venlafaxine: a population-based study. J Clin Psychiatry. 2014;75:e552–8.
100. Shah S, Iqbal Z, White A, White S. Heart and mind: (2) psychotropic and cardiovascular therapeutics. Postgrad Med J. 2005;81:33–40.
101. Mackin P. Cardiac side effects of psychiatric drugs. Hum Psychopharmacol Clin Exp. 2008;23(S1):3–14.
102. Kovacs D, Arora R. Cardiovascular effects of psychotropic drugs. Am J Ther. 2008;15:474–83.
103. Giardina E-GV, Johnson LL, Vita J, Bigger JT Jr, Brem RF. Effect of imipramine and nortriptyline on left ventricular function and blood pressure in patients treated for arrhythmias. Am Heart J. 1985;109:992–8.
104. Roose SP, Dalack GW. Cardiovascular effects of bupropion in depressed patients with heart disease. Am J Psychiatry. 1991;148:512.
105. Roose SP, Glassman AH, Giardina EG, Johnson LL, Walsh BT, Bigger JT Jr. Cardiovascular effects of imipramine and bupropion in depressed patients with congestive heart failure. J Clin Psychopharmacol. 1987;7:247–51.
106. Vitullo RN, Wharton JM, Allen NB, Pritchett EL. Trazodone-related exercise-induced non-sustained ventricular tachycardia. Chest. 1990;98:247–8.
107. Boschmans S, Perkin M, Terblanche S, Opie L. The effects of imipramine, mianserin and trazodone on the chronotropic, inotropic and coronary vascular responses in the isolated perfused rat heart. Gen Pharmacol. 1989;20:233–7.
108. Mazur A, Strasberg B, Kusniec J, Sclarovsky S. QT prolongation and polymorphous ventricular tachycardia associated with trazodone amiodarone combination. Int J Cardiol. 1995;52:27–9.
109. Libert J, Amoros C, Muzet A, Ehrhart J, Di Nisi J. Effects of triazolam on heart rate level and on phasic cardiac response to noise during sleep. Psychopharmacology. 1988;96:188–93.
110. Lapane KL, Zierler S, Lasater TM, Barbour MM, Carleton R, Hume AL. Is the use of psychotropic drugs associated with increased risk of ischemic heart disease? Epidemiology. 1995;6:376–81.

111. Kim YH, Kim HB, Kim DH, Kim JY, Shin HY. Use of hypnotics and the risk of or mortality from heart disease: a meta-analysis of observational studies. Korean J Intern Med. 2017;33(4):727–36. [E-pub ahead of print].
112. Schneier FR. Social anxiety disorder. N Engl J Med. 2006;355:1029–36.
113. Hoogwegt MT, Kupper N, Theuns DA, Jordaens L, Pedersen SS. Beta-blocker therapy is not associated with symptoms of depression and anxiety in patients receiving an implantable cardioverter-defibrillator. Europace. 2011;14:74–80.
114. Hammond DC. What is neurofeedback: an update. J Neurother. 2011;15:305–36.
115. Scott WC, Kaiser D, Othmer S, Sideroff SI. Effects of an EEG biofeedback protocol on a mixed substance abusing population. Am J Drug Alcohol Abuse. 2005;3:1455–69.
116. Kaiser DA, Othmer S. Effect of neurofeedback on variables of attention in a large multi-center trial. J Neurother. 2000;4(1):5–28.
117. Demos JN. Getting started with neurofeedback. New York/London: Norton & company; 2005.
118. Gunkelman JD, Johnstone J. Neurofeedback and the brain. J Adult Dev. 2005;12:93–100.
119. Kropotov JD, Grin-Yatsenko VA, Ponomarev VA, Chutko LS, Yakovenko EA, Nikishena IS. Changes in EEG spectrograms, event-related potentials and event-related desynchronization induced by relative beta training in ADHD children. J Neurother. 2007;11(2):3–11.
120. Strehl U, Leins U, Goth G, Klinger C, Hinterberger T, Birbaumer N. Self-regulation of slow cortical potentials: a new treatment for children with attention-deficit/hyperactivity disorder. J Pediatr. 2006;118:1530–40.
121. Rossiter T. The effectiveness of neurofeedback and stimulant drugs in treating AD/HD: part I. Review of methodological issues. Appl Psychophysiol Biofeedback. 2004;29(2):95–112.
122. Fuchs T, Birbaumer N, Lutzenberger W, Gruzelier JH, Kaiser J. Neurofeedback treatment for attention-deficit/hyperactivity disorder in children: a comparison with methylphenidate. Appl Psychophysiol Biofeedback. 2003;28(1):1–12.
123. Kotchoubey B, Strehl U, Uhlmann C, Holzapfel S, Konig M, Froscher W, et al. Modification of slow cortical potentials in patients with refractory epilepsy: a controlled outcome study. Epilepsies. 2001;42(3):406–16.
124. Putman JA. EEG biofeedback on a female patient stroke patient with depression: a case study. J Neurother. 2001;5(3):27–38.
125. Hammond DC. Neurofeedback with anxiety and affective disorders. Child Adolesc Psychiatr. 2005;14(1):105–23.
126. Vanathy S, Sharma PSVN, Kumar KB. The efficacy of alpha and theta neurofeedback training in treatment of generalized anxiety disorder. Indian J Clin Psychol. 1998;25(2):136–43.
127. Muller HH, Donaldson CCS, Nelson DV, Layman M. Treatment of fibromyalgia incorporating EEG-driven stimulation: a clinical study. J Clin Psychol. 2001;57(7):925–33.
128. Hammond DC. QEEG-guided neurofeedback in the treatment of obsessive compulsive disorder. J Neurother. 2003;7(2):25–52.
129. Wilson VE, Peper E, Moss D. Professional issue "the mind room" in Italian soccer training: the use of biofeedback and neurofeedback for optimum performance. Biofeedback. 2006;34:79–810.
130. Hanslmayr S, Sauseng P, Doppelmayr M, Schabus M, Klimesch W. Increasing individual upper alpha power by neurofeedback improves cognitive performance in human subjects. Appl Psychophysiol Biofeedback. 2005;30(1):1–10.
131. Egner T, Strawson E, Gruzelier JH. EEG signature and phenomenology of alpha-theta neurofeedback training versus mock feedback. Appl Psychophysiol Biofeedback. 2002;27:4–18.
132. Vernon D, Egner T, Nick C, et al. The effect of training distinct neurofeedback protocols on aspects of cognitive performance. J Psychophysiol. 2003;47(1):75–85.
133. Sokhadze TM, Cannon RL, Trudeau DL. EEG biofeedback as a treatment for substance use disorders: review, rating of efficacy, and recommendations for further research. Appl Psychophysiol Biofeedback. 2008;33(1):1–28.
134. Frederick JA, Timmermann DL, Russell HL, Lubar JF. EEG coherence effects of audio-visual stimulation (AVS) at dominant alpha frequency. J Neurother. 2005;8(4):25–42.
135. Burkett VS, Cummins JM, Dickson RM, Skolnick MH. Treatment effects related to EEG-biofeedback for crack cocaine dependency in a faith-based homeless mission. J Neurother. 2004;8(2):138–40.
136. Masterpasqua F, Healey KN. Neurofeedback in psychological practice. Prof Psychol Res Pract. 2003;34(6):652–6.
137. Kaiser DA, Othmer S, Scott B. Effect of neurofeedback on chemical dependency treatment. Biofeedback Self Regul. 1999;20(3):304–5.
138. Peniston EG, Saxby E. Alpha-theta brainwave neurofeedback training: an effective treatment for male and female alcoholics with depression symptoms. Biofeedback Cent. 1995;51(5):685–93.
139. Hammond DC. The need for individualization in neurofeedback: heterogeneity in qEEG patterns associated with diagnoses and symptoms. Appl Psychophysiol Biofeedback. 2010;35(1):31–6.
140. Ross SM. Neurofeedback: an integrative treatment of substance use disorders. Holist Nurs Pract. 2013;27(4):246–50.
141. Dehghani-Arani F, Rostami R, Nadali H. Neurofeedback training for opiate addiction: improvement of mental health and craving. Appl Psychophysiol Biofeedback. 2013;38:133–41. https://doi.org/10.1007/s10484-013-9218-5.

142. Peniston EG, Kulkosky PJ. Alpha-theta brainwave training and beta endorphin levels in alcoholics. Alcohol Clin Exp Res. 1989;13:271–9.
143. Peniston EG, Kulkosky PJ. Alcoholic personality and alpha-theta brainwave training. Med Psychother. 1990;2:37–55.
144. Peniston EG, Marriman DA, Deming WA, Kulkosky PG. EEG alpha theta brain wave synchronization in Vietnam theater veterans with combat related post traumatic stress disorder and alcohol abuse. Adv Med Psychol. 1993;6:37–49.
145. Gruzelier J, Egner T. Critical validation studies of neurofeedback. Child Adolesc Psychiatr Clin N Am. 2005;14:83–104.
146. Singer W, Spies JM, McArthur J, Low J, Griffin JW, Nickander KK, Gordon V, Low PA. Prospective evaluation of somatic and autonomic small fibers in selected autonomic neuropathies. Neurology. 2004;62:612–8.
147. Dabby R, Vaknine H, Gilad R, Djaldetti R, Sadeh M. Evaluation of cutaneous autonomic innervation in idiopathic sensory small-fiber neuropathy. J Peripher Nerv Syst. 2007;12:98–101.
148. Lauria G, Bakkers M, Schmitz C, Lombardi R, Penza P, Devigili G, Smith AG, Hsieh ST, Mellgren SI, Umapathi T, Ziegler D, Faber CG, Merkies IS. Intraepidermal nerve fiber density at the distal leg: a worldwide normative reference study. J Peripher Nerv Syst. 2010;15:202–7.
149. Jacobs AM, Cheng D. Management of diabetic small-fiber neuropathy with combination L-methylfolate, methylcobalamin, and pyridoxal 5′-phosphate. Rev Neurol Dis. 2011;8(1–2):39–47.
150. Hovaguimian A, Gibbons CH. Diagnosis and treatment of pain in small fiber neuropathy. Curr Pain Headache Rep. 2011;15(3):193–200. https://doi.org/10.1007/s11916-011-0181-7.
151. Brannagan TH 3rd, Hays AP, Chin SS, Sander HW, Chin RL, Magda P, Green PH, Latov N. Small-fiber neuropathy/neuronopathy associated with celiac disease: skin biopsy findings. Arch Neurol. 2005;62(10):1574–8.
152. Ho TW, Backonja M, Ma J, Leibensperger H, Froman S, Polydefkis M. Efficient assessment of neuropathic pain drugs in patients with small fiber sensory neuropathies. Pain. 2009;141:19–24.
153. Ametov AS, Barinov A, Dyck PJ, Hermann R, Kozlova N, Litchy WJ, Low PA, Nehrdich D, Novosadova M, O'Brien PC, Reljanovic M, Samigullin R, Schuette K, Strokov I, Tritschler HJ, Wessel K, Yakhno N, Ziegler D, SYDNEY Trial Study Group. The sensory symptoms of diabetic polyneuropathy are improved with alpha-lipoic acid: the SYDNEY trial. Diabetes Care. 2003;26(3):770–6. Erratum in: Diabetes Care. 2003 Jul;26(7):2227.
154. Ziegler D, Nowak H, Kempler P, Vargha P, Low PA. Treatment of symptomatic diabetic polyneuropathy with the antioxidant alpha-lipoic acid: a meta-analysis. Diabet Med. 2004;21(2):114–21.
155. Ziegler D, Ametov A, Barinov A, Dyck PJ, Gurieva I, Low PA, Munzel U, Yakhno N, Raz I, Novosadova M, Maus J, Samigullin R. Oral treatment with alpha-lipoic acid improves symptomatic diabetic polyneuropathy: the SYDNEY 2 trial. Diabetes Care. 2006;29(11):2365–70.
156. Vinik AI. A medicinal food provides food for thought in managing diabetic neuropathy. Am J Med. 2013;126(2):95–6. https://doi.org/10.1016/j.amjmed.2012.08.008.
157. Head KA. Peripheral neuropathy: pathogenic mechanisms and alternative therapies. Altern Med Rev. 2006;11:294–329.
158. Zhang YF, Ning G. Mecobalamin. Expert Opin Ivestigat Drugs. 2008;17:953–64.
159. Schrezenmaier C, Singer W, Muenter Swift N, Sletten D, Tanabe J, Low PA. Adrenergic and vagal baroreflex sensitivity in autonomic failure. Arch Neurol. 2007;64:381–6.
160. Boulton AJM, Vinik AI, Arrezzo JC, Bril V, Feldman EI, Freeman R, Malik RA, Maser RE, Sosenko JM, Ziegler D. Diabetic neuropathies: a statement by the American Diabetes Association. Diabetes Care. 2005;28(4):956–62.
161. Curtis BM, O'Keefe JH. Autonomic tone as a cardiovascular risk factor: the dangers of chronic fight or flight. Mayo Clin Proc. 2002;77:45–54.
162. Low PA, The Therapeutics and Technology Assessment Subcommittee Assessment. Clinical autonomic testing report of the Therapeutics and Technology Assessment Subcommittee of the American Academy of Neurology. Neurology. 1996;46:873–80.
163. Joint Editorial Statement by the American Diabetes Association; the National Heart, Lung, and Blood Institute; the Juvenile Diabetes Foundation International; the National Institute of Diabetes and Digestive and Kidney Diseases; and the American Heart Association. Diabetes mellitus: a major risk factor for cardiovascular disease. Circulation. 1999;100:1132–3.
164. Grundy SM, Benjamin IJ, Burke GL, Chait A. AHA scientific statement: diabetes and cardiovascular disease, a statement for healthcare professionals from the American Heart Association. Circulation. 1999;100:1134–46.
165. Aring AM, Jones DE, Falko JM. Evaluation and prevention of diabetic neuropathy. Am Fam Physicians. 2005;71:2123–30.
166. Vinik AI, Maser RE, Nakave AA. Diabetic cardiovascular autonomic nerve dysfunction. US Endocr Dis. 2007;2:2–9.
167. Vinik A, Ziegler D. Diabetic cardiovascular autonomic neuropathy. Circulation. 2007;115:387–97.
168. Arora RR, Bulgarelli RJ, Ghosh-Dastidar S, Colombo J. Autonomic mechanisms and therapeutic implications of postural diabetic cardiovascular abnormalities. J Diabetes Sci Technol. 2008;2(4):568–71.
169. Arora RR, Ghosh Dastidar S, Colombo J Autonomic balance is associated with decreased morbidity. American Autonomic Society, 17th International Symposium, Kauai; 29 Oct–1 Nov 2008.
170. Waheed A, Ali MA, Jurivich DA, et al. Gender differences in longevity and autonomic function.

Presented at the Geriatric Medicine Society Meeting, Chicago; 3–7 May 2006.
171. Arora RR, Aysin E, Aysin B, Colombo J. Therapeutic implications of Sympathetic stimulus in orthostatic patients: measured by spectral domain analysis. AHA Scientific Sessions, Orlando; 4–7 Nov 2007.
172. Vinik AI, Murray GL. Autonomic neuropathy is treatable. US Endocrinol. 2008;2:82–4.
173. Nemechek P, Ghosh Dastidar S, Colombo J. Early autonomic dysfunction is associated with secondary hypertension in HIV/AIDS patients. American Autonomic Society, St. Thomas, Virgin Islands; 31 Oct–3 Nov 2009.
174. Nemechek P, Ghosh Dastidar S, Colombo J. HIV/AIDS leads to early cardiovascular autonomic neuropathy. American Autonomic Society, St. Thomas, Virgin Islands, 31 Oct–3 Nov 2009.
175. Arora RR, Bulgarelli RJ, Hearyman M, Ghosh Dastidar S, Colombo J. Carvedilol reverses standing parasympathetic excess in non-diabetics. American Autonomic Society, St. Thomas, Virgin Islands; 31 Oct–3 Nov 2009.
176. Nanavati SH, Bulgarelli RJ, Vazquez-Tanus J, Ghosh-Dastidar S, Colombo J, Arora RR. Altered autonomic activity with atrial fibrillation as demonstrated by non-invasive autonomic monitoring. US Cardiol. 2010;7(1):47–50.
177. Vinik AI, Aysin B, Colombo J. Differentiation of autonomic dysfunction by enhanced frequency domain analysis reveals additional stages in the progression of autonomic decline in diabetics. Diabetes Technology Conference, San Francisco; 10–12 Nov 2005.
178. Boyd GL, Taylor JA, Ovalle F, Stout DG, Aultman M, Garner VM, Morris RE, Witherspoon CD, Albert M, Vetter TR. Prevalence of advanced autonomic dysfunction in patients presenting for retinal surgery. Submitted, Anesthesiology; 2013.
179. Wani AL, Bhat SA, Ara A. Omega-3 fatty acids and the treatment of depression: a review of scientific evidence. Integr Med Res. 2015;4(3):132–41.
180. Boulton AJM, Vinik AI, Arrezzo JC, Bril V, Feldman EI, Freeman R, Malik RA, Maser RE, Sosenko JM, Ziegler D. Diabetic neuropathies: a statement by the American Diabetes Association. Diabetes Care. 2005;28(4):956–62.
181. Boulton AJM, Vinik AI, Arrezzo JC, Bril V, Feldman EI, Freeman R, Malik RA, Maser RE, Sosenko JM, Ziegler D. Diabetic neuropathies: a statement by the American Diabetes Association. Diabetes Care. 2005;28(4):956–62.
182. Aring AM, Jones DE, Falko JM. Evaluation and prevention of diabetic neuropathy. Am Fam Physicians. 2005;71:2123–30.
183. Chen J, Long JB, Hurria A, Owusu C, Steingart RM, Gross CP. Incidence of heart failure or cardiomyopathy after adjuvant trastuzumab therapy for breast cancer. J Am Coll Cardiol. 2012;60:2504–12.
184. Bowles EJA, Wellman R, Feigelson HS, et al. Risk of heart failure in breast cancer patients after anthracycline and trastuzumab treatment: a retrospective cohort study. J Natl Cancer Inst. 2012;104:1293–305.
185. Lenihan DJ, Cardinale DM. Late cardiac effects of cancer treatment [published correction appears in J Clin Oncol 2012;30:4590]. J Clin Oncol. 2012;30:3657–64.
186. Mukhopadhyay P, Rajesh M, Bátkai S, et al. Role of superoxide, nitric oxide, and peroxynitrite in doxorubicin-induced cell death in vivo and in vitro. Am J Physiol Heart Circ Physiol. 2009;296:1466–83.
187. Weinstein DM, Mihm MJ, Bauer JA. Cardiac peroxynitrite formation and left ventricular dysfunction following doxorubicin treatment in mice. J Pharmacol Exp Ther. 2000;294:396–401.
188. Fogli S, Nieri P, Breschi MC. The role of nitric oxide in anthracycline toxicity and prospects for pharmacologic prevention of cardiac damage. FASEB J. 2004;18:664–75.
189. Ky B, Putt M, Sawaya H, et al. Early increases in multiple biomarkers predict subsequent cardiotoxicity in patients with breast cancer treated with doxorubicin, taxanes, and trastuzumab [published correction appears in J Am Coll Cardiol 2016;67:1385]. J Am Coll Cardiol. 2014;63:809–16.
190. Zhang S, Liu X, Bawa-Khalfe T, et al. Identification of the molecular basis of doxorubicin induced cardiotoxicity. Nat Med. 2012;18:1639–42.
191. Wan A, Rodrigues B. Endothelial cell cardiomyocyte crosstalk in diabetic cardiomyopathy. Cardiovasc Res. 2016;111:172–83.
192. Hahn VS, Lenihan DJ, Ky B. Cancer therapy induced cardiotoxicity: basic mechanisms and potential cardioprotective therapies. J Am Heart Assoc. 2014;3:e000665.
193. Versari D, Daghini E, Virdis A, Ghiadoni L, Taddei S. Endothelium-dependent contractions and endothelial dysfunction in human hypertension. Br J Pharmacol. 2009;157:527–36.
194. Milano G, Raucci A, Scopece A, et al. Doxorubicin and trastuzumab regimen induces biventricular failure in mice. J Am Soc Echocardiogr. 2014;27:568–79.
195. Aghajanian H, Cho YK, Manderfield LJ, et al. Coronary vasculature patterning requires a novel endothelial ErbB2 holoreceptor. Nat Commun. 2016;7:12038.
196. Wolf MB, Baynes JW. The anti-cancer drug, doxorubicin, causes oxidant stress-induced endothelial dysfunction. Biochim Biophys Acta. 1760;2006:267–71.
197. Finkelman BS, Putt M, Wang T, Wang L, Narayan H, Domchek S, DeMichele A, Fox K, Matro J, Shah P, Clark A, Bradbury A, Narayan V, Carver JR, Tang WHW, Ky B. Arginine-nitric oxide metabolites and cardiac dysfunction in patients with breast cancer. J Am Coll Cardiol. 2017;70(2):152–62. https://doi.org/10.1016/j.jacc.2017.05.019. Erratum in: J Am Coll Cardiol. 2017 Nov 28;70(21):2738.
198. Toya T, Hakuno D, Shiraishi Y, Kujiraoka T, Adachi T. Arginase inhibition augments nitric oxide production and facilitates left ventricular systolic function

in doxorubicin-induced cardiomyopathy in mice. Physiol Rep. 2014;2:e12130.
199. Hammond J, Balligand J. Nitric oxide synthase and cyclic GMP signaling in cardiac myocytes: from contractility to remodeling. J Mol Cell Cardiol. 2012;52:330–40.
200. Meinitzer A, Seelhorst U, Wellnitz B, et al. Asymmetrical dimethylarginine independently predicts total and cardiovascular mortality in individuals with angiographic coronary artery disease (the Ludwigshafen Risk and Cardiovascular Health Study). Clin Chem. 2007;53:273–83.
201. Boger RH, Sullivan LM, Schwedhelm E, et al. Plasma asymmetric dimethylarginine and incidence of cardiovascular disease and death in the community. Circulation. 2009;119:1592–600.
202. Dückelmann C, Mittermayer F, Haider DG, Altenberger J, Eichinger J, Wolzt M. Asymmetric dimethylarginine enhances cardiovascular risk prediction in patients with chronic heart failure. Arterioscler Thromb Vasc Biol. 2007;27:2037–42.
203. Liu X, Hou L, Xu D, et al. Effect of asymmetric dimethylarginine (ADMA) on heart failure development. Nitric Oxide. 2016;54:73–81.
204. Myalgic encephalomyelitis, chronic fatigue syndrome. Centers for Disease Control and Prevention; 3 July 2007.
205. Carruthers BM, van de Sande MI, De Meirleir KL, Klimas NG, Broderick G, Mitchell T, Staines D, Powles AC, Speight N, Vallings R, Bateman L, Baumgarten-Austrheim B, Bell DS, Carlo-Stella N, Chia J, Darragh A, Jo D, Lewis D, Light AR, Marshall-Gradisbik S, Mena I, Mikovits JA, Miwa K, Murovska M, Pall ML, Stevens S. Myalgic encephalomyelitis: international consensus criteria. J Intern Med. 2011;270(4):327–38. https://doi.org/10.1111/j.1365-2796.2011.02428.x. Epub 2011 Aug 22. Review. Erratum in: J Intern Med. 2017 Oct;282(4):353. PMID: 21777306.
206. Carruthers BM. Definitions and aetiology of myalgic encephalomyelitis: how the Canadian consensus clinical definition of myalgic encephalomyelitis works. J Clin Pathol. 2007;60(2):117–9. Epub 2006 Aug 25.
207. Barnden LR, Kwiatek R, Crouch B, Burnet R, Del Fante P. Autonomic correlations with MRI are abnormal in the brainstem vasomotor centre in Chronic Fatigue Syndrome. Neuroimage Clin. 2016;11:530–7. https://doi.org/10.1016/j.nicl.2016.03.017. eCollection 2016. PMID: 27114901.
208. Bested AC, Marshall LM. Review of Myalgic Encephalomyelitis/Chronic Fatigue Syndrome: an evidence-based approach to diagnosis and management by clinicians. Rev Environ Health. 2015;30(4):223–49. https://doi.org/10.1515/reveh-2015-0026. Review. PMID: 26613325.
209. Tanaka M, Tajima S, Mizuno K, Ishii A, Konishi Y, Miike T, Watanabe Y. Frontier studies on fatigue, autonomic nerve dysfunction, and sleep-rhythm disorder. J Physiol Sci. 2015;65(6):483–98. https://doi.org/10.1007/s12576-015-0399-y. Epub 2015 Sept 29. Review. PMID: 26420687.
210. Van Cauwenbergh D, Nijs J, Kos D, Van Weijnen L, Struyf F, Meeus M. Malfunctioning of the autonomic nervous system in patients with chronic fatigue syndrome: a systematic literature review. Eur J Clin Investig. 2014;44(5):516–26. https://doi.org/10.1111/eci.12256.
211. Lewis I, Pairman J, Spickett G, Newton JL. Clinical characteristics of a novel subgroup of chronic fatigue syndrome patients with postural orthostatic tachycardia syndrome. J Intern Med. 2013;273(5):501–10. https://doi.org/10.1111/joim.12022. Epub 2013 Jan 7. PMID: 23206180.
212. Myhill S, Booth NE, McLaren-Howard J. Targeting mitochondrial dysfunction in the treatment of Myalgic Encephalomyelitis/Chronic Fatigue Syndrome (ME/CFS) – a clinical audit. Int J Clin Exp Med. 2013;6(1):1–15. Epub 2012 Nov 20. PMID: 23236553.
213. Booth NE, Myhill S, McLaren-Howard J. Mitochondrial dysfunction and the pathophysiology of Myalgic Encephalomyelitis/Chronic Fatigue Syndrome (ME/CFS). Int J Clin Exp Med. 2012;5(3):208–20. Epub 2012 Jun 15. PMID: 22837795.
214. Myhill S, Booth NE, McLaren-Howard J. Chronic fatigue syndrome and mitochondrial dysfunction. Int J Clin Exp Med. 2009;2(1):1–16. Epub 2009 Jan 15. PMID: 19436827.
215. World Health Association International Statistics Classification Disease and Related Health Problems, 10th revision, ICD-10, 2010, cited 2014, available from http/APPS.WHO.International Classifications, ICD-10, Brown, 2010, G90–G99. https://icd.who.int/browse10/2014/en#/
216. Morris G, Maes M. Myalgic encephalomyelitis/chronic fatigue syndrome and encephalomyelitis disseminata/multiple sclerosis show remarkable levels of similarity in phenomenology and neuroimmune characteristics. BMC Med. 2013;11:205. https://doi.org/10.1186/1741-7015-11-205. Review. PMID: 24229326.
217. Agarwal AK, Garg R, Ritch A, Sarkar P. Postural orthostatic tachycardia syndrome. Postgrad Med J. 2007;83(981):478–80. Review. PMID: 17621618.
218. Tomas C, Newton J, Watson S. A review of hypothalamic-pituitary-adrenal axis function in chronic fatigue syndrome. ISRN Neurosci. 2013;2013:784520. https://doi.org/10.1155/2013/784520. eCollection 2013. PMID: 24959566.
219. Jason L, Sorenson M, Sebally K, Alkazemi D, Lerch A, Porter N, Kubow S. Increased HDAC in association with decreased plasma cortisol in older adults with chronic fatigue syndrome. Brain Behav Immun. 2011;25(8):1544–7. https://doi.org/10.1016/j.bbi.2011.04.007. Epub 2011 Apr 28. PMID: 21549189.
220. Crofford LJ, Young EA, Engleberg NC, Korszun A, Brucksch CB, McClure LA, Brown MB, Demitrack

MA. Basal circadian and pulsatile ACTH and cortisol secretion in patients with fibromyalgia and/or chronic fatigue syndrome. Brain Behav Immun. 2004;18(4):314–25.

221. Cairns R, Hotopf M. A systematic review describing the prognosis of chronic fatigue syndrome. Occup Med (Lond). 2005;55(1):20–31.
222. Newton JL, Okonkwo O, Sutcliffe K, Seth A, Shin J, Jones DE. Symptoms of autonomic dysfunction in chronic fatigue syndrome. QJM. 2007;100(8):519–26. Epub 2007 Jul 7.
223. Costigan A, Elliott C, McDonald C, Newton JL. Orthostatic symptoms predict functional capacity in chronic fatigue syndrome: implications for management. QJM. 2010;103(8):589–95. https://doi.org/10.1093/qjmed/hcq094. Epub 2010 Jun 9.
224. Woltjer HH, Bogaard HJ, de Vries PM. The technique of impedance cardiography. Eur Heart J. 1997;18(9):1396–403.
225. Jones DE, Gray J, Frith J, Newton JL. Fatigue severity remains stable over time and independently associated with orthostatic symptoms in chronic fatigue syndrome: a longitudinal study. J Intern Med. 2011;269(2):182–8. https://doi.org/10.1111/j.1365--2796.2010.02306.x. Epub 2010 Nov 14. PMID: 21073560.
226. Hollingsworth KG, Jones DE, Taylor R, Blamire AM, Newton JL. Impaired cardiovascular response to standing in chronic fatigue syndrome. Eur J Clin Investig. 2010;40(7):608–15. https://doi.org/10.1111/j.1365-2362.2010.02310.x. Epub 2010 May 23. PMID: 20497461.
227. Okamoto LE, Raj SR, Peltier A, Gamboa A, Shibao C, Diedrich A, Black BK, Robertson D, Biaggioni I. Neurohumoral and haemodynamic profile in postural tachycardia and chronic fatigue syndromes. Clin Sci (Lond). 2012;122(4):183–92. https://doi.org/10.1042/CS20110200. PMID: 21906029.
228. Naschitz J, Dreyfuss D, Yeshurun D, Rosner I. Midodrine treatment for chronic fatigue syndrome. Postgrad Med J. 2004;80(942):230–2. PMID: 15082846.
229. Naschitz JE, Rosner I, Rozenbaum M, Naschitz S, Musafia-Priselac R, Shaviv N, Fields M, Isseroff H, Zuckerman E, Yeshurun D, Sabo E. The head-up tilt test with haemodynamic instability score in diagnosing chronic fatigue syndrome. QJM. 2003;96(2):133–42.
230. DuBois RE. Gamma globulin therapy for chronic mononucleosis syndrome. AIDS Res. 1986;2(Suppl 1):S191–5. PMID: 2435296.
231. Fluge Ø, Risa K, Lunde S, Alme K, Rekeland IG, Sapkota D, Kristoffersen EK, Sørland K, Bruland O, Dahl O, Mella O. B-lymphocyte depletion in myalgic encephalopathy/chronic fatigue syndrome. An open-label phase ii study with rituximab maintenance treatment. PLoS One. 2015;10(7):e0129898. https://doi.org/10.1371/journal.pone.0129898. eCollection 2015. PMID: 26132314.
232. Fluge Ø, Bruland O, Risa K, Storstein A, Kristoffersen EK, Sapkota D, Næss H, Dahl O, Nyland H, Mella O. Benefit from B-lymphocyte depletion using the anti-CD20 antibody rituximab in chronic fatigue syndrome. A double-blind and placebo-controlled study. PLoS One. 2011;6(10):e26358. https://doi.org/10.1371/journal.pone.0026358. Epub 2011 Oct 19. PMID: 22039471.
233. Papadopoulos A, Ebrecht M, Roberts AD, Poon L, Rohleder N, Cleare AJ. Glucocorticoid receptor mediated negative feedback in chronic fatigue syndrome using the low dose (0.5 mg) dexamethasone suppression test. J Affect Disord. 2009;112(1–3):289–94. https://doi.org/10.1016/j.jad.2008.05.001. Epub 2008 Jun 24. PMID: 18573538.
234. Filler K, Lyon D, Bennett J, McCain N, Elswick R, Lukkahatai N, Saligan LN. Association of mitochondrial dysfunction and fatigue: a review of the literature. BBA Clin. 2014;1:12–23.
235. Gerdle B, Forsgren MF, Bengtsson A, Leinhard OD, Sören B, Karlsson A, Brandejsky V, Lund E, Lundberg P. Decreased muscle concentrations of ATP and PCR in the quadriceps muscle of fibromyalgia patients – a 31P-MRS study. Eur J Pain. 2013;17(8):1205–15. https://doi.org/10.1002/j.1532-2149.2013.00284.x. Epub 2013 Jan 30.
236. Castro-Marrero J, Cordero MD, Sáez-Francas N, Jimenez-Gutierrez C, Aguilar-Montilla FJ, Aliste L, Alegre-Martin J. Could mitochondrial dysfunction be a differentiating marker between chronic fatigue syndrome and fibromyalgia? Antioxid Redox Signal. 2013;19(15):1855–60. https://doi.org/10.1089/ars.2013.5346. Epub 2013 May 29.
237. Singh B, Singh R. Mitochondrial dysfunction and chronic fatigue syndromes: issues in clinical care. IOSR-JDMS. 2014;13(5):30–3. e-ISSN: 2279-0853, p-ISSN: 2279-0861.
238. Sarzi-Puttini P, Atzeni F, Mease PJ. Chronic widespread pain: from peripheral to central evolution. Best Pract Res Clin Rheumatol. 2011;25(2):133–9. https://doi.org/10.1016/j.berh.2011.04.001.
239. Heidenreich PA, Albert NM, Allen LA, et al. Forecasting the impact of heart failure in the United States: a policy statement from the American Heart Association. Circ Heart Fail. 2013;6:606–19.
240. Go AS, Mozaffarian D, Roger VL, et al. Heart disease and stroke statistics – 2014 update: a report from the American Heart Association. Circulation. 2014;129(3):e 28–292.
241. Shah SJ, Kitzman DW, Borlaug BA, et al. Phenotype – specific treatment of heart failure with preserved ejection fraction: a multiorgan roadmap. Circulation. 2006;134:73–90.
242. Zhang Y, Guallar E, Ashar FN, Longchamps RJ, Castellani CA, Lane J, Grove ML, Coresh J, Sotoodehnia N, Ilkhanoff L, Boerwinkle E, Pankratz N, Arking DE. Association between mitochondrial DNA copy number and sudden cardiac death: find-

ings from the Atherosclerosis Risk in Communities study (ARIC). Eur Heart J. 2017. https://doi.org/10.1093/eurheartj/ehx354. [Epub ahead of print].
243. Packer M, Kitzman DW. Obesity-related heart failure with a preserved ejection fraction: the mechanistic rationale for combining inhibitors of aldosterone, neprilysin, and sodium-glucose cotransporter. JACC Heart Fail. 2018;6(8):633–9.
244. Adabag AS, Luepker RV, Roger VL, Gersh BJ. Sudden cardiac death: epidemiology and risk factors. Nat Rev Cardiol. 2010;7(4):216–25. https://doi.org/10.1038/nrcardio.2010.3.
245. Haykowsky MJ, et al. Regional adipose distribution and its relation to excess intolerance in older obese patients who has heart failure with preserved ejection fraction. JACC Heart Fail. 2018;6(9):642–9.
246. Bharadwaj MS, et al. Relationship between mitochondrial content and bioenergetics with obesity, body composition and fat distribution to healthy older adults. BMC Obes. 2015;2:40.
247. Forman DE, Goodpasture BH. Weighty matters in HFpEF and aging. JACC Heart Fail. 2018;6(8):650–2.
248. Paulus WJ, Tschope C. A novel paradigm for heart failure with preserved ejection fraction: comorbidities drive myocardial dysfunction and remodeling through coronary microvascular endothelial dysfunction. J Am Coll Cardiol. 2013;62:263–71.
249. Schmidt-Wilcke T, Clauw DJ. Fibromyalgia: from pathophysiology to therapy. Nat Rev Rheumatol. 2011;7(9):518–27. https://doi.org/10.1038/nrrheum.2011.98.
250. Fatima G, Das SK, Mahdi AA. Oxidative stress and antioxidative parameters and metal ion content in patients with fibromyalgia syndrome: implications in the pathogenesis of the disease. Clin Exp Rheumatol. 2013;31(6 Suppl 79):S128–33. Epub 2013 Dec 16.
251. Ohnishi H, Saito Y. Eicosapentaenoic acid (EPA) reduces cardiovascular events: relationship with the EPA/arachidonic acid ratio. J Atheroscler Thromb. 2013;20(12):861–77. Epub 2013 Sept 18. Review.
252. El-Sawya N, El-Tantawia G, Achmawib GAH, Sultana H, Younisa S. Autonomic changes in fibromyalgia: clinical and electrophysiological study. Alexandria J Med. 2012;48(3):215–22.
253. Solano C, Martinez A, Becerril L, Vargas A, Figueroa J, Navarro C, Ramos-Remus C, Martinez-Lavin M. Autonomic dysfunction in fibromyalgia assessed by the Composite Autonomic Symptoms Scale (COMPASS). J Clin Rheumatol. 2009;15(4):172–6. https://doi.org/10.1097/RHU.0b013e3181a1083d.
254. Kadetoff D, Kosek E. The effects of static muscular contraction on blood pressure, heart rate, pain ratings and pressure pain thresholds in healthy individuals and patients with fibromyalgia. Eur J Pain. 2007;11(1):39–47. Epub 2006 Feb 9.
255. Ramírez M, Martínez-Martínez LA, Hernández-Quintela E, Velazco-Casapía J, Vargas A, Martínez-Lavín M. Small fiber neuropathy in women with fibromyalgia. An in vivo assessment using corneal confocal bio-microscopy. Semin Arthritis Rheum. 2015;45(2):214–9. https://doi.org/10.1016/j.semarthrit.2015.03.003. Epub 2015 Mar 19.
256. Clauw DJ. Fibromyalgia: a clinical review. JAMA. 2014;311(15):1547–55. https://doi.org/10.1001/jama.2014.3266.
257. Goldenberg DL, Burckhardt C, Crofford L. Management of fibromyalgia syndrome. JAMA. 2004;292(19):2388–95.
258. Dell'Osso L, Bazzichi L, Baroni S, Falaschi V, Conversano C, Carmassi C, Marazziti D. The inflammatory hypothesis of mood spectrum broadened to fibromyalgia and chronic fatigue syndrome. Clin Exp Rheumatol. 2015;33(1 Suppl 88):S109–16. Epub 2015 Mar 18.
259. Giles TD, Materson BJ, Cohn JN, Kostis JB. Definition and classification of hypertension: an update. J Clin Hypertens (Greenwich). 2009;11(11):611–4. https://doi.org/10.1111/j.1751--7176.2009.00179.x. Erratum in: J Clin Hypertens (Greenwich). 2010 Jan;12(1):13.
260. Lüscher TF, Mahfoud F. Renal nerve ablation after SYMPLICITY HTN-3: confused at the higher level? Eur Heart J. 2014;35(26):1706–11. https://doi.org/10.1093/eurheartj/ehu195. Epub 2014 May 14.
261. DePace NL, Bateman JA, Yayac M, Oh J, Siddique M. Acosta C, Pinales JM, Vinik AI, Bloom HL. Improved patient outcomes by normalizing sympathovagal balance: differentiating syncope – precise subtype differentiation leads to improved outcomes. Cardiol Res Pract. 2018, Article ID 9532141, 8 pages. https://doi.org/10.1155/2018/953214.
262. Murray GL, Colombo J. (R)alpha lipoic acid is a safe, effective pharmacologic therapy of chronic orthostatic hypotension associated with low sympathetic tone. Int J Angiol. 2019 (eFirst);1. https://doi.org/10.1055/s-0038-1676957.
263. Mohammadi V, Dehghani S, Askari G. Does alpha-lipoic acid supplement regulate blood pressure? A systematic review of randomized, double-blind placebo-controlled clinical trials. Int J Prev Med. 2017;8:33–8.
264. Bangalore S, Messerlli F, Wun C, Zuckerman A, DeMicco D, Kostis J, et al. J-curve revisited: an analysis of blood pressure and cardiovascular events in the Treating to New Targets (TNT) trial. Eur Heart J. 2010;31(23):2897–908.
265. Queiroz T, Guimaraes D, Medndes-Junior L, Braga V. α-lipoic acid reduces hypertension and increases baroreflex sensitivity in renovascular hypertensive rats. Molecules. 2012;17(11):13357–67.
266. Gouty S, Regalia J, Cai F, Helke C. Alpha-lipoic acid treatment prevents the diabetes-induced attenuation of the afferent limb of the baroreceptor reflex in rats. Auton Neurosci. 2003;108(1–2):32–44.

267. Wray D, Nishiyama S, Harris R, Zhao J, McDaniel J, Fjeldstad A, et al. Acute reversal of endothelial dysfunction in the elderly after antioxidant consumption. Hypertension. 2012;59(4):818–24.
268. Rahman S, Merchant N, Haque T, Wahi J, Bhaheetharan S, Ferdinand K, Khan B. The impact of lipoic acid on endothelial function and proteinuria in quinapril-treated diabetic patients with stage 1 hypertension: results from the QUALITY study. J Cardiovasc Pharmacol Ther. 2012;17(2):139–45.
269. Xiang G, Pu J, Yue L, Hou J, Sun H. α-lipoic acid can improve endothelial dysfunction in subjects with impaired fasting glucose. Metabolism. 2011;60(4):480–5.
270. Tardif J, Rheaume E. Lipoic acid supplementation and endothelial function. Br J Pharmacol. 2008;153:1587–8.
271. Charles A. Advances in the basic and clinical science of migraine. Ann Neurol. 2009;65(5):491–8. https://doi.org/10.1002/ana.21691.
272. Leão AA. Spreading depression. Funct Neurol. 1986;1(4):363–6.
273. Headache classification committee of the international headache society IHS, The international classification headache disorders. 3rd ed, beta version, Cephalgia. 2013;33: 629–808.
274. Yorns WR Jr, Hardison HH. Mitochondrial dysfunction in migraine. Semin Pediatr Neurol. 2013;20(3):188–93. https://doi.org/10.1016/j.spen.2013.09.002.
275. Stuart S, Griffiths LR. A possible role for mitochondrial dysfunction in migraine. Mol Gen Genomics. 2012;287(11–12):837–44. https://doi.org/10.1007/s00438-012-0723-7. Epub 2012 Oct 7.
276. Millichap JG. Migraine and autonomic nervous system dysfunction. Pediatr Neurol Briefs. 2002;16(2):15–6.
277. Vetvik KG, MacGregor EA. Sex differences in the epidemiology, clinical features, and pathophysiology of migraine. Lancet Neurol. 2017;16(1):76–87. https://doi.org/10.1016/S1474-4422(16)30293-9. Epub 2016 Nov 9.
278. Shechter A, Stewart WF, Silberstein SD, Lipton RB. Migraine and autonomic nervous system function: a population-based, case-control study. Neurology. 2002;58(3):422–7.
279. Millichap JG, Yee MM. The diet factor in pediatric and adolescent migraine. Pediatr Neurol. 2003;28(1):9–15.
280. Charles A. Migraine. N Engl J Med. 2017;377(17):1698–9. https://doi.org/10.1056/NEJMc1711803.
281. Natoli JL, Manack A, Dean B, Butler Q, Turkel CC, Stovner L, Lipton RB. Global prevalence of chronic migraine: a systematic review. Cephalalgia. 2010;30(5):599–609. https://doi.org/10.1111/j.1468-2982.2009.01941.x.
282. Minen MT, Begasse De Dhaem O, Kroon Van Diest A, Powers S, Schwedt TJ, Lipton R, Silbersweig D. Migraine and its psychiatric comorbidities. J Neurol Neurosurg Psychiatry. 2016;87(7):741–9. https://doi.org/10.1136/jnnp-2015-312233. Epub 2016 Jan 5.
283. Bigal ME, Lipton RB. Excessive acute migraine medication use and migraine progression. Neurology. 2008;71(22):1821–8. https://doi.org/10.1212/01.wnl.0000335946.53860.1d.
284. Pieczenik SR, Neustadt J. Mitochondrial dysfunction and molecular pathways of disease. Exp Mol Pathol. 2007;83(1):84–92. Epub 2007 Jan 18.
285. Kelman L. The triggers or precipitants of the acute migraine attack. Cephalalgia. 2007;27(5):394–402. Epub 2007 Mar 30.
286. Elmenshawy E, Sakr S. Autonomic dysfunction in migraine; what do we need to know? Egypt J Neurol Psychiatr Neurosur. 2009;46:489–96.
287. Gaul C, Diener HC, Danesch U, Migravent® Study Group. Improvement of migraine symptoms with a proprietary supplement containing riboflavin, magnesium and Q10: a randomized, placebo-controlled, double-blind, multicenter trial. J Headache Pain. 2015;16:516. https://doi.org/10.1186/s10194-015-0516-6. Epub 2015 Apr 3.
288. Reeve AK, Simcox EM, Duchen MR, Turnbull DM, editors. Mitochondrial dysfunction in neurodegenerative disorders. 2nd ed. Cham: Springer International Publishing; 2016.
289. Vos M, Lauwers E, Verstreken P. Synaptic mitochondria in synaptic transmission and organization of vesicle pools in health and disease Front Synaptic Neurosci. 2010. https://doi.org/10.3389/fnsyn.2010.00139
290. Lambert AJ, Brand MD. Reactive oxygen species production by mitochondria. Methods Mol Biol. 2009;554:165–81. https://doi.org/10.1007/978-1-59745-521-3_11.
291. Balaban RS, Nemoto S, Finkel T. Mitochondria, oxidants, and aging. Cell. 2005;120(4):483–95.
292. Papadopoulos V, Miller WL. Role of mitochondria in steroidogenesis. Best Pract Res Clin Endocrinol Metab. 2012;26(6):771–90. https://doi.org/10.1016/j.beem.2012.05.002. Epub 2012 Jun 16.
293. Glancy B, Balaban RS. Role of mitochondrial Ca2+ in the regulation of cellular energetics. Biochemistry. 2012;51(14):2959–73. https://doi.org/10.1021/bi2018909. Epub 2012 Mar 29.
294. Chrysostomou A, Turnbull DM. Mitochondria, the synapse, and neurodegeneration. In: Reeve A, Simcox E, Duchen M, Turnbull D, editors. Mitochondrial dysfunction in neurodegenerative disorders. https://doi.org/10.1007/978-3-319-28637-2_9.
295. Marland JRK, Hasel P, Bonnycastle K, Cousin MA. Mitochondrial calcium uptake modulates synaptic vesicle endocytosis in central nerve terminals. J Biol Chem. 2016;291(5):2080–6. https://doi.org/10.1074/jbc.M115.686956.
296. Rizzuto R, De Stefani D, Raffaello A, Mammucari C. Mitochondria as sensors and regulators of calcium signalling. Nat Rev Mol Cell Biol. 2012;13(9):566–78. https://doi.org/10.1038/nrm3412. Epub 2012 Aug 1.

297. Kasahara A, Scorrano L. Mitochondria: from cell death executioners to regulators of cell differentiation. Trends Cell Biol. 2014;24(12):761–70. https://doi.org/10.1016/j.tcb.2014.08.005. Epub 2014 Sept 2.
298. Ahuja M, Muallem S. The gatekeepers of mitochondrial calcium influx: MICU1 and MICU2. EMBO Rep. 2014;15(3):205–6. https://doi.org/10.1002/embr.201438446. Epub 2014 Feb 14.
299. Lagouge M, Argmann C, Gerhart-Hines Z, Meziane H, Lerin C, Daussin F, Messadeq N, Milne J, Lambert P, Elliott P, Geny B, Laakso M, Puigserver P, Auwerx J. Resveratrol improves mitochondrial function and protects against metabolic disease by activating SIRT1 and PGC-1alpha. Cell. 2006;127(6):1109–22. Epub 2006 Nov 16.
300. Baur JA, Pearson KJ, Price NL, Jamieson HA, Lerin C, Kalra A, Prabhu VV, Allard JS, Lopez-Lluch G, Lewis K, Pistell PJ, Poosala S, Becker KG, Boss O, Gwinn D, Wang M, Ramaswamy S, Fishbein KW, Spencer RG, Lakatta EG, Le Couteur D, Shaw RJ, Navas P, Puigserver P, Ingram DK, de Cabo R, Sinclair DA. Resveratrol improves health and survival of mice on a high-calorie diet. Nature. 2006;444(7117):337–42. Epub 2006 Nov 1.
301. Shalev A, Liberzon I, Marmar C. Post traumatic stress disorder. (Longo DL, ed) NEJM. 2017;376:2459–69. https://doi.org/10.1056/NEJMra1612499.
302. American Psychiatric Association. Diagnostic and statistical manual of mental disorders. 5th ed. Washington, DC; 2000.
303. Brudey C, Park J, Wiaderkiewicz J, Kobayashi I, Mellman TA, Marvar PJ. Autonomic and inflammatory consequences of posttraumatic stress disorder and the link to cardiovascular disease. Am J Physiol Regul Integr Comp Physiol. 2015;309:R315–21.
304. Nance DM, Sanders VM. Autonomic innervation and regulation of the immune system (1987–2007). Brain Behav Immun. 2007;21:736–45.
305. Kanel von R, Hepp U, Kraemer B, Traber R, Keel M, Mica L, Schnyder U. Evidence for low-grade systemic proinflammatory activity in patients with posttraumatic stress disorder. J Psychiatr Res. 2007;41:744–52.
306. Ridker PM. Clinical application of C-reactive protein for cardiovascular disease detection and prevention. Circulation. 2003;107:363–9.
307. Miller AH, Haroon E, Raison CL, Felger JC. Cytokine targets in the brain: impact on neurotransmitters and neurocircuits. Depress Anxiety. 2013;30:297–306.
308. Song C, Phillips AG, Leonard B. Interleukin 1β enhances conditioned fear memory in rats: possible involvement of glucocorticoids. Eur J Neurosci. 2003;18:1739–43.
309. Wohleb ES, Patterson JM, Sharma V, Quan N, Godbout JP, Sheridan JF. Knockdown of interleukin-1 receptor type-1 on endothelial cells attenuated stress-induced neuroinflammation and prevented anxiety-like behavior. J Neurosci. 2014;34:2583–91.
310. Oosthuizen F, Wegener G, Harvey BH. Nitric oxide as inflammatory mediator in post-traumatic stress disorder (PTSD): evidence from an animal model. Neuropsychiatr Dis Treat. 2005;1:109–23.
311. de Lange T. Protection of mammalian telomeres. Oncogene. 2002;21:532–40.
312. Roake CM, Artandi SE. Control of cellular aging, tissue function, and cancer by p53 downstream of telomeres. Cold Spring Harb Perspect Med. 2017;7(5):a026088. https://doi.org/10.1101/cshperspect.a026088.
313. Vera E, Blasco MA. Beyond average: potential for measurement of short telomeres. Aging (Albany NY). 2012;4(6):379–92.
314. Harley CB, Futcher AB, Greider CW. Telomeres shorten during ageing of human fibroblasts. Nature. 1990;345:458–60.
315. Blackburn EH. Switching and signaling at the telomere. Cell. 2001;106:661–73.
316. Collins K, Mitchell JR. Telomerase in the human organism. Oncogene. 2002;21:564–79.
317. Canela A, Vera E, Klatt P, Blasco MA. High-throughput telomere length quantification by FISH and its application to human population studies. Proc Natl Acad Sci U S A. 2007;104:5300–5.
318. Flores I, Canela A, Vera E, Tejera A, Cotsarelis G, Blasco MA. The longest telomeres: a general signature of adult stem cell compartments. Genes Dev. 2008;22:654–67.
319. Yui J, Chiu CP, Lansdorp PM. Telomerase activity in candidate stem cells from fetal liver and adult bone marrow. Blood. 1998;91:3255–62.
320. Deng Y, Chan SS, Chang S. Telomere dysfunction and tumour suppression: the senescence connection. Nat Rev Cancer. 2008;8:450–8.
321. Collado M, Blasco MA, Serrano M. Cellular senescence in cancer and aging. Cell. 2007;130:223–33.
322. Blasco MA. Telomere length, stem cells and aging. Nat Chem Biol. 2007;3:640–9.
323. de Cabo R, Carmona-Gutierrez D, Bernier M, Hall MN, Madeo F. The search for antiaging interventions: from elixirs to fasting regimens. Cell. 2014;157(7):1515–26.
324. Aviv A. Genetics of leukocyte telomere length and its role in atherosclerosis. Mutat Res. 2012;730:68–74.
325. Levy D, Neuhausen SL, Hunt SC, Kimura M, Hwang SJ, Chen W, Bis JC, Fitzpatrick AL, Smith E, Johnson AD, Gardner JP, Srinivasan SR, Schork N, Rotter JI, Herbig U, Psaty BM, Sastrasinh M, Murray SS, Vasan RS, Province MA, Glazer NL, Lu X, Cao X, Kronmal R, Mangino M, Soranzo N, Spector TD, Berenson GS, Aviv A. Genome-wide association identifies OBFC1 as a locus involved in human leukocyte telomere biology. Proc Natl Acad Sci U S A. 2010;107:9293–8.
326. Mangino M, Hwang SJ, Spector TD, Hunt SC, Kimura M, Fitzpatrick AL, Christiansen L, Petersen I, Elbers CC, Harris T, Chen W, Srinivasan SR, Kark JD, Benetos A, El Shamieh S, Visvikis-Siest S, Christensen K, Berenson GS, Valdes AM, Viñuela A, Garcia M, Arnett DK, Broeckel U, Province MA, Pankow JS, Kammerer C, Liu Y, Nalls M,

Tishkoff S, Thomas F, Ziv E, Psaty BM, Bis JC, Rotter JI, Taylor KD, Smith E, Schork NJ, Levy D, Aviv A. Genome-wide meta-analysis points to CTC1 and ZNF676 as genes regulating telomere homeostasis in humans. Hum Mol Genet. 2012;21: 5385–94.
327. Codd V, Nelson CP, Albrecht E, Mangino M, Deelen J, Buxton JL, et al. Identification of seven loci affecting mean telomere length and their association with disease. Nat Genet. 2013;45:422–7.
328. Armanios M, Blackburn EH. The telomere syndromes. Nat Rev Genet. 2012;13:693–704.
329. Guarante L. The Franklin H. Epstein lecture: sirtuins, aging, and medicine. N Engl J Med. 2011;364:2235–44.
330. Cardus A, Uryga AK, Walters G, Erusalimsky JD. SIRT6 protects human endothelial cells from DNA damage, telomere dysfunction, and senescence. Cardiovasc Res. 2013;97:571–9.
331. Wang JC, Bennett M. Aging and atherosclerosis: mechanisms, functional consequences, and potential therapeutics for cellular senescence. Circ Res. 2012;111:245–59.
332. Tzanetakou IP, Nzietchueng R, Perrea DN, Benetos A. Telomeres and their role in aging and longevity. Curr Vasc Pharmacol. 2014;12:726–34.
333. Kovacic JC, Moreno P, Nabel EG, Hachinski V, Fuster V. Cellular senescence, vascular disease, and aging: part 2 of a 2-part review. Circulation. 2011;123:1990–2010.
334. Fyhrquist F, Saijonmaa O, Strandberg T. The roles of senescence and telomere shortening in cardiovascular disease. Nat Rev Cardiol. 2013;10:274–83.
335. Nilsson PM, Tufvesson H, Leosdottir M, Melander O. Telomeres and cardiovascular disease risk: an update 2013. Transl Res. 2013;162:371–80.
336. de Lange T. Shelterin: the protein complex that shapes and safeguards human telomeres. Genes Dev. 2005;19:2001–10.
337. Blackburn EH, Greider CW, Szostak JW. Telomeres and telomerase: the path from maize, Tetrahymena and yeast to human cancer and aging. Nat Med. 2006;12:1133–8.
338. Campisi J. Cellular senescence: putting the paradoxes in perspective. Curr Opin Genet Dev. 2011;21:107–12.
339. von Zglinicki T, Saretzki G, Ladhoff J, d'Adda di Fagagna F, Jackson SP. Human cell senescence as a DNA damage response. Mech Ageing Dev. 2005;126:111–7.
340. von Zglinicki T. Oxidative stress shortens telomeres. Trends Biochem Sci. 2002;27:339–44.
341. Jurk D, Wilson C, Passos JF, Oakley F, Correia-Melo C, Greaves L, Saretzki G, Fox C, Lawless C, Anderson R, Hewitt G, Pender SL, Fullard N, Nelson G, Mann J, van de Sluis B, Mann DA, von Zglinicki T. Chronic inflammation induces telomere dysfunction and accelerates ageing in mice. Nat Commun. 2014;2:4172.
342. Correia-Melo C, Hewitt G, Passos JF. Telomeres, oxidative stress and inflammatory factors: partners in cellular senescence? Longev Healthspan. 2014;3(1):1.
343. Erusalimsky JD, Kurz DJ. Cellular senescence in vivo: its relevance in ageing and cardiovascular disease. Exp Gerontol. 2005;40:634–42.
344. Savage SA, Stewart BJ, Eckert A, Kiley M, Liao JS, Channock SJ. Genetic variation, nucleotide diversity, and linkage disequilibrium in seven telomere stability genes suggest that these genes may be under constraint. Hum Mutat. 2005;26:343–50.
345. Blasco MA. Telomeres and human disease: ageing, cancer and beyond. Nat Rev Genet. 2005;6:611–22.
346. Kosmadaki MG, Gilchrest BA. The role of telomeres in skin aging/photoaging. Micron. 2004;35:155–9.
347. de Jesus BB, Schneeberger K, Vera E, Tejera A, Harley CB, Blasco MA. The telomerase activator TA-65 elongates short telomeres and increases health span of adult/old mice without increasing cancer incidence. Aging Cell. 2011;10:604–21.
348. Kyo S, Takakura M, Kanaya T, Zhuo W, Fujimoto K, Nishio Y, Orimo A, Inoue M. Estrogen activates telomerase. Cancer Res. 1999;59:5917–21.
349. Valdes AM, Andrew T, Gardner JP, Kimura M, Oelsner E, Cherkas LF, Aviv A, Spector TD. Obesity, cigarette smoking, and telomere length in women. Lancet. 2005;366:662–720.
350. Strandberg TE, Strandberg AY, Saijonmaa O, Tilvis RS, Pitkälä KH, Fyhrquist F. Association of telomere length in older men with mortality and midlife body mass index and smoking. J Gerontol A Biol Sci Med Sci. 2011;66:815–20.
351. Gellert C, Schöttker B, Brenner H. Smoking and all-cause mortality in older people: systematic review and meta-analysis. Arch Intern Med. 2012;172:837–44.
352. Strandberg TE, Strandberg AY, Saijonmaa O, Tilvis RS, Pitkälä KH, Fyhrquist F. Association between alcohol consumption in healthy midlife and telomere length in older men. The Helsinki Businessmen Study. Eur J Epidemiol. 2012;27:815–22.
353. Müezzinler A, Zaineddin AK, Brenner H. Body mass index and leukocyte telomere length in adults: a systematic review and meta-analysis. Obes Rev. 2014;15:192–201.
354. Donato AJ, Morgan RG, Walker AE, Lesniewski LA. Cellular and molecular biology of aging endothelial cells. J Mol Cell Cardiol. 2015;89:122–35.
355. Cherkas LF, Hunkin JL, Kato BS, Richards JB, Gardner JP, Surdulescu GL, Kimura M, Lu X, Spector TD, Aviv A. The association between physical activity in leisure time and leukocyte telomere length. Arch Intern Med. 2008;168:154–8.
356. Njajou OT, Hsueh WC, Blackburn EH, Newman AB, Wu SH, Li R, Simonsick EM, Harris TM, Cummings SR, Cawthon RM. Association between telomere length, specific causes of death, and years of healthy life in health, aging, and body composi-

tion, a population-based cohort study. J Gerontol A Biol Sci Med Sci. 2009;64(8):860–4.
357. Kennedy BK, et al. Geroscience; linking aging to chronic disease. Cell. 2014;159:709–13.
358. Epel ES, Blackburn EH, Lin J, Dhabhar FS, Adler NE, Morrow JD, Cawthon RM. Accelerated telomere shortening in response to life stress. Proc Natl Acad Sci U S A. 2004;101:17312–5.
359. Shalev I, Entringer S, Wadhwa PD, Wolkowitz OM, Puterman E, Lin J, Epel ES. Stress and telomere biology: a lifespan perspective. Psychoneuroendocrinology. 2013;38:1835–42.
360. Krauss J, Farzaneh-Far R, Puterman E, Na B, Lin J, Epel E, Blackburn E, Whooley MA. Physical fitness and telomere length in patients with coronary heart disease: findings from the heart and soul study. PLoS One. 2011;6:e26983.
361. Ornish D, Lin J, Daubenmier J, Weidner G, Epel E, Kemp C, Magbanua MJ, Marlin R, Yglecias L, Carroll PR, Blackburn EH. Increased telomerase activity and comprehensive lifestyle changes: a pilot study. Lancet Oncol. 2008;9:1048–57.
362. Fontana L, Hu FB. Optimal body weight for health and longevity: bridging basic, clinical, and population research. Aging Cell. 2014;14:391–400.
363. Ornish D, Lin J, Chan JM, Epel E, Kemp C, Weidner G, Marlin R, Frenda SJ, Magbanua MJ, Daubenmier J, Estay I, Hills NK, Chainani-Wu N, Carroll PR, Blackburn EH. Effect of comprehensive lifestyle changes on telomerase activity and telomere length in men with biopsy-proven low-risk prostate cancer: 5-year follow-up of a descriptive pilot study. Lancet Oncol. 2013;14:1112–20.
364. Rizzuto D, Fratiglioni L. Life style factors related to mortality and survival: a mini-review. Gerontology. 2014;60:327–35.
365. Werner C, Fürster T, Widmann T, Pöss J, Roggia C, Hanhoun M, Scharhag J, Büchner N, Meyer T, Kindermann W, Haendeler J, Böhm M, Laufs U. Physical exercise prevents cellular senescence in circulating leukocytes and in the vessel wall. Circulation. 2009;120:2438–47.
366. Richards BJ, Valdes AM, Gardner JP, Paximadas D, Kimura M, Nessa A, Lu X, Surdulescu GL, Swaminathan R, Spector TD, Aviv A. Higher vitamin D concentrations are associated with longer leukocyte telomere length in women. Am J Clin Nutr. 2007;86:1420–5.
367. Xu Q, Parks CG, DeRoo LA, Cawthon RM, Sandler DP, Chen H. Multivitamin use and telomere length in women. Am J Clin Nutr. 2009;89:1857–63.
368. Sen A, Marsche G, Freudenberger P, Schallert M, Toeglhofer AM, Nagl C, Schmidt R, Launer LJ, Schmidt H. Association between higher plasma lutein, zeaxanthin, and vitamin C concentrations and longer telomere length: results of the Austrian Stroke Prevention Study. J Am Geriatr Soc. 2014;62(2):222–9.
369. Farzaneh-Far R, Lin J, Epel ES, Harris WS, Blackburn EH, Whooley MA. Association of marine omega-3 fatty acid levels with telomeric aging in patients with coronary heart disease. JAMA. 2010;303:250–7.
370. Paul L. Diet, nutrition and telomere length. J Nutr Biochem. 2011;20:895–901.
371. Boccardi V, Esposito A, Rizzo MR, Marfella R, Barbieri M, Polisso G. Mediterranean diet, telomere maintenance and health status among elderly. PLoS One. 2013;8:1–6.
372. Crous-Bou M, Fung TF, Prescott J, Julin B, Du M, Sun Q, Rexrode KM, Hu FB, De Vivo I. Mediterranean diet and telomere length in Nurses' health study: population based cohort study. BMJ. 2014;349:6674.
373. Saliques S, Teyssier J-R, Vergely C, Lorgis L, Lorin J. Circulating leukocyte telomere length and oxidative stress: a new target for statin therapy. Atherosclerosis. 2011;219:753–60.
374. Rode L, Nordestgaard BG, Bojesen SE. Peripheral blood leukocyte telomere length and mortality among 64 637 individuals from the general population. J Natl Cancer Inst. 2015;107(6):107.
375. Guarante L. The Franklin H. Epstein lecture: sirtuins, aging, and medicine. N Engl J Med. 2011;364:2235–44.
376. Armanios M, Alder JK, Parry EM, Karim B, Strong MA, Greider CW. Short telomeres are sufficient to cause the degenerative defects associated with aging. Am J Hum Genet. 2009;85(6):823–32.
377. Shimamoto A, Koutaro Y, Tahara H. Werner-syndrome-specific induced pluripotent stem cells: recovery of telomere function by reprogramming. Front Genet. 2015.
378. Bär C, Blasco MA. Telomeres and telomerase as therapeutic targets to prevent and treat age-related diseases. F1000 Research. 2016;5:F1000 Faculty Rev-89. https://doi.org/10.12688/f1000research.7020.1.
379. López-Otín C, Blasco MA, Partridge L, et al. The hallmarks of aging. Cell. 2013;153(6):1194–217. https://doi.org/10.1016/j.cell.2013.05.039.
380. Collado M, Blasco MA, Serrano M. Cellular senescence in cancer and aging. Cell. 2007;130(2):223–33. https://doi.org/10.1016/j.cell.2007.07.003.
381. Muñoz-Espín D, Serrano M. Cellular senescence: from physiology to pathology. Nat Rev Mol Cell Biol. 2014;15(7):482–96. https://doi.org/10.1038/nrm3823.
382. Flores I, Cayuela ML, Blasco MA. Effects of telomerase and telomere length on epidermal stem cell behavior. Science. 2005;309(5738):1253–6. https://doi.org/10.1126/science.1115025.
383. Sharpless NE, DePinho RA. How stem cells age and why this makes us grow old. Nat Rev Mol Cell Biol. 2007;8(9):703–13. https://doi.org/10.1038/nrm2241.
384. Calado RT, Young NS. Telomere diseases. N Engl J Med. 2009;361(24):2353–65. https://doi.org/10.1056/NEJMra0903373.

385. Armanios M, Blackburn EH. The telomere syndromes. Nat Rev Genet. 2012;13(10):693–704. https://doi.org/10.1038/nrg3246.
386. Holohan B, Wright WE, Shay JW. Cell biology of disease: telomeropathies: an emerging spectrum disorder. J Cell Biol. 2014;205(3):289–99. https://doi.org/10.1083/jcb.201401012.
387. Townsley DM, Dumitriu B, Young NS. Bone marrow failure and the telomeropathies. Blood. 2014;124(18):2775–83. https://doi.org/10.1182/blood-2014-05-526285.
388. Counter CM, Avilion AA, LeFeuvre CE, et al. Telomere shortening associated with chromosome instability is arrested in immortal cells which express telomerase activity. EMBO J. 1992;11(5):1921–9.
389. Chin L, Artandi SE, Shen Q, et al. p53 deficiency rescues the adverse effects of telomere loss and cooperates with telomere dysfunction to accelerate carcinogenesis. Cell. 1999;97(4):527–38. https://doi.org/10.1016/S0092-8674(00)80762-X.
390. Sahin E, Colla S, Liesa M, et al. Telomere dysfunction induces metabolic and mitochondrial compromise. Nature. 2011;470(7334):359–65. https://doi.org/10.1038/nature09787.
391. Slagboom PE, Droog S, Boomsma DI. Genetic determination of telomere size in humans: a twin study of three age groups. Am J Hum Genet. 1994;55(5):876–82.
392. Canela A, Klatt P, Blasco MA. Telomere length analysis. Methods Mol Biol. 2007;371:45–72. https://doi.org/10.1007/978-1-59745-361-5_5.
393. von Zglinicki T. Oxidative stress shortens telomeres. Trends Biochem Sci. 2002;27(7):339–44. https://doi.org/10.1016/S0968-0004(02)02110-2.
394. Valdes AM, Andrew T, Gardner JP, et al. Obesity, cigarette smoking, and telomere length in women. Lancet. 2005;366(9486):662–4. https://doi.org/10.1016/S0140-6736(05)66630-5.
395. Strandberg TE, Saijonmaa O, Tilvis RS, et al. Association of telomere length in older men with mortality and midlife body mass index and smoking. J Gerontol A Biol Sci Med Sci. 2011;66(7):815–20. https://doi.org/10.1093/gerona/glr064.
396. Verde Z, Reinoso-Barbero L, Chicharro L, et al. Effects of cigarette smoking and nicotine metabolite ratio on leukocyte telomere length. Environ Res. 2015;140:488–94. https://doi.org/10.1016/j.envres.2015.05.008.
397. Révész D, Milaneschi Y, Verhoeven JE, et al. Longitudinal associations between metabolic syndrome components and telomere shortening. J Clin Endocrinol Metab. 2015;100(8):3050–9. https://doi.org/10.1210/JC.2015-1995.
398. Strandberg TE, Strandberg AY, Saijonmaa O, et al. Association between alcohol consumption in healthy midlife and telomere length in older men. The Helsinki Businessmen Study. Eur J Epidemiol. 2012;27(10):815–22. https://doi.org/10.1007/s10654-012-9728-0.
399. Müezzinler A, Mons U, Dieffenbach AK, et al. Smoking habits and leukocyte telomere length dynamics among older adults: results from the ESTHER cohort. Exp Gerontol. 2015;70:18–25. https://doi.org/10.1016/j.exger.2015.07.002.
400. Wolkowitz OM, Mellon SH, Epel ES, et al. Leukocyte telomere length in major depression: correlations with chronicity, inflammation and oxidative stress – preliminary findings. PLoS One. 2011;6(3):e17837. https://doi.org/10.1371/journal.pone.0017837.
401. Karabatsiakis A, Kolassa IT, Kolassa S, et al. Telomere shortening in leukocyte subpopulations in depression. BMC Psychiatry. 2014;14:192. https://doi.org/10.1186/1471-244X-14-192.
402. O'Donovan A, Epel E, Lin J, et al. Childhood trauma associated with short leukocyte telomere length in posttraumatic stress disorder. Biol Psychiatry. 2011;70(5):465–71. https://doi.org/10.1016/j.biopsych.2011.01.035.
403. Lin J, Epel E, Blackburn E. Telomeres and lifestyle factors: roles in cellular aging. Mutat Res. 2012;730(1–2):85–9. https://doi.org/10.1016/j.mrfmmm.2011.08.003.
404. Kinser PA, Lyon DE. Major depressive disorder and measures of cellular aging: an integrative review. Nurs Res Pract. 2013;2013:469070. https://doi.org/10.1155/2013/469070.
405. Lindqvist D, Epel ES, Mellon SH, et al. Psychiatric disorders and leukocyte telomere length: underlying mechanisms linking mental illness with cellular aging. Neurosci Biobehav Rev. 2015;55:333–64. https://doi.org/10.1016/j.neubiorev.2015.05.007.
406. Simon NM, Smoller JW, McNamara KL, et al. Telomere shortening and mood disorders: preliminary support for a chronic stress model of accelerated aging. Biol Psychiatry. 2006;60(5):432–5. https://doi.org/10.1016/j.biopsych.2006.02.004.
407. Elvsåshagen T, Vera E, Bøen E, et al. The load of short telomeres is increased and associated with lifetime number of depressive episodes in bipolar II disorder. J Affect Disord. 2011;135(1–3):43–50. https://doi.org/10.1016/j.jad.2011.08.006.
408. Canela A, Vera E, Klatt P, et al. High-throughput telomere length quantification by FISH and its application to human population studies. Proc Natl Acad Sci U S A. 2007;104(13):5300–5. https://doi.org/10.1073/pnas.0609367104.
409. De Jesus BB, Blasco MA. Telomerase at the intersection of cancer and aging. Trends Genet. 2013;29(9):513–20. https://doi.org/10.1016/j.tig.2013.06.007.
410. Kovacic JC, Moreno P, Hachinski V, et al. Cellular senescence, vascular disease, and aging: part 1 of a 2-part review. Circulation. 2011;123:1650–60.
411. Sanders JL, Newman AB. Telomere length in epidemiology: a biomarker of aging, age-related disease, both, or neither? Epidemiol Rev. 2013;35:112–31.
412. D'Mello MJ, Ross SA, Briel M, et al. Association between shortened leukocyte telomere length and

cardiometabolic outcomes: systematic review and meta-analysis. Circ Cardiovasc Genet. 2015;8:82–90.
413. Haycock PC, Heydon EE, Kaptoge S, et al. Leucocyte telomere length and risk of cardiovascular disease: systematic review and meta-analysis. BMJ. 2014;349:g4227.
414. Fernández-Alvira JM, Fuster V, Dorado B, Soberón N, Flores I, Gallardo M, Pocock S, Blasco MA, Andrés V. Short telomere load, telomere length, and subclinical atherosclerosis. J Am Coll Cardiol. 2016;67(21):2467–76. https://doi.org/10.1016/j.jacc.2016.03.530.
415. Rietzschel ER, Bekaert S, De Meyer T. Telomeres and atherosclerosis: the attrition of an attractive hypothesis. J Am Coll Cardiol. 2016;67(21):2477–9. https://doi.org/10.1016/j.jacc.2016.03.541.
416. Slagboom PE, Droog S, Boomsma DI. Genetic determination of telomere size in humans: a twin study of three age groups. Am J Hum Genet. 1994;55(5):876–82.
417. Bischoff C, Graakjaer J, Petersen HC, et al. The heritability of telomere length among the elderly and oldest-old. Twin Res Hum Genet. 2005;8(5):433–9. https://doi.org/10.1375/183242705774310141.
418. Andrew T, Aviv A, Falchi M, et al. Mapping genetic loci that determine leukocyte telomere length in a large sample of unselected female sibling pairs. Am J Hum Genet. 2006;78(3):480–6. https://doi.org/10.1086/500052.
419. Broer L, Codd V, Nyholt DR, et al. Meta-analysis of telomere length in 19,713 subjects reveals high heritability, stronger maternal inheritance and a paternal age effect. Eur J Hum Genet. 2013;21(10):1163–8. https://doi.org/10.1038/ejhg.2012.303.
420. von Zglinicki T. Oxidative stress shortens telomeres. Trends Biochem Sci. 2002;27(7):339–44. https://doi.org/10.1016/S0968-0004(02)02110-2.
421. Farzaneh-Far R, Lin J, Epel ES, et al. Association of marine omega-3 fatty acid levels with telomeric aging in patients with coronary heart disease. JAMA. 2010;303(3):250–7. https://doi.org/10.1001/jama.2009.2008.
422. Werner C, Fürster T, Widmann T, et al. Physical exercise prevents cellular senescence in circulating leukocytes and in the vessel wall. Circulation. 2009;120(24):2438–47. https://doi.org/10.1161/CIRCULATIONAHA.109.861005.
423. Song Z, von Figura G, Liu Y, et al. Lifestyle impacts on the aging-associated expression of biomarkers of DNA damage and telomere dysfunction in human blood. Aging Cell. 2010;9(4):607–15. https://doi.org/10.1111/j.1474-9726.2010.00583.x.
424. Soares-Miranda L, Imamura F, Siscovick D, et al. Physical activity, physical fitness, and leukocyte telomere length: the Cardiovascular Health Study. Med Sci Sports Exerc. 2015;47(12):2525–34. https://doi.org/10.1249/MSS.0000000000000720.

# Frequently Asked Questions

## The P&S (Autonomic) Nervous Systems

**Question 1: What Is the Autonomic Nervous System (ANS)?**

**Answer**: Anatomically, the body's nervous system consists of two parts: (1) the central nervous system (CNS, inside the skull and spine) and (2) peripheral nervous system (PNS, outside the skull and spine). Functionally (physiologically), the body's nervous system consists of three parts: (1) the sensory nervous system (taking input from the outside world through the eyes, ears, nose, tongue, skin, etc.), (2) the motor nervous system (the nerves that control all muscles in order to respond to the input from the outside world, sometimes known as the voluntary nervous system), and (3) the autonomic nervous system (ANS, the nerves that take input from inside and control everything inside, virtually every cell in the body, and it is sometimes known as the involuntary nervous system). It influences and modifies the function of all internal organs. The ANS, with its two branches: the Parasympathetic and Sympathetic branches, acts as the control system and functions without conscious knowledge. We classify the Enteric Nervous System as part of the Parasympathetic Nervous System. That is to say it functions unconsciously or involuntarily. It regulates bodily functions such as heart rate, blood pressure, breathing, digestion, urination, sexual function, sweating, eye blink, and pupil reaction to light.

**Question 2: What Are the Two Branches of the ANS?**

**Answer**: The ANS is composed of two parts. These two parts control all of the systems of the body and coordinate them. They are the parasympathetic nervous system (P) and the sympathetic nervous system (S).

The parasympathetic nervous system is commonly referred to as the "rest and digest nervous system." It is responsible for conserving energy and establishing metabolic baselines. In many situations, it acts like the brakes on a car. It is the "protective" nervous system. The sympathetic nervous system is commonly referred to as the "fight or flight" nervous system. In many situations, it acts as the accelerator of a car. It is the "reactionary" nervous system. The P&S nervous systems are one of the main human systems responsible for this capability and adaptability. The interplay between the P&S branches underlies this ability.

Collectively, the P&S nervous systems are the regulatory branches of the nervous system. Anatomically and physiologically, they exist in both the central and peripheral portions of the nervous system. Together the P&S nervous systems control bodily functions. To properly affect this control in two components, P&S need to be in balance. The specific P&S balance required varies from individual to individual, time to time, and activity to activity and is affected by a person's genetics. It also varies with age, lifestyle, environment, and medical history. P&S dysfunctions result


N. L. DePace, J. Colombo, *Clinical Autonomic and Mitochondrial Disorders*,
https://doi.org/10.1007/978-3-030-17016-5

when there is an imbalance between the P&S nervous systems.

**Question 3: What Are the Main Chemical Messengers, or Neurotransmitters, Used to Communicate Within the Autonomic Nervous System and Between the ANS and the Rest of the Body?**

**Answer**: The main chemical messengers or neurotransmitters are acetylcholine (Ach) and norepinephrine (NE). The nerve fibers that secrete Ach are called cholinergic fibers, whereas the fibers that secrete NE are called adrenergic fibers. Generally, Ach has parasympathetic effects, and NE has sympathetic effects. Note, parasympathetic effects are typically thought of as inhibitory (slowing things down or decreasing them), and sympathetic effects are thought of as excitatory (speeding things up or increasing them), things like heart rate and blood pressure (the so-called "push-pull" effect); however, that is mainly for the heart and most other organs and organ systems outside the brain. P&S function in the brain is more complicated.

**Question 4: Only Two Chemical Messengers, or Neurotransmitters, Affect the Whole Body?**

**Answer**: Yes, only two. This is so that the whole body may have a totally coordinated response to a single (important) stimulus. Think about it. If you are scared and need to run away or fight, many different systems of the body need to act in concert so that you have a chance of running away or fighting. Just standing up engages several different systems doing several different things all together, as coordinated by the sympathetic nervous system: the vasculature needs to constrict in the periphery to move more blood to the heart to help the heart get blood to the brain, which means the core vasculature must dilate and heart rate and blood pressure must increase for a few seconds, breathing must increase for a few seconds, the fluid systems in the central nervous system must compensate for the pressure changes, and even though they have constricted, the peripheral vasculature needs to supply more blood to the leg muscles, so they may work to support standing. This additional work also requires additional "fuel," so insulin must be released from the pancreas to open the muscle cells to receive more glucose (sugar), and the glucose and nutrients stored in the liver must be released to supply the muscle cells.

Simple pharmacological drugs can relieve symptoms of P&S dysfunction, some of which work like or through NE or Ach or some which oppose NE or Ach. P&S testing may provide guidance of how to treat a certain disorder by evaluating which P&S branch is responsible: for example, whether there is an S-dominance or a P-dominance.

**Question 5: How Do the Two Chemical Messengers, or Neurotransmitters, Affect the Brain?**

**Answer**:

- More parasympathetic activity in the brain and people become more sleepy, and with even more, people begin to become fatigued or depressed (depression is too much parasympathetic activity and is the start of many of the psychological symptoms of today, including anxiety, ADD/ADHD, bipolar disorders, manic depression, major depressive disorders, obsessive-compulsive disorders, etc.).
- Less parasympathetic activity in the brain and people become less sleepy or less depressed.
- More sympathetic activity in the brain and people become more awake, and with even more, people begin to become hyperaroused and may experience anxiety (including palpitations), ADD/ADHD, obsessive-compulsive disorders, etc. It is hard to focus and learn because that is more a parasympathetic-mediated function.
  - Note, the reason why both too much parasympathetic and too much sympathetic activity may lead to anxiety,

ADD/ADHD, and OCD, etc. is because these symptoms are caused by too much sympathetic activity (sympathetic excess or SE). SE may happen on its own (where SE is a primary response) or may be forced due to a parasympathetic excess (where SE is a secondary response). Therefore, the symptoms of SE are possible in both situations.

- Less sympathetic activity in the brain and people become less awake less aroused.

**Question 6: The Answer to Question 3 Describes the "Push-Pull" Effect of the P&S Systems on the Heart, But That Does Not Seem to Be the Case in the Brain. What Other Systems of the Body Are Under the Influence of Both P&S with the "Push-Pull" Effects?**

**Answer**: All organs and organ systems, in fact, almost all cells of the body, are under the influence of the P&S nervous systems. For example:

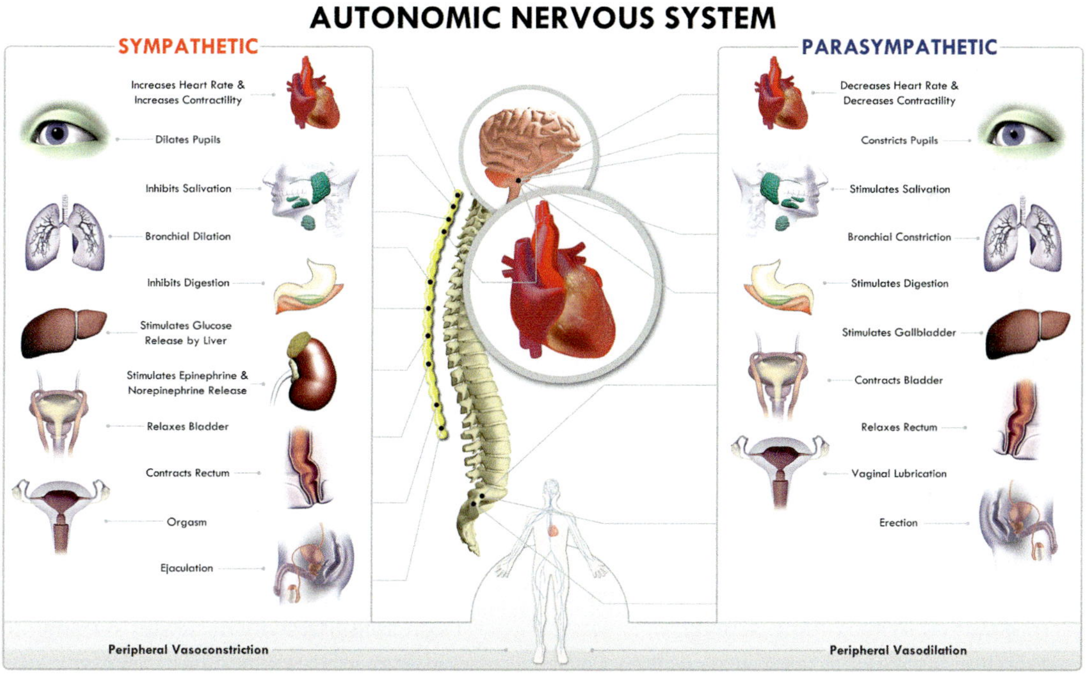


- The diameter of the iris of the eye opens with sympathetic activation to let in more light (e.g., to run or fight), and the opposite happens with parasympathetic activation to let in less light.
- Thyroid gland: S-activity increases thyroid activity, SE causes hyperthyroidism, P-activity decreases thyroid activity, and PE causes hypothyroidism.
- Insulin release from the pancreas is increased with S-activity and decreased with P-activity.
- Liver function: glucose and nutrients are released from the liver with S-activity and stored in the liver with P-activity (note, P-activity controls digestion, see Question 12, and the storage of the glucose and nutrients from digestion is part of this operation).

- Kidneys: S-activity decreases volume to prevent excessive blood loss if injured while fleeing or fighting, and P-activity increases volume to ensure all cells of the body are properly perfused (receive proper amounts of blood).
- Bladder: S-activity increases sphincter tone to prevent emptying. SE causes a persistent "full-feeling." P-activity decreases sphincter tone to urge emptying. PE causes the feeling of needing to empty often.
- Estrogen and testosterone increase with S-activity and decrease with P-activity. Too much testosterone, due to SE, leads to rage. Too little P-activity is associated with too little estrogen or too little testosterone and is associated with perimenopause or impotence, respectively.

**Question 7: What Systems of the Body Are *Not* Under the Influence of Both P&S Systems and Their "Push-Pull" Effects?**

**Answer**:

- Hormones are typically controlled by only one autonomic branch: more or less adrenaline or cortisol is from more or less S-activity. More or less growth hormone is from more or less P-activity.
- Tearing (lachrymal gland activity) and salivation are increased or decreased with increases or decreases in P-activity. Sjögren's disease (dry eyes and dry mouth) is caused by too little P-activity.
- While breathing is controlled by both P&S branches, ventilation (diaphragm) movement is controlled by P-activity, and the diameter of the bronchi is controlled by S-activity.
- The entire gastrointestinal tract is controlled uniquely by P-activity. More P-activity increases motility, including gastric emptying and bowel motility and vice versa. PE leads to GERD due to excessive gastric motility and diarrhea with or without IBS. Too little P-activity leads to gastroparesis (which may also lead to GERD due to food backing up gastric juices into the Esophagus and constipation with or without IBS. As a corollary, the splanchnic system is also uniquely controlled by P-activity. To collect the nutrients from digestion when P-activity increases to facilitate digestion, P-activity opens the splanchnic system and vice versa. PE can lead to hypovolemia.
- The vasculature throughout the body is uniquely controlled by S-activity. More αS-activity constricts the peripheral vasculature (increasing blood pressure) and vice versa. As a corollary, the angiotensin-renin system is also controlled by S-activity to also help control fluid volume within the body. Increased S-activity increases angiotensin-renin activity, thereby increasing volume and causing thirst. Decreased S-activity decreases angiotensin-renin activity, thereby decreasing volume. SE overstimulates angiotensin-renin activity and leads to hypertension. S-insufficiency does not stimulate enough angiotensin-renin activity and leads to hypotension.
- Different aspects of sex function are controlled by only one or the other P&S systems. P-activation leads to vaginal lubrication and erection, and S-activation leads to orgasm and ejaculation. S-insufficiency is associated with impotence, and SE is associated with premature ejaculation.
- Sweat glands are uniquely controlled by S-activity. Increased S-activity increases sweating to reduce core temperature. Decreased S-activity decreases sweating to conserve core temperature. Occasionally, Ach has S-effects as well, such as stimulating sweating or piloerection, where the hair stands up on end.

## Dysfunction of the P&S Nervous Systems

**Question 8: What Is P&S or Autonomic Dysfunction?**

**Answer**: Autonomic dysfunction, also called dysautonomia, occurs when the nerves of the autonomic nervous system are damaged or not working normally. Oftentimes, this is called autonomic neuropathy or, as mentioned, dysautonomia. It can range from life-threatening to only a minor problem. It can affect the entire autonomic nervous system or only parts of it.

Regardless of the cause, autonomic dysfunction is a result of a persistent imbalance between the P&S nervous systems. Again, the P&S nerves control actions such as heartbeat, involuntary breathing, blood vessel size, and blood delivery to all parts of the body, especially the brain. As a result, any dysregulation can cause serious problems, especially with blood pressure or heart rhythm. In the case of blood flow to the brain, P&S dysfunction may cause light-headedness or dizziness, which may be debilitating, or it may cause cognitive difficulties or "brain fog." Also, sexual function could be adversely affected, as can digestive, bowel, or urinary function. Basically, any organ system in the body may be adversely affected when there is a dysfunction of the P&S nervous systems.

## Question 9: What May Cause P&S or Autonomic Dysfunction?

**Answer**: The P&S nerves that control and coordinate the organs are small, type C fibers and are typically more fragile than other nerves. As a result, they are more sensitive to insult and attack. They are oftentimes damaged by other disease entities such as diabetes, Parkinson's, amyloid, or autoimmune processes. Occasionally, toxic substances or conditions such as alcohol, high blood acid levels such as from too much sugar in the blood, or infectious agents such as viruses or bacteria can cause damage to the P&S nerves. Further, nerves have some of the highest cellular metabolic rates in the body and as a result are very sensitive to low oxygen or nutrient levels which may be damaging. Simple aging can cause degeneration of the P&S nerve fibers. Some individuals have accelerated aging of their nerve fibers, typically due to persistent imbalances between the P&S systems caused by disease, injury, adverse lifestyle, poor genetics, etc.

## Question 10: What Is the Typical P&S or Autonomic Dysfunction?

**Answer**: Again, all P&S dysfunctions are P&S imbalances, and actually, there are two general types of imbalances: a resting imbalance and a dynamic or challenge imbalance. The typical imbalance is a resting imbalance and is due to the fact that the P-nervous system (the majority of which, outside the central nervous system, is the vagus nerve) is a longer and a more exposed portion of the ANS and therefore more vulnerable to insult or attack. The balance then suffers, and the P-nervous system declines faster than the S-nervous system. Ultimately this is like the "brakes" failing faster than the "accelerator" on a car. The problem is that once the "brakes" inside fail, they cannot be replaced. This progression (see insert below) includes (1) peripheral autonomic neuropathy (PAN or peripheral autonomic dysfunction[1]), (2) advanced autonomic dysfunction (AAD, indicating increased morbidity risk – the risk of more secondary symptoms) or diabetic autonomic neuropathy (DAN, which is ADD with the complications of abnormal insulin and blood glucose levels due to diabetes), and finally (3) cardiovascular autonomic neuropathy (CAN, indicating increased mortality risk, the risk of sudden death or other major adverse cardiac event, aka MACE).

[1]At this stage "neuropathy" is a misnomer and has led to the misperception that P&S imbalance cannot be treated. As a result many people have suffered unnecessarily. "Neuropathy" implies "dead nerves." The nerves are not dead, just damaged, and they can be healed and their function normalized for their age. This is why "dysfunction" is the preferred term.

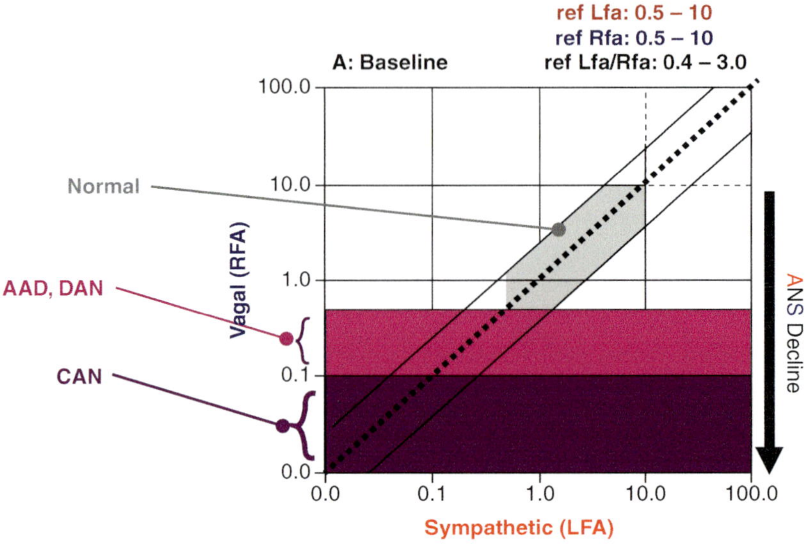


Some types of P&S dysfunctions are temporary and may recover over time, such as functional CAN (CAN that is reversed with therapy, as opposed to structural CAN that is not reversed with therapy). Identification and treatment is therefore important. Some types of P&S dysfunction cannot recover completely but can recover only partially. Ultimately, all that may be done is delay continued deterioration of P&S nerve fibers (in effect delay the aging effect) with several measures, including the Mind-Body Wellness Program.

**Question 11: What Are Dynamic P&S or Autonomic Dysfunctions?**

**Answer**: The clinical P&S (or ANSAR) test includes three dynamic challenges (see insert below) that simulate common, daily activities: deep breathing challenge (which stimulates the P-nervous system), Valsalva challenge (which stimulates the S-nervous system), and the postural change or stand challenge (which stimulates both the P&S systems and tests the coordination between the P&S systems). Dynamic balances by definition require one branch to be significantly higher than the other, but there are limits, both lower and upper limits to how much higher.

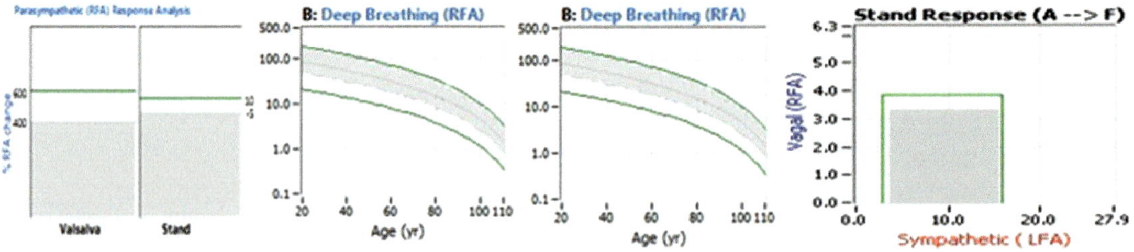


Dynamic imbalances contribute significantly to quality of life (QoL) dysfunctions, as well as PAN and AAD (or DAN). Even though the primary issue in CAN is minimizing the risk of MACE, once CAN is minimized by normalizing P&S balance (sympathovagal balance), normalizing remaining dynamic imbalances may help to improve QoL. Oftentimes, when P&S dysfunction is secondary to a disease entity, the autonomics will improve when the underlying disease gets treated and improved. When no cause of P&S

dysfunction is identified, this is called idiopathic. In many instances, treatment can improve the symptoms and abnormalities. There may be no cure, but treatment often improves QoL. In these cases, the goal of therapy, including lifestyle changes (such as those in the Mind-Body Wellness Program), is to have more better days than bad days in treating patients with these illnesses.

**Question 12: What Common Disorders Involve P&S Nervous System Dysfunction?**

**Answer**: There are many disorders involving P&S nervous system dysfunction. These include anxiety, chronic fatigue, fibromyalgia, persistent headache, and various forms of fainting or pre-fainting (involving light-headedness or dizziness), which is, respectively, termed "syncope" and "near syncope." Digestive problems such as gastroparesis, gastroesophageal reflux disease (GERD), and irritable bowel syndrome are also affected by P&S nervous system dysfunction. Most importantly, a large percentage of patients in the world have what is termed "orthostatic dysfunction," commonly manifested as "orthostatic intolerance." This form of light-headedness or dizziness is arguably the most debilitating symptom of ANS dysfunction or autonomic neuropathy. Usually, orthostatic dysfunction occurs when people are in the upright position, standing, or walking and develop evidence of lack of proper cerebral perfusion, which is blood flow to the brain. It can cause visual effects such as black spots.

Up to 90% of the time, this orthostatic intolerance syndrome is associated with chronic fatigue syndrome (CFS), which is defined as 6 months of significant exhaustion associated with, oftentimes, unrefreshing sleep, daytime somnolence, swollen lymph nodes, sore throat, depression, and an inability to function. It is felt that many of these disorders, including anxiety, migraines, and neurodegenerative diseases such as Parkinson's disease and Alzheimer's dementia, may be the result of, or contributed to by, P&S dysfunction.

**Question 13: How Do I Know I Have ANS Dysfunction?**

**Answer**: First, note that "if you can feel it, it is not autonomic dysfunction." In other words, "pins and needles," pain (the other small type C fibers), weakness, numbness, etc. are sensory (somatic) and motor dysfunctions, not autonomic dysfunctions. Typically, by the time these sensory and motor dysfunctions present, P&S dysfunction has already presented. For example, P&S dysfunction first causes vascular disorder which causes poor perfusion of the tissues in that area (like hands and feet or legs), including the other nerves in that area, which is what leads to the sensory and motor dysfunction.

Diabetes is a sign of P&S dysfunction. According to the American Diabetes Association, by the time a patient is diagnosed with type 2 diabetes, they have had the disease for 5–7 years, and the early stages of autonomic decline already began (see Question 13 with Fig. 7.6).

Light-headedness or dizziness is a common first symptom of P&S dysfunction, as is fatigue, malaise, and exercise intolerance, but there are a number of other potential reasons for these symptoms as well. Light-headedness or dizziness may include postural orthostatic tachycardia syndrome (POTS) or syncope, with or without fainting. P&S monitoring helps to identify P&S dysfunction as a reason for these symptoms. Compromise of the QoL functions is also an indicator, including stomach (GI) upset, sleep disorders, bowel and bladder dysfunction, and sex dysfunction. Also, difficult to control blood pressure, blood sugar (even without diabetes), and hormones (e.g., estrogen and thyroid) are signs of P&S dysfunction, as are unexplained seizures or palpitations, excessive sweating or no sweating, and frequent headache or migraine. Depression, anxiety, PTSD, and Ehlers-Danlos syndrome are conditions that typically involve P&S dysfunction.

### Question 14: What Symptoms Are Indicators of Autonomic Dysfunction?

**Answer**: As indicated in the answer to Question 13, early symptoms are difficult to detect, and by the time symptoms present, it is later in the progression of autonomic decline. The reason for this is that the P&S nervous systems are "hidden" behind the organs. In fact, the job of the P&S nervous systems is to maintain normal organ function, as long as possible, even if they themselves are abnormal or dysfunctional. Symptoms are caused by the organs. So by the time the organs become symptomatic, the P&S nervous systems may have been dysfunctional for a while.

In addition to the symptoms listed in the answer to Question 13, other questions to ask include the following: (1) "Do I have erectile dysfunction?", (2) urinary tract questions such as "Does one pass urine involuntarily such as urinary incontinence?", or (3) "Does one have difficulty emptying urine such as urinary retention?" While structural abnormalities may be the etiology, oftentimes autonomic dysfunction may be the problem.

The 25 point "Simplified Autonomic Questionnaire" (Chap. 9) above is used to help determine if P&S monitoring is to be considered. The more positive items answered, the higher the possibility an individual will test positive for P&S dysfunction.

### Question 15: Are There Different Degrees of Abnormality or Gradation to Autonomic Dysfunction?

**Answer**: Autonomic dysfunction can be mild, moderate, or severe. It is really a continuum. There is no dichotomy. The most advanced form is known as cardiac autonomic neuropathy (CAN). CAN is a serious medical condition because the heart rate is unstable and there are problems with essential and peripheral vascular control. CAN has been linked to greater risks of sudden cardiac death and mortality, heart attack, and silent ischemia. Patients with CAN may be diabetics and have silent ischemia, but many patients do not have diabetes. Basically, CAN should be suspected if an individual has orthostatic hypotension, resting tachycardia, neurocardiogenic syncope, exercise intolerance, postural orthostatic tachycardia, or silent myocardial ischemia. P&S Monitoring is considered one of the earliest and first signs and symptoms to suggest CAN. Testing can be done in a laboratory or even in a doctor's office by looking at changes and beat-to-beat heart rate intervals to see if a person has evidence of CAN. If CAN is detected, a full noninvasive cardiac work-up is recommended, even in patients who are asymptomatic, if they have not recently had one.

As noted, autonomic dysfunction occurs when the autonomic nerves are damaged. CAN appears to be a rather advanced stage of autonomic dysfunction. It is believed that there are measures that can be instituted when patients have autonomic dysfunction prior to developing CAN. Oftentimes, the patient does have a sinus tachycardia at rest because they have low vagal tone and the vagal function or parasympathetic function is greatly impaired. Testing with Valsalva maneuvers, deep breathing, and standing and tilt response can yield calculations and reflect if a person has cardiac autonomic neuropathy or not.

A less advanced but still significant form of autonomic nervous system dysfunction is advanced autonomic nervous system dysfunction (AAD). This is a stage that precedes CAN. If it is associated with diabetes, this is labeled diabetic autonomic neuropathy (DAN). In DAN, patients may also have resting heart rates that are high. Usually, the same testing that is done to detect CAN is done to detect AAD or DAN, namely, heart rate variable intervals with different maneuvers. Many patients with DAN also will have peripheral neuropathy which is common in diabetics. It is hoped that by detecting patients in AAD stages, treatment may be instituted, especially with antioxidant therapy, and try to balance the P&S nervous systems with other measures to prevent progression to CAN. Aggressive risk factor modification as in CAN is also important, that is, controlling cholesterol, BP, and blood sugar if the patient is diabetic. Also, if one smokes, they should stop smoking. If they drink alcohol excessively, they should stop drinking alcohol entirely in these instances. Exercising daily maintains a good healthy condition. Drinking plenty of fluids, exercising regularly, and avoiding stress may also be important in treating autonomic dysfunction.

Mild autonomic neuropathy oftentimes can be diagnosed also with assessing heart rate variable intervals based on the electrocardiogram changes and heart rate with response to the maneuvers of Valsalva, which is bearing against a closed glottis maneuver as though you were bearing down, and deep breathing responses along with standing or tilt responses. With mild autonomic neuropathy, one sees abnormalities mainly just with deep breathing or with Valsalva or both. There are calculations and a format that is relied upon called time domain variables in which three different measurements are taken from individuals when assessing heart rate variability. If they have one out of three abnormalities, autonomic neuropathy is usually mild, two out of three abnormalities are usually moderate or advanced, and three abnormalities suggest they may have CAN. Again, risk factor reduction is most important along with antioxidant therapy approaches as outlined above.

## Tests of the P&S Nervous Systems and for Autonomic (P&S) Dysfunction

### Question 16: Are There Lab Tests to Determine the Presence of Autonomic Dysfunction?

**Answer**: There are lab tests that may be useful in assessing if an individual has autonomic dysfunction. Norepinephrine levels are often drawn while one is lying and standing. Cortisol levels are drawn to rule out Addison's disease, an adrenal disorder. Oftentimes, a 24-hour urine for prostaglandins and metabolites of histamine are assessed to rule out a mast cell activation syndrome which may have autonomic dysfunction components associated with it. Also, blood tryptase levels are drawn for individuals suspected of mast cell activation syndrome.

There are many tests which can also assess for autonomic dysfunction that can be done in a doctor's office or in an outpatient laboratory setting. One is a tilt test, which is a special type of evaluation in which a person is exposed to passive tilt at 45° or 60° and the feet are unsupported. Blood pressure and heart rate monitoring are done, and certain maneuvers are performed to see how their vital signs respond. Computer printouts and waveforms are also analyzed. There are also tests which require respiration and EKG heart rate monitoring in which cardiorespiratory testing can be employed to test an individual's heart rate responses to certain maneuvers such as a Valsalva maneuver (bearing down as though someone was moving their bowels), a stand-up or orthostatic posture assumption, or a passive tilt. Also, deep breathing is a maneuver used to assess for vagal autonomic function. There are also machines which can test for one's sweating function. This may be important, and an abnormal test may indicate peripheral autonomic nervous system dysfunction.

### Question 17: What Tests Are Available to Determine if I Have P&S or Autonomic Dysfunction?

**Answer**: Over the years several noninvasive tests have been developed to assess the P&S nervous systems, including tilt-table testing, heart rate variability, beat-to-beat blood pressure, quantitative sudomotor axon reflex test (Q-SART), and a simplified version of Q-SART, Q-Sweat. However, the one most preferred is P&S monitoring, which is most able to quantify the P&S branches, simultaneously and without assumption or approximation. This is preferred because "simultaneously and without assumption or approximation" is unique to P&S monitoring [11].

**Question 18: Why Is P&S Monitoring, or Autonomic Testing in General, Not Well Understood?**

**Answer**: There are various tests that can test for types of disorders of the somatic nervous system (a part of the peripheral nervous system separate from the autonomic nervous system). Usually, a neurologist can address the work-up of various types of peripheral neuropathies which are non-autonomic but somatic. Unfortunately, because of the difficulty measuring the P&S nervous systems (because they are "hidden" behind the organs), there was very little data on them until relatively recently, and the data that was available was on total (the sum of P&S) autonomic function, which was not specific enough.

Where it is more well-known was (and is) in the diabetes world. Autonomic (diabetic autonomic neuropathy), as well as somatosensory, neuropathies are very commonly found in diabetics. Oftentimes, an individual can have both peripheral autonomic neuropathy and peripheral somatic neuropathy coexisting. In patients who present with neuropathy symptoms, e.g., burning and tingling in their hands and feet, oftentimes they will be tested and concomitant autonomic nervous system dysfunction will also be indicated. Remember, both types of small fibers known as type C nerve fibers are affected and get disease in these types of peripheral nervous system disorders.

**Question 19: Why May P&S Monitoring Discover and Document Things Most Other Physicians or Tests Cannot?**

**Answer**: The P&S nervous systems are dynamic systems. Except for stress tests (on treadmills), most other tests are administered while you are at rest (sitting or lying on the exam table). To that end, most patients present after having seen several physicians, who by that time all say that the patient is "normal." Yet the patient is still complaining of symptoms. When a patient is tested, they are tested at rest and dynamically (in response to challenges). This is what makes the test more complicated both for the physician and the patient. However this dynamic feature is important, because most often that is where the patients' disorders are found and documented. So patients are shown both the fact that (1) often they are normal at rest (they should be normal at rest; a number of doctors have worked on them a number of years to get them, and keep them, that way!) and (2) they have abnormal responses to challenges. Furthermore, these abnormalities are also treatable, and in treating them, they may be relieved.

**Question 20: Why Is P&S Monitoring a Complex Test Both for the Patient and the Physician?**

**Answer**: As stated in the Answer to Question 17, the P&S nervous systems are dynamic systems and as such require more testing to document. In addition, a doctor's evaluation is important. Blood pressure and heart rate responses to different stresses and sitting and standing need to be taken and require up to 5 minutes to document. A weak blood pressure response (increase) to Valsalva (the stress response) or too great a blood pressure response (decrease) to deep breathing (the relaxation response) may cause light-headedness and other symptoms (including "brain fog" and anxiety-depression syndromes). A drop in systolic blood pressure of more than 20 millimeters of mercury or 10 millimeters of mercury drop in diastolic upon standing may be seen in orthostatic hypotension. This is another potential cause of light-headedness and other symptoms, as are its related diseases: orthostatic intolerance and orthostatic hypertension. Another is postural orthostatic tachycardia syndrome (POTS), which is characterized by a rise in heart rate greater than 30 beats per minute within 3 minutes of standing. Syncope, including vasovagal syncope, is another fairly common disorder that requires a dynamic test to elucidate. These are yet other potential causes of light-headedness and other symptoms. None of these abnormal responses common to P&S dysfunction may be detected at rest.

Questions are also important including: "Do you feel full prematurely after eating?" "Do you feel that your stomach empties slowly or that you have to vomit or you get nauseous quite easily?" This may represent gastroparesis. While one is thought to be a purely gastrointestinal disorder, this may reflect abnormalities in autonomic system dysfunction and also may be a clue that an individual has autonomic system dysfunction.

## Light-Headedness ("Dizziness") Due to Autonomic Dysfunction

**Question 21: What Autonomic Dysfunctions Underlie Light-Headedness?**

**Answer**: As mentioned in Question 12, light-headedness (also characterized as "dizziness"[2]) is a common (first) symptom of P&S (autonomic) dysfunction. The postural change (stand) portion of the P&S monitoring test helps to differentiate the underlying cause of light-headedness. There are three possible, abnormal, P&S results: sympathetic withdrawal (SW), sympathetic excess (SE), and parasympathetic excess (PE).

- SW is associated with orthostatic dysfunctions, i.e., orthostatic intolerance, orthostatic hypotension, orthostatic hypertension, and postural orthostatic tachycardia syndrome (POTS).
  - PE may mask SW, especially if there is a decrease blood pressure response to stand.
- SE is associated with (pre-)Syncope, i.e., neurogenic syncope, vasovagal syncope, cardiogenic syncope, and neurocardiogenic syncope (yes, patients may have both a neurological and cardiological dysfunction that both may cause syncope).
  - PE with SE is associated with (pre-) vasovagal syncope.
- PE is associated with poor brain perfusion, not associated with orthostatic dysfunction (SW) or syncope (SE).

**Question 22: Why Is Sympathetic Withdrawal Associated with Orthostatic Dysfunction?**

**Answer**: In 1980, Williams and coworkers described episodes of low blood pressure associated with sympathetic withdrawal (SW). Normally upon standing, the (alpha-) sympathetic nervous system increases activity to cause vasoconstriction in the legs to help move blood to the abdomen to help the heart pump blood to the brain upon assuming an upright (head-up) posture. This is a compensatory mechanism, compensating for the effects of gravity upon standing. Sympathetic withdrawal (SW) is the failing of the increase due to autonomic dysfunction (possibly due to disease, aging, or injury), where the sympathetics do not respond properly, and due to the lack of vasoconstriction, blood pressure may not increase sufficiently, or may decrease, and orthostatic dysfunction may result.

Note, SW is more information and may be used to indicate preliminary (aka., pre-clinical) forms of orthostatic dysfunction prior to symptoms or the demonstration of full clinical symptoms. This may help to prevent full clinical symptoms or enable earlier treatment, helping to promote prevention and wellness.

SW has been observed in patients with orthostatic intolerance symptoms without having rises in heart rate consistent with POTS or drops in blood pressure consistent with orthostatic hypotension. These patients have been monitored with heart rate variability and cardiorespiratory testing, a form of testing that can identify if an individual's compensatory increase in sympathetics on rising from a sitting to standing position occurs too slowly or is inadequate. This prevents the leg veins from getting their blood squeezed from increasing sympathetic tone and propelling blood to the brain. SW can cause brain fog and orthostatic intolerance-type symptoms. Occasionally, they have small drops in blood pressures, but

[2]Physicians differentiate light-headedness from dizziness by associating dizziness specifically to vestibular disorders and light-headedness to non-vestibular causes of "dizziness." Patients, especially the elderly, frequently have both vestibular and at least one non-vestibular cause of light-headedness or dizziness.

do not have the appropriate stand response, which is a 5 mmHg rise in diastolic blood pressure and usually no change in systolic blood pressure. Also, the heart rate usually increased by less than 10 beats per minute in individuals with SW.

**Question 23: Is SW Treatable?**

**Answer**: The treatment of SW is the same as that for any orthostatic intolerant symptomatic patient (see "Light-Headedness ("Dizziness") Due to Autonomic"); usually fluids, salt, compression stockings, and occasionally midodrine are needed. Rarely is Florinef needed. Also, rarely is combination therapy of mineralocorticoids or alpha-adrenergic agonists, such as midodrine, indicated. Although, occasionally this combination is prescribed when patients are found with OH or POTS syndrome. It appears that SW is a mild form of autonomic dysfunction, although patients can have syncopal episodes when their blood volume is down, such as times of dehydration or hypovolemia. It is important to recognize since patients are told to well hydrate, consume enough salt, and use compression stockings as needed.

**Question 24: What Causes Fainting (Syncope) or Near Fainting (Pre-syncope)?**

**Answer**: Fainting or syncope occurs when there is self-limited loss of consciousness caused by lack of blood flow and oxygen delivery to the brain resulting in reduced cerebral perfusion. Pre-syncope is near loss of consciousness by the same mechanism. Blood loss and dehydration are common causes which precipitate syncope or pre-syncope. Sympathetic excess upon standing is associated with (pre-) syncope and is believed to be the result of the brain using the sympathetic nervous system to signal for more blood (by increasing heart rate or blood pressure, thereby increasing cardiac output, expecting to drive more blood to the brain).

Syncope can be caused by cardiac abnormalities, abnormalities of the vessels within the lungs, or abnormalities within the large blood vessel which leads to the heart (the aorta). An electrical abnormality in the heart or a cardiac arrhythmia is extremely important to exclude as this oftentimes can be life-threatening. When cardiovascular diseases (structural or electrical) are excluded, most causes of syncope are usually benign, albeit potentially debilitating. The remaining causes of syncope are neural.

Note, the most commonly diagnosed form of syncope is neurocardiogenic syncope, meaning both of neural and cardiac origins. While both may cause syncope at the same time in a patient, this is more often a guess due to the fact that most autonomic measures cannot differentiate P&S without assumption or approximation. The most common cause of syncope is due to an abnormal neural reflex known as vasovagal syncope (VVS). This neural (vagal) reflex can be situational to cough, post-micturitional (after urination), status post-emotional (like seeing blood or like the excitement experienced after one's football team scores a touchdown), or post-prandial (after a large meal) or as a reaction to pain or extreme heat.

**Question 25: Do All Forms of Syncope Occur Only While Standing?**

**Answer**: Some forms of syncope occur only on assuming the upright position, either immediately or in a delayed fashion. Vasovagal syncope may occur sitting or standing for a prolonged period of time but usually not immediately.

**Question 26: What Is the Difference Between Syncope and Orthostatic Dysfunction, Including POTS?**

**Answer**: As mentioned in the answer to Question 20, some forms of syncope (i.e., vasovagal syncope) may occur anytime (while sitting or standing), whereas orthostatic dysfunctions occur only upon assuming the upright position and usually occur more immediately. The orthostatic causes of syncope are due to a considerable drop in the blood pressure that can be induced by drugs or other disorders that affect the autonomic nervous system. Such disorders include diabetes, viruses, Parkinson's disease, amyloidosis, and rarely other forms of autonomic central nervous system abnormalities such as multiple system atrophy (MSA). There is also a disorder known as primary autonomic dysfunction with pure autonomic failure, which affects the peripheral autonomic nervous system. Parkinson's, although it is a central nervous system disease, affects the peripheral autonomic nerves.

A cardiologist and a neurologist are often required to identify the cause of syncope if one is not clearly evident. A cardiac arrhythmia and structural heart disease must be ruled out before addressing non-cardiac causes of syncope. Cardiologists will use Holter monitors, long-term monitors up to 30 days, and even implantable loop recorders for years to search for arrhythmias which may be causing fainting episodes. Echocardiograms, which are ultrasounds of the heart, stress tests, and even more advanced cardiac testing including electrophysiology assessment in a laboratory oftentimes can be required to exclude arrhythmias.

When a cardiac cause of syncope is excluded, but one is not sure if the patient is having a syncopal episode due to a vasovagal or an orthostatic issue, a tilt test is oftentimes indicated to differentiate between the two entities. There are some other noninvasive tests which can be done in the office and use standing responses without tilt testing which may also be helpful, such as P&S (aka cardiorespiratory) testing. You should seek out a trained physician, preferably a neurologist, cardiologist, or occasionally an endocrinologist, who may have specialized training in using these various forms of equipment.

## Question 27: What Is Vasovagal Syncope (VVS)?

**Answer**: Vasovagal syncope is also known as the "simple fainting spell." This is a neurally mediated type of syncope. Vasovagal syncope involves a temporary loss of consciousness by a neurological reflex due to sudden dilatation of blood vessels of the legs and/or a slow heart rate or both. Vasovagal syncope is also known as neurocardiogenic syncope.

Vasovagal syncope is usually benign and may be recurrent. It also may be chronic. It can go into crescendo phases of flare-ups. Usually, it is caused by blood pooling in the legs due to sudden vasodilatation of the venous blood vessels. Vasovagal syncope can be precipitated by emotional stress or prolonged upright posture or even prolonged sitting. It is oftentimes situational and can be caused by cough, heat, urination, emotion, a large meal, pain, and alcohol. A tilt test may be necessary to differentiate vasovagal syncope from an orthostatic type of fainting such as orthostatic hypotension. A tilt test may also be needed to confirm that the syncope is reflexed by showing first a progressive early drop in blood pressure gradual in onset without symptoms with the passive or head-up tilt test procedure. This is later followed by a rapid drop in blood pressure and finally a slow heart rate. Oftentimes, nausea, excessive fatigue, and sweating precede episodes of vasovagal syncope. These are warning symptoms and allow the patient to preemptively lie down.

## Question 28: There Are Warning Signs to Vasovagal Syncope (VVS)?

**Answer**: Warning symptoms, when they occur, are often helpful in having a patient lie down to avoid an overt fainting episode. These symptoms consist of light-headedness, ringing in the ears, visual disturbances, sweating, and nausea. As mentioned, symptoms of vasovagal syncope may occur sporadically and may not occur for long periods of time. One out of three individuals will experience an episode of vasovagal syncope during their lifetime. Some may not have recurrence. Individuals who have recurrent episodes at times can go into a crescendo or a frequent and disabling time period when they have very frequent episodes of vasovagal syncope. These patients oftentimes require intensive pharmacology to attempt to put these reflex syncope episodes in remission.

**Question 29: What Is Therapy for Vasovagal Syncope (VVS)?**

**Answer**: Pacemaker therapy is rarely warranted and is usually discouraged in patients with frequent vasovagal syncope. However, it may be helpful in older individuals over the age of 40 when documented periods of asystole (a pause in the heart rate) or very slow heart rates are recorded, oftentimes with Holter monitors or loop recorders.

Treatment for vasovagal syncope is typically supportive. An individual should avoid circumstances that precipitate fainting episodes such as a crowded room or drinking alcohol in a hot environment. Medications may also be helpful in treating episodes, especially when there are flare-ups. Anticholinergic therapy (to treat the vagal or parasympathetic component) in individuals who test positive for high vagal tone may be useful. In the past, individuals have used anticholinergics such as Norpace (which is actually an antiarrhythmic drug). Some people have used scopolamine (another anticholinergic). With P&S monitoring, oftentimes the low-dose tricyclic agent, nortriptyline, is prescribed. Nortriptyline has strong anticholinergic mechanisms. SSRIs and SNRIs, which are also antidepressants, oftentimes have some anticholinergic effect and often are useful in people who have high anxiety syndromes or are very tense.

It is useful to hydrate and use salt loading frequently in patients who have frequent vasovagal syncope, especially with low blood pressures. Compression stockings are often useful in addition. In terms of pharmacological treatment, mineralocorticoids such as fludrocortisone are also useful. These retain water within the blood vessel system, building or maintaining blood volume to help properly perfuse the brain. Beta-blockers, once thought to be very effective, have now been found not to be extremely effective. They may be beneficial in patients older than 40 years of age, but they have limited efficacy.

Midodrine is often helpful and may be taken up to three to four times a day, usually starting at a 2.5 mg low dose and titrating upwards. In fact, midodrine has been shown to be the most effective agent in patients who have flare-ups.

**Question 30: If Midodrine Is So Useful for VVS, Why Is It Not Used More Often and by More Physicians?**

**Answer**: While midodrine is usually well tolerated, it is not recommended in patients with hypertension or heart failure. It is also contraindicated for people with supine hypertension or high resting blood pressure. Midodrine is an adrenergic agonist, a potent vasoconstrictor, that constricts the veins in the lower extremities. It was approved by the Food and Drug Administration in 1996 for treatment of dysautonomia and orthostatic hypotension. Midodrine is a prodrug which forms an active metabolite desglymidodrine, which is an alpha-receptor agonist. It does not stimulate heart rate. Because it does not cross into the central nervous system, it does not cause any central effects. Individuals who take midodrine, however, do complain of piloerection or goose bumps, sometimes paresthesias and tingling, especially over the scalp; occasionally men will have symptoms attributed to urinary frequency, and occasional headache can occur. Titrating very low doses up slowly makes it much easier for people to tolerate this medication, and if a pure autonomic dysfunction, it may not need the higher doses. Midodrine is a very inexpensive and very effective agent in all types of autonomic nervous system dysfunction whether they are vasovagal or orthostatic, such as orthostatic hypotension and postural orthostatic tachycardia syndrome. The key is to start the medication very slowly at a low dose and slowly titrate it upward and give the patient time so that they can adapt to some of the minor side effects.

A new pharmacologic agent, ivabradine (Corlanor), is a new sodium-potassium channel blocking agent which affects the sinus node and thereby heart rate. It slows the heart rate down. As vasovagal syncope may involve an increase in heart rate prior to when the blood pressure drops further, there is a decrease. This medication may blunt the initial heart rate rise in the early part of the reflex. While more research is being done on this agent, it has been found that Corlanor (ivabradine) is very effective in various types of fainting disorders and even in treating patients with POTS who have pre-syncope and not actual syncope.

**Question 31: What Is Orthostatic Intolerance (OI)?**

**Answer**: Orthostatic intolerance affects millions of Americans at all ages. It is a condition that is triggered when the body changes position (e.g., assumes an upright posture); dizziness, light-headedness, nausea, sweating, fainting, or near fainting may occur. Lying down improves symptoms. It is often related to improper regulation of the ANS, typically the alpha-sympathetic nerves that innervate the peripheral vasculature. These alpha-sympathetic nerves do not communicate properly to the blood vessels, which do not constrict upon standing, causing blood to pool in the legs and making it hard for the heart to properly pump blood to the brain.

"Brain fog" (aka brain fatigue) can be caused by prolonged standing in a patient with orthostatic intolerance. This is due to an abnormality of cerebral blood flow, where not enough blood is delivered and oxygen demand is not met in the brain tissue. Brain fog can (a) cause a lack of focus, (b) cause poor memory recall, and (c) reduce mental acuity and (d) is often associated with light-headedness and near syncope. It is also associated with significant levels of (physiologic) fatigue. After episodes of brain fog and orthostatic intolerance, individuals have to lie down and often have debilitating fatigue for hours and possibly days.

Orthostatic intolerance is predominantly due to three mechanisms: (1) withdrawal of the (alpha-) sympathetic nervous system input into the legs while assuming the upright position; (2) a more advanced form is actual orthostatic hypotension, where the blood pressure drops more than 20 millimeters systolic or 10 millimeters diastolic and this can cause dramatic effects, including syncope; (3) postural orthostatic tachycardia can also result from orthostatic intolerance. This is because there is a significant increase in the sympathetic nervous system outpouring on standing and the heart rate response becomes very rapid and impairs blood flow to the brain. Young women tend to have POTS due to their smaller heart size, whereas men and older women tend to have OH.

**Question 32: Why Do Some People Have Orthostatic Intolerance (OI) Only Occasionally and in Others It Is Debilitating?**

**Answer**: In some people, OI may be masked by elevated or high blood pressure. This may be a compensatory mechanism, where the body sets the resting pressure high enough to sustain the drop and still provide enough blood to the brain. In others, their hearts are strong enough to compensate, but it may only be short-lived. Regardless of the disease entity associated with orthostatic intolerance, the mechanism is a failure of delivery of enough blood to the brain via the cerebral vessels leading to "brain fog," fatigue, visual acuity issues, memory issues, and a lack of focus. These issues become very important and are treated independently, oftentimes to the exclusion of recognizing and treating the underlying cause. By not recognizing the underlying cause, symptom therapy is often ineffective. It is a very disabling problem and requires medical attention.

One needs to understand the pathophysiology of upright posture to understand why orthostatic intolerance occurs. Normally, when a person stands, about one-half liter of blood leaves their chest and goes into their lower abdomen, buttocks, and legs. Also, 10–15% of the plasma volume leaks out of blood vessels and goes into interstitial tissues. To compensate for this, there is a transient increased heart rate of 10–20 beats a minute (over about the first 30 seconds after assuming an upright position), a negligible change in systolic blood pressure, and a 5 millimeter increase in diastolic blood pressure. People with orthostatic intolerance have abnormal compensatory mechanisms for this one-half liter of blood which goes from the chest into the lower extremities. This causes a lack of appropriate blood flow to the brain and, hence, the symptoms of brain fog.

### Question 33: What Is the Treatment for Orthostatic Intolerance?

**Answer**: Simple measures such as elevating the feet of the bed may help patients who have orthostatic intolerance. Patients are also encouraged to drink six to eight glasses of water a day or more if possible. Adding sodium to the diet is also helpful. Usually, cardiac patients have their sodium restricted for blood pressure or heart failure reasons. However, adding sodium in people who are not hypertensive or have heart failure may be beneficial. Gentle isometric exercise to build muscle tone is also helpful. Wearing compression stockings is a very important non-pharmacological measure. Therapy is started with compression stockings below the knees at 20 millimeters, but they do leave indentations and oftentimes need to do them up to the waist. Also, changing positions slowly is important. Medicines such as midodrine in low doses have also been effective in people who are quite symptomatic from orthostatic intolerance. Frequent small meals may also be helpful. Avoiding alcohol or heat may be helpful. Patients have learned countermeasures such as crossing their legs and tensing their leg muscles or whole body to relieve symptoms of orthostatic intolerance.

Drinking water rapidly does improve symptoms of orthostatic intolerance. It was initially thought that this was due to increasing volume; however, drinking fluids rapidly also increases sympathetic activity by a reflex mechanism. Also, in addition to gentle isometric exercises, water aerobics and water jogging may be useful. Often people with orthostatic intolerance find using a recumbent bike initially before embarking on more upright exercises is helpful in adapting. Some people do postural training measures where they stand erect against a wall or other surface for longer periods of time. Using an inversion table has also been found helpful, where having the head down and legs up for prolonged periods of time may also be helpful in relieving ongoing symptoms of orthostatic intolerance with patients.

### Question 34: What Is Postural Orthostatic Tachycardia Syndrome (POTS)?

**Answer**: POTS is a condition where there is an excessive increase in heart rate in the upright position usually seen soon after standing, within 10 minutes. A heart rate of greater than 30 beats per minute in adults and 40 beats per minute in children is usually required. There is no drop in blood pressure. There usually has to be accompanying symptoms such as those due to orthostatic intolerance that are occurring for more than 6 months to make this diagnosis. These are symptoms of chest discomfort, light-headedness, tachycardia, anxiety, palpitations, exercise intolerance, extreme fatigue, headache, brain fog, mental clouding, blurred vision, tunnel vision, tremulousness, and nausea. Headaches and fatigue are often non-positional. Symptoms are relieved with lying down. It is difficult to make a diagnosis of POTS without having orthostatic intolerance symptoms that are lasting more than 6 months despite the heart rate rising with standing position as described above.

Symptoms can be mild to severe, and the spectrum at times can lead people to severe exhaustion and disability. One in four people may not be able to work. Almost all patients with POTS have some degree of fatigue.

### Question 35: Who May Postural Orthostatic Tachycardia Syndrome (POTS) Affect?

**Answer**: POTS can affect children, teenagers, and adults. It is five times more common in women than in men and usually affects women in their childbearing years. It is more common than expected, and it is estimated to affect 1–3 million people in the United States. Interestingly, 30% of people with POTS also have reflux or vasovagal syncope (see Question 22). Patients with POTS do not have syncopal episodes, but have pre-fainting or pre-syncope. However, if 30% of them do have a vasovagal syndrome, they can have fainting and that needs to be determined.

POTS is seen oftentimes in patients with Ehlers-Danlos syndrome, which is a hypermobility-type disorder. Oftentimes, an orthopedic physician or a rheumatologist can diagnose these hypermobility syndromes which run in families. Also, POTS is seen in patients who have a high incidence of irritable bowel syndrome.

**Question 36: What Are the Symptoms of Postural Orthostatic Tachycardia Syndrome (POTS)?**

**Answer**: Patients with POTS on standing have a marked decrease in their stroke volume or the amount of blood ejected from the heart. Normally, when people stand, they initially have a small drop in the stroke volume or blood that is ejected from the heart, but in POTS, this is exaggerated, and there is an extremely small amount of blood ejected from the heart, and the heart becomes very small in size. This causes an overcompensation of the sympathetic nervous system where it becomes extremely hyperactive ("revved up"). With this sympathetic hyperactivity, heart rate becomes extremely high on standing. There is no drop in blood pressure. Therefore, this is characterized by a hypersympathetic state.

POTS is a heterogeneous type of disorder. There are several different types of POTS, and oftentimes patients are not tested to find out what type of POTS syndrome a patient is in because there can be overlaps. Initially, it was said that there can be a type of POTS that involves dysfunction or denervation of the sympathetic nerves to the lower extremities which prevents blood from going from the leg up to the heart. There are other types of POTS which involve chronic hyper-adrenergic activity where norepinephrine levels increase on standing. Other types of POTS patients are chronically hypovolemic or have a low blood volume. Hypovolemia may be confirmed by nuclear testing, although it has become a rare requirement. Other types of POTS are associated with mast cell disorders where histamine is released into the blood system and hives, anaphylaxis, and flushing can occur. Histamine may induce a form of hypovolemia. There is also a genetic type where there is a norepinephrine reuptake transporter defect which is very rarely seen.

**Question 37: What Is the Treatment for POTS?**

**Answer**: Regardless of the type of POTS, usually the treatment requires fluid hydration to increase blood volume, and drink the water very rapidly along with taking salt tablets. Doing this immediately before arising in the morning is very beneficial. Compression stockings are also useful.

Exercise training has been found to be highly beneficial, improving symptoms in POTS, and many POTS patients go into remissions at various times for prolonged periods. Also, females have exacerbations of POTS in the premenstrual cycle. Oftentimes, fluids are increased and midodrine prescribed specifically during this time of the month for females who have symptomatic POTS.

Patients with POTS can be quite disabled. Because of this, pharmacology may be necessary:

- Fludrocortisone: A volume expander. Fludrocortisone has been effective in many patients with POTS who have a hypovolemic-type syndrome. Plasma volume is expanded through enhanced kidney sodium retention. However, one can lose potassium and become hypokalemic or have a low potassium, and this should be monitored. Also, edema occasionally is seen with fludrocortisone.
- Propranolol: Low doses of beta-blocker such as propranolol 10–20 mg by mouth several times a day have also been shown to be effective in keeping the heart rate from rising.
- Clonidine: Is a blood pressure medicine which also acts centrally in the brain to prevent increases from sympathetic nervous system activation, and it is often given at

night as it can make patients drowsy. This also blunts the heart rate response.

- Midodrine: A vasoconstrictor. Vasoconstrictor therapy with midodrine has been found to be extremely effective, especially with fluid loading in patients with POTS. Midodrine is an alpha-sympathetic agonist which constricts the venous blood vessels in the lower extremities and promotes blood flow to the brain.
- Pyridostigmine: Increasing vagal tone with pyridostigmine 30–60 mg by mouth several times a day is also important. Pyridostigmine is a peripheral acetylcholinesterase inhibitor, and by increasing the Ach, it prevents the heart rate response to standing in patients with POTS. It is very effective in combination with low-dose beta-blockers. However, it can cause diarrhea and is usually better tolerated in people who have significant constipation and not diarrhea-predominant irritable bowel syndrome if they have POTS.
- Ivabradine (Corlanor): Ivabradine is prescribed to treat the inappropriate sinus tachycardia that occurs with POTS with great success. It has been found to be more successful than beta-blockers. It does not affect blood pressure. As mentioned, it blocks the ion channels of the sodium-potassium membrane. It is a proven treatment of angina pectoris and heart failure in patients but has been used off-label in dysautonomia, especially in patients with vasovagal syncope and in patients with POTS. This medicine is preferred over beta-blockers, but it is expensive and it needs to be pre-certified.
- Modafinil (Provigil): Occasionally, the central nervous system is stimulated with modafinil to treat the significant brain fog which occurs with patients with POTS. However, this may aggravate blood pressure and arrhythmias and needs to be watched carefully if prescribed. Usually, this medication is used for patients who are refractory to conventional treatment for sleep apnea. It does have alert-producing properties. This drug is not preferred, unless it is an extreme last resort in a patient who is very disabled.

## Question 38: What Is Orthostatic Hypotension (OH)?

**Answer**: Orthostatic hypotension is sometimes called neurogenic orthostatic hypotension (NOH) if there is no identifying cause such as dehydration, blood loss, or medications. Idiopathic or NOH is defined as a blood pressure drop greater than 20 millimeters systolic or 10 millimeters diastolic within 3 minutes of one standing from a lying or sitting position. Usually, this drop in blood pressure occurs earlier. If someone is severely hypertensive, the diagnosis may be based on a systolic blood pressure drop of 30 millimeters rather than 20. There are delayed forms of OH, but often these patients are not very symptomatic.

OH occurs with increasing frequency as one ages or suffers from prolonged or chronic diseases (the aging and disease effects correlate with the progression of autonomic decline). It is estimated to have a prevalence greater than 20% in individuals over the age of 60. It is also a very strong adverse prognostic factor for cardiovascular events such as heart attacks and strokes.

Orthostatic hypotension can be a primary disorder. It could also be associated with other neurological disorders such as dementia and with Lewy bodies and Parkinson's disease. There is a pure autonomic failure type which was identified back in the 1920s. A severe, very aggressive form of autonomic dysfunction known as multiple system atrophy can also occur but is rarely seen.

## Question 39: What Are the Symptoms of Orthostatic Hypotension (OH)?

**Answer**: The mechanism for OH is that on standing, the stroke volume goes down in normal amounts as it does in a normal individual. However, there is a failure of the compensatory sympathetic nervous system to increase, and it remains level or decreases. This causes a drop in blood pressure without an increase in heart rate since the sympathetic nervous system has not been activated appropriately in a compensatory fashion. (In POTS, the situation is the reverse. The heart rate goes up because of too much sympathetic reactivity, and the blood pressure does not drop.) In OH, the heart rate does not go up because there is a lack of sympathetic activation, and the blood pressure goes down because without compensatory sympathetic activation of any type, one cannot get blood from the veins up to the upper extremities and brain.

Oftentimes, people who faint with OH are difficult to differentiate from individuals with vasovagal syncope, as the drop in blood pressure can occur sporadically. In these instances, a tilt test may be useful. In a hemodynamic head-up tilt test, there is usually a sudden drop in blood pressure and heart rate with vasovagal syncope during the examination in a laboratory, whereas patients with OH will have an early and progressive decline in blood pressure without a drop in heart rate.

OH is also a very disabling disorder and oftentimes requires hospitalization as patients fall and can have trauma, especially as they get older. It is usually important to exclude causes of OH such as anemia, blood loss, dehydration, and medication, which can be easily reversed, before concluding that a person has an autonomic or idiopathic type of OH disorder.

**Question 40: What Is Treatment for Orthostatic Hypotension?**

**Answer**: In addition to conventional treatment of orthostatic intolerance, which involves hydration or reversing dehydration, increasing salt, bolus of water ingestion, and waist-high garments are often required. However, pharmacology is usually required as a system worsens:

- Midodrine (Proamatine): is a mainstay of treatment started at a low dose; however, midodrine is contraindicated in patients with supine hypertension, and in elderly men, especially, midodrine may cause urinary retention. One should not lie down for several hours after taking midodrine. If a person is extremely hypertensive, their blood pressure must be reduced first with pharmacological therapy which does not induce orthostasis prior to giving it.
- Pyridostigmine (Mestinon): is an alternative to midodrine in people who are hypertensive. Pyridostigmine is an acetylcholinesterase inhibitor that prolongs the effects of acetylcholine and increases sympathetic tone. However, it can cause diarrhea, nausea, vomiting, and excessive salivation but does not cause blood pressure elevations when lying down and, therefore, is a rather safe medicine to give in patients who have underlying supine hypertension or resting hypertension, and one does not want to give midodrine. Initial reports in studies in 2004 showed its efficacy in treating OH.
- Fludrocortisone (Florinef): is occasionally given but again can cause blood pressure elevations when lying down, headaches, low potassium, and swelling of the legs. One has to follow the potassium closely on an individual on Florinef. Salt tablets and fluid loading orally are preferred.
- Droxidopa (Northera): recently Northera has been approved for treatment of OH. It is the synthetic amino acid precursor which acts as a prodrug to the neural transmitter norepinephrine. Unlike norepinephrine, however, it does cross the blood-brain barrier and converts norepinephrine in the brain. It has few side effects except for maybe mild headache, nausea, some hypertension, some dizziness, and fatigue. It has been found to be extremely effective in treating this disorder and even more efficacious than midodrine without the worries of significant supine hypertension, although Northera can increase the blood pressure while lying down. Northera induces a peripheral venous constriction which maintains blood flow to the brain. However, it is extremely expensive and requires special pre-certification, and the cost is thousands

of dollars a month if one does not have proper insurance, although compassionate care can be obtained.
- Some people have attempted to use a caffeine and ergotamine combination as they use in migraines for treatment of orthostatic hypotension, although this has not been found to be very effective.
- There are other medications which have been used off-label to treat orthostatic hypotension which may require consulting with a specialist in autonomics regarding their use as some cannot be obtained in the United States. Others require subcutaneous use and have significant side effects.

## Diseases that Result from Dysfunction of the P&S (Autonomic) Nervous Systems

**Question 41: What Is Multiple System Atrophy (MSA)?**

**Answer**: MSA is a progressive disease which involves degeneration of the nervous system, usually involving the autonomic nervous system (ANS) and areas of the central nervous systems (CNS) such as the cerebellum or basal ganglia/striato-nigral pathways. When involving the cerebellum, gait issues are evident. Ocular movement disorders may also occur. The striato-nigral pathways produce Parkinson-like symptoms. These involve tremor, rigidity, slow movement, and irregular, jerky, postural, and intentional tremors. Speech can be affected in both types of MSA, as can swallowing.

MSA usually presents itself with an individual in their 50s. The autonomic dysfunction, which occurs later, encompasses urinary incontinence and retention, erectile dysfunction in men, and orthostatic hypotension, which is usually more than 30 millimeters on standing.

It may be difficult to differentiate true Parkinson's disease from MSA, especially early. Usually, patients with Parkinson's disease respond to the medicine levodopa, and patients with MSA do not respond. In general, patients with MSA loose sympathetic innervation of the heart, whereas those with Parkinson's do not.

**Question 42: How Do I Get Checked for MSA?**

**Answer**: A good board-certified neurologist should be sought out first. Also, a good clinical evaluation and brain imaging are helpful. MRI may suggest a patient has MSA and not Parkinson's disease by showing atrophy of certain parts of the brain known as putamen and cerebellum. This, however, is not conclusive. Positron emission tomography (PET) may be suggestive of MSA if metabolism of glucose is low in the areas of the brain affected. Most imaging techniques are still experimental, however.

Usually, MSA occurs at a younger age and progresses more rapidly than Parkinson's disease, which it can mimic. Some investigators measure supine and standing norepinephrine levels. ANS testing and sweat testing may be useful. In MSA, pseudo-motor testing for sweat testing may be normal. This is because MSA is a central autonomic failure and not peripheral.

There are specialized university centers which have expertise in the diagnosis of MSA. Your neurologist or autonomic specialist may refer you to one for further testing, especially some of the new state-of-the-art imaging techniques which are helping to narrow the diagnosis.

**Question 43: What Autonomic Findings Can You See in Parkinson's Disease?**

**Answer**: Autonomic dysfunction is a peripheral type in Parkinson's disease, whereas in MSA it is an essential type. Similar autonomic dysfunction features are seen in Parkinson's disease as in MSA, but they are more severe in MSA. Also, MSA patients do not respond to levodopa, a drug used to improve symptoms in Parkinson's disease.

Symptoms in Parkinson's disease which reflect autonomic dysfunction include orthostatic hypotension, which is a significant drop in blood pressure on standing, urinary symptoms such as urgency and incontinence due to diminished bladder capacity, diaphoresis, constipation, sexual dysfunction, and swallowing difficulties.

It should be noted that Parkinsonian patients are usually older in age than patients who develop MSA. Treatment of orthostatic hypotension in Parkinson's disease along with other autonomic dysfunction symptoms is similar to the treatment of other disorders which cause orthostatic hypotension or idiopathic orthostatic hypotension.

### Question 44: What Is Ehlers-Danlos Syndrome?

**Answer**: Ehlers-Danlos syndrome is a group of disorders that affect the connective tissue or the supportive tissue in the body that is found in the skin, bones, blood vessels, and virtually every organ. The connective tissue is loose or stretched, causing vessels to be "leaky" and structures more loose than normal. Usually, individuals with Ehlers-Danlos syndrome have very loose joints, but they could have life-threatening complications, especially from the vascular standpoint. There are six types of Ehlers-Danlos syndromes that have been described. There is the (1) classical type, the (2) hypermobility type, the (3) vascular type, the (4) kyphoscoliosis type, the (5) arthrochalasia type, and the (6) dermatosparaxis type. Different genetic causes and patterns of inheritance are noted. The skin is oftentimes affected, it can be lax or also very hypermobile. Usually large joints can become hypermobile with most forms of Ehlers-Danlos syndrome. The hypermobility type has the most excessive movement of joints. Many of these joints become dislocated or pop out. Patients will complain of their hips, knees, elbows, and even jaw dislocating oftentimes. Even the cervical spine can dislocate. Patients get quite accustomed to putting their joints back in position themselves.

Many patients with Ehlers-Danlos syndrome have a velvety-type skin that is highly stretchable or elastic. Some types of Ehlers-Danlos syndrome have poor wound healing, largely due to poor peripheral circulation, in part, due to P&S dysfunction. This leaves scars that are the so-called cigarette paper-type scars. Life-threatening rupture of blood vessels can occur in the vascular type of Ehlers-Danlos syndrome. P&S dysfunction is often found in the hypermobility-type Ehlers-Danlos syndromes.

### Question 45: What Symptoms Are Associated with Ehlers-Danlos Syndrome?

**Answer**: Typical symptoms include fast heartbeat or tachycardia, low blood pressure, gastrointestinal (GI) motility problems, bladder problems, and sweating regulation abnormalities. Postural change abnormalities are common in patients, including orthostatic intolerance, orthostatic hypotension, postural orthostatic tachycardia syndrome, or vasovagal syncope.

Some patients with Ehlers-Danlos syndromes excrete an excessive amount of histamine which can cause low blood pressure and tachycardia. Mast cell activation syndromes have been noted in high frequency in some of these patients in studies. It has been postulated that high circulating levels of histamine, causing inflammation and abnormal blood volume changes, may be a mechanism for contributing to cardiovascular dysfunction in patients with Ehlers-Danlos syndrome.

Interestingly, mitral valve prolapse, a disorder of the mitral valve with excessive motion of the valve, has been shown to be associated with excessive catecholamine and orthostatic intolerance syndromes. Literature suggests that it is not very common in patients with Ehlers-Danlos syndrome, but empirically it has been seen in more than 10% of patients (the literature suggests 6%). While screening for mitral valve prolapse in Ehlers-Danlos syndrome is not indicated, if auscultatory (stethoscope) features reveal a murmur or a click or a patient has significant palpitations or chest pain, echocardiographic evaluation is considered. This is especially true if the electrocardiogram is abnormal.

### Question 46: What Autonomic Dysfunction Is Associated with Ehlers-Danlos Syndrome?

**Answer**: The typical symptoms of fast heartbeat or tachycardia, low blood pressure, gastrointestinal (GI) motility problems, bladder problems, and sweating regulation abnormalities are associated with autonomic dysfunction (both branches, P&S). Postural change abnormalities (including orthostatic intolerance, orthostatic hypotension, postural orthostatic tachycardia syndrome (POTS), or vasovagal syncope) are also associated with P&S dysfunction. An overlap has been found between reflex and vagal-dominant autonomic dysfunction and postural orthostatic abnormalities.

To test for P&S dysfunction and differentiate the specific postural change abnormality for the individual patient (e.g., orthostatic hypotension or POTS), a stand test may be ordered. Usually, this should be done for at least 5 minutes or up to 10 minutes. Usually, changes are seen within 3–5 minutes; however, some take longer. The patient should rest supine for 5 minutes before testing to establish a baseline. HR, BP, and P&S measurements are taken during the two postural positions of the stand test.

Individual patients who have autonomic symptoms are recommended to be checked for Ehlers-Danlos syndrome (EDS), especially the hypermobile type. They should be checked by an experienced rheumatologist or orthopedic physician if they have abnormalities of their joints with subluxation, dislocation, or extreme flexibility or double-jointed features.

### Question 47: What Therapies Are Typical for Ehlers-Danlos Syndrome?

**Answer**: P&S dysfunction is treated to address the autonomic imbalances that may underlie the cardiovascular, GI, bladder, sweating, and light-headedness (due to postural change abnormalities) symptoms. Treatment of P&S dysfunction in Ehlers-Danlos syndrome is not different than treatment for the various categories of orthostatic disorders and reflex disorders. The underlying P&S imbalances often exacerbate the pain associated with Ehlers-Danlos syndrome and lead to anxiety and depressive symptoms. As a result, stimulants such as methylphenidate and dextroamphetamine are avoided, especially because there is some incidence of vascular abnormalities in some of these patients.

Understandably, many of these patients have significant disabilities and require neck braces, knee braces, and whole-body braces at times because of significant subluxation (joint dislocations). Anxiety and depression levels can be quite high. Selective serotonin reuptake inhibitors (SSRIs) or serotonin-norepinephrine reuptake inhibitors (SNRIs) are helpful in these patients, especially with orthostatic intolerance and in the setting of coexisting pain and the anxiety and depressive symptoms.

### Question 48: Why Are Diabetics More Susceptible to Neuropathies, Including Peripheral Sensory Neuropathies and Peripheral Autonomic Neuropathies?

**Answer**: When a diabetic develops neuropathy, they are more at risk of heart disease than a diabetic who does not have neuropathy. However, the odds of a diabetic developing neuropathy are very high, and the heart disease is a result of the associated increases in morbidity (the stage known as diabetic autonomic neuropathy or DAN) and mortality risks (the stage known as cardiovascular autonomic neuropathy or CAN), significantly affecting QoL and longevity, respectively.

Regardless of diabetes, any person can develop neuropathy of the sensory nerves which can leave one with a burning sensation, tingling sensation, and pain in the extremities. However, it is more common in diabetics. The reason that neuropathy is more common in diabetics has not been fully elucidated. However, it is believed to significantly involve the effects of sugar acidosis due to excess sugars remaining in the blood stream turning the blood more acid. The more acid the blood the more likely it is to damage tissues, especially the highly fragile P&S nerves. Once the P&S nerves are compromised, blood flow becomes compromised. Compromised blood flow means less blood to the periphery, meaning less oxygen delivered to the periphery. So now, not only are the nerves being damaged by the acid in the blood, there is less oxygen being delivered to support the remaining function. Less oxygen also means a slowing of the repair processes, which are slow enough naturally in nerves.

**Question 49: What Are DAN and CAN?**

**Answer**: DAN is diabetic autonomic neuropathy. It is an indication of increased morbidity risk. It is the diabetic form of advanced autonomic dysfunction (AAD), including the insulin and blood glucose issues. DAN is a serious complication of diabetes. It often leads to cardiovascular autonomic neuropathy (CAN). CAN is an indication of increased mortality risk. CAN is a more severe form of P&S nerve dysfunction than DAN. Both CAN and DAN in diabetics leave patients at a higher risk of having cardiac events such as heart attacks and sudden cardiac death. CAN may be characterized as very high risk. In fact, if a person is found to demonstrate CAN, and they have not recently had a cardiac work-up, then the cardiac work-up is highly recommended as soon as possible. An aggressive approach to diagnosing CAN and treating these patients is highly recommended.

**Question 50: How Might I Know that I May Have DAN or CAN?**

**Answer**: DAN and CAN are painless since they affect the nerves that would let you sense the associated pain or discomfort. So it is difficult to know without P&S testing. This is why P&S testing is recommended shortly after diagnosis. Many people associated the fatigue and malaise with "getting older and slowing down." This may not be the case. Clinical manifestations of DAN and CAN include orthostatic dysfunction. Many times, these patients have orthostatic hypotension. They experience an increase in heart rate, or resting tachycardia, with exercise intolerance. This is a result of the imbalance between the P&S nervous systems, in which P-activity declines faster than S-activity. A lack of P-activity means that the body, including the heart, is not properly protected. A common effect of CAN is silent myocardial ischemia (a lack of blood supply to the heart without chest pain due to a lack of the nerves that enable one to feel the heart attack).

The lack of P-activity may cause GI motility problems, including gastroparesis (a disorder of the stomach in which the weak parasympathetics do not move the stomach contents through the stomach into the intestines at a quick enough rate). This leaves the patient with nausea, vomiting, and early satiety. Constipation or diarrhea can be a manifestation of DAN, as can actual incontinence of stool. Oftentimes, the bladder becomes neurogenic, and this is labeled diabetic cystopathy. Erectile dysfunction and retrograde ejaculation can occur in men. Women may have sexual dysfunction with loss of vaginal lubrication. There is also lack of sweating and heat intolerance which can be associated along with dry skin in diabetics who develop advanced neuropathy, as can any person who develops advanced neuropathy. Gallbladder enlargement and contraction of gallbladder has also been described in patients with DAN.

**Question 51: What Are the Clinical Manifestations of DAN or CAN?**

**Answer**: Microvascular or small vessel blood flow is under the control of the autonomic nervous system (ANS) and is regulated both by the central and peripheral parts of the ANS. In diabetics, the contraction of the small blood vessels is disordered, and microvascular insufficiency results. Therefore, it is believed that a blood flow phenomenon, especially with diabetics who are susceptible to this, could be the potential cause of diabetic neuropathy. Microvascular blood flow can be accurately measured noninvasively in a laboratory utilizing various Doppler techniques. It is important that diabetics have a good blood flow, especially to the skin, since dry skin, loss of sweating, and development of fissures and cracks can lead to infections with microorganisms which can cause cellulitis and eventually even gangrene of the extremities. This is why foot care is extremely important. Interestingly, autonomic neuropathy can also lead to increased activity of osteoclasts, which are cells which can cause reduction in bone density and osteoporosis.

As mentioned, HR response to various maneuvers can be important to determine dysfunction of the ANS. A HR response in deep breathing is an important function of P-activity. Light-headedness due to sympathetic withdrawal is a common, early, clinical manifestation leading to orthostatic dysfunction. HR responses to Valsalva maneuver and stand are influenced by both P&S activity. To assess S-responses, measurements of BP, HR, and P&S activity, and sometimes to sustained hand grip, are used.

The danger with DAN, and especially CAN, is that there may be the inability to get warning signals of when the blood sugar drops, that is, when hypoglycemia occurs. This is an extremely important problem which easily induces silent heart attacks. A physician trained in autonomic assessment can do simple noninvasive tests in the office to determine if there are abnormalities in the P&S nervous systems and to what severity.

## Question 52: In What Areas Has Targeting the Autonomic Nervous System with Therapy Been Most Supported by Research Data and Applied Clinically?

**Answer**: Historically, diabetes is arguably the area that has been most supported by research, the results of which are mentioned in Question 48 through Question 51. Heart failure is another area that has been well targeted. A manipulation of the ANS has been a tremendous breakthrough in heart failure. Major advances in heart failure management have been achieved over the past three decades by targeting two main pathways activated in heart failure, namely, the renin-angiotensin-aldosterone system and the sympathetic nervous system.

It appears that heart failure progresses when the sympathetic nervous system is activated. This sympathetic activation causes myocardial dysfunction and fibrosis. In fact, the current pharmacotherapies are drugs used to treat heart failure by targeting the ANS. For example, beta-blockers and renin-angiotensin system inhibitors reduce morbidity and mortality by targeting aspects of the ANS, specifically those that involve the sympathetic nervous system. Even recently in animal studies, renal sympathetic denervation, which is a non-pharmacological measure, has been shown to protect failing hearts. There is a recent article in the Journal of the American College of Cardiology by Dr. Polhemus and coworkers out of New Orleans that explains how aspects of manipulating the ANS, particularly the sympathetics, are most effective in treating heart failure patients: "Modulation of the Autonomic Nervous System is a treatment for Heart Failure, but has been limited mostly to pharmacological therapies" [1932]. This is the culmination of research that has proven that blunting the sympathetic nervous system, or modulating it, can improve the most advanced forms of heart disease, that is, those patients with heart failure.

For several decades, it has been evident that by blunting the effects of the sympathetic nervous system by various means [24], whether using beta-blockers or in some cases angiotensin receptor blockers (what are labeled ACE inhibitors), heart failure patients improve their heart function and extend their life expectancy. There is recent data that there are other methods that will modulate the ANS in a beneficial way. Recent data has looked at enhancing the parasympathetic nervous system activity in heart patients to afford them a protection from such things as sudden cardiac death and cardiac events.

Autonomic dysfunction, however, can affect other organs besides the heart. It can affect the blood vessels, the brain, the kidneys, the GI tract, the urinary tract, the lungs, and so on. Modulation of the P&S nervous systems is not only beneficial, but it may also be beneficially influenced by the significant ongoing research that is evolving in this area.

The tendency is to treat autonomic dysfunction pharmacologically when feasible and to correct excesses of what is believed to be due to P&S problems or deficiencies. An example of this is the use of midodrine to promote the possible relief in some cases of depression, chronic fatigue, fibromyalgia, and migraine, as examples. However, it is also noted that pharmacological therapies are often insufficient, leaving gaps. In these cases, lifestyle and supplement therapy are also recommended to support the pharmacological therapy and sometimes to "fill the gaps." The lifestyle and supplement recommendations are contained in the Mind-Body Wellness Program.

In summary, therefore, tremendous evidence with diabetes and heart failure and modulating the P&S nervous system by pharmacology which blocks the sympathetic activation has shown the most evidence-based data to date, but data forthcoming with other organ systems is becoming more supportive that the heart is not the only organ benefited by modulating the ANS.

## Mitochondria and Mitochondrial Disorders

### Question 53: What Are Mitochondria?

**Answer**: Mitochondria are small components known as organelles of most cells in the body, the most notable exception being red blood cells. Mitochondria are the power factories of the body. They produce the energy molecule adenosine triphosphate (ATP). The production of energy or ATP is somewhat complex and critical to good health, well-being, and life itself. There are several biochemical cycles in the body which help produce the ATP. One cycle is known as the Krebs or citric acid cycle. The other is the electron transport chain. There are cofactors and enzymes in these biochemical pathways that are crucial for production of the energy molecule ATP. There is also the pyruvate dehydrogenase complex that is a substrate for the transition reaction going into the Krebs cycle. While these types of biochemical terms appear to be quite formidable, what they basically state is that nature has a way of transforming things that are consumed such as sugars, fats, and proteins into the energy molecule going through these pathways. Most of the reactions take place in the mitochondria which are the power factories of the cells.

The biochemical reactions involved with mitochondrial dysfunction are beyond the scope of this question and answer section. However, when mitochondrial damaged ATP production is diminished, energy is diminished, and fatigue is a major factor. The immune system is compromised, and inflammation becomes more widespread in the body. The autonomic (P&S) nervous system is very susceptible to injury when mitochondrial dysfunction occurs as the neurons (nerve cells) are some of the highest consumers of energy in the body.

### Question 54: What Are Mitochondrial Disorders?

**Answer**: Mitochondrial disorders were initially described as genetic disorders that involve ocular and neurological abnormalities from birth. However, it has recently been noted that the mitochondria can become diseased with the aging process and develop acquired myocardial and P&S dysfunction disorders.

As one ages, the mitochondria become smaller in size and less in number. With certain illnesses, mitochondrial number and size can drop dramatically. For example, in chronic fatigue syndrome and fibromyalgia, some researchers have noted very small and decreased numbers of mitochondria.

When mitochondria are diseased or decreased in number, they produce less of the energy molecule of the body known as ATP (adenosine triphosphate). Fewer ATPs mean less fuel (energy) to support nerve, heart, and muscle activities, which causes fatigue and patients tire much more easily. Also, mitochondria are very important in extinguishing free radicals which are actually produced by the mitochondria themselves. (See the "Energy Production" section of this book (Chap. 2), and note that the few free radicals that normal mitochondrial function does produce are used by the immune system to attack and destroy invading bacteria and viruses.)

As mitochondria become dysfunctional, such as in aging or with chronic disease, all body parts and organs are affected. Persistent oxidative stress also destroys mitochondria. Chronic diseases are noted to occur, and this includes slowing of the immune system. Slowing of the immune system could also promote tumorigenesis (cancer).

**Question 55: How Does Mitochondrial Disorder Affect Me?**

**Answer**: Mitochondrial dysfunction affects many organs and may cause chronic fatigue, fibromyalgia, and migraines. It has also been associated with many neurodegenerative disorders such as Friedreich's ataxia, brain ischemia, and spinal cord injury. It also has been linked to Parkinson's disease and various dementias. Mitochondrial dysfunction may be linked to myocardial infarction, atherosclerosis, and diabetes complications. In the liver, one can see abnormalities of liver function and even steatosis, or fatty liver. In the kidneys, one can see glomerulonephritis, ischemic injury, and potentially even renal stones. This is because the mitochondria, when they are damaged and diseased, produce excess free radicals and reactive oxygen species which, if there are not enough antioxidants in the body, can go unopposed to cause more tissue damage.

**Question 56: How Is Mitochondrial Disorder Treated?**

**Answer**: One method of treating mitochondrial dysfunction is to promote a strong antioxidant atmosphere (milieu) throughout the body. Another is to promote an anti-inflammatory milieu throughout the body. A third would be increased nitric oxide throughout the body, especially for anti-atherosclerotic effects. These are some of the goals of the Mind-Body Wellness Program. Many patients with autonomic dysfunction do respond to this cocktail of antioxidants which is also helpful in mitochondrial dysfunction based on the fact that some of these substances are actually seen in the chemical pathways of the Krebs and electron transport chain. Specifically, these substances include alpha-lipoic acid and coenzyme Q10. Other cofactors such as B vitamins, manganese, and magnesium are important. The nitric oxide pathway is also important to preserve, and it is felt that using precursors to nitric oxide such as L-citrulline, L-arginine, and even beet root extract, in which inorganic nitrates go to nitric oxide, is very helpful. Also Omega-3 is found useful in strengthening myelin sheaths and in acting as an anti-inflammatory molecule. An interesting point is that atherosclerosis requires oxidation of LDL molecules to be incorporated into the plaque of atherosclerotic lesions of the artery walls and many of the compounds in the cocktail have antioxidant effects which retard oxidation of LDL particles.

The Mind-Body Wellness Program cocktail regimen has been given to patients in whole or in part as an adjunct to treat certain diseases which may have a basis of mitochondrial dysfunction. There are other such cocktails that one can research in the medical literature that have been proposed to be beneficial also. Individuals are encouraged to research the medical literature to see what supplements and lifestyle modifications are best for them. Typical lifestyle modifications include (1) a healthy diet (the Mediterranean diet is preferred), (2) a healthy exercise program (a minimum of 150 minutes of exercise a week is strongly recommended), and (3) a stress reduction program (exercise or meditation is preferred for stress reduction). Typical supplement programs include anti-inflammatories, antioxidants, and nitric oxide boosting compounds. Many patients on this program have noted a significant increase in energy and diminishing of autonomic dysfunction symptoms when on these regimens, while others have not.

# References


1. Olshansky B, Sabbah HH, Hauptman PJ, Colucci WS. Parasympathetic nervous system and heart failure. Circulation. 2008;118:863–871, originally published August 18, 2008. https://doi.org/10.1161/CIRCULATIONAHA.107.760405.
2. Maser R, Mitchell B, Vinik AI, Freeman R. The association between cardiovascular autonomic neuropathy and mortality in individuals with diabetes, a meta-analysis. Diabetes Care. 2003;26(6):1895–901.
3. Ashar FN, Zhang Y, Longchamps RJ, Lane J, Moes A, Grove ML, Mychaleckyj JC, Taylor KD, Coresh J, Rotter JI, Boerwinkle E, Pankratz N, Guallar E, Arking DE. Association of mitochondrial DNA copy number with cardiovascular disease. JAMA Cardiol. 2017. https://doi.org/10.1001/jamacardio.2017.3683. [Epub ahead of print].
4. Zhang Y, Guallar E, Ashar FN, Longchamps RJ, Castellani CA, Lane J, Grove ML, Coresh J, Sotoodehnia N, Ilkhanoff L, Boerwinkle E, Pankratz N, Arking DE. Association between mitochondrial DNA copy number and sudden cardiac death: findings from the Atherosclerosis Risk in Communities study (ARIC). Eur Heart J. 2017. https://doi.org/10.1093/eurheartj/ehx354. [Epub ahead of print].
5. Adabag AS, Luepker RV, Roger VL, Gersh BJ. Sudden cardiac death: epidemiology and risk factors. Nat Rev Cardiol. 2010;7(4):216–25. https://doi.org/10.1038/nrcardio.2010.3.
6. Boulton AJM, Vinik AI, Arrezzo JC, Bril V, Feldman EI, Freeman R, Malik RA, Maser RE, Sosenko JM, Ziegler D. Diabetic neuropathies: a statement by the American Diabetes Association. Diabetes Care. 2005;28(4):956–62.
7. Berkson B. Alpha lipoic acid breakthrough: the superb antioxidant that may slow aging, repair liver damage, and reduce the risk of cancer, heart disease, and diabetes. New York: Three Rivers Press; 1998.
8. Hargreaves IP. Coenzyme Q10: from fact to fiction. New York: Nova Science Publishing, Inc.; 2015.
9. Ferrier DP. Biochemistry. 6th ed. Philadelphia: Lippincott, Williams & Williams, a Wolters Kluwer Business; 2014.
10. DePace NL, Dowinsky SK, Sherman M. The heart repair manual. New York: WW Norton and Co; 1993.
11. Colombo J, Arora RR, DePace NL, Vinik AI. Clinical autonomic dysfunction: measurement, indications, therapies, and outcomes. New York: Springer Science + Business Media; 2014.
12. Tsuji H, Venditti FJ Jr, Manders ES, Evans JC, Larson MG, Feldman CL, Levy D. Reduced heart rate variability and mortality risk in an elderly cohort. The Framingham Heart Study. Circulation. 1994;90(2):878–83.
13. D'Agostino RB, Vasan RS, Pencina MJ, Wolf PA, Cobain M, Massaro JM, Kannel WB. General cardiovascular risk profile for use in primary care: the Framingham Heart Study. Circulation. 2008;117(6):743–53. https://doi.org/10.1161/CIRCULATIONAHA.107.699579. Epub 2008 Jan 22.
14. DePace NL, Colombo J. Autonomic and mitochondrial dysfunction in clinical diseases: diagnostic, prevention, and therapy. New York: Springer Science + Business Media, (In Press).
15. Vinik A, Ziegler D. Diabetic cardiovascular autonomic neuropathy. Circulation. 2007;115:387–97.
16. Vinik AI, Maser RE, Nakave AA. Diabetic cardiovascular autonomic nerve dysfunction. US Endocr Dis. 2007;2:2–9.
17. Jay SJ. Orthostatic hypotension and chronic fatigue syndrome. JAMA. 2001;285(11):1441–3. https://doi.org/10.1001/jama.285.11.1441.
18. https://my.clevelandclinic.org/health/articles/what-are-mitochondrial-diseases
19. Zhang ZW, Cheng J, Xu F, Chen YE, Du JB, Yuan M, Zhu F, Xu XC, Yuan S. Red blood cell extrudes nucleus and mitochondria against oxidative stress. IUBMB Life. 2011;63(7):560–5. https://doi.org/10.1002/iub.490.
20. Tobias H, Vinitsky A, Bulgarelli RJ, Ghosh-Dastidar S, Colombo J. Autonomic nervous system monitoring of patients with excess parasympathetic responses to sympathetic challenges – clinical observations. US Neurol. 2010;5(2):62–6.
21. Arora RR, Bulgarelli RJ, Ghosh-Dastidar S, Colombo J. Autonomic mechanisms and therapeutic implications of postural diabetic cardiovascular abnormalities. J Diabetes Sci Technol. 2008;2(4):568–71.

22. Nanavati SH, Bulgarelli RJ, Vazquez-Tanus J, Ghosh-Dastidar S, Colombo J, Arora RR. Altered autonomic activity with atrial fibrillation as demonstrated by non-invasive autonomic monitoring. US Cardiol. 2010;7(1):47–50.
23. Vinik AI, Maser RE, Mitchell BD, Freeman R. Diabetic autonomic neuropathy. Diabetes Care. 2003;26(5):1553–79.
24. Curtis BM, O'Keefe JH. Autonomic tone as a cardiovascular risk factor: the dangers of chronic fight or flight. Mayo Clin Proc. 2002;77:45–54.
25. DePace NL, Mears JP, Yayac M, Colombo J. Cardiac autonomic testing and diagnosing heart disease. "A clinical perspective". Heart Int. 2014;9(2):37–44. https://doi.org/10.5301/heartint.5000218; published online 12/5/2014 12:29:58 PM.
26. DePace NL, Mears JP, Yayac M, Colombo J. Cardiac autonomic testing and treating heart disease. "A clinical perspective". Heart Int. 2014;9(2):45–52. https://doi.org/10.5301/heartint.5000216; published online 11/19/2014 1:16:08 PM.
27. Bullinga JR, Alharethi R, Schram MS, Bristow MR, Gilbert EM. Changes in heart rate variability are correlated to hemodynamic improvement with chronic CARVEDILOL therapy in heart failure. J Card Fail. 2005;11(9):693–9.
28. Fatoni C, Raffa S, Regoli F, Giraldi F, La Rovere MT, Prentice J, Pastori F, Fratini S, Salerno-Uriarte JA, Klein HU, Auricchio A. Cardiac resynchronization therapy improves heart rate profile and heart rate variability of patients with moderate to severe heart failure. J Am Coll Cardiol. 2005;46(10):1875–82.
29. Fathizadeh P, Shoemaker WC, Woo CCJ, Colombo J. Autonomic activity in trauma patients based on variability of heart rate and respiratory rate. Crit Care Med. 2004;32(5):1300–5.
30. Chen JY, Fung JW, Yu CM. The mechanisms of atrial fibrillation. J Cardiovasc Electrophysiol. 2006;17(Suppl 3):S2–7.
31. Copie X, Lamaison D, Salvador M, Sadoul N, DaCosta A, Faucher L, Legal F, Le Heuzey JY, VALID Investigators. Heart rate variability before ventricular arrhythmias in patients with coronary artery disease and an implantable cardioverter defibrillator. Ann Noninvasive Electrocardiol. 2003;8(3):179–84.
32. Alter P, Grimm W, Vollrath A, Czerny F, Maisch B. Heart rate variability in patients with cardiac hypertrophy – relation to left ventricular mass and etiology. Am Heart J. 2006;151(4):829–36.
33. Debono M, Cachia E. The impact of cardiovascular autonomic neuropathy in diabetes: is it associated with left ventricular dysfunction? Auton Neurosci. 2007;132(1–2):1–7.
34. Just H. Peripheral adaptations in congestive heart failure: a review. Am J Med. 1991;90:23S–6S.
35. Nakamura K, Matsumura K, Kobayashi S, Kaneko T. Sympathetic premotor neurons mediating thermoregulatory functions. Neurosci Res. 2005;51(1):1–8.
36. Manfrini O, Morgagni G, Pizzi C, Fontana F, Bugiardini R. Changes in autonomic nervous system activity: spontaneous versus balloon-induced myocardial ischemia. Eur Heart J. 2004;25(17):1502–8.
37. Clarke B, Ewing D, Campbell I. Diabetic autonomic neuropathy. Diabetologia. 1979;17:195–212.
38. Litchman JH, Bigger JT Jr, Blumenthal JA, et al. Depression and coronary heart disease recommendations for screening, referral, and treatment: a science advisory from the American Heart Association Prevention Committee of the Council on Cardiovascular Nursing, Council on Clinical Cardiology, Council on Epidemiology and Prevention, and Interdisciplinary Council on Quality of Care and Outcomes Research: endorsed by the American Psychiatric Association. Circulation. 2008;118:1768–75.
39. Murphy MP. How mitochondria produce reactive oxygen species. Biochem J. 2009;417:1–13 (Printed in Great Britain). https://doi.org/10.1042/BJ20081386.
40. National Institute of Standards and Technology.
41. Novo E, Parola M. Redox mechanisms in hepatic chronic wound healing and fibrogenesis. Fibrogenesis Tissue Repair. 2008;1:5; 1–58. http://www.fibrogenesis.com/content/1/1/5
42. Gerschman R, Gilbert DL, Nye SW, Dwyer P, Fenn WO. Oxygen poisoning and X-irradiation: a mechanism in common. Science. 1954;119:623–6.
43. Gerschman R, Gilbert DL, Nye SW, Fenn WO. Influence of x-irradiation on oxygen poisoning in mice. Proc Soc Exp Biol Med. 1954;86(1):27–9.
44. Halliwell B, Gutteridge JMC. Free radicals in biology and medicine. 4th ed. Oxford: Oxford University Press; 2007.
45. Finkel T, Holbrook NJ. Oxidants, oxidative stress and the biology of aging. Nature. 2000;408:239–47.
46. Dickinson BC, Chang CJ. Chemistry and biology of reactive oxygen species in signaling or stress responses. Nat Chem Biol. 2011;7(8):504–11.
47. Dröge W. Free radicals in the physiological control of cell function. Physiol Rev. 2002;82(1):47–95.
48. Barnham KJ, Masters CL, Bush AI. Neurodegenerative diseases and oxidative stress. Nat Rev Drug Discov. 2004;3(3):205–14.
49. Finkel T, Serrano M, Blasco MA. The common biology of cancer and aging. Nature. 2007;448(7155):767–74.
50. Harman D. Aging: a theory based on free radical and radiation chemistry. J Gerontol. 1956;11(3):298–300.
51. Harman D. Free radical theory of aging. Mutat Res, DNAging. 1992;275:257–66.
52. Apel K, Hirt H. Reactive oxygen species: metabolism, oxidative stress, and signal transduction. Annu Rev Plant Biol. 2004;55:373–99.
53. Rhee SG. Cell signaling. H2O2, a necessary evil for cell signaling. Science. 2006;312(5782):1882–3.
54. Kagan VE, Quinn PJ. Toward oxidative lipidomics of cell signaling. Antioxid Redox Signal. 2004;6(2):199–202.
55. West JD, Marnett LJ. Endogenous reactive intermediates as modulators of cell signaling and cell death. Chem Res Toxicol. 2006;19(2):173–94.
56. Krumova K, Cosa G. Overview of reactive oxygen species. In: Nonell S, Flors C, editors. Singlet

oxygen: applications in biosciences and nanosciences, vol. 1. Cambridge: RSC Publishing; 2016. http://pubs.rsc.org/en/content/chapterhtml/2016/bk9781782620389-00001?isbn=978-1-78262-038-9.
57. Nathan C, Cunningham-Bussel A. Beyond oxidative stress: an immunologist's guide to reactive oxygen species. Nat Rev Immunol. 2013;13(3):349–61.
58. Nathan C, Ding A. SnapShot: reactive oxygen intermediates (ROI). Cell. 2010;140(6):951.
59. Yin H, Xu L, Porter NA. Free radical lipid peroxidation: mechanisms and analysis. Chem Rev. 2011;111(10):5944–72.
60. D'Autreaux B, Toledano MB. ROS as signaling molecules: mechanisms that generate specificity in ROS homeostasis. Nat Rev Mol Cell Biol. 2007;8(10):813–24.
61. Nishii W, Kukimoto-Niino M, Terada T, Shirouzu M, Muramatsu T, Kojima M, Kihara H, Yokoyama S. A redox switch shapes the Lon protease exit pore to facultatively regulate proteolysis. Nat Chem Biol. 2015;11(1):46–51.
62. Finkel T, Holbrook NJ. Oxidants, oxidative stress and the biology of aging. Nature. 2000;408(6809):239–47.
63. Stadtman ER. Protein oxidation and aging. Free Radic Res. 2006;40(12):1250–8.
64. Niki E, Noguchi N. Dynamics of antioxidant action of vitamin E. Acc Chem Res. 2004;37(1):45–51.
65. Cardinali DP. Autonomic nervous system: basic and clinical aspects. Cham: Springer International Publishing AG; 2018.
66. Menotti A, Keys A, Blackburn H, Kromhout D, Karvonen M, Nissinen A, Pekkanen J, Punsar S, Fidanza F, Giampaoli S, Seccareccia F, Buzina R, Mohacek I, Nedeljkovic S, Aravanis C, Dontas A, Toshima H, Lanti M. Comparison of multivariate predictive power of major risk factors for coronary heart diseases in different countries: results from eight nations of the Seven Countries Study, 25-year follow-up. J Cardiovasc Risk. 1996;3(1):69–75.
67. Menotti A, Seccareccia F, Blackburn H, Keys A. Coronary mortality and its prediction in samples of US and Italian railroad employees in 25 years within the Seven Countries Study of cardiovascular diseases. Int J Epidemiol. 1995;24(3):515–21.
68. Toshima H, Koga Y, Menotti A, Keys A, Blackburn H, Jacobs DR, Seccareccia F. The Seven Countries Study in Japan. Twenty-five-year experience in cardiovascular and all-causes deaths. Jpn Heart J. 1995;36(2):179–89.
69. Kostka T, Drai J, Berthouze SE, Lacour JR, Bonnefoy M. Physical activity, aerobic capacity and selected markers of oxidative stress and the anti-oxidant defense system in healthy active elderly men. Clin Physiol. 2000;20(3):185–90.
70. Santos-Parker JR, LaRocca TJ, Seals DR. Aerobic exercise and other healthy lifestyle factors that influence vascular aging. Adv Physiol Educ. 2014;38(4):296–307. https://doi.org/10.1152/advan.00088.2014.
71. Seals DR, Edward F. Adolph Distinguished Lecture: the remarkable anti-aging effects of aerobic exercise on systemic arteries. J Appl Physiol. 2014;117(5):425–39. https://doi.org/10.1152/japplphysiol.00362.2014.
72. Rosengren A, Hawken S, Ounpuu S, Sliwa K, Zubaid M, Almahmeed WA, Blackett KN, Sitthi-amorn C, Sato H, Yusuf S, INTERHEART investigators. Association of psychosocial risk factors with risk of acute myocardial infarction in 11119 cases and 13648 controls from 52 countries (the INTERHEART study): case-control study. Lancet. 2004;364(9438):953–62.
73. David JKS, DePace N, Noval J, Reichie FA. Cholesterol lowering mechanism of fish oil rich in ω-3 fatty acids in cardiac patients. Arteriosclerosis. 1987;7(5):512A.
74. Crawford MH, DiMarco JP, editors. Cardiology. London: Mosby; 2001.
75. Chen M, Nagase M, Fujita T, Narumiya S, Masaki T, Sawamura T. Diabetes enhances lectin-like oxidized LDL receptor-1 (LOX-1) expression in the vascular endothelium: possible role of LOX-1 ligand and AGALE. Biophys Res Commun. 2001;287:962–8.
76. Pothineni NVK, Karathanasis SK, Ding Z, Arulandu A, Varughese KI, Mehta JL. LOX-1 in atherosclerosis and myocardial ischemia: biology, genetics, and modulation. J Am Coll Cardiol. 2017;69(22):2759–68. https://doi.org/10.1016/j.jacc.2017.04.010. Review.
77. Deanfield JE, Halcox JP, Rabelink TJ. Endothelial function and dysfunction: testing and clinical relevance. Circulation. 2007;115(10):1285–95. Review.
78. Ding Z, et al. Mitochondrial DNA damage in NLRP-3 inflammation activation and macrophages implication in atherogenesis. Cardiovasc Res. 2014;103:619–28.
79. Marwali MR, Hu CP, Mohandas B, Dandapat A, Deonikar P, Chen J, Cawich I, Sawamura T, Kavdia M, Mehta JL. Modulation of ADP-induced platelet activation by aspirin and pravastatin: role of lectin-like oxidized low-density lipoprotein receptor-1, nitric oxide, oxidative stress, and inside-out integrin signaling. J Pharmacol Exp Ther. 2007;322(3):1324–32. Epub 2007 May 30.
80. Niwa Y, Iwai N. Nanomaterials induce oxidized low-density lipoprotein cellular uptake in macrophages and platelet aggregation. Circ J. 2007;71(3):437–44.
81. Hayashida K, et al. Serum soluble lectin-like oxidized low-density lipoprotein receptor-1 levels are elevated in acute coronary syndrome, a novel marker for early diagnosis. Circulation. 2005;112:812–8.
82. Besler C, et al. Mechanisms underlying adverse effects of HDL on eNOS-activating pathways in patients with coronary artery disease. J Clin Invest. 2011;121:2693–708.
83. Mehta JL. Aspirin inhibits oxidized LDL-mediated LOX-1 expression and metalloproteinase- 1 in human coronary endothelial cells. Cardiovasc Res. 2004;64(2):243–9.
84. Oz HS. Chronic inflammatory diseases and green tea polyphenols. Nutrients. 2017;9(6). pii: E561. https://doi.org/10.3390/nu9060561.
85. Kohli P, Levy BD. Resolvins and protectins: mediating solutions to inflammation. Br J Pharmacol. 2009;158(4):960–71. https://doi.org/10.1111/j.1476-5381.2009.00290.x.

86. Chandrasekharan JA, Sharma-Walia N. Lipoxins: nature's way to resolve inflammation. J Inflamm Res. 2015;8:181–92. Published online 2015 Sep 30. https://doi.org/10.2147/JIR.S90380.
87. Serhan CN, Yang R, Martinod K, Kasuga K, Pillai PS, Porter TF, Oh SF, Spite M. Maresins: novel macrophage mediators with potent anti-inflammatory and pro-resolving actions. J Exp Med. 2009;206(1):15–23. https://doi.org/10.1084/jem.20081880.
88. Ridker PM, Everett BM, Thuren T, MacFadyen JG, Chang WH, Ballantyne C, Fonseca F, Nicolau J, Koenig W, Anker SD, Kastelein JJP, Cornel JH, Pais P, Pella D, Genest J, Cifkova R, Lorenzatti A, Forster T, Kobalava Z, Vida-Simiti L, Flather M, Shimokawa H, Ogawa H, Dellborg M, Rossi PRF, Troquay RPT, Libby P, Glynn RJ, CANTOS Trial Group. Anti-inflammatory therapy with canakinumab for atherosclerotic disease. N Engl J Med. 2017;377(12):1119–31. https://doi.org/10.1056/NEJMoa1707914. Epub 2017 Aug 27.
89. Hu PJ, Pittet JF, Kerby JD, Bosarge PL, Wagener BM. Acute brain trauma, lung injury and pneumonia: more than just altered mental status and decreased airway protection. Am J Physiol Lung Cell Mol Physiol. 2017. https://doi.org/10.1152/ajplung.00485.2016. [Epub ahead of print].
90. Kromhout D, Bosschieter EB, de Lezenne Coulander C. The inverse relation between fish consumption and 20-year mortality from coronary heart disease. N Engl J Med. 1985;312(19):1205–9.
91. Kenny D, Warltier DC, Pleuss JA, Hoffmann RG, Goodfriend TL, Egan BM. Effect of omega-3 fatty acids on the vascular response to angiotensin in normotensive men. Am J Cardiol. 1992;70(15):1347–52.
92. Chin JP, Gust AP, Nestel PJ, Dart AM. Marine oils dose-dependently inhibit vasoconstriction of forearm resistance vessels in humans. Hypertension. 1993;21(1):22–8.
93. Bjerregaard P, Mulvad G, Pedersen HS. Cardiovascular risk factors in Inuit of Greenland. Int J Epidemiol. 1997;26(6):1182–90.
94. Nordøy A. Fish consumption and cardiovascular diseases. Eur Heart J Suppl. 2001;3(Suppl D):D4–7.
95. Leaf A, Kang JX, Xiao YF, Billman GE. Clinical prevention of sudden death by n-3 polyunsaturated fatty acids and mechanism of prevention of arrhythmias by n-3 fish oils. Circulation. 2003;107(21):2646–52. Review.
96. Kris-Etherton PM, Harris WS, Appel LJ, American Heart Association. Nutrition Committee. Fish consumption, fish oil, omega-3 fatty acids, and cardiovascular disease. Circulation. 2002;106(21):2747–57. No abstract available. Erratum in: Circulation. 2003 Jan 28;107(3):512.
97. Wang C, Harris WS, Chung M, Lichtenstein AH, Balk EM, Kupelnick B, Jordan HS, Lau J. n-3 Fatty acids from fish or fish-oil supplements, but not alpha-linolenic acid, benefit cardiovascular disease outcomes in primary- and secondary-prevention studies: a systematic review. Am J Clin Nutr. 2006;84(1):5–17. Review.
98. Chrysohoou C, Panagiotakos DB, Pitsavos C, Skoumas J, Krinos X, Chloptsios Y, Nikolaou V, Stefanadis C. Long-term fish consumption is associated with protection against arrhythmia in healthy persons in a Mediterranean region – the ATTICA study. Am J Clin Nutr. 2007;85(5):1385–91.
99. Mozaffarian D, Rimm EB. Fish intake, contaminants, and human health: evaluating the risks and the benefits. JAMA. 2006;296(15):1885–99. Review. Erratum in: JAMA. 2007 Feb 14;297(6):590.
100. O'Keefe JH Jr, Abuissa H, Sastre A, Steinhaus DM, Harris WS. Effects of omega-3 fatty acids on resting heart rate, heart rate recovery after exercise, and heart rate variability in men with healed myocardial infarctions and depressed ejection fractions. Am J Cardiol. 2006;97(8):1127–30. Epub 2006 Mar 3.
101. von Schacky C, Harris WS. Cardiovascular benefits of omega-3 fatty acids. Cardiovasc Res. 2007;73(2):310–5. Epub 2006 Sept 1. Review.
102. Artham SM, Lavie CJ, Milani RV, Anand RG, O'Keefe JH, Ventura HO. Fish oil in primary and secondary cardiovascular prevention. Ochsner J. 2008;8(2):49–60.
103. Weitz D, Weintraub H, Fisher E, Schwartzbard AZ. Fish oil for the treatment of cardiovascular disease. Cardiol Rev. 2010;18(5):258–63. https://doi.org/10.1097/CRD.0b013e3181ea0de0. Review.
104. Kromhout D, Yasuda S, Geleijnse JM, Shimokawa H. Fish oil and omega-3 fatty acids in cardiovascular disease: do they really work? Eur Heart J. 2012;33(4):436–43. https://doi.org/10.1093/eurheartj/ehr362. Epub 2011 Sept 19. Review.
105. Moertl D, Hammer A, Steiner S, Hutuleac R, Vonbank K, Berger R. Dose-dependent effects of omega-3-polyunsaturated fatty acids on systolic left ventricular function, endothelial function, and markers of inflammation in chronic heart failure of nonischemic origin: a double-blind, placebo-controlled, 3-arm study. Am Heart J. 2011;161(5):915.e1–9. https://doi.org/10.1016/j.ahj.2011.02.011.
106. Albert CM. Omega-3 fatty acids, ventricular arrhythmias, and sudden cardiac death: antiarrhythmic, proarrhythmic, or neither. Circ Arrhythm Electrophysiol. 2012;5(3):456–9. https://doi.org/10.1161/CIRCEP.112.971416.
107. Güttler N, Zheleva K, Parahuleva M, Chasan R, Bilgin M, Neuhof C, Burgazli M, Niemann B, Erdogan A, Böning A. Omega-3 fatty acids and vitamin d in cardiology. Cardiol Res Pract. 2012, Article ID: 729670, 11 pages. https://doi.org/10.1155/2012/729670. Epub 2012 Dec 31.
108. Kotwal S1, Jun M, Sullivan D, Perkovic V, Neal B. Omega 3 fatty acids and cardiovascular outcomes: systematic review and meta-analysis. Circ Cardiovasc Qual Outcomes. 2012;5(6):808–18. https://doi.org/10.1161/CIRCOUTCOMES.112.966168. Epub 2012 Oct 30.
109. Kwak SM, Myung SK, Lee YJ, Seo HG, Korean Meta-analysis Study Group. Efficacy of omega-3 fatty acid supplements (eicosapentaenoic acid and

docosahexaenoic acid) in the secondary prevention of cardiovascular disease: a meta-analysis of randomized, double-blind, placebo-controlled trials. Arch Intern Med. 2012;172(9):686–94. https://doi.org/10.1001/archinternmed.2012.262. Review.

110. Rizos EC, Ntzani EE, Bika E, Kostapanos MS, Elisaf MS. Association between omega-3 fatty acid supplementation and risk of major cardiovascular disease events: a systematic review and meta-analysis. JAMA. 2012;308(10):1024–33. https://doi.org/10.1001/2012.jama.11374. Review.
111. Ohnishi H, Saito Y. Eicosapentaenoic acid (EPA) reduces cardiovascular events: relationship with the EPA/arachidonic acid ratio. J Atheroscler Thromb. 2013;20(12):861–77. Epub 2013 Sept 18. Review.
112. Casula M, Soranna D, Catapano AL, Corrao G. Long-term effect of high dose omega-3 fatty acid supplementation for secondary prevention of cardiovascular outcomes: a meta-analysis of randomized, placebo controlled trials [corrected]. Atheroscler Suppl. 2013;14(2):243–51. https://doi.org/10.1016/S1567-5688(13)70005-9. Review. Erratum in: Atheroscler Suppl. 2014 Mar;233(1):122.
113. Nosaka K, Miyoshi T, Iwamoto M, Kajiya M, Okawa K, Tsukuda S, Yokohama F, Sogo M, Nishibe T, Matsuo N, Hirohata S, Ito H, Doi M. Early initiation of eicosapentaenoic acid and statin treatment is associated with better clinical outcomes than statin alone in patients with acute coronary syndromes: 1-year outcomes of a randomized controlled study. Int J Cardiol. 2017;228:173–9. https://doi.org/10.1016/j.ijcard.2016.11.105. Epub 2016 Nov 9.
114. Watanabe Y, Tatsuno I. Omega-3 polyunsaturated fatty acids for cardiovascular diseases: present, past and future. Expert Rev Clin Pharmacol. 2017;29:1–9. https://doi.org/10.1080/17512433.2017.1333902. [Epub ahead of print].
115. Siscovick DS, Barringer TA, Fretts AM, Wu JH, Lichtenstein AH, Costello RB, Kris-Etherton PM, Jacobson TA, Engler MB, Alger HM, Appel LJ, Mozaffarian D, American Heart Association Nutrition Committee of the Council on Lifestyle and Cardiometabolic Health; Council on Epidemiology and Prevention; Council on Cardiovascular Disease in the Young; Council on Cardiovascular and Stroke Nursing; and Council on Clinical Cardiology. Omega-3 polyunsaturated fatty acid (fish oil) supplementation and the prevention of clinical cardiovascular disease: a science advisory from the American Heart Association. Circulation. 2017;135(15):e867–84. https://doi.org/10.1161/CIR.0000000000000482. Epub 2017 Mar 13. Review.
116. Bjerregaard P, Pedersen HS, Mulvad G. The associations of a marine diet with plasma lipids, blood glucose, blood pressure and obesity among the inuit in Greenland. Eur J Clin Nutr. 2000;54(9):732–7.
117. Yamagishi K, Iso H, Date C, Fukui M, Wakai K, Kikuchi S, Inaba Y, Tanabe N, Tamakoshi A, Japan Collaborative Cohort Study for Evaluation of Cancer Risk Study Group. Fish, omega-3 polyunsaturated fatty acids, and mortality from cardiovascular diseases in a nationwide community-based cohort of Japanese men and women the JACC (Japan Collaborative Cohort Study for evaluation of cancer risk) study. J Am Coll Cardiol. 2008;52(12):988–96. https://doi.org/10.1016/j.jacc.2008.06.018.
118. Nakamura Y, Hozawa A, Turin TC, Takashima N, Okamura T, Hayakawa T, Kita Y, Okayama A, Miura K, Ueshima H, NIPPON DATA80 Research Group. Dietary habits in middle age and future changes in activities of daily living – NIPPON DATA80. Gerontology. 2009;55(6):707–13. https://doi.org/10.1159/000235906. Epub 2009 Aug 28.
119. Hirai Y, Geleijnse JM, Adachi H, Imaizumi T, Kromhout D. Systolic blood pressure predicts cardiovascular mortality in farming but not in a fishing community. -A 40-year follow up of the Japanese cohorts of the Seven Countries Study. Circ J. 2011;75(8):1890–6. Epub 2011 Jun 15.
120. Eguchi E, Iso H, Tanabe N, Wada Y, Yatsuya H, Kikuchi S, Inaba Y, Tamakoshi A, Japan Collaborative Cohort Study Group. Healthy lifestyle behaviors and cardiovascular mortality among Japanese men and women: the Japan Collaborative Cohort Study. Eur Heart J. 2012;33(4):467–77. https://doi.org/10.1093/eurheartj/ehr429.
121. Tsugane S, Sawada N. The JPHC study: design and some findings on the typical Japanese diet. Jpn J Clin Oncol. 2014;44(9):777–82. https://doi.org/10.1093/jjco/hyu096. Epub 2014 Aug 7.
122. Nakamura Y, Okuda N, Okamura T, Kadota A, Miyagawa N, Hayakawa T, Kita Y, Fujiyoshi A, Nagai M, Takashima N, Ohkubo T, Miura K, Okayama A, Ueshima H, NIPPON DATA Research Group. Low-carbohydrate diets and cardiovascular and total mortality in Japanese: a 29-year follow-up of NIPPON DATA80. Br J Nutr. 2014;112(6):916–24. https://doi.org/10.1017/S0007114514001627.
123. Menotti A, Puddu PE. How the Seven Countries Study contributed to the definition and development of the Mediterranean diet concept: a 50-year journey. Nutr Metab Cardiovasc Dis. 2015;25(3):245–52. https://doi.org/10.1016/j.numecd.2014.12.001. Epub 2014 Dec 12.
124. Nanri A, Mizoue T, Shimazu T, Ishihara J, Takachi R, Noda M, Iso H, Sasazuki S, Sawada N, Tsugane S, Japan Public Health Center-Based Prospective Study Group. Dietary patterns and all-cause, cancer, and cardiovascular disease mortality in Japanese men and women: the Japan public health center-based prospective study. PLoS One. 2017;12(4):e0174848. https://doi.org/10.1371/journal.pone.0174848. eCollection 2017.
125. Oomen CM, Feskens EJ, Räsänen L, Fidanza F, Nissinen AM, Menotti A, Kok FJ, Kromhout D. Fish consumption and coronary heart disease mortality in Finland, Italy, and The Netherlands. Am J Epidemiol. 2000;151(10):999–1006.

126. Oomen CM, Ocké MC, Feskens EJ, van Erp-Baart MA, Kok FJ, Kromhout D. Association between trans fatty acid intake and 10-year risk of coronary heart disease in the Zutphen Elderly Study: a prospective population-based study. Lancet. 2001;357(9258):746–51.
127. Streppel MT, Ocké MC, Boshuizen HC, Kok FJ, Kromhout D. Long-term fish consumption and n-3 fatty acid intake in relation to (sudden) coronary heart disease death: the Zutphen study. Eur Heart J. 2008;29(16):2024–30. https://doi.org/10.1093/eurheartj/ehn294. Epub 2008 Jul 18.
128. Keli SO, Feskens EJ, Kromhout D. Fish consumption and risk of stroke. The Zutphen Study. Stroke. 1994;25(2):328–32.
129. Woodside JV, Kromhout D. Fatty acids and CHD. Proc Nutr Soc. 2005;64(4):554–64.
130. Alexander DD, Miller PE, Van Elswyk ME, Kuratko CN, Bylsma LC. A meta-analysis of randomized controlled trials and prospective cohort studies of eicosapentaenoic and docosahexaenoic long-chain omega-3 fatty acids and coronary heart disease risk. Mayo Clin Proc. 2017;92(1):15–29. https://doi.org/10.1016/j.mayocp.2016.10.018. Review.
131. Gorder DD, Dolecek TA, Coleman GG, Tillotson JL, Brown HB, Lenz-Litzow K, Bartsch GE, Grandits G. Dietary intake in the Multiple Risk Factor Intervention Trial (MRFIT): nutrient and food group changes over 6 years. J Am Diet Assoc. 1986;86(6):744–51.
132. Miura K, Greenland P, Stamler J, Liu K, Daviglus ML, Nakagawa H. Relation of vegetable, fruit, and meat intake to 7-year blood pressure change in middle-aged men: the Chicago Western Electric Study. Am J Epidemiol. 2004;159(6):572–80.
133. Daviglus ML, Stamler J, Orencia AJ, Dyer AR, Liu K, Greenland P, Walsh MK, Morris D, Shekelle RB. Fish consumption and the 30-year risk of fatal myocardial infarction. N Engl J Med. 1997;336(15):1046–53.
134. Orencia AJ, Daviglus ML, Dyer AR, Shekelle RB, Stamler J. Fish consumption and stroke in men. 30-year findings of the Chicago Western Electric Study. Stroke. 1996;27(2):204–9.
135. Liu XQ, Li YH. Epidemiological and nutritional research on prevention of cardiovascular disease in China. Br J Nutr. 2000;84(Suppl 2):S199–203.
136. Hunter DJ, Kazda I, Chockalingam A, Fodor JG. Fish consumption and cardiovascular mortality in Canada: an inter-regional comparison. Am J Prev Med. 1988;4(1):5–10.
137. McLaughlin J, Middaugh J, Boudreau D, Malcom G, Parry S, Tracy R, Newman W. Adipose tissue triglyceride fatty acids and atherosclerosis in Alaska Natives and non-Natives. Atherosclerosis. 2005;181(2):353–62.
138. Shay CM, Stamler J, Dyer AR, Brown IJ, Chan Q, Elliott P, Zhao L, Okuda N, Miura K, Daviglus ML, Van Horn L. Nutrient and food intakes of middle-aged adults at low risk of cardiovascular disease: the international study of macro-/micronutrients and blood pressure (INTERMAP). Eur J Nutr. 2012;51(8):917–26. https://doi.org/10.1007/s00394-011-0268-2. Epub 2011 Nov 6.
139. Menotti A, Puddu PE. How the Seven Countries Study contributed to the definition and development of the Mediterranean diet concept: a 50-year journey. Nutr Metab Cardiovasc Dis. 2015;25(3):245–52. https://doi.org/10.1016/j.numecd.2014.12.001. Epub 2014 Dec 12.
140. McVeigh GE, Brennan GM, Johnston GD, McDermott BJ, McGrath LT, Henry WR, Andrews JW, Hayes JR. Dietary fish oil augments nitric oxide production or release in patients with type 2 (non-insulin-dependent) diabetes mellitus. Diabetologia. 1993;36(1):33–8.
141. Rossi E, Costa M. Fish oil derivatives as a prophylaxis of recurrent miscarriage associated with antiphospholipid antibodies (APL): a pilot study. Lupus. 1993;2(5):319–23.
142. Belluzzi A, Brignola C, Campieri M, Pera A, Boschi S, Miglioli M. Effect of an enteric-coated fish-oil preparation on relapses in Crohn's disease. N Engl J Med. 1996;334(24):1557–60.
143. Teitelbaum JE, Allan Walker W. Review: the role of omega 3 fatty acids in intestinal inflammation. J Nutr Biochem. 2001;12(1):21–32.
144. Nemets B, Stahl Z, Belmaker RH. Addition of omega-3 fatty acid to maintenance medication treatment for recurrent unipolar depressive disorder. Am J Psychiatry. 2002;159(3):477–9.
145. MacLean CH, Newberry SJ, Mojica WA, Khanna P, Issa AM, Suttorp MJ, Lim YW, Traina SB, Hilton L, Garland R, Morton SC. Effects of omega-3 fatty acids on cancer risk: a systematic review. JAMA. 2006;295(4):403–15. Review. Erratum in: JAMA. 2006 Apr 26;295(16):1900.
146. Reisman J, Schachter HM, Dales RE, Tran K, Kourad K, Barnes D, Sampson M, Morrison A, Gaboury I, Blackman J. Treating asthma with omega-3 fatty acids: where is the evidence? A systematic review. BMC Complement Altern Med. 2006;6:26. Review.
147. Mita T, Watada H, Ogihara T, Nomiyama T, Ogawa O, Kinoshita J, Shimizu T, Hirose T, Tanaka Y, Kawamori R. Eicosapentaenoic acid reduces the progression of carotid intima-media thickness in patients with type 2 diabetes. Atherosclerosis. 2007;191(1):162–7. Epub 2006 Apr 17.
148. Brunborg LA, Madland TM, Lind RA, Arslan G, Berstad A, Frøyland L. Effects of short-term oral administration of dietary marine oils in patients with inflammatory bowel disease and joint pain: a pilot study comparing seal oil and cod liver oil. Clin Nutr. 2008;27(4):614–22. https://doi.org/10.1016/j.clnu.2008.01.017. Epub 2008 Apr 18.
149. Caughey GE, James MJ, Proudman SM, Cleland LG. Fish oil supplementation increases the cyclooxygenase inhibitory activity of paracetamol in rheumatoid arthritis patients. Complement Ther Med.

2010;18(3–4):171–4. https://doi.org/10.1016/j.ctim.2010.05.032.

150. Gogus U, Smith C. n-3 Omega fatty acids: a review of current knowledge. Int J Food Sci Technol. 2010;45:417–36. Review.
151. Huang TL. Omega-3 fatty acids, cognitive decline, and Alzheimer's disease: a critical review and evaluation of the literature. J Alzheimers Dis. 2010;21(3):673–90. https://doi.org/10.3233/JAD-2010-090934. Review.
152. Masterton GS, Plevris JN, Hayes PC. Review article: omega-3 fatty acids – a promising novel therapy for non-alcoholic fatty liver disease. Aliment Pharmacol Ther. 2010;31(7):679–92. https://doi.org/10.1111/j.1365-2036.2010.04230.x. Review.
153. Naqvi AZ, Buettner C, Phillips RS, Davis RB, Mukamal KJ. n-3 fatty acids and periodontitis in US adults. J Am Diet Assoc. 2010;110(11):1669–75. https://doi.org/10.1016/j.jada.2010.08.009.
154. Aghdassi E, Ma DW, Morrison S, Hillyer LM, Clarke S, Gladman DD, Urowitz MB, Fortin PR. Alterations in circulating fatty acid composition in patients with systemic lupus erythematosus: a pilot study. JPEN J Parenter Enteral Nutr. 2011;35(2):198–208. https://doi.org/10.1177/0148607110386378.
155. Bloch MH, Qawasmi A. Omega-3 fatty acid supplementation for the treatment of children with attention-deficit/hyperactivity disorder symptomatology: systematic review and meta-analysis. J Am Acad Child Adolesc Psychiatry. 2011;50(10):991–1000. https://doi.org/10.1016/j.jaac.2011.06.008. Epub 2011 Aug 12. Review.
156. Kiecolt-Glaser JK, Belury MA, Andridge R, Malarkey WB, Glaser R. Omega-3 supplementation lowers inflammation and anxiety in medical students: a randomized controlled trial. Brain Behav Immun. 2011;25(8):1725–34. https://doi.org/10.1016/j.bbi.2011.07.229. Epub 2011 Jul 19.
157. Sublette ME, Ellis SP, Geant AL, Mann JJ. Meta-analysis of the effects of eicosapentaenoic acid (EPA) in clinical trials in depression. J Clin Psychiatry. 2011;72(12):1577–84. https://doi.org/10.4088/JCP.10m06634. Epub 2011 Sept 6.
158. Swanson D, Block R, Mousa SA. Omega-3 fatty acids EPA and DHA: health benefits throughout life. Adv Nutr. 2012;3(1):1–7. https://doi.org/10.3945/an.111.000893. Epub 2012 Jan 5.
159. Wu JH, Micha R, Imamura F, Pan A, Biggs ML, Ajaz O, Djousse L, Hu FB, Mozaffarian D. Omega-3 fatty acids and incident type 2 diabetes: a systematic review and meta-analysis. Br J Nutr. 2012;107(Suppl 2):S214–27. https://doi.org/10.1017/S0007114512001602. Review.
160. Desbois AP, Lawlor KC. Antibacterial activity of long-chain polyunsaturated fatty acids against Propionibacterium acnes and Staphylococcus aureus. Mar Drugs. 2013;11(11):4544–57. https://doi.org/10.3390/md11114544.
161. Robinson LE, Mazurak VC. N-3 polyunsaturated fatty acids: relationship to inflammation in healthy adults and adults exhibiting features of metabolic syndrome. Lipids. 2013;48(4):319–32. https://doi.org/10.1007/s11745-013-3774-6. Epub 2013 Mar 1. Review.
162. Skilton MR, Mikkilä V, Würtz P, Ala-Korpela M, Sim KA, Soininen P, Kangas AJ, Viikari JS, Juonala M, Laitinen T, Lehtimäki T, Taittonen L, Kähönen M, Celermajer DS, Raitakari OT. Fetal growth, omega-3 (n-3) fatty acids, and progression of subclinical atherosclerosis: preventing fetal origins of disease? The Cardiovascular Risk in Young Finns Study. Am J Clin Nutr. 2013;97(1):58–65. https://doi.org/10.3945/ajcn.112.044198. Epub 2012 Nov 14.
163. Bauer I, Hughes M, Rowsell R, Cockerell R, Pipingas A, Crewther S, Crewther D. Omega-3 supplementation improves cognition and modifies brain activation in young adults. Hum Psychopharmacol. 2014;29(2):133–44.
164. Hawkey E, Nigg JT. Omega-3 fatty acid and ADHD: blood level analysis and meta-analytic extension of supplementation trials. Clin Psychol Rev. 2014;34(6):496–505. https://doi.org/10.1016/j.cpr.2014.05.005. Epub 2014 Jun 2.
165. Pappalardo G, Almeida A, Ravasco P. Eicosapentaenoic acid in cancer improves body composition and modulates metabolism. Nutrition. 2015;31(4):549–55. https://doi.org/10.1016/j.nut.2014.12.002. Epub 2014 Dec 12. Review.
166. Yang P, Jiang Y, Fischer SM. Prostaglandin E3 metabolism and cancer. Cancer Lett. 2014;348(1–2):1–11. https://doi.org/10.1016/j.canlet.2014.03.010. Epub 2014 Mar 18. Review.
167. Brinton EA, Ballantyne CM, Bays HE, Kastelein JJ, Braeckman RA, Soni PN. Effects of icosapent ethyl on lipid and inflammatory parameters in patients with diabetes mellitus-2, residual elevated triglycerides (200–500 mg/dL), and on statin therapy at LDL-C goal: the ANCHOR study. Cardiovasc Diabetol. 2013;12:100. https://doi.org/10.1186/1475-2840-12-100. Erratum in: Cardiovasc Diabetol. 2015 Jul–Aug;9(4):618.
168. Proudman SM, Cleland LG, Metcalf RG, Sullivan TR, Spargo LD, James MJ. Plasma n-3 fatty acids and clinical outcomes in recent-onset rheumatoid arthritis. Br J Nutr. 2015;114(6):885–90. https://doi.org/10.1017/S0007114515002718. Epub 2015 Aug 18.
169. Wani AL, Bhat SA, Ara A. Omega-3 fatty acids and the treatment of depression: a review of scientific evidence. Integr Med Res. 2015;4(3):132–41.
170. Bradberry JC, Hilleman DE. Overview of omega-3 fatty acid therapies. P T. 2013;38(11):681–91.
171. Patterson E, Wall R, Fitzgerald GF, Ross RP, Stanton C. Health implications of high dietary omega-6 polyunsaturated fatty acids. Published online 2012 Apr 5. https://doi.org/10.1155/2012/539426.
172. Bagga D, Wang L, Farias-Eisner R, Glaspy JA, Reddy ST. Differential effects of prostaglandin derived from omega-6 and omega-3 polyunsaturated

fatty acids on COX-2 expression and IL-6 secretion. Proc Natl Acad Sci U S A. 2003;100(4):1751–6. Epub 2003 Feb 10.
173. Simopoulos AP. An increase in the omega-6/omega-3 fatty acid ratio increases the risk for obesity. Nutrients. 2016;8(3):128. Published online 2016 Mar 2. https://doi.org/10.3390/nu8030128.
174. Macartney MJ, Hingley L, Brown MA, Peoples GE, McLennan PL. Intrinsic heart rate recovery after dynamic exercise is improved with an increased omega-3 index in healthy males. Br J Nutr. 2014;112(12):1984–92. https://doi.org/10.1017/S0007114514003146. Epub 2014 Oct 30.
175. Ali MA, Waheed A, Jurivich DA, Colombo J, Singer DH. Short-term time domain HRV measures: comparisons with 24-hr Holter monitoring. Chicago: Geriatric Medicine Society Meeting; 2006.
176. Umetani K, Singer DH, McCraty R, Atkinson M. Twenty-four hour time domain heart rate variability and heart rate: relations to age and gender over nine decades. J Am Coll Cardiol. 1998;31(3):593–601.
177. Rovelli F, De Vita C, Feruglio GA, Lotto A, Selvini A, Tognoni G. GISSI trial: early results and late follow-up. Gruppo Italiano per la Sperimentazione della Streptochinasi nell'Infarto Miocardico. J Am Coll Cardiol. 1987;10(5 Suppl B):33B–9B.
178. Fresco C, Franzosi MG, Maggioni AP, Tognoni G. The GISSI-2 trial: premises, results, epidemiological (and other) implications. Gruppo Italiano per lo Studio delia Sopravvivenza nell'Infarto Miocardico. Clin Cardiol. 1990;13(8 Suppl 8):VIII32–6.
179. Marchioli R, Barzi F, Bomba E, Chieffo C, Di Gregorio D, Di Mascio R, Franzosi MG, Geraci E, Levantesi G, Maggioni AP, Mantini L, Marfisi RM, Mastrogiuseppe G, Mininni N, Nicolosi GL, Santini M, Schweiger C, Tavazzi L, Tognoni G, Tucci C, Valagussa F, GISSI-Prevenzione Investigators. Early protection against sudden death by n-3 polyunsaturated fatty acids after myocardial infarction: time-course analysis of the results of the Gruppo Italiano per lo Studio della Sopravvivenza nell'Infarto Miocardico (GISSI)-Prevenzione. Circulation. 2002;105(16):1897–903.
180. Yokoyama M, Origasa H, JELIS Investigators. Effects of eicosapentaenoic acid on cardiovascular events in Japanese patients with hypercholesterolemia: rationale, design, and baseline characteristics of the Japan EPA Lipid Intervention Study (JELIS). Am Heart J. 2003;146(4):613–20.
181. Yokoyama M, Origasa H, Matsuzaki M, Matsuzawa Y, Saito Y, Ishikawa Y, Oikawa S, Sasaki J, Hishida H, Itakura H, Kita T, Kitabatake A, Nakaya N, Sakata T, Shimada K, Shirato K, Japan EPA lipid intervention study (JELIS) Investigators. Effects of eicosapentaenoic acid on major coronary events in hypercholesterolemia patients (JELIS): a randomized open-label, blinded endpoint analysis. Lancet. 2007;369(9567):1090–8. Erratum in: Lancet. 2007 Jul 21;370(9583):220.
182. Cleland JG, Freemantle N, Coletta AP, Clark AL. Clinical trials update from the American Heart Association: REPAIR-AMI, ASTAMI, JELIS, MEGA, REVIVE-II, SURVIVE, and PROACTIVE. Eur J Heart Fail. 2006;8(1):105–10. Review.
183. http://news.heart.org/fish-oil-supplements-provide-some-benefit-after-heart-attack-heart-failure/
184. Tong X, Christian P, Zhao M, Wang H, Moreau R, Su Q. Activation of hepatic CREBH and Insig signaling in the anti-hypertriglyceridemic mechanism of R-α-lipoic acid. J Nutr Biochem. 2015;26(9):921–8. https://doi.org/10.1016/j.jnutbio.2015.03.011. Epub 2015 May 7.
185. http://www.heart.org/HEARTORG/HealthyLiving/HealthyEating/HealthyDietGoals/Fish-and-Omega-3-Fatty-Acids_UCM_303248_Article.jsp#.WUKmyMq7qpo
186. McVeigh GE, Brennan GM, Johnston GD, McDermott BJ, McGrath LT, Henry WR, Andrews JW, Hayes JR. Dietary fish oil augments nitric oxide production or release in patients with type 2 (non-insulin-dependent) diabetes mellitus. Diabetologia. 1993;36(1):33–8.
187. Omura M, Kobayashi S, Mizukami Y, Mogami K, Todoroki-Ikeda N, Miyake T, Matsuzaki M. Eicosapentaenoic acid (EPA) induces Ca(2+)-independent activation and translocation of endothelial nitric oxide synthase and endothelium-dependent vasorelaxation. FEBS Lett. 2001;487(3):361–6.
188. De Caterina R, Liao JK, Libby P. Fatty acid modulation of endothelial activation. Am J Clin Nutr. 2000;71(1 Suppl):213S–23S. Review.
189. Curtis BM, O'Keefe JH. Autonomic tone as a cardiovascular risk factor: the dangers of chronic fight or flight. Mayo Clin Proc. 2002;77:45–54.
190. Pu H, Guo Y, Zhang W, Huang L, Wang G, Liou AK, Zhang J, Zhang P, Leak RK, Wang Y, Chen J, Gao Y. Omega-3 polyunsaturated fatty acid supplementation improves neurologic recovery and attenuates white matter injury after experimental traumatic brain injury. J Cereb Blood Flow Metab. 2013;33(9):1474–84. https://doi.org/10.1038/jcbfm.2013.108. Epub 2013 Jun 26.
191. Ohnishi H, Saito Y. Eicosapentaenoic acid (EPA) reduces cardiovascular events: relationship with the EPA/arachidonic acid ratio. J Atheroscler Thromb. 2013;20(12):861–77. Epub 2013 Sept 18.
192. Calder PC. Omega-3 fatty acids and inflammatory processes. Nutrients. 2010;2(3):355–74. https://doi.org/10.3390/nu2030355. Epub 2010 Mar 18.
193. Calder PC. Omega-3 fatty acids and inflammatory processes: from molecules to man. Biochem Soc Trans. 2017;45(5):1105–15. https://doi.org/10.1042/BST20160474. Epub 2017 Sept 12.
194. Arnold LE, Young AS, Belury MA, Cole RM, Gracious B, Seidenfeld AM, Wolfson H, Fristad MA. Omega-3 fatty acid plasma levels before and after supplementation: correlations with mood and clinical outcomes in the omega-3 and therapy studies.

J Child Adolesc Psychopharmacol. 2017;27(3):223–33. https://doi.org/10.1089/cap.2016.0123. Epub 2017 Feb 3.

195. Pompili M, Longo L, Dominici G, Serafini G, Lamis DA, Sarris J, Amore M, Girardi P. Polyunsaturated fatty acids and suicide risk in mood disorders: a systematic review. Prog Neuro-Psychopharmacol Biol Psychiatry. 2017;74:43–56. https://doi.org/10.1016/j.pnpbp.2016.11.007. Epub 2016 Dec 8. Review.
196. Abdulrazaq M, Innes JK, Calder PC. Effect of ω-3 polyunsaturated fatty acids on arthritic pain: asystematic review. Nutrition. 2017;39–40:57–66. https://doi.org/10.1016/j.nut.2016.12.003. Epub 2016 Dec 21. Review.
197. Senftleber NK, Nielsen SM, Andersen JR, Bliddal H, Tarp S, Lauritzen L, Furst DE, Suarez-Almazor ME, Lyddiatt A, Christensen R. Marine oil supplements for arthritis pain: a systematic review and meta-analysis of randomized trials. Nutrients. 2017;9(1). pii: E42. https://doi.org/10.3390/nu9010042. Review.
198. Beermann C, Neumann S, Fußbroich D, Zielen S, Schubert R. Combinations of distinct long-chain polyunsaturated fatty acid species for improved dietary treatment against allergic bronchial asthma. Nutrition. 2016;32(11–12):1165–70. https://doi.org/10.1016/j.nut.2016.04.004. Epub 2016 May 6. Review.
199. Barnadas MA, Díaz Encarnación MM. Refractory cutaneous IgA vasculitis treated with omega-3 fatty acids. Case Rep Dermatol. 2016;8(3):333–40. https://doi.org/10.1159/000452320. eCollection 2016 Sept–Dec.
200. Chauhan S, Kodali H, Noor J, Ramteke K, Gawai V. Role of omega-3 fatty acids on lipid profile in diabetic dyslipidemia: single blind, randomized clinical trial. J Clin Diagn Res. 2017;11(3):OC13–6. https://doi.org/10.7860/JCDR/2017/20628.9449. Epub 2017 Mar 1.
201. Ebrahimi M, Ghayour-Mobarhan M, Rezaiean S, Hoseini M, Parizade SM, Farhoudi F, Hosseininezhad SJ, Tavallaei S, Vejdani A, Azimi-Nezhad M, Shakeri MT, Rad MA, Mobarra N, Kazemi-Bajestani SM, Ferns GA. Omega-3 fatty acid supplements improve the cardiovascular risk profile of subjects with metabolic syndrome, including markers of inflammation and auto-immunity. Acta Cardiol. 2009;64(3):321–7.
202. Ong HT, Cheah JS. Statin alternatives or just placebo: an objective review of omega-3, red yeast rice and garlic in cardiovascular therapeutics. Chin Med J. 2008;121(16):1588–94. Review.
203. Zhao YT, Chen Q, Sun YX, Li XB, Zhang P, Xu Y, Guo JH. Prevention of sudden cardiac death with omega-3 fatty acids in patients with coronary heart disease: a meta-analysis of randomized controlled trials. Ann Med. 2009;41(4):301–10. https://doi.org/10.1080/07853890802698834.
204. Artham SM, Lavie CJ, Milani RV, Anand RG, O'Keefe JH, Ventura HO. Fish oil in primary and secondary cardiovascular prevention. Ochsner J. 2008;8(2):49–60.
205. Christensen JH. n-3 fatty acids and the risk of sudden cardiac death. Emphasis on heart rate variability. Dan Med Bull. 2003;50(4):347–67. Review.
206. Katsi V, Georgiopoulos G, Laina A, Koutli E, Parissis J, Tsioufis C, Nihoyannopoulos P, Tousoulis D. Left ventricular ejection fraction as therapeutic target: is it the ideal marker? Heart Fail Rev. 2017. https://doi.org/10.1007/s10741-017-9624-5. [Epub ahead of print] Review.
207. Khoueiry G, Abi Rafeh N, Sullivan E, Saiful F, Jaffery Z, Kenigsberg DN, Krishnan SC, Khanal S, Bekheit S, Kowalski M. Do omega-3 polyunsaturated fatty acids reduce risk of sudden cardiac death and ventricular arrhythmias? A meta-analysis of randomized trials. Heart Lung. 2013;42(4):251–6. https://doi.org/10.1016/j.hrtlng.2013.03.006. Epub 2013 May 25.
208. Harris WS, Del Gobbo L, Tintle NL. The omega-3 index and relative risk for coronary heart disease mortality: estimation from 10 cohort studies. Atherosclerosis. 2017;262:51–4. https://doi.org/10.1016/j.atherosclerosis.2017.05.007. Epub 2017 May 6.
209. Davis W, Rockway S, Kwasny M. Effect of a combined therapeutic approach of intensive lipid management, omega-3 fatty acid supplementation, and increased serum 25 (OH) vitamin D on coronary calcium scores in asymptomatic adults. Am J Ther. 2009;16(4):326–32. https://doi.org/10.1097/MJT.0b013e31817a8f3c.
210. Mazahery H, Stonehouse W, Delshad M, Kruger MC, Conlon CA, Beck KL, von Hurst PR. Relationship between long chain n-3 polyunsaturated fatty acids and autism spectrum disorder: systematic review and meta-analysis of case-control and randomised controlled trials. Nutrients. 2017;9(2). pii: E155. https://doi.org/10.3390/nu9020155. Review.
211. Stirban A, Nandrean S, Götting C, Tamler R, Pop A, Negrean M, Gawlowski T, Stratmann B, Tschoepe D. Effects of n-3 fatty acids on macro- and microvascular function in subjects with type 2 diabetes mellitus. Am J Clin Nutr. 2010;91(3):808–13. https://doi.org/10.3945/ajcn.2009.28374. Epub 2010 Jan 13
212. Nishizaki Y, Shimada K, Daida H. The balance of omega-3 polyunsaturated fatty acids for -reducing residual risks in patients with coronary artery disease. Acta Cardiol. 2017;21:1–9. https://doi.org/10.1080/00015385.2017.1305174. [Epub ahead of print].
213. Drudi LM, Schaller MS, Hiramoto J, Gasper W, Harris WS, Hills NK, Grenon SM. Predictors of change in omega-3 index with fish oil supplementation in peripheral artery disease. J Surg Res. 2017;210:124–31. https://doi.org/10.1016/j.jss.2016.11.011. Epub 2016 Nov 11.
214. Woodcock BE, Smith E, Lambert WH, Jones WM, Galloway JH, Greaves M, Preston FE. Beneficial effect of fish oil on blood viscosity in periph-

eral vascular disease. Br Med J (Clin Res Ed). 1984;288(6417):592–4.
215. Enns JE, Yeganeh A, Zarychanski R, Abou-Setta AM, Friesen C, Zahradka P, Taylor CG. The impact of omega-3 polyunsaturated fatty acid supplementation on the incidence of cardiovascular events and complications in peripheral arterial disease: a systematic review and meta-analysis. BMC Cardiovasc Disord. 2014;14:70. https://doi.org/10.1186/1471-2261-14-70. Review.
216. Arriens C, Hynan LS, Lerman RH, Karp DR, Mohan C. Placebo-controlled randomized clinical trial of fish oil's impact on fatigue, quality of life, and disease activity in systemic lupus erythematosus. Nutr J. 2015;14:82. https://doi.org/10.1186/s12937-015-0068-2.
217. Sun Q, Ma J, Campos H, Rexrode KM, Albert CM, Mozaffarian D, Hu FB. Blood concentrations of individual long-chain n-3 fatty acids and risk of nonfatal myocardial infarction. Am J Clin Nutr. 2008;88(1):216–23.
218. Hu FB, Bronner L, Willett WC, Stampfer MJ, Rexrode KM, Albert CM, Hunter D, Manson JE. Fish and omega-3 fatty acid intake and risk of coronary heart disease in women. JAMA. 2002;287(14):1815–21.
219. Hu FB, Stampfer MJ, Manson JE, Rimm EB, Wolk A, Colditz GA, Hennekens CH, Willett WC. Dietary intake of alpha-linolenic acid and risk of fatal ischemic heart disease among women. Am J Clin Nutr. 1999;69(5):890–7.
220. Ghule AE, Kandhare AD, Jadhav SS, Zanwar AA, Bodhankar SL. Omega-3-fatty acid adds to the protective effect of flax lignan concentrate in pressure overload-induced myocardial hypertrophy in rats via modulation of oxidative stress and apoptosis. Int Immunopharmacol. 2015;28(1):751–63. https://doi.org/10.1016/j.intimp.2015.08.005. Epub 2015 Aug 14.
221. Song TJ, Chang Y, Shin MJ, Heo JH, Kim YJ. Low levels of plasma omega 3-polyunsaturated fatty acids are associated with cerebral small vessel diseases in acute ischemic stroke patients. Nutr Res. 2015;35(5):368–74. https://doi.org/10.1016/j.nutres.2015.04.008. Epub 2015 Apr 16.
222. Virtanen JK, Siscovick DS, Lemaitre RN, Longstreth WT, Spiegelman D, Rimm EB, King IB, Mozaffarian D. Circulating omega-3 polyunsaturated fatty acids and subclinical brain abnormalities on MRI in older adults: the cardiovascular health study. J Am Heart Assoc. 2013;2(5):e000305. https://doi.org/10.1161/JAHA.113.000305.
223. Bo Y, Zhang X, Wang Y, You J, Cui H, Zhu Y, Pang W, Liu W, Jiang Y, Lu Q. The n-3 polyunsaturated fatty acids supplementation improved the cognitive function in the Chinese elderly with mild cognitive impairment: a double-blind randomized controlled trial. Nutrients. 2017;9(1). pii: E54. https://doi.org/10.3390/nu9010054.
224. Molina-Leyva I, Molina-Leyva A, Bueno-Cavanillas A. Efficacy of nutritional supplementation with omega-3 and omega-6 fatty acids in dry eye syndrome: a systematic review of randomized clinical trials. Acta Ophthalmol. 2017; https://doi.org/10.1111/aos.13428. [Epub ahead of print].
225. Mohammadpour M, Mehrabi S, Hassanpoor N, Mirshahi R. Effects of adjuvant omega-3 fatty acid supplementation on dry eye syndrome following cataract surgery: a randomized clinical trial. J Curr Ophthalmol. 2016;29(1):33–8. https://doi.org/10.1016/j.joco.2016.05.006. eCollection 2017 Mar.
226. Königs A, Kiliaan AJ. Critical appraisal of omega-3 fatty acids in attention-deficit/hyperactivity disorder treatment. Neuropsychiatr Dis Treat. 2016;12:1869–82. https://doi.org/10.2147/NDT.S68652. eCollection 2016. Review.
227. Kalupahana NS, Claycombe K, Newman SJ, Stewart T, Siriwardhana N, Matthan N, Lichtenstein AH, Moustaid-Moussa N. Eicosapentaenoic acid prevents and reverses insulin resistance in high-fat diet-induced obese mice via modulation of adipose tissue inflammation. J Nutr. 2010;140(11):1915–22. https://doi.org/10.3945/jn.110.125732. Epub 2010 Sept 22.
228. Best K, Makrides M. Possible protective effect of prenatal omega-3 long-chain polyunsaturated fatty acids supplementation on persistent wheeze and asthma in early childhood. Evid Based Med. 2017;22(3):104. https://doi.org/10.1136/ebmed-2017-110696. Epub 2017 May 12.
229. Oliveira V, Marinho R, Vitorino D, Santos GA, Moraes JC, Dragano N, Sartori-Cintra A, Pereira L, Catharino RR, da Silva AS, Ropelle ER, Pauli JR, De Souza CT, Velloso LA, Cintra DE. Diets containing α-linolenic (ω3) or oleic (ω9) fatty acids rescues obese mice from insulin resistance. Endocrinology. 2015;156(11):4033–46. https://doi.org/10.1210/en.2014-1880. Epub 2015 Aug 17.
230. Best KP, Sullivan T, Palmer D, Gold M, Kennedy DJ, Martin J, Makrides M. Prenatal fish oil supplementation and allergy: 6-year follow-up of a randomized controlled trial. Pediatrics. 2016;137(6). pii: e20154443. https://doi.org/10.1542/peds.2015-4443.
231. Galarraga B, Ho M, Youssef HM, Hill A, McMahon H, Hall C, Ogston S, Nuki G, Belch JJ. Cod liver oil (n-3 fatty acids) as an non-steroidal anti-inflammatory drug sparing agent in rheumatoid arthritis. Rheumatology (Oxford). 2008;47(5):665–9. https://doi.org/10.1093/rheumatology/ken024. Epub 2008 Mar 24.
232. Proudman SM, Cleland LG, James MJ. Dietary omega-3 fats for treatment of inflammatory joint disease: efficacy and utility. Rheum Dis Clin N Am. 2008;34(2):469–79. https://doi.org/10.1016/j.rdc.2008.03.003.
233. Chhetry BT, Hezghia A, Miller JM, Lee S, Rubin-Falcone H, Cooper TB, Oquendo MA, Mann JJ,

Sublette ME. Omega-3 polyunsaturated fatty acid supplementation and white matter changes in major depression. J Psychiatr Res. 2016;75:65–74. https://doi.org/10.1016/j.jpsychires.2015.12.007. Epub 2016 Jan 11.

234. Souied EH, Delcourt C, Querques G, Bassols A, Merle B, Zourdani A, Smith T, Benlian P, Nutritional AMD Treatment 2 Study Group. Oral docosahexaenoic acid in the prevention of exudative age-related macular degeneration: the Nutritional AMD Treatment 2 study. Ophthalmology. 2013;120(8):1619–31. https://doi.org/10.1016/j.ophtha.2013.01.005. Epub 2013 Feb 8.
235. Widmer RJ, Lerman A. Endothelial dysfunction and cardiovascular disease. Glob Cardiol Sci Pract. 2014;2014(3):291–308. https://doi.org/10.5339/gcsp.2014.43. eCollection 2014. Review.
236. Endemann DH, Schiffrin EL. Endothelial dysfunction. J Am Soc Nephrol. 2004;15(8):1983–92. Review.
237. Hadi HA, Carr CS, Al SJ. Endothelial dysfunction: cardiovascular risk factors, therapy, and outcome. Vasc Health Risk Manag. 2005;1(3):183–98. Review.
238. Michel T, Vanhoutte PM. Cellular signaling and NO production. Pflugers Arch. 2010;459(6):807–16. https://doi.org/10.1007/s00424-009-0765-9. Epub 2010 Jan 16. Review.
239. Snyder SH. Nitric oxide: first in a new class of neurotransmitters. Science. 1992;257(5069):494–6.
240. Groneberg D, Voussen B, Friebe A. Integrative control of gastrointestinal motility by nitric oxide. Curr Med Chem. 2016;23(24):2715–35. Review.
241. Hibbs JB Jr, Taintor RR, Vavrin Z, Rachlin EM. Nitric oxide: a cytotoxic activated macrophage effector molecule. Biochem Biophys Res Commun. 1988;157(1):87–94. Erratum in: Biochem Biophys Res Commun 1989 Jan 31;158(2):624.
242. Hibbs JB Jr. Synthesis of nitric oxide from L-arginine: a recently discovered pathway induced by cytokines with antitumour and antimicrobial activity. Res Immunol. 1991;142(7):565–9; discussion 596–8. Review.
243. Nathan CF, Hibbs JB Jr. Role of nitric oxide synthesis in macrophage antimicrobial activity. Curr Opin Immunol. 1991;3(1):65–70. Review.
244. Margel D, Mizrahi M, Regev-Shoshani G, Ko M, Moshe M, Ozalvo R, Shavit-Grievink L, Baniel J, Kedar D, Yossepowitch O, Lifshitz D, Nadu A, Greenberg D, Av-Gay Y. Nitric oxide charged catheters as a potential strategy for prevention of hospital acquired infections. PLoS One. 2017;12(4):e0174443. https://doi.org/10.1371/journal.pone.0174443. eCollection 2017.
245. Tsukiyama Y, Ito T, Nagaoka K, Eguchi E, Ogino K. Effects of exercise training on nitric oxide, blood pressure and antioxidant enzymes. J Clin Biochem Nutr. 2017;60(3):180–6. https://doi.org/10.3164/jcbn.16-108. Epub 2017 Apr 7.
246. Faraci FM. Reactive oxygen species: influence on cerebral vascular tone. J Appl Physiol (1985). 2006;100(2):739–43. Review.
247. Faraci FM, Brian JE Jr. Nitric oxide and the cerebral circulation. Stroke. 1994;25(3):692–703.
248. Musicki B, Lagoda G, Goetz T, La Favor JD, Burnett AL. Transnitrosylation: a factor in nitric oxide-mediated penile erection. J Sex Med. 2016;13(5):808–14. https://doi.org/10.1016/j.jsxm.2016.03.003.
249. Elder JA, Braver Y. Female sexual dysfunction. http://www.clevelandclinicmeded.com/medicalpubs/diseasemanagement/womens-health/female-sexual-dysfunction/
250. Brown GC. Regulation of mitochondrial respiration by nitric oxide inhibition of cytochrome c oxidase. Biochim Biophys Acta. 2001;1504(1):46–57. Review.
251. Damodaran VB, Leszczak V, Wold KA, Lantvit SM, Popat KC, Reynolds MM. Anti-thrombogenic properties of a nitric oxide-releasing dextran derivative: evaluation of platelet activation and whole blood clotting kinetics. RSC Adv. 2013;3(46). https://doi.org/10.1039/C3RA45521A.
252. Lefer AM. Nitric oxide: nature's naturally occurring leukocyte inhibitor. Circulation. 1997;95(3):553–4. Review.
253. Lefer AM, Lefer DJ. Nitric oxide. II. Nitric oxide protects in intestinal inflammation. Am J Phys. 1999;276(3 Pt 1):G572–5. Review.
254. Predonzani A, Calì B, Agnellini AH, Molon B. Spotlights on immunological effects of reactive nitrogen species: when inflammation says nitric oxide. World J Exp Med. 2015;5(2):64–76.
255. Korhonen R, Korpela R, Saxelin M, Mäki M, Kankaanranta H, Moilanen E. Induction of nitric oxide synthesis by probiotic lactobacillus rhamnosus GG in J774 macrophages and human T84 intestinal epithelial cells. Inflammation. 2001;25(4):223–32.
256. Geiger R, Rieckmann JC, Wolf T, Basso C, Feng Y, Fuhrer T, Kogadeeva M, Picotti P, Meissner F, Mann M, Zamboni N, Sallusto F, Lanzavecchia A. L-arginine modulates T cell metabolism and enhances survival and anti-tumor activity. Cell. 2016;167(3):829–842.e13. https://doi.org/10.1016/j.cell.2016.09.031. Epub 2016 Oct 13.
257. Niedbala W, Cai B, Liew FY. Role of nitric oxide in the regulation of T cell functions. Ann Rheum Dis. 2006;65(Suppl 3):iii37–40. Review.
258. Niedbala W, Besnard AG, Jiang HR, Alves-Filho JC, Fukada SY, Nascimento D, Mitani A, Pushparaj P, Alqahtani MH, Liew FY. Nitric oxide-induced regulatory T cells inhibit Th17 but not Th1 cell differentiation and function. J Immunol. 2013;191(1):164–70. https://doi.org/10.4049/jimmunol.1202580. Epub 2013 May 29.
259. Winkler MS, Kluge S, Holzmann M, Moritz E, Robbe L, Bauer A, Zahrte C, Priefler M, Schwedhelm E, Böger RH, Goetz AE, Nierhaus

A, Zoellner C. Markers of nitric oxide are associated with sepsis severity: an observational study. Crit Care. 2017;21(1):189. https://doi.org/10.1186/s13054-017-1782-2.

260. Predonzani A, Calì B, Agnellini AH, Molon B. Spotlights on immunological effects of reactive nitrogen species: when inflammation says nitric oxide. World J Exp Med. 2015;5(2):64–76.
261. Ying L, Hofseth LJ. An emerging role for endothelial nitric oxide synthase in chronic inflammation and cancer. Cancer Res. 2007;67:1407–10.
262. Choudhari SK, Chaudhary M, Bagde S, Gadbail AR, Joshi V. Nitric oxide and cancer: a review. World J Surg Oncol. 2013;11:118. https://doi.org/10.1186/1477-7819-11-118. Review.
263. Li LM, Kibourn RG, Adams J, Filder IJ. Role of NO in lysis of tumor cells by cytokine activated endothelial cells. Cancer Res. 1991;51:2531–5.
264. Shang ZJ, Li JR. Expression of endothelial nitric oxide synthase and vascular endothelial growth factor in oral squamous cell carcinoma: its correlation with angiogenesis and disease progression. J Oral Pathol Med. 2005;4:134–9.
265. Lechner M, Lirk P, Rieder J. Inducible nitric oxide synthase (iNOS) in tumor biology: the two sides of the same coin. Semin Cancer Biol. 2005;15:277–89.
266. Rapozzi V, Della Pietra E, Bonavida B. Dual roles of nitric oxide in the regulation of tumor cell response and resistance to photodynamic therapy. Redox Biol. 2015;6:311–7. https://doi.org/10.1016/j.redox.2015.07.015. Epub 2015 Jul 31. Review.
267. Reveneau S, Arnould L, Jolimoy G, Hilpert S, Lejeune P, Saint-Giorgio V, Belichard C, Jeannin JF. Nitric oxide synthase in human breast cancer is associated with tumor grade, proliferation rate, and expression of progesterone receptor. Lab Investig. 1999;79:1215–25.
268. Seabra AB, de Lima R, Calderón M. Nitric oxide releasing nanomaterials for cancer treatment: current status and perspectives. Curr Top Med Chem. 2015;15(4):298–308. Review.
269. Brown GC. Regulation of mitochondrial respiration by nitric oxide inhibition of cytochrome c oxidase. Review. Biochim Biophys Acta Bioenerg. 2001;1504(1):46–57.
270. Brown GC. Regulation of mitochondrial respiration by nitric oxide inhibition of cytochrome c oxidase. Review. Biochim Biophys Acta Bioenerg. 2001;1504(1):46–57.
271. Chakraborty S, Ain R. Nitric-oxide synthase trafficking inducer is a pleiotropic regulator of endothelial cell function and signaling. J Biol Chem. 2017;292(16):6600–20. https://doi.org/10.1074/jbc.M116.742627. Epub 2017 Feb 24.
272. Siegel C, McCullough LD. NAD+ depletion or PAR polymer formation: which plays the role of executioner in ischemic cell death? Acta Physiol (Oxf). 2011;203(1):225–34. https://doi.org/10.1111/j.1748-1716.2010.02229.x.
273. Siegel C, McCullough LD. NAD+ depletion or PAR polymer formation: which plays the role of executioner in ischemic cell death? Acta Physiol (Oxf). 2011;203(1):225–34. https://doi.org/10.1111/j.1748-1716.2010.02229.x.
274. Morbidelli L, Chang CH, Douglas JG, Granger HJ, Ledda F, Ziche M. Nitric oxide mediates mitogenic effect of VEGF on coronary venular endothelium. Am J Phys. 1996;270(1 Pt 2):H411–5.
275. Ziche M, Morbidelli L, Choudhuri R, Zhang HT, Donnini S, Granger HJ, Bicknell R. Nitric oxide synthase lies downstream from vascular endothelial growth factor-induced but not basic fibroblast growth factor-induced angiogenesis. J Clin Invest. 1997;99(11):2625–34.
276. Uhlmann S, Friedrichs U, Eichler W, Hoffmann S, Wiedemann P. Direct measurement of VEGF-induced nitric oxide production by choroidal endothelial cells. Microvasc Res. 2001;62(2):179–89.
277. Kimura H, Esumi H. Reciprocal regulation between nitric oxide and vascular endothelial growth factor in angiogenesis. Acta Biochim Pol. 2003;50(1):49–59. Review.
278. Zhang HH, Chen JC, Sheibani L, Lechuga TJ, Chen DB. Pregnancy augments VEGF-stimulated in vitro angiogenesis and vasodilator (NO and H2S) production in human uterine artery endothelial cells. J Clin Endocrinol Metab. 2017. https://doi.org/10.1210/jc.2017-00437.
279. Estrada C, Murillo-Carretero M. Nitric oxide and adult neurogenesis in health and disease. Neuroscientist. 2005;11(4):294.
280. Wimalawansa SJ. Nitric oxide and bone. Ann N Y Acad Sci. 2010;1192:391–403. https://doi.org/10.1111/j.1749-6632.2009.05230.x. Review.
281. Yu Q, Li T, Li J, Zhong L, Mao X. Nitricoxidesynthase in male urological and andrologic functions. Nitric oxide synthase – simple enzyme-complex roles. 113–36. http://www.intechopen.com/books/nitric-oxide-synthase-simpleenzyme-complex-roles
282. Gad MZ. Anti-aging effects of L-arginine. J Adv Res. 2010;1:169–77. Review.
283. Yeboah J, Folsom AR, Burke GL, Johnson C, Polak JF, Post W, Lima JA, Crouse JR, Herrington DM. Predictive value of brachial flow-mediated dilation for incident cardiovascular events in a population-based study: the multi-ethnic study of atherosclerosis. Circulation. 2009;120(6):502–9.
284. Huang A, Silver AE, Shvenke E, Schopfer DW, Jahangir E, Titas MA, Shpilman A, Menzoian JO, Watkins MT, Raffetto JD, Gibbons G, Woodson J, Shaw PM, Dhadly M, Eberhardt RT, Keaney JF Jr, Gokce N, Vita JA. Predictive value of reactive hyperemia for cardiovascular events in patients with peripheral arterial disease undergoing vascular surgery. Arterioscler Thromb Vasc Biol. 2007;27(10):2113–9.
285. Anderson T, Charbonneau F, Title LM, Buithieu J, Rose MS, Conradson H, Hildebrand K, Fung M, Verma S, Lonn EM. Microvascular function predicts

cardiovascular events in primary prevention: long-term results from the firefighters and their endothelium (FATE) study. Circulation. 2011;123(2):163–9.

286. Lind L, Berglund L, Larsson A, Sundström J. Endothelial function in resistance and conduit arteries and 5-year risk of cardiovascular disease. Circulation. 2011;123(14):1545–51.
287. Gorren AC, Mayer B. Tetrahydrobiopterin in nitric oxide synthesis: a novel biological role for pteridines. Curr Drug Metab. 2002;3(2):133–57. Review.
288. Michel T. NO way to relax: the complexities of coupling nitric oxide synthase pathways in the heart. Circulation. 2010;121(4):484–6. https://doi.org/10.1161/CIR.0b013e3181d1e24e. Epub 2010 Jan 18.
289. Channon KM. Tetrahydrobiopterin: a vascular redox target to improve endothelial function. Curr Vasc Pharmacol. 2012;10(6):705–8. Review.
290. Zhang Y, Janssens SP, Wingler K, Schmidt HH, Moens AL. Modulating endothelial nitric oxide synthase: a new cardiovascular therapeutic strategy. Am J Physiol Heart Circ Physiol. 2011;301(3):H634–46. https://doi.org/10.1152/ajpheart.01315.2010. Epub 2011 May 27. Review. Erratum in: Am J Physiol Heart Circ Physiol. 2012 Jul 15;303(2):H241.
291. Menzel D, Haller H, Wilhelm M, et al. L-arginine and B vitamins improve endothelial function in subjects with mild to moderate blood pressure elevation. Eur J Nutr. 2018;57(2):557–68. https://doi.org/10.1007/s00394-016-1342-6 (Springer Berlin Heidelberg).
292. Stuehr DJ. Enzymes of the L-arginine to nitric oxide pathway. J Nutr. 2004;134(10 Suppl):2748S–51S; discussion 2765S–2767S. Review
293. Scalera F, Bode-Böger SM. Nitric oxide–asymmetric dimethylarginine system in endothelial cell senescence. In: Ignarro LJ, editor. Nitric oxide biology and pathobiology. 2nd ed. San Diego: Elsevier; 2010.
294. Moyzis RK, Buckingham JM, Cram LS, Dani M, Deaven LL, Jones MD, Meyne J, Ratliff RL, Wu JR. A highly conserved repetitive DNA sequence, (TTAGGG)n, present at the telomeres of human chromosomes. Proc Natl Acad Sci U S A. 1988;85(18):6622–6.
295. Blackburn EH. Telomere states and cell fates. Nature. 2000;408:53–6.
296. Blackburn EH. Switching and signaling at the telomere. Cell. 2001;106:661–73.
297. Blasco MA. Mammalian telomeres and telomerase: why they matter for cancer and aging. Eur J Cell Biol. 2003;82:441–6.
298. Bode-Böger SM, Martens-Lobenhoffer J, Täger M, Schröder H, Scalera F. Aspirin reduces endothelial cell senescence. Biochem Biophys Res Commun. 2005;334:1226–32.
299. Scalera F, Martens-Lobenhoffer J, Bukowska A, Lendeckel U, Täger M, Bode-Böger SM. Effect of telmisartan on nitric oxide-asymmetrical dimethylarginine system. Role of angiotensin II type 1 receptor and peroxisome proliferator activated receptor γ signaling during endothelial aging. Hypertension. 2008;51:696–703.
300. Jin ZG. Where is endothelial nitric oxide synthase more critical: plasma membrane or Golgi? Arterioscler Thromb Vasc Biol. 2006;26(5):959–61.
301. Petruson K, Stalfors J, Jacobsson KE, Ny L, Petruson B. Nitric oxide production in the sphenoidal sinus by the inducible and constitutive isozymes of nitric oxide synthase. Rhinology. 2005;43(1):18–23.
302. Fleming I, Busse R. Molecular mechanisms involved in the regulation of the endothelial nitric oxide synthase. Am J Physiol Regul Integr Comp Physiol. 2003;284(1):R1–12.
303. Ostrom RS, Bundey RA, Insel PA. Nitric oxide inhibition of adenylyl cyclase type 6 activity is dependent upon lipid rafts and caveolin signaling complexes. J Biol Chem. 2004;279(19):19846–53.
304. Minshall RD, Sessa WC, Stan RV, Anderson RG, Malik AB. Caveolin regulation of endothelial function. Am J Physiol Lung Cell Mol Physiol. 2003;285(6):L1179–83.
305. Ho FM, Lin WW, Chen BC, Chao CM, Yang CR, Lin LY, Lai CC, Liu SH, Liau CS. High glucose-induced apoptosis in human vascular endothelial cells is mediated through NF-kappaB and c-Jun NH(2)-terminal kinase pathway and prevented by PI3K/Akt/eNOS pathway. Cell Signal. 2006;18(3):391–9. Epub 2005 Jun 20.
306. Boo YC, Jo H. Flow-dependent regulation of endothelial nitric oxide synthase: role of protein kinases. Am J Physiol Cell Physiol. 2003;285(3):C499–508.
307. Goubareva I, Gkaliagkousi E, Shah A, Queen L, Ritter J, Ferro A. Age decreases nitric oxide synthesis and responsiveness in human platelets and increases formation of monocyte-platelet aggregates. Cardiovasc Res. 2007;75(4):793–802. Epub 2007 May 24.
308. Eggebeen J, Kim-Shapiro DB, Haykowsky M, Morgan TM, Basu S, Brubaker P, Rejeski J, Kitzman DW. One week of daily dosing with beetroot juice improves submaximal endurance and blood pressure in older patients with heart failure and preserved ejection fraction. JACC Heart Fail. 2016;4(6):428–37. https://doi.org/10.1016/j.jchf.2015.12.013. Epub 2016 Feb 10.
309. Shaltout HA, Eggebeen J, Marsh AP, Brubaker PH, Laurienti PJ, Burdette JH, Basu S, Morgan A, Dos Santos PC, Norris JL, Morgan TM, Miller GD, Rejeski WJ, Hawfield AT, Diz DI, Becton JT, Kim-Shapiro DB, Kitzman DW. Effects of supervised exercise and dietary nitrate in older adults with controlled hypertension and/or heart failure with preserved ejection fraction. Nitric Oxide. 2017;69:78–90. https://doi.org/10.1016/j.niox.2017.05.005. Epub 2017 May 23.
310. Woessner MN, McIlvenna LC, Ortiz de Zevallos J, Neil C, Allen JD. Dietary nitrate supplementation in cardiovascular health: an ergogenic aid or exercise therapeutic? Am J Physiol Heart Circ Physiol. 2017. https://doi.org/10.1152/ajpheart.00414.2017.

311. Notay K, Incognito AV, Millar PJ. Acute beetroot juice supplementation on sympathetic nerve activity: a randomized, double-blind, placebo-controlled proof-of-concept study. Am J Physiol Heart Circ Physiol. 2017;313(1):H59–65. https://doi.org/10.1152/ajpheart.00163.2017. Epub 2017 May 5.
312. Ashor AW, Lara J, Siervo M. Medium-term effects of dietary nitrate supplementation on systolic and diastolic blood pressure in adults: a systematic review and meta-analysis. J Hypertens. 2017;35(7):1353–9. https://doi.org/10.1097/HJH.0000000000001305.
313. Clements WT, Lee SR, Bloomer RJ. Nitrate ingestion: a review of the health and physical performance effects. Nutrients. 2014;6(11):5224–64. https://doi.org/10.3390/nu6115224. Review.
314. Siervo M, Lara J, Ogbonmwan I, Mathers JC. Inorganic nitrate and beetroot juice supplementation reduces blood pressure in adults: a systematic review and meta-analysis. J Nutr. 2013;143(6):818–26. https://doi.org/10.3945/jn.112.170233. Epub 2013 Apr 17. Review.
315. Coles LT, Clifton PM. Effect of beetroot juice on lowering blood pressure in free-living, disease-free adults: a randomized, placebo-controlled trial. Nutr J. 2012;11:106. https://doi.org/10.1186/1475-2891-11-106.
316. Hobbs DA, Goulding MG, Nguyen A, Malaver T, Walker CF, George TW, Methven L, Lovegrove JA. Acute ingestion of beetroot bread increases endothelium-independent vasodilation and lowers diastolic blood pressure in healthy men: a randomized controlled trial. J Nutr. 2013;143(9):1399–405. https://doi.org/10.3945/jn.113.175778. Epub 2013 Jul 24.
317. Jajja A, Sutyarjoko A, Lara J, Rennie K, Brandt K, Qadir O, Siervo M. Beetroot supplementation lowers daily systolic blood pressure in older, overweight subjects. Nutr Res. 2014;34(10):868–75. https://doi.org/10.1016/j.nutres.2014.09.007. Epub 2014 Sept 28.
318. Wong RH, Garg ML, Wood LG, Howe PR. Antihypertensive potential of combined extracts of olive leaf, green coffee bean and beetroot: a randomized, double-blind, placebo-controlled crossover trial. Nutrients. 2014;6(11):4881–94. https://doi.org/10.3390/nu6114881.
319. Clements WT, Lee SR, Bloomer RJ. Nitrate ingestion: a review of the health and physical performance effects. Nutrients. 2014;6(11):5224–64. https://doi.org/10.3390/nu6115224. Review.
320. Lara J, Ashor AW, Oggioni C, Ahluwalia A, Mathers JC, Siervo M. Effects of inorganic nitrate and beetroot supplementation on endothelial function: a systematic review and meta-analysis. Eur J Nutr. 2016;55(2):451–9. https://doi.org/10.1007/s00394-015-0872-7. Epub 2015 Mar 13. Review.
321. Lee JS, Stebbins CL, Jung E, Nho H, Kim JK, Chang MJ, Choi HM. Effects of chronic dietary nitrate supplementation on the hemodynamic response to dynamic exercise. Am J Physiol Regul Integr Comp Physiol. 2015;309(5):R459–66. https://doi.org/10.1152/ajpregu.00099.2015. Epub 2015 Jun 17.
322. Clifford T, Howatson G, West DJ, Stevenson EJ. The potential benefits of red beetroot supplementation in health and disease. Nutrients. 2015;7(4):2801–22. https://doi.org/10.3390/nu7042801. Review.
323. Bondonno CP, Liu AH, Croft KD, Ward NC, Shinde S, Moodley Y, Lundberg JO, Puddey IB, Woodman RJ, Hodgson JM. Absence of an effect of high nitrate intake from beetroot juice on blood pressure in treated hypertensive individuals: a randomized controlled trial. Am J Clin Nutr. 2015;102(2):368–75. https://doi.org/10.3945/ajcn.114.101188. Epub 2015 Jul 1.
324. Kelly J, Vanhatalo A, Wilkerson DP, Wylie LJ, Jones AM. Effects of nitrate on the power-duration relationship for severe-intensity exercise. Med Sci Sports Exerc. 2013;45(9):1798–806. https://doi.org/10.1249/MSS.0b013e31828e885c.
325. Muggeridge DJ, Howe CC, Spendiff O, Pedlar C, James PE, Easton C. The effects of a single dose of concentrated beetroot juice on performance in trained flatwater kayakers. Int J Sport Nutr Exerc Metab. 2013;23(5):498–506. Epub 2013 Apr 9. Erratum in: Int J Sport Nutr Exerc Metab. 2013 Dec;23 (6):642.
326. Hoon MW, Jones AM, Johnson NA, Blackwell JR, Broad EM, Lundy B, Rice AJ, Burke LM. The effect of variable doses of inorganic nitrate-rich beetroot juice on simulated 2,000-m rowing performance in trained athletes. Int J Sports Physiol Perform. 2014;9(4):615–20. https://doi.org/10.1123/ijspp.2013-0207. Epub 2013 Sept 30.
327. Breese BC, McNarry MA, Marwood S, Blackwell JR, Bailey SJ, Jones AM. Beetroot juice supplementation speeds O2 uptake kinetics and improves exercise tolerance during severe-intensity exercise initiated from an elevated metabolic rate. Am J Physiol Regul Integr Comp Physiol. 2013;305(12):R1441–50. https://doi.org/10.1152/ajpregu.00295.2013. Epub 2013 Oct 2.
328. Lowery RP, Joy JM, Dudeck JE, Oliveira de Souza E, McCleary SA, Wells S, Wildman R, Wilson JM. Effects of 8 weeks of Xpand® 2X pre workout supplementation on skeletal muscle hypertrophy, lean body mass, and strength in resistance trained males. J Int Soc Sports Nutr. 2013;10(1):44. https://doi.org/10.1186/1550-2783-10-44.
329. Thompson KG, Turner L, Prichard J, Dodd F, Kennedy DO, Haskell C, Blackwell JR, Jones AM. Influence of dietary nitrate supplementation on physiological and cognitive responses to incremental cycle exercise. Respir Physiol Neurobiol. 2014;193:11–20. https://doi.org/10.1016/j.resp.2013.12.015. Epub 2013 Dec 31.
330. Pinna M, Roberto S, Milia R, Marongiu E, Olla S, Loi A, Migliaccio GM, Padulo J, Orlandi C, Tocco F, Concu A, Crisafulli A. Effect of beetroot juice

supplementation on aerobic response during swimming. Nutrients. 2014;6(2):605–15. https://doi.org/10.3390/nu6020605.

331. Flanagan SD, Looney DP, Miller MJ, DuPont WH, Pryor L, Creighton BC, Sterczala AJ, Szivak TK, Hooper DR, Maresh CM, Volek JS, Ellis LA, Kraemer WJ. The effects of nitrate-rich supplementation on neuromuscular efficiency during heavy resistance exercise. J Am Coll Nutr. 2016;35(2):100–7. https://doi.org/10.1080/07315724.2015.1081572. Epub 2016 Feb 17.
332. Petrie M, Rejeski WJ, Basu S, Laurienti PJ, Marsh AP, Norris JL, Kim-Shapiro DB, Burdette JH. Beet root juice: an ergogenic aid for exercise and the aging brain. J Gerontol A Biol Sci Med Sci. 2016. https://doi.org/10.1093/gerona/glw219. [Epub ahead of print].
333. Domínguez R, Cuenca E, Maté-Muñoz JL, García-Fernández P, Serra-Paya N, Estevan MC, Herreros PV, Garnacho-Castaño MV. Effects of beetroot juice supplementation on cardiorespiratory endurance in athletes. A systematic review. Nutrients. 2017;9(1). pii: E43. https://doi.org/10.3390/nu9010043. Review.
334. Montenegro CF, Kwong DA, Minow ZA, Davis BA, Lozada CF, Casazza GA. Betalain-rich concentrate supplementation improves exercise performance and recovery in competitive triathletes. Appl Physiol Nutr Metab. 2017;42(2):166–72. https://doi.org/10.1139/apnm-2016-0452. Epub 2016 Oct 14.
335. Vanhatalo A, Jones AM, Blackwell JR, Winyard PG, Fulford J. Dietary nitrate accelerates postexercise muscle metabolic recovery and O2 delivery in hypoxia. J Appl Physiol (1985). 2014;117(12):1460–70. https://doi.org/10.1152/japplphysiol.00096.2014. Epub 2014 Oct 9.
336. Kim JK, Moore DJ, Maurer DG, Kim-Shapiro DB, Basu S, Flanagan MP, Skulas-Ray AC, Kris-Etherton P, Proctor DN. Acute dietary nitrate supplementation does not augment submaximal forearm exercise hyperemia in healthy young men. Appl Physiol Nutr Metab. 2015;40(2):122–8. https://doi.org/10.1139/apnm-2014-0228. Epub 2014 Oct 15.
337. MacLeod KE, Nugent SF, Barr SI, Koehle MS, Sporer BC, MacInnis MJ. Acute beetroot juice supplementation does not improve cycling performance in normoxia or moderate hypoxia. Int J Sport Nutr Exerc Metab. 2015;25(4):359–66. https://doi.org/10.1123/ijsnem.2014-0129. Epub 2015 Mar 26.
338. Arnold JT, Oliver SJ, Lewis-Jones TM, Wylie LJ, Macdonald JH. Beetroot juice does not enhance altitude running performance in well-trained athletes. Appl Physiol Nutr Metab. 2015;40(6):590–5. https://doi.org/10.1139/apnm-2014-0470. Epub 2015 Feb 4.
339. Flueck JL, Bogdanova A, Mettler S, Perret C. Is beetroot juice more effective than sodium nitrate? The effects of equimolar nitrate dosages of nitrate-rich beetroot juice and sodium nitrate on oxygen consumption during exercise. Appl Physiol Nutr Metab. 2016;41(4):421–9. https://doi.org/10.1139/apnm-2015-0458. Epub 2015 Dec 23.
340. Chirinos JA, Akers SR, Trieu L, Ischiropoulos H, Doulias PT, Tariq A, Vassim I, Koppula MR, Syed AA, Soto-Calderon H, Townsend RR, Cappola TP, Margulies KB, Zamani P. Heart failure, left ventricular remodeling, and circulating nitric oxide metabolites. J Am Heart Assoc. 2016;5(10). pii: e004133. Erratum in: J Am Heart Assoc. 2017 Feb 14;6(2).
341. Zamani P, Tan V, Soto-Calderon H, Beraun M, Brandimarto JA, Trieu L, Varakantam S, Doulias PT, Townsend RR, Chittams J, Margulies KB, Cappola TP, Poole DC, Ischiropoulos H, Chirinos JA. Pharmacokinetics and pharmacodynamics of inorganic nitrate in heart failure with preserved ejection fraction. Circ Res. 2017;120(7):1151–61. https://doi.org/10.1161/CIRCRESAHA.116.309832. Epub 2016 Dec 7.
342. Jacob T, Ascher E, Vorsanger M, Hingorani A, Kallakuri S, Yorkovich W, Schuzter R. Decreased production of nitric oxide by peripheral blood mononuclear cells of patients with peripheral vascular disease. Vasc Endovasc Surg. 2005;39(2):175–81.
343. Tapiero H, Mathé G, Couvreur P, Tew KD. L-Arginine. Biomed Pharmacother. 2002;56(9):439–45.
344. Dhanakoti SN, Brosnan JT, Herzberg GR, Brosnan ME. Renal arginine synthesis: studies in vitro and in vivo. Am J Phys. 1990;259(3 Pt1):E437–42.
345. Watford M. The urea cycle: a two-compartment system. Essays Biochem. 1991;26:49–58.
346. Fritz JH. Arginine cools the inflamed gut. Infect Immun. 2013;81(10):3500–2. https://doi.org/10.1128/IAI.00789-13. Epub 2013 Jul 29.
347. Patel VB, Preedy VR, Rajendram R, editors. L-arginine in clinical nutrition. Cham: Humana Press, Springer International Publishing; 2017.
348. Pahlavani N, Jafari M, Sadeghi O, Rezaei M, Rasad H, Rahdar HA, Entezari MH. L-arginine supplementation and risk factors of cardiovascular diseases in healthy men: a double-blind randomized clinical trial. Version 2. F1000Res. 2014 [revised 2017 Jun 1];3:306. https://doi.org/10.12688/f1000research.5877.2. eCollection 2014.
349. Clifford T, Howatson G, West DJ, Stevenson EJ. The potential benefits of red beetroot supplementation in health and disease. Nutrients. 2015;7(4):2801–22. https://doi.org/10.3390/nu7042801. Review.
350. Flanagan SD, Looney DP, Miller MJ, DuPont WH, Pryor L, Creighton BC, Sterczala AJ, Szivak TK, Hooper DR, Maresh CM, Volek JS, Ellis LA, Kraemer WJ. The effects of nitrate-rich supplementation on neuromuscular efficiency during heavy resistance exercise. J Am Coll Nutr. 2016;35(2):100–7. https://doi.org/10.1080/07315724.2015.1081572. Epub 2016 Feb 17.
351. Domínguez R, Cuenca E, Maté-Muñoz JL, García-Fernández P, Serra-Paya N, Estevan MC, Herreros PV, Garnacho-Castaño MV. Effects of beetroot juice supplementation on cardiorespiratory endurance in athletes. A systematic review. Nutrients. 2017;9(1).

pii: E43. https://doi.org/10.3390/nu9010043. Review.

352. Bondonno CP, Liu AH, Croft KD, Ward NC, Shinde S, Moodley Y, Lundberg JO, Puddey IB, Woodman RJ, Hodgson JM. Absence of an effect of high nitrate intake from beetroot juice on blood pressure in treated hypertensive individuals: a randomized controlled trial. Am J Clin Nutr. 2015;102(2):368–75. https://doi.org/10.3945/ajcn.114.101188. Epub 2015 Jul 1.
353. Arnold JT, Oliver SJ, Lewis-Jones TM, Wylie LJ, Macdonald JH. Beetroot juice does not enhance altitude running performance in well-trained athletes. Appl Physiol Nutr Metab. 2015;40(6):590–5. https://doi.org/10.1139/apnm-2014-0470. Epub 2015 Feb 4.
354. Boger RH, Bode Boger SM. The clinical pharmacology of L-arginine. Annu Rev Pharmacol Toxicol. 2001;41:79–99.
355. Kamada Y, Nagaretani H, Tamura S, Ohama T, Maruyama T, Hiraoka H, et al. Vascular endothelial dysfunction resulting from L-arginine deficiency in a patient with lysinuric protein intolerance. J Clin Invest. 2001;108(5):717–24.
356. Boger RH, Ron ES. L-arginine improves vascular function by overcoming deleterious effects of ADMA, a novel cardiovascular risk factor. Altern Med Rev. 2005;10(1):14–23.
357. Holt LE Jr, Albanese AA. Observations on amino acid deficiencies in man. Trans Assoc Am Phys. 1944;58:143–56.
358. Tanimura J. Studies on arginine in human semen. II. The effects of medication with L-arginine-HCL on male infertility. Bull Osaka Med Sch. 1967;13(2):84–9.
359. Schwentker A, Vodovotz Y, Weller R, Billiar TR. Nitric oxide and wound repair: role of cytokines? Nitric Oxide. 2002;7(1):1–10.
360. Seifter E, Rettura G, Barbul A, Levenson SM. Arginine: an essential amino acid for injured rats. Surgery. 1978;84(2):224–30.
361. Kirk SJ, Hurson M, Regan MC, Holt DR, Wasserkrug HL, Barbul A. Arginine stimulates wound healing and immune function in elderly human beings. Surgery. 1993;114(2):155–9.
362. Arbss MA, Ferrando JM, Vidal J, Quiles MT, Huguet P, Castells J, et al. Early effects of exogenous arginine after the implantation of prosthetic material into the rat abdominal wall. Life Sci. 2000;67(20):2493–512.
363. Albina JE, Mills CD, Henry WL Jr, Caldwell MD. Temporal expression of different pathways of L-arginine metabolism in healing wounds. J Immunol. 1990;144(10):3877–80.
364. Shi HP, Efron DT, Most D, Tantry US, Barbul A. Supplemental dietary arginine enhances wound healing in normal but not inducible nitric oxide synthase knockout mice. Surgery. 2000;128(2):374–8.
365. Angele MK, Nitsch SM, Hatz RA, Angele P, Hernandez Richter T, Wichmann MW, et al. L-arginine: a unique amino acid for improving depressed wound immune function following hemorrhage. Eur Surg Res. 2002;34(1–2):53–60.
366. Chen X, Li Y, Cai X, Xu W, Lu S, Shi J. Dose–effect of dietary L-arginine supplementation on burn wound healing in rats. Chin Med J. 1999;112(9):828–31.
367. Yu YM, Ryan CM, Castillo L, Lu XM, Beaumier L, Tompkins RG, et al. Arginine and ornithine kinetics in severely burned patients: increased rate of arginine disposal. Am J Physiol Endocrinol Metab. 2001;280(3):E509–17.
368. Pieper GM, Siebeneich W, Dondlinger LA. Short-term oral administration of L-arginine reverses defective endothelium-dependent relaxation and cGMP generation in diabetes. Eur J Pharmacol. 1996;317(2–3):317–20.
369. Abbasi F, Asagmi T, Cooke JP, Lamendola C, McLaughlin T, Reaven GM, et al. Plasma concentrations of asymmetric dimethylarginine are increased in patients with type 2 diabetes mellitus. Am J Cardiol. 2001;88(10):1201–3.
370. Giugliano D, Marfella R, Verrazzo G, Acampora R, Nappo F, Ziccardi P, et al. L-arginine for testing endothelium-dependent vascular functions in health and disease. Am J Phys. 1997;273(3 Pt 1):E606–12.
371. Wascher TC, Graier WF, Dittrich P, Hussain MA, Bahadori B, Wallner S, et al. Effects of low-dose L-arginine on insulin-mediated vasodilatation and insulin sensitivity. Eur J Clin Investig. 1997;27(8):690–5.
372. Lubec B, Hayn M, Kitzmuller E, Vierhapper H, Lubec G. L-arginine reduces lipid peroxidation in patients with diabetes mellitus. Free Radic Biol Med. 1997;22(1–2):355–7.
373. Piatti PM, Monti LD, Valsecchi G, Magni F, Setola E, Marchesi F, et al. Long-term oral L-arginine administration improves peripheral and hepatic insulin sensitivity in type 2 diabetic patients. Diabetes Care. 2001;24(5):875–80.
374. Bohme GA, Bon C, Stutzmann JM, Doble A, Blanchard JC. Possible involvement of nitric oxide in long-term potentiation. Eur J Pharmacol. 1991;199(3):379–81.
375. Moncada S, Higgs A. The L-arginine–nitric oxide pathway. N Engl J Med. 1993;329(27):2002–12. [73] Campbell BI, La Bounty PM, Roberts M. The ergogenic potential of arginine. J Int Soc Sports Nutr 2004;1(2):35–8.
376. Campbell BI, La Bounty PM, Roberts M. The ergogenic potential of arginine. J Int Soc Sports Nutr. 2004;1(2):35–8.
377. Fossel ET. Improvement of temperature and flow in feet of subjects with diabetes with use of a transdermal preparation of L-arginine: a pilot study. Diabetes Care. 2004;27(1):284–5.
378. Klahr S. Can L-arginine manipulation reduce renal disease? Semin Nephrol. 1999;19(3):304–9.
379. Park KG, Hayes PD, Garlick PJ, Sewell H, Eremin O. Stimulation of lymphocyte natural cytotoxicity by L-arginine. Lancet. 1991;337(8742):645–6.

380. Gupta V, Gupta A, Saggu S, Divekar HM, Grover SK, Kumar R. Antistress and adaptogenic activity of L-arginine supplementation. Evid Based Complement Alternat Med. 2005;2(1):93–7.
381. Collier SR, Casey DP, Kanaley JA. Growth hormone responses to varying doses of oral arginine. Growth Hormon IGF Res. 2005;15(2):136–9.
382. Boger RH, Bode Boger SM. The clinical pharmacology of L-arginine. Annu Rev Pharmacol Toxicol. 2001;41:79–99.
383. Boger RH, Bode Boger SM, Mugge A, Kienke S, Brandes R, Dwenger A, et al. Supplementation of hypercholesterolaemic rabbits with L-arginine reduces the vascular release of superoxide anions and restores NO production. Atherosclerosis. 1995;117(2):273–84.
384. Grasemann H, Kurtz F, Ratjen F. Inhaled L-arginine improves exhaled nitric oxide and pulmonary function in patients with cystic fibrosis. Am J Respir Crit Care Med. 2006;174(2):208–12.
385. Shindel AW, Kishore S, Lue TF. Drugs designed to improve endothelial function: effects on erectile dysfunction. Curr Pharm Des. 2008;14(35):3758–67. Review.
386. Enzlin P, Mathieu C, Vanderschueren D, Demyttenaere K. Diabetes mellitus and female sexuality: a review of 25 years' research. Diabet Med. 1998;15(10):809–15.
387. Ryan JJ, Fang JC. Taking NO for an answer: exploring the therapeutic potential of nitrite in HFpEF. Circ Res. 2016;119(7):782–4. https://doi.org/10.1161/CIRCRESAHA.116.309623.
388. Gevaert AB, Shakeri H, Leloup AJ, Van Hove CE, De Meyer GRY, Vrints CJ, Lemmens K, Van Craenenbroeck EM. Endothelial senescence contributes to heart failure with preserved ejection fraction in an aging mouse model. Circ Heart Fail. 2017;10(6). pii: e003806. https://doi.org/10.1161/CIRCHEARTFAILURE.116.003806.
389. Octavia Y, Kararigas G, de Boer M, Chrifi I, Kietadisorn R, Swinnen M, Duimel H, Verheyen FK, Brandt MM, Fliegner D, Cheng C, Janssens S, Duncker DJ, Moens AL. Folic acid reduces doxorubicin-induced cardiomyopathy by modulating endothelial nitric oxide synthase. J Cell Mol Med. 2017. https://doi.org/10.1111/jcmm.13231. [Epub ahead of print].
390. Lahera V. Nitric oxide: a possible new biomarker in heart failure? Relationship with pulmonary hypertension secondary to left heart failure. Clin Investig Arterioscler. 2017;29(3):127–8. https://doi.org/10.1016/j.arteri.2017.04.001.
391. Kraehling JR, Sessa WC. Contemporary approaches to modulating the nitric oxide-cGMP pathway in cardiovascular disease. Circ Res. 2017;120(7):1174–82. https://doi.org/10.1161/CIRCRESAHA.117.303776. Review.
392. Ritchie RH, Drummond GR, Sobey CG, De Silva TM, Kemp-Harper BK. The opposing roles of NO and oxidative stress in cardiovascular disease. Pharmacol Res. 2017;116:57–69. https://doi.org/10.1016/j.phrs.2016.12.017. Epub 2016 Dec 15.
393. Sharma NM, Patel KP. Post-translational regulation of neuronal nitric oxide synthase: implications for sympathoexcitatory states. Expert Opin Ther Targets. 2017;21(1):11–22. Epub 2016 Dec 2. Review.
394. Zhang YH. Neuronal nitric oxide synthase in hypertension – an update. Clin Hypertens. 2016;22:20. eCollection 2016. Review.
395. Simon MA, Vanderpool RR, Nouraie M, Bachman TN, White PM, Sugahara M, Gorcsan J 3rd, Parsley EL, Gladwin MT. Acute hemodynamic effects of inhaled sodium nitrite in pulmonary hypertension associated with heart failure with preserved ejection fraction. JCI Insight. 2016;1(18):e89620.
396. Forte M, Conti V, Damato A, Ambrosio M, Puca AA, Sciarretta S, Frati G, Vecchione C, Carrizzo A. Targeting nitric oxide with natural derived compounds as a therapeutic strategy in vascular diseases. Oxidative Med Cell Longev. 2016;2016:7364138. https://doi.org/10.1155/2016/7364138. Epub 2016 Aug 29. Review.
397. Shabeeh H, Seddon M, Brett S, Melikian N, Casadei B, Shah AM, Chowienczyk P. Sympathetic activation increases NO release from eNOS but neither eNOS nor nNOS play an essential role in exercise hyperemia in the human forearm. Am J Physiol Heart Circ Physiol. 2013;304(9):H1225–30. https://doi.org/10.1152/ajpheart.00783.2012. Epub 2013 Feb 22.
398. Zhang YH, Jin CZ, Jang JH, Wang Y. Molecular mechanisms of neuronal nitric oxide synthase in cardiac function and pathophysiology. J Physiol. 2014;592(15):3189–200. https://doi.org/10.1113/jphysiol.2013.270306. Epub 2014 Apr 22. Review.
399. Mohan RM, Choate JK, Golding S, Herring N, Casadei B, Paterson DJ. Peripheral pre-synaptic pathway reduces the heart rate response to sympathetic activation following exercise training: role of NO. Cardiovasc Res. 2000;47:90–8.
400. Choate JK, Danson EJ, Morris JF, Paterson DJ. Peripheral vagal control of heart rate is impaired in neuronal NOS knockout mice. Am J Physiol Heart Circ Physiol. 2001;281:H2310–7.
401. Danson EJ, Choate JK, Paterson DJ. Cardiac nitric oxide: emerging role for nNOS in regulating physiological function. Pharmacol Ther. 2005;106:57–74.
402. Han G, Ma H, Chintala R, Miyake K, Fulton DJ, Barman SA, White RE. Nongenomic, endothelium-independent effects of estrogen on human coronary smooth muscle are mediated by type I (neuronal) NOS and PI3-kinase-Akt signalling. Am J Physiol Heart Circ Physiol. 2007;293:H314–21.
403. Seddon M, Melikian N, Dworakowski R, Shabeeh H, Jiang B, Byrne J, Casadei B, Chowienczyk P, Shah AM. Effects of neuronal nitric oxide synthase on human coronary artery diameter and blood flow in vivo. Circulation. 2009;119:2656–62.

404. Wang Y, Golledge J. Neuronal nitric oxide synthase and sympathetic nerve activity in neurovascular and metabolic systems. Curr Neurovasc Res. 2013;10(1):81–9. Review.
405. Pyner S. The paraventricular nucleus and heart failure. Exp Physiol. 2014;99(2):332–9. https://doi.org/10.1113/expphysiol.2013.072678. Epub 2013 Dec 6. Review.
406. Rocha BML, Cunha GJL, Menezes Falcão LF. The burden of iron deficiency in heart failure: therapeutic approach. J Am Coll Cardiol. 2018;71(7):782–93.
407. Hu PJ, Pittet JF, Kerby JD, Bosarge PL, Wagener BM. Acute brain trauma, lung injury and pneumonia: more than just altered mental status and decreased airway protection. Am J Physiol Lung Cell Mol Physiol. 2017. https://doi.org/10.1152/ajplung.00485.2016. [Epub ahead of print].
408. Pacher P, Beckman JS, Liaudet L. Nitric oxide and peroxynitrite in health and disease. Physiol Rev. 2007;87(1):315–424. Review.
409. Spanagel R. Alcoholism: a systems approach from molecular physiology to addictive behavior. Physiol Rev. 2009;89(2):649–705. https://doi.org/10.1152/physrev.00013.2008. Review.
410. Lee RH, Tseng TY, Wu CY, Chen PY, Chen MF, Kuo JS, Lee TJ. Memantine inhibits α3β2-nAChRs-mediated nitrergic neurogenic vasodilation in porcine basilar arteries. PLoS One. 2012;7(7):e40326. https://doi.org/10.1371/journal.pone.0040326. Epub 2012 Jul 5.
411. Filiano AJ, Gadani SP, Kipnis J. Interactions of innate and adaptive immunity in brain development and function. Brain Res. 2015;1617:18–27. https://doi.org/10.1016/j.brainres.2014.07.050. PMC 4320678. PMID 25110235.
412. Bowerman M, Vincent T, Scamps F, Perrin FE, Camu W, Raoul C. Neuroimmunity dynamics and the development of therapeutic strategies for amyotrophic lateral sclerosis. Front Cell Neurosci. 2013;7:214. https://doi.org/10.3389/fncel.2013.00214. Review.
413. Gehrmann J, Matsumoto Y, Kreutzberg GW. Microglia: intrinsic immuneffector cell of the brain. Brain Res Rev. 1995;20(3):269–87.
414. Mukherjee P, Cinelli MA, Kang S, Silverman RB. Development of nitric oxide synthase inhibitors for neurodegeneration and neuropathic pain. Chem Soc Rev. 2014;43(19):6814–38. https://doi.org/10.1039/c3cs60467e. Review.
415. Streit WJ. Microglial senescence: does the brain's immune system have an expiration date? Trends Neurosci. 2006;29(9):506–10.
416. Wood P. Neuroinflammation: mechanisms and management. Totowa: Humana Press; 2003.
417. Clark AK, Staniland AA, Marchand F, Kaan TKY, McMahon SB, Malcangio M. P2X7-dependent release of interleukin-1 and nociception in the spinal cord following lipopolysaccharide. J Neurosci. 2010;30(2):573–82.
418. Shigemoto-Mogami Y, Koizumi S, Tsuda M, Ohsawa K, Kohsaka S, Inoue K. Mechanisms underlying extracellular ATP-evoked interleukin-6 release in mouse microglial cell line, MG-5. J Neurochem. 2001;78(6):1339–49.
419. Hide I, Tanaka M, Inoue A, Nakajima K, Kohsaka S, Inoue K, Nakata Y. Extracellular ATP triggers tumor necrosis factor-α release from rat microglia. J Neurochem. 2002;75(3):965–72.
420. Gokce N. L-arginine and hypertension. J Nutr. 2004;134(10 Suppl):2807S–11S; discussion 2818S–2819S.
421. Higashi Y, Oshima T, Ozono R, et al. Aging and severity of hypertension attenuate endothelium-dependent renal vascular relaxation in humans. Hypertension. 1997;30(2 Pt 1):252–8.
422. Clarkson P, Adams MR, Powe AJ, et al. Oral L-arginine improves endothelium-dependent dilation in hypercholesterolemic young adults. J Clin Invest. 1996;97(8):1989–94.
423. Kawano H, Motoyama T, Hirai N, et al. Endothelial dysfunction in hypercholesterolemia is improved by L-arginine administration: possible role of oxidative stress. Atherosclerosis. 2002;161(2):375–80.
424. Adams MR, McCredie R, Jessup W, et al. Oral L-arginine improves endothelium-dependent dilatation and reduces monocyte adhesion to endothelial cells in young men with coronary artery disease. Atherosclerosis. 1997;129(2):261–9.
425. Sydow K, Mondon CE, Cooke JP. Insulin resistance: potential role of the endogenous nitric oxide synthase inhibitor ADMA. Vasc Med. 2005;10(Suppl 1):S35–43.
426. Piatti PM, Monti LD, Valsecchi G, et al. Long-term oral L-arginine administration improves peripheral and hepatic insulin sensitivity in type 2 diabetic patients. Diabetes Care. 2001;24(5):875–80.
427. Pieper GM, Siebeneich W, Dondlinger LA. Short-term oral administration of L-arginine reverses defective endothelium-dependent relaxation and cGMP generation in diabetes. Eur J Pharmacol. 1996;317(2–3):317–20.
428. Bode-Boger SM, Muke J, Surdacki A, et al. Oral L-arginine improves endothelial function in healthy individuals older than 70 years. Vasc Med. 2003;8(2):77–81.
429. Alvares TS, Meirelles CM, Bhambhani YN, et al. L-arginine as a potential ergogenic aid in healthy subjects. Sports Med. 2011;41(3):233–48.
430. Vallance P, Chan N. Endothelial function and nitric oxide: clinical relevance. Heart. 2001;85(3):342–50.
431. Boger RH, Cooke JP, Vallance P. ADMA: an emerging cardiovascular risk factor. Vasc Med. 2005;10(Suppl 1):S1–2.
432. Cooke JP. ADMA: its role in vascular disease. Vasc Med. 2005;10(Suppl 1):S11–7.
433. Boger RH. Asymmetric dimethylarginine, an endogenous inhibitor of nitric oxide synthase, explains the "L-arginine paradox" and acts as a novel cardiovascular risk factor. J Nutr. 2004;134(10 Suppl):2842S–7S; discussion 2853S.

434. Sibal L, Agarwal SC, Home PD, et al. The role of asymmetric dimethylarginine (ADMA) in endothelial dysfunction and cardiovascular disease. Curr Cardiol Rev. 2010;6(2):82–90.
435. Cooke JP. Asymmetrical dimethylarginine: the Uber marker? Circulation. 2004;109(15):1813–8.
436. Tran CT, Leiper JM, Vallance P. The DDAH/ADMA/NOS pathway. Atheroscler Suppl. 2003;4(4):33–40.
437. Hensley K, Floyd RA, editors. Methods in biological oxidative stress. Methods in pharmacology and toxicology. Totowa: Humana Press; 2010.
438. Rahal A, Kumar A, Singh V, Yadev B, Tiwari R, Chakraborty S, Dhama K. Oxidative stress, Prooxidants, and antioxidants: The interplay. Biomed Res Int. 2014, Article ID 761264, 19 pages.
439. Nicolson G. Mitochondrial dysfunction and chronic disease: treatment with natural supplements. Altern Ther Health Med. 2014;20(Suppl 1):18–25.
440. Parikh S, Goldstein A, Karaa A, Koenig MK, Anselm I, Brunel-Guitton C, Christodoulou J, Cohen BH, Dimmock D, Enns GM, Falk MJ, Feigenbaum A, Frye RE, Ganesh J, Griesemer D, Haas R, Horvath R, Korson M, Kruer MC, Mancuso M, McCormack S, Raboisson MJ, Reimschisel T, Salvarinova R, Saneto RP, Scaglia F, Shoffner J, Stacpoole PW, Sue CM, Tarnopolsky M, Van Karnebeek C, Wolfe LA, Cunningham ZZ, Rahman S, Chinnery PF. Patient care standards for primary mitochondrial disease: a consensus statement from the mitochondrial medicine society. Genet Med. 2017. https://doi.org/10.1038/gim.2017.107. [Epub ahead of print] Review.
441. Mammucari C, Gherardi G, Rizzuto R. Structure, activity regulation, and role of the mitochondrial calcium uniporter in health and disease. Front Oncol. 2017;7:139. https://doi.org/10.3389/fonc.2017.00139. eCollection 2017. Review.
442. Picca A, Lezza AMS, Leeuwenburgh C, Pesce V, Calvani R, Landi F, Bernabei R, Marzetti E. Fueling inflamm-aging through mitochondrial dysfunction: mechanisms and molecular targets. Int J Mol Sci. 2017;18(5). pii: E933. https://doi.org/10.3390/ijms18050933. Review.
443. Vatansever F, de Melo WC, Avci P, Vecchio D, Sadasivam M, Gupta A, Chandran R, Karimi M, Parizotto NA, Yin R, Tegos GP, Hamblin MR. Antimicrobial strategies centered around reactive oxygen species – bactericidal antibiotics, photodynamic therapy, and beyond. FEMS Microbiol Rev. 2013;37(6):955–89. https://doi.org/10.1111/1574-6976.12026. Epub 2013 Jul 25. Review.
444. Brynildsen MP, Winkler JA, Spina CS, MacDonald IC, Collins JJ. Potentiating antibacterial activity by predictably enhancing endogenous microbial ROS production. Nat Biotechnol. 2013;31(2):160–5. https://doi.org/10.1038/nbt.2458. Epub 2013 Jan 6.
445. Dizaj SM, Lotfipour F, Barzegar-Jalali M, Zarrintan MH, Adibkia K. Antimicrobial activity of the metals and metal oxide nanoparticles. Mater Sci Eng C Mater Biol Appl. 2014;44:278–84. https://doi.org/10.1016/j.msec.2014.08.031. Epub 2014 Aug 16. Review.
446. Dan Dunn J, Alvarez LA, Zhang X, Soldati T. Reactive oxygen species and mitochondria: a nexus of cellular homeostasis. Redox Biol. 2015;6:472–85. https://doi.org/10.1016/j.redox.2015.09.005. Epub 2015 Sept 10. Review.
447. D'Autréaux B, Toledano MB. ROS as signalling molecules: mechanisms that generate specificity in ROS homeostasis. Nat Rev Mol Cell Biol. 2007;8(10):813–24. Review.
448. Liou GY, Storz P. Reactive oxygen species in cancer. Free Radic Res. 2010;44(5):479–96. https://doi.org/10.3109/10715761003667554. Review.
449. Hafstad AD, Nabeebaccus AA, Shah AM. Novel aspects of ROS signalling in heart failure. Basic Res Cardiol. 2013;108(4):359. https://doi.org/10.1007/s00395-013-0359-8. Epub 2013 Jun 6. Review.
450. Zhang M, Shah AM. ROS signalling between endothelial cells and cardiac cells. Cardiovasc Res. 2014;102(2):249–57. https://doi.org/10.1093/cvr/cvu050. Epub 2014 Mar 3. Review.
451. Meeus M, Nijs J, Hermans L, Goubert D, Calders P. The role of mitochondrial dysfunctions due to oxidative and nitrosative stress in the chronic pain or chronic fatigue syndromes and fibromyalgia patients: peripheral and central mechanisms as therapeutic targets? Expert Opin Ther Targets. 2013;17(9):1081–9. https://doi.org/10.1517/14728222.2013.818657. Epub 2013 Jul 9. Review.
452. Tanaka M, Tajima S, Mizuno K, Ishii A, Konishi Y, Miike T, Watanabe Y. Frontier studies on fatigue, autonomic nerve dysfunction, and sleep-rhythm disorder. J Physiol Sci. 2015;65(6):483–98. https://doi.org/10.1007/s12576-015-0399-y. Epub 2015 Sept 29. Review.
453. Van Cauwenbergh D, Nijs J, Kos D, Van Weijnen L, Struyf F, Meeus M. Malfunctioning of the autonomic nervous system in patients with chronic fatigue syndrome: a systematic literature review. Eur J Clin Investig. 2014;44(5):516–26. https://doi.org/10.1111/eci.12256. Review.
454. El-Hattab AW, Scaglia F. Mitochondrial cardiomyopathies. Front Cardiovasc Med. 2016;3:25. https://doi.org/10.3389/fcvm.2016.00025. eCollection 2016. Review.
455. Sharafati-Chaleshtori R, Shirzad H, Rafieian-Kopaei M, Soltani A. Melatonin and human mitochondrial diseases. J Res Med Sci. 2017;22:2. https://doi.org/10.4103/1735-1995.199092. eCollection 2017. Review.
456. Frye RE, Rossignol DA. Mitochondrial dysfunction can connect the diverse medical symptoms associated with autism spectrum disorders. Pediatr Res. 2011;69(5 Pt 2):41R–7R. https://doi.org/10.1203/PDR.0b013e318212f16b. Review.
457. Martínez-Martínez LA, Mora T, Vargas A, Fuentes-Iniestra M, Martínez-Lavín M. Sympathetic nervous system dysfunction in fibromyalgia, chronic fatigue syndrome, irritable bowel syndrome, and

interstitial cystitis: a review of case-control studies. J Clin Rheumatol. 2014;20(3):146–50. https://doi.org/10.1097/RHU.0000000000000089. Review.
458. Zsurka G, Kunz WS. Mitochondrial dysfunction and seizures: the neuronal energy crisis. Lancet Neurol. 2015;14(9):956–66. https://doi.org/10.1016/S1474-4422(15)00148-9. Review.
459. Murphy MP. Understanding and preventing mitochondrial oxidative damage. Biochem Soc Trans. 2016;44(5):1219–26. Review.
460. Li AN, Li S, Zhang YJ, Xu XR, Chen YM, Li HB. Resources and biological activities of natural polyphenols. Nutrients. 2014;6:6020–47.
461. Feng Y, Wang N, Ye X, Li H, Feng Y, Cheung F, Nagamatsu T. Hepatoprotective effect and its possible mechanism of Coptidis rhizoma aqueous extract on carbon tetrachloride-induced chronic liver hepatotoxicity in rats. J Ethnopharmacol. 2011;138:683–90.
462. Singal AK, Jampana SC, Weinman SA. Antioxidants as therapeutic agents for liver disease. Liver Int. 2011;31:1432–48.
463. Medina J, Moreno-Otero R. Pathophysiological basis for antioxidant therapy in chronic liver disease. Drugs. 2005;65:2445–61.
464. Li S, Tan HY, Wang N, Zhang ZJ, Lao L, Wong CW, Feng Y. The role of oxidative stress and antioxidants in liver diseases. Int J Mol Sci. 2015;16(11):26087–124. https://doi.org/10.3390/ijms161125942. Review.
465. Al-Dalaen SM, Al-Qtaitat AI. Review article: oxidative stress versus antioxidants. Am J Biosci Bioeng. 2014;2(5):60–71.
466. Sindhi V, Gupta V, Sharma K, Bhatnagar S, Kumari R, Dhaka N. Potential applications of antioxidants – a review. J Pharm Res. 2013;7(9):828–835. ISSN 0974-6943. https://doi.org/10.1016/j.jopr.2013.10.001.
467. Villamena FA. Molecular basis of oxidative stress: chemistry, mechanisms, and disease pathogenesis. Hoboken: John Wiley & Sons, Inc.; 2013.
468. Carr AC, McCall MR, Frei B. Oxidation of LDL by myeloperoxidase and reactive nitrogen species: reaction pathways and antioxidant protection. Arterioscler Thromb Vasc Biol. 2000;20:1716–23.
469. Daugherty A, Dunn JL, Rateri DL, Heinecke JW. Myeloperoxidase, a catalyst for lipoprotein oxidation, is expressed in human atherosclerotic lesions. J Clin Invest. 1994;94:437–44.
470. Adly AAM. Oxidative stress and disease: an updated review. Res J Immunol. 2010;3:129–45.
471. Ho E, Karimi Galougahi K, Liu CC, Bhindi R, Figtree GA. Biological markers of oxidative stress: applications to cardiovascular research and practice. Redox Biol. 2013;1:483–91. https://doi.org/10.1016/j.redox.2013.07.006. Review.
472. Kirkman HN, Gaetani GF. Mammalian catalase: a venerable enzyme with new mysteries. Trends Biochem Sci. 2007;32(1):44–50. Epub 2006 Dec 8. Review.
473. Sonoda J, Pei L, Evans RM. Nuclear receptors: decoding metabolic disease. FEBS Lett. 2008;582(1):2–9.
474. Cai D. NFkappaB-mediated metabolic inflammation in peripheral tissues versus central nervous system. Cell Cycle. 2009;8:2542–8.
475. Lumeng CN, Saltiel AR. Inflammatory links between obesity and metabolic disease. J Clin Invest. 2011;121(6):2111–7.
476. Cai D, Liu T. Inflammatory cause of metabolic syndrome via brain stress and NF-κB. Aging. 2012;4(2):98–115.
477. Zhang X, Zhang G, Zhang H, Karin M, Bai H, Cai D. Hypothalamic IKKbeta/NF-kappaB and ER stress link overnutrition to energy imbalance and obesity. Cell. 2008;135:61–73.
478. DeSouza CT, Araujo EP, Bordin S, et al. Consumption of a fat-rich diet activates a proinflammatory response and induces insulin resistance in the hypothalamus. Endocrinology. 2005;146(10):4192–9.
479. Belgardt BF, Mauer J, Wunderlich FT, et al. Hypothalamic and pituitary c-Jun N-terminal kinase 1 signaling coordinately regulates glucose metabolism. Proc Natl Acad Sci U S A. 2010;107(13):6028–33.
480. Ozcan U, Yilmaz E, Ozcan L, et al. Chemical chaperones reduce ER stress and restore glucose homeostasis in a mouse model of type 2 diabetes. Science. 2006;313(5790):1137–40.
481. Lin MT, Beal MF. Mitochondrial dysfunction and oxidative stress in neurodegenerative diseases. Nature. 2006;443(7113):787–95.
482. Brown MK, Naidoo N. The endoplasmic reticulum stress response in aging and age-related diseases. Front Physiol. 2012;3:263.
483. Cadenas E, Davies KJA. Mitochondrial free radical generation, oxidative stress, and aging. Free Radic Biol Med. 2000;29(3–4):222–30.
484. Hotamisligil GS. Endoplasmic reticulum stress and the inflammatory bas is of metabolic disease. Cell. 2010;140(6):900–17.
485. Tabas I, Ron D. Integrating the mechanisms of apoptosis induced by endoplasmic reticulum stress. Nat Cell Biol. 2011;13(3):184–90.
486. Meng Y, Yong Y, Yang G, et al. Autophagy alleviates neurodegeneration caused by mild impairment of oxidative metabolism. J Neurochem. 2013;126(6):805–18.
487. Rao RV, Ellerby HM, Bredesen DE. Coupling endoplasmic reticulum stress to the cell death program. Cell Death Differ. 2004;11(4):372–80.
488. Purkayastha S, Zhang G, Cai D. Uncoupling the mechanisms of obesity and hypertension by targeting hypothalamic IKK-beta and NF-kappaB. Nat Med. 2011;17:883–7.
489. Cullinan SB, Diehl JA. Coordination of ER and oxidative stress signaling: the PERK/Nrf2 signaling pathway. Int J Biochem Cell Biol. 2006;38(3):317–32.
490. Muriach M, Flores-Bellver M, Romero FJ, Barcia JM. Diabetes and the brain: oxidative stress,

inflammation, and autophagy. Oxidative Med Cell Longev. 2014;2014:102158. https://doi.org/10.1155/2014/102158. Epub 2014 Aug 24. Review.
491. Halliwell B, Gutteridge J. Free radicals in biology and medicine. Oxford: Oxford University Press; 2007.
492. Powers SK, Jackson MJ. Exercise-induced oxidative stress: cellular mechanisms and impact on muscle force production. Physiol Rev. 2008;88(4):1243–76. https://doi.org/10.1152/physrev.00031.2007. Review.
493. Alam MN, Bristi NJ, Rafiquzzaman M. Review on in vivo and in vitro methods evaluation of antioxidant activity. Saudi Pharm J. 2013;21(2):143–52. https://doi.org/10.1016/j.jsps.2012.05.002. Epub 2012 Jun 15.
494. Davies MJ, Fu S, Wang H, Dean RT. Stable markers of oxidant damage to proteins and their application in the study of human disease. Free Radic Biol Med. 1999;27:1151–63.
495. Diplock AT. Introduction: markers of oxidative damage and antioxidant modulation. Free Radic Res. 2000;33(Suppl):S21–6.
496. Han D, Loukianoff S, McLaughlin L. Oxidative stress indices: analytical aspects and significance. In: Sen CK, Packer L, Hanninen O, editors. Handbook of oxidants and antioxidants in exercise. Amsterdam: Elsevier; 2000. p. 433–83.
497. Hwang ES, Kim GH. Biomarkers for oxidative stress status of DNA, lipids, proteins in vitro and in vivo cancer research. Toxicology. 2007;229:1–10.
498. Jones DP. Redefining oxidative stress. Antioxid Redox Signal. 2006;8:1865–79.
499. Lawson JA, Rokach J, FitzGerald GA. Isoprostanes: formation, analysis and use as indices of lipid peroxidation in vivo. J Biol Chem. 1999;274:24441–4.
500. Roberts LJ, Morrow JD. Measurement of F(2)-isoprostanes as an index of oxidative stress in vivo. Free Radic Biol Med. 2000;28:505–13.
501. Sachdev S, Davies KJ. Production, detection, adaptive responses to free radicals in exercise. Free Radic Biol Med. 2008;44:215–23.
502. Kasai H. Analysis of a form of oxidative DNA damage, 8-hydroxy-2′-deoxyguanosine, as a marker of cellular oxidative stress during carcinogenesis. Mutat Res. 1997;387:147–63.
503. Cheng J, Wang F, Yu DF, Wu PF, Chen JG. The cytotoxic mechanism of malondialdehyde and protective effect of carnosine via protein crosslinking/mitochondrial dysfunction/reactive oxygen species/AMPK pathway in neurons. Eur J Pharmacol. 2011;650:184–94.
504. Long EK, Murphy TC, Leiphon LJ, Watt J, Morrow JD, Milne GL, Howard JRH, Picklo MJ. Trans-4-hydroxy-2-hexenal is a neurotoxic product of docosahexaenoic (22:6; n-3) acid oxidation. J Neurochem. 2008;105:714–24.
505. Bae EH, Cho S, Joo SY, Ma SK, Kim SH, Lee J, Kim SW. 4-Hydroxy-2-hexenalinduced apoptosis in human renal proximal tubular epithelial cells. Nephrol Dial Transplant. 2011;26:3866–73.
506. Uchida K, Shiraishi M, Naito Y, Torii Y, Nakamura Y, Osawa T. Activation of stress signaling pathways by the end product of lipid peroxidation. 4-hydroxy-2-nonenal is a potential inducer of intracellular peroxide production. J Biol Chem. 1999;274:2234–42.
507. Lee JY, Jung GY, Heo HJ, Yun MR, Park JY, Bae SS, Hong KW, Lee WS, Kim CD. 4-Hydroxynonenal induces vascular smooth muscle cell apoptosis through mitochondrial generation of reactive oxygen species. Toxicol Lett. 2006;166:212–21.
508. Pillon NJ, Croze ML, Vella RE, Soulère L, Lagarde M, Soulage CO. The lipid peroxidation by-product 4-hydroxy-2-nonenal (4-HNE) induces insulin resistance in skeletal muscle through both carbonyl and oxidative stress. Endocrinology. 2012;153:2099–111.
509. Luo J, Robinson JP, Shi R. Acrolein-induced cell death in PC12 cells: role of mitochondria-mediated oxidative stress. Neurochem Int. 2005;47:449–57.
510. Kostyuk V, Potapovich A, Cesareo E, Brescia S, Guerra L, Valacchi G, Pecorelli A, Raskovic D, De Luca C, Pastore S, Korkina L. Dysfunction of glutathione S-transferase leads to excess 4-hydroxy-2-nonenal and H2O2 and impaired cytokine pattern in cultured keratinocytes and blood of vitiligo patients. Antioxid Redox Signal. 2010. https://doi.org/10.1089/ars.2009.2976.
511. Curtis JM, Grimsrud PA, Wright WS, Xu X, Foncea RE, Graham DW, Brestoff JR, Wiczer BM, Ilkayeva O, Cianflone K, Muoio DE, Arriaga EA, Bernlohr DA. Downregulation of adipose glutathione S-transferase A4 leads to increased protein carbonylation, oxidative stress, and mitochondrial dysfunction. Diabetes. 2010;59:1132–42.
512. Furukawa S, Fujita T, Shimabukuro M, Iwaki M, Yamada Y, Nakajima Y, Nakayama O, Makishima M, Matsuda M, Shimomura I. Increased oxidative stress in obesity and its impact on metabolic syndrome. J Clin Invest. 2004;114:1752–61.
513. Wellen KE, Hotamisligil GS. Obesity-induced inflammatory changes in adipose tissue. J Clin Invest. 2003;112:1785–8.
514. Soares AF, Guichardant M, Cozzone D, Bernoud-Hubac N, Bouzaidi-Tiali N, Lagarde M, Geloen A. Effects of oxidative stress on adiponectin secretion and lactate production in 3T3-L1 adipocytes. Free Radic Biol Med. 2005;38:882–9.
515. Wang Z, Dou X, Gu D, Shen C, Yao T, Nguyen V, Braunschweig C, Song Z. 4-Hydroxynonenal differentially regulates adiponectin gene expression and secretion via activating PPARγ and accelerating ubiquitin-proteasome degradation. Mol Cell Endocrinol. 2012;349:222–31.
516. Trevisan M, Browne R, Ram M, Muti P, Freudenheim J, Carosella AM, Armstrong D. Correlates of markers of oxidative status in the general population. Am J Epidemiol. 2001;154:348–56.

517. Menon V, Ram M, Dorn J, Armstrong D, Muti P, Freudenheim JL, Browne R, Schunemann H, Trevisan M. Oxidative stress and glucose levels in a population-based sample. Diabet Med. 2004;21:1346–52.
518. Maxwell SR, Thomason H, Sandler D, Leguen C, Baxter MA, Thorpe GH, Jones AF, Barnett AH. Antioxidant status in patients with uncomplicated insulin-dependent and non-insulin-dependent diabetes mellitus. Eur J Clin Investig. 1997;27:484–90.
519. Dierckx N, Horvath G, van Gils C, Vertommen J, van de Vliet J, De Leeuw I, Manuel-y-Keenoy B. Oxidative stress status in patients with diabetes mellitus: relationship to diet. Eur J Clin Nutr. 2003;57:999–1008.
520. Kamenova P. Improvement of insulin sensitivity in patients with type 2 diabetes mellitus after oral administration of alpha-lipoic acid. Hormones (Athens). 2006;5:251–8.
521. Vincent HK, Bourguignon CM, Weltman AL, Vincent KR, Barrett E, Innes KE, Taylor AG. Effects of antioxidant supplementation on insulin sensitivity, endothelial adhesion molecules, and oxidative stress in normal-weight and overweight young adults. Metab Clin Exp. 2009;58:254–62.
522. Bashan N, Kovsan J, Kachko I, Ovadia H, Rudich A. Positive and negative regulation of insulin signaling by reactive oxygen and nitrogen species. Physiol Rev. 2009;89:27–71.
523. Zimniak P. 4-Hydroxynonenal and fat storage: a paradoxical pro-obesity mechanism? Cell Cycle. 2010;9:3393–4.
524. Jacob S, Streeper RS, Fogt DL, Hokama JY, Tritschler HJ, Dietze GJ, Henriksen EJ. The antioxidant alpha-lipoic acid enhances insulin-stimulated glucose metabolism in insulin-resistant rat skeletal muscle. Diabetes. 1996;45:1024–9.
525. Ziegler D, Gries F. Alpha-lipoic acid and the treatment of diabetic peripheral autonomic cardiac neuropathy. Diabetes. 1997;46(Suppl 2):S62–6.
526. Prendergast JJ. Diabetic autonomic neuropathy: part 1. Early detection. Pract Diabetol. 2001;20(1):7–14.
527. Prendergast JJ. Diabetic autonomic neuropathy: part 2. Treatment. Pract Diabetol. 2001:30–6.
528. Ziegler D, Ametov A, Barinov A, Dyck PJ, Gurieva I, Low PA, Munzel U, Yakhno N, Raz I, Novosadova M, Maus J, Samigullin R. Oral treatment with alpha-lipoic acid improves symptomatic diabetic polyneuropathy: The SYDNEY 2 trial. Diabetes Care. 2006;29(11):2365–70.
529. Ametov AS, Barinov A, Dyck PJ, Hermann R, Kozlova N, Litchy WJ, Low PA, Nehrdich D, Novosadova M, O'Brien PC, Reljanovic M, Samigullin R, Schuette K, Strokov I, Tritschler HJ, Wessel K, Yakhno N, Ziegler D, SYDNEY Trial Study Group. The sensory symptoms of diabetic polyneuropathy are improved with alpha-lipoic acid. The SYDNEY trial. Diabetes Care. 2003;26(3):770–6.
530. Ziegler D, Low PA, Litchy WJ, Boulton AJM, Vinik AI, Freeman R, The NATHAN 1 Trial Group. Efficacy and safety of antioxidant treatment with α-lipoic acid over 4 years in diabetic polyneuropathy. Diabetes Care. 2011;34:2054–60.
531. Manning PJ, Sutherland WHF, Walker RJ, Williams SM, De Jong SA, Ryalls AR, Berry EA. Effect of high-dose vitamin E on insulin resistance and associated parameters in overweight subjects. Diabetes Care. 2004;27:2166–71.
532. Rudich A, Tirosh A, Potashnik R, Khamaisi M, Bashan N. Lipoic acid protects against oxidative stress induced impairment in insulin stimulation of protein kinase B and glucose transport in 3T3-L1 adipocytes. Diabetologia. 1999;42:949–57.
533. Maddux BA, See W, Lawrence JC Jr, Goldfine AL, Goldfine ID, Evans JL. Protection against oxidative stress-induced insulin resistance in rat L6 muscle cells by micromolar concentrations of alpha-lipoic acid. Diabetes. 2001;50:404–10.
534. Jungas T, Motta I, Duffieux F, Fanen P, Stoven V, Ojcius DM. Glutathione levels and BAX activation during apoptosis due to oxidative stress in cells expressing wild-type and mutant cystic fibrosis transmembrane conductance regulator. J Biol Chem. 2002;277:27912–8.
535. Dominy JE, Hwang J, Stipanuk MH. Overexpression of cysteine dioxygenase reduces intracellular cysteine and glutathione pools in HepG2/C3A cells. Am J Physiol Endocrinol Metab. 2007;293:E62–9.
536. Miyata T, Izuhara Y, Sakai H, Kurokawa K. Carbonyl stress: increased carbonyl modification of tissue and cellular proteins in uremia. Perit Dial Int. 1999;19(Suppl 2):S58–61.
537. Kirkham PA, Barnes PJ. Oxidative stress in COPD. Chest. 2013;144(1):266–73. https://doi.org/10.1378/chest.12-2664. Review.
538. Ziegler D, Gries F. Alpha-lipoic acid and the treatment of diabetic peripheral autonomic cardiac neuropathy. Diabetes. 1997;46(Suppl 2):S62–6.
539. Ziegler D, Ametov A, Barinov A, Dyck PJ, Gurieva I, Low PA, Munzel U, Yakhno N, Raz I, Novosadova M, Maus J, Samigullin R. Oral treatment with alpha-lipoic acid improves symptomatic diabetic polyneuropathy: the SYDNEY 2 trial. Diabetes Care. 2006;29(11):2365–70.
540. Ametov AS, Barinov A, Dyck PJ, Hermann R, Kozlova N, Litchy WJ, Low PA, Nehrdich D, Novosadova M, O'Brien PC, Reljanovic M, Samigullin R, Schuette K, Strokov I, Tritschler HJ, Wessel K, Yakhno N, Ziegler D, SYDNEY Trial Study Group. The sensory symptoms of diabetic polyneuropathy are improved with alpha-lipoic acid. The SYDNEY trial. Diabetes Care. 2003;26(3):770–6.
541. Ziegler D, Low PA, Litchy WJ, Boulton AJM, Vinik AI, Freeman R, The NATHAN 1 Trial Group. Efficacy and safety of antioxidant treatment with α-lipoic acid over 4 years in diabetic polyneuropathy. Diabetes Care. 2011;34:2054–60.

542. Ali AM, Awad TG, Al-Adl NM. Efficacy of combined topiramate/thioctic acid therapy in migraine prophylaxis. Saudi Pharm J. 2010;18(4):239–43. https://doi.org/10.1016/j.jsps.2010.07.006. Epub 2010 Jul 30.
543. Mahboob A, Farhat SM, Iqbal G, Babar MM, Zaidi NU, Nabavi SM, Ahmed T. Alpha-lipoic acid-mediated activation of muscarinic receptors improves hippocampus- and amygdala-dependent memory. Brain Res Bull. 2016;122:19–28. https://doi.org/10.1016/j.brainresbull.2016.02.014. Epub 2016 Feb 18.
544. Kuhla A, Derbenev M, Shih HY, Vollmar B. Prophylactic and abundant intake of α-lipoic acid causes hepatic steatosis and should be reconsidered in usage as an anti-aging drug. Biofactors. 2016;42(2):179–89. https://doi.org/10.1002/biof.1262. Epub 2016 Feb 15.
545. Logan AC, Wong C. Chronic fatigue syndrome: oxidative stress and dietary modifications. Altern Med Rev. 2001;6(5):450–9. Review.
546. Hiller S, DeKroon R, Hamlett ED, Xu L, Osorio C, Robinette J, Winnik W, Simington S, Maeda N, Alzate O, Yi X. Alpha-lipoic acid supplementation protects enzymes from damage by nitrosative and oxidative stress. Biochim Biophys Acta. 2016;1860(1 Pt A):36–45. https://doi.org/10.1016/j.bbagen.2015.09.001. Epub 2015 Sept 4.
547. Wollen KA. Alzheimer's disease: the pros and cons of pharmaceutical, nutritional, botanical, and stimulatory therapies, with a discussion of treatment strategies from the perspective of patients and practitioners. Altern Med Rev. 2010;15(3):223–44. Review.
548. Ajith TA, Padmajanair G. Mitochondrial pharmaceutics: a new therapeutic strategy to ameliorate oxidative stress in Alzheimer's disease. Curr Aging Sci. 2015;8(3):235–40. Review.
549. Li YH, He Q, Yu JZ, Liu CY, Feng L, Chai Z, Wang Q, Zhang HZ, Zhang GX, Xiao BG, Ma CG. Lipoic acid protects dopaminergic neurons in LPS-induced Parkinson's disease model. Metab Brain Dis. 2015;30(5):1217–26. https://doi.org/10.1007/s11011-015-9698-5. Epub 2015 Jun 19.
550. Zhao H, Zhao X, Liu L, Zhang H, Xuan M, Guo Z, Wang H, Liu C. Neurochemical effects of the R form of α-lipoic acid and its neuroprotective mechanism in cellular models of Parkinson's disease. Int J Biochem Cell Biol. 2017;87:86–94. https://doi.org/10.1016/j.biocel.2017.04.002. Epub 2017 Apr 6.
551. Zhao H, Zhao X, Liu L, Zhang H, Xuan M, Guo Z, Wang H, Liu C. Neurochemical effects of the R form of α-lipoic acid and its neuroprotective mechanism in cellular models of Parkinson's disease. Int J Biochem Cell Biol. 2017;87:86–94. https://doi.org/10.1016/j.biocel.2017.04.002. Epub 2017 Apr 6.
552. Namazi N, Larijani B, Azadbakht L. Alpha-lipoic acid supplement in obesity treatment: a systematic review and meta-analysis of clinical trials. Clin Nutr. 2017. pii: S0261-5614(17)30212-1. https://doi.org/10.1016/j.clnu.2017.06.002. [Epub ahead of print] Review.
553. DePace NL, Mears JP, Yayac M, Colombo J. Cardiac autonomic testing and diagnosing heart disease. "A clinical perspective.". Heart Int. 2014;9(2):37–44. https://doi.org/10.5301/heartint.5000218; published online 12/5/2014 12:29:58 PM.
554. DePace NL, Mears JP, Yayac M, Colombo J. Cardiac autonomic testing and treating heart disease. "A clinical perspective.". Heart Int. 2014;9(2):45–52. https://doi.org/10.5301/heartint.5000216; published online 11/19/2014 1:16:08 PM.
555. Sorescu D, Weiss D, Lassegue B, Clempus RE, Szocs K, Sorescu GP, Valppu L, Quinn MT, Lambeth JD, Vega JD, Taylor WR, Griendling KK. Superoxide production and expression of Nox family proteins in human atherosclerosis. Circulation. 2002;105:1429–35.
556. Li H, Wallerath T, Münzel T, Förstermann U. Regulation of endothelial-type NO synthase expression in pathophysiology and in response to drugs. Nitric Oxide Biol Chem. 2002;7:149–64.
557. Drummond GR, Cai H, Davis ME, Ramasamy S, Harrison DG. Transcriptional and posttranscriptional regulation of endothelial nitric oxide synthase expression by hydrogen peroxide. Circ Res. 2000;86:347–54.
558. Förstermann U, Münzel T. Endothelial nitric oxide synthase in vascular disease: from marvel to menace. Circulation. 2006;113:1708–14.
559. Riha RL, Diefenbach K, Jennum P, et al. Genetic aspects of hypertension and metabolic disease in the obstructive sleep apnoea-hypopnoea syndrome. Sleep Med Rev. 2008;12:49–63.
560. Goldbart AD, Row BW, Kheirandish-Gozal L, et al. High fat/refined carbohydrate diet enhances the susceptibility to spatial learning deficits in rats exposed to intermittent hypoxia. Brain Res. 2006;1090:190–6.
561. Somers VK, Mark AL, Abboud FM. Sympathetic activation by hypoxia and hypercapnia – implications for sleep apnea. Clin Exp Hypertens A. 1988;10(Suppl. 1):413–22.
562. Hedner J, Darpo B, Ejnell H, et al. Reduction in sympathetic activity after long-term CPAP treatment in sleep apnoea: cardiovascular implications. Eur Respir J. 1995;8:222–9.
563. Carlson JT, Hedner J, Elam M, et al. Augmented resting sympathetic activity in awake patients with obstructive sleep apnea. Chest. 1993;103:1763–8.
564. Narkiewicz K, Somers VK. Obstructive sleep apnea as a cause of neurogenic hypertension. Curr Hypertens Rep. 1999;1:268–73.
565. Lavie L, Lavie P. Molecular mechanisms of cardiovascular disease in OSAHS: the oxidative stress link. Eur Respir J. 2009;33:1467–84.
566. Tsuji H, Venditti FJ Jr, Manders ES, Evans JC, Larson MG, Feldman CL, Levy D. Reduced heart rate variability and mortality risk in an elderly

cohort. The Framingham Heart Study. Circulation. 1994;90(2):878–83.

567. Vinik AI, Maser RE, Mitchell BD, Freeman R. Diabetic autonomic neuropathy. Diabetes Care. 2003;26(5):1553–79.
568. Maser R, Mitchell B, Vinik AI, Freeman R. The association between cardiovascular autonomic neuropathy and mortality in individuals with diabetes, a meta-analysis. Diabetes Care. 2003;26(6):1895–901.
569. Bullinga JR, Alharethi R, Schram MS, Bristow MR, Gilbert EM. Changes in heart rate variability are correlated to hemodynamic improvement with chronic CARVEDILOL therapy in heart failure. J Card Fail. 2005;11(9):693–9.
570. Fatoni C, Raffa S, Regoli F, Giraldi F, La Rovere MT, Prentice J, Pastori F, Fratini S, Salerno-Uriarte JA, Klein HU, Auricchio A. Cardiac resynchronization therapy improves heart rate profile and heart rate variability of patients with moderate to severe heart failure. J Am Coll Cardiol. 2005;46(10):1875–82.
571. Fathizadeh P, Shoemaker WC, Woo CCJ, Colombo J. Autonomic activity in trauma patients based on variability of heart rate and respiratory rate. Crit Care Med. 2004;32(5):1300–5.
572. Chen JY, Fung JW, Yu CM. The mechanisms of atrial fibrillation. J Cardiovasc Electrophysiol. 2006;17(Suppl 3):S2–7.
573. Copie X, Lamaison D, Salvador M, Sadoul N, DaCosta A, Faucher L, Legal F, Le Heuzey JY, VALID Investigators. Heart rate variability before ventricular arrhythmias in patients with coronary artery disease and an implantable cardioverter defibrillator. Ann Noninvasive Electrocardiol. 2003;8(3):179–84.
574. Alter P, Grimm W, Vollrath A, Czerny F, Maisch B. Heart rate variability in patients with cardiac hypertrophy – relation to left ventricular mass and etiology. Am Heart J. 2006;151(4):829–36.
575. Debono M, Cachia E. The impact of cardiovascular autonomic neuropathy in diabetes: is it associated with left ventricular dysfunction? Auton Neurosci. 2007;132(1–2):1–7.
576. Just H. Peripheral adaptations in congestive heart failure: a review. Am J Med. 1991;90:23S–6S.
577. Nakamura K, Matsumura K, Kobayashi S, Kaneko T. Sympathetic premotor neurons mediating thermoregulatory functions. Neurosci Res. 2005;51(1):1–8.
578. Manfrini O, Morgagni G, Pizzi C, Fontana F, Bugiardini R. Changes in autonomic nervous system activity: spontaneous versus balloon-induced myocardial ischemia. Eur Heart J. 2004;25(17):1502–8.
579. Clarke B, Ewing D, Campbell I. Diabetic autonomic neuropathy. Diabetologia. 1979;17:195–212.
580. Arora R. Recent insights into the role of the autonomic nervous system in the creation of substrate for atrial fibrillation. Implications for therapies targeting the atrial autonomic nervous system. Circ Arrhythm Electrophysiol. 2012;5:850–9.
581. Ng J, Villuendas R, Cokic I, Schliamser JE, Gordon D, Koduri H, Benefield B, Simon J, Murthy SN, Lomasney JW, Wasserstrom JA, Goldberger JJ, Aistrup GL, Arora R. Autonomic remodeling in the left atrium and pulmonary veins in heart failure: creation of a dynamic substrate for atrial fibrillation. Circ Arrhythm Electrophysiol. 2011;4:388–96.
582. Kishi T, Hirooks Y. Oxidative stress in the brain causes hypertension via sympathoexcitation. Front Physiol. 2012;17:335. https://doi.org/10.3389/fphys.2012.00335. eCollection 2012.
583. Kishi T, Hirooka Y, Sakai K, Shigematsu H, Shimokawa H, Takeshita A. Overexpression of eNOS in the RVLM causes hypotension and bradycardia via GABA release. Hypertension. 2001;38:896–901.
584. Patel K, Li YF, Hirooka Y. Role of nitric oxide in central sympathetic outflow. Exp Biol Med. 2001;226:814–24.
585. Li DP, Chen SR, Pan HL. Nitric oxide inhibits spinally projecting paraventricular neurons through potentiation of presynaptic GABA release. J Neurophysiol. 2002;88:2664–74.
586. Garthwaite J. Concepts of neural nitric oxide-mediated transmission. Eur J Neurosci. 2008;27:2783–802.
587. Kimura Y, Hirooka Y, Sagara Y, Ito K, Kishi T, Shimokawa H, Takeshita A, Sunagawa K. Overexpression of inducible nitric oxide synthase in rostral ventrolateral medulla causes hypertension and sympathoexcitation via an increase in oxidative stress. Circ Res. 2005;96:252–60.
588. Oliveira-Sales EB, Colombari DSA, Davisson RL, Kasparov S, Hirata AE, Campos RR, Paton JFR. Kidney-induced hypertension depends on superoxide signaling in the rostral ventrolateral medulla. Hypertension. 2010;56:290–6.
589. Golbidi S, Frisbee JC, Laher XI. Chronic stress impacts the cardiovascular system: animal models and clinical outcomes. Review. Am J Physiol Heart Circ Physiol. 2015;308:H1476–98.
590. Gao L, Mao Q, Cao J, Wang Y, Zhou X, Fan L. Effects of coenzyme Q10 on vascular endothelial function in humans: a meta-analysis of randomized controlled trials. Atherosclerosis. 2012;221(2):311–6. https://doi.org/10.1016/j.atherosclerosis.2011.
591. Zhou M, Zhi Q, Tang Y, Yu D, Han J. Effects of coenzyme Q10 on myocardial protection during cardiac valve replacement and scavenging free radical activity in vitro. J Cardiovasc Surg. 1999;40(3):355–61.
592. Rosenfeldt F, Marasco S, Lyon W, Wowk M, Sheeran F, Bailey M, Esmore D, Davis B, Pick A, Rabinov M, Smith J, Nagley P, Pepe S. Coenzyme Q10 therapy before cardiac surgery improves mitochondrial function and in vitro contractility of myocardial tissue. J Thorac Cardiovasc Surg. 2005;129(1):25–32.
593. Mordente A, Martorana GE, Santini SA, Miggiano GA, Petitti T, Giardina B, Battino M, Littarru GP. Antioxidant effect of coenzyme Q on hydrogen peroxide-activated myoglobin. Clin Investig. 1993;71(8 Suppl):S92–6.
594. Folkers K, Littarru GP, Ho L, Runge TM, Havanonda S, Cooley D. Evidence for a deficiency of coenzyme

Q10 in human heart disease. Int Z Vitaminforsch. 1970;40(3):380–90.
595. Folkers K, Vadhanavikit S, Mortensen SA. Biochemical rationale and myocardial tissue data on the effective therapy of cardiomyopathy with coenzyme Q10. Proc Natl Acad Sci U S A. 1985;82(3):901–4.
596. Mortensen SA. Overview on coenzyme Q10 as adjunctive therapy in chronic heart failure. Rationale, design and end-points of "Q-symbio" – a multinational trial. Biofactors. 2003;18(1–4):79–89.
597. Rosenfeldt F, Hilton D, Pepe S, Krum H. Systematic review of effect of coenzyme Q10 in physical exercise, hypertension and heart failure. Biofactors. 2003;18(1–4):91–100.
598. Sander S, Coleman CI, Patel AA, Kluger J, White CM. The impact of coenzyme Q10 on systolic function in patients with chronic heart failure. J Card Fail. 2006;12(6):464–72.
599. Kumar A, Singh RB, Saxena M, Niaz MA, Josh SR, Chattopadhyay P, Mechirova V, Pella D, Fedacko J. Effect of carni Q-gel (ubiquinol and carnitine) on cytokines in patients with heart failure in the Tishcon study. Acta Cardiol. 2007;62(4):349–54.
600. Hargreaves IP, Hargreaves AK. Coenzyme Q10 from fact to fiction. New York: Nova Science Publishers Inc; 2015. p. 67.
601. Morisco C, Trimarco B, Condorelli M. Effect of coenzyme Q10 therapy in patients with congestive heart failure: a long-term multicenter randomized study. Clin Investig. 1993;71(8 Suppl):S134–6.
602. Tarnopolsky MA, Beal MF. Potential for creatine and other therapies targeting cellular energy dysfunction in neurological disorders. Ann Neurol. 2001;49(5):561–74.
603. Matthews RT, Yang L, Browne S, Baik M, Beal MF. Coenzyme Q10 administration increases brain mitochondrial concentrations and exerts neuroprotective effects. Proc Natl Acad Sci U S A. 1998;95(15):8892–7.
604. Rustin P, von Kleist-Retzow JC, Chantrel-Groussard K, Sidi D, Munnich A, Rötig A. Effect of idebenone on cardiomyopathy in Friedreich's ataxia: a preliminary study. Lancet. 1999;354(9177):477–9.
605. Lodi R, Schapira AH, Manners D, Styles P, Wood NW, Taylor DJ, Warner TT. Abnormal in vivo skeletal muscle energy metabolism in Huntington's disease and dentatorubropallidoluysian atrophy. Ann Neurol. 2000;48(1):72–6.
606. Huntington Study Group. A randomized, placebo-controlled trial of coenzyme Q10 and remacemide in Huntington's disease. Neurology. 2001;57(3):397–404.
607. Sack MN, Fyhrquist FY, Saijonmaa OJ, Fuster V, Kovacic JC. Basic biology of oxidative stress and the cardiovascular system: part 1 of a 3-part series. J Am Coll Cardiol. 2017;70(2):196–211. https://doi.org/10.1016/j.jacc.2017.05.034.
608. Schaper J, Meiser E, Stämmler G. Ultrastructural morphometric analysis of myocardium from dogs, rats, hamsters, mice, and from human hearts. Circ Res. 1985;56(3):377–91.
609. Sack MN. Type 2 diabetes mitochondrial biology in the heart. J Mol Cell Cardiol. 2009;46:842–9.
610. Munzel T, Gori T, Keaney JF Jr, Macck C, Daiver A. Pathophysiologic role of oxidative stress in systolic and diastolic heart failure and the therapeutic implications. Eur Heart J. 2015;36:2555–64.
611. Sack MN. Mitochondrial depolarization in the role of uncoupling proteins and ischemia tolerance. Cardiovasc Res. 2006;72:210–9.
612. Oka T, Hikoso S, Yamaguchi G, et al. Mitochondrial DNA that escapes from autophagy cause inflammation and heart failure. Nature. 2012;485:251–5.
613. Blikseen M, Maierlo H, Omh IK, et al. Precirculating mitochondrial DNA after myocardial infarction. Int J Cardiol. 2012;158:132–4.
614. Okonko DO, Shah AM. Heart failure: mitochondrial dysfunction and oxidative stress in CHF. Nat Rev Cardiol. 2015;12(1):6–8. https://doi.org/10.1038/nrcardio.2014.189. Epub 2014 Nov 25.
615. Smith RA, Murphy MP. Animal and human studies with the mitochondria-targeted antioxidant MitoQ. Ann N Y Acad Sci. 2010;1201:96–103. https://doi.org/10.1111/j.1749-6632.2010.05627.x.
616. von Zglinicki T. Oxidative stress shortens telomeres. Trends Biochem Sci. 2002;27(7):339–44. PMID: 12114022.
617. Song Z, von Figura G, Liu Y, Kraus JM, Torrice C, Dillon P, Rudolph-Watabe M, Ju Z, Kestler HA, Sanoff H, Lenhard Rudolph K. Lifestyle impacts on the aging-associated expression of biomarkers of DNA damage and telomere dysfunction in human blood. Aging Cell. 2010;9(4):607–15. https://doi.org/10.1111/j.1474-9726.2010.00583.x. Epub 2010 Jun 17.
618. Njajou OT, Hsueh WC, Blackburn EH, Newman AB, Wu SH, Li R, Simonsick EM, Harris TM, Cummings SR, Cawthon RM, Health ABC study. Association between telomere length, specific causes of death, and years of healthy life in health, aging, and body composition, a population-based cohort study. J Gerontol A Biol Sci Med Sci. 2009;64(8):860–4. https://doi.org/10.1093/gerona/glp061. Epub 2009 May 12.
619. Ornish D, Lin J, Chan JM, Epel E, Kemp C, Weidner G, Marlin R, Frenda SJ, Magbanua MJ, Daubenmier J, Estay I, Hills NK, Chainani-Wu N, Carroll PR, Blackburn EH. Effect of comprehensive lifestyle changes on telomerase activity and telomere length in men with biopsy-proven low-risk prostate cancer: 5-year follow-up of a descriptive pilot study. Lancet Oncol. 2013;14(11):1112–20. https://doi.org/10.1016/S1470-2045(13)70366-8. Epub 2013 Sept 17.
620. Farzaneh-Far R, Lin J, Epel ES, Harris WS, Blackburn EH, Whooley MA. Association of marine omega-3 fatty acid levels with telomeric aging in patients with coronary heart disease. JAMA. 2010;303(3):250–7. https://doi.org/10.1001/jama.2009.2008.

621. Saliques S, Teyssier JR, Vergely C, Lorgis L, Lorin J, Farnier M, Donzel A, Sicard P, Berchoud J, Lagrost AC, Touzery C, Ragot S, Cottin Y, Rochette L, Zeller M. Circulating leukocyte telomere length and oxidative stress: a new target for statin therapy. Atherosclerosis. 2011;219(2):753–60. https://doi.org/10.1016/j.atherosclerosis.2011.09.011. Epub 2011 Sept 16.
622. de Kreutzenberg SV, Ceolotto G, Cattelan A, Pagnin E, Mazzucato M, Garagnani P, Borelli V, Bacalini MG, Franceschi C, Fadini GP, Avogaro A. Metformin improves putative longevity effectors in peripheral mononuclear cells from subjects with prediabetes. A randomized controlled trial. Nutr Metab Cardiovasc Dis. 2015;25(7):686–93. https://doi.org/10.1016/j.numecd.2015.03.007. Epub 2015 Mar 24.
623. Cherkas LF, Hunkin JL, Kato BS, Richards JB, Gardner JP, Surdulescu GL, Kimura M, Lu X, Spector TD, Aviv A. The association between physical activity in leisure time and leukocyte telomere length. Arch Intern Med. 2008;168(2):154–8. https://doi.org/10.1001/archinternmed.2007.39.
624. Laimer M, Melmer A, Lamina C, Raschenberger J, Adamovski P, Engl J, Ress C, Tschoner A, Gelsinger C, Mair L, Kiechl S, Willeit J, Willeit P, Stettler C, Tilg H, Kronenberg F, Ebenbichler C. Telomere length increase after weight loss induced by bariatric surgery: results from a 10 year prospective study. Int J Obes. 2016;40(5):773–8. https://doi.org/10.1038/ijo.2015.238. Epub 2015 Nov 26.
625. Correia-Melo C, Hewitt G, Passos JF. Telomeres, oxidative stress and inflammatory factors: partners in cellular senescence? Longev Healthspan. 2014;3(1):1. https://doi.org/10.1186/2046-2395-3-1.
626. Bayne S, Liu JP. Hormones and growth factors regulate telomerase activity in ageing and cancer. Mol Cell Endocrinol. 2005;240(1–2):11–22.
627. Münzel T, Camici GG, Maack C, Bonetti NR, Fuster V, Kovacic JC. Impact of oxidative stress on the heart and vasculature: part 2 of a 3-part series. J Am Coll Cardiol. 2017;70(2):212–29. https://doi.org/10.1016/j.jacc.2017.05.035.
628. Maack C, Kartes T, Kilter H, et al. Oxygen free radical release in human failing myocardium is associated with increased activity of rac1-GTPase and represents a target for statin treatment. Circulation. 2003;108:1567–74.
629. Mollnau H, Oelze M, August M, et al. Mechanisms of increased vascular superoxide production in an experimental model of idiopathic dilated cardiomyopathy. Arterioscler Thromb Vasc Biol. 2005;25:2554–9.
630. Belch JJ, Bridges AB, Scott N, Chopra M. Oxygen free radicals and congestive heart failure. Br Heart J. 1991;65:245–8.
631. Heart Outcomes Prevention Evaluation Study Investigators. Effects of an angiotensin converting-enzyme inhibitor, ramipril, on cardiovascular events in high-risk patients. N Engl J Med. 2000;342:145–53.
632. Lonn E, Bosch J, Yusuf S, et al., HOPE and HOPE-TOO Trial Investigators. Effects of longterm vitamin E supplementation on cardiovascular events and cancer: a randomized controlled trial. JAMA. 2005;293:1338–47.
633. Förstermann U. Nitric oxide and oxidative stress in vascular disease. Pflugers Arch. 2010;459:923–39.
634. Förstermann U, Münzel T. Endothelial nitric oxide synthase in vascular disease: from marvel to menace. Circulation. 2006;113:1708–14.
635. Gryglewski RJ, Palmer RM, Moncada S. Superoxide anion is involved in the breakdown of endothelium-derived vascular relaxing factor. Nature. 1986;320:454–6.
636. Li H, Horke S, Förstermann U. Vascular oxidative stress, nitric oxide and atherosclerosis. Atherosclerosis. 2014;237:208–19.
637. Libby P. Inflammatory and immune mechanisms in atherogenesis. In: Leaf A, Weber P, editors. Atheroclerosis reviews. New York: Raven Press; 1990. p. 79–89.
638. Libby P, Ridker PM, Hansson GK. Inflammation in atherosclerosis: from pathophysiology to practice. J Am Coll Cardiol. 2009;54:2129–38.
639. Lichtman AH, Binder CJ, Tsimikas S, Witztum JL. Adaptive immunity in atherogenesis: new insights and therapeutic approaches. J Clin Invest. 2013;123:27–36.
640. Hansson GK, Libby P, Tabas I. Inflammation and plaque vulnerability. J Intern Med. 2015;278:483–93.
641. Libby P, Hansson GK. Inflammation and immunity in diseases of the arterial tree: players and layers. Circ Res. 2015;116:307–11.
642. Nus M, Mallat Z. Immune-mediated mechanisms of atherosclerosis and implications for the clinic. Expert Rev Clin Immunol. 2016;12:1217–37.
643. Weber C, Shantsila E, Hristov M, et al. Role and analysis of monocyte subsets in cardiovascular disease. Joint consensus document of the European Society of Cardiology (ESC) Working Groups "Atherosclerosis and Vascular Biology" and "Thrombosis.". Thromb Haemost. 2016;116:626–37.
644. Libby P. History of discovery: inflammation in atherosclerosis. Arterioscler Thromb. 2012;32:2045–51.
645. Cook NR, Paynter NP, Eaton CB, et al. Comparison of the Framingham and Reynolds Risk scores for global cardiovascular risk prediction in the multiethnic Women's Health Initiative. Circulation. 2012;125:1748–56, S1741–11.
646. Ridker PM. A test in context: high-sensitivity c-reactive protein. J Am Coll Cardiol. 2016;67:712–23.
647. Ridker PM, Danielson E, Fonseca FA, et al. Rosuvastatin to prevent vascular events in men and women with elevated C-reactive protein. N Engl J Med. 2008;359:2195–207.
648. Schonbeck U, Libby P. Inflammation, immunity, and HMG-CoA reductase inhibitors: statins as antiinflammatory agents? Circulation. 2004;109:II18–26.

649. Ridker PM, Cannon CP, Morrow D, et al. C-reactive protein levels and outcomes after statin therapy. N Engl J Med. 2005;352:20–8.
650. Jain MK, Sangwung P, Hamik A. Regulation of an inflammatory disease: Kruppel-like factors and atherosclerosis. Arterioscler Thromb. 2014;34:499–508.
651. Libby P. The forgotten majority: unfinished business in cardiovascular risk reduction. J Am Coll Cardiol. 2005;46:1225–8.
652. Jernberg T, Asvold P, Henriksson M, Hjelm H, Thuresson M, Janzon M. Cardiovascular risk in post-myocardial infarction patients: nationwide real world data demonstrate the importance of a long-term perspective. Eur Heart J. 2015;36:1163–70.
653. Masoudi FA, Ponirakis A, de Lemos JA, et al. Trends in U.S. cardiovascular care: 2016 report from 4 ACC national cardiovascular data registries. J Am Coll Cardiol. 2017;69:1427–50.
654. Libby P. Interleukin-1 Beta as a target for atherosclerosis therapy: biological basis of CANTOS and beyond. J Am Coll Cardiol. 2017;70(18):2278–89. https://doi.org/10.1016/j.jacc.2017.09.028.
655. Evrard SM, Lecce L, Michelis KC, Nomura-Kitabayashi A, Pandey G, Purushothaman KR, d'Escamard V, Li JR, Hadri L, Fujitani K, Moreno PR, Benard L, Rimmele P, Cohain A, Mecham B, Randolph GJ, Nabel EG, Hajjar R, Fuster V, Boehm M, Kovacic JC. Endothelial to mesenchymal transition is common in atherosclerotic lesions and is associated with plaque instability. Nat Commun. 2016;7:11853. https://doi.org/10.1038/ncomms11853.
656. Camici GG, Savarese G, Akhmedov A, Lüscher TF. Molecular mechanism of endothelial and vascular aging: implications for cardiovascular disease. Eur Heart J. 2015;36(48):3392–403. https://doi.org/10.1093/eurheartj/ehv587. Epub 2015 Nov 4. PMID: 26543043.
657. Bjelakovic G, Nikolova D, Gluud LL, Simonetti RG, Gluud C. Mortality in randomized trials of antioxidant supplements for primary and secondary prevention: systematic review and meta-analysis. JAMA. 2007;297:842–57.
658. Touyz RM. Reactive oxygen species, vascular oxidative stress, and redox signaling in hypertension: what is the clinical significance? Hypertension. 2004;44:248–52.
659. Steinberg D, Witztum JL. Is the oxidative modification hypothesis relevant to human atherosclerosis? Do the antioxidant trials conducted to date refute the hypothesis? Circulation. 2002;105:2107–11.
660. Lopaschuk GD, Ussher JR, Folmes CD, Jaswal JS, Stanley WC. Myocardial fatty acid metabolism in health and disease. Physiol Rev. 2010;90:207–58.
661. Niemann B, Rohrbach S, Miller MR, Newby DE, Fuster V, Kovacic JC. Oxidative stress and cardiovascular risk: obesity, diabetes, smoking, and pollution: part 3 of a 3-part series. J Am Coll Cardiol. 2017;70(2):230–51. https://doi.org/10.1016/j.jacc.2017.05.043.
662. Anderson EJ, Kypson AP, Rodriguez E, Anderson CA, Lehr EJ, Neufer PD. Substrate specific derangements in mitochondrial metabolism and redox balance in the atrium of the type 2 diabetic human heart. J Am Coll Cardiol. 2009;54:1891–8.
663. Brownlee M. Biochemistry and molecular cell biology of diabetic complications. Nature. 2001;414:813–20.
664. Salonen JT, Nyyssönen K, Tuomainen TP, et al. Increased risk of non-insulin dependent diabetes mellitus at low plasma vitamin E concentrations: a four year follow up study in men. BMJ. 1995;311:1124–7.
665. Itoh K, Mimura J, Yamamoto M. Discovery of the negative regulator of Nrf2, Keap1: a historical overview. Antioxid Redox Signal. 2010;13:1665–78.
666. Wegner M, Neddermann D, Piorunska-Stolzmann M, Jagodzinski PP. Role of epigenetic mechanisms in the development of chronic complications of diabetes. Diabetes Res Clin Pract. 2014;105:164–75.
667. Kayama Y, Raaz U, Jagger A, et al. Diabetic cardiovascular disease induced by oxidative stress. Int J Mol Sci. 2015;16:25234–63.
668. Aurich AC, Niemann B, Pan R, et al. Age dependent effects of high fat-diet on murine left ventricles: role of palmitate. Basic Res Cardiol. 2013;108:369.
669. Ghosh S, Rodrigues B. Cardiac cell death in early diabetes and its modulation by dietary fatty acids. Biochim Biophys Acta. 1761;2006:1148–62.
670. van de Weijer T, Schrauwen-Hinderling VB, Schrauwen P. Lipotoxicity in type 2 diabetic cardiomyopathy. Cardiovasc Res. 2011;92:10–8.
671. Niemann B, Chen Y, Teschner M, Li L, Silber RE, Rohrbach S. Obesity induces signs of premature cardiac aging in younger patients: the role of mitochondria. J Am Coll Cardiol. 2011;57:577–85.
672. The Heart Outcomes Prevention Evaluation Study Investigators. Vitamin E supplementation and cardiovascular events in high-risk patients. N Engl J Med. 2000;342:154–60.
673. Centers for Disease Control and Prevention (US), National Center for Chronic Disease Prevention and Health Promotion (US), Office on Smoking and Health (US). How tobacco smoke causes disease: the biology and behavioral basis for smoking-attributable disease: a report of the Surgeon General. Atlanta: Centers for Disease Control and Prevention; 2010. Available at: http://www.ncbi.nlm.nih.gov/books/NBK53014. Accessed 15 May 2017.
674. Cesaroni G, Forastiere F, Stafoggia M, et al. Long term exposure to ambient air pollution and incidence of acute coronary events: prospective cohort study and meta-analysis in 11 European cohorts from the ESCAPE project. BMJ. 2014;348:f7412.
675. Chen H, Goldberg MS, Burnett RT, Jerrett M, Wheeler AJ, Villeneuve PJ. Long-term exposure to traffic-related air pollution and cardiovascular mortality. Epidemiology. 2013;24:35–43.
676. Miller KA, Siscovick DS, Sheppard L, et al. Long-term exposure to air pollution and incidence of

cardiovascular events in women. N Engl J Med. 2007;356:447–58.
677. Pope CA III, Verrier RL, Lovett EG, et al. Heart rate variability associated with particulate air pollution. Am Heart J. 1999;138:890–9.
678. Hoffmann B, Moebus S, Kröger K, et al. Residential exposure to urban air pollution, ankle brachial index, and peripheral arterial disease. Epidemiology. 2009;20:280–8.
679. Fowkes FG, Aboyans V, Fowkes FJ, McDermott MM, Sampson UK, Criqui MH. Peripheral artery disease: epidemiology and global perspectives. Nat Rev Cardiol. 2017;14:156–70.
680. Atkinson RW, Carey IM, Kent AJ, van Staa TP, Anderson HR, Cook DG. Long-term exposure to outdoor air pollution and incidence of cardiovascular diseases. Epidemiology. 2013;24:44–53.
681. Shah AS, Langrish JP, Nair H, et al. Global association of air pollution and heart failure: a systematic review and meta-analysis. Lancet. 2013;382:1039–48.
682. Shah AS, Lee KK, McAllister DA, et al. Short term exposure to air pollution and stroke: systematic review and meta-analysis. BMJ. 2015;350:h1295.
683. Stafoggia M, Cesaroni G, Peters A, et al. Long-term exposure to ambient air pollution and incidence of cerebrovascular events: results from 11 European cohorts within the ESCAPE project. Environ Health Perspect. 2014;122:919–25.
684. Low RB, Bielory L, Qureshi AI, Dunn V, Stuhlmiller DF, Dickey DA. The relation of stroke admissions to recent weather, airborne allergens, air pollution, seasons, upper respiratory infections, and asthma incidence, September 11, 2001, and day of the week. Stroke. 2006;37:951–7.
685. Raza A, Bellander T, Bero-Bedada G, et al. Short-term effects of air pollution on out-of hospital cardiac arrest in Stockholm. Eur Heart J. 2014;35:861–8.
686. D'Alessandro A, Boeckelmann I, Hammwhösner M, Goette A. Nicotine, cigarette smoking and cardiac arrhythmia: an overview. Eur J Prev Cardiol. 2012;19:297–305.
687. Baccarelli A, Martinelli I, Pegoraro V, et al. Living near major traffic roads and risk of deep vein thrombosis. Circulation. 2009;119:3118–24.
688. Messner B, Bernhard D. Smoking and cardiovascular disease: mechanisms of endothelial dysfunction and early atherogenesis. Arterioscler Thromb Vasc Biol. 2014;34:509–15.
689. Mills NL, Donaldson K, Hadoke PW, et al. Adverse cardiovascular effects of air pollution. Nat Clin Pract Cardiovasc Med. 2009;6:36–44.
690. Brook RD, Rajagopalan S. Particulate matter, air pollution, and blood pressure. J Am Soc Hypertens. 2009;3:332–50.
691. Liang R, Zhang B, Zhao X, Ruan Y, Lian H, Fan Z. Effect of exposure to PM2.5 on blood pressure: a systematic review and meta-analysis. J Hypertens. 2014;32:2130–40, discussion 2141.
692. Wauters A, Dreyfuss C, Pochet S, et al. Acute exposure to diesel exhaust impairs nitric oxide mediated endothelial vasomotor function by increasing endothelial oxidative stress. Hypertension. 2013;62:352–8.
693. Brook RD, Rajagopalan S, Pope CA III, et al. Particulate matter air pollution and cardiovascular disease: an update to the scientific statement from the American Heart Association. Circulation. 2010;121:2331–78.
694. Forbes LJ, Patel MD, Rudnicka AR, et al. Chronic exposure to outdoor air pollution and markers of systemic inflammation. Epidemiology. 2009;20:245–53.
695. Goodman JE, Prueitt RL, Sax SN, et al. Ozone exposure and systemic biomarkers: evaluation of evidence for adverse cardiovascular health impacts. Crit Rev Toxicol. 2015;45:412–52.
696. Yatera K, Hsieh J, Hogg JC, et al. Particulate matter air pollution exposure promotes recruitment of monocytes into atherosclerotic plaques. Am J Physiol Heart Circ Physiol. 2008;294:H944–53.
697. Bartoli CR, Wellenius GA, Coull BA, et al. Concentrated ambient particles alter myocardial blood flow during acute ischemia in conscious canines. Environ Health Perspect. 2009;117:333–7.
698. Campen MJ, Babu NS, Helms GA, et al. Nonparticulate components of diesel exhaust promote constriction in coronary arteries from ApoE_/_ mice. Toxicol Sci. 2005;88:95–102.
699. Cherng TW, Campen MJ, Knuckles TL, Gonzalez Bosc L, Kanagy NL. Impairment of coronary endothelial cell ETB receptor function after short-term inhalation exposure to whole diesel emissions. Am J Physiol Regul Integr Comp Physiol. 2009;297:R640–7.
700. Lemos M, Mohallen SV, Macchione M, et al. Chronic exposure to urban air pollution induces structural alterations in murine pulmonary and coronary arteries. Inhal Toxicol. 2006;18:247–53.
701. Brucker N, Moro AM, Charão MF, et al. Biomarkers of occupational exposure to air pollution, inflammation and oxidative damage in taxi drivers. Sci Total Environ. 2013;463–464:884–93.
702. Sørensen M, Daneshvar B, Hansen M, et al. Personal PM2.5 exposure and markers of oxidative stress in blood. Environ Health Perspect. 2003;111:161–6.
703. Li W, Wilker EH, Dorans KS, et al. Short-term exposure to air pollution and biomarkers of oxidative stress: the Framingham Heart Study. J Am Heart Assoc. 2016;5:e002742.
704. Bagryantseva Y, Novotna B, Rossner P Jr, et al. Oxidative damage to biological macromolecules in Prague bus drivers and garagemen: impact of air pollution and genetic polymorphisms. Toxicol Lett. 2010;199:60–8.
705. Ren C, Fang S, Wright RO, Suh H, Schwartz J. Urinary 8-hydroxy-20-deoxyguanosine as a biomarker of oxidative DNA damage induced by ambient pollution in the Normative Aging Study. Occup Environ Med. 2011;68:562–9.

706. Rossner P Jr, Rossnerova A, Sram RJ. Oxidative stress and chromosomal aberrations in an environmentally exposed population. Mutat Res. 2011;707:34–41.
707. Huang W, Wang G, Lu SE, et al. Inflammatory and oxidative stress responses of healthy young adults to changes in air quality during the Beijing Olympics. Am J Respir Crit Care Med. 2012;186:1150–9.
708. Pell JP, Haw S, Cobbe S, et al. Smoke-free legislation and hospitalizations for acute coronary syndrome. N Engl J Med. 2008;359:482–91.
709. Bondy SC, Campbell A, editors. Inflammation, aging, and oxidative stress. Oxidative stress in applied basic research and clinical practice. Cham: Springer International Publishing; 2016.
710. Vinik AI, Arora RR, Colombo J. Age matched attenuation of both autonomic branches in chronic disease: II. Diabetes mellitus. Cleveland Clinic Heart-Brain Summit, Cleveland Clinic Lou Ruvo Center for Brain Health, Las Vegas, 23–24 Sept 2010.
711. American Diabetes Association. Standards of medical care in diabetes – 2008. Diabetes Care. 2008;31(Suppl 1):S12–54.
712. American Diabetes Association. Standards of medical care in diabetes – 2013. Diabetes Care. 2013;36(Suppl 1):S11–66.
713. Umetani K, Singer DH, McCraty R, Atkinson M. Twenty-four hour time domain heart rate variability and heart rate: relations to age and gender over nine decades. J Am Coll Cardiol. 1998;31(3):593–601.
714. Cheyuo C, Jacob A, Wu R, Zhou M, Coppa GF, Wang P. The parasympathetic nervous system in the quest for stroke therapeutics. J Cereb Blood Flow Metab. 2011;31(5):1187–95. https://doi.org/10.1038/jcbfm.2011.24. Epub 2011 Mar 2. Review.
715. Hayflick L. Biological aging is no longer an unsolved problem. Ann N Y Acad Sci. 2007;1100:1–13.
716. Kirkwood TB. Understanding the odd science of aging. Cell. 2005;120:437–47.
717. Beckman KB, Ames BN. The free radical theory of aging matures. Physiol Rev. 1998;78:547–81.
718. Lee CK, Klopp RG, Weindruch R, Prolla TA. Gene expression profile of aging and its retardation by caloric restriction. Science. 1999;285:1390–3.
719. Stadtman ER. Protein oxidation and aging. Science. 1992;257:1220–4.
720. Balaban RS, Nemoto S, Finkel T. Mitochondria, oxidants, and aging. Cell. 2005;120:483–95.
721. Cencioni C, Spallotta F, Martelli F, Valente S, Mai A, Zeiher AM, Gaetano C. Oxidative stress and epigenetic regulation in aging and age-related diseases. Int J Mol Sci. 2013;14(9):17643–63. https://doi.org/10.3390/ijms140917643. Review.
722. Haigis MC, Yankner BA. The aging stress response. Mol Cell. 2010;40:333–44.
723. Sohal RS, Weindruch R. Oxidative stress, caloric restriction, and aging. Science. 1996;273:59–63.
724. Davies KJ. Oxidative stress, antioxidant defenses, and damage removal, repair, and replacement systems. IUBMB Life. 2000;50:279–89.
725. Finkel T, Holbrook NJ. Oxidants, oxidative stress and the biology of aging. Nature. 2000;408:239–47.
726. Stadtman ER. Protein oxidation in aging and age-related diseases. Ann N Y Acad Sci. 2001;928:22–38.
727. Ben-Avraham D, Muzumdar RH, Atzmon G. Epigenetic genome-wide association methylation in aging and longevity. Epigenomics. 2012;4:503–9.
728. Boon RA, Iekushi K, Lechner S, Seeger T, Fischer A, Heydt S, Kaluza D, Treguer K, Carmona G, Bonauer A, et al. MicroRNA-34a regulates cardiac aging and function. Nature. 2013;495:107–10.
729. North BJ, Sinclair DA. The intersection between aging and cardiovascular disease. Circ Res. 2012;110:1097–108.
730. Oxenham H, Sharpe N. Cardiovascular aging and heart failure. Eur J Heart Fail. 2003;5:427–34.
731. Versari D, Daghini E, Virdis A, Ghiadoni L, Taddei S. The aging endothelium, cardiovascular risk and disease in man. Exp Physiol. 2009;94:317–21.
732. Strait JB, Lakatta EG. Aging-associated cardiovascular changes and their relationship to heart failure. Heart Fail Clin. 2012;8:143–64.
733. Ota H, Tokunaga E, Chang K, Hikasa M, Iijima K, Eto M, Kozaki K, Akishita M, Ouchi Y, Kaneki M. SIRT1 inhibitor, Sirtinol, induces senescence-like growth arrest with attenuated Ras-MAPK signaling in human cancer cells. Oncogene. 2006;25:176–85.
734. Ota H, Eto M, Kano MR, Kahyo T, Setou M, Ogawa S, Iijima K, Akishita M, Ouchi Y. Induction of endothelial nitric oxide synthase, SIRT1, and catalase by statins inhibits endothelial senescence through the Akt pathway. Arterioscler Thromb Vasc Biol. 2010;30:2205–11.
735. Rahman I, Marwick J, Kirkham P. Redox modulation of chromatin remodeling: impact on histone acetylation and deacetylation, NF-kappaB and pro-inflammatory gene expression. Biochem Pharmacol. 2004;68:1255–67.
736. Repine JE, Bast A, Lankhorst I. The oxidative stress study group. Oxidative stress in chronic obstructive pulmonary disease. Am J Respir Crit Care Med. 1997;156:341–57.
737. Tuder RM, Kern JA, Miller YE. Senescence in chronic obstructive pulmonary disease. Proc Am Thorac Soc. 2012;9:62–3.
738. Yao H, Rahman I. Role of histone deacetylase 2 in epigenetics and cellular senescence: implications in lung inflammaging and COPD. Am J Physiol Lung Cell Mol Physiol. 2012;303:L557–66.
739. Sundar IK, Yao H, Rahman I. Oxidative stress and chromatin remodeling in chronic obstructive pulmonary disease and smoking-related diseases. Antioxid Redox Signal. 2012;18:1956–71.
740. Adenuga D, Yao H, March TH, Seagrave J, Rahman I. Histone deacetylase 2 is phosphorylated, ubiquitinated, and degraded by cigarette smoke. Am J Respir Cell Mol Biol. 2009;40:464–73.

741. Marwick JA, Kirkham PA, Stevenson CS, Danahay H, Giddings J, Butler K, Donaldson K, Macnee W, Rahman I. Cigarette smoke alters chromatin remodeling and induces proinflammatory genes in rat lungs. Am J Respir Cell Mol Biol. 2004;31:633–42.
742. Moodie FM, Marwick JA, Anderson CS, Szulakowski P, Biswas SK, Bauter MR, Kilty I, Rahman I. Oxidative stress and cigarette smoke alter chromatin remodeling but differentially regulate NF-κB activation and proinflammatory cytokine release in alveolar epithelial cells. FASEB J. 2004;18:1897–9.
743. Rajendrasozhan S, Yang SR, Kinnula VL, Rahman I. SIRT1, an antiinflammatory and antiaging protein, is decreased in lungs of patients with chronic obstructive pulmonary disease. Am J Respir Crit Care Med. 2008;177:861–70.
744. Yang SR, Chida AS, Bauter MR, Shafiq N, Seweryniak K, Maggirwar SB, Kilty I, Rahman I. Cigarette smoke induces proinflammatory cytokine release by activation of NF-κB and posttranslational modifications of histone deacetylase in macrophages. Am J Physiol Lung Cell Mol Physiol. 2006;291:L46–57.
745. Kedar NP. Can we prevent Parkinson's and Alzheimer's disease? J Postgrad Med. 2003;49:236–45.
746. Coppede F, Migliore L. Evidence linking genetics, environment, and epigenetics to impaired DNA repair in Alzheimer's disease. J Alzheimers Dis. 2010;20:953–66.
747. Myung NH, Zhu X, Kruman II, Castellani RJ, Petersen RB, Siedlak SL, Perry G, Smith MA, Lee HG. Evidence of DNA damage in Alzheimer disease: phosphorylation of histone H2AX in astrocytes. Age. 2008;30:209–15.
748. Zawia NH, Lahiri DK, Cardozo-Pelaez F. Epigenetics, oxidative stress, and Alzheimer disease. Free Radic Biol Med. 2009;46:1241–9.
749. Rimm EB. Folate and vitamin B6 from diet and supplements in relation to risk of coronary heart disease among women. Bibl Nutr Dieta. 2001;55:42–5. Review.
750. Gupta A, Moustapha A, Jacobsen DW, Goormastic M, Tuzcu EM, Hobbs R, Young J, James K, McCarthy P, van Lente F, Green R, Robinson K. High homocysteine, low folate, and low vitamin B6 concentrations: prevalent risk factors for vascular disease in heart transplant recipients. Transplantation. 1998;65(4):544–50.
751. Rimm EB, Willett WC, Hu FB, Sampson L, Colditz GA, Manson JE, Hennekens C, Stampfer MJ. Folate and vitamin B6 from diet and supplements in relation to risk of coronary heart disease among women. JAMA. 1998;279(5):359–64.
752. Saito A, Kaseda R, Hosojima M, Sato H. Proximal tubule cell hypothesis for cardiorenal syndrome in diabetes. Int J Nephrol. 2010;2011:957164. https://doi.org/10.4061/2011/957164.
753. Alkaitis MS, Crabtree MJ. Recoupling the cardiac nitric oxide synthases: tetrahydrobiopterin synthesis and recycling. Curr Heart Fail Rep. 2012;9(3):200–10. https://doi.org/10.1007/s11897-012-0097-5. Review.
754. Moustafa AA, Hewedi DH, Eissa AM, Frydecka D, Błażej M. Homocysteine levels in schizophrenia and affective disorders – focus on cognition. Front Behav Neurosci. 2014;8:343–55.
755. Wald DS, Wald NJ, Morris JK, Law M. Folic acid, homocysteine, and cardiovascular disease: judging causality in the face of inconclusive trial evidence. BMJ. 2006;333(7578):1114–7. Review.
756. Jenkins DJA, Spence JD, Giovannucci EL, Kim YI, Josse R, Vieth R, Blanco Mejia S, Viguiliouk E, Nishi S, Sahye-Pudaruth S, Paquette M, Patel D, Mitchell S, Kavanagh M, Tsirakis T, Bachiri L, Maran A, Umatheva N, McKay T, Trinidad G, Bernstein D, Chowdhury A, Correa-Betanzo J, Del Principe G, Hajizadeh A, Jayaraman R, Jenkins A, Jenkins W, Kalaichandran R, Kirupaharan G, Manisekaran P, Qutta T, Shahid R, Silver A, Villegas C, White J, Kendall CWC, Pichika SC, Sievenpiper JL. Supplemental vitamins and minerals for CVD prevention and treatment. J Am Coll Cardiol. 2018;71(22):2570–84. https://doi.org/10.1016/j.jacc.2018.04.020.
757. Clarke R, Bennett DA, Parish S, Verhoef P, Dötsch-Klerk M, Lathrop M, Xu P, Nordestgaard BG, Holm H, Hopewell JC, Saleheen D, Tanaka T, Anand SS, Chambers JC, Kleber ME, Ouwehand WH, Yamada Y, Elbers C, Peters B, Stewart AF, Reilly MM, Thorand B, Yusuf S, Engert JC, Assimes TL, Kooner J, Danesh J, Watkins H, Samani NJ, Collins R, Peto R, MTHFR Studies Collaborative Group. Homocysteine and coronary heart disease: meta-analysis of MTHFR case-control studies, avoiding publication bias. PLoS Med. 2012;9(2):e1001177. https://doi.org/10.1371/journal.pmed.1001177. Epub 2012 Feb 21.
758. Abrahaham JM, et al. The homocysteine hypothesis: still relevant to the prevention and treatment of cardiovascular disease? Cleve Clin J Med. 2010;77(12):911–8.
759. Soinio M, Marniemi J, Laakso M, Lehto S, Rönnemaa T. Elevated plasma homocysteine level is an independent predictor of coronary heart disease events in patients with type 2 diabetes mellitus. Ann Intern Med. 2004;140:94–100.
760. Kong X, Huang X, Zhao M, Xu B, Xu R, Song Y, Yu Y, Yang W, Zhang J, Liu L, Zhang Y, Tang G, Wang B, Hou FF, Li P, Cheng X, Zhao S, Wang X, Qin X, Li J, Huo Y. Platelet count affects efficacy of folic acid in preventing first stroke. J Am Coll Cardiol. 2018;71(19):2136–46. https://doi.org/10.1016/j.jacc.2018.02.072.
761. Glynn SA, Albanes D. Folate and cancer: a review of the literature. Nutr Cancer. 1994;22(2):101–19. Review.

762. Common questions about diet and cancer: folate and folic acid. American Cancer Society. 2017. https://www.cancer.org/healthy/eat-healthy-get-active/acs-guidelines-nutrition-physical-activity-cancer-prevention/common-questions.html
763. Wien TN, Pike E, Wisløff T, Staff A, Smeland S, Klemp M. Cancer risk with folic acid supplements: a systematic review and meta-analysis. BMJ Open. 2012;2(1):e000653. https://doi.org/10.1136/bmjopen-2011-000653. Print 2012.
764. Wang R, Zheng Y, Huang JY, Zhang AQ, Zhou YH, Wang JN. Folate intake, serum folate levels, and prostate cancer risk: a meta-analysis of prospective studies. BMC Public Health. 2014;14:1326. https://doi.org/10.1186/1471-2458-14-1326.
765. Stott DJ, MacIntosh G, Lowe GD, Rumley A, McMahon AD, Langhorne P, Tait RC, O'Reilly DS, Spilg EG, MacDonald JB, MacFarlane PW, Westendorp RG. Randomized controlled trial of homocysteine-lowering vitamin treatment in elderly patients with vascular disease. Am J Clin Nutr. 2005;82(6):1320–6.
766. Clarke R. Lowering blood homocysteine with folic acid-based supplements: meta-analysis of randomised trials. Indian Heart J. 2000;52(7 Suppl):S59–64.
767. Huo Y, Li J, Qin X, Huang Y, Wang X, Gottesman RF, Tang G, Wang B, Chen D, He M, Fu J, Cai Y, Shi X, Zhang Y, Cui Y, Sun N, Li X, Cheng X, Wang J, Yang X, Yang T, Xiao C, Zhao G, Dong Q, Zhu D, Wang X, Ge J, Zhao L, Hu D, Liu L, Hou FF, CSPPT Investigators. Efficacy of folic acid therapy in primary prevention of stroke among adults with hypertension in China: the CSPPT randomized clinical trial. JAMA. 2015;313(13):1325–35. https://doi.org/10.1001/jama.2015.2274.
768. Xu X, Qin X, Li Y, Sun D, Wang J, Liang M, Wang B, Huo Y, Hou FF, Investigators of the Renal Substudy of the China Stroke Primary Prevention Trial (CSPPT). Efficacy of folic acid therapy on the progression of chronic kidney disease: the renal substudy of the China stroke primary prevention trial. JAMA Intern Med. 2016;176(10):1443–50. https://doi.org/10.1001/jamainternmed.2016.4687.
769. Mandaviya PR, Stolk L, Heil SG. Homocysteine and DNA methylation: a review of animal and human literature. Mol Genet Metab. 2014;113(4):243–52. https://doi.org/10.1016/j.ymgme.2014.10.006. Epub 2014 Oct 14. Review.
770. Antoniades C, Shirodaria C, Warrick N, Cai S, de Bono J, Lee J, Leeson P, Neubauer S, Ratnatunga C, Pillai R, Refsum H, Channon KM. 5-methyltetrahydrofolate rapidly improves endothelial function and decreases superoxide production in human vessels: effects on vascular tetrahydrobiopterin availability and endothelial nitric oxide synthase coupling. Circulation. 2006;114(11):1193–201. Epub 2006 Aug 28.
771. Joshi R, Adhikari S, Patro BS, Chattopadhyay S, Mukherjee T. Free radical scavenging behavior of folic acid: evidence for possible antioxidant activity. Free Radic Biol Med. 2001;30(12):1390–9.
772. Zhao M, Chen YH, Dong XT, Zhou J, Chen X, Wang H, Wu SX, Xia MZ, Zhang C, Xu DX. Folic acid protects against lipopolysaccharide-induced preterm delivery and intrauterine growth restriction through its anti-inflammatory effect in mice. PLoS One. 2013;8(12):e82713. https://doi.org/10.1371/journal.pone.0082713. eCollection 2013.
773. Majewski M, Kozlowska A, Thoene M, Lepiarczyk E, Grzegorzewski WJ. Overview of the role of vitamins and minerals on the kynurenine pathway in health and disease. J Physiol Pharmacol. 2016;67(1):3–19. Review.
774. Cantó C, Menzies KJ, Auwerx J. NAD(+) metabolism and the control of energy homeostasis: a balancing act between mitochondria and the nucleus. Cell Metab. 2015;22:31–53.
775. Huang J-Y, Hirschey MD, Shimazu T, Ho L, Verdin E. Mitochondrial sirtuins. Biochim Biophys Acta. 2010;1804:1645–51.
776. Correia M, Perestrelo T, Rodrigues AS, et al. Sirtuins in metabolism, stemness and differentiation. Biochim Biophys Acta. 2017;1861(1 Pt A):3444–55.
777. Cheng H-L, Mostoslavsky R, Saito S, et al. Developmental defects and p53 hyperacetylation in Sir2 homolog (SIRT1)-deficient mice. Proc Natl Acad Sci U S A. 2003;100:10794–9.
778. Kirkland JB. Niacin requirements for genomic stability. Mutat Res. 2012;733:14–20.
779. Shi H, Enriquez A, Rapadas M, Martin EMMA, Wang R, Moreau J, Lim CK, Szot JO, Ip E, Hughes JN, Sugimoto K, Humphreys DT, McInerney-Leo AM, Leo PJ, Maghzal GJ, Halliday J, Smith J, Colley A, Mark PR, Collins F, Sillence DO, Winlaw DS, Ho JWK, Guillemin GJ, Brown MA, Kikuchi K, Thomas PQ, Stocker R, Giannoulatou E, Chapman G, Duncan EL, Sparrow DB, Dunwoodie SL. NAD deficiency, congenital malformations, and niacin supplementation. N Engl J Med. 2017;377(6):544–52. https://doi.org/10.1056/NEJMoa1616361.
780. Celinski K, Konturek PC, Slomka M, Cichoz-Lach H, Brzozowski T, Konturek SJ, Korolczuk A. Effects of treatment with melatonin and tryptophan on liver enzymes, parameters of fat metabolism and plasma levels of cytokines in patients with non-alcoholic fatty liver disease – 14 months follow up. J Physiol Pharmacol. 2014;65(1):75–82.
781. Vinik AI, Maser RE, Nakave AA. Diabetic cardiovascular autonomic nerve dysfunction. US Endocr Dis. 2007;2:2–9.
782. Vinik A, Ziegler D. Diabetic cardiovascular autonomic neuropathy. Circulation. 2007;115:387–97.
783. Vinik AI, Freeman R, Erbas T. Diabetic autonomic neuropathy. Semin Neurol. 2003;23:365–72.
784. Vinik A, Erbas T, Pfeifer M, Feldman E, Stevens M, Russell J. Diabetic autonomic neuropathy. In: Zucchi SE, editor. The diabetes mellitus manual: a primary care companion to Ellenberg and

Rifkin's. 6th ed. New York: McGraw Hill; 2004. p. 351.
785. Ziegler D, Low PA, Litchy WJ, Boulton AJM, Vinik AI, Freeman R, The NATHAN 1 Trial Group. Efficacy and safety of antioxidant treatment with α-lipoic acid over 4 years in diabetic polyneuropathy. Diabetes Care. 2011;34:2054–60.
786. Vinik AI, Maser RE, Ziegler D. Neuropathy. The crystal ball for cardiovascular disease. Diabetes Care. 2010;33(7):1688–90.
787. Vinik AI, Maser RE, Ziegler D. Autonomic imbalance: prophet of doom or scope for hope? Diabet Med. 2011;28:643–51.
788. Vinik AI. The conductor of the autonomic orchestra. Front Endocrinol. 2012;3(71):1–13.
789. Vinik AI, Nevoret ML, Casellini CM, Parson H. Diabetic neuropathy. Endocrinol Metab Clin N Am. 2013;42(4):747–87. https://doi.org/10.1016/j.ecl.2013.06.001. Review.
790. Maser RE, Mitchell BD, Vinik AI, et al. The association between cardiovascular autonomic neuropathy and mortality in individuals with diabetes: A meta-analysis. Diabetes Care. 2003;26:1895–901.
791. Vinik AI, Erbas T, Casellini CM. Diabetic cardiac autonomic neuropathy, inflammation and cardiovascular disease. J Diab Invest. 2013;4(1):4–18.
792. Vinik AI, Mehrabyan A. Diabetic neuropathies. Med Clin N Am. 2004;88:947–99.
793. Vinik AI, Strotmeyer ES, Nakave AA, Patel CV. Diabetic neuropathy in older adults. Clin Geriatr Med. 2008;24:407–35.
794. Vinik AI, Erbas T. Cardiovascular autonomic neuropathy: diagnosis and management. Curr Diab Rep. 2006;6:424–30.
795. Feldman EL. Oxidative stress and diabetic neuropathy: a new understanding of an old problem. J Clin Invest. 2003;111(4):431–3.
796. Tsuji H, Venditti FJ Jr, Manders ES, Evans JC, Larson MG, Feldman CL, Levy D. Reduced heart rate variability and mortality risk in an elderly cohort. The Framingham Heart Study. Circulation. 1994;90(2):878–83.
797. Vallianou N, Evangelopoulos A, Koutalas P. Alpha-lipoic acid and diabetic neuropathy. Rev Diabet Stud. 2009;6(4):230–6. https://doi.org/10.1900/RDS.2009.6.230. Epub 2009 Dec 30.
798. Vinik AI, Casellini C, Nakave A, Patel C. Diabetic neuropathies. Endotext.com. http://diabetesmanager.pbworks.com/w/page/17680180/Diabetic%20Neuropathies#Oxidativestress; Last edited by Rushakoff R. 2009.
799. Ziegler D, Sohr CG, Nourooz-Zadeh J. Oxidative stress and antioxidant defense in relation to the severity of diabetic polyneuropathy and cardiovascular autonomic neuropathy. Diabetes Care. 2004;27:2178–83.
800. Ziegler D, Gries F. Alpha-lipoic acid and the treatment of diabetic peripheral autonomic cardiac neuropathy. Diabetes. 1997;46(Suppl 2):S62–6.
801. Prendergast JJ. Diabetic autonomic neuropathy: part 2. Treatment. Pract Diabetol. 2001:30–6.
802. Ziegler D, Ametov A, Barinov A, Dyck PJ, Gurieva I, Low PA, Munzel U, Yakhno N, Raz I, Novosadova M, Maus J, Samigullin R. Oral treatment with alpha-lipoic acid improves symptomatic diabetic polyneuropathy: The SYDNEY 2 trial. Diabetes Care. 2006;29(11):2365–70.
803. Ametov AS, Barinov A, Dyck PJ, Hermann R, Kozlova N, Litchy WJ, Low PA, Nehrdich D, Novosadova M, O'Brien PC, Reljanovic M, Samigullin R, Schuette K, Strokov I, Tritschler HJ, Wessel K, Yakhno N, Ziegler D, SYDNEY Trial Study Group. The sensory symptoms of diabetic polyneuropathy are improved with alpha-lipoic acid. The SYDNEY trial. Diabetes Care. 2003;26(3):770–6.
804. Ziegler D, Low PA, Litchy WJ, Boulton AJM, Vinik AI, Freeman R, The NATHAN 1 Trial Group. Efficacy and safety of antioxidant treatment with α-lipoic acid over 4 years in diabetic polyneuropathy. Diabetes Care. 2011;34:2054–60.
805. Serhiyenko VA, Serhiyenko AA. Diabetic cardiac autonomic neuropathy: do we have any treatment perspectives? World J Diabetes. 2015;6(2):245–58. https://doi.org/10.4239/wjd.v6.i2.245. Review.
806. Keen H, Payan J, Allawi J, Walker J, Jamal GA, Weir AI, Henderson LM, Bissessar EA, Watkins PJ, Sampson M, Gale EA, Scarpello J, Boddie HG, Hardy KJ, Thomas PK, Misra P, Halonen JP. Treatment of diabetic neuropathy with gamma-linolenic acid. Diabetes Care. 1993;16:8–15.
807. Uribarri J, Tuttle KR. Advanced glycation end products and nephrotoxicity of high-protein diets. Clin J Am Soc Nephrol. 2006;1(6):1293–9. Epub 2006 Sept 27.
808. De Marchi E, Baldassari F, Bononi A, Wieckowski MR, Pinton P. Oxidative stress in cardiovascular diseases and obesity: role of p66Shc and protein kinase C. Oxidative Med Cell Longev. 2013;2013:564961. https://doi.org/10.1155/2013/564961. Epub 2013 Mar 27. Review.
809. Pittenger G, Vinik A. Nerve growth factor and diabetic neuropathy. Exp Diabesity Res. 2003;4:271–85.
810. Rivard A, Silver M, Chen D, Kearney M, Magner M, Annex B, Peters K, Isner JM. Rescue of diabetes-related impairment of angiogenesis by intramuscular gene therapy with adeno-VEGF. Am J Pathol. 1999;154:355–63.
811. Tam J, Rosenberg L, Maysinger D. INGAP peptide improves nerve function and enhances regeneration in streptozotocin-induced diabetic C57BL/6 mice. FASEB J. 2004;18:1767–9.
812. Milicevic Z, Newlon PG, Pittenger GL, Stansberry KB, Vinik AI. Anti-ganglioside GM1 antibody and distal symmetric "diabetic polyneuropathy" with dominant motor features. Diabetologia. 1997;40:1364–5.

813. Sharma K, Cross J, Farronay O, Ayyar D, Sheber R, Bradley W. Demyelinating neuropathy in diabetes mellitus. Arch Neurol. 2002;59:758–65.
814. Krendel DA, Costigan DA, Hopkins LC. Successful treatment of neuropathies in patients with diabetes mellitus. Arch Neurol. 1995;52:1053–61.
815. Pfeifer MA, Weinberg CR, Cook DL, Reenan A, Halter JB, Ensinck JW. Autonomic neural dysfunction in recently diagnosed diabetic subjects. Diabetes Care. 1984;7:447–53.
816. Stansberry KB, Hill MA, Shapiro SA, McNitt PM, Bhatt BA, Vinik AI. Impairment of peripheral blood flow responses in diabetes resembles an enhanced aging effect. Diabetes Care. 1997;20:1711–6.
817. Stansberry KB, Shapiro SA, Hill MA, McNitt PM, Meyer MD, Vinik AI. Impaired peripheral vasomotion in diabetes. Diabetes Care. 1996;19:715–21.
818. Stansberry KB, Hill MA, Shapiro SA, McNitt PM, Bhatt BA, Vinik AI. Impairment of peripheral blood flow responses in diabetes resembles an enhanced aging effect. Diabetes Care. 1997;20:1711–6.
819. Stansberry KB. Primary nociceptive afferents mediate the blood flow dysfunction in non-glabrous (hairy) skin of type 2 diabetes. Diabetes Care. 1999;22:1549–54.
820. Haak ES, Usadel KH, Kohleisen M, Yilmaz A, Kusterer K, Haak T. The effect of alpha-lipoic on the neurovascular reflex arc in patients with diabetic neuropathy assessed by capillary microscopy. Microvasc Res. 1999;58:28–34.
821. Ziegler D. Diabetic cardiovascular autonomic neuropathy: prognosis, diagnosis and treatment. Diabetes Metab Rev. 1994;10:339–83.
822. Valensi P. Diabetic autonomic neuropathy: what are the risks? Diabetes Metab. 1998;24:66–72.
823. Levitt NS, Stansberry KB, Wychanck S, Vinik AI. Natural progression of autonomic neuropathy and autonomic function tests in a cohort of IDDM. Diabetes Care. 1996;19:751–4.
824. Gaede P, Vedel P, Larsen N, Jensen GV, Parving HH, Pedersen O. Multifactorial intervention and cardiovascular disease in patients with type 2 diabetes. N Engl J Med. 2003;348:383–93.
825. Gaede P, Lund-Andersen H, Parving HH, Pedersen O. Effect of a multifactorial intervention on mortality in type 2 diabetes. N Engl J Med. 2008;358:580–91.
826. Dimitropoulos G, Tahrani AA, Stevens MJ. Cardiac autonomic neuropathy in patients with diabetes mellitus. World J Diabetes. 2014;5(1):17–39. Published online Feb 15, 2014. https://doi.org/10.4239/wjd.v5.i1.17.
827. Edwards JL, Vincent AM, Cheng HT, Feldman EL. Diabetic neuropathy: mechanisms to management. Pharmacol Ther. 2008;120:1–34.
828. Vinik AI, Freeman R, Erbas T. Diabetic autonomic neuropathy. Semin Neurol. 2003;23:365–72.
829. Leinninger GM, Edwards JL, Lipshaw MJ, Feldman EL. Mechanisms of disease: mitochondria as new therapeutic targets in diabetic neuropathy. Nat Clin Pract Neurol. 2006;2:620–8.
830. Soriano FG, Virág L, Szabó C. Diabetic endothelial dysfunction: role of reactive oxygen and nitrogen species production and poly(ADP-ribose) polymerase activation. J Mol Med (Berl). 2001;79:437–48.
831. Obrosova IG, Julius UA. Role for poly(ADP-ribose) polymerase activation in diabetic nephropathy, neuropathy and retinopathy. Curr Vasc Pharmacol. 2005;3:267–83.
832. Yamagishi S, Uehara K, Otsuki S, Yagihashi S. Differential influence of increased polyol pathway on protein kinase C expressions between endoneurial and epineurial tissues in diabetic mice. J Neurochem. 2003;87:497–507.
833. Giacco F, Brownlee M. Oxidative stress and diabetic complications. Circ Res. 2010;107:1058–70.
834. Williams B, Gallacher B, Patel H, Orme C. Glucose-induced protein kinase C activation regulates vascular permeability factor mRNA expression and peptide production by human vascular smooth muscle cells in vitro. Diabetes. 1997;46:1497–503.
835. Russell JW, Sullivan KA, Windebank AJ, Herrmann DN, Feldman EL. Neurons undergo apoptosis in animal and cell culture models of diabetes. Neurobiol Dis. 1999;6:347–63.
836. Ramasamy R, Vannucci SJ, Yan SS, Herold K, Yan SF, Schmidt AM. Advanced glycation end products and RAGE: a common thread in aging, diabetes, neurodegeneration, and inflammation. Glycobiology. 2005;15:16R–28R.
837. Kolm-Litty V, Sauer U, Nerlich A, Lehmann R, Schleicher ED. High glucose-induced transforming growth factor beta1 production is mediated by the hexosamine pathway in porcine glomerular mesangial cells. J Clin Invest. 1998;101:160–9.
838. Wada R, Yagihashi S. Role of advanced glycation end products and their receptors in development of diabetic neuropathy. Ann N Y Acad Sci. 2005;1043:598–604.
839. Sayeski PP, Kudlow JE. Glucose metabolism to glucosamine is necessary for glucose stimulation of transforming growth factor-alpha gene transcription. J Biol Chem. 1996;271:15237–43.
840. Narkiewicz K, Somers VK. Sympathetic nerve activity in obstructive sleep apnoea. Acta Physiol Scand. 2003;177:385–90.
841. Bradley TD, Floras JS. Obstructive sleep apnoea and its cardiovascular consequences. Lancet. 2009;373:82–93.
842. Tahrani AA, Ali A, Raymond NT, Begum S, Dubb K, Mughal S, Jose B, Piya MK, Barnett AH, Stevens MJ. Obstructive sleep apnea and diabetic neuropathy: a novel association in patients with type 2 diabetes. Am J Respir Crit Care Med. 2012;186:434–41.
843. Ficker JH, Dertinger SH, Siegfried W, König HJ, Pentz M, Sailer D, Katalinic A, Hahn EG. Obstructive sleep apnoea and diabetes mellitus: the role of car-

diovascular autonomic neuropathy. Eur Respir J. 1998;11(1):14–9.
844. Janovsky CC, Rolim LC, de Sá JR, Poyares D, Tufik S, Silva AB, Dib SA. Cardiovascular autonomic neuropathy contributes to sleep apnea in young and lean type 1 diabetes mellitus patients. Front Endocrinol (Lausanne). 2014;5:119. https://doi.org/10.3389/fendo.2014.00119. eCollection 2014.
845. Axelrod S, Lishner M, Oz O, Bernheim J, Ravid M. Spectral analysis of fluctuations in heart rate: an objective evaluation of autonomic nervous control in chronic renal failure. Nephron. 1987;45:202–6.
846. Felten SY, Peterson RG, Shea PA, Besch HR, Felten DL. Effects of streptozotocin diabetes on the noradrenergic innervation of the rat heart: a longitudinal histofluorescence and neurochemical study. Brain Res Bull. 1982;8:593–607.
847. Poulsen PL, Hansen KW, Mogensen CE. Increase in nocturnal blood pressure and progression to microalbuminuria in diabetes. N Engl J Med. 2003;348:260–24; author reply 260–24.
848. Hirabara SM, Silveira LR, Alberici LC, Leandro CV, Lambertucci RH, Polimeno GC, Cury Boaventura MF, Procopio J, Vercesi AE, Curi R. Acute effect of fatty acids on metabolism and mitochondrial coupling in skeletal muscle. Biochim Biophys Acta. 2006;1757:57–66.
849. Schrauwen P, Hoeks J, Hesselink MK. Putative function and physiological relevance of the mitochondrial uncoupling protein-3: involvement in fatty acid metabolism. Prog Lipid Res. 2006;45:17–41.
850. Collins-Nakai RL, Noseworthy D, Lopaschuk GD. Epinephrine increases ATP production in hearts by preferentially increasing glucose metabolism. Am J Phys. 1994;267:H1862–71.
851. Francis GS. Diabetic cardiomyopathy: fact or fiction. Heart. 2001;85:247–8.
852. Frustaci A, Kajstura J, Chimenti C, Jakoniuk I, Leri A, Maseri A, Nadal-Ginard B, Anversa P. Myocardial cell death in human diabetes. Circ Res. 2000;87:1123–32.
853. Katz AM. Potential deleterious effects of inotropic agents in the therapy of chronic heart failure. Circulation. 1986;73:III184–90.
854. Eichhorn EJ, Bristow MR. Medical therapy can improve the biological properties of the chronically failing heart. A new era in the treatment of heart failure. Circulation. 1996;94:2285–96.
855. Yaplito-Lee J, Weintraub R, Jamsen K, Chow CW, Thorburn DR, Boneh A. Cardiac manifestations in oxidative phosphorylation disorders of childhood. J Pediatr. 2007;150:407–11.
856. Givertz MM, Sawyer DB, Colucci WS. Antioxidants and myocardial contractility: illuminating the "dark side" of beta-adrenergic receptor activation. Circulation. 2001;103:782–3.
857. Scacco S, Vergari R, Scarpulla RC, Technikova-Dobrova Z, Sardanelli A, Lambo R, Lorusso V, Papa S. cAMP-dependent phosphorylation of the nuclear encoded 18-kDa (IP) subunit of respiratory complex I and activation of the complex in serum-starved mouse fibroblast cultures. J Biol Chem. 2000;275:17578–82.
858. An D, Rodrigues B. Role of changes in cardiac metabolism in development of diabetic cardiomyopathy. Am J Physiol Heart Circ Physiol. 2006;291:H1489–506.
859. Iwai-Kanai E, Hasegawa K, Araki M, Kakita T, Morimoto T, Sasayama S. Alpha- and beta-adrenergic pathways differentially regulate cell type-specific apoptosis in rat cardiac myocytes. Circulation. 1999;100:305–11. Communal C, Singh K, Pimentel DR, Colucci WS. Norepinephrine stimulates apoptosis in adult rat ventricular myocytes by activation of the beta-adrenergic pathway. Circulation. 1998;98:1329–1334.
860. Communal C, Singh K, Pimentel DR, Colucci WS. Norepinephrine stimulates apoptosis in adult rat ventricular myocytes by activation of the beta-adrenergic pathway. Circulation. 1998;98:1329–34.
861. Carnethon MR, Prineas RJ, Temprosa M, Zhang ZM, Uwaifo G, Molitch ME. The association among autonomic nervous system function, incident diabetes, and intervention arm in the Diabetes Prevention Program. Diabetes Care. 2006;29:914–9.
862. Maser RE, Lenhard MJ. An overview of the effect of weight loss on cardiovascular autonomic function. Curr Diabetes Rev. 2007;3:204–11.
863. Voulgari C, Pagoni S, Vinik A, Poirier P. Exercise improves cardiac autonomic function in obesity and diabetes. Metabolism. 2013;62:609–21.
864. Yarandi S, Srinivasan S. Diabetic gastrointestinal motility disorders and the role of enteric nervous system: current status and future directions. Neurogastroenterol Motil. 2014;26(5):611–24. Published online 2014 Mar 24. https://doi.org/10.1111/nmo.12330.
865. Golbidi S, Ebadi SA, Laher I. Antioxidants in the treatment of diabetes. Curr Diabetes Rev. 2011;7:106–25.
866. Rhee SH, Pothoulakis C, Mayer EA. Principles and clinical implications of the brain-gut-enteric microbiota axis. Nat Rev Gastroenterol Hepatol. 2009;6:306–14.
867. Czesnikiewicz-Guzik M, Konturek SJ, Loster B, Wisniewska G, Majewski S. Melatonin and its role in oxidative stress related diseases of oral cavity. J Physiol Pharmacol. 2007;58(Suppl 3):5–19. Review.
868. Finaud J, Lac G, Filaire E. Oxidative stress. Sports Med. 2006;36:327–58.
869. Powers SK, Talbert EE, Adhihetty PJ. Reactive oxygen and nitrogen species as intracellular signals in skeletal muscle. J Physiol. 2011;589:2129–38.
870. Newsholme P, Cruzat VF, Keane KN, Carlessi R, de Bittencourt PIH. Molecular mechanisms of ROS production and oxidative stress in diabetes. Biochem J. 2016;473(24):4527–50.
871. Silvestri S, Orlando P, Armeni T, Padella L, Brugè F, Seddaiu G, Littarru GP, Tiano L. Coenzyme

Q10 and α-lipoic acid: antioxidant and pro-oxidant effects in plasma and peripheral blood lymphocytes of supplemented subjects. J Clin Biochem Nutr. 2015;57(1):21–6. Published online 2015 Apr 16. https://doi.org/10.3164/jcbn.14-130.
872. Dröge W. Free radicals in the physiological control of cell function. Physiol Rev. 2002;82:47–95.
873. Niess AM. Generation and disposal of reactive oxygen and nitrogen species. In: Mooren FC, Volker K, editors. Molecular and cellular exercise physiology. Champaign: Human Kinetics; 2005. p. 179–97.
874. Powers SK, Deruisseau KC, Quindry J, Hamilton KL. Dietary antioxidants and exercise. J Sports Sci. 2004;22:81–94.
875. Christofidou-Solomidou M, Muzykantov VR. Antioxidant strategies in respiratory medicine. Treat Respir Med. 2006;5(1):47–78. Review.
876. Halliwell B. Oxidative stress and neurodegeneration: where are we now? J Neurochem. 2006;97(6):1634–58. Review.
877. Sies H. Oxidative stress: oxidants and antioxidants. Exp Physiol. 1997;82(2):291–5. Review.
878. Ilie M, Margină D. Trends in the evaluation of lipid peroxidation processes. In: Catala A, editor. Lipid peroxidation, Ch 5; 2012. p. 111–30. http://www.intechopen.com/books/lipid-peroxidation
879. Aruoma OI, Halliwell B, Laughton MJ, Quinlan GJ, Gutteridge JM. The mechanism of initiation of lipid peroxidation. Evidence against a requirement for an iron(II)-iron(III) complex. Biochem J. 1989;258(2):617–20.
880. Elroy-Stein O, Bernstein Y, Groner Y. Overproduction of human Cu/Zn-superoxide dismutase in transfected cells: extenuation of paraquat-mediated cytotoxicity and enhancement of lipid peroxidation. EMBO J. 1986;5(3):615–22.
881. Freinbichler W, Colivicchi MA, Stefanini C, Bianchi L, Ballini C, Misini B, Weinberger P, Linert W, Varešlija D, Tipton KF, Della CL. Highly reactive oxygen species: detection, formation, and possible functions. Cell Mol Life Sci. 2011;68(12):2067–79. https://doi.org/10.1007/s00018-011-0682-x. Epub 2011 May 2. Review.
882. Halliwell B, Gutteridge JM. Role of iron in oxygen radical reactions. Methods Enzymol. 1984;105:47–56.
883. Velayutham M, Hemann C, Zweier JL. Removal of $H_2O_2$ and generation of superoxide radical: role of cytochrome c and NADH. Free Radic Biol Med. 2011;51(1):160–70. https://doi.org/10.1016/j.freeradbiomed.2011.04.007. Epub 2011 Apr 13.
884. Gordon MH. Significance of dietary antioxidants for health. Int J Mol Sci. 2012;13(1):173–9. https://doi.org/10.3390/ijms13010173. Epub 2011 Dec 23. Review.
885. Halliwell B. Reactive species and antioxidants. Redox biology is a fundamental theme of aerobic life. Plant Physiol. 2006;141(2):312–22.
886. Halliwell B. Phagocyte-derived reactive species: salvation or suicide? Trends Biochem Sci. 2006;31(9):509–15. Epub 2006 Aug 4. Review.
887. Powers SK, Lennon SL. Analysis of cellular responses to free radicals: focus on exercise and skeletal muscle. Proc Nutr Soc London. 1999;58:1025–33.
888. Seifried HE, Anderson DE, Fisher EI, Milner JA. A review of the interaction among dietary antioxidants and reactive oxygen species. J Nutr Biochem. 2007;18:567–79.
889. MacRae HS, Mefferd KM. Dietary antioxidant supplementation combined with quercetin improves cycling time trial performance. Int J Sport Nutr Exerc Metab. 2006;16:405–19.
890. Oh J, Shin Y, Yoon J, et al. Effect of supplementation with Ecklonia cava polyphenol on endurance performance of college students. Int J Sport Nutr Exerc Metab. 2010;20:72–9.
891. Villegas L, Stidham T, Nozik-Grayck E. Oxidative stress and therapeutic development in lung diseases. J Pulm Respir Med. 2014;4(4). pii: 194. Epub 2014 Jul 15.
892. Chapple SJ, Cheng X, Mann GE. Effects of 4-hydroxynonenal on vascular endothelial and smooth muscle cell redox signaling and function in health and disease. Redox Biol. 2013;1:319–31.
893. Ushio-Fukai M. VEGF signaling through NADPH oxidase-derived ROS. Antioxid Redox Signal. 2007;9:731–9.
894. Urao N, Ushio-Fukai M. Redox regulation of stem/progenitor cells and bone marrow niche. Free Radic Biol Med. 2013;54:26–39.
895. Baran CP, Zeigler MM, Tridandapani S, Marsh CB. The role of ROS and RNS in regulating life and death of blood monocytes. Curr Pharm Des. 2004;10:855–66.
896. Fialkow L, Wang Y, Downey GP. Reactive oxygen and nitrogen species as signaling molecules regulating neutrophil function. Free Radic Biol Med. 2007;42:153–64.
897. Birukov KG. Cyclic stretch, reactive oxygen species, and vascular remodeling. Antioxid Redox Signal. 2009;11:1651–67.
898. Frazziano G, Champion HC, Pagano PJ. NADPH oxidase-derived ROS and the regulation of pulmonary vessel tone. Am J Physiol Heart Circ Physiol. 2012;302:H2166–77.
899. Knock GA, Ward JP. Redox regulation of protein kinases as a modulator of vascular function. Antioxid Redox Signal. 2011;15:1531–47.
900. Janssen LJ. Isoprostanes and lung vascular pathology. Am J Respir Cell Mol Biol. 2008;39:383–9.
901. Janssen LJ, Catalli A, Helli P. The pulmonary biology of isoprostanes. Antioxid Redox Signal. 2005;7:244–55.
902. Ckless K. Redox proteomics: from bench to bedside. Adv Exp Med Biol. 2014;806:301–17.
903. Matsuo M, Kaneko T. The chemistry of reactive oxygen species and related free radicals. In: Radak Z, editor. Free radicals in exercise and aging. Leeds: Human Kinetics; 2000. p. 1–34.
904. Sawka MN, Burke LM, Eichner ER, Maughan RJ, Montain SJ, et al. American College of Sports

Medicine position stand. Exercise and fluid replacement. Med Sci Sports Exerc. 2007;39(2):377–90. PMID: 17277604.
905. Paik IY, Jeong MH, Jin HE, Kim YI, Suh AR, et al. Fluid replacement following dehydration reduces oxidative stress during recovery. Biochem Biophys Res Commun. 2009;383(1):103–7. https://doi.org/10.1016/j.bbrc.2009.03.135.
906. Ziegler D, Schatz H, Conrad F, Gries FA, Ulrich H, Reichel G. Effects of treatment with the antioxidant alpha-lipoic acid on cardiac autonomic neuropathy in NIDDM patients. A 4-month randomized controlled multicenter trial (DEKAN Study). Deutsche Kardiale Autonome Neuropathy. Diabetes Care. 1997;20:369–73.
907. Spallone V, Ziegler D, Freeman R, Bernardi L, Frontoni S, Pop-Busui R, Stevens M, Kempler P, Hilsted J, Tesfaye S, Low P, Valensi P; On Behalf of the Toronto Consensus Panel on Diabetic Neuropathy*. Cardiovascular autonomic neuropathy in diabetes: clinical impact, assessment, diagnosis, and management. Diabetes Metab Res Rev. 2011;27(7):639–53; Epub ahead of print.
908. Manzella D, Barbieri M, Ragno E, Paolisso G. Chronic administration of pharmacologic doses of vitamin E improves the cardiac autonomic nervous system in patients with type 2 diabetes. Am J Clin Nutr. 2001;73:1052–7.
909. Ametov AS, Barinov A, Dyck PJ, Hermann R, Kozlova N, Litchy WJ, Low PA, Nehrdich D, Novosadova M, O'Brien PC, Reljanovic M, Samigullin R, Schuette K, Strokov I, Tritschler HJ, Wessel K, Yakhno N, Ziegler D. The sensory symptoms of diabetic polyneuropathy are improved with alpha-lipoic acid: the SYDNEY trial. Diabetes Care. 2003;26:770–6.
910. Ruhnau KJ, Meissner HP, Finn R, Reljanovic M, Lobisch M, Schutte K, Nehrdich D, Tritschler H, Mehnert H, Ziegler D. Effects of 3-week oral treatment with the antioxidant thioctic acid (alpha-lipoic acid) in symptomatic diabetic polyneuropathy. Diabet Med. 1999;16(12):1040–3.
911. Ziegler D, Hanefeld M, Ruhnau KJ, Meissner HP, Lobisch M, Schutte K, Gries FA. Treatment of symptomatic diabetic peripheral neuropathy with the anti-oxidant alpha-lipoic acid. A 3-week multicentre randomized controlled trial (ALADIN Study). Diabetologia. 1995;38:1425–33.
912. Reljanovic M, Reichel G, Rett K, Lobisch M, Schuette K, Moller W, Tritschler HJ, Mehnert H. Treatment of diabetic polyneuropathy with the antioxidant thioctic acid (alpha-lipoic acid): a two year multicenter randomized double-blind placebo-controlled trial (ALADIN II). Alpha Lipoic Acid in Diabetic Neuropathy. Free Radic Res. 1999;31(3):171–9.
913. Ziegler D, Nowak H, Kempler P, Vargha P, Low PA. Treatment of symptomatic diabetic polyneuropathy with the antioxidant alpha-lipoic acid: a meta-analysis. Diabet Med. 2004;21:114–21.
914. Mortensen SA, Rosenfeldt F, Kumar A, Dolliner P, Filipiak KJ, Pella D, Alehagen U, Steurer G, Littarru GP, Q-SYMBIO Study Investigators. The effect of coenzyme Q10 on morbidity and mortality in chronic heart failure: results from Q-SYMBIO: a randomized double-blind trial. JACC Heart Fail. 2014;2(6):641–9. https://doi.org/10.1016/j.jchf.2014.06.008. Epub 2014 Oct 1.
915. Rosenfeldt FL, Haas SJ, Krum H, Hadj A, Ng K, Leong JY, Watts GF. Coenzyme Q10 in the treatment of hypertension: a meta-analysis of the clinical trials. J Hum Hypertens. 2007;21(4):297–306. Epub 2007 Feb 8.
916. Rosenfeldt F, Hilton D, Pepe S, Krum H. Systematic review of effect of coenzyme Q10 in physical exercise, hypertension and heart failure. Biofactors. 2003;18(1–4):91–100. Review.
917. Deichmann R, Lavie C, Andrews S. Coenzyme q10 and statin-induced mitochondrial dysfunction. Ochsner J. 2010;10(1):16–21.
918. Greene DA, Arezzo JC, Brown MB. Effect of aldose reductase inhibition on nerve conduction and morphometry in diabetic neuropathy. Zenarestat Study Group. Neurology. 1999;53:580–91.
919. Hotta N, Toyota T, Matsuoka K, Shigeta Y, Kikkawa R, Kaneko T, Takahashi A, Sugimura K, Koike Y, Ishii J, Sakamoto N, The SNK-860 Diabetic Neuropathy Study Group. Clinical efficacy of fidarestat, a novel aldose reductase inhibitor, for diabetic peripheral neuropathy. Diabetes Care. 2001;24:1776–82.
920. Hotta N, Shigeta Y, Sakamoto N. Long-term effects of epalrestat, an aldose reductase inhibitor, on diabetic peripheral neuropathy: A 3-y multicenter comparative study, ARI-diabetes complications trial (ADCT) (abstract). Diabetes. 2005;54:A213.
921. Vinik AI, Mehrabyan A. Diabetic neuropathies. Med Clin North Am. 2004;88:947–99, xi.
922. Vinik AI, Bril V, Litchy WJ, Price KL, Bastyr EJ III. Sural sensory action potential identifies diabetic peripheral neuropathy responders to therapy. Muscle Nerve. 2005;32(5):619–25.
923. Casellini CM, Barlow PM, Rice AL, Casey M, Simmons K, Pittenger G, Bastyr EJ III, Wolka AM, Vinik AI. A 6-month, randomized, double-masked, placebo-controlled study evaluating the effects of the protein kinase C-{beta} inhibitor ruboxistaurin on skin microvascular blood flow and other measures of diabetic peripheral neuropathy. Diabetes Care. 2007;30:896–902.
924. Myung SK, Ju W, Cho B, Oh SW, Park SM, Koo BK, Park BJ. Efficacy of vitamin and antioxidant supplements in prevention of cardiovascular disease: systematic review and meta-analysis of randomised controlled trials. BMJ. 2013;346:f10. Published online 2013 Jan 18. https://doi.org/10.1136/bmj.f10
925. Granata S, Dalla Gassa A, Tomei P, Lupo A, Zaza G. Mitochondria: a new therapeutic target in chronic kidney disease. Nutr Metab (Lond). 2015;12:49. https://doi.org/10.1186/s12986-015-0044-z. eCollection 2015. Review.

926. Esteban Zubero E, García-Gil FA, López-Pingarrón L, Alatorre-Jiménez MA, Ramirez JM, Tan DX, García JJ, Reiter RJ. Melatonin role preventing steatohepatitis and improving liver transplantation results. Cell Mol Life Sci. 2016;73(15):2911–27. https://doi.org/10.1007/s00018-016-2185-2.
927. Abilés J, de la Cruz AP, Castaño J, Rodríguez-Elvira M, Aguayo E, Moreno-Torres R, Llopis J, Aranda P, Argüelles S, Ayala A, de la Quintana AM, Planells EM. Oxidative stress is increased in critically ill patients according to antioxidant vitamins intake, independent of severity: a cohort study. Crit Care. 2006;10(5):R146.
928. Therond P, Bonnefont-Rousselout D, Davit-Sparaul A, Conti M, Legrand A. Biomarkers of oxidative stress: an analytical approach. Curr Opin Clin Nutr Metab Care. 2000;3:373–84. https://doi.org/10.1097/00075197-200009000-00009.
929. Alonso de la Vega JM, Díaz J, Serrano E, Carbonell LF. Plasma redox status relates to severity in critically ill patients. Crit Care Med. 2000;28:1812–4. https://doi.org/10.1097/00003246-200006000-00021.
930. Motoyama T, Okamoto K, Kukita I, Hamaguchi M, Kinoshita Y, Ogawa H. Possible role of increase oxidant stress in multiple organ failure after systemic inflammatory response syndrome. Crit Care Med. 2003;31:1048–52. https://doi.org/10.1097/01.CCM.0000055371.27268.36.
931. Goode HF, Cowley HC, Walker BE, Howdle PD, Webster NR. Decreased antioxidant status and increased lipid peroxidation in patients with septic shock and secondary organ dysfunction. Crit Care Med. 1995;23:646–51. https://doi.org/10.1097/00003246-199504000-00011.
932. Grimble RF. Nutrition antioxidants and the modulation of inflammation theory and practice. New Horiz. 1994;2:175–85.
933. Hammerman C, Kaplan M. Ischemia and reperfusion injury. Clin Perinatol. 1998;25:757–77.
934. Yu BP. Cellular defenses against damage from reactive species. Physiol Rev. 1994;74:139–62.
935. Jeevanandam M, Begay CK, Shahbazian LM, Scott R, Petersen MD. Altered plasma cytokines and total glutathione levels in parenterally fed critically ill trauma patients with adjuvant recombinant human growth hormone therapy. Crit Care Med. 2000;28:324–9. https://doi.org/10.1097/00003246-200002000-00006.
936. Nathens AB, Neff MJ, Jurkavich GJ. Randomized, prospective trial of antioxidant supplementation in critically ill surgical patients. Ann Surg. 2002;236:814–22. https://doi.org/10.1097/00000658-200212000-00014.
937. Preiser JC, Gossum AV, Berré J, Vincent JL, Carpentier Y. Enteral feeding with a solution enriched with antioxidant vitamins A, C and E enhances the resistance to oxidative stress. Crit Care Med. 2000;28:3828–32. https://doi.org/10.1097/00003246-200012000-00013.
938. Crimi E, Liguori A, Condorelli M, Cioffi M, Astuto M, Bontempo P, Pignalosa O, Viteri MT, Molinari AM, Sica V, et al. The beneficial effects of antioxidant supplementation in enteral feeding in critically ill patients: a prospective, randomized, double-blind, placebo-controlled trial. Anesth Analg. 2004;99:857–63. https://doi.org/10.1213/01.ANE.0000133144.60584.F6.
939. Rahman I, Biswas SK, Kode A. Oxidant and antioxidant balance in the airways and airway diseases. Eur J Pharmacol. 2006;533(1–3):222–39. Epub 2006 Feb 28. Review.
940. Spickett CM, Forman HJ, editors. Lipid oxidation in health and disease. Oxidative stress and disease. Boca Raton: CRC Press; 2015.
941. Freeman R, Abuzinadah A, Gibbons C, Jones P, Miglis M, Sinn,D. Orthostatic hypotension. J Am Coll Cardiol State Art Rev 2018; 22(7); 1294–1309.
942. Liu G, Zhang C, Yin J, Li X, Cheng F, Li Y, Yang H, Uéda K, Chan P, Yu S. Alpha-synuclein is differentially expressed in mitochondria from different rat brain regions and dose-dependently down-regulates complex I activity. Neurosci Lett. 2009;454(3):187–92. https://doi.org/10.1016/j.neulet.2009.02.056.
943. Zhang H, Jia H, Liu J, Ao N, Yan B, Shen W, Wang X, et al. Combined R-alpha-lipoic acid and acetyl-L-carnitine exerts efficient preventative effects in a cellular model of Parkinson's disease. J Cell Mol Med. 2010;14(1–2):215–25.
944. Biosa A, Outiero T, Bubacco L, Bisaglia M. Diabetes mellitus as a risk factor for Parkinson's disease: a molecular point of view. Mol Neurobiol. 2018;28:1025–9. https://doi.org/10.1007/s12035-018-1025-9.
945. Lee W, Kim S, Kim G, Han S, Won J, Jung C, et al. Alpha-lipoic acid activates dimethylaminohydrolase in cultured endothelial cells. Biochem Biophys Res Commun. 2010;398(4):653–8.
946. Goudy S, Regalia J, Cai F, Helke C. Alpha-lipoic acid treatment prevents the diabetes-induced attenuation of the afferent limb of the baroreceptor reflex in rats. Auton Neurosci. 2003;108(1–2):32–44.
947. Queiroz TM, Guimarães DD, Mendes-Junior LG, Braga VA. α-lipoic acid reduces hypertension and increases baroreflex sensitivity in renovascular hypertensive rats. Molecules. 2012;17(11):13357–67.
948. Mohammadi V, Khorvash F, Feizi A, Askari G. Does alpha-lipoic acid supplementation modulate cardiovascular risk factors in patients with stroke? A randomized, double-blind clinical trial. Int J Prev Med. 2018;9:34.
949. Tardif J, Rheaume E. Lipoic acid supplementation and endothelial function. Br J Pharmacol. 2008;153(8):1587–8.
950. Bavarsad Shahripour R, Harrigan MR, Alexandrov AV. N-acetylcysteine (NAC) in neurological disorders: mechanisms of action and therapeutic opportunities. Brain Behav. 2014;4(2):108–22. https://doi.org/10.1002/brb3.208. Epub 2014 Jan 13. Review.

951. Berk M, Malhi GS, Gray LJ, Dean OM. The promise of N-acetylcysteine in neuropsychiatry. Trends Pharmacol Sci. 2013;34(3):167–77. https://doi.org/10.1016/j.tips.2013.01.001. Epub 2013 Jan 29. Review.
952. Dean O, Giorlando F, Berk M. N-acetylcysteine in psychiatry: current therapeutic evidence and potential mechanisms of action. J Psychiatry Neurosci. 2011;36(2):78–86. https://doi.org/10.1503/jpn.100057. Review.
953. Smaga I, Pomierny B, Krzyżanowska W, Pomierny-Chamioło L, Miszkiel J, Niedzielska E, Ogórka A, Filip M. N-acetylcysteine possesses antidepressant-like activity through reduction of oxidative stress: behavioral and biochemical analyses in rats. Prog Neuro-Psychopharmacol Biol Psychiatry. 2012;39(2):280–7. https://doi.org/10.1016/j.pnpbp.2012.06.018. Epub 2012 Jul 20.
954. Maes M, Galecki P, Chang YS, Berk M. A review on the oxidative and nitrosative stress (O&NS) pathways in major depression and their possible contribution to the (neuro)degenerative processes in that illness. Prog Neuro-Psychopharmacol Biol Psychiatry. 2011;35(3):676–92. https://doi.org/10.1016/j.pnpbp.2010.05.004. Epub 2010 May 12. Review.
955. Bilici M, Efe H, Köroğlu MA, Uydu HA, Bekaroğlu M, Değer O. Antioxidative enzyme activities and lipid peroxidation in major depression: alterations by antidepressant treatments. J Affect Disord. 2001;64(1):43–51.
956. Altuntas I, Aksoy H, Coskun I, Cayköylü A, Akçay F. Erythrocyte superoxide dismutase and glutathione peroxidase activities, and malondialdehyde and reduced glutathione levels in schizophrenic patients. Clin Chem Lab Med. 2000;38(12):1277–81.
957. Circu ML, Aw TY. Glutathione and apoptosis. Free Radic Res. 2008;42(8):689–706. https://doi.org/10.1080/10715760802317663. Review.
958. Franco R, Cidlowski JA. Apoptosis and glutathione: beyond an antioxidant. Cell Death Differ. 2009;16(10):1303–14. https://doi.org/10.1038/cdd.2009.107. Epub 2009 Aug 7. Review.
959. Circu ML, Aw TY. Glutathione and modulation of cell apoptosis. Biochim Biophys Acta. 2012;1823(10):1767–77. https://doi.org/10.1016/j.bbamcr.2012.06.019. Epub 2012 Jun 23. Review.
960. Franco R, Cidlowski JA. Glutathione efflux and cell death. Antioxid Redox Signal. 2012;17(12):1694–713. https://doi.org/10.1089/ars.2012.4553. Epub 2012 Jul 16. Review.
961. Konradi C, Eaton M, MacDonald ML, Walsh J, Benes FM, Heckers S. Molecular evidence for mitochondrial dysfunction in bipolar disorder. Arch Gen Psychiatry. 2004;61(3):300–8. Erratum in: Arch Gen Psychiatry. 2004 Jun;61(6):538.
962. Chen AT, Chibnall JT, Nasrallah HA. Placebo-controlled augmentation trials of the antioxidant NAC in schizophrenia: a review. Ann Clin Psychiatry. 2016;28(3):190–6.
963. Vavilin VA, Safronova OG, Manankin NA, Kaznacheeva LF, Lyakhovich VV. Glutathione-S-transferase polymorphism and clinical features of acute drug poisoning in children. Bull Exp Biol Med. 2005;139(4):431–3.
964. Morris G, Anderson G, Dean O, Berk M, Galecki P, Martin-Subero M, Maes M. The glutathione system: a new drug target in neuroimmune disorders. Mol Neurobiol. 2014;50(3):1059–84. https://doi.org/10.1007/s12035-014-8705-x. Epub 2014 Apr 22. Review.
965. Yeligar SM, Harris FL, Hart CM, Brown LA. Glutathione attenuates ethanol-induced alveolar macrophage oxidative stress and dysfunction by downregulating NADPH oxidases. Am J Physiol Lung Cell Mol Physiol. 2014;306(5):L429–41. https://doi.org/10.1152/ajplung.00159.2013. Epub 2014 Jan 17.
966. Kodama Y, Kishimoto Y, Muramatsu Y, Tatebe J, Yamamoto Y, Hirota N, Itoigawa Y, Atsuta R, Koike K, Sato T, Aizawa K, Takahashi K, Morita T, Homma S, Seyama K, Ishigami A. Antioxidant nutrients in plasma of Japanese patients with chronic obstructive pulmonary disease (COPD), asthma-COPD overlap syndrome, and bronchial asthma. Clin Respir J. 2015. https://doi.org/10.1111/crj.12436. [Epub ahead of print].
967. Vicentini GE, Fracaro L, de Souza SR, Martins HA, Guarnier FA, Zanoni JN. Experimental cancer cachexia changes neuron numbers and peptide levels in the intestine: partial protective effects after dietary supplementation with L-glutamine. PLoS One. 2016;11(9):e0162998. https://doi.org/10.1371/journal.pone.0162998. eCollection 2016.
968. Lott J. The mother of all antioxidants: how health gurus are misleading you and what you should know about glutathione. Archangel Ink; 2014.
969. Jason LA, Boulton A, Porter NS, Jessen T, Njoku MG, Friedberg F. Classification of myalgic encephalomyelitis/chronic fatigue syndrome by types of fatigue. Behav Med. 2010;36(1):24–31. https://doi.org/10.1080/08964280903521370.
970. Mathew SJ. Treatment-resistant depression: recent developments and future directions. Depress Anxiety. 2008;25(12):989–92. https://doi.org/10.1002/da.20540.
971. Kato T, Kubota M, Kasahara T. Animal models of bipolar disorder. Neurosci Biobehav Rev. 2007;31(6):832–42. Epub 2007 Mar 27. Review.
972. Baxter LR Jr, Phelps ME, Mazziotta JC, Schwartz JM, Gerner RH, Selin CE, Sumida RM. Cerebral metabolic rates for glucose in mood disorders. Studies with positron emission tomography and fluorodeoxyglucose F 18. Arch Gen Psychiatry. 1985;42(5):441–7.
973. Caliyurt O, Altiay G. Resting energy expenditure in manic episode. Bipolar Disord. 2009;11(1):102–6. https://doi.org/10.1111/j.1399-5618.2008.00649.x.
974. Shao L, Martin MV, Watson SJ, Schatzberg A, Akil H, Myers RM, Jones EG, Bunney WE, Vawter MP. Mitochondrial involvement in psychiatric dis-

orders. Ann Med. 2008;40(4):281–95. https://doi.org/10.1080/07853890801923753. Review. Erratum in: Ann Med. 2011 Jun;43(4):329.

975. Konradi C, Eaton M, MacDonald ML, Walsh J, Benes FM, Heckers S. Molecular evidence for mitochondrial dysfunction in bipolar disorder. Arch Gen Psychiatry. 2004;61(3):300–8. Erratum in: Arch Gen Psychiatry. 2004 Jun;61(6):538.
976. Berk M, Bodemer W, van Oudenhove T, Butkow N. Dopamine increases platelet intracellular calcium in bipolar affective disorder and controls. Int Clin Psychopharmacol. 1994;9(4):291–3.
977. Berk M, Kapczinski F, Andreazza AC, Deana OM, Giorlando F, Maes M, Yücelb M, Gama CS, Dodd S, Dean B, Magalhãesa PVS, Amminger P, McGorry P, Malhi GS. Pathways underlying neuroprogression in bipolar disorder: focus on inflammation, oxidative stress and neurotrophic factors. Neurosci Biobehav Rev. 2011;35:804–17.
978. Andreazza AC, Kapczinski F, Kauer-Sant'Anna M, Walz JC, Bond DJ, Gonçalves CA, Young LT, Yatham LN. 3-Nitrotyrosine and glutathione antioxidant system in patients in the early and late stages of bipolar disorder. J Psychiatry Neurosci. 2009;34(4):263–71.
979. Maurer IC, Schippel P, Volz HP. Lithium-induced enhancement of mitochondrial oxidative phosphorylation in human brain tissue. Bipolar Disord. 2009;11(5):515–22. https://doi.org/10.1111/j.1399-5618.2009.00729.x.
980. Machado-Vieira R, Andreazza AC, Viale CI, Zanatto V, Cereser V Jr, da Silva Vargas R, Kapczinski F, Portela LV, Souza DO, Salvador M, Gentil V. Oxidative stress parameters in unmedicated and treated bipolar subjects during initial manic episode: a possible role for lithium antioxidant effects. Neurosci Lett. 2007;421(1):33–6. Epub 2007 May 22.
981. Rosa AR, Frey BN, Andreazza AC, Cerésr KM, Cunha AB, Quevedo J, Santin A, Gottfried C, Gonçalves CA, Vieta E, Kapczinski F. Increased serum glial cell line-derived neurotrophic factor immunocontent during manic and depressive episodes in individuals with bipolar disorder. Neurosci Lett. 2006;407(2):146–50. Epub 2006 Sept 7.
982. Cui J, Shao L, Young LT, Wang JF. Role of glutathione in neuroprotective effects of mood stabilizing drugs lithium and valproate. Neuroscience. 2007;144(4):1447–53. Epub 2006 Dec 19.
983. Dodd S, Dean O, Copolov DL, Malhi GS, Berk M. N-acetylcysteine for antioxidant therapy: pharmacology and clinical utility. Expert Opin Biol Ther. 2008;8(12):1955–62. https://doi.org/10.1517/14728220802517901. Review.
984. Laux I, Nel A. Evidence that oxidative stress-induced apoptosis by menadione involves Fas-dependent and Fas-independent pathways. Clin Immunol. 2001;101(3):335–44.
985. Pacher P, Beckman JS, Liaudet L. Nitric oxide and peroxynitrite in health and disease. Physiol Rev. 2007;87(1):315–424. Review.
986. Triposkiadis F, Karayannis G, Giamouzis G, Skoularigis J, Louridas G, Butler J. The sympathetic nervous system in heart failure physiology, pathophysiology, and clinical implications. J Am Coll Cardiol. 2009;54(19):1747–62. https://doi.org/10.1016/j.jacc.2009.05.015. Review.
987. Olshansky B, Sabbah HN, Hauptman PJ, Colucci WS. Parasympathetic nervous system and heart failure: pathophysiology and potential implications for therapy. Circulation. 2008;118(8):863–71. https://doi.org/10.1161/CIRCULATIONAHA.107.760405. Review.
988. Kinugawa T, Dibner-Dunlap ME. Altered vagal and sympathetic control of heart rate in left ventricular dysfunction and heart failure. Am J Phys. 1995;268:R317–23.
989. Newton GE, Parker AB, Landzberg JS, Colucci WS, Parker JD. Muscarinic receptor modulation of basal and beta-adrenergic stimulated function of the failing human left ventricle. J Clin Invest. 1996;98:2756–63.
990. Dunlap ME, Bibevski S, Rosenberry TL, Ernsberger P. Mechanisms of altered vagal control in heart failure: influence of muscarinic receptors and acetylcholinesterase activity. Am J Physiol Heart Circ Physiol. 2003;285:H1632–40.
991. Zhao G, Shen W, Xu X, Ochoa M, Bernstein R, Hintze TH. Selective impairment of vagally mediated, nitric oxide-dependent coronary vasodilation in conscious dogs after pacing-induced heart failure. Circulation. 1995;91:2655–63.
992. Dibner-Dunlap ME, Thames MD. Control of sympathetic nerve activity by vagal mechanoreflexes is blunted in heart failure. Circulation. 1992;86:1929–34.
993. Eschenhagen T, Mende U, Nose M, Schmitz W, Scholz H, Schulte am Esch J, Sempell R, Warnholtz A, Wustel JM. Regulation and possible functional implications of G-protein mRNA expression in nonfailing and failing ventricular myocardium. Basic Res Cardiol. 1992;87:51–64.
994. Ferramosca A, Di Giacomo M, Zara V. Antioxidant dietary approach in treatment of fatty liver: new insights and updates. World J Gastroenterol. 2017;23(23):4146–57. https://doi.org/10.3748/wjg.v23.i23.4146.
995. Reddy JK, Rao MS. Lipid metabolism and liver inflammation. II. Fatty liver disease and fatty acid oxidation. Am J Physiol Gastrointest Liver Physiol. 2006;290(5):G852–8.
996. Angulo P. Nonalcoholic fatty liver disease. N Engl J Med. 2002;346(16):1221–31.
997. Bayard M, Holt J, Boroughs E. Nonalcoholic fatty liver disease. Am Fam Physician. 2006;73(11):1961–8.
998. Medina J, Fernández-Salazar LI, García-Buey L, Moreno-Otero R. Approach to the pathogenesis and treatment of non-alcoholic steatohepatitis. Diabetes Care. 2004;27(8):2057–66.

999. Day CP, James OF. Steatohepatitis: a tale of two "hits"? Gastroenterology. 1998;114(4):842–5.
1000. Gramlich T, Kleiner DE, McCullough AJ, Matteoni CA, Boparai N, Younossi ZM. Pathologic features associated with fibrosis in nonalcoholic fatty liver disease. Hum Pathol. 2004;35(2):196–9.
1001. Zafrani ES. Non-alcoholic fatty liver disease: an emerging pathological spectrum. Virchows Arch. 2004;444(1):3–12.
1002. Ma J, Hennein R, Liu C, Long MT, Hoffmann U, Jacques PF, Lichtenstein AH, Hu FB, Levy D. Improved diet quality associates with reduction in liver fat, particularly in individuals with high genetic risk scores for nonalcoholic fatty liver disease. Gastroenterology. 2018. pii: S0016-5085(18)30345-7. https://doi.org/10.1053/j.gastro.2018.03.038. [Epub ahead of print].
1003. Valent P. Mast cell activation syndromes: definition and classification. Allergy. 2013;68(4):417–24.
1004. Akin C, Valent P, Metcalfe DD. Mast cell activation syndrome: proposed diagnostic criteria. J Allergy Clin Immunol. 2010;126:1099–104.
1005. Akin C. Mast cell activation syndromes presenting as anaphylaxis. Immunol Allergy Clin N Am. 2015;35(2):277–85.
1006. Milner J. Research update: POTS, EDS, MCAS Genetics. Dysautonomia International Conference & CME. Washington, DC. Dysautonomia International Research Update: POTS, EDS, MCAS Genetics. Web; 2015.
1007. Szczawinska-Poplonyk A. An overlapping syndrome of allergy and immune deficiency in children. J Allergy. 2012;2012:1–9.
1008. Talkington J, Nickell SP. Borrelia burgdorferi spirochetes induce mast cell activation and cytokine release. Infect Immun. 1999;67(3):1107–15.
1009. Christy AL, Brown MA. The multitasking mast cell: positive and negative roles in the progression of autoimmunity. J Immunol. 2007;179(5):2673–9.
1010. Gao L, Mao Q, Cao J, Wang Y, Zhou X, Fan L. Effects of coenzyme Q10 on vascular endothelial function in humans: a meta-analysis of randomized controlled trials. Atherosclerosis. 2012;221(2):311–6. https://doi.org/10.1016/j.atherosclerosis.2011.10.027. Epub 2011 Oct 25. Review.
1011. Yoritaka A, Kawajiri S, Yamamoto Y, Nakahara T, Ando M, Hashimoto K, Nagase M, Saito Y, Hattori N. Randomized, double-blind, placebo-controlled pilot trial of reduced coenzyme Q10 for Parkinson's disease. Parkinsonism Relat Disord. 2015;21(8):911–6. https://doi.org/10.1016/j.parkreldis.2015.05.022. Epub 2015 May 29.
1012. Butt JH, Franzmann U, Kruuse C. Endothelial function in migraine with aura – a systematic review. Headache. 2015;55(1):35–54. https://doi.org/10.1111/head.12494. Epub 2014 Dec 24. Review.
1013. Dalla Volta G, Carli D, Zavarise P, Ngonga G, Vollaro S. P026. Pilot study on the use of coenzyme Q10 in a group of patients with episodic migraine without aura. J Headache Pain. 2015;16(Suppl 1):A186. https://doi.org/10.1186/1129-2377-16-S1-A186.
1014. Shoeibi A, Olfati N, Soltani Sabi M, Salehi M, Mali S, Akbari Oryani M. Effectiveness of coenzyme Q10 in prophylactic treatment of migraine headache: an open-label, add-on, controlled trial. Acta Neurol Belg. 2017;117(1):103–9. https://doi.org/10.1007/s13760-016-0697-z. Epub 2016 Sept 26.
1015. Scapagnini G, Davinelli S, Drago F, De Lorenzo A, Oriani G. Antioxidants as antidepressants: fact or fiction? CNS Drugs. 2012;26(6):477–90. https://doi.org/10.2165/11633190-000000000-00000. Review.
1016. Morris G, Anderson G, Berk M, Maes M. Coenzyme Q10 depletion in medical and neuropsychiatric disorders: potential repercussions and therapeutic implications. Mol Neurobiol. 2013;48(3):883–903. https://doi.org/10.1007/s12035-013-8477-8. Epub 2013 Jun 13. Review.
1017. Maurya PK, Noto C, Rizzo LB, Rios AC, Nunes SO, Barbosa DS, Sethi S, Zeni M, Mansur RB, Maes M, Brietzke E. The role of oxidative and nitrosative stress in accelerated aging and major depressive disorder. Prog Neuro-Psychopharmacol Biol Psychiatry. 2016;65:134–44. https://doi.org/10.1016/j.pnpbp.2015.08.016. Epub 2015 Sept 6. Review.
1018. Forester BP, Harper DG, Georgakas J, Ravichandran C, Madurai N, Cohen BM. Antidepressant effects of open label treatment with coenzyme Q10 in geriatric bipolar depression. J Clin Psychopharmacol. 2015;35(3):338–40. https://doi.org/10.1097/JCP.0000000000000326.
1019. Sanoobar M, Dehghan P, Khalili M, Azimi A, Seifar F. Coenzyme Q10 as a treatment for fatigue and depression in multiple sclerosis patients: a double blind randomized clinical trial. Nutr Neurosci. 2016;19(3):138–43. https://doi.org/10.1179/1476830515Y.0000000002. Epub 2015 Jan 20.
1020. Salviati L, Trevisson E, Doimo M, Navas P. Primary coenzyme Q10 deficiency. In: Pagon RA, Adam MP, Ardinger HH, Wallace SE, Amemiya A, Bean LJH, Bird TD, Ledbetter N, Mefford HC, Smith RJH, Stephens K, editors. GeneReviews® [Internet]. Seattle: University of Washington; 2017. p. 1993–2017.
1021. Mitsui J, Matsukawa T, Yasuda T, Ishiura H, Tsuji S. Plasma coenzyme Q10 levels in patients with multiple system atrophy. JAMA Neurol. 2016;73(8):977–80. https://doi.org/10.1001/jamaneurol.2016.1325.
1022. Singh RB, Kartik C, Otsuka K, Pella D, Pella J. Brain-heart connection and the risk of heart attack. Biomed Pharmacother. 2002;56(Suppl 2):257s–65s.
1023. Li Z, Wang P, Yu Z, Cong Y, Sun H, Zhang J, Zhang J, Sun C, Zhang Y, Ju X. The effect of creatine and coenzyme q10 combination therapy on mild cognitive impairment in Parkinson's disease.

Eur Neurol. 2015;73(3–4):205–11. https://doi.org/10.1159/000377676. Epub 2015 Mar 10.
1024. Atalay Guzel N, Erikoglu Orer G, Sezen Bircan F, Coskun Cevher S. Effects of acute L-carnitine supplementation on nitric oxide production and oxidative stress after exhaustive exercise in young soccer players. J Sports Med Phys Fitness. 2015;55(1–2):9–15. Epub 2014 Oct 7.
1025. Lim HB, Smith M. Systemic complications after head injury: a clinical review. Anaesthesia. 2007;62(5):474–82. Review.
1026. Tobias H, Vinitsky A, Bulgarelli RJ, Ghosh-Dastidar S, Colombo J. Autonomic nervous system monitoring of patients with excess parasympathetic responses to sympathetic challenges – clinical observations. US Neurology. 2010;5(2):62–6.
1027. Procaccini C, Pucino V, De Rosa V, Marone G, Matarese G. Neuro-endocrine networks controlling immune system in health and disease. Front Immunol. 2014;5:143. https://doi.org/10.3389/fimmu.2014.00143. eCollection 2014. Review.
1028. Gunnars K. 5 Studies on the Mediterranean diet – does it really work? https://authoritynutrition.com/5-studies-on-the-mediterranean-diet
1029. Davis C, Bryan J, Hodgson J, Murphy K. Definition of the Mediterranean diet; a literature review. Nutrients. 2015;7(11):9139–53. https://doi.org/10.3390/nu7115459. Review.
1030. Castro-Quezada I, Román-Viñas B, Serra-Majem L. The Mediterranean diet and nutritional adequacy: a review. Nutrients. 2014;6(1):231–48. https://doi.org/10.3390/nu6010231. Review.
1031. Sofi F, Macchi C, Abbate R, Gensini GF, Casini A. Mediterranean diet and health status: an updated meta-analysis and a proposal for a literature-based adherence score. Public Health Nutr. 2014;17(12):2769–82. https://doi.org/10.1017/S1368980013003169. Epub 2013 Nov 29. Review.
1032. Mancini JG, Filion KB, Atallah R, Eisenberg MJ. Systematic review of the Mediterranean diet for long-term weight loss. Am J Med. 2016;129(4):407–415.e4. https://doi.org/10.1016/j.amjmed.2015.11.028. Epub 2015 Dec 22. Review.
1033. Widmer RJ, Flammer AJ, Lerman LO, Lerman A. The Mediterranean diet, its components, and cardiovascular disease. Am J Med. 2015;128(3):229–38. https://doi.org/10.1016/j.amjmed.2014.10.014. Epub 2014 Oct 15. Review.
1034. Liyanage T, Ninomiya T, Wang A, Neal B, Jun M, Wong MG, Jardine M, Hillis GS, Perkovic V. Effects of the Mediterranean diet on cardiovascular outcomes-a systematic review and meta-analysis. PLoS One. 2016;11(8):e0159252. https://doi.org/10.1371/journal.pone.0159252. eCollection 2016. Review.
1035. Grosso G, Marventano S, Yang J, Micek A, Pajak A, Scalfi L, Galvano F, Kales SN. A comprehensive meta-analysis on evidence of Mediterranean diet and cardiovascular disease: are individual components equal? Crit Rev Food Sci Nutr. 2017;57(15):3218–32. https://doi.org/10.1080/10408398.2015.1107021.
1036. Nordmann AJ, Suter-Zimmermann K, Bucher HC, Shai I, Tuttle KR, Estruch R, Briel M. Meta-analysis comparing Mediterranean to low-fat diets for modification of cardiovascular risk factors. Am J Med. 2011;124(9):841–51.e2. https://doi.org/10.1016/j.amjmed.2011.04.024.
1037. Satija A, Bhupathiraju SN, Spiegelman D, Chiuve SE, Manson JE, Willett W, Rexrode KM, Rimm EB, Hu FB. Healthful and unhealthful plant-based diets and the risk of coronary heart disease in U.S. adults. J Am Coll Cardiol. 2017;70(4):411–22. https://doi.org/10.1016/j.jacc.2017.05.047.
1038. Ros E, Martínez-González MA, Estruch R, Salas-Salvadó J, Fitó M, Martínez JA, Corella D. Mediterranean diet and cardiovascular health: teachings of the PREDIMED study. Adv Nutr. 2014;5(3):330S–6S. https://doi.org/10.3945/an.113.005389. Print 2014 May. Review.
1039. Estruch R, Ros E, Salas-Salvadó J, Covas MI, Corella D, Arós F, Gómez-Gracia E, Ruiz-Gutiérrez V, Fiol M, Lapetra J, et al. Primary prevention of cardiovascular disease with a Mediterranean diet. N Engl J Med. 2013;368:1279–90.
1040. Khera AV, Emdin CA, Drake I, Natarajan P, Bick AG, Cook NR, Chasman DI, Baber U, Mehran R, Rader DJ, Fuster V, Boerwinkle E, Melander O, Orho-Melander M, Ridker PM, Kathiresan S. Genetic risk, adherence to a healthy lifestyle, and coronary disease. N Engl J Med. 2016;375(24):2349–58. Epub 2016 Nov 13.
1041. Fuentes F, López-Miranda J, Sánchez E, Sánchez F, Paez J, Paz-Rojas E, Marín C, Gómez P, Jimenez-Perepérez J, Ordovás JM, Pérez-Jiménez F. Mediterranean and low-fat diets improve endothelial function in hypercholesterolemic men. Ann Intern Med. 2001;134(12):1115–9.
1042. Ludwig DS. Lowering the bar on the low-fat diet. JAMA. 2016;316(20):2087–8. https://doi.org/10.1001/jama.2016.15473.
1043. Nissensohn M, Román-Viñas B, Sánchez-Villegas A, Piscopo S, Serra-Majem L. The effect of the Mediterranean diet on hypertension: a systematic review and meta-analysis. J Nutr Educ Behav. 2016;48(1):42–53.e1. https://doi.org/10.1016/j.jneb.2015.08.023. Epub 2015 Oct 21. Review.
1044. Wang Q, Afshin A, Yakoob MY, Singh GM, Rehm CD, Khatibzadeh S, Micha R, Shi P, Mozaffarian D, Global Burden of Diseases Nutrition and Chronic Diseases Expert Group (NutriCoDE). Impact of nonoptimal intakes of saturated, polyunsaturated, and trans fat on global burdens of coronary heart disease. J Am Heart Assoc. 2016;5(1). pii: e002891. https://doi.org/10.1161/JAHA.115.002891.
1045. Kris-Etherton P, Eckel RH, Howard BV, St Jeor S, Bazzarre TL; Nutrition Committee Population Science Committee and Clinical Science Committee of the American Heart Association. AHA Science Advisory: Lyon Diet Heart Study. Benefits of

a Mediterranean-style, National Cholesterol Education Program/American Heart Association Step I Dietary Pattern on Cardiovascular Disease. Circulation. 2001;103(13):1823–5. http://circ.ahajournals.org/content/103/13/1823.long
1046. Estruch R, Ros E, Salas-Salvadó J, Covas MI, Corella D, Arós F, Gómez-Gracia E, Ruiz-Gutiérrez V, Fiol M, Lapetra J, Lamuela-Raventos RM, Serra-Majem L, Pintó X, Basora J, Muñoz MA, Sorlí JV, Martínez JA, Martínez-González MA, PREDIMED Study Investigators. Primary prevention of cardiovascular disease with a Mediterranean diet. N Engl J Med. 2013;368(14):1279–90. https://doi.org/10.1056/NEJMoa1200303. Epub 2013 Feb 25. Erratum in: N Engl J Med. 2014 Feb 27;370(9):886.
1047. Gay HC, Rao SG, Vaccarino V, Ali MK. Effects of different dietary interventions on blood pressure: systematic review and meta-analysis of randomized controlled trials. Hypertension. 2016;67(4):733–9. https://doi.org/10.1161/HYPERTENSIONAHA.115.06853. Epub 2016 Feb 22. Review.
1048. Bloomfield HE, Koeller E, Greer N, MacDonald R, Kane R, Wilt TJ. Effects on health outcomes of a Mediterranean diet with no restriction on fat intake: a systematic review and meta-analysis. Ann Intern Med. 2016;165(7):491–500. https://doi.org/10.7326/M16-0361. Epub 2016 Jul 19. Review.
1049. Sofi F, Cesari F, Abbate R, Gensini GF, Casini A. Adherence to Mediterranean diet and health status: meta-analysis. BMJ. 2008;337:a1344. https://doi.org/10.1136/bmj.a1344. Review.
1050. Esposito K, Maiorino MI, Bellastella G, Chiodini P, Panagiotakos D, Giugliano D. A journey into a Mediterranean diet and type 2 diabetes: a systematic review with meta-analyses. BMJ Open. 2015;5(8):e008222. https://doi.org/10.1136/bmjopen-2015-008222. Review.
1051. Ros E, Hu FB. Consumption of plant seeds and cardiovascular health: epidemiologic and clinical trial evidence. Circulation. 2013;128:553–65.
1052. Salas-Salvadó J, Guasch-Ferré M, Lee CH, Estruch R, Clish CB, Ros E. Protective effects of the Mediterranean diet on type 2 diabetes and metabolic syndrome. J Nutr. 2016. pii: jn218487. [Epub ahead of print] Review.
1053. Schwingshackl L, Missbach B, König J, Hoffmann G. Adherence to a Mediterranean diet and risk of diabetes: a systematic review and meta-analysis. Public Health Nutr. 2015;18(7):1292–9. https://doi.org/10.1017/S1368980014001542. Epub 2014 Aug 22. Review.
1054. Koloverou E, Esposito K, Giugliano D, Panagiotakos D. The effect of Mediterranean diet on the development of type 2 diabetes mellitus: a meta-analysis of 10 prospective studies and 136,846 participants. Metabolism. 2014;63(7):903–11. https://doi.org/10.1016/j.metabol.2014.04.010. Epub 2014 Apr 24. Review.
1055. Esposito K, Maiorino MI, Ceriello A, Giugliano D. Prevention and control of type 2 diabetes by Mediterranean diet: a systematic review. Diabetes Res Clin Pract. 2010;89(2):97–102. https://doi.org/10.1016/j.diabres.2010.04.019. Epub 2010 May 23. Review.
1056. Garcia M, Bihuniak JD, Shook J, Kenny A, Kerstetter J, Huedo-Medina TB. The effect of the traditional Mediterranean-style diet on metabolic risk factors: a meta-analysis. Nutrients. 2016;8(3):168. https://doi.org/10.3390/nu8030168. Review.
1057. Godos J, Zappalà G, Bernardini S, Giambini I, Bes-Rastrollo M, Martinez-Gonzalez M. Adherence to the Mediterranean diet is inversely associated with metabolic syndrome occurrence: a meta-analysis of observational studies. Int J Food Sci Nutr. 2017;68(2):138–48. https://doi.org/10.1080/09637486.2016.1221900. Epub 2016 Aug 25. Review.
1058. Esposito K, Kastorini CM, Panagiotakos DB, Giugliano D. Mediterranean diet and metabolic syndrome: an updated systematic review. Rev Endocr Metab Disord. 2013;14(3):255–63. https://doi.org/10.1007/s11154-013-9253-9. Review.
1059. Schwingshackl L, Hoffmann G. Adherence to Mediterranean diet and risk of cancer: an updated systematic review and meta-analysis of observational studies. Cancer Med. 2015;4(12):1933–47. https://doi.org/10.1002/cam4.539. Epub 2015 Oct 16. Review.
1060. D'Alessandro A, De Pergola G, Silvestris F. Mediterranean diet and cancer risk: an open issue. Int J Food Sci Nutr. 2016;67(6):593–605. https://doi.org/10.1080/09637486.2016.1191444. Epub 2016 Jun 2. Review.
1061. Song M, Giovannucci E. Preventable incidence and mortality of carcinoma associated with lifestyle factors among white adults in the United States. JAMA Oncol. 2016;2(9):1154–61. https://doi.org/10.1001/jamaoncol.2016.0843.
1062. La Vecchia C. Mediterranean diet and cancer. Public Health Nutr. 2004;7(7):965–8. Review.
1063. Fabiani R, Minelli L, Bertarelli G, Bacci S. A western dietary pattern increases prostate cancer risk: a systematic review and meta-analysis. Nutrients. 2016;8(10). pii: E626. Review.
1064. van den Brandt PA, Schulpen M. Mediterranean diet adherence and risk of postmenopausal breast cancer: results of a cohort study and meta-analysis. Int J Cancer. 2017;140(10):2220–31. https://doi.org/10.1002/ijc.30654. Epub 2017 Mar 5.
1065. Neale EP, Batterham MJ, Tapsell LC. Consumption of a healthy dietary pattern results in significant reductions in C-reactive protein levels in adults: a meta-analysis. Nutr Res. 2016;36(5):391–401. https://doi.org/10.1016/j.nutres.2016.02.009. Epub 2016 Feb 22. Review.
1066. Cao L, Tan L, Wang HF, Jiang T, Zhu XC, Lu H, Tan MS, Yu JT. Dietary patterns and risk of dementia: a systematic review and meta-analysis of cohort

studies. Mol Neurobiol. 2016;53(9):6144–54. https://doi.org/10.1007/s12035-015-9516-4. Epub 2015 Nov 9.
1067. Stephan BCM, Harrison SL, Keage HAD, Babateen A, Robinson L, Siervo M. Cardiovascular disease, the nitric oxide pathway and risk of cognitive impairment and dementia. Curr Cardiol Rep. 2017;19(9):87. https://doi.org/10.1007/s11886-017-0898-y. Review.
1068. Cuello AC. Early and late CNS inflammation in Alzheimer's disease: two extremes of a continuum? Trends Pharmacol Sci. 2017. pii: S0165-6147(17)30144-X. https://doi.org/10.1016/j.tips.2017.07.005. [Epub ahead of print] Review.
1069. Lourida I, Soni M, Thompson-Coon J, Purandare N, Lang IA, Ukoumunne OC, Llewellyn DJ. Mediterranean diet, cognitive function, and dementia: a systematic review. Epidemiology. 2013;24(4):479–89. https://doi.org/10.1097/EDE.0b013e3182944410. Review.
1070. Wu L, Sun D. Adherence to Mediterranean diet and risk of developing cognitive disorders: an updated systematic review and meta-analysis of prospective cohort studies. Sci Rep. 2017;7:41317. https://doi.org/10.1038/srep41317.
1071. Loughrey DG, Lavecchia S, Brennan S, Lawlor BA, Kelly ME. The impact of the Mediterranean diet on the cognitive functioning of healthy older adults: a systematic review and meta-analysis. Adv Nutr. 2017;8(4):571–86. https://doi.org/10.3945/an.117.015495. Print 2017 Jul. Review. PMID: 28710144.
1072. Kunutsor SK, Laukkanen JA, Whitehouse MR, Blom AW. Adherence to a Mediterranean-style diet and incident fractures: pooled analysis of observational evidence. Eur J Nutr. 2017; https://doi.org/10.1007/s00394-017-1432-0.
1073. Malmir H, Saneei P, Larijani B, Esmaillzadeh A. Adherence to Mediterranean diet in relation to bone mineral density and risk of fracture: a systematic review and meta-analysis of observational studies. Eur J Nutr. 2017. https://doi.org/10.1007/s00394-017-1490-3.
1074. Papamichael MM, Itsiopoulos C, Susanto NH, Erbas B. Does adherence to the Mediterranean dietary pattern reduce asthma symptoms in children? A systematic review of observational studies. Public Health Nutr. 2017;14:1–13. https://doi.org/10.1017/S1368980017001823.
1075. Sainani GS. Role of diet, exercise and drugs in modulation of endothelial cell dysfunction. J Assoc Physicians India. 2012;60:14–9.
1076. Pandey KB, Rizvi SI. Plant polyphenols as dietary antioxidants in human health and disease. Oxidative Med Cell Longev. 2009;2(5):270–8. https://doi.org/10.4161/oxim.2.5.9498. Review.
1077. Graf BA, Milbury PE, Blumberg JB. Flavonols, favonones, flavanones and human health: epidemiological evidence. J Med Food. 2005;8:281–90.
1078. Arts ICW, Hollman PCH. Polyphenols and disease risk in epidemiologic studies. Am J Clin Nutr. 2005;81:317–25.
1079. García-Lafuente A, Guillamón E, Villares A, Rostagno MA, Martínez JA. Flavonoids as anti-inflammatory agents: implications in cancer and cardiovascular disease. Inflamm Res. 2009;58:537–52.
1080. Pirola L, Frojdo S. Resveratrol: one molecule, many targets. IUBMB Life. 2008;60:323–32.
1081. Kamaraj S, Vinodhkumar R, Anandakumar P, Jagan S, Ramakrishnan G, Devaki T. The effects of quercetin on antioxidant status and tumor markers in the lung and serum of mice treated with benzo(a)pyrene. Biol Pharm Bull. 2007;30:2268–73.
1082. Scarmeas N, Luchsinger JA, Mayeux R, Stern Y. Mediterranean diet and Alzheimer disease mortality. Neurology. 2007;69:1084–93.
1083. Aquilano K, Baldelli S, Rotilio G, Ciriolo MR. Role of nitric oxide synthases in Parkinson's disease: a review on the antioxidant and anti-inflammatory activity of polyphenols. Neurochem Res. 2008;33:2416–26.
1084. Rossi L, Mazzitelli S, Arciello M, Capo CR, Rotilio G. Benefits from dietary polyphenols for brain aging and Alzheimer's disease. Neurochem Res. 2008;33:2390–400.
1085. Kiritsakis A. Olive oil- from the tree to the table. 2nd ed. Trumbull: Food and Nutrition Press, Inc; 1998. p. 006611.
1086. Visioli F, Poli A, Gall C. Antioxidant and other biological activities of phenols from olives and olive oil. Med Res Rev. 2002;22(1):65–75.
1087. Baldioli M, Servili M, Perretti G, Montedoro GF. Antioxidant activity of tocopherols and phenolic compounds of virgin olive oil. J Am Oil Chem Soc. 1996;73(11):1589–93.
1088. Han X, Shen T, Lou H. Dietary polyphenols and their biological significance. Int J Mol Sci. 2007;8(9):950–88. https://doi.org/10.3390/i8090950. Review.
1089. Estruch R, Ros E, Salas-Salvadó J, Covas MI, Corella D, Arós F, Gómez-Gracia E, Ruiz-Gutiérrez V, Fiol M, Lapetra J, Lamuela-Raventos RM, Serra-Majem L, Pintó X, Basora J, Muñoz MA, Sorlí JV, Martínez JA, Martínez-González MA, PREDIMED Study Investigators. Primary prevention of cardiovascular disease with a Mediterranean diet. N Engl J Med. 2013;368(14):1279–90. https://doi.org/10.1056/NEJMoa1200303. Epub 2013 Feb 25. Erratum in: N Engl J Med. 2014 Feb 27;370(9):886.
1090. Escribá PV, Halver JE. How Oleic acid in olive oil reduces blood pressure. www.pitt.edu/~super4/33011-34001/33541.ppt
1091. Seeram NP, Aviram M, Zhang Y, Henning SM, Feng L, Dreher M, Heber D. Comparison of antioxidant potency of commonly consumed polyphenol-rich beverages in the United States. J Agric Food Chem. 2008;56(4):1415–22.

1092. Durak I, Avci A, Kacmaz M, Büyükkoçak S, Cimen MY, Elgün S, Oztürk HS. Comparison of antioxidant potentials of red wine, white wine, grape juice and alcohol. Curr Med Res Opin. 1999;15(4):316–20.
1093. Keevil JG, Osman HE, Reed JD, Folts JD. Grape juice, but not orange juice or grapefruit juice, inhibits human platelet aggregation. J Nutr. 2000;130(1):53–6.
1094. Folts JD. Antithrombotic potential of grape juice and red wine for preventing heart attacks. Pharm Biol. 1998;36(Supplement 1):21–7.
1095. O'Byrne DJ, Devaraj S, Grundy SM, Jialal I. Comparison of the antioxidant effects of Concord grape juice flavonoids alpha-tocopherol on markers of oxidative stress in healthy adults. Am J Clin Nutr. 2002;76(6):1367–74.
1096. Stein JH, Keevil JG, Wiebe DA, Aeschlimann S, Folts JD. Purple grape juice improves endothelial function and reduces the susceptibility of LDL cholesterol to oxidation in patients with coronary artery disease. Circulation. 1999;100(10):1050–5.
1097. Park YK, Kim JS, Kang MH. Concord grape juice supplementation reduces blood pressure in Korean hypertensive men: double-blind, placebo controlled intervention trial. Biofactors. 2004;22(1–4):145–7.
1098. Mark D, Maki K. Concord grape juice reduces blood pressure in men with high systolic blood pressure. Experimental biology. San Diego. 11–15 Apr 2003.
1099. Dohadwala MM, Hamburg NM, Holbrook M, Kim BH, Duess M, Levit A, Titas M, Chung WB, Vincent FB, Caiano T, Frame AA, Keaney JF Jr, Vita JA. Effects of Concord grape juice on ambulatory blood pressure in prehypertension and stage 1 hypertension. Am J Clin Nutr. 2010;91(5):1052–9.
1100. Dohadwala MM, Vita JA. Grapes and cardiovascular disease. J Nutr. 2009;139(9):1788S–93S.
1101. Chou EJ, Keevil JG, Aeschlimann S, Wiebe DA, Folts JD, Stein JH. Effect of ingestion of purple grape juice on endothelial function in patients with coronary heart disease. Am J Cardiol. 2001;88(5):553–5.
1102. Freedman JE, Parker C 3rd, Li L, Perlman JA, Frei B, Ivanov V, Deak LR, Iafrati MD, Folts JD. Select flavonoids and whole juice from purple grapes inhibit platelet function and enhance nitric oxide release. Circulation. 2001;103(23):2792–8.
1103. Anselm E, Chataigneau M, Ndiaye M, Chataigneau T, Schini-Kerth VB. Grape juice causes endothelium-dependent relaxation via a redox-sensitive Src- and Akt-dependent activation of eNOS. Cardiovasc Res. 2007;73(2):404–13.
1104. Fitzpatrick DF, Hirschfield SL, Coffey RG. Endothelium-dependent vasorelaxing activity of wine and other grape products. Am J Physiol Heart Circ Physiol. 1993;265(34):H774–8.
1105. Albers AR, Varghese S, Vitseva O, Vita JA, Freedman JE. The antiinflammatory effects of purple grape juice consumption in subjects with stable coronary artery disease. Arterioscler Thromb Vasc Biol. 2004;24(Nov):e179–80.
1106. Vislocky LM, Fernandez MLF. Biomedical effects of grape products. Nutr Rev. 2010;68(11):656–70.
1107. Krikorian R, Nash TA, Shidler MD, Shukitt-Hale B, Joseph JA. Concord grape juice supplementation improves memory function in older adults with mild cognitive impairment. Br J Nutr. 2010;103(5):730–4.
1108. Shukitt-Hale B, Carey A, Simon L, Mark DA, Joseph JA. Effects of Concord grape juice on cognitive and motor deficits in aging. Nutrition. 2006;22(3):295–302.
1109. Ho L, Ferruzzi MG, Janle EM, Lobo J, Chen TY, Talcott ST, Simon J, Wu QL, Wang J, Cheng A, Weaver CM, Percival SS, Pasinetti GM. Bioavailability of grape-derived polyphenolics and implications in Alzheimer's disease prevention and therapy. Presented at Experimental Biology; 2010 Apr 24–28; Anaheim;2010.
1110. Joseph JA, Shukitt-Hale B, Casadesus G. Reversing the deleterious effects of aging on neuronal communication and behavior: beneficial properties of fruit polyphenolic compounds. Am J Clin Nutr. 2005;81(1 Suppl):313S–6S.
1111. Lipson SM, Cohen P, Zhou J, Burdowski A, Stotzky G. Cranberry cocktail juice, cranberry concentrates, and proanthocyanidins reduce reovirus infectivity titers in African green monkey kidney epithelial cell cultures. Mol Nutr Food Res. 2007;51(6):752–8.
1112. Mallol J, Crane J, von Mutius E, Odhiambo J, Keil U, Stewart A, ISAAC Phase Three Study Group. The International Study of Asthma and Allergies in Childhood (ISAAC) phase three: a global synthesis. Allergol Immunopathol (Madr). 2013;41(2):73–85. https://doi.org/10.1016/j.aller.2012.03.001. Epub 2012 Jul 6.
1113. Fremont L. Biological effects of resveratrol. Life Sci. 2000;66(8):663–73.
1114. Khakimov B, Engelsen SB. Resveratrol in the foodomics era: 1:25,000. Ann N Y Acad Sci. 2017. https://doi.org/10.1111/nyas.13425. [Epub ahead of print] Review.
1115. Higdon J, Drake VJ, Steward WP. Resveratrol. Corvallis: Micronutrient Information Center. Linus Pauling Institute, Oregon State University; 2016.
1116. Schwager J, Richard N, Widmer F, Raederstorff D. Resveratrol distinctively modulates the inflammatory profiles of immune and endothelial cells. BMC Complement Altern Med. 2017;17(1):309. https://doi.org/10.1186/s12906-017-1823-z.
1117. Kulkarni SS, Cantó C. The molecular targets of resveratrol. Biochim Biophys Acta. 2015;1852(6):1114–23. https://doi.org/10.1016/j.bbadis.2014.10.005. Epub 2014 Oct 12. Review.
1118. Kim I, He YY. Targeting the AMP-activated protein kinase for cancer prevention and therapy. Front Oncol. 2013;3:175. https://doi.org/10.3389/fonc.2013.00175. eCollection 2013.

1119. Wang S, Wang J, Zhao A, Li J. SIRT1 activation inhibits hyperglycemia-induced apoptosis by reducing oxidative stress and mitochondrial dysfunction in human endothelial cells. Mol Med Rep. 2017;16(3):3331–8. https://doi.org/10.3892/mmr.2017.7027. Epub 2017 Jul 17.
1120. Teixeira J, Chavarria D, Borges F, Wojtczak L, Wieckowski MR, Karkucińska-Wieckowska A, Oliveira PJ. Dietary polyphenols and mitochondrial function: role in health and disease. Curr Med Chem. 2017. https://doi.org/10.2174/0929867324666170529101810. [Epub ahead of print].
1121. Yousuf S, Atif F, Ahmad M, Hoda N, Ishrat T, Khan B, Islam F. Resveratrol exerts its neuroprotective effect by modulating mitochondrial dysfunctions and associated cell death during cerebral ischemia. Brain Res. 2009;1250:242–53. https://doi.org/10.1016/j.brainres.2008.10.068. Epub 2008 Nov 11.
1122. Bhandari R, Kuhad A. Resveratrol suppresses neuroinflammation in the experimental paradigm of autism spectrum disorders. Neurochem Int. 2017;103:8–23. https://doi.org/10.1016/j.neuint.2016.12.012. Epub 2016 Dec 23.
1123. Hermann DM, Zechariah A, Kaltwasser B, Bosche B, Caglayan AB, Kilic E, Doeppner TR. Sustained neurological recovery induced by resveratrol is associated with angioneurogenesis rather than neuroprotection after focal cerebral ischemia. Neurobiol Dis. 2015;83:16–25. https://doi.org/10.1016/j.nbd.2015.08.018. Epub 2015 Aug 24.
1124. Pang C, Cao L, Wu F, Wang L, Wang G, Yu Y, Zhang M, Chen L, Wang W, Lv W, Chen L, Zhu J, Pan J, Zhang H, Xu Y, Ding L. The effect of trans-resveratrol on post-stroke depression via regulation of hypothalamus-pituitary-adrenal axis. Neuropharmacology. 2015;97:447–56. https://doi.org/10.1016/j.neuropharm.2015.04.017. Epub 2015 Apr 29.
1125. Zhang F, Wang H, Wu Q, Lu Y, Nie J, Xie X, Shi J. Resveratrol protects cortical neurons against microglia-mediated neuroinflammation. Phytother Res. 2013;27(3):344–9. https://doi.org/10.1002/ptr.4734. Epub 2012 May 14.
1126. Anekonda TS. Resveratrol – a boon for treating Alzheimer's disease? Brain Res Rev. 2006;52(2):316–26. Review.
1127. Ferrières J. The French paradox: lessons for other countries. Heart. 2004;90(1):107–11.
1128. Webb AJ, Patel N, Loukogeorgakis S, Okorie M, Aboud Z, Misra S, Rashid R, Miall P, Deanfield J, Benjamin N, MacAllister R, Hobbs AJ, Ahluwalia A. Acute blood pressure lowering, vasoprotective, and antiplatelet properties of dietary nitrate via bioconversion to nitrite. Hypertension. 2008;51(3):784–90. https://doi.org/10.1161/HYPERTENSIONAHA.107.103523. Epub 2008 Feb 4.
1129. Lock K, Promerleau J, Causer L, Altman DR, McKee M. The global burden of disease attributable to low consumption of fruit and vegetables: implications for the global strategy of diet. Bull World Health Organ. 2005;83:100–8.
1130. Quin X, Huo Y, Langman CB, Hou F, Chen Y, Matossin D, et al. Folic acid therapy and cardiovascular disease in end-stage renal disease or advanced chronic kidney disease: a metaanalysis. Clin J Am Soc Nephrol. 2011;6:482–8.
1131. Lee M, Hong KS, Chang SC, Saver JL. Efficiency of homocysteine lowering therapy with folic acid and stroke prevention: a metaanalysis. Stroke. 2010;41:1205–12.
1132. Potter JD. Cancer prevention: epidemiology and experiment. Cancer Lett. 1997;114(1–2):7–9.
1133. Faraci FM, Heistad DD. Regulation of the cerebral circulation: role of endothelium and potassium channels. Physiol Rev. 1998;78(1):53–97.
1134. Rubinshtein R, Kuvin JT, Soffler M, Lennon RJ, Lavi S, Nelson RE, Pumper GM, Lerman LO, Lerman A. Assessment of endothelial function by non-invasive peripheral arterial tonometry predicts late cardiovascular adverse events. Eur Heart J. 2010;31(9):1142–8. https://doi.org/10.1093/eurheartj/ehq010. Epub 2010 Feb 24.
1135. Benbaibeche H, Haffaf el M, Kacimi G, Oudjit B, Khan NA, Koceïr EA. Implication of corticotropic hormone axis in eating behaviour pattern in obese and type 2 diabetic participants. Br J Nutr. 2015;113(8):1237–43. https://doi.org/10.1017/S0007114515000549. Epub 2015 Mar 18.
1136. García-Prieto MD, Tébar FJ, Nicolás F, Larqué E, Zamora S, Garaulet M. Cortisol secretary pattern and glucocorticoid feedback sensitivity in women from a Mediterranean area: relationship with anthropometric characteristics, dietary intake and plasma fatty acid profile. Clin Endocrinol. 2007;66(2):185–91.
1137. Kanauchi M, Kanauchi K. Development of a Mediterranean diet score adapted to Japan and its relation to obesity risk. Food Nutr Res. 2016;60:32172. https://doi.org/10.3402/fnr.v60.32172. eCollection 2016.
1138. Zhang R, Wang Z, Fei Y, Zhou B, Zheng S, Wang L, Huang L, Jiang S, Liu Z, Jiang J, Yu Y. The difference in nutrient intakes between Chinese and Mediterranean, Japanese and American diets. Nutrients. 2015;7(6):4661–88. https://doi.org/10.3390/nu7064661.
1139. Verberne L, Bach-Faig A, Buckland G, Serra-Majem L. Association between the Mediterranean diet and cancer risk: a review of observational studies. Nutr Cancer. 2010;62(7):860–70. https://doi.org/10.1080/01635581.2010.509834. Review.
1140. Tyrovolas S, Panagiotakos DB. The role of Mediterranean type of diet on the development of cancer and cardiovascular disease, in the elderly: a systematic review. Maturitas. 2010;65(2):122–30. https://doi.org/10.1016/j.maturitas.2009.07.003. Epub 2009 Aug 4. Review.
1141. Pelucchi C, Bosetti C, Rossi M, Negri E, La Vecchia C. Selected aspects of Mediterranean diet and can-

cer risk. Nutr Cancer. 2009;61(6):756–66. https://doi.org/10.1080/01635580903285007. Review.

1142. La Vecchia C. Mediterranean diet and cancer. Public Health Nutr. 2004;7(7):965–8. Review.

1143. La Vecchia C. Estrogen and combined estrogen-progestogen therapy in the menopause and breast cancer. Breast. 2004;13(6):515–8. Review.

1144. Giacosa A, Barale R, Bavaresco L, Gatenby P, Gerbi V, Janssens J, Johnston B, Kas K, La Vecchia C, Mainguet P, Morazzoni P, Negri E, Pelucchi C, Pezzotti M, Rondanelli M. Cancer prevention in Europe: the Mediterranean diet as a protective choice. Eur J Cancer Prev. 2013;22(1):90–5. https://doi.org/10.1097/CEJ.0b013e328354d2d7. Review.

1145. Dalvi TB, Canchola AJ, Horn-Ross PL. Dietary patterns, Mediterranean diet, and endometrial cancer risk. Cancer Causes Control. 2007;18(9):957–66. Epub 2007 Jul 19.

1146. Kontou N, Psaltopoulou T, Panagiotakos D, Dimopoulos MA, Linos A. The Mediterranean diet in cancer prevention: a review. J Med Food. 2011;14(10):1065–78. https://doi.org/10.1089/jmf.2010.0244. Epub 2011 Jun 11. Review.

1147. Sacchi R, Paduano A, Savarese M, Vitaglione P, Fogliano V. Extra virgin olive oil: from composition to "molecular gastronomy". Cancer Treat Res. 2014;159:325–38. https://doi.org/10.1007/978-3-642-38007-5_19. Review.

1148. Kang BY. Curcumin reduces angiotensin to mediated cardiomyocyte growth via LOX-1 inhibition. J Cardiovasc Pharmacol. 2010;55:417–24.

1149. Xi B, Veeranki SP, Zhao M, Ma C, Yan Y, Mi J. Relationship of alcohol consumption to all-cause, cardiovascular, and cancer-related mortality in U.S. adults. J Am Coll Cardiol. 2017;70(8):913–22. https://doi.org/10.1016/j.jacc.2017.06.054.

1150. de Gaetano G, Costanzo S. Alcohol and health: praise of the J curves. J Am Coll Cardiol. 2017;70(8):923–5. https://doi.org/10.1016/j.jacc.2017.07.710.

1151. Plunk AD, Syed-Mohammed H, Cavazos-Rehg P, Bierut LJ, Grucza RA. Alcohol consumption, heavy drinking and mortality: re-thinking the J-shaped curve. Alcohol Clin Exp Res. 2014;38(2):471–8. https://doi.org/10.1111/acer.12250.

1152. Plowman SA, Smith DL. Exercise physiology: for health, fitness, and performance. Philadelphia: Lippincott, Williams and Wilkins; 2014.

1153. Potteiger JA. ACSM's introduction to exercise science. Philadelphia: Lippincott, Williams and Wilkins; 2014.

1154. Williams KA, Patel H. Healthy plant-based diet: what does it really mean? J Am Coll Cardiol. 2017;70(4):423–5.

1155. Mueller PJ. Physical (in)activity-dependent alterations at the rostral ventrolateral medulla: influence on sympathetic nervous system regulation. Am J Physiol Regul Integr Comp Physiol. 2010;298:R1468–74.

1156. Mischel NA, Subramanian M, Dombrowski MD, Llewellyn-Smith IJ, Mueller PJ. Inactivity-related neuroplasticity in brainstem control of sympathetic outflow: unraveling underlying molecular, cellular, and anatomical mechanisms. Am J Physiol Heart Circ Physiol. 2015;309:H235–43. https://doi.org/10.1152/ajpheart.00929.2014. Epub 2015 May 8.

1157. Fisher JP, Young CN, Fadel PJ. Central sympathetic overactivity: maladies and mechanisms. Auton Neurosci. 2009;148:5–15.

1158. Go AS, Mozaffarian D, Roger VL, et al. Executive summary: heart disease and stroke statistics – 2013 update: a report from the American Heart Association. Circulation. 2013;127:143–52.

1159. Lindberg FA. The GI Mediterranean diet: the glycemic index-based life-saving diet of the Greeks. Berkley: Ulysses Press; 2009.

1160. Matsuo M, Kaneko T. The chemistry of reactive oxygen species and related free radicals. In: Radak Z, editor. Free radicals in exercise and aging. Leeds: Human Kinetics; 2000. p. 1–34.

1161. Sudano I, Spreker LE, Hermam F, Flammer A, Corti R, Noli G, et al. Protection of endothelial function targets for nutritional and pharmacologic intervention. J Cardiovasc Pharmacol. 2006;47(suppl 2):S136–50.

1162. Powers SK, Jackson MJ. Exercise-induced oxidative stress: cellular mechanisms and impact on muscle force production. Physiol Rev. 2008;88:1243–76.

1163. Zembroń-Łacny A, Szyszka K, Hübner-Woźniak E. The pro-antioxidant-oxidant balance in the blood of middle – distance runners. Biol Sport. 1998;16:51–9.

1164. Alessio HM, Hagerman AE, Fulkerson BK, Ambrose J, Rice RE, et al. Generation of reactive oxygen species after exhaustive aerobic and isometric exercise. Med Sci Sports Exerc. 2000;32(9):1576–81.

1165. Goto C, Higashi Y, Kimura M, Noma K, Hara K, et al. Effect of different intensities of exercise on endothelium-dependent vasodilation in humans: role of endothelium-dependent nitric oxide and oxidative stress. Circulation. 2003;108(5):530–5.

1166. Knez WL, Jenkins DG, Coombes JS. Oxidative stress in half and full ironman triathletes. Med Sci Sports Exerc. 2007;39(2):283–8.

1167. Pilch W, Szygula Z, Tyka AK, Palka T, Tyka A, Cison T, Pilch P, Teleglow A. Disturbances in pro-antioxidant-oxidant balance after passive body overheating and after exercise in elevated ambient temperatures in athletes and untrained men. PLoS One. 2014;9(1):e85320. https://doi.org/10.1371/journal.pone.0085320. eCollection 2014.

1168. Sengupta P. Health impacts of yoga and pranayama: a state-of-the-art review. Int J Prev Med. 2012;3(7):444–58.

1169. Traub O, Berk BC. Laminar shear stress: mechanisms by which endothelial cells transducer an atheroprotective force. Arterioscler Thromb Vasc Biol. 1998;18:677–85.

1170. Garcia-Cardenia G, Fan R, Shah V, Sorrentino R, Cinno G, Papapetriopoulas A, Sessa WC. Dynamic activation of endothelial nitric oxide synthase by Hsp90. Nature. 1998;392:821–4.
1171. Fleming I, Busse R. Signal transduction of eNOS activation. Cardiovasc Res. 1999;43:532–41.
1172. Russell KS, Haynes MP, Caulin-Glaser T, Rosneck J, Sessa WC, Bender JR. Estrogen stimulates heat shock protein 90 binding to endothelial nitric oxide synthase in human vascular endothelial cells. Effects on calcium sensitivity and NO release. J Biol Chem. 2000;275:5026–30.
1173. Hudicka O, Brown M, Egginton S. Angiogenesis in skeletal and cardiac muscle. Physiol Rev. 1992;72:369–417.
1174. Lee JS, Feldman AM. Gene therapy for therapeutic myocardial angiogenesis a promising synthesis of two emerging technologies. Nat Med. 1998;4:739–42.
1175. Dijhorst-Oci LT, Stores ES, Koomans HA, Rabelink TJ. Acute simultaneous stimulation of nitric oxide and oxygen radicals by angiotensin II in humans in vivo. J Cardiovasc Pharmacol. 1999;33:420–4.
1176. Romero JC, Reckelhoff JE. Role of angiotensin and oxidative stress in essential hypertension. Hypertension. 1999;34:943–9.
1177. Cai H, Harrison DG. Endothelial dysfunction in cardiovascular diseases: the role of oxidant stress. Circ Res. 2000;87:840–4.
1178. Sowers JR. Hypertension angiotensin II and oxidative stress. N Engl J Med. 2002;346:1999–2001.
1179. Martin JE, Dubbert PM, Cushman WC. Controlled trial of aerobic exercise in hypertension. Circulation. 1990;81:1560–7.
1180. Wood PD, Statanick ML, Williams PT, Haskell WL. The effects on plasma lipoproteins of a prudent weight-reducing diet with or without exercise in overweight men and women. N Engl J Med. 1991;325:461–6.
1181. Arakawa K. Antihypertensive mechanism of exercise. J Hypertens. 1993;11:223–9.
1182. Paffenbarger RS, Hyde RT, Wing AL, et al. The association of changes in physical-activity level and other lifestyle characteristics with mortality among men. N Engl J Med. 1993;328:538–45.
1183. Higashi Y, Yoshizumi M. Exercise and endothelial function: role of endothelium derived nitric oxide and oxidative stress in healthy subjects and hypertensive patients. Pharmacol Ther. 2004;102:87–96.
1184. Griffin KL, Laughlin MH, Parker JL. Exercise training improves endothelium-mediated vasorelaxation after chronic coronary occlusion. J Appl Physiol. 1999;87:1948–56.
1185. Mancini GB, Henry GC, Macaya C, O'Neil BJ, Pucilo AL, Carere RG, et al. Angiotensin-converting enzyme inhibition with quinapril improves endothelial vasomotor dysfunction in patients with coronary artery disease. The TREND (Trial on Reversing Endothelial Dysfunction) study. Circulation. 1996;94:258–65.
1186. Ghadoni L, Virdis A, Magagna A, Taddei S, Salvetti A. Effects of the angiotensin II type 1 receptor blocker candesartan on endothelial function in patients with essential hypertension. Hypertension. 2000;35:501–6.
1187. The long term intervention with Pravastatin in ischaemic Disease (LIPID) Study Group. Prevention of cardiovascular events and death with pravastatin in patients with coronary heart disease and a broad range of mitral cholesterol levels. N Engl J Med. 1998;339:1349–57.
1188. Fryer LG, Hajduch E, Rencurel F, Salt IS, Hundal HS, Hardie DG, et al. Activation of glucose transport by AMP-activated protein kinase via stimulation of nitric oxide synthase. Diabetes. 2000;49:1978–85.
1189. Calvert JW, Lefer DJ. Role of β-adrenergic receptors and nitric oxide signaling in exercise-mediated cardioprotection. Physology. 2013;28(4):216–24. https://doi.org/10.1152/physiol.00011.2013.
1190. Abraham P, Saumet JL, Chevalier JM. External iliac artery endofibrosis in athletes. Sports Med. 1997;24:221–6.
1191. Bergholm R, Makimattila S, Valkomen M, Liu ML, Lahdempera S, Taskinen MR, Sovijarvi A, Malmberg P, Yki-Jarvinen H. Intense physical training decreases circulating antioxidants and endothelium-dependent vasodilation in vivo. Atherosclerosis. 1999;145:341–9.
1192. Nichols S, Gleadall-Siddall DO, Antony R, Clark AL, Cleland JGF, Carroll S, Ingle L. Estimated peak functional capacity: an accurate method for assessing change in peak oxygen consumption after cardiac rehabilitation? Clin Physiol Funct Imaging. 2017. https://doi.org/10.1111/cpf.12468.
1193. Palermo P, Corrà U. Exercise prescriptions for training and rehabilitation in patients with heart and lung disease. Ann Am Thorac Soc. 2017;14(Supplement_1):S59–66. https://doi.org/10.1513/AnnalsATS.201702-160FR.
1194. Abdul-Jawad Altisent O, Puri R, Regueiro A, Chamandi C, Rodriguez-Gabella T, Del Trigo M, Campelo-Parada F, Couture T, Marsal JR, Côté M, Paradis JM, DeLarochellière R, Doyle D, Mohammadi S, Dumont E, Rodés-Cabau J. Predictors and association with clinical outcomes of the changes in exercise capacity after transcatheter aortic valve replacement. Circulation. 2017;136(7):632–43. https://doi.org/10.1161/CIRCULATIONAHA.116.026349. Epub 2017 Jun 6.
1195. Talwar A, Sahni S, Verma S, Khan SZ, Dhar S, Kohn N. Exercise tolerance improves after pulmonary rehabilitation in pulmonary hypertension patients. J Exerc Rehabil. 2017;13(2):214–7. https://doi.org/10.12965/jer.1732872.436. eCollection 2017 Apr. PMID: 28503536.
1196. Cheng ST, Wu YK, Yang MC, Huang CY, Huang HC, Chu WH, Lan CC. Pulmonary rehabilitation improves heart rate variability at peak exercise, exercise capacity and health-related quality

of life in chronic obstructive pulmonary disease. Heart Lung. 2014;43(3):249–55. https://doi.org/10.1016/j.hrtlng.2014.03.002. Epub 2014 Mar 29. PMID: 24685394.

1197. Karssemeijer EGA, Aaronson JA, Bossers WJ, Smits T, Olde Rikkert MGM, Kessels RPC. Positive effects of combined cognitive and physical exercise training on cognitive function in older adults with mild cognitive impairment or dementia: a meta-analysis. Ageing Res Rev. 2017. pii: S1568-1637(17)30114-9. https://doi.org/10.1016/j.arr.2017.09.003. [Epub ahead of print] Review.

1198. Ebrahimi K, Majdi A, Baghaiee B, Hosseini SH, Sadigh-Eteghad S. Physical activity and beta-amyloid pathology in Alzheimer's disease: a sound mind in a sound body. EXCLI J. 2017;16:959–72. https://doi.org/10.17179/excli2017-475. eCollection 2017. Review. PMID: 28900376.

1199. Cheng ST. Cognitive reserve and the prevention of dementia: the role of physical and cognitive activities. Curr Psychiatry Rep. 2016;18(9):85. https://doi.org/10.1007/s11920-016-0721-2. Review.

1200. Richter EA, Ruderman NB. AMPK and the biochemistry of exercise: implications for human health and disease. Biochem J. 2009;418(2):261–75. https://doi.org/10.1042/BJ20082055. Review.

1201. Segev D, Hellerstein D, Dunsky A. Physical activity – does it really increase bone density in postmenopausal women? A review of articles published between 2001–2016. Curr Aging Sci. 2017. https://doi.org/10.2174/1874609810666170918170744.

1202. Swedish Council on Health Technology Assessment. Osteoporosis – prevention, diagnosis and treatment: a systematic review [Internet]. Stockholm: Swedish Council on Health Technology Assessment (SBU); 2003.

1203. Senderovich H, Tang H, Belmont S. The role of exercises in osteoporotic fracture prevention and current care gaps. Where are we now? Recent updates. Rambam Maimonides Med J. 2017;8(3). https://doi.org/10.5041/RMMJ.10308. Review.

1204. Loeser RF, Beavers DP, Bay-Jensen AC, Karsdal MA, Nicklas BJ, Guermazi A, Hunter DJ, Messier SP. Effects of dietary weight loss with and without exercise on interstitial matrix turnover and tissue inflammation biomarkers in adults with knee osteoarthritis: the Intensive Diet and Exercise for Arthritis trial (IDEA). Osteoarthr Cartil. 2017. pii: S1063-4584(17)31107-X. https://doi.org/10.1016/j.joca.2017.07.015.

1205. Feldman BM. Exercise as medicine for children with arthritis. J Rheumatol. 2017;44(8):1103–5. https://doi.org/10.3899/jrheum.170461.

1206. Gordon BR, McDowell CP, Lyons M, Herring MP. The effects of resistance exercise training on anxiety: a meta-analysis and meta-regression analysis of randomized controlled trials. Sports Med. 2017. https://doi.org/10.1007/s40279-017-0769-0. [Epub ahead of print] Review.

1207. Yeh HP, Stone JA, Churchill SM, Brymer E, Davids K. Physical and emotional benefits of different exercise environments designed for treadmill running. Int J Environ Res Public Health. 2017;14(7). pii: E752. https://doi.org/10.3390/ijerph14070752.

1208. Awick EA, Ehlers DK, Aguiñaga S, Daugherty AM, Kramer AF, McAuley E. Effects of a randomized exercise trial on physical activity, psychological distress and quality of life in older adults. Gen Hosp Psychiatry. 2017. pii: S0163-8343(17)30101-9. https://doi.org/10.1016/j.genhosppsych.2017.06.005. [Epub ahead of print].

1209. Hearing CM, Chang WC, Szuhany KL, Deckersbach T, Nierenberg AA, Sylvia LG. Physical Exercise for treatment of mood disorders: a critical review. Curr Behav Neurosci Rep. 2016;3(4):350–9. https://doi.org/10.1007/s40473-016-0089-y. Epub 2016 Oct 14.

1210. Kovacevic A, Mavros Y, Heisz JJ, Fiatarone Singh MA. The effect of resistance exercise on sleep: a systematic review of randomized controlled trials. Sleep Med Rev. 2017. pii: S1087-0792(16)30152-6. https://doi.org/10.1016/j.smrv.2017.07.002. [Epub ahead of print] Review.

1211. S Delevatti R, Schuch FB, Kanitz AC, Alberton CL, Marson EC, Lisboa SC, Pinho CDF, Bregagnol LP, Becker MT, Kruel LFM. Quality of life and sleep quality are similarly improved after aquatic or dry-land aerobic training in patients with type 2 diabetes: a randomized clinical trial. J Sci Med Sport. 2017. pii: S1440-2440(17)31029-0. https://doi.org/10.1016/j.jsams.2017.08.024. [Epub ahead of print].

1212. Koo P, Gjelsvik A, Choudhary G, Wu WC, Wang W, McCool FD, Eaton CB. Prospective association of physical activity and heart failure hospitalizations among black adults with normal ejection fraction: The Jackson Heart Study. J Am Heart Assoc. 2017;6(9). pii: e006107. https://doi.org/10.1161/JAHA.117.006107.

1213. Torell MF, Strömsöe A, Zagerholm E, Herlitz J, Claesson A, Svensson L, Börjesson M. Higher survival rates in exercise-related out-of-hospital cardiac arrests, compared to non-exercise-related – a study from the Swedish Register of Cardiopulmonary Resuscitation. Eur J Prev Cardiol. 2017;1:2047487317729251. https://doi.org/10.1177/2047487317729251.

1214. Maessen MF, Eijsvogels TM, Stevens G, van Dijk AP, Hopman MT. Benefits of lifelong exercise training on left ventricular function after myocardial infarction. Eur J Prev Cardiol. 2017;1:2047487317728765. https://doi.org/10.1177/2047487317728765.

1215. Campkin LM, Boyd JM, Campbell DJT. Coronary artery disease patient perspectives on exercise participation. J Cardiopulm Rehabil Prev. 2017;37(5):305–14. https://doi.org/10.1097/HCR.0000000000000195.

1216. Nichols S, Gleadall-Siddall DO, Antony R, Clark AL, Cleland JGF, Carroll S, Ingle L. Estimated peak functional capacity: an accurate method for assessing change in peak oxygen consumption after cardiac rehabilitation? Clin Physiol Funct Imaging. 2017. https://doi.org/10.1111/cpf.12468.
1217. Piña IL, Apstein CS, Balady GJ, Belardinelli R, Chaitman BR, Duscha BD, Fletcher BJ, Fleg JL, Myers JN, Sullivan MJ, American Heart Association Committee on exercise, rehabilitation, and prevention. Exercise and heart failure: a statement from the American Heart Association Committee on exercise, rehabilitation, and prevention. Circulation. 2003;107(8):1210–25. Review.
1218. Myers J. Cardiology patient pages. Exercise and cardiovascular health. Circulation. 2003;107(1):e2–5.
1219. Tinlin L, Fini N, Bernhardt J, Lewis LK, Olds T, English C. Best practice guidelines for the measurement of physical activity levels in stroke survivors: a secondary analysis of an observational study. Int J Rehabil Res. 2017. https://doi.org/10.1097/MRR.0000000000000253.
1220. Oberlin LE, Waiwood AM, Cumming TB, Marsland AL, Bernhardt J, Erickson KI.Effects of physical activity on poststroke cognitive function: a meta-analysis of randomized controlled trials. Stroke. 2017. pii: STROKEAHA.117.017319. https://doi.org/10.1161/STROKEAHA.117.017319.
1221. Yfanti C, Tsiokanos A, Fatouros IG, Theodorou AA, Deli CK, Koutedakis Y, Jamurtas AZ. Chronic eccentric exercise and antioxidant supplementation: effects on lipid profile and insulin sensitivity. J Sports Sci Med. 2017;16(3):375–82. eCollection 2017 Sept.
1222. Mendes R, Sousa N, Reis VM, Themudo-Barata JL. Implementing low-cost, community-based exercise programs for middle-aged and older patients with type 2 diabetes: what are the benefits for glycemic control and cardiovascular risk? Int J Environ Res Public Health. 2017;14(9). pii: E1057. https://doi.org/10.3390/ijerph14091057. PMID: 28902144.
1223. Miele EM, Headley SAE, Germain M, Joubert J, Herrick S, Milch C, Evans E, Cornelius A, Brewer B, Taylor B, Wood RJ. High-density lipoprotein particle pattern and overall lipid responses to a short-term moderate-intensity aerobic exercise training intervention in patients with chronic kidney disease. Clin Kidney J. 2017;10(4):524–31. https://doi.org/10.1093/ckj/sfx006. Epub 2017 Mar 27. PMID: 28852492.
1224. Villafaina S, Collado-Mateo D, Fuentes JP, Merellano-Navarro E, Gusi N. Physical exercise improves heart rate variability in patients with type 2 diabetes: a systematic review. Curr Diab Rep. 2017;17(11):110. https://doi.org/10.1007/s11892-017-0941-9. Review.
1225. Ostman C, Smart NA, Morcos D, Duller A, Ridley W, Jewiss D. The effect of exercise training on clinical outcomes in patients with the metabolic syndrome: a systematic review and meta-analysis. Cardiovasc Diabetol. 2017;16(1):110. https://doi.org/10.1186/s12933-017-0590-y. PMID: 28854979.
1226. Myers J, Atwood JE, Froelicher V. Active lifestyle and diabetes. Circulation. 2003;107(19):2392–4.
1227. Brown JC, Zemel BS, Troxel AB, Rickels MR, Damjanov N, Ky B, Rhim AD, Rustgi AK, Courneya KS, Schmitz KH. Dose-response effects of aerobic exercise on body composition among colon cancer survivors: a randomised controlled trial. Br J Cancer. 2017. https://doi.org/10.1038/bjc.2017.339.
1228. Brown JC, Troxel AB, Ky B, Damjanov N, Zemel BS, Rickels MR, Rhim AD, Rustgi AK, Courneya KS, Schmitz KH. Dose-response effects of aerobic exercise among colon cancer survivors: a randomized phase II trial. Clin Colorectal Cancer. 2017. pii: S1533-0028(16)30168-2. https://doi.org/10.1016/j.clcc.2017.06.001.
1229. Hartman SJ, Nelson SH, Myers E, Natarajan L, Sears DD, Palmer BW, Weiner LS, Parker BA, Patterson RE. Randomized controlled trial of increasing physical activity on objectively measured and self-reported cognitive functioning among breast cancer survivors: the memory & motion study. Cancer. 2017. https://doi.org/10.1002/cncr.30987.
1230. Livsey L, Lewis K. Breast cancer survivors' perceptions of participating in a supervised exercise intervention: an exploratory review of the literature. Women Health. 2017. https://doi.org/10.1080/03630242.2017.1372844.
1231. Vashistha V, Singh B, Kaur S, Prokop LJ, Kaushik D. The effects of exercise on fatigue, quality of life, and psychological function for men with prostate cancer: systematic review and meta-analyses. Eur Urol Focus. 2016;2(3):284–95. https://doi.org/10.1016/j.euf.2016.02.011. Epub 2016 Mar 9. Review.
1232. Daly RM. Exercise and nutritional approaches to prevent frail bones, falls and fractures: an update. Climacteric. 2017;20(2):119–24. https://doi.org/10.1080/13697137.2017.1286890. Epub 2017 Feb 8. Review.
1233. Greenway KG, Walkley JW, Rich PA. Impact exercise and bone density in premenopausal women with below average bone density for age. Eur J Appl Physiol. 2015;115(11):2457–69. https://doi.org/10.1007/s00421-015-3225-6. Epub 2015 Aug 1.
1234. Fuchs RK, Kersh ME, Carballido-Gamio J, Thompson WR, Keyak JH, Warden SJ. Physical activity for strengthening fracture prone regions of the proximal femur. Curr Osteoporos Rep. 2017;15(1):43–52. https://doi.org/10.1007/s11914-017-0343-6. Review.
1235. Turner JE, Brum PC. Does regular exercise counter T cell immunosenescence reducing the risk

of developing cancer and promoting successful treatment of malignancies? Oxidative Med Cell Longev. 2017;2017:4234765. https://doi.org/10.1155/2017/4234765. Epub 2017 Jul 2. Review.

1236. Hojman P. Exercise protects from cancer through regulation of immune function and inflammation. Biochem Soc Trans. 2017;45(4):905–11. https://doi.org/10.1042/BST20160466. Epub 2017 Jul 3. Review.

1237. Gustafson MP, DiCostanzo AC, Wheatley CM, Kim CH, Bornschlegl S, Gastineau DA, Johnson BD, Dietz AB. A systems biology approach to investigating the influence of exercise and fitness on the composition of leukocytes in peripheral blood. J Immunother Cancer. 2017;5:30. https://doi.org/10.1186/s40425-017-0231-8.

1238. Ackland GL, Minto G, Clark M, Whittle J, Stephens RCM, Owen T, Prabhu P, Del Arroyo AG. Autonomic regulation of systemic inflammation in humans: a multi-center, blinded observational cohort study. Brain Behav Immun. 2017. pii: S0889-1591(17)30398-7. https://doi.org/10.1016/j.bbi.2017.08.010.

1239. Jafariyan S, Monazzami A, Nikosefat Z, Nobahar M, Yari K. Inflammatory and immune responses to a 3-day period of downhill running in active females. Cell Mol Biol (Noisy-le-Grand). 2017;63(7):76–83. https://doi.org/10.14715/cmb/2017.63.7.13.

1240. Bartlett DB, Shepherd SO, Wilson OJ, Adlan AM, Wagenmakers AJM, Shaw CS, Lord JM. Neutrophil and monocyte bactericidal responses to 10 weeks of low-volume high-intensity interval or moderate-intensity continuous training in sedentary adults. Oxidative Med Cell Longev. 2017;2017:8148742. https://doi.org/10.1155/2017/8148742. Epub 2017 Jun 1.

1241. Clark LV, Buckland M, Murphy G, Taylor N, Vleck V, Mein C, Wozniak E, Smuk M, White PD. Cytokine responses to exercise and activity in patients with chronic fatigue syndrome: case control study. Clin Exp Immunol. 2017. https://doi.org/10.1111/cei.13023.

1242. Monteiro Junior RS, de Tarso Maciel-Pinheiro P, da Matta M, Portugal E, da Silva Figueiredo LF, Terra R, Carneiro LSF, Rodrigues VD, Nascimento OJM, Deslandes AC, Laks J. Effect of exercise on inflammatory profile of older persons: systematic review and meta-analyses. J Phys Act Health. 2017;3:1–24. https://doi.org/10.1123/jpah.2016-0735.

1243. Zimmer P, Schenk A, Kieven M, Holthaus M, Lehmann J, Lövenich L, Bloch W. Exercise induced alterations in NK-cell cytotoxicity – methodological issues and future perspectives. Exerc Immunol Rev. 2017;23:66–81.

1244. Moore SC, Lee IM, Weiderpass E, Campbell PT, Sampson JN, Kitahara CM, Keadle SK, Arem H, Berrington de Gonzalez A, Hartge P, Adami HO, Blair CK, Borch KB, Boyd E, Check DP, Fournier A, Freedman ND, Gunter M, Johannson M, Khaw KT, Linet MS, Orsini N, Park Y, Riboli E, Robien K, Schairer C, Sesso H, Spriggs M, Van Dusen R, Wolk A, Matthews CE, Patel AV. Association of leisure-time physical activity with risk of 26 types of cancer in 1.44 million adults. JAMA Intern Med. 2016;176(6):816–25. https://doi.org/10.1001/jamainternmed.2016.1548.

1245. O'Donovan G, Lee IM, Hamer M, Stamatakis E. Association of "weekend warrior" and other leisure time physical activity patterns with risks for all-cause, cardiovascular disease, and cancer mortality. JAMA Intern Med. 2017;177(3):335–42. https://doi.org/10.1001/jamainternmed.2016.8014.

1246. Song M, Giovannucci E. Preventable incidence and mortality of carcinoma associated with lifestyle factors among white adults in the United States. JAMA Oncol. 2016;2(9):1154–61. https://doi.org/10.1001/jamaoncol.2016.0843.

1247. Manson JE, Hu FB, Rich-Edwards JW, Colditz GA, Stampfer MJ, Willett WC, Speizer FE, Hennekens CH. A prospective study of walking as compared with vigorous exercise in the prevention of coronary heart disease in women. N Engl J Med. 1999;341(9):650–8.

1248. Hu FB, Sigal RJ, Rich-Edwards JW, Colditz GA, Solomon CG, Willett WC, Speizer FE, Manson JE. Walking compared with vigorous physical activity and risk of type 2 diabetes in women: a prospective study. JAMA. 1999;282(15):1433–9.

1249. US Public Health Service, Office of the Surgeon General. Physical activity and health: a report of the surgeon general. Atlanta: US Department of Health and Human Services, Centers for Disease Control and Prevention, National Center for Chronic Disease Prevention and Health Promotion; 1996.

1250. Fletcher GF, Balady GJ, Amsterdam EA, et al. Exercise standards for testing and training: a statement for healthcare professionals from the American Heart Association. Circulation. 2001;104:1694–740.

1251. Pate RR, Pratt MP, Blair SN, et al. Physical activity and public health: a recommendation from the Centers for Disease Control and Prevention and the American College of Sports Medicine. JAMA. 1995;273:402–7.

1252. American College of Sports Medicine. Guidelines for exercise testing and prescription. 6th ed. Baltimore: Lippincott Williams & Wilkins; 2000.

1253. Myers J. Cardiology patient pages. Exercise and cardiovascular health. Circulation. 2003;107(1):e2–5.

1254. Pop-Busui R, Evans GW, Gerstein HC, Fonseca V, Fleg JL, Hoogwerf BJ, Genuth MS, Grimm RH, Corson MA, Prineas R, The ACCORD Study Group. Effects of cardiac autonomic dysfunction on mortality risk in the action to control cardiovascular risk in diabetes (ACCORD) trial. Diabetes Care. 2010;33:1578–84.

1255. Vinik AI, Maser RE, Ziegler D. Neuropathy. The crystal ball for cardiovascular disease. Diabetes Care. 2010;33(7):1688–90.

1256. Dinas PC, Valente A, Granzotto M, Rossato M, Vettor R, Zacharopoulou A, Carrillo AE, Davies NA, Gkiata P, Jamurtas AZ, Koutedakis Y, Metsios GS, Flouris AD. Browning formation markers of subcutaneous adipose tissue in relation to resting energy expenditure, physical activity and diet in humans. Horm Mol Biol Clin Invest. 2017. pii: /j/hmbci.2017.31.issue-1/hmbci-2017-0008/hmbci-2017-0008.xml. https://doi.org10.1515/hmbci-2017-0008.
1257. Høydal MA, Stølen TO, Kettlewell S, Maier LS, Brown JH, Sowa T, Catalucci D, Condorelli G, Kemi OJ, Smith GL, Wisløff U. Exercise training reverses myocardial dysfunction induced by CaMKIIδC overexpression by restoring Ca2+ homeostasis. J Appl Physiol (1985). 2016;121(1):212–20. https://doi.org/10.1152/japplphysiol.00188.2016. Epub 2016 May 26.
1258. Khera AV, Emdin CA, Drake I, Natarajan P, Bick AG, Cook NR, Chasman DI, Baber U, Mehran R, Rader DJ, Fuster V, Boerwinkle E, Melander O, Orho-Melander M, Ridker PM, Kathiresan S. Genetic risk, adherence to a healthy lifestyle, and coronary disease. N Engl J Med. 2016;375(24):2349–58. Epub 2016 Nov 13.
1259. Nicolson GL. Mitochondrial dysfunction and chronic disease: treatment with natural supplements. Integr Med (Encinitas). 2014;13(4):35–43.
1260. Carling D, Viollet B. Beyond energy homeostasis: the expanding role of AMP-activated protein kinase in regulating metabolism. Cell Metab. 2015;21(6):799–804. https://doi.org/10.1016/j.cmet.2015.05.005. Review.
1261. Towler MC, Hardie DG. AMP-activated protein kinase in metabolic control and insulin signaling. Circ Res. 2007;100(3):328–41. Review.
1262. Nakano M, Inui A. Metformin and incretin-based therapies up-regulate central and peripheral Adenosine monophosphate-activated protein affecting appetite and metabolism. Indian J Endocrinol Metab. 2012;16(Suppl S3):529–31.
1263. UK Prospective Diabetes Study (UKPDS) Group. Intensive blood-glucose control with sulphonylureas or insulin compared with conventional treatment and risk of complications in patients with type 2 diabetes (UKPDS 33). Lancet. 1998;352:837–53.
1264. Ruiter R, Visser LE, van Herk-Sukel MP, Coebergh JW, Haak HR, Geelhoed-Duijvestijn PH, Straus SM, Herings RM, Stricker BH. Lower risk of cancer in patients on metformin in comparison with those on sulfonylurea derivatives: results from a large population-based follow-up study. Diabetes Care. 2012;35(1):119–24. https://doi.org/10.2337/dc11-0857. Epub 2011 Nov 18.
1265. Tennen RI, Michishita-Kioi E, Chua KF. Finding a target for resveratrol. Cell. 2012;148(3):387–9. https://doi.org/10.1016/j.cell.2012.01.032.
1266. Zhang QJ, McMillin SL, Tanner JM, Palionyte M, Abel ED, Symons JD. Endothelial nitric oxide synthase phosphorylation in treadmill-running mice: role of vascular signalling kinases. J Physiol. 2009;587(Pt 15):3911–20. https://doi.org/10.1113/jphysiol.2009.172916. Epub 2009 Jun 8.
1267. Bavarsad Shahripour R, Harrigan MR, Alexandrov AV. N-acetylcysteine (NAC) in neurological disorders: mechanisms of action and therapeutic opportunities. Brain Behav. 2014;4(2):108–22. https://doi.org/10.1002/brb3.208. Epub 2014 Jan 13. Review.
1268. Berk M, Malhi GS, Gray LJ, Dean OM. The promise of N-acetylcysteine in neuropsychiatry. Trends Pharmacol Sci. 2013;34(3):167–77. https://doi.org/10.1016/j.tips.2013.01.001. Epub 2013 Jan 29. Review.
1269. Dean O, Giorlando F, Berk M. N-acetylcysteine in psychiatry: current therapeutic evidence and potential mechanisms of action. J Psychiatry Neurosci. 2011;36(2):78–86. https://doi.org/10.1503/jpn.100057. Review.
1270. Fernandes BS, Dean OM, Dodd S, Malhi GS, Berk M. N-acetylcysteine in depressive symptoms and functionality: a systematic review and meta-analysis. J Clin Psychiatry. 2016;77(4):e457–66. https://doi.org/10.4088/JCP.15r09984.
1271. Harrington R. Stress, health & well-being: thriving in the 21st century. Belmont: Wadsworth Cengage Learning; 2013.
1272. Hjemdahl P, Rosengren A, Steptoe A, editors. Stress and cardiovascular disease. London: Springer-Verlag; 2012.
1273. Bot I, Kuiper J. Stressed brain, stressed heart? Lancet. 2017;389(10071):770–1. https://doi.org/10.1016/S0140-6736(17)30044-2. Epub 2017 Jan 12.
1274. Chi JS, Kloner RA. Stress and myocardial infarction. Heart. 2003;89(5):475–6.
1275. Pignalberi C, Patti G, Chimenti C, Pasceri V, Maseri A. Role of different determinants of psychological distress in acute coronary syndromes. J Am Coll Cardiol. 1998;32(3):613–9.
1276. Yusuf S, Hawken S, Ounpuu S, Dans T, Avezum A, Lanas F, McQueen M, Budaj A, Pais P, Varigos J, Lisheng L, INTERHEART Study Investigators. Effect of potentially modifiable risk factors associated with myocardial infarction in 52 countries (the INTERHEART study): case-control study. Lancet. 2004;364(9438):937–52.
1277. Ohlin B, Nilsson PM, Nilsson JA, Berglund G. Chronic psychosocial stress predicts long-term cardiovascular morbidity and mortality in middle-aged men. Eur Heart J. 2004;25(10):867–73.
1278. Tofler GH, Stone PH, Maclure M, Edelman E, Davis VG, Robertson T, Antman EM, Muller JE. Analysis of possible triggers of acute myocardial infarction (the MILIS study). Am J Cardiol. 1990;66(1):22–7.
1279. Brezinka V, Kittel F. Psychosocial factors of coronary heart disease in women: a review. Soc Sci Med. 1996;42(10):1351–65. Review.
1280. Gonzales TK, Yonker JA, Chang V, Roan CL, Herd P, Atwood CS. Myocardial infarction in the Wisconsin Longitudinal Study: the interaction

among environmental, health, social, behavioural and genetic factors. BMJ Open. 2017;7(1):e011529. https://doi.org/10.1136/bmjopen-2016-011529.
1281. Bunker SJ, Colquhoun DM, Esler MD, Hickie IB, Hunt D, Jelinek VM, Oldenburg BF, Peach HG, Ruth D, Tennant CC, Tonkin AM. "Stress" and coronary heart disease: psychosocial risk factors. Med J Aust. 2003;178(6):272–6. Review.
1282. Kuper H, Adami HO, Theorell T, Weiderpass E. Psychosocial determinants of coronary heart disease in middle-aged women: a prospective study in Sweden. Am J Epidemiol. 2006;164(4):349–57. Epub 2006 Jun 20.
1283. Welin C, Lappas G, Wilhelmsen L. Independent importance of psychosocial factors for prognosis after myocardial infarction. J Intern Med. 2000;247(6):629–39.
1284. Rosengren A, Hawken S, Ounpuu S, Sliwa K, Zubaid M, Almahmeed WA, Blackett KN, Sitthi-amorn C, Sato H, Yusuf S, INTERHEART investigators. Association of psychosocial risk factors with risk of acute myocardial infarction in 11119 cases and 13648 controls from 52 countries (the INTERHEART study): case-control study. Lancet. 2004;364(9438):953–62.
1285. Smyth A, O'Donnell M, Lamelas P, Teo K, Rangarajan S, Yusuf S, INTERHEART Investigators. Physical activity and anger or emotional upset as triggers of acute myocardial infarction: The INTERHEART study. Circulation. 2016;134(15):1059–67.
1286. Tawakol A, Ishai A, Takx RA, Figueroa AL, Ali A, Kaiser Y, Truong QA, Solomon CJ, Calcagno C, Mani V, Tang CY, Mulder WJ, Murrough JW, Hoffmann U, Nahrendorf M, Shin LM, Fayad ZA, Pitman RK. Relation between resting amygdalar activity and cardiovascular events: a longitudinal and cohort study. Lancet. 2017;389(10071):834–45. https://doi.org/10.1016/S0140-6736(16)31714-7. Epub 2017 Jan 12.
1287. Selye H. The stress of life. 2nd ed. New York: McGraw-Hill; 1956.
1288. Ulrich-Lai YM, Herman JP. Neural regulation of endocrine and autonomic stress responses. Nat Rev Neurosci. 2009;10:397–409.
1289. Bamberger CM, Schulte HM, Chrousos GP. Molecular determinants of glucocorticoid receptor function and tissue sensitivity to glucocorticoids. Endocr Rev. 1996;17:245–61.
1290. McEwen BS. The neurobiology of stress: from serendipity to clinical relevance. Brain Res. 2000;886:172–89.
1291. Chrousos GP. Stress and disorders of the stress system. Nat Rev Endocrinol. 2009;5:374–81.
1292. Stratakis CA, Chrousos GP. Neuroendocrinology and pathophysiology of the stress system. Ann N Y Acad Sci. 1995;771:1–18.
1293. Taggart P, Lambiase P. Anger, emotion, and arrhythmias: from brain to heart. Front Physiol. 2011;19(2):67–72.
1294. Tait AS, Butts CL, Sternberg EM. The role of glucocorticoids and progestins in inflammatory, autoimmune, and infectious disease. J Leukoc Biol. 2008;84(4):924–31. https://doi.org/10.1189/jlb.0208104.
1295. Butts CL, Sternberg EM. Neuroendocrine factors alter host defense by modulating immune function. Cell Immunol. 2008;252(1–2):7–15.
1296. Thayer JF, Loerbroks A, Sternberg EM. Inflammation and cardiorespiratory control: the role of the vagus nerve. Respir Physiol Neurobiol. 2011;178(3):387–94. https://doi.org/10.1016/j.resp.2011.05.016. Epub 2011 May 27. Review.
1297. Felton DL. Neural influence on immune responses: underlying suppositions and basic principles of neural-immune signaling. Prog Brain Res. 2000;122:381–9.
1298. Bär K-J, Boettger MK, Berger S, Baier V, Sauer H, Yeragani VK, Voss A. Decreased baroreflex sensitivity in acute schizophrenia. J Appl Physiol. 2007;102(3):1051–6.
1299. Craig AD. Forebrain emotional asymmetry: a neuroanatomical basis? Trends Cogn Sci. 2005;9:566–71.
1300. Akashi YJ, Goldstein DS, Barbaro G, Ueyama T. Takotsubo cardiomyopathy: a new form of acute, reversible heart failure. Circulation. 2008;118:2754–62.
1301. Nalivaiko E. Animal models of psychogenic cardiovascular disorders: what we can learn from them and what we cannot. Clin Exp Pharmacol Physiol. 2011;38:115–25.
1302. Pelliccia F, Greco C, Vitale C, Rosano G, Gaudio C, Kaski JC. Takotsubo syndrome (stress cardiomyopathy): an intriguing clinical condition in search of its identity. Am J Med. 2014;127:699–704.
1303. Terefe YG, Niraj A, Pradhan J, Kondur A, Afonso L. Myocardial infarction with angiographically normal coronary arteries in the contemporary era. Coron Artery Dis. 2007;18:621–6.
1304. Pelliccia F, Greco C, Vitale C, Rosano G, Gaudio C, Kaski JC. Takotsubo syndrome (stress cardiomyopathy): an intriguing clinical condition in search of its identity. Am J Med. 2014;127:699–704.
1305. Kurisu S, Sato H, Kawagoe T, Ishihara M, Shimatani Y, Nishioka K, Kono Y, Umemura T, Nakamura S. Tako-tsubo-like left ventricular dysfunction with ST-segment elevation: a novel cardiac syndrome mimicking acute myocardial infarction. Am Heart J. 2002;143:448–55.
1306. Sharkey SW, Lesser JR, Zenovich AG, Maron MS, Lindberg J, Longe TF, Maron BJ. Acute and reversible cardiomyopathy provoked by stress in women from the United States. Circulation. 2005;111:472–9.
1307. Mori H, Ishikawa S, Kojima S, Hayashi J, Watanabe Y, Hoffman JI, Okino H. Increased responsiveness of left ventricular apical myocardium to adrenergic stimuli. Cardiovasc Res. 1993;27:192–8.
1308. Gullette EC, Blumenthal JA, Babyak M, Jiang W, Waugh RA, Frid DJ, O'Connor CM, Morris

JJ, Krantz DS. Effects of mental stress on myocardial ischemia during daily life. JAMA. 1997;277:1521–6.
1309. Pimple P, Shah A, Rooks C, Bremner JD, Nye J, Ibeanu I, Murrah N, Shallenberger L, Kelley M, Raggi P, Vaccarino V. Association between anger and mental stress-induced myocardial ischemia. Am Heart J. 2015;169:115–21.
1310. Boyle SH, Williams RB, Mark DB, Brummett BH, Siegler IC, Barefoot JC. Hostility, age, and mortality in a sample of cardiac patients. Am J Cardiol. 2005;96:64–6.
1311. Reich P, DeSilva RA, Lown B, Murawski BJ. Acute psychological disturbances preceding life-threatening ventricular arrhythmias. JAMA. 1981;246:233–5.
1312. Lampert R, Shusterman V, Burg MM, Lee FA, Earley C, Goldberg A, McPherson CA, Batsford WP, Soufer R. Effects of psychologic stress on repolarization and relationship to autonomic and hemodynamic factors. J Cardiovasc Electrophysiol. 2005;16:372–7.
1313. Lampert R. Anger and ventricular arrhythmias. Curr Opin Cardiol. 2010;25:46–52.
1314. Tan AY, Verrier RL. The role of the autonomic nervous system in cardiac arrhythmias. Handb Clin Neurol. 2013;117:135–45.
1315. Alfano KM, Cimino CR. Alteration of expected hemispheric asymmetries: valence and arousal effects in neuropsychological models of emotion. Brain Cogn. 2008;66:213–20.
1316. Hagemann D, Waldstein SR, Thayer JF. Central and autonomic nervous system integration in emotion. Brain Cogn. 2003;52:79–87.
1317. Taggart P, Boyett MR, Logantha S, Lambiase PD. Anger, emotion, and arrhythmias: from brain to heart. Front Physiol. 2011;2:67.
1318. Cannon WB, Mendenhall WL. Factors affecting the coagulation time of blood. IV. The hastening of coagulation in pain and emotional excitement. Am J Phys. 1914;34:251–61.
1319. Steptoe A, Kivimäki M. Stress and cardiovascular disease: an update on current knowledge. Annu Rev Public Health. 2013;34:337–54.
1320. von Känel R, Mills PJ, Fainman C, Dimsdale JE. Effects of psychological stress and psychiatric disorders on blood coagulation and fibrinolysis: a biobehavioral pathway to coronary artery disease? Psychosom Med. 2001;63:531–44.
1321. Wirtz PH, Ehlert U, Emini L, Rüdisüli K, Groessbauer S, Gaab J, Elsenbruch S, von Känel R. Anticipatory cognitive stress appraisal and the acute procoagulant stress response in men. Psychosom Med. 2006;68:851–8.
1322. Shimbo D, Child J, Davidson K, Geer E, Osende JI, Reddy S, Dronge A, Fuster V, Badimon JJ. Exaggerated serotonin-mediated platelet reactivity as a possible link in depression and acute coronary syndromes. Am J Cardiol. 2002;89:331–3.
1323. Zafar MU, Paz-Yepes M, Shimbo D, Vilahur G, Burg MM, Chaplin W, Fuster V, Davidson KW, Badimon JJ. Anxiety is a better predictor of platelet reactivity in coronary artery disease patients than depression. Eur Heart J. 2010;31:1573–82.
1324. Lesch KP, Wolozin BL, Murphy DL, Reiderer P. Primary structure of the human platelet serotonin uptake site: identity with the brain serotonin transporter. J Neurochem. 1993;60:2319–22.
1325. Becker RC. Editor's page: fundamentals in neurocardiology: the brain-platelet-coronary artery interface. J Thromb Thrombolysis. 2008;26:74–7.
1326. Wirtz PH, Redwine LS, Baertschi C, Spillmann M, Ehlert U, von Känel R. Coagulation activity before and after acute psychosocial stress increases with age. Psychosom Med. 2008;70:476–81.
1327. Jern C, Eriksson E, Tengborn L, Risberg B, Wadenvik H, Jern S. Changes of plasma coagulation and fibrinolysis in response to mental stress. Thromb Haemost. 1989;62:767–71.
1328. von Känel R, Bellingrath S, Kudielka BM. Association between burnout and circulating levels of pro- and anti-inflammatory cytokines in schoolteachers. J Psychosom Res. 2008;65:51–9.
1329. von Känel R, Dimsdale JE, Ziegler MG, Mills PJ, Patterson TL, Lee SK, Grant I. Effect of acute psychological stress on the hypercoagulable state in subjects (spousal caregivers of patients with Alzheimer's disease) with coronary or cerebrovascular disease and/or systemic hypertension. Am J Cardiol. 2001;87:1405–8.
1330. Steptoe A, Wardle J, Marmot M. Positive affect and health-related neuroendocrine, cardiovascular, and inflammatory processes. Proc Natl Acad Sci U S A. 2005;102:6508–12.
1331. Preckel D, von Känel R. Regulation of hemostasis by the sympathetic nervous system: any contribution to coronary artery disease? Heart. 2004;4:123–30.
1332. von Känel R, Dimsdale JE. Effects of sympathetic activation by adrenergic infusions on hemostasis in vivo. Eur J Haematol. 2000;65:357–69.
1333. von Känel R, Mills PJ, Ziegler MG, Dimsdale JE. Effect of beta2-adrenergic receptor functioning and increased norepinephrine on the hypercoagulable state with mental stress. Am Heart J. 2002;144:68–72.
1334. Stämpfli SF, Camici GG, Keller S, Rozenberg I, Arras M, Schuler B, Gassmann M, Garcia I, Lüscher TF, Tanner FC. Restraint stress enhances arterial thrombosis in vivo – role of the sympathetic nervous system. Stress. 2014;17:126–32.
1335. Allen MT, Patterson SM. Hemoconcentration and stress: a review of physiological mechanisms and relevance for cardiovascular disease risk. Biol Psychol. 1995;41:1–27.
1336. Austin AW, Patterson SM, von Känel R. Hemoconcentration and hemostasis during acute stress: interacting and independent effects. Ann Behav Med. 2011;42:153–73.

1337. Nater UM, Skoluda N, Strahler J. Biomarkers of stress in behavioural medicine. Curr Opin Psychiatry. 2013;26:440–5.

1338. Sojka P, Stålnacke BM, Björnstig U, Karlsson K. One-year follow-up of patients with mild traumatic brain injury: occurrence of post-traumatic stress-related symptoms at follow-up and serum levels of cortisol, S-100B and neuron-specific enolase in acute phase. Brain Inj. 2006;20:613–20.

1339. Michaud K, Matheson K, Kelly O, Anisman H. Impact of stressors in a natural context on release of cortisol in healthy adult humans: a meta-analysis. Stress. 2008;11:177–97.

1340. Poll EM, Kreitschmann-Andermahr I, Langejuergen Y, Stanzel S, Gilsbach JM, Gressner A, Yagmur E. Saliva collection method affects predictability of serum cortisol. Clin Chim Acta. 2007;382:15–9.

1341. Bozovic D, Racic M, Ivkovic N. Salivary cortisol levels as a biological marker of stress reaction. Med Arh. 2013;67:374–7.

1342. Elenkov IJ, Chrousos GP. Stress hormones, Th1/Th2 patterns, pro/anti-inflammatory cytokines and susceptibility to disease. Trends Endocrinol Metab. 1999;10:359–68.

1343. Moretti M, Colla A, de Oliveira BG, dos Santos DB, Budni J, de Freitas AE, Farina M, Severo Rodrigues AL. Ascorbic acid treatment, similarly to fluoxetine, reverses depressive-like behavior and brain oxidative damage induced by chronic unpredictable stress. J Psychiatr Res. 2012;46:331–40.

1344. Bertone-Johnson ER, Whitcomb BW, Missmer SA, Karlson EW, Rich-Edwards JW. Inflammation and early-life abuse in women. Am J Prev Med. 2012;43:611–20.

1345. Chavda N, Kantharia ND, Jaykaran. Effects of fluoxetine and escitalopram on C-reactive protein in patients of depression. J Pharmacol Pharmacother. 2011;2:11–6.

1346. Antoni MH, Lutgendorf SK, Blomberg B, Carver CS, Lechner S, Diaz A, Stagl J, Arevalo JM, Cole SW. Cognitive-behavioral stress management reverses anxiety-related leukocyte transcriptional dynamics. Biol Psychiatry. 2012;71:366–72.

1347. Lu XT, Zhao YX, Zhang Y, Jiang F. Psychological stress, vascular inflammation, and atherogenesis: potential roles of circulating cytokines. J Cardiovasc Pharmacol. 2013;62:6–12.

1348. Skurk T, van Harmelen V, Hauner H. Angiotensin II stimulates the release of interleukin-6 and interleukin-8 from cultured human adipocytes by activation of NF-kappaB. Arterioscler Thromb Vasc Biol. 2004;24:1199–203.

1349. Tsuchiya K, Yoshimoto T, Hirono Y, Tateno T, Sugiyama T, Hirata Y. Angiotensin II induces monocyte chemoattractant protein-1 expression via a nuclear factor kappaB- dependent pathway in rat preadipocytes. Am J Physiol Endocrinol Metab. 2006;291:E771–8.

1350. Lu XT, Zhao YX, Zhang Y, Jiang F. Psychological stress, vascular inflammation, and atherogenesis: potential roles of circulating cytokines. J Cardiovasc Pharmacol. 2013;62:6–12.

1351. Hapuarachchi JR, Chalmers AH, Winefield AH, Blake-Mortimer JS. Changes in clinically relevant metabolites with psychological stress parameters. Behav Med. 2003;29:52–9.

1352. Tyagi N, Sedoris KC, Steed M, Ovechkin AV, Moshal KS, Tyagi SC. Mechanisms of homocysteine-induced oxidative stress. Am J Physiol Heart Circ Physiol. 2005;289:H2649–56.

1353. Hiroki J, Shimokawa H, Higashi M, Morikawa K, Kandabashi T, Kawamura N, Kubota T, Ichiki T, Amano M, Kaibuchi K, Takeshita A. Inflammatory stimuli upregulate Rho-kinase in human coronary vascular smooth muscle cells. J Mol Cell Cardiol. 2004;37:537–46.

1354. Bierhaus A, Wolf J, Andrassy M, Rohleder N, Humpert PM, Petrov D, Ferstl R, von Eynatten M, Wendt T, Rudofsky G, Joswig M, Morcos M, Schwaninger M, McEwen B, Kirschbaum C, Nawroth PP. A mechanism converting psychosocial stress into mononuclear cell activation. Proc Natl Acad Sci U S A. 2003;100:1920–5.

1355. Sivonová M, Zitnanová I, Hlincíková L, Skodácek I, Trebatická J, Duracková Z. Oxidative stress in university students during examinations. Stress. 2004;7:183–8.

1356. Mauck HP, Hockman CH. Central nervous system mechanisms mediating cardiac rate and rhythm. Am Heart J. 1967;74:106–9.

1357. Engel GL. Sudden and rapid death during psychological stress. Ann Intern Med. 1971;74:771–82.

1358. Trichopoulos D, Katsoutanni K, Zavitsanos X, Tronou A, Dalla-Vorgia P. Psychological stress and fatal heart attack: the Athens earthquake natural experiment. Lancet. 1983;1:441–3.

1359. Meisel SR, Kutz I, Dayan KI, Pauzner H, Chetbourg I, Arbel Y, David D. Effect of Iraqi missile war on incidence of acute myocardial infarction and sudden death in Israeli civilians. Lancet. 1991;338:660–1.

1360. Leor J, Poole WK, Kloner RA. Sudden cardiac death triggered by an earthquake. N Engl J Med. 1996;334:413–9.

1361. Steinberg JS, Arshad A, Kowalski M, Kukar A, Suma V, Vloka M, Eklert F, Herweg B, Donelly J, Phillip J, Reed G, Rozanski A. Increased incidence of life threatening arrhythmias in implantable defibrillator patients after the World Trade Centre attack. J Am Coll Cardiol. 2004;44:1261–4.

1362. Lampert R, Jain D, Burg MM, Batsford WP, McPherson CA. Destabilising effects of mental stress on ventricular arrhythmias in patients with implantable cardio-verter defibrillators. Circulation. 2000;101:158–64.

1363. Toivonen L, Helenius K, Vitasalo M. Electrocardiographic repolarization during stress from awakening on alarm call. J Am Coll Cardiol. 1997;30:774–7.

1364. James PR, Taggart P, McNally ST, Newman SP, Sporton SC, Hardman SMC. Acute psychological stress and the propensity to ventricular arrhythmias. Eur Heart J. 2000;21:1023–8.
1365. Kop WJ, Krantz DS, Nearing BD, Gottdiener JS, Quigley JF, O'Callahan M, DelNegro AA, Friehling TD, Karasik P, Suchday S, Levine J, Verrier RL. Effects of acute mental stress and exercise on T-wave alternans in patients with implantable cardioverter defibrillators and controls. Circulation. 2004;109:1864–9.
1366. Taggart P, Sutton P, Redfern C, Batchvarov VN, Hnatkova K, Malik M, James U, Joseph A. The effect of mental stress on the non-dipolar components of the T wave: modulation by hypnosis. Psychosom Med. 2005;67:376–83.
1367. Lampert R, Shusterman V, Burg M, McPherson C, Batsford W, Goldberg A, Soufer R. Anger induced T wave alternans predicts future ventricular arrhythmias in patients with implantable cardioverter defibrillators. J Am Coll Cardiol. 2009;53:774–8.
1368. Zipes DP, Rubart M. Neural modulation of cardiac arrhythmias and sudden cardiac death. Heart Rhythm. 2006;3:108–13.
1369. Coote JH. Landmarks in understanding the central nervous control of the cardiovascular system. Exp Physiol. 2007;92:3–18.
1370. Schwartz PJ. The rationale and the role of left stellectomy for the prevention of malignant arrhythmias. Ann N Y Acad Sci. 1984;427:199–221.
1371. Schwartz PJ, Zipes DP. Autonomic modulation of cardiac arrhythmias. In: Zipes DP, Jalife J, editors. Cardiac electrophysiology. From cell to bedside. 4th ed. Philadelphia: W. B. Saunders; 2004. p. 300–14.
1372. Umetani K, Singer DH, McCraty R, Atkinson M. Twenty-four hour time domain heart rate variability and heart rate: relations to age and gender over nine decades. J Am Coll Cardiol. 1998;31(3):593–601.
1373. Leenen FHH. Brain mechanisms contributing to sympathetic hyperactivity & heart failure. Circ Res. 2007;101:221–3.
1374. Ajijola OA, Lux RL, Khahera A, Kwon O, Aliotta E, Ennis DB, Fishbein MC, Ardell JL, Shivkumar K. Sympathetic modulation of electrical activation in normal and infarcted myocardium: implications for arrhythmogenesis. Am J Physiol Heart Circ Physiol. 2017;312(3):H608–21. https://doi.org/10.1152/ajpheart.00575.2016. Epub 2017 Jan 13
1375. La Rovere MT, Bigger JT, Marcus FI, Mortara A, Schwartz PJ. Baroreflex sensitivity and heart rate variability in prediction of total cardiac mortality after myocardial infarction. Lancet. 1998;351:478–84.
1376. Gottlieb SS, McCarter RJ, Vogel RA. Effect of beta blockade on mortality among high-risk and low risk patients after myocardial infarction. N Engl J Med. 1998;339:489–97.
1377. Schwartz PJ, De Ferrari GM. Sympathetic-parasympathetic interaction in health and disease:abnormalities and relevance in heart failure. Heart Fail Rev. 2011;16:101–7.
1378. Koizumi K, Kollai M. Control of reciprocal and non reciprocal action of vagal and sympathetic efferents: study of centrally induced reactions. J Auton Nerv Syst. 1981;3:483–501.
1379. Zipes DP, Miyazaki T. The autonomic nervous system and the heart: basis for understanding interactions and effects on arrhythmia development. In: Zipes DP, Jalife J, editors. Cardiac electrophysiology: from cell to bedside. Philadelphia: W. B. Saunders; 1990. p. 312–30.
1380. Paton JFR, Boscan P, Pickering AE, Nalivaiko E. The yin and yang of cardiac autonomic control: vago-sympathetic interactions revisited. Brain Res Rev. 2005;49:555–65.
1381. Lane RD, Jennings JR. Hemispheric asymmetry, autonomic asymmetry and the problem of sudden death. In: Davidson RJ, Hugdahl K, editors. Brain asymmetry. Cambridge, MA: The MIT Press; 1995. p. 271–304.
1382. Porges SW. The polyvagal theory: neurophysiological foundations of emotions, attachment, communication, and self-regulation. New York: WW Norton & Co., Inc; 2011.
1383. Randall WC, Szentivanyi M, Pace JB, Wechsler JS, Kaye MP. Patterns of sympathetic nerve projections onto the canine heart. Circ Res. 1968;22(3):315–23.
1384. Katritsis DG, Pokushalov E, Romanov A, et al. Autonomic denervation added to pulmonary vein isolation for paroxysmal atrial fibrillation: a randomized clinical trial. J Am Coll Cardiol. 2013;62:2318–25.
1385. Wu J, Wu J, Zipes DP. Mechanisms of initiation of ventricular tachyarrhythmias. In: Zipes DP, Jalife J, editors. Cardiac electrophysiology; from cell to bedside. 4th ed. Philadelphia: Saunders; 2004. p. 380–9.
1386. Levy MN, Ng ML, Zieske H. Functional distribution of the peripheral sympathetic pathways. Circ Res. 1966;14:650–61.
1387. Yanowitz F, Preston JB, Abildskov JA. Functional distribution of right and left stellate innervation to the ventricles: production of neurogenic electrocardiographic changes by unilateral alteration of sympathetic tone. Circ Res. 1966;28:416–28.
1388. Randall WC, Ardell JL. Nervous control of the heart: anatomy and pathophysiology. In: Zipes DP, Jalife J, editors. Cardiac electrophysiology: from cell to bedside. Philadelphia: W. B. Saunders; 1990. p. 291–9.
1389. Kralios FA, Martin L, Burgess MJ, Millar K. Local ventricular repolarization changes due to sympathetic nerve-branch stimulation. Am J Phys. 1975;228:1621–6.
1390. Chen PS, Chen LS, Cao JM, Sharifi B, Karagueuzian HS, Fishbein MS. Sympathetic nerve sprouting, electrical remodeling and the mechanisms of sudden death. Cardiovasc Res. 2001;50:409–16.
1391. Chen LS, Chen PS. Nerve sprouting and cardiac arrhythmias. In: Zipes DP, Jalife J, editors.

Cardiac electrophysiology: from cell to bedside. Philadelphia: W. B. Saunders; 2004. p. 299–305.
1392. Schwartz PJ. The rationale and the role of left stellectomy for the prevention of malignant arrhythmias. Ann N Y Acad Sci. 1984;427:199–221.
1393. McNeill EM, Roos KP, Moechars D, Clagett-Dame M. Nav2 is necessary for cranial nerve development and blood pressure regulation. Neural Dev. 2010;5:6. https://doi.org/10.1186/1749-8104-5-6.
1394. Malpas SC. The rhythmicity of sympathetic nerve activity. Prog Neurobiol. 1998;56:65–96.
1395. Hainsworth R. Reflexes from the heart. Am J Physiol. 1991;71:617–58.
1396. Longhurst JC, Tjen-A-Looi S, Fu L-W. Cardiac sympathetic afferent activation provoked by myocardial ischemia and reperfusion: mechanisms and reflexes. Ann N Y Acad Sci. 2001;940:74–95.
1397. Critchley HD. Psychophysiology of neural, cognitive and affective integration: fMRI and autonomic indicants Int. J Psychophysiol. 2009;73:88–94.
1398. Patterson E, Po SS, Scherlag BJ, Lazzara R. Triggered firing in pulmonary veins initiated by in vitro autonomic nerve stimulation. Heart Rhythm. 2005;2:624–31.
1399. Pope ML, Smith TW. Cortisol excretion in high and low cynically hostile men. Psychosom Med. 1991;53:386–92.
1400. Suarez EC, Shiller AD, Kuhn CM, Schanberg SM, Williams RB Jr, Zimmerman EA. The relationship between hostility and beta adrenergic receptor physiology in healthy males. Psychosom Med. 1997;59:481–7.
1401. Mattioli AV, Bonatti S, Zennaro M, Melotti R, Mattioli G. Effect of coffee consumption, lifestyle and acute life stress in the development of acute lone atrial fibrillation. J Cardiovasc Med. (Hagerstown). 2008;9:794–8.
1402. James W. What is an emotion? Mind. 1884;9:188–205.
1403. Cannon WB. The James-Lange theory of emotions: a critical examination and an alternative theory. Am J Psychol. 1927;39:106–24.
1404. Lampert R, Joska T, Burg MM, Batsford WP, McPherson CA, Jain D. Emotional and physical precipitants of ventricular arrhythmias. Circulation. 2002;106:1800–5.
1405. Narayan SM. T-wave alternans and the susceptibility to ventricular arrhythmias. J Am Coll Cardiol. 2006;47(2):269–81. Epub 2006 Jan 4. Review.
1406. Ekman P, Levenson RW, Friesen WV. Autonomic nervous system activity distinguishes among emotions. Science. 1983;221:1208–10.
1407. Levenson RW, Ekman P, Friesen WV. Voluntary facial action generates emotion-specific autonomic nervous system activity. Psychophysiology. 1990;27:363–84.
1408. Christie IC, Friedman BH. Autonomic specificity of discrete emotion and dimensions of affective space: a multivariate approach. Int J Psychophysiol. 2004;51:143–53.
1409. Rainville P, Bechara A, Naqvi N, Damasio AR. Basic emotions are associated with distinct patterns of cardiorespiratory activity. Int J Psychophysiol. 2006;61:5–18.
1410. McCraty R, Atkinson M, Tiller WA, Rein G, Watkins AD. The effects of emotions on short-term power spectrum analysis of heart rate variability. Am J Cardiol. 1995;76:1089–93.
1411. Lampert R, Shusterman V, Burg MM, Jee FA, Earley C, Goldberg A, McPherson CA, Batsford WP, Soufer R. Effects of psychological stress on repolarization and relationship to autonomic and haemodynamic factors. J Cardiovasc Electrophysiol. 2005;16:372–7.
1412. Bernardi L, Wdowczyk-Szulc J, Valenti C, Castoldi S, Passino C, Spadacine G, Sleight P. Effects of controlled breathing, mental activity, and mental stress with or without verbalisation on heart rate variability. J Am Coll Cardiol. 2000;35:1462–9.
1413. Stopper M, Joska T, Burg MM, Batsford WP, McPherson CA, Jain D, Lampert R. Electrophysiologic characteristics of anger–triggered arrhythmias. Heart Rhythm. 2007;4:268–73.
1414. Friedman BH, Thayer JF. Autonomic balance revisited: panic anxiety and heart rate variability. J Psychosom Res. 1998;44:133–51.
1415. Taggart P, Carruthers M, Somerville W. Some effects of emotion on the normal and abnormal heart. Curr Probl Cardiol. 1983;12:1–29.
1416. Golbidi S, Frisbee JC, Laher I. Chronic stress impacts the cardiovascular system: animal models and clinical outcomes. Am J Physiol Heart Circ Physiol. 2015;308:H1476–98.
1417. Thayera JF, Sternberg EM. Neural aspects of immunomodulation: focus on the vagus nerve. Brain Behav Immun. 2010;24(8):1223–8.
1418. Huston M, Tracey KJ. The pulse of inflammation: heart rate variability, the cholinergic anti-inflammatory pathway and implications for therapy. J Intern Med. 2011;269(1):45–53.
1419. Cohen S, Janicki-Deverts D, Doyle WJ, Miller GE, Frank E, Rabin BS, Turner RB. Chronic stress, glucocorticoid receptor resistance, inflammation, and disease risk. Proc Natl Acad Sci U S A. 2012;109(16):5995–9. https://doi.org/10.1073/pnas.1118355109. Epub 2012 Apr 2.
1420. Critchley HD, Corfield DR, Chandler MP. Cerebral correlates of autonomic cardiovascular arousal: a functional neuroimaging investigation. J Physiol (Lond). 2000;523:259–70.
1421. Napadow V, Dhond R, Conti G, Makris N, Brown EN, Barberi R. Brain correlates of autonomic modulation: combining heart rate variability with fmri. NeuroImage. 2008;42:169–77.
1422. Xavier CH, Nalivaiko E, Beig MI, Menezes GB, Cara DC, Campagnole-Santos MJ, Fontes MAP. Functional asymmetry in the descending cardiovascular pathways from dorsomedial hypothalamic nucleus. Neuroscience. 2009;164:1360–8.

1423. Mujica-Parodi LR, Korgaonkar M, Ravindranath B, Greenberg T, Tomasi D, Wagshul M, Ardekani B, Guilfoyle D, Khan S, Zhong Y, Chon K, Malaspina D. Limbic dysregulation is associated with lowered heart rate variability and increased trait anxiety in healthy adults. Hum Brain Mapp. 2009;30:47–58.
1424. Oppenheimer SM, Gelb AW, Girvin JP, Hachinski VC. Cardiovascular effects of human insular cortex stimulation. Neurology. 1992;42:1727–32.
1425. Wittling W. Brain asymmetry in the control of autonomic-physiologic activity. In: Davidson RJ, Hugdahl KJ, editors. Brain asymmetry. Cambridge, MA: The MIT Press; 1995. p. 305–57.
1426. Rozanski A, Bairey CN, Krantz DS, Friedman J, Ressler KJ, Morell M, Hilton-Chalfen S, Hestrin L, Bietendorf J, Berman DS. Mental stress and the induction of silent myocardial ischemia in patients with coronary artery disease. N Engl J Med. 1988;318:1005–12.
1427. Burg MM, Soufer JD, Kerns RD, Zaret BL. Role of behavioural and psychological factors in mental stress induced silent left ventricular dysfunction in coronary artery disease. J Am Coll Cardiol. 1993;22:440–8.
1428. Gottdiener JS, Krantz DS, Howell RH, Hecht GM, Klein J, Falconer JJ, Rozanski A. Induction of silent myocardial ischemia with mental stress testing: relation to the triggers of ischemia during daily life activities and to ischemia functional severity. J Am Coll Cardiol. 1994;24:1645–51.
1429. Goldberg AD, Becker LC, Bonsall R, Cohen JD, Ketterer MW, Kaufman PG, Krantz DS, Light KC, McMahon RP, Noreuil T, Pepine CJ, Raczynski J, Stone PH, Strother D, Taylor H, Sheps DS. Ischemic, haemodynamic and neurohumoral responses to mental and exercise stress. Circulation. 1996;94:2402–9.
1430. Raadsheer FC, Hoogendijk WJ, Stam FC, Tilders FJ, Swaab DF. Increased numbers of corticotropin-releasing hormone expressing neurons in the hypothalamic paraventricular nucleus of depressed patients. Neuroendocrinology. 1994;6:436–44.
1431. Purba JS, Raadsheer FC, Hofman MA, Ravid R, Polman CH, Kamphorst W, Swaab DF. Increased number of corticotropin-releasing hormone expressing neurons in the hypothalamic paraventricular nucleus of patients with multiple sclerosis. Neuroendocrinology. 1995;62:62–70.
1432. Frasure-Smith N, Lespérance F, Gravel G, Masson A, Juneau M, Talajic M, Bourassa MG. Depression and health-care costs during the first year following myocardial infarction. J Psychosom Res. 2000;48(4–5):471–8.
1433. Sternberg EM. Neural regulation of innate immunity: a coordinated nonspecific host response to pathogens. Nat Rev Immunol. 2006;6(4):318–28. Review.
1434. Hintsa T, Puttonen S, Toivonen L, Kontula K, Swan H, Keltikangas-Jarvinen L. A history of stressful life events, prolonged mental stress and arrhythmic events in inherited long QT syndrome. Heart. 2010;96:1281–6.
1435. Dyson KS, Shoemaker JK, Hughson RL. Effect of acute sympathetic nervous system activation on flow-mediated dilation of brachial artery. Am J Physiol Heart Circ Physiol. 2006;290:H1446–53.
1436. Poitras VJ, Pyke KE. The impact of acute mental stress on vascular endothelial function: evidence, mechanisms and importance. Int J Psychophysiol. 2013;88:124–35.
1437. Hijmering ML, Stroes ES, Olijhoek J, Hutten BA, Blankestijn PJ, Rabelink TJ. Sympathetic activation markedly reduces endothelium-dependent, flow-mediated vasodilation. J Am Coll Cardiol. 2002;39:683–8.
1438. Eriksson M, Johansson K, Sarabi M, Lind L. Mental stress impairs endothelial vasodilatory function by a beta-adrenergic mechanism. Endothelium. 2007;14:151–6.
1439. Black PH, Garbutt LD. Stress, inflammation and cardiovascular disease. J Psychosom Res. 2002;52:1–23.
1440. Kaplan JR, Manuck SB, Clarkson TB, Lusso FM, Taub DM. Social stress and atherosclerosis in normocholesterolemic monkeys. Science. 1983;220:733–5.
1441. Manuck SB, Adams MR, McCaffery JM, Kaplan JR. Behaviorally elicited heart rate reactivity and atherosclerosis in ovariectomized cynomolgus monkeys (Macaca fascicularis). Arterioscler Thromb Vasc Biol. 2000;17:1774–9.
1442. Groeschel M, Braam B. Connecting chronic and recurrent stress to vascular dysfunction: no relaxed role for the renin-angiotensin system. Am J Physiol Renal Physiol. 2011;300:F1–F10.
1443. Spieker LE, Hürlimann D, Ruschitzka F, Corti R, Enseleit F, Shaw S, Hayoz D, Deanfield JE, Lüscher TF, Noll G. Mental stress induces prolonged endothelial dysfunction via endothelin-A receptors. Circulation. 2002;105:2817–20.
1444. Seya Y, Fukuda T, Isobe K, Kawakami Y, Takekoshi K. Effect of norepinephrine on RhoA, MAP kinase, proliferation and VEGF expression in human umbilical vein endothelial cells. Eur J Pharmacol. 2006;553:54–60.
1445. Ghiadoni L, Donald AE, Cropley M, Mullen MJ, Oakley G, Taylor M, O'Connor G, Betteridge J, Klein N, Steptoe A, Deanfield JE. Mental stress induces transient endothelial dysfunction in humans. Circulation. 2000;102:2473–8.
1446. Uji M, Yoshida K, Shitani-Ishida K, Morimoto K. Sex difference in norepinephrine surge in response to psychological stress through nitric oxide in rats. Life Sci. 2007;80:860–6.
1447. Toda N, Nakanishi-Toda M. How mental stress affects endothelial function. Pflügers Arch. 2011;462:779–94.
1448. Aberg G, Ferrer P. Effects of captopril on atherosclerosis in cynomolgus monkeys. J Cardiovasc Pharmacol. 1990;15:s65–72.

1449. Keidar S, Kaplan M, Hoffman A, Aviram M. Angiotensin II stimulates macrophage-mediated oxidation of low density lipoproteins. Atherosclerosis. 1995;115:201–15.
1450. Kaplan M, Aviram M, Knopf C, Keidar S. Angiotensin II reduces macrophage cholesterol efflux: a role for the AT-1 receptor but not for the ABC1 transporter. Biochem Biophys Res Commun. 2002;290:1529–34.
1451. Keidar S, Heinrich R, Kaplan M, Hayek T, Aviram M. Angiotensin II administration to atherosclerotic mice increases macrophage uptake of oxidized LDL: a possible role for interleukin-6. Arterioscler Thromb Vasc Biol. 2001;21:1464–9.
1452. Mateo T, Abu Nabah YN, Abu Taha M, Mata M, Cerda-Nicolas M, Proudfoot AE, Stahl RA, Issekutz AC, Cortijo J, Morcillo EJ, Jose PJ, Sanz MJ. Angiotensin II-induced mononuclear leukocyte interactions with arteriolar and venular endothelium are mediated by the release of different CC chemokines. J Immunol. 2006;176:5577–86.
1453. Mateo T, Naim Abu Nabah Y, Losada M, Estelles R, Company C, Bedrina B, Cerda-Nicolas JM, Poole S, Jose PJ, Cortijo J, Morcillo EJ, Sanz MJ. A critical role for TNFalpha in the selective attachment of mononuclear leukocytes to angiotensin-II-stimulated arterioles. Blood. 2007;110:1895–902.
1454. Piqueras L, Kubes P, Alvarez A, O'Connor E, Issekutz AC, Esplugues JV, Sanz MJ. Angiotensin II induces leukocyte-endothelial cell interactions in vivo via AT1 and AT2 receptor-mediated P-selectin upregulation. Circulation. 2000;102:2118–23.
1455. Zhao Q, Ishibashi M, Hiasa K, Tan C, Takeshita A, Egashira K. Essential role of vascular endothelial growth factor in angiotensin II induced vascular inflammation and remodeling. Hypertension. 2004;44:264–470.
1456. Chan YC, Leung PS. Angiotensin II type 1 receptor-dependent nuclear factor-kappaB activation-mediated proinflammatory actions in a rat model of obstructive acute pancreatitis. J Pharmacol Exp Ther. 2007;323:10–8.
1457. Hsu YH, Chen JJ, Chang NC, Chen CH, Liu JC, Chen TH, Jeng CJ, Chao HH, Cheng TH. Role of reactive oxygen species-sensitive extracellular signal-regulated kinase pathway in angiotensin II-induced endothelin-1 gene expression in vascular endothelial cells. J Vasc Res. 2004;41:64–74.
1458. Liu HQ, Wei XB, Sun R, Cai YW, Lou HY, Wang JW, Chen AF, Zhang XM. Angiotensin II stimulates intercellular adhesion molecule-1 via an AT1 receptor/nuclear factor-kappaB pathway in brain microvascular endothelial cells. Life Sci. 2006;78:1293–8.
1459. Pueyo ME, Gonzalez W, Nicoletti A, Savoie F, Arnal JF, Michel JB. Angiotensin II stimulates endothelial vascular cell adhesion molecule-1 via nuclear factor-kappaB activation induced by intracellular oxidative stress. Arterioscler Thromb Vasc Biol. 2000;20:645–51.
1460. Ruiz-Ortega M, Lorenzo O, Ruperez M, Suzuki Y, Egido J. Angiotensin II activates nuclear transcription factor-kappaB in aorta of normal rats and in vascular smooth muscle cells of AT1 knockout mice. Nephrol Dial Transplant. 2001;16:S27–33.
1461. Suzuki Y, Ruiz-Ortega M, Lorenzo O, Ruperez M, Esteban V, Egido J. Inflammation and angiotensin II. Int J Biochem Cell Biol. 2003;35:881–900.
1462. Kaplan JR, Adams MR, Clarkson TB, Manuck SB, Shively CA, Williams JK. Psychosocial factors, sex differences, and atherosclerosis: lessons from animal models. Psychosom Med. 1996;58:598–611.
1463. Wassmann S, Czech T, van Eickels M, Fleming I, Bohm M, Nickenig G. Inhibition of diet-induced atherosclerosis and endothelial dysfunction in apolipoprotein E/angiotensin II type 1A receptor double-knockout mice. Circulation. 2004;110:3062–7.
1464. Fukuda D, Sata M, Ishizaka N, Nagai R. Critical role of bone marrow angiotensin II type 1 receptor in the pathogenesis of atherosclerosis in apolipoprotein E deficient mice. Arterioscler Thromb Vasc Biol. 2008;28:90–6.
1465. Pavel J, Benicky J, Murakami Y, Sanchez-Lemus E, Saavedra JM. Peripherally administered angiotensin II AT1 receptor antagonists are anti-stress compounds in vivo. Ann N Y Acad Sci. 2008;1148:360–6.
1466. Schiavone MT, Santos RA, Brosnihan KB, Khosla MC, Ferrario CM. Release of vasopressin from the rat hypothalamo-neurohypophysial system by angiotensin (1–7) heptapeptide. Proc Natl Acad Sci U S A. 1988;85:4095–8.
1467. Benter IF, Yousif MH, Anim JT, Cojocel C, Diz DI. Angiotensin-(1–7) prevents development of severe hypertension and end-organ damage in spontaneously hypertensive rats treated with l-NAME. Am J Physiol Heart Circ Physiol. 2006;290:H684–91.
1468. Grobe JL, Mecca AP, Lingis M, Shenoy V, Bolton TA, Machado JM, Speth RC, Raizada MK, Katovich MJ. Prevention of angiotensin II-induced cardiac remodeling by angiotensin-(1–7). Am J Physiol Heart Circ Physiol. 2007;292:H736–42.
1469. Gilsanz P, Mayeda ER, Glymour MM, Quesenberry CP, Mungas DM, DeCarli C, Dean A, Whitmer RA. Female sex, early-onset hypertension, and risk of dementia. Neurology. 2017;89(18):1886–93.
1470. Otite FO, Liaw N, Khandelwal P, Malik AM, Romano JG, Rundek T, Sacco RL, Chaturvedi S. Increasing prevalence of vascular risk factors in patients with stroke: a call to action. Neurology. 2017;89(19):1985–94.
1471. Otite FO, Liaw N, Khandelwal P, Malik AM, Romano JG, Rundek T, Sacco RL, Chaturvedi S. Increasing prevalence of vascular risk factors in patients with stroke: a call to action. Neurology. 2017;89(19):1985–94.

1472. Clancy JA, Mary DA, Witte KK, Greenwood JP, Deuchars SA, Deuchars J. Non-invasive vagus nerve stimulation in healthy humans reduces sympathetic nerve activity. Brain Stimul. 2014;7(6):871–7. https://doi.org/10.1016/j.brs.2014.07.031. Epub 2014 Jul 16.
1473. Andersson U, Tracey KJ. Neural reflexes in inflammation and immunity. J Exp Med. 2012;209(6):1057–68. https://doi.org/10.1084/jem.20120571.
1474. Pavlov VA, Tracey KJ. The vagus nerve and the inflammatory reflex – linking immunity and metabolism. Nat Rev Endocrinol. 2012;8(12):743–54. https://doi.org/10.1038/nrendo.2012.189.
1475. Borovikova LV, et al. Vagus nerve stimulation attenuates the systemic inflammatory response to endotoxin. Nature. 2000;405:458. https://doi.org/10.1038/35013070.
1476. Gold MR, Van Veldhuisen DJ, Hauptman PJ, Borggrefe M, Kubo SH, Lieberman RA, Milasinovic G, Berman BJ, Djordjevic S, Neelagaru S, Schwartz PJ, Starling RC, Mann DL. Vagus nerve stimulation for the treatment of heart failure: the INOVATE-HF trial. J Am Coll Cardiol. 2016;68(2):149–58. https://doi.org/10.1016/j.jacc.2016.03.525. Epub 2016 Apr 4.
1477. Hauptman PJ, Schwartz PJ, Gold MR, Borggrefe M, Van Veldhuisen DJ, Starling RC, Mann DL. Rationale and study design of the increase of vagal tone in heart failure study: INOVATE-HF. Am Heart J. 2012;163(6):954–962.e1. https://doi.org/10.1016/j.ahj.2012.03.021.
1478. Van Wagoner DR. Chronic vagal nerve stimulation for the treatment of human heart failure: progress in translating a vision into reality. Eur Heart J. 2011;32(7):788–90. https://doi.org/10.1093/eurheartj/ehq424. Epub 2010 Nov 18.
1479. De Ferrari GM, Crijns HJ, Borggrefe M, Milasinovic G, Smid J, Zabel M, Gavazzi A, Sanzo A, Dennert R, Kuschyk J, Raspopovic S, Klein H, Swedberg K, Schwartz PJ, CardioFit Multicenter Trial Investigators. Chronic vagus nerve stimulation: a new and promising therapeutic approach for chronic heart failure. Eur Heart J. 2011;32(7):847–55. https://doi.org/10.1093/eurheartj/ehq391. Epub 2010 Oct 28.
1480. Premchand RK, Sharma K, Mittal S, Monteiro R, Dixit S, Libbus I, DiCarlo LA, Ardell JL, Rector TS, Amurthur B, KenKnight BH, Anand IS. Autonomic regulation therapy via left or right cervical vagus nerve stimulation in patients with chronic heart failure: results of the ANTHEM-HF trial. J Card Fail. 2014;20(11):808–16. https://doi.org/10.1016/j.cardfail.2014.08.009. Epub 2014 Sept 1.
1481. Zannad F, De Ferrari GM, Tuinenburg AE, Wright D, Brugada J, Butter C, Klein H, Stolen C, Meyer S, Stein KM, Ramuzat A, Schubert B, Daum D, Neuzil P, Botman C, Castel MA, D'Onofrio A, Solomon SD, Wold N, Ruble SB. Chronic vagal stimulation for the treatment of low ejection fraction heart failure: results of the Neural Cardiac Therapy for Heart Failure (NECTAR-HF) randomized controlled trial. Eur Heart J. 2015;36(7):425–33. https://doi.org/10.1093/eurheartj/ehu345. Epub 2014 Aug 31.
1482. De Ferrari G, et al. Chronic vagus nerve stimulation: a new and promising therapeutic approach for chronic heart failure. Eur Heart J. 2011;32:847. https://doi.org/10.1093/eurheartj/ehq391.
1483. Yu L, et al. Low-level vagosympathetic nerve stimulation inhibits atrial fibrillation inducibility: direct evidence by neural recordings from intrinsic cardiac ganglia. J Cardiovasc Electrophysiol. 2011;22:455. https://doi.org/10.1111/j.1540-8167.2010.01908.x.
1484. Stavrakis S, et al. Low-level transcutaneous electrical vagus nerve stimulation suppresses atrial fibrillation. J Am Coll Cardiol. 2015;65:867. https://doi.org/10.1016/j/jack.2014.12.026.
1485. Galbarriatu L, et al. Vagus nerve stimulation therapy for treatment-resistant epilepsy: a 15-year experience at a single institution. Clin Neurol Neurosurg. 2015;137:89. https://doi.org/10.1016/j.clineuro.2015.06.023.
1486. Bonaz B, et al. Vagus nerve stimulation: from epilepsy to the cholinergic anti-inflammatory pathway. Neurogastroenterol Motil. 2013. https://doi.org/10.1111/nmo.12076.
1487. Grimonprez A, et al. The antidepressant-like effect of vagus nerve stimulation is mediated through the locus coeruleus. J Psychiatr Res. 2015;68:1. https://doi.org/10.1016/j.psychires.2015.05.002.
1488. Premchand R, et al. Autonomic regulation therapy via left or right cervical vagus nerve stimulation in patients with chronic heart failure: results of the ANTHEM-HF trial. J Card Fail. 2014;20:808. https://doi.org/10.1016/j.cardfail.2014.08.009.
1489. Jacobs H, et al. Transcutaneous vagus nerve stimulation boosts associative memory in older individuals. Neurobiol Aging. 2015;36:1860. https://doi.org/10.1016/j.neurobiolaging.2015.02.023.
1490. Gaul C, et al. Non-invasive vagus nerve stimulation for PREVention and Acute treatment of chronic cluster headache (PREVA): a randomised controlled study. Cephalalgia. Published online September 21, 2015. https://doi.org/10.1177/0333102415607070.
1491. Wang S, et al. Transcutaneous vagus nerve stimulation induces tidal melatonin secretion and has an antidiabetic effect in Zucker fatty rats. PLOS One. Published online April 16, 2015. https://doi.org/10.1371/journal.pone.0124195.
1492. Groves DA, Brown VJ. Vagal nerve stimulation: a review of its applications and potential mechanisms that mediate its clinical effects. Neurosci Biobehav Rev. 2005;29:493. https://doi.org/10.1016/j.neubiorev.2005.01.004.
1493. Jacobs HI, Riphagen JM, Razat CM, Wiese S, Sack AT. Transcutaneous vagus nerve stimulation boosts associative memory in older individuals. Neurobiol Aging. 2015;36(5):1860–7. https://doi.

org/10.1016/j.neurobiolaging.2015.02.023. Epub 2015 Feb 28.
1494. Yuan H, Silberstein SD. Vagus nerve and vagus nerve stimulation, a comprehensive review: part III. Headache. 2016;56(3):479–90. https://doi.org/10.1111/head.12649. Epub 2015 Sept 14. Review.
1495. Ben-Menachem E, Revesz D, Simon BJ, Silberstein S. Surgically implanted and non-invasive vagus nerve stimulation: a review of efficacy, safety and tolerability. Eur J Neurol. 2015;22(9):1260–8. https://doi.org/10.1111/ene.12629.
1496. Grazzi L, Egeo G, Liebler E, Padovan AM, Barbanti P. Non-invasive vagus nerve stimulation (nVNS) as symptomatic treatment of migraine in young patients: a preliminary safety study. Neurol Sci. 2017;38(Suppl 1):197–9. https://doi.org/10.1007/s10072-017-2942-5.
1497. Larkum ME, Launey T, Dityatev A, Lüscher H-R. Integration of excitatory postsynaptic potentials in dendrites of motoneurons of rat spinal cord slice cultures. J Neurophysiol. 1998;80(2):924–35.
1498. Myers B, Greenwood-Van MB. Role of anxiety in the pathophysiology of irritable bowel syndrome: importance of the amygdala. Front Neurosci. 2009;3:47. https://doi.org/10.3389/neuro.21.002.2009. eCollection 2009.
1499. Jezova D, Makatsori A, Smriga M, Morinaga Y, Duncko R. Subchronic treatment with amino acid mixture of L-lysine and L-arginine modifies neuroendocrine activation during psychosocial stress in subjects with high trait anxiety. Nutr Neurosci. 2005;8(3):155–60.
1500. Sherwood A, Hinderliter AL, Watkins LL, Waugh RA, Blumenthal JA. Impaired endothelial function in coronary heart disease patients with depressive symptomatology. J Am Coll Cardiol. 2005;46(4):656–9.
1501. Hatcher S, Arroll B. Newer antidepressants for the treatment of depression in adults. BMJ. 2012;344:d8300. https://doi.org/10.1136/bmj.d8300.
1502. Jolly K, Langman MJS. Psychotropic medication: curing illness or creating problems? Heart. 2009;95:1893–4. https://doi.org/10.1136/hrt.2009.179127.
1503. Olfson M, Marcus SC. National patterns in antidepressant medication treatment. Arch Gen Psychiatry. 2009;66:848–56. https://doi.org/10.1001/archgenpsychiatry.2009.81.
1504. Lockhart P, Guthrie B. Trends in primary care antidepressant prescribing 1995–2007: a longitudinal population database analysis. Br J Gen Pract. 2011;61:e565–72. https://doi.org/10.3399/bjgp11X593848.
1505. Stephenson CP, Karanges E, McGregor IS. Trends in the utilisation of psychotropic medications in Australia from 2000 to 2011. Aust N Z J Psychiatry. 2013;47:74–87. https://doi.org/10.1177/0004867412466595.
1506. Cohn JN, Tognoni G, for the Valsartan Heart Failure Trial Investigators. A randomized trial of the angiotensin-receptor blocker valsartan in chronic heart failure. N Engl J Med. 2001;345:1667–75.
1507. Lachmann J, Banerjee A, Davoudi M, Aragon D, Talerja A, Sonnenblick EH, Shirani J, LeJemtel TH. Withdrawal of angiotensin receptor blocker (ARB) from triple neurohormonal therapy partially restores sympathetic activity in patients with chronic congestive heart failure. Am Heart Assoc. Scientific Sessions. Circulation. 2001;104:e9051–e9052.
1508. US Food and Drug Administration. FDA Drug Safety Communication. FDA Drug Safety Communication: abnormal heart rhythms associated with high doses of Celexa (citalopram hydrobromide). 2011. www.fda.gov/Drugs/DrugSafety/ucm269086.htm
1509. Castro VM, Clements CC, Murphy SN, et al. QT interval and antidepressant use: a cross sectional study of electronic health records. BMJ. 2013;346:f288. https://doi.org/10.1136/bmj.f288.
1510. Girardin FR, Gex-Fabry M, Berney P, Shah D, Gaspoz JM, Dayer P. Drug-induced long QT in adult psychiatric inpatients: the 5-year cross-sectional ECG screening outcome in psychiatry study. Am J Psychiatry. 2013;170:1468–76. https://doi.org/10.1176/appi.ajp.2013.12060860.
1511. El-Sherif N, Turitto G. Torsade de pointes. Curr Opin Cardiol. 2003;18:6–13. https://doi.org/10.1097/00001573-200301000-00002.
1512. Coupland C, Hill T, Morriss R, Moore M, Arthur A, Hippisley-Cox J. Antidepressant use and risk of cardiovascular outcomes in people aged 20 to 64: cohort study using primary care database. BMJ. 2016;352:i1350. https://doi.org/10.1136/bmj.i1350.
1513. Cadegiani FA, Kater CE. Adrenal fatigue does not exist: a systematic review. BMC Endocr Disord. 2016;16(1):48. https://doi.org/10.1186/s12902-016-0128-4.
1514. Rosengren A, Hawken S, Ounpuu S, Sliwa K, Zubaid M, Almahmeed WA, Blackett KN, Sitthi-amorn C, Sato H, Yusuf S, INTERHEART investigators. Association of psychosocial risk factors with risk of acute myocardial infarction in 11119 cases and 13648 controls from 52 countries (the INTERHEART study): case-control study. Lancet. 2004;364(9438):953–62.
1515. Landsbergis PA, Schnall PL, Pickering TG, et al. Life-course exposure to job strain and ambulatory blood pressure in men. Am J Epidemiol. 2003;157:998–1006.
1516. Vrijkotte TG, van Doornen LJ, de Geus EJ. Effects of work stress on ambulatory blood pressure, heart rate, and heart rate variability. Hypertension. 2000;35:880–6.
1517. Herd JA. Cardiovascular response to stress. Physiol Rev. 1991;71:305–30.
1518. Malik M, The Task Force of the European Society of Cardiology and the North American Society

of Pacing and Electrophysiology. Heart rate variability, standards of measurement, physiological interpretation, and clinical use. Circulation. 1996;93:1043–65.
1519. Malik M, The Task Force of the European Society of Cardiology and the North American Society of Pacing and Electrophysiology. Heart rate variability, standards of measurement, physiological interpretation, and clinical use. Eur Heart J. 1996;17:354–81.
1520. Gawaz M, Langer H, May AE. Platelets in inflammation atherogenesis. J Clin Invest. 2005;115:3378–84.
1521. von Känel R, Mills PJ, Fainman C, Dimsdale JE. Effects of psychological stress and psychiatric disorders on blood coagulation and fibrinolysis: a biobehavioral pathway to coronary artery disease? Psychosom Med. 2001;63(4):531–44.
1522. Kessler R, et al. Posttraumatic stress disorders in a national comorbidity survey. Arch Gen Psychiatry. 1995;52:1048–60.
1523. Kubzanski LD, et al. Prospective study of the posttraumatic stress disorder symptom in coronary artery disease and normative aging study. Arch Gen Psychiatry. 2007;64:109–16.
1524. Mewisse ML, et al. Cortisol and posttraumatic stress disorder in adults: systemic review of meta-analysis. Br J Psychiatry. 2007;191:387–92.
1525. Sack M, et al. Low respiratory sinus arrhythmia and prolonged psychophysiological arousal in posttraumatic disorder: heart rate dynamics and individual differences in arousal regulation. Biol Psychiatry. 2004:55, 284–290.
1526. Tracy KD. Physiology and immunology of the cholinergic antiinflammatory pathway. J Clin Invest. 2007;117:289–96.
1527. Bhaskar L, Kharya C, Deepak KK, Kochupillai V. Assessment of cardiac autonomic tone following Long Sudarshan Kriya yoga in art of living practitioners. J Altern Complement Med. 2017;23(9):705–12. https://doi.org/10.1089/acm.2016.0391. Epub 2017 Jul 10.
1528. Gothe NP, Keswani RK, McAuley E. Yoga practice improves executive function by attenuating stress levels. Biol Psychol. 2016;121(Pt A):109–16. https://doi.org/10.1016/j.biopsycho.2016.10.010. Epub 2016 Oct 26.
1529. Jones SM, Guthrie KA, Reed SD, Landis CA, Sternfeld B, LaCroix AZ, Dunn A, Burr RL, Newton KM. A yoga & exercise randomized controlled trial for vasomotor symptoms: effects on heart rate variability. Complement Ther Med. 2016;26:66–71. https://doi.org/10.1016/j.ctim.2016.03.001. Epub 2016 Mar 4.
1530. Doufesh H, Ibrahim F, Ismail NA, Wan Ahmad WA. Effect of Muslim prayer (Salat) on α electroencephalography and its relationship with autonomic nervous system activity. J Altern Complement Med. 2014;20(7):558–62. https://doi.org/10.1089/acm.2013.0426. Epub 2014 May 14.
1531. Tyagi A, Cohen M. Yoga and hypertension: a systematic review. Altern Ther Health Med. 2014;20(2):32–59.
1532. Berntson GG, Norman GJ, Hawkley LC, Cacioppo JT. Spirituality and autonomic cardiac control. Ann Behav Med. 2008;35(2):198–208. https://doi.org/10.1007/s12160-008-9027-x. Epub 2008 Mar 21.
1533. Ajabshir S, Asif A, Nayer A. The effects of vitamin D on the renin-angiotensin system. J Nephropathol. 2014;3(2):41–3. https://doi.org/10.12860/jnp.2014.09.
1534. Pieczenik SR, Neustadt J. Mitochondrial dysfunction and molecular pathways of disease. Exp Mol Pathol. 2007;83(1):84–92. Epub 2007 Jan 18.
1535. Vanderplasschen W, et al. Poly substance use and mental health among individuals presenting for substance abuse treatment. Science and society series. Ghent: Academia Press; 2012.
1536. Yankey BA, Rothenberg R, Strasser S, Ramsey-White K, Okosun IS. Effect of marijuana use on cardiovascular and cerebrovascular mortality: a study using the National Health and Nutrition Examination Survey linked mortality file. Eur J Prev Cardiol. 2017;24(17):1833–40. https://doi.org/10.1177/2047487317723212. Epub 2017 Aug 8.
1537. Desbois AC, Cacoub P. Cannabis-associated arterial disease. Ann Vasc Surg. 2013;27(7):996–1005. https://doi.org/10.1016/j.avsg.2013.01.002. Epub 2013 Jul 10. Review.
1538. Thomas G, Kloner RA, Rezkalla S. Adverse cardiovascular, cerebrovascular, and peripheral vascular effects of marijuana inhalation: what cardiologists need to know. Am J Cardiol. 2014;113(1):187–90. https://doi.org/10.1016/j.amjcard.2013.09.042. Epub 2013 Oct 5. Review.
1539. Gorelick DA, Heishman SJ, Preston KL, Nelson RA, Moolchan ET, Huestis MA. The cannabinoid CB1 receptor antagonist rimonabant attenuates the hypotensive effect of smoked marijuana in male smokers. Am Heart J. 2006;151(3):754.e1–5.
1540. Mittleman MA, Lewis RA, Maclure M, Sherwood JB, Muller JE. Triggering myocardial infarction by marijuana. Circulation. 2001;103(23):2805–9.
1541. Mukamal KJ, Maclure M, Muller JE, Mittleman MA. An exploratory prospective study of marijuana use and mortality following acute myocardial infarction. Am Heart J. 2008;155(3):465–70. https://doi.org/10.1016/j.ahj.2007.10.049.
1542. Mehra R, Moore BA, Crothers K, Tetrault J, Fiellin DA. The association between marijuana smoking and lung cancer: a systematic review. Arch Intern Med. 2006;166(13):1359–67. Review.
1543. Korantzopoulos P, Liu T, Papaioannides D, Li G, Goudevenos JA. Atrial fibrillation and marijuana smoking. Int J Clin Pract. 2008;62(2):308–13. Epub 2007 Nov 21. Review.
1544. Korantzopoulos P. Marijuana smoking is associated with atrial fibrillation. Am J Cardiol.

2014;113(6):1085–6. https://doi.org/10.1016/j.amjcard.2014.01.001. Epub 2014 Jan 8.

1545. Hackam DG. Cannabis and stroke: systematic appraisal of case reports. Stroke. 2015;46(3):852–6. https://doi.org/10.1161/STROKEAHA.115.008680. Review.
1546. Desbois AC, Cacoub P. Cannabis-associated arterial disease. Ann Vasc Surg. 2013;27(7):996–1005. https://doi.org/10.1016/j.avsg.2013.01.002. Epub 2013 Jul 10. Review.
1547. Vander Heiden MG. Metabolism and congenital malformations – NAD's effects on development. N Engl J Med. 2017;377(6):509–11. https://doi.org/10.1056/NEJMp1707487.
1548. Sletten DM, Suarez GA, Low PA, Mandrekar J, Singer W. COMPASS 31: a refined and abbreviated composite autonomic symptom score. Mayo Clin Proc. 2012;87(12):1196–201. https://doi.org/10.1016/j.mayocp.2012.10.013.
1549. Sletten DM, Suarez GA, Low PA, Mandrekar J, Singer W. COMPASS 31: a refined and abbreviated composite autonomic symptom score. Mayo Clin Proc. 2012;87(12):1196–201. https://doi.org/10.1016/j.mayocp.2012.10.013.
1550. Treister R, O'Neil K, Downs HM, Oaklander AL. Validation of the composite autonomic symptom scale 31 (COMPASS-31) in patients with and without small fiber polyneuropathy. Eur J Neurol. 2015;22(7):1124–30. https://doi.org/10.1111/ene.12717. Epub 2015 Apr 23.
1551. Bowling A, Bond M, Jenkinson C, Lamping DL. Short Form 36 (SF-36) health survey questionnaire: which normative data should be used? Comparisons between the norms provided by the Omnibus Survey in Britain, the Health Survey for England and the Oxford Healthy Life Survey. J Public Health Med. 1999;21(3):255–70.
1552. Hunt SM, McKenna SP, McEwen J, Backett EM, Williams J, Papp E. A quantitative approach to perceived health status: a validation study. J Epidemiol Community Health. 1980;34(4):281–6.
1553. https://www.ehlers-danlos.com/assessing-joint-hypermobility/
1554. Naal FD, Hatzung G, Müller A, Impellizzeri F, Leunig M. Validation of a self-reported Beighton score to assess hypermobility in patients with femoroacetabular impingement. Int Orthop. 2014;38(11):2245–50. https://doi.org/10.1007/s00264-014-2424-9. Epub 2014 Jul 5.
1555. Smits-Engelsman B, Klerks M, Kirby A. Beighton score: a valid measure for generalized hypermobility in children. J Pediatr. 2011;158(1):119–23, 123.e1–4. https://doi.org/10.1016/j.jpeds.2010.07.021. Epub 2010 Sep 17.
1556. Low PA. Composite autonomic scoring scale for laboratory quantification of generalized autonomic failure. Mayo Clin Proc. 1993;68(8):748–52.
1557. Nabavi SM, Daglia M, Braidy N, Nabavi SF. Natural products, micronutrients, and nutraceuticals for the treatment of depression: a short review. Nutr Neurosci. 2017;20(3):180–94. https://doi.org/10.1080/1028415X.2015.1103461. Epub 2015 Nov 27.
1558. Deepmala, Slattery J, Kumar N, Delhey L, Berk M, Dean O, Spielholz C, Frye R. Clinical trials of N-acetylcysteine in psychiatry and neurology: a systematic review. Neurosci Biobehav Rev. 2015;55:294–321. https://doi.org/10.1016/j.neubiorev.2015.04.015. Epub 2015 May 6.
1559. Kumar A, Chanana P. Role of nitric oxide in stress-induced anxiety: from pathophysiology to therapeutic target. Vitam Horm. 2017;103:147–67. https://doi.org/10.1016/bs.vh.2016.09.004. Epub 2016 Dec 2.
1560. Müller CP, Reichel M, Mühle C, Rhein C, Gulbins E, Kornhuber J. Brain membrane lipids in major depression and anxiety disorders. Biochim Biophys Acta. 2015;1851(8):1052–65. https://doi.org/10.1016/j.bbalip.2014.12.014. Epub 2014 Dec 24.
1561. Hennebelle M, Champeil-Potokar G, Lavialle M, Vancassel S, Denis I. Omega-3 polyunsaturated fatty acids and chronic stress-induced modulations of glutamatergic neurotransmission in the hippocampus. Nutr Rev. 2014;72(2):99–112. https://doi.org/10.1111/nure.12088. Epub 2014 Jan 13.
1562. Appleton KM, Sallis HM, Perry R, Ness AR, Churchill R. ω-3 fatty acids for major depressive disorder in adults: an abridged Cochrane. BMJ Open. 2016;6(3):e010172. https://doi.org/10.1136/bmjopen-2015-010172.
1563. Vesco AT, Lehmann J, Gracious BL, Arnold LE, Young AS, Fristad MA. Omega-3 supplementation for psychotic mania and comorbid anxiety in children. J Child Adolesc Psychopharmacol. 2015;25(7):526–34. https://doi.org/10.1089/cap.2013.0141. Epub 2015 Aug 19.
1564. Ball J, Carrington MJ, McMurray JJ, Stewart S. Atrial fibrillation: profile and burden of an evolving epidemic in the 21st century. Int J Cardiol. 2013;167:1807–24.
1565. Lloyd-Jones DM, Wang TJ, Leip EP, et al. Lifetime risk for development of atrial fibrillation: the Framingham Heart Study. Circulation. 2004;110:1042–6.
1566. Fenger-Grøn M, Overvad K, Tjønneland A, Frost L. Lean body mass is the predominant anthropometric risk factor for atrial fibrillation. J Am Coll Cardiol. 2017;69(20):2488–97. https://doi.org/10.1016/j.jacc.2017.03.558.
1567. Schnabel RB, Yin X, Gona P, et al. 50 year trends in atrial fibrillation prevalence, incidence, risk factors, and mortality in the Framingham Heart Study: a cohort study. Lancet. 2015;386:154–62.
1568. Nattel S. Atrial fibrillation and body composition: is it fat or lean that ultimately determines the risk? J Am Coll Cardiol. 2017;69(20):2498–501. https://doi.org/10.1016/j.jacc.2017.03.566.

1569. Garrey WE. The nature of fibrillatory contraction of the heart: its relation to tissue mass and form. Am J Phys. 1914;33:397–414.
1570. Moore EN, Spear JF. Electrophysiological studies on atrial fibrillation. Heart Vessels Suppl. 1987;2:32–9.
1571. Zou R, Kneller J, Leon LJ, Nattel S. Substrate size as a determinant of fibrillatory activity maintenance in a mathematical model of canine atrium. Am J Physiol Heart Circ Physiol. 2005;289:H1002–12.
1572. Poirier P, Giles TD, Bray GA, et al. Obesity and cardiovascular disease: pathophysiology, evaluation, and effect of weight loss: an update of the 1997 American Heart Association Scientific Statement on Obesity and Heart Disease from the Obesity Committee of the Council on Nutrition, Physical Activity, and Metabolism. Circulation. 2006;113:898–918.
1573. https://www.psychiatry.org/psychiatrists/practice/dsm
1574. Rowney J, Hermida T, Malone D. Definition and etiology. 2010. http://www.clevelandclinicmeded.com/medicalpubs/diseasemanagement/psychiatry-psychology/anxiety-disorder/
1575. Weissman M, Wickramaratne P, Nomura Y, et al. Offspring of depressed parents: 20 years later. Am J Psychiatry. 2006;163:1001–8.
1576. Grases G, Colom MA, Fernandez RA, Costa-Bauzá A, Grases F. Evidence of higher oxidative status in depression and anxiety. Oxidative Med Cell Longev. 2014;2014:430216. https://doi.org/10.1155/2014/430216. Epub 2014 Apr 29.
1577. McIntyre RS, Soczynska JK, Lewis GF, MacQueen GM, Konarski JZ, Kennedy SH. Managing psychiatric disorders with antidiabetic agents: translational research and treatment opportunities. Expert Opin Pharmacother. 2006;7(10):1305–21.
1578. Kinrys G, Coleman E, Rothstein E. Natural remedies for anxiety disorders: potential use and clinical applications. Depress Anxiety. 2009;26(3):259–65. https://doi.org/10.1002/da.20460.
1579. Lakhan SE, Vieira KF. Nutritional and herbal supplements for anxiety and anxiety-related disorders: systematic review. Nutr J. 2010;9:42. https://doi.org/10.1186/1475-2891-9-42.
1580. Smaga I, Niedzielska E, Gawlik M, Moniczewski A, Krzek J, Przegaliński E, Pera J, Filip M. Oxidative stress as an etiological factor and a potential treatment target of psychiatric disorders. Part 2. Depression, anxiety, schizophrenia and autism. Pharmacol Rep. 2015;67(3):569–80. https://doi.org/10.1016/j.pharep.2014.12.015. Epub 2015 Jan 5.
1581. Gulati K, Rai N, Ray A. Nitric oxide and anxiety. Vitam Horm. 2017;103:169–92. https://doi.org/10.1016/bs.vh.2016.09.001. Epub 2016 Oct 31.
1582. Qato DM, Ozenberger K, Olfson M. Prevalence of prescription medications with depression as a potential adverse effect among adults in the United States. JAMA. 2018;319(22):2289. https://doi.org/10.1001/jama.2018.6741.
1583. Haas H, Panula P. The role of histamine and the tuberomammillary nucleus in the nervous system. Nat Rev Neurosci. 2003;4:121–30.
1584. Piña IL, Di Palo KE, Ventura HO. Psychopharmacology and cardiovascular disease. J Am Coll Cardiol. 2018;71(20):2346–59.
1585. American Heart Association Nutrition Committee, Lichtenstein AH, Appel LJ, Brands M, Carnethon M, Daniels S, Franch HA, Franklin B, Kris-Etherton P, Harris WS, Howard B, Karanja N, Lefevre M, Rudel L, Sacks F, Van Horn L, Winston M, Wylie-Rosett J. Diet and lifestyle recommendations revision 2006: a scientific statement from the American Heart Association Nutrition Committee. Circulation. 2006;114(1):82–96. Epub 2006 Jun 19. Erratum in: Circulation. 2006 Dec 5;114(23):e629. Circulation. 2006 Jul 4;114(1):e27.
1586. Nemeroff CB, Evans DL. Correlation between the dexamethasone suppression test in depressed patients and clinical response. Am J Psychiatry. 1984;141:247–9.
1587. Nemeroff CB, Widerlov E, Bissette G, et al. Elevated concentrations of CSF corticotropin releasing factor-like immunoreactivity in depressed patients. Science. 1984;226:1342–4.
1588. Musselman DL, Tomer A, Manatunga AK, et al. Exaggerated platelet reactivity in major depression. Am J Psychiatry. 1996;153:1313–7.
1589. Carney RM, Saunders RD, Freedland KE, Stein P, Rich MW, Jaffe AS. Association of depression with reduced heart rate variability in coronary artery disease. Am J Cardiol. 1995;76(8):562–4.
1590. Rozanski A, Blumenthal JA, Kaplan J. Impact of psychological factors on the pathogenesis of cardiovascular disease and implications for therapy. Circulation. 1999;99(16):2192–217.
1591. Khan SG, Melikian N, Shabeeh H, Cabaco AR, Martin K, Khan F, O'Gallagher K, Chowienczyk PJ, Shah AM. The human coronary vasodilatory response to acute mental stress is mediated by neuronal nitric oxide synthase. Am J Physiol Heart Circ Physiol. 2017;313(3):H578–83. https://doi.org/10.1152/ajpheart.00745.2016. Epub 2017 Jun 23.
1592. Preisig M, Waeber G, Mooser V, Vollenweider P. PsyCoLaus: mental disorders and cardiovascular diseases: spurious association? Rev Med Suisse. 2011;7:2127–9.
1593. Chaddha A, Robinson EA, Kline-Rogers E, Alexandris-Souphis T, Rubenfire M. Mental health and cardiovascular disease. Am J Med. 2016;129:1145–8.
1594. Rugulies R. Depression as a predictor for coronary heart disease: a review and meta-analysis1. Am J Prev Med. 2002;23:51–61.
1595. Denollet J, Maas K, Knottnerus A, Keyzer JJ, Pop VJ. Anxiety predicted premature all-cause and car-

diovascular death in a 10-year follow-up of middle-aged women. J Clin Epidemiol. 2009;62:452–6.
1596. Blumenthal JA, Babyak MA, O'Connor C, Keteyian S, Landzberg J, Howlett J, et al. Effects of exercise training on depressive symptoms inpatients with chronic heart failure: the HF-ACTION randomized trial. JAMA. 2012;308:465–74.
1597. Janszky I, Ahnve S, Lundberg I, Hemmingsson T. Early-onset depression, anxiety, and risk of subsequent coronary heart disease: 37- year follow-up of 49,321 young Swedish men. J Am Coll Cardiol. 2010;56:31–7.
1598. Roest AM, Martens EJ, de Jonge P, Denollet J. Anxiety and risk of incident coronary heart disease: a meta-analysis. J Am Coll Cardiol. 2010;56:38–46.
1599. Phillips AC, Batty GD, Gale CR, et al. Generalized anxiety disorder, major depressive disorder, and their comorbidity as predictors of all-cause and cardiovascular mortality: the Vietnam experience study. Psychosom Med. 2009;71:395–403.
1600. Rutledge T, Linke SE, Krantz DS, et al. Comorbid depression and anxiety symptoms as predictors of cardiovascular events: results from the NHLBI-sponsored Women's Ischemia Syndrome Evaluation (WISE) study. Psychosom Med. 2009;71:958–64.
1601. Chida Y, Steptoe A. The association of anger and hostility with future coronary heart disease: a meta-analytic review of prospective evidence. J Am Coll Cardiol. 2009;53:936–46.
1602. Lampert R, Joska T, Burg MM, Batsford WP, McPherson CA, Jain D. Emotional and physical precipitants of ventricular arrhythmia. Circulation. 2002;106:1800–5.
1603. Krantz DS, Kop WJ, Santiago HT, Gottdiener JS. Mental stress as a trigger of myocardial ischemia and infarction. Cardiol Clin. 1996;14(2):271–87.
1604. Krantz DS, McCeney MK. Effects of psychological and social factors on organic disease: a critical assessment of research on coronary heart disease. Annu Rev Psychol. 2002;53:341–69.
1605. Karasek R, Baker D, Marxer F, Ahlbom A, Theorell T. Job decision latitude, job demands, and cardiovascular disease: a prospective study of Swedish men. Am J Public Health. 1981;71:694–705.
1606. Greenlund KJ, Kiefe CI, Giles WH, Liu K. Associations of job strain and occupation with subclinical atherosclerosis: the CARDIA study. Ann Epidemiol. 2010;20:323–31.
1607. Eller NH, Netterstrøm B, Gyntelberg F, et al. Work-related psychosocial factors and the development of ischemic heart disease: a systematic review. Cardiol Rev. 2009;17:83–97.
1608. Leor J, Poole WK, Kloner RA. Sudden cardiac death triggered by an earthquake. N Engl J Med. 1996;334:413–9.
1609. Ader R, Felten DL, Cohen N, editors. Psychoneuroimmunology, vol. 2. Waltham Abbey: Academic Press; 2000. ISBN 978-0-12-0443147.
1610. Rosengren A, Hawken S, Ôunpuu S, et al. Association of psychosocial risk factors with risk of acute myocardial infarction in 11 119 cases and 13 648 controls from 52 countries (the INTERHEART study): case-control study. Lancet. 2004;364:953–62.
1611. Orth-Gomer K, Wamala SP, Horsten M, Schenck-Gustafsson K, Schneiderman N, Mittleman MA. Marital stress worsens prognosis in women with coronary heart disease: the Stockholm Female Coronary Risk Study. JAMA. 2000;284:3008–14.
1612. Gabbay FH, Krantz DS, Kop WJ, et al. Triggers of myocardial ischemia during daily life in patients with coronary artery disease: physical and mental activities, anger and smoking. J Am Coll Cardiol. 1996;27:585–92.
1613. Gullette EC, Blumenthal JA, Babyak M, et al. Effects of mental stress on myocardial ischemia during daily life. JAMA. 1997;277:1521–6.
1614. Jiang W, Babyak M, Krantz DS, et al. Mental stress–induced myocardial ischemia and cardiac events. JAMA. 1996;275:1651–6.
1615. Williams RB, Haney TL, Lee KL, Kong Y-H, Blumenthal JA, Whalen RE. Type A behavior, hostility, and coronary atherosclerosis. Psychosom Med. 1980;42:539–49.
1616. Tindle HA, Chang YF, Kuller LH, et al. Optimism, cynical hostility, and incident coronary heart disease and mortality in the Women's Health Initiative. Circulation. 2009;120:656–62.
1617. Mc Donnell CG, Shorten G, Van Pelt FN. Effect of atorvastatin and fluvastatin on the metabolism of midazolam by cytochrome P450 in vitro. Anaesthesia. 2005;60:747–53.
1618. Jiang W, O'Connor C, Silva SG, et al. Safety and efficacy of sertraline for depression in patients with CHF (SADHART-CHF): a randomized, double-blind, placebo-controlled trial of sertraline for major depression with congestive heart failure. Am Heart J. 2008;156:437–44.
1619. Pizzi C, Mancini S, Angeloni L, Fontana F, Manzoli L, Costa G. Effects of selective serotonin reuptake inhibitor therapy on endothelial function and inflammatory markers in patients with coronary heart disease. Clin Pharmacol Ther. 2009;86:527–32.
1620. Beach SR, Kostis WJ, Celano CM, et al. Metaanalysis of selective serotonin reuptake inhibitor associated QTc prolongation. J Clin Psychiatry. 2014;75:e441–9.
1621. Pizzi C, Rutjes AWS, Costa GM, Fontana F, Mezzetti A, Manzoli L. Meta-analysis of selective serotonin reuptake inhibitors in patients with depression and coronary heart disease. Am J Cardiol. 2011;107:972–9.
1622. Ho JM, Gomes T, Straus SE, Austin PC, Mamdani M, Juurlink DN. Adverse cardiac events in older patients receiving venlafaxine: a population-based study. J Clin Psychiatry. 2014;75:e552–8.

1623. Shah S, Iqbal Z, White A, White S. Heart and mind: (2) psychotropic and cardiovascular therapeutics. Postgrad Med J. 2005;81:33–40.
1624. Mackin P. Cardiac side effects of psychiatric drugs. Hum Psychopharmacol Clin Exp. 2008;23(S1):3–14.
1625. Kovacs D, Arora R. Cardiovascular effects of psychotropic drugs. Am J Ther. 2008;15:474–83.
1626. Giardina E-GV, Johnson LL, Vita J, Bigger JT Jr, Brem RF. Effect of imipramine and nortriptyline on left ventricular function and blood pressure in patients treated for arrhythmias. Am Heart J. 1985;109:992–8.
1627. Roose SP, Dalack GW. Cardiovascular effects of bupropion in depressed patients with heart disease. Am J Psychiatry. 1991;148:512.
1628. Roose SP, Glassman AH, Giardina EG, Johnson LL, Walsh BT, Bigger JT Jr. Cardiovascular effects of imipramine and bupropion in depressed patients with congestive heart failure. J Clin Psychopharmacol. 1987;7:247–51.
1629. Vitullo RN, Wharton JM, Allen NB, Pritchett EL. Trazodone-related exercise-induced nonsustained ventricular tachycardia. Chest. 1990;98:247–8.
1630. Boschmans S, Perkin M, Terblanche S, Opie L. The effects of imipramine, mianserin and trazodone on the chronotropic, inotropic and coronary vascular responses in the isolated perfused rat heart. Gen Pharmacol. 1989;20:233–7.
1631. Mazur A, Strasberg B, Kusniec J, Sclarovsky S. QT prolongation and polymorphous ventricular tachycardia associated with trazodone amiodarone combination. Int J Cardiol. 1995;52:27–9.
1632. Libert J, Amoros C, Muzet A, Ehrhart J, Di Nisi J. Effects of triazolam on heart rate level and on phasic cardiac response to noise during sleep. Psychopharmacology. 1988;96:188–93.
1633. Lapane KL, Zierler S, Lasater TM, Barbour MM, Carleton R, Hume AL. Is the use of psychotropic drugs associated with increased risk of ischemic heart disease? Epidemiology. 1995;6:376–81.
1634. Kim YH, Kim HB, Kim DH, Kim JY, Shin HY. Use of hypnotics and the risk of or mortality from heart disease: a meta-analysis of observational studies. Korean J Intern Med. 2017;33(4):727–36. [E-pub ahead of print].
1635. Schneier FR. Social anxiety disorder. N Engl J Med. 2006;355:1029–36.
1636. Hoogwegt MT, Kupper N, Theuns DA, Jordaens L, Pedersen SS. Beta-blocker therapy is not associated with symptoms of depression and anxiety in patients receiving an implantable cardioverter-defibrillator. Europace. 2011;14:74–80.
1637. Hammond DC. What is neurofeedback: an update. J Neurother. 2011;15:305–36.
1638. Scott WC, Kaiser D, Othmer S, Sideroff SI. Effects of an EEG biofeedback protocol on a mixed substance abusing population. Am J Drug Alcohol Abuse. 2005;3:1455–69.
1639. Kaiser DA, Othmer S. Effect of neurofeedback on variables of attention in a large multi-center trial. J Neurother. 2000;4(1):5–28.
1640. Demos JN. Getting started with neurofeedback. New York/London: Norton & company; 2005.
1641. Gunkelman JD, Johnstone J. Neurofeedback and the brain. J Adult Dev. 2005;12:93–100.
1642. Kropotov JD, Grin-Yatsenko VA, Ponomarev VA, Chutko LS, Yakovenko EA, Nikishena IS. Changes in EEG spectrograms, event-related potentials and event-related desynchronization induced by relative beta training in ADHD children. J Neurother. 2007;11(2):3–11.
1643. Strehl U, Leins U, Goth G, Klinger C, Hinterberger T, Birbaumer N. Self-regulation of slow cortical potentials: a new treatment for children with attention-deficit/hyperactivity disorder. J Pediatr. 2006;118:1530–40.
1644. Rossiter T. The effectiveness of neurofeedback and stimulant drugs in treating AD/HD: part I. Review of methodological issues. Appl Psychophysiol Biofeedback. 2004;29(2):95–112.
1645. Fuchs T, Birbaumer N, Lutzenberger W, Gruzelier JH, Kaiser J. Neurofeedback treatment for attention-deficit/hyperactivity disorder in children: a comparison with methylphenidate. Appl Psychophysiol Biofeedback. 2003;28(1):1–12.
1646. Kotchoubey B, Strehl U, Uhlmann C, Holzapfel S, Konig M, Froscher W, et al. Modification of slow cortical potentials in patients with refractory epilepsy: a controlled outcome study. Epilepsies. 2001;42(3):406–16.
1647. Putman JA. EEG biofeedback on a female patient stroke patient with depression: a case study. J Neurother. 2001;5(3):27–38.
1648. Hammond DC. Neurofeedback with anxiety and affective disorders. Child Adolesc Psychiatr. 2005;14(1):105–23.
1649. Vanathy S, Sharma PSVN, Kumar KB. The efficacy of alpha and theta neurofeedback training in treatment of generalized anxiety disorder. Indian J Clin Psychol. 1998;25(2):136–43.
1650. Muller HH, Donaldson CCS, Nelson DV, Layman M. Treatment of fibromyalgia incorporating EEG-driven stimulation: a clinical study. J Clin Psychol. 2001;57(7):925–33.
1651. Hammond DC. QEEG-guided neurofeedback in the treatment of obsessive compulsive disorder. J Neurother. 2003;7(2):25–52.
1652. Wilson VE, Peper E, Moss D. Professional issue "the mind room" in Italian soccer training: the use of biofeedback and neurofeedback for optimum performance. Biofeedback. 2006;34:79–810.
1653. Hanslmayr S, Sauseng P, Doppelmayr M, Schabus M, Klimesch W. Increasing individual upper alpha power by neurofeedback improves cognitive performance in human subjects. Appl Psychophysiol Biofeedback. 2005;30(1):1–10.
1654. Egner T, Strawson E, Gruzelier JH. EEG signature and phenomenology of alpha-theta neurofeedback

training versus mock feedback. Appl Psychophysiol Biofeedback. 2002;27:4–18.

1655. Vernon D, Egner T, Nick C, et al. The effect of training distinct neurofeedback protocols on aspects of cognitive performance. J Psychophysiol. 2003;47(1):75–85.
1656. Sokhadze TM, Cannon RL, Trudeau DL. EEG biofeedback as a treatment for substance use disorders: review, rating of efficacy, and recommendations for further research. Appl Psychophysiol Biofeedback. 2008;33(1):1–28.
1657. Scott WC, Kaiser D, Othmer S, Sideroff SI. Effects of an EEG biofeedback protocol on a mixed substance abusing population. Am J Drug Alcohol Abuse. 2005;3:1455–69.
1658. Frederick JA, Timmermann DL, Russell HL, Lubar JF. EEG coherence effects of audio-visual stimulation (AVS) at dominant alpha frequency. J Neurother. 2005;8(4):25–42.
1659. Burkett VS, Cummins JM, Dickson RM, Skolnick MH. Treatment effects related to EEG-biofeedback for crack cocaine dependency in a faith-based homeless mission. J Neurother. 2004;8(2):138–40.
1660. Masterpasqua F, Healey KN. Neurofeedback in psychological practice. Prof Psychol Res Pract. 2003;34(6):652–6.
1661. Kaiser DA, Othmer S, Scott B. Effect of neurofeedback on chemical dependency treatment. Biofeedback Self Regul. 1999;20(3):304–5.
1662. Peniston EG, Saxby E. Alpha-theta brainwave neurofeedback training: an effective treatment for male and female alcoholics with depression symptoms. Biofeedback Cent. 1995;51(5):685–93.
1663. Hammond DC. The need for individualization in neurofeedback: heterogeneity in qEEG patterns associated with diagnoses and symptoms. Appl Psychophysiol Biofeedback. 2010;35(1):31–6.
1664. Ross SM. Neurofeedback: an integrative treatment of substance use disorders. Holist Nurs Pract. 2013;27(4):246–50.
1665. Dehghani-Arani F, Rostami R, Nadali H. Neurofeedback training for opiate addiction: improvement of mental health and craving. Appl Psychophysiol Biofeedback. 2013;38:133–41. https://doi.org/10.1007/s10484-013-9218-5.
1666. Peniston EG, Kulkosky PJ. Alpha-theta brainwave training and beta endorphin levels in alcoholics. Alcohol Clin Exp Res. 1989;13:271–9.
1667. Peniston EG, Kulkosky PJ. Alcoholic personality and alpha-theta brainwave training. Med Psychother. 1990;2:37–55.
1668. Peniston EG, Marriman DA, Deming WA, Kulkosky PG. EEG alpha theta brain wave synchronization in Vietnam theater veterans with combat related post traumatic stress disorder and alcohol abuse. Adv Med Psychol. 1993;6:37–49.
1669. Gruzelier J, Egner T. Critical validation studies of neurofeedback. Child Adolesc Psychiatr Clin N Am. 2005;14:83–104.
1670. Singer W, Spies JM, McArthur J, Low J, Griffin JW, Nickander KK, Gordon V, Low PA. Prospective evaluation of somatic and autonomic small fibers in selected autonomic neuropathies. Neurology. 2004;62:612–8.
1671. Dabby R, Vaknine H, Gilad R, Djaldetti R, Sadeh M. Evaluation of cutaneous autonomic innervation in idiopathic sensory small-fiber neuropathy. J Peripher Nerv Syst. 2007;12:98–101.
1672. Lauria G, Bakkers M, Schmitz C, Lombardi R, Penza P, Devigili G, Smith AG, Hsieh ST, Mellgren SI, Umapathi T, Ziegler D, Faber CG, Merkies IS. Intraepidermal nerve fiber density at the distal leg: a worldwide normative reference study. J Peripher Nerv Syst. 2010;15:202–7.
1673. Jacobs AM, Cheng D. Management of diabetic small-fiber neuropathy with combination L-methylfolate, methylcobalamin, and pyridoxal 5′-phosphate. Rev Neurol Dis. 2011;8(1–2):39–47.
1674. Hovaguimian A, Gibbons CH. Diagnosis and treatment of pain in small fiber neuropathy. Curr Pain Headache Rep. 2011;15(3):193–200. https://doi.org/10.1007/s11916-011-0181-7.
1675. Brannagan TH 3rd, Hays AP, Chin SS, Sander HW, Chin RL, Magda P, Green PH, Latov N. Small-fiber neuropathy/neuronopathy associated with celiac disease: skin biopsy findings. Arch Neurol. 2005;62(10):1574–8.
1676. Ho TW, Backonja M, Ma J, Leibensperger H, Froman S, Polydefkis M. Efficient assessment of neuropathic pain drugs in patients with small fiber sensory neuropathies. Pain. 2009;141:19–24.
1677. Ametov AS, Barinov A, Dyck PJ, Hermann R, Kozlova N, Litchy WJ, Low PA, Nehrdich D, Novosadova M, O'Brien PC, Reljanovic M, Samigullin R, Schuette K, Strokov I, Tritschler HJ, Wessel K, Yakhno N, Ziegler D, SYDNEY Trial Study Group. The sensory symptoms of diabetic polyneuropathy are improved with alpha-lipoic acid: the SYDNEY trial. Diabetes Care. 2003;26(3):770–6. Erratum in: Diabetes Care. 2003 Jul;26(7):2227.
1678. Ziegler D, Nowak H, Kempler P, Vargha P, Low PA. Treatment of symptomatic diabetic polyneuropathy with the antioxidant alpha-lipoic acid: a meta-analysis. Diabet Med. 2004;21(2):114–21.
1679. Ziegler D, Ametov A, Barinov A, Dyck PJ, Gurieva I, Low PA, Munzel U, Yakhno N, Raz I, Novosadova M, Maus J, Samigullin R. Oral treatment with alpha-lipoic acid improves symptomatic diabetic polyneuropathy: the SYDNEY 2 trial. Diabetes Care. 2006;29(11):2365–70.
1680. Vinik AI. A medicinal food provides food for thought in managing diabetic neuropathy. Am J Med. 2013;126(2):95–6. https://doi.org/10.1016/j.amjmed.2012.08.008.
1681. Head KA. Peripheral neuropathy: pathogenic mechanisms and alternative therapies. Altern Med Rev. 2006;11:294–329.

1682. Zhang YF, Ning G. Mecobalamin. Expert Opin Ivestigat Drugs. 2008;17:953–64.
1683. Schrezenmaier C, Singer W, Muenter Swift N, Sletten D, Tanabe J, Low PA. Adrenergic and vagal baroreflex sensitivity in autonomic failure. Arch Neurol. 2007;64:381–6.
1684. Low PA, The Therapeutics and Technology Assessment Subcommittee Assessment. Clinical autonomic testing report of the Therapeutics and Technology Assessment Subcommittee of the American Academy of Neurology. Neurology. 1996;46:873–80.
1685. Joint Editorial Statement by the American Diabetes Association; the National Heart, Lung, and Blood Institute; the Juvenile Diabetes Foundation International; the National Institute of Diabetes and Digestive and Kidney Diseases; and the American Heart Association. Diabetes mellitus: a major risk factor for cardiovascular disease. Circulation. 1999;100:1132–3.
1686. Grundy SM, Benjamin IJ, Burke GL, Chait A. AHA scientific statement: diabetes and cardiovascular disease, a statement for healthcare professionals from the American Heart Association. Circulation. 1999;100:1134–46.
1687. Aring AM, Jones DE, Falko JM. Evaluation and prevention of diabetic neuropathy. Am Fam Physicians. 2005;71:2123–30.
1688. Arora RR, Ghosh Dastidar S, Colombo J Autonomic balance is associated with decreased morbidity. American Autonomic Society, 17th International Symposium, Kauai; 29 Oct–1 Nov 2008.
1689. Waheed A, Ali MA, Jurivich DA, et al. Gender differences in longevity and autonomic function. Presented at the Geriatric Medicine Society Meeting, Chicago; 3–7 May 2006.
1690. Arora RR, Aysin E, Aysin B, Colombo J. Therapeutic implications of Sympathetic stimulus in orthostatic patients: measured by spectral domain analysis. AHA Scientific Sessions, Orlando; 4–7 Nov 2007.
1691. Vinik AI, Murray GL. Autonomic neuropathy is treatable. US Endocrinol. 2008;2:82–4.
1692. Nemechek P, Ghosh Dastidar S, Colombo J. Early autonomic dysfunction is associated with secondary hypertension in HIV/AIDS patients. American Autonomic Society, St. Thomas, Virgin Islands; 31 Oct–3 Nov 2009.
1693. Nemechek P, Ghosh Dastidar S, Colombo J. HIV/AIDS leads to early cardiovascular autonomic neuropathy. American Autonomic Society, St. Thomas, Virgin Islands, 31 Oct–3 Nov 2009.
1694. Arora RR, Bulgarelli RJ, Hearyman M, Ghosh Dastidar S, Colombo J. Carvedilol reverses standing parasympathetic excess in non-diabetics. American Autonomic Society, St. Thomas, Virgin Islands; 31 Oct–3 Nov 2009.
1695. Nanavati SH, Bulgarelli RJ, Vazquez-Tanus J, Ghosh-Dastidar S, Colombo J, Arora RR. Altered autonomic activity with atrial fibrillation as demonstrated by non-invasive autonomic monitoring. US Cardiol. 2010;7(1):47–50.
1696. Vinik AI, Aysin B, Colombo J. Differentiation of autonomic dysfunction by enhanced frequency domain analysis reveals additional stages in the progression of autonomic decline in diabetics. Diabetes Technology Conference, San Francisco; 10–12 Nov 2005.
1697. Boyd GL, Taylor JA, Ovalle F, Stout DG, Aultman M, Garner VM, Morris RE, Witherspoon CD, Albert M, Vetter TR. Prevalence of advanced autonomic dysfunction in patients presenting for retinal surgery. Submitted, Anesthesiology; 2013.
1698. Boulton AJM, Vinik AI, Arrezzo JC, Bril V, Feldman EI, Freeman R, Malik RA, Maser RE, Sosenko JM, Ziegler D. Diabetic neuropathies: a statement by the American Diabetes Association. Diabetes Care. 2005;28(4):956–62.
1699. Boulton AJM, Vinik AI, Arrezzo JC, Bril V, Feldman EI, Freeman R, Malik RA, Maser RE, Sosenko JM, Ziegler D. Diabetic neuropathies: a statement by the American Diabetes Association. Diabetes Care. 2005;28(4):956–62.
1700. Malik M, editor. Clinical guide to cardiac autonomic tests. Dordrecht: Kluwer Academic Publishers; 1998.
1701. Vinik AI, Camacho PM, Davidson JA, Handelsman Y, Lando HM, Leddy AL, Reddy SK, Cook R, Spallone V, Tesfaye S, Ziegler D, Task Force to Develop an AACE Position Statement on Autonomic Testing. American Association of Clinical Endocrinologists and American College of Endocrinology position statement on testing for autonomic and somatic nerve dysfunction. Endocr Pract. 2017;23(12):1472–8. https://doi.org/10.4158/EP-2017-0053.
1702. Aring AM, Jones DE, Falko JM. Evaluation and prevention of diabetic neuropathy. Am Fam Physicians. 2005;71:2123–30.
1703. Chen J, Long JB, Hurria A, Owusu C, Steingart RM, Gross CP. Incidence of heart failure or cardiomyopathy after adjuvant trastuzumab therapy for breast cancer. J Am Coll Cardiol. 2012;60:2504–12.
1704. Bowles EJA, Wellman R, Feigelson HS, et al. Risk of heart failure in breast cancer patients after anthracycline and trastuzumab treatment: a retrospective cohort study. J Natl Cancer Inst. 2012;104:1293–305.
1705. Lenihan DJ, Cardinale DM. Late cardiac effects of cancer treatment [published correction appears in J Clin Oncol 2012;30:4590]. J Clin Oncol. 2012;30:3657–64.
1706. Mukhopadhyay P, Rajesh M, Bátkai S, et al. Role of superoxide, nitric oxide, and peroxynitrite in doxorubicin-induced cell death in vivo and in vitro. Am J Physiol Heart Circ Physiol. 2009;296:1466–83.
1707. Weinstein DM, Mihm MJ, Bauer JA. Cardiac peroxynitrite formation and left ventricular dysfunction following doxorubicin treatment in mice. J Pharmacol Exp Ther. 2000;294:396–401.

1708. Fogli S, Nieri P, Breschi MC. The role of nitric oxide in anthracycline toxicity and prospects for pharmacologic prevention of cardiac damage. FASEB J. 2004;18:664–75.

1709. Ky B, Putt M, Sawaya H, et al. Early increases in multiple biomarkers predict subsequent cardiotoxicity in patients with breast cancer treated with doxorubicin, taxanes, and trastuzumab [published correction appears in J Am Coll Cardiol 2016;67:1385]. J Am Coll Cardiol. 2014;63:809–16.

1710. Zhang S, Liu X, Bawa-Khalfe T, et al. Identification of the molecular basis of doxorubicin induced cardiotoxicity. Nat Med. 2012;18:1639–42.

1711. Wan A, Rodrigues B. Endothelial cell cardiomyocyte crosstalk in diabetic cardiomyopathy. Cardiovasc Res. 2016;111:172–83.

1712. Hahn VS, Lenihan DJ, Ky B. Cancer therapy induced cardiotoxicity: basic mechanisms and potential cardioprotective therapies. J Am Heart Assoc. 2014;3:e000665.

1713. Versari D, Daghini E, Virdis A, Ghiadoni L, Taddei S. Endothelium-dependent contractions and endothelial dysfunction in human hypertension. Br J Pharmacol. 2009;157:527–36.

1714. Milano G, Raucci A, Scopece A, et al. Doxorubicin and trastuzumab regimen induces biventricular failure in mice. J Am Soc Echocardiogr. 2014;27:568–79.

1715. Aghajanian H, Cho YK, Manderfield LJ, et al. Coronary vasculature patterning requires a novel endothelial ErbB2 holoreceptor. Nat Commun. 2016;7:12038.

1716. Wolf MB, Baynes JW. The anti-cancer drug, doxorubicin, causes oxidant stress-induced endothelial dysfunction. Biochim Biophys Acta. 1760;2006:267–71.

1717. Toya T, Hakuno D, Shiraishi Y, Kujiraoka T, Adachi T. Arginase inhibition augments nitric oxide production and facilitates left ventricular systolic function in doxorubicin-induced cardiomyopathy in mice. Physiol Rep. 2014;2:e12130.

1718. Hammond J, Balligand J. Nitric oxide synthase and cyclic GMP signaling in cardiac myocytes: from contractility to remodeling. J Mol Cell Cardiol. 2012;52:330–40.

1719. Meinitzer A, Seelhorst U, Wellnitz B, et al. Asymmetrical dimethylarginine independently predicts total and cardiovascular mortality in individuals with angiographic coronary artery disease (the Ludwigshafen Risk and Cardiovascular Health Study). Clin Chem. 2007;53:273–83.

1720. Boger RH, Sullivan LM, Schwedhelm E, et al. Plasma asymmetric dimethylarginine and incidence of cardiovascular disease and death in the community. Circulation. 2009;119:1592–600.

1721. Dückelmann C, Mittermayer F, Haider DG, Altenberger J, Eichinger J, Wolzt M. Asymmetric dimethylarginine enhances cardiovascular risk prediction in patients with chronic heart failure. Arterioscler Thromb Vasc Biol. 2007;27:2037–42.

1722. Liu X, Hou L, Xu D, et al. Effect of asymmetric dimethylarginine (ADMA) on heart failure development. Nitric Oxide. 2016;54:73–81.

1723. Myalgic encephalomyelitis, chronic fatigue syndrome. Centers for Disease Control and Prevention; 3 July 2007. https://www.cdc.gov/me-cfs/index.html.

1724. Carruthers BM, van de Sande MI, De Meirleir KL, Klimas NG, Broderick G, Mitchell T, Staines D, Powles AC, Speight N, Vallings R, Bateman L, Baumgarten-Austrheim B, Bell DS, Carlo-Stella N, Chia J, Darragh A, Jo D, Lewis D, Light AR, Marshall-Gradisbik S, Mena I, Mikovits JA, Miwa K, Murovska M, Pall ML, Stevens S. Myalgic encephalomyelitis: international consensus criteria. J Intern Med. 2011;270(4):327–38. https://doi.org/10.1111/j.1365-2796.2011.02428.x. Epub 2011 Aug 22. Review. Erratum in: J Intern Med. 2017 Oct;282(4):353. PMID: 21777306.

1725. Carruthers BM. Definitions and aetiology of myalgic encephalomyelitis: how the Canadian consensus clinical definition of myalgic encephalomyelitis works. J Clin Pathol. 2007;60(2):117–9. Epub 2006 Aug 25.

1726. Barnden LR, Kwiatek R, Crouch B, Burnet R, Del Fante P. Autonomic correlations with MRI are abnormal in the brainstem vasomotor centre in Chronic Fatigue Syndrome. Neuroimage Clin. 2016;11:530–7. https://doi.org/10.1016/j.nicl.2016.03.017. eCollection 2016. PMID: 27114901.

1727. Bested AC, Marshall LM. Review of Myalgic Encephalomyelitis/Chronic Fatigue Syndrome: an evidence-based approach to diagnosis and management by clinicians. Rev Environ Health. 2015;30(4):223–49. https://doi.org/10.1515/reveh-2015-0026. Review. PMID: 26613325.

1728. Tanaka M, Tajima S, Mizuno K, Ishii A, Konishi Y, Miike T, Watanabe Y. Frontier studies on fatigue, autonomic nerve dysfunction, and sleep-rhythm disorder. J Physiol Sci. 2015;65(6):483–98. https://doi.org/10.1007/s12576-015-0399-y. Epub 2015 Sept 29. Review. PMID: 26420687.

1729. Van Cauwenbergh D, Nijs J, Kos D, Van Weijnen L, Struyf F, Meeus M. Malfunctioning of the autonomic nervous system in patients with chronic fatigue syndrome: a systematic literature review. Eur J Clin Investig. 2014;44(5):516–26. https://doi.org/10.1111/eci.12256.

1730. Lewis I, Pairman J, Spickett G, Newton JL. Clinical characteristics of a novel subgroup of chronic fatigue syndrome patients with postural orthostatic tachycardia syndrome. J Intern Med. 2013;273(5):501–10. https://doi.org/10.1111/joim.12022. Epub 2013 Jan 7. PMID: 23206180.

1731. Myhill S, Booth NE, McLaren-Howard J. Targeting mitochondrial dysfunction in the treatment of Myalgic Encephalomyelitis/Chronic Fatigue Syndrome (ME/CFS) – a clinical audit. Int J Clin Exp Med. 2013;6(1):1–15. Epub 2012 Nov 20. PMID: 23236553.

1732. Booth NE, Myhill S, McLaren-Howard J. Mitochondrial dysfunction and the pathophysiology of Myalgic Encephalomyelitis/Chronic Fatigue Syndrome (ME/CFS). Int J Clin Exp Med. 2012;5(3):208–20. Epub 2012 Jun 15. PMID: 22837795.

1733. Myhill S, Booth NE, McLaren-Howard J. Chronic fatigue syndrome and mitochondrial dysfunction. Int J Clin Exp Med. 2009;2(1):1–16. Epub 2009 Jan 15. PMID: 19436827.

1734. World Health Association International Statistics Classification Disease and Related Health Problems, 10th revision, ICD-10, 2010, cited 2014, available from https://icd.who.int/browse10/2014/en#/.

1735. Morris G, Maes M. Myalgic encephalomyelitis/chronic fatigue syndrome and encephalomyelitis disseminata/multiple sclerosis show remarkable levels of similarity in phenomenology and neuroimmune characteristics. BMC Med. 2013;11:205. https://doi.org/10.1186/1741-7015-11-205. Review. PMID: 24229326.

1736. Agarwal AK, Garg R, Ritch A, Sarkar P. Postural orthostatic tachycardia syndrome. Postgrad Med J. 2007;83(981):478–80. Review. PMID: 17621618.

1737. Tomas C, Newton J, Watson S. A review of hypothalamic-pituitary-adrenal axis function in chronic fatigue syndrome. ISRN Neurosci. 2013;2013:784520. https://doi.org/10.1155/2013/784520. eCollection 2013. PMID: 24959566.

1738. Papadopoulos AS, Cleare AJ. Hypothalamic-pituitary-adrenal axis dysfunction in chronic fatigue syndrome. Nat Rev Endocrinol. 2011;8(1):22–32. https://doi.org/10.1038/nrendo.2011.153.

1739. Jason L, Sorenson M, Sebally K, Alkazemi D, Lerch A, Porter N, Kubow S. Increased HDAC in association with decreased plasma cortisol in older adults with chronic fatigue syndrome. Brain Behav Immun. 2011;25(8):1544–7. https://doi.org/10.1016/j.bbi.2011.04.007. Epub 2011 Apr 28. PMID: 21549189.

1740. Crofford LJ, Young EA, Engleberg NC, Korszun A, Brucksch CB, McClure LA, Brown MB, Demitrack MA. Basal circadian and pulsatile ACTH and cortisol secretion in patients with fibromyalgia and/or chronic fatigue syndrome. Brain Behav Immun. 2004;18(4):314–25.

1741. Cairns R, Hotopf M. A systematic review describing the prognosis of chronic fatigue syndrome. Occup Med (Lond). 2005;55(1):20–31.

1742. Newton JL, Okonkwo O, Sutcliffe K, Seth A, Shin J, Jones DE. Symptoms of autonomic dysfunction in chronic fatigue syndrome. QJM. 2007;100(8):519–26. Epub 2007 Jul 7.

1743. Costigan A, Elliott C, McDonald C, Newton JL. Orthostatic symptoms predict functional capacity in chronic fatigue syndrome: implications for management. QJM. 2010;103(8):589–95. https://doi.org/10.1093/qjmed/hcq094. Epub 2010 Jun 9.

1744. Woltjer HH, Bogaard HJ, de Vries PM. The technique of impedance cardiography. Eur Heart J. 1997;18(9):1396–403.

1745. Jones DE, Gray J, Frith J, Newton JL. Fatigue severity remains stable over time and independently associated with orthostatic symptoms in chronic fatigue syndrome: a longitudinal study. J Intern Med. 2011;269(2):182–8. https://doi.org/10.1111/j.1365-2796.2010.02306.x. Epub 2010 Nov 14. PMID: 21073560.

1746. Hollingsworth KG, Jones DE, Taylor R, Blamire AM, Newton JL. Impaired cardiovascular response to standing in chronic fatigue syndrome. Eur J Clin Investig. 2010;40(7):608–15. https://doi.org/10.1111/j.1365-2362.2010.02310.x. Epub 2010 May 23. PMID: 20497461.

1747. Okamoto LE, Raj SR, Peltier A, Gamboa A, Shibao C, Diedrich A, Black BK, Robertson D, Biaggioni I. Neurohumoral and haemodynamic profile in postural tachycardia and chronic fatigue syndromes. Clin Sci (Lond). 2012;122(4):183–92. https://doi.org/10.1042/CS20110200. PMID: 21906029.

1748. Naschitz J, Dreyfuss D, Yeshurun D, Rosner I. Midodrine treatment for chronic fatigue syndrome. Postgrad Med J. 2004;80(942):230–2. PMID: 15082846.

1749. Naschitz JE, Rosner I, Rozenbaum M, Naschitz S, Musafia-Priselac R, Shaviv N, Fields M, Isseroff H, Zuckerman E, Yeshurun D, Sabo E. The head-up tilt test with haemodynamic instability score in diagnosing chronic fatigue syndrome. QJM. 2003;96(2):133–42.

1750. DuBois RE. Gamma globulin therapy for chronic mononucleosis syndrome. AIDS Res. 1986;2(Suppl 1):S191–5. PMID: 2435296.

1751. Fluge Ø, Risa K, Lunde S, Alme K, Rekeland IG, Sapkota D, Kristoffersen EK, Sørland K, Bruland O, Dahl O, Mella O. B-lymphocyte depletion in myalgic encephalopathy/chronic fatigue syndrome. An open-label phase ii study with rituximab maintenance treatment. PLoS One. 2015;10(7):e0129898. https://doi.org/10.1371/journal.pone.0129898. eCollection 2015. PMID: 26132314.

1752. Fluge Ø, Bruland O, Risa K, Storstein A, Kristoffersen EK, Sapkota D, Næss H, Dahl O, Nyland H, Mella O. Benefit from B-lymphocyte depletion using the anti-CD20 antibody rituximab in chronic fatigue syndrome. A double-blind and placebo-controlled study. PLoS One. 2011;6(10):e26358. https://doi.org/10.1371/journal.pone.0026358. Epub 2011 Oct 19. PMID: 22039471.

1753. Papadopoulos A, Ebrecht M, Roberts AD, Poon L, Rohleder N, Cleare AJ. Glucocorticoid receptor mediated negative feedback in chronic fatigue syndrome using the low dose (0.5 mg) dexamethasone suppression test. J Affect Disord. 2009;112(1–3):289–94. https://doi.org/10.1016/j.jad.2008.05.001. Epub 2008 Jun 24. PMID: 18573538.

1754. Filler K, Lyon D, Bennett J, McCain N, Elswick R, Lukkahatai N, Saligan LN. Association of mitochondrial dysfunction and fatigue: a review of the literature. BBA Clin. 2014;1:12–23.
1755. Gerdle B, Forsgren MF, Bengtsson A, Leinhard OD, Sören B, Karlsson A, Brandejsky V, Lund E, Lundberg P. Decreased muscle concentrations of ATP and PCR in the quadriceps muscle of fibromyalgia patients – a 31P-MRS study. Eur J Pain. 2013;17(8):1205–15. https://doi.org/10.1002/j.1532-2149.2013.00284.x. Epub 2013 Jan 30.
1756. Castro-Marrero J, Cordero MD, Sáez-Francas N, Jimenez-Gutierrez C, Aguilar-Montilla FJ, Aliste L, Alegre-Martin J. Could mitochondrial dysfunction be a differentiating marker between chronic fatigue syndrome and fibromyalgia? Antioxid Redox Signal. 2013;19(15):1855–60. https://doi.org/10.1089/ars.2013.5346. Epub 2013 May 29.
1757. Singh B, Singh R. Mitochondrial dysfunction and chronic fatigue syndromes: issues in clinical care. IOSR-JDMS. 2014;13(5):30–3. e-ISSN: 2279-0853, p-ISSN: 2279-0861.
1758. Sarzi-Puttini P, Atzeni F, Mease PJ. Chronic widespread pain: from peripheral to central evolution. Best Pract Res Clin Rheumatol. 2011;25(2):133–9. https://doi.org/10.1016/j.berh.2011.04.001.
1759. Heidenreich PA, Albert NM, Allen LA, et al. Forecasting the impact of heart failure in the United States: a policy statement from the American Heart Association. Circ Heart Fail. 2013;6:606–19.
1760. Go AS, Mozaffarian D, Roger VL, et al. Heart disease and stroke statistics – 2014 update: a report from the American Heart Association. Circulation. 2014;129(3):e 28–292.
1761. Shah SJ, Kitzman DW, Borlaug BA, et al. Phenotype – specific treatment of heart failure with preserved ejection fraction: a multiorgan roadmap. Circulation. 2006;134:73–90.
1762. Packer M, Kitzman DW. Obesity-related heart failure with a preserved ejection fraction: the mechanistic rationale for combining inhibitors of aldosterone, neprilysin, and sodium-glucose cotransporter. JACC Heart Fail. 2018;6(8):633–9.
1763. Haykowsky MJ, et al. Regional adipose distribution and its relation to excess intolerance in older obese patients who has heart failure with preserved ejection fraction. JACC Heart Fail. 2018;6(9):642–9.
1764. Bharadwaj MS, et al. Relationship between mitochondrial content and bioenergetics with obesity, body composition and fat distribution to healthy older adults. BMC Obes. 2015;2:40.
1765. Forman DE, Goodpasture BH. Weighty matters in HFpEF and aging. JACC Heart Fail. 2018;6(8):650–2.
1766. Paulus WJ, Tschope C. A novel paradigm for heart failure with preserved ejection fraction: comorbidities drive myocardial dysfunction and remodeling through coronary microvascular endothelial dysfunction. J Am Coll Cardiol. 2013;62:263–71.
1767. Schmidt-Wilcke T, Clauw DJ. Fibromyalgia: from pathophysiology to therapy. Nat Rev Rheumatol. 2011;7(9):518–27. https://doi.org/10.1038/nrrheum.2011.98.
1768. Fatima G, Das SK, Mahdi AA. Oxidative stress and antioxidative parameters and metal ion content in patients with fibromyalgia syndrome: implications in the pathogenesis of the disease. Clin Exp Rheumatol. 2013;31(6 Suppl 79):S128–33. Epub 2013 Dec 16.
1769. El-Sawya N, El-Tantawia G, Achmawib GAH, Sultana H, Younisa S. Autonomic changes in fibromyalgia: clinical and electrophysiological study. Alexandria J Med. 2012;48(3):215–22.
1770. Solano C, Martinez A, Becerril L, Vargas A, Figueroa J, Navarro C, Ramos-Remus C, Martinez-Lavin M. Autonomic dysfunction in fibromyalgia assessed by the Composite Autonomic Symptoms Scale (COMPASS). J Clin Rheumatol. 2009;15(4):172–6. https://doi.org/10.1097/RHU.0b013e3181a1083d.
1771. Kadetoff D, Kosek E. The effects of static muscular contraction on blood pressure, heart rate, pain ratings and pressure pain thresholds in healthy individuals and patients with fibromyalgia. Eur J Pain. 2007;11(1):39–47. Epub 2006 Feb 9.
1772. Ramírez M, Martínez-Martínez LA, Hernández-Quintela E, Velazco-Casapía J, Vargas A, Martínez-Lavín M. Small fiber neuropathy in women with fibromyalgia. An in vivo assessment using corneal confocal bio-microscopy. Semin Arthritis Rheum. 2015;45(2):214–9. https://doi.org/10.1016/j.semarthrit.2015.03.003. Epub 2015 Mar 19.
1773. Clauw DJ. Fibromyalgia: a clinical review. JAMA. 2014;311(15):1547–55. https://doi.org/10.1001/jama.2014.3266.
1774. Goldenberg DL, Burckhardt C, Crofford L. Management of fibromyalgia syndrome. JAMA. 2004;292(19):2388–95.
1775. Dell'Osso L, Bazzichi L, Baroni S, Falaschi V, Conversano C, Carmassi C, Marazziti D. The inflammatory hypothesis of mood spectrum broadened to fibromyalgia and chronic fatigue syndrome. Clin Exp Rheumatol. 2015;33(1 Suppl 88):S109–16. Epub 2015 Mar 18.
1776. Giles TD, Materson BJ, Cohn JN, Kostis JB. Definition and classification of hypertension: an update. J Clin Hypertens (Greenwich). 2009;11(11):611–4.https://doi.org/10.1111/j.1751--7176.2009.00179.x. Erratum in: J Clin Hypertens (Greenwich). 2010 Jan;12(1):13.
1777. Lüscher TF, Mahfoud F. Renal nerve ablation after SYMPLICITY HTN-3: confused at the higher level? Eur Heart J. 2014;35(26):1706–11. https://doi.org/10.1093/eurheartj/ehu195. Epub 2014 May 14.
1778. DePace NL, Bateman JA, Yayac M, Oh J, Siddique M. Acosta C, Pinales JM, Vinik AI, Bloom HL. Improved patient outcomes by normalizing sympathovagal balance: differentiating syncope – precise subtype differentiation leads to improved out-

comes. Cardiol Res Pract. 2018, Article ID 9532141, 8 pages. https://doi.org/10.1155/2018/953214.
1779. Murray GL, Colombo J. (R)alpha lipoic acid is a safe, effective pharmacologic therapy of chronic orthostatic hypotension associated with low sympathetic tone. Int J Angiol. 2019 (eFirst); 1. https://doi.org/10.1055/s-0038-1676957.
1780. Mohammadi V, Dehghani S, Askari G. Does alpha-lipoic acid supplement regulate blood pressure? A systematic review of randomized, double-blind placebo-controlled clinical trials. Int J Prev Med. 2017;8:33–8.
1781. Bangalore S, Messerlli F, Wun C, Zuckerman A, DeMicco D, Kostis J, et al. J-curve revisited: an analysis of blood pressure and cardiovascular events in the Treating to New Targets (TNT) trial. Eur Heart J. 2010;31(23):2897–908.
1782. Queiroz T, Guimaraes D, Medndes-Junior L, Braga V. α-lipoic acid reduces hypertension and increases baroreflex sensitivity in renovascular hypertensive rats. Molecules. 2012;17(11):13357–67.
1783. Gouty S, Regalia J, Cai F, Helke C. Alpha-lipoic acid treatment prevents the diabetes-induced attenuation of the afferent limb of the baroreceptor reflex in rats. Auton Neurosci. 2003;108(1–2):32–44.
1784. Wray D, Nishiyama S, Harris R, Zhao J, McDaniel J, Fjeldstad A, et al. Acute reversal of endothelial dysfunction in the elderly after antioxidant consumption. Hypertension. 2012;59(4):818–24.
1785. Rahman S, Merchant N, Haque T, Wahi J, Bhaheetharan S, Ferdinand K, Khan B. The impact of lipoic acid on endothelial function and proteinuria in quinapril-treated diabetic patients with stage 1 hypertension: results from the QUALITY study. J Cardiovasc Pharmacol Ther. 2012;17(2):139–45.
1786. Xiang G, Pu J, Yue L, Hou J, Sun H. α-lipoic acid can improve endothelial dysfunction in subjects with impaired fasting glucose. Metabolism. 2011;60(4):480–5.
1787. Tardif J, Rheaume E. Lipoic acid supplementation and endothelial function. Br J Pharmacol. 2008;153:1587–8.
1788. Charles A. Advances in the basic and clinical science of migraine. Ann Neurol. 2009;65(5):491–8. https://doi.org/10.1002/ana.21691.
1789. Leão AA. Spreading depression. Funct Neurol. 1986;1(4):363–6.
1790. Headache classification committee of the international headache society IHS, The international classification headache disorders. 3rd ed, beta version, Cephalgia. 2013;33: 629–808.
1791. Yorns WR Jr, Hardison HH. Mitochondrial dysfunction in migraine. Semin Pediatr Neurol. 2013;20(3):188–93. https://doi.org/10.1016/j.spen.2013.09.002.
1792. Stuart S, Griffiths LR. A possible role for mitochondrial dysfunction in migraine. Mol Gen Genomics. 2012;287(11–12):837–44. https://doi.org/10.1007/s00438-012-0723-7. Epub 2012 Oct 7.
1793. Millichap JG. Migraine and autonomic nervous system dysfunction. Pediatr Neurol Briefs. 2002;16(2):15–6.
1794. Vetvik KG, MacGregor EA. Sex differences in the epidemiology, clinical features, and pathophysiology of migraine. Lancet Neurol. 2017;16(1):76–87. https://doi.org/10.1016/S1474-4422(16)30293-9. Epub 2016 Nov 9.
1795. Shechter A, Stewart WF, Silberstein SD, Lipton RB. Migraine and autonomic nervous system function: a population-based, case-control study. Neurology. 2002;58(3):422–7.
1796. Millichap JG, Yee MM. The diet factor in pediatric and adolescent migraine. Pediatr Neurol. 2003;28(1):9–15.
1797. Charles A. Migraine. N Engl J Med. 2017;377(17):1698–9. https://doi.org/10.1056/NEJMc1711803.
1798. Natoli JL, Manack A, Dean B, Butler Q, Turkel CC, Stovner L, Lipton RB. Global prevalence of chronic migraine: a systematic review. Cephalalgia. 2010;30(5):599–609. https://doi.org/10.1111/j.1468-2982.2009.01941.x.
1799. Minen MT, Begasse De Dhaem O, Kroon Van Diest A, Powers S, Schwedt TJ, Lipton R, Silbersweig D. Migraine and its psychiatric comorbidities. J Neurol Neurosurg Psychiatry. 2016;87(7):741–9. https://doi.org/10.1136/jnnp-2015-312233. Epub 2016 Jan 5.
1800. Bigal ME, Lipton RB. Excessive acute migraine medication use and migraine progression. Neurology. 2008;71(22):1821–8. https://doi.org/10.1212/01.wnl.0000335946.53860.1d.
1801. Pieczenik SR, Neustadt J. Mitochondrial dysfunction and molecular pathways of disease. Exp Mol Pathol. 2007;83(1):84–92. Epub 2007 Jan 18.
1802. Kelman L. The triggers or precipitants of the acute migraine attack. Cephalalgia. 2007;27(5):394–402. Epub 2007 Mar 30.
1803. Elmenshawy E, Sakr S. Autonomic dysfunction in migraine; what do we need to know? Egypt J Neurol Psychiatr Neurosur. 2009;46:489–96.
1804. Gaul C, Diener HC, Danesch U, Migravent® Study Group. Improvement of migraine symptoms with a proprietary supplement containing riboflavin, magnesium and Q10: a randomized, placebo-controlled, double-blind, multicenter trial. J Headache Pain. 2015;16:516. https://doi.org/10.1186/s10194-015-0516-6. Epub 2015 Apr 3.
1805. Reeve AK, Simcox EM, Duchen MR, Turnbull DM, editors. Mitochondrial dysfunction in neurodegenerative disorders. 2nd ed. Cham: Springer International Publishing; 2016.
1806. Vos M, Lauwers E, Verstreken P. Synaptic mitochondria in synaptic transmission and organization of vesicle pools in health and disease Front Synaptic Neurosci. 2010. https://doi.org/10.3389/fnsyn.2010.00139
1807. Lambert AJ, Brand MD. Reactive oxygen species production by mitochondria. Methods

Mol Biol. 2009;554:165–81. https://doi.org/10.1007/978-1-59745-521-3_11.
1808. Balaban RS, Nemoto S, Finkel T. Mitochondria, oxidants, and aging. Cell. 2005;120(4):483–95.
1809. Papadopoulos V, Miller WL. Role of mitochondria in steroidogenesis. Best Pract Res Clin Endocrinol Metab. 2012;26(6):771–90. https://doi.org/10.1016/j.beem.2012.05.002. Epub 2012 Jun 16.
1810. Glancy B, Balaban RS. Role of mitochondrial Ca2+ in the regulation of cellular energetics. Biochemistry. 2012;51(14):2959–73. https://doi.org/10.1021/bi2018909. Epub 2012 Mar 29.
1811. Marland JRK, Hasel P, Bonnycastle K, Cousin MA. Mitochondrial calcium uptake modulates synaptic vesicle endocytosis in central nerve terminals. J Biol Chem. 2016;291(5):2080–6. https://doi.org/10.1074/jbc.M115.686956.
1812. Rizzuto R, De Stefani D, Raffaello A, Mammucari C. Mitochondria as sensors and regulators of calcium signalling. Nat Rev Mol Cell Biol. 2012;13(9):566–78. https://doi.org/10.1038/nrm3412. Epub 2012 Aug 1.
1813. Kasahara A, Scorrano L. Mitochondria: from cell death executioners to regulators of cell differentiation. Trends Cell Biol. 2014;24(12):761–70. https://doi.org/10.1016/j.tcb.2014.08.005. Epub 2014 Sept 2.
1814. Ahuja M, Muallem S. The gatekeepers of mitochondrial calcium influx: MICU1 and MICU2. EMBO Rep. 2014;15(3):205–6. https://doi.org/10.1002/embr.201438446. Epub 2014 Feb 14.
1815. Lagouge M, Argmann C, Gerhart-Hines Z, Meziane H, Lerin C, Daussin F, Messadeq N, Milne J, Lambert P, Elliott P, Geny B, Laakso M, Puigserver P, Auwerx J. Resveratrol improves mitochondrial function and protects against metabolic disease by activating SIRT1 and PGC-1alpha. Cell. 2006;127(6):1109–22. Epub 2006 Nov 16.
1816. Baur JA, Pearson KJ, Price NL, Jamieson HA, Lerin C, Kalra A, Prabhu VV, Allard JS, Lopez-Lluch G, Lewis K, Pistell PJ, Poosala S, Becker KG, Boss O, Gwinn D, Wang M, Ramaswamy S, Fishbein KW, Spencer RG, Lakatta EG, Le Couteur D, Shaw RJ, Navas P, Puigserver P, Ingram DK, de Cabo R, Sinclair DA. Resveratrol improves health and survival of mice on a high-calorie diet. Nature. 2006;444(7117):337–42. Epub 2006 Nov 1.
1817. Shalev A, Liberzon I, Marmar C. Post traumatic stress disorder. (Longo DL, ed) NEJM. 2017;376:2459–69. https://doi.org/10.1056/NEJMra1612499.
1818. American Psychiatric Association. Diagnostic and statistical manual of mental disorders. 5th ed. Washington, DC; 2000.
1819. Brudey C, Park J, Wiaderkiewicz J, Kobayashi I, Mellman TA, Marvar PJ. Autonomic and inflammatory consequences of posttraumatic stress disorder and the link to cardiovascular disease. Am J Physiol Regul Integr Comp Physiol. 2015;309:R315–21.
1820. Nance DM, Sanders VM. Autonomic innervation and regulation of the immune system (1987–2007). Brain Behav Immun. 2007;21:736–45.
1821. Kanel von R, Hepp U, Kraemer B, Traber R, Keel M, Mica L, Schnyder U. Evidence for low-grade systemic proinflammatory activity in patients with posttraumatic stress disorder. J Psychiatr Res. 2007;41:744–52.
1822. Ridker PM. Clinical application of C-reactive protein for cardiovascular disease detection and prevention. Circulation. 2003;107:363–9.
1823. Miller AH, Haroon E, Raison CL, Felger JC. Cytokine targets in the brain: impact on neurotransmitters and neurocircuits. Depress Anxiety. 2013;30:297–306.
1824. Song C, Phillips AG, Leonard B. Interleukin 1β enhances conditioned fear memory in rats: possible involvement of glucocorticoids. Eur J Neurosci. 2003;18:1739–43.
1825. Wohleb ES, Patterson JM, Sharma V, Quan N, Godbout JP, Sheridan JF. Knockdown of interleukin-1 receptor type-1 on endothelial cells attenuated stress-induced neuroinflammation and prevented anxiety-like behavior. J Neurosci. 2014;34:2583–91.
1826. Oosthuizen F, Wegener G, Harvey BH. Nitric oxide as inflammatory mediator in post-traumatic stress disorder (PTSD): evidence from an animal model. Neuropsychiatr Dis Treat. 2005;1:109–23.
1827. Vera E, Blasco MA. Beyond average: potential for measurement of short telomeres. Aging (Albany NY). 2012;4(6):379–92.
1828. de Lange T. Protection of mammalian telomeres. Oncogene. 2002;21:532–40.
1829. Harley CB, Futcher AB, Greider CW. Telomeres shorten during ageing of human fibroblasts. Nature. 1990;345:458–60.
1830. Blackburn EH. Switching and signaling at the telomere. Cell. 2001;106:661–73.
1831. Collins K, Mitchell JR. Telomerase in the human organism. Oncogene. 2002;21:564–79.
1832. Canela A, Vera E, Klatt P, Blasco MA. High-throughput telomere length quantification by FISH and its application to human population studies. Proc Natl Acad Sci U S A. 2007;104:5300–5.
1833. Flores I, Canela A, Vera E, Tejera A, Cotsarelis G, Blasco MA. The longest telomeres: a general signature of adult stem cell compartments. Genes Dev. 2008;22:654–67.
1834. Yui J, Chiu CP, Lansdorp PM. Telomerase activity in candidate stem cells from fetal liver and adult bone marrow. Blood. 1998;91:3255–62.
1835. Deng Y, Chan SS, Chang S. Telomere dysfunction and tumour suppression: the senescence connection. Nat Rev Cancer. 2008;8:450–8.
1836. Collado M, Blasco MA, Serrano M. Cellular senescence in cancer and aging. Cell. 2007;130:223–33.
1837. Blasco MA. Telomere length, stem cells and aging. Nat Chem Biol. 2007;3:640–9.
1838. de Cabo R, Carmona-Gutierrez D, Bernier M, Hall MN, Madeo F. The search for antiaging interventions: from elixirs to fasting regimens. Cell. 2014;157(7):1515–26.

1839. Aviv A. Genetics of leukocyte telomere length and its role in atherosclerosis. Mutat Res. 2012;730:68–74.

1840. Levy D, Neuhausen SL, Hunt SC, Kimura M, Hwang SJ, Chen W, Bis JC, Fitzpatrick AL, Smith E, Johnson AD, Gardner JP, Srinivasan SR, Schork N, Rotter JI, Herbig U, Psaty BM, Sastrasinh M, Murray SS, Vasan RS, Province MA, Glazer NL, Lu X, Cao X, Kronmal R, Mangino M, Soranzo N, Spector TD, Berenson GS, Aviv A. Genome-wide association identifies OBFC1 as a locus involved in human leukocyte telomere biology. Proc Natl Acad Sci U S A. 2010;107:9293–8.

1841. Mangino M, Hwang SJ, Spector TD, Hunt SC, Kimura M, Fitzpatrick AL, Christiansen L, Petersen I, Elbers CC, Harris T, Chen W, Srinivasan SR, Kark JD, Benetos A, El Shamieh S, Visvikis-Siest S, Christensen K, Berenson GS, Valdes AM, Viñuela A, Garcia M, Arnett DK, Broeckel U, Province MA, Pankow JS, Kammerer C, Liu Y, Nalls M, Tishkoff S, Thomas F, Ziv E, Psaty BM, Bis JC, Rotter JI, Taylor KD, Smith E, Schork NJ, Levy D, Aviv A. Genome-wide meta-analysis points to CTC1 and ZNF676 as genes regulating telomere homeostasis in humans. Hum Mol Genet. 2012;21:5385–94.

1842. Codd V, Nelson CP, Albrecht E, Mangino M, Deelen J, Buxton JL, et al. Identification of seven loci affecting mean telomere length and their association with disease. Nat Genet. 2013;45:422–7.

1843. Armanios M, Blackburn EH. The telomere syndromes. Nat Rev Genet. 2012;13:693–704.

1844. Guarante L. The Franklin H. Epstein lecture: sirtuins, aging, and medicine. N Engl J Med. 2011;364:2235–44.

1845. Cardus A, Uryga AK, Walters G, Erusalimsky JD. SIRT6 protects human endothelial cells from DNA damage, telomere dysfunction, and senescence. Cardiovasc Res. 2013;97:571–9.

1846. Wang JC, Bennett M. Aging and atherosclerosis: mechanisms, functional consequences, and potential therapeutics for cellular senescence. Circ Res. 2012;111:245–59.

1847. Tzanetakou IP, Nzietchueng R, Perrea DN, Benetos A. Telomeres and their role in aging and longevity. Curr Vasc Pharmacol. 2014;12:726–34.

1848. Kovacic JC, Moreno P, Nabel EG, Hachinski V, Fuster V. Cellular senescence, vascular disease, and aging: part 2 of a 2-part review. Circulation. 2011;123:1990–2010.

1849. Fyhrquist F, Saijonmaa O, Strandberg T. The roles of senescence and telomere shortening in cardiovascular disease. Nat Rev Cardiol. 2013;10:274–83.

1850. Nilsson PM, Tufvesson H, Leosdottir M, Melander O. Telomeres and cardiovascular disease risk: an update 2013. Transl Res. 2013;162:371–80.

1851. de Lange T. Shelterin: the protein complex that shapes and safeguards human telomeres. Genes Dev. 2005;19:2001–10.

1852. Blackburn EH, Greider CW, Szostak JW. Telomeres and telomerase: the path from maize, Tetrahymena and yeast to human cancer and aging. Nat Med. 2006;12:1133–8.

1853. Campisi J. Cellular senescence: putting the paradoxes in perspective. Curr Opin Genet Dev. 2011;21:107–12.

1854. von Zglinicki T, Saretzki G, Ladhoff J, d'Adda di Fagagna F, Jackson SP. Human cell senescence as a DNA damage response. Mech Ageing Dev. 2005;126:111–7.

1855. von Zglinicki T. Oxidative stress shortens telomeres. Trends Biochem Sci. 2002;27:339–44.

1856. Jurk D, Wilson C, Passos JF, Oakley F, Correia-Melo C, Greaves L, Saretzki G, Fox C, Lawless C, Anderson R, Hewitt G, Pender SL, Fullard N, Nelson G, Mann J, van de Sluis B, Mann DA, von Zglinicki T. Chronic inflammation induces telomere dysfunction and accelerates ageing in mice. Nat Commun. 2014;2:4172.

1857. Correia-Melo C, Hewitt G, Passos JF. Telomeres, oxidative stress and inflammatory factors: partners in cellular senescence? Longev Healthspan. 2014;3(1):1.

1858. Erusalimsky JD, Kurz DJ. Cellular senescence in vivo: its relevance in ageing and cardiovascular disease. Exp Gerontol. 2005;40:634–42.

1859. Savage SA, Stewart BJ, Eckert A, Kiley M, Liao JS, Channock SJ. Genetic variation, nucleotide diversity, and linkage disequilibrium in seven telomere stability genes suggest that these genes may be under constraint. Hum Mutat. 2005;26:343–50.

1860. Blasco MA. Telomeres and human disease: ageing, cancer and beyond. Nat Rev Genet. 2005;6:611–22.

1861. Kosmadaki MG, Gilchrest BA. The role of telomeres in skin aging/photoaging. Micron. 2004;35:155–9.

1862. de Jesus BB, Schneeberger K, Vera E, Tejera A, Harley CB, Blasco MA. The telomerase activator TA-65 elongates short telomeres and increases health span of adult/old mice without increasing cancer incidence. Aging Cell. 2011;10:604–21.

1863. Kyo S, Takakura M, Kanaya T, Zhuo W, Fujimoto K, Nishio Y, Orimo A, Inoue M. Estrogen activates telomerase. Cancer Res. 1999;59:5917–21.

1864. Valdes AM, Andrew T, Gardner JP, Kimura M, Oelsner E, Cherkas LF, Aviv A, Spector TD. Obesity, cigarette smoking, and telomere length in women. Lancet. 2005;366:662–720.

1865. Strandberg TE, Strandberg AY, Saijonmaa O, Tilvis RS, Pitkälä KH, Fyhrquist F. Association of telomere length in older men with mortality and midlife body mass index and smoking. J Gerontol A Biol Sci Med Sci. 2011;66:815–20.

1866. Gellert C, Schöttker B, Brenner H. Smoking and all-cause mortality in older people: systematic review and meta-analysis. Arch Intern Med. 2012;172:837–44.

1867. Strandberg TE, Strandberg AY, Saijonmaa O, Tilvis RS, Pitkälä KH, Fyhrquist F. Association between alcohol consumption in healthy midlife and telo-

mere length in older men. The Helsinki Businessmen Study. Eur J Epidemiol. 2012;27:815–22.
1868. Müezzinler A, Zaineddin AK, Brenner H. Body mass index and leukocyte telomere length in adults: a systematic review and meta-analysis. Obes Rev. 2014;15:192–201.
1869. Donato AJ, Morgan RG, Walker AE, Lesniewski LA. Cellular and molecular biology of aging endothelial cells. J Mol Cell Cardiol. 2015;89:122–35.
1870. Cherkas LF, Hunkin JL, Kato BS, Richards JB, Gardner JP, Surdulescu GL, Kimura M, Lu X, Spector TD, Aviv A. The association between physical activity in leisure time and leukocyte telomere length. Arch Intern Med. 2008;168:154–8.
1871. Njajou OT, Hsueh WC, Blackburn EH, Newman AB, Wu SH, Li R, Simonsick EM, Harris TM, Cummings SR, Cawthon RM. Association between telomere length, specific causes of death, and years of healthy life in health, aging, and body composition, a population-based cohort study. J Gerontol A Biol Sci Med Sci. 2009;64(8):860–4.
1872. Kennedy BK, et al. Geroscience; linking aging to chronic disease. Cell. 2014;159:709–13.
1873. Epel ES, Blackburn EH, Lin J, Dhabhar FS, Adler NE, Morrow JD, Cawthon RM. Accelerated telomere shortening in response to life stress. Proc Natl Acad Sci U S A. 2004;101:17312–5.
1874. Shalev I, Entringer S, Wadhwa PD, Wolkowitz OM, Puterman E, Lin J, Epel ES. Stress and telomere biology: a lifespan perspective. Psychoneuroendocrinology. 2013;38:1835–42.
1875. Krauss J, Farzaneh-Far R, Puterman E, Na B, Lin J, Epel E, Blackburn E, Whooley MA. Physical fitness and telomere length in patients with coronary heart disease: findings from the heart and soul study. PLoS One. 2011;6:e26983.
1876. Ornish D, Lin J, Daubenmier J, Weidner G, Epel E, Kemp C, Magbanua MJ, Marlin R, Yglecias L, Carroll PR, Blackburn EH. Increased telomerase activity and comprehensive lifestyle changes: a pilot study. Lancet Oncol. 2008;9:1048–57.
1877. Fontana L, Hu FB. Optimal body weight for health and longevity: bridging basic, clinical, and population research. Aging Cell. 2014;14:391–400.
1878. Ornish D, Lin J, Chan JM, Epel E, Kemp C, Weidner G, Marlin R, Frenda SJ, Magbanua MJ, Daubenmier J, Estay I, Hills NK, Chainani-Wu N, Carroll PR, Blackburn EH. Effect of comprehensive lifestyle changes on telomerase activity and telomere length in men with biopsy-proven low-risk prostate cancer: 5-year follow-up of a descriptive pilot study. Lancet Oncol. 2013;14:1112–20.
1879. Rizzuto D, Fratiglioni L. Life style factors related to mortality and survival: a mini-review. Gerontology. 2014;60:327–35.
1880. Werner C, Fürster T, Widmann T, Pöss J, Roggia C, Hanhoun M, Scharhag J, Büchner N, Meyer T, Kindermann W, Haendeler J, Böhm M, Laufs U. Physical exercise prevents cellular senescence in circulating leukocytes and in the vessel wall. Circulation. 2009;120:2438–47.
1881. Richards BJ, Valdes AM, Gardner JP, Paximadas D, Kimura M, Nessa A, Lu X, Surdulescu GL, Swaminathan R, Spector TD, Aviv A. Higher vitamin D concentrations are associated with longer leukocyte telomere length in women. Am J Clin Nutr. 2007;86:1420–5.
1882. Xu Q, Parks CG, DeRoo LA, Cawthon RM, Sandler DP, Chen H. Multivitamin use and telomere length in women. Am J Clin Nutr. 2009;89:1857–63.
1883. Sen A, Marsche G, Freudenberger P, Schallert M, Toeglhofer AM, Nagl C, Schmidt R, Launer LJ, Schmidt H. Association between higher plasma lutein, zeaxanthin, and vitamin C concentrations and longer telomere length: results of the Austrian Stroke Prevention Study. J Am Geriatr Soc. 2014;62(2):222–9.
1884. Farzaneh-Far R, Lin J, Epel ES, Harris WS, Blackburn EH, Whooley MA. Association of marine omega-3 fatty acid levels with telomeric aging in patients with coronary heart disease. JAMA. 2010;303:250–7.
1885. Paul L. Diet, nutrition and telomere length. J Nutr Biochem. 2011;20:895–901.
1886. Boccardi V, Esposito A, Rizzo MR, Marfella R, Barbieri M, Polisso G. Mediterranean diet, telomere maintenance and health status among elderly. PLoS One. 2013;8:1–6.
1887. Crous-Bou M, Fung TF, Prescott J, Julin B, Du M, Sun Q, Rexrode KM, Hu FB, De Vivo I. Mediterranean diet and telomere length in Nurses' health study: population based cohort study. BMJ. 2014;349:6674.
1888. Saliques S, Teyssier J-R, Vergely C, Lorgis L, Lorin J. Circulating leukocyte telomere length and oxidative stress: a new target for statin therapy. Atherosclerosis. 2011;219:753–60.
1889. Rode L, Nordestgaard BG, Bojesen SE. Peripheral blood leukocyte telomere length and mortality among 64 637 individuals from the general population. J Natl Cancer Inst. 2015;107(6):107.
1890. Guarante L. The Franklin H. Epstein lecture: sirtuins, aging, and medicine. N Engl J Med. 2011;364:2235–44.
1891. Armanios M, Alder JK, Parry EM, Karim B, Strong MA, Greider CW. Short telomeres are sufficient to cause the degenerative defects associated with aging. Am J Hum Genet. 2009;85(6):823–32.
1892. Shimamoto A, Koutaro Y, Tahara H. Werner-syndrome-specific induced pluripotent stem cells: recovery of telomere function by reprogramming. Front Genet. 2015.
1893. Roake CM, Artandi SE. Control of cellular aging, tissue function, and cancer by p53 downstream of telomeres. Cold Spring Harb Perspect Med. 2017;7(5):a026088. https://doi.org/10.1101/cshperspect.a026088.
1894. Bär C, Blasco MA. Telomeres and telomerase as therapeutic targets to prevent and treat age-related

diseases. F1000Research. 2016;5:F1000 Faculty Rev-89. https://doi.org/10.12688/f1000research.7020.1.
1895. López-Otín C, Blasco MA, Partridge L, et al. The hallmarks of aging. Cell. 2013;153(6):1194–217. https://doi.org/10.1016/j.cell.2013.05.039.
1896. Collado M, Blasco MA, Serrano M. Cellular senescence in cancer and aging. Cell. 2007;130(2):223–33. https://doi.org/10.1016/j.cell.2007.07.003.
1897. Muñoz-Espín D, Serrano M. Cellular senescence: from physiology to pathology. Nat Rev Mol Cell Biol. 2014;15(7):482–96. https://doi.org/10.1038/nrm3823.
1898. Flores I, Cayuela ML, Blasco MA. Effects of telomerase and telomere length on epidermal stem cell behavior. Science. 2005;309(5738):1253–6. https://doi.org/10.1126/science.1115025.
1899. Sharpless NE, DePinho RA. How stem cells age and why this makes us grow old. Nat Rev Mol Cell Biol. 2007;8(9):703–13. https://doi.org/10.1038/nrm2241.
1900. Calado RT, Young NS. Telomere diseases. N Engl J Med. 2009;361(24):2353–65. https://doi.org/10.1056/NEJMra0903373.
1901. Armanios M, Blackburn EH. The telomere syndromes. Nat Rev Genet. 2012;13(10):693–704. https://doi.org/10.1038/nrg3246.
1902. Holohan B, Wright WE, Shay JW. Cell biology of disease: telomeropathies: an emerging spectrum disorder. J Cell Biol. 2014;205(3):289–99. https://doi.org/10.1083/jcb.201401012.
1903. Townsley DM, Dumitriu B, Young NS. Bone marrow failure and the telomeropathies. Blood. 2014;124(18):2775–83. https://doi.org/10.1182/blood-2014-05-526285.
1904. Counter CM, Avilion AA, LeFeuvre CE, et al. Telomere shortening associated with chromosome instability is arrested in immortal cells which express telomerase activity. EMBO J. 1992;11(5):1921–9.
1905. Chin L, Artandi SE, Shen Q, et al. p53 deficiency rescues the adverse effects of telomere loss and cooperates with telomere dysfunction to accelerate carcinogenesis. Cell. 1999;97(4):527–38. https://doi.org/10.1016/S0092-8674(00)80762-X.
1906. Sahin E, Colla S, Liesa M, et al. Telomere dysfunction induces metabolic and mitochondrial compromise. Nature. 2011;470(7334):359–65. https://doi.org/10.1038/nature09787.
1907. Slagboom PE, Droog S, Boomsma DI. Genetic determination of telomere size in humans: a twin study of three age groups. Am J Hum Genet. 1994;55(5):876–82.
1908. Canela A, Klatt P, Blasco MA. Telomere length analysis. Methods Mol Biol. 2007;371:45–72. https://doi.org/10.1007/978-1-59745-361-5_5.
1909. von Zglinicki T. Oxidative stress shortens telomeres. Trends Biochem Sci. 2002;27(7):339–44. https://doi.org/10.1016/S0968-0004(02)02110-2.
1910. Valdes AM, Andrew T, Gardner JP, et al. Obesity, cigarette smoking, and telomere length in women. Lancet. 2005;366(9486):662–4. https://doi.org/10.1016/S0140-6736(05)66630-5.
1911. Strandberg TE, Saijonmaa O, Tilvis RS, et al. Association of telomere length in older men with mortality and midlife body mass index and smoking. J Gerontol A Biol Sci Med Sci. 2011;66(7):815–20. https://doi.org/10.1093/gerona/glr064.
1912. Verde Z, Reinoso-Barbero L, Chicharro L, et al. Effects of cigarette smoking and nicotine metabolite ratio on leukocyte telomere length. Environ Res. 2015;140:488–94. https://doi.org/10.1016/j.envres.2015.05.008.
1913. Révész D, Milaneschi Y, Verhoeven JE, et al. Longitudinal associations between metabolic syndrome components and telomere shortening. J Clin Endocrinol Metab. 2015;100(8):3050–9. https://doi.org/10.1210/JC.2015-1995.
1914. Strandberg TE, Strandberg AY, Saijonmaa O, et al. Association between alcohol consumption in healthy midlife and telomere length in older men. The Helsinki Businessmen Study. Eur J Epidemiol. 2012;27(10):815–22. https://doi.org/10.1007/s10654-012-9728-0.
1915. Müezzinler A, Mons U, Dieffenbach AK, et al. Smoking habits and leukocyte telomere length dynamics among older adults: results from the ESTHER cohort. Exp Gerontol. 2015;70:18–25. https://doi.org/10.1016/j.exger.2015.07.002.
1916. Wolkowitz OM, Mellon SH, Epel ES, et al. Leukocyte telomere length in major depression: correlations with chronicity, inflammation and oxidative stress – preliminary findings. PLoS One. 2011;6(3):e17837. https://doi.org/10.1371/journal.pone.0017837.
1917. Karabatsiakis A, Kolassa IT, Kolassa S, et al. Telomere shortening in leukocyte subpopulations in depression. BMC Psychiatry. 2014;14:192. https://doi.org/10.1186/1471-244X-14-192.
1918. O'Donovan A, Epel E, Lin J, et al. Childhood trauma associated with short leukocyte telomere length in posttraumatic stress disorder. Biol Psychiatry. 2011;70(5):465–71. https://doi.org/10.1016/j.biopsych.2011.01.035.
1919. Lin J, Epel E, Blackburn E. Telomeres and lifestyle factors: roles in cellular aging. Mutat Res. 2012;730(1–2):85–9. https://doi.org/10.1016/j.mrfmmm.2011.08.003.
1920. Kinser PA, Lyon DE. Major depressive disorder and measures of cellular aging: an integrative review. Nurs Res Pract. 2013;2013:469070. https://doi.org/10.1155/2013/469070.
1921. Lindqvist D, Epel ES, Mellon SH, et al. Psychiatric disorders and leukocyte telomere length: underlying mechanisms linking mental illness with cellular aging. Neurosci Biobehav Rev. 2015;55:333–64. https://doi.org/10.1016/j.neubiorev.2015.05.007.
1922. Simon NM, Smoller JW, McNamara KL, et al. Telomere shortening and mood disorders: preliminary support for a chronic stress model of accel-

erated aging. Biol Psychiatry. 2006;60(5):432–5. https://doi.org/10.1016/j.biopsych.2006.02.004.
1923. Elvsåshagen T, Vera E, Bøen E, et al. The load of short telomeres is increased and associated with lifetime number of depressive episodes in bipolar II disorder. J Affect Disord. 2011;135(1–3):43–50. https://doi.org/10.1016/j.jad.2011.08.006.
1924. Canela A, Vera E, Klatt P, et al. High-throughput telomere length quantification by FISH and its application to human population studies. Proc Natl Acad Sci U S A. 2007;104(13):5300–5. https://doi.org/10.1073/pnas.0609367104.
1925. De Jesus BB, Blasco MA. Telomerase at the intersection of cancer and aging. Trends Genet. 2013;29(9):513–20. https://doi.org/10.1016/j.tig.2013.06.007.
1926. Kovacic JC, Moreno P, Hachinski V, et al. Cellular senescence, vascular disease, and aging: part 1 of a 2-part review. Circulation. 2011;123:1650–60.
1927. Sanders JL, Newman AB. Telomere length in epidemiology: a biomarker of aging, age-related disease, both, or neither? Epidemiol Rev. 2013;35:112–31.
1928. D'Mello MJ, Ross SA, Briel M, et al. Association between shortened leukocyte telomere length and cardiometabolic outcomes: systematic review and meta-analysis. Circ Cardiovasc Genet. 2015;8:82–90.
1929. Haycock PC, Heydon EE, Kaptoge S, et al. Leucocyte telomere length and risk of cardiovascular disease: systematic review and meta-analysis. BMJ. 2014;349:g4227.
1930. Fernández-Alvira JM, Fuster V, Dorado B, Soberón N, Flores I, Gallardo M, Pocock S, Blasco MA, Andrés V. Short telomere load, telomere length, and subclinical atherosclerosis. J Am Coll Cardiol. 2016;67(21):2467–76. https://doi.org/10.1016/j.jacc.2016.03.530.
1931. Rietzschel ER, Bekaert S, De Meyer T. Telomeres and atherosclerosis: the attrition of an attractive hypothesis. J Am Coll Cardiol. 2016;67(21):2477–9. https://doi.org/10.1016/j.jacc.2016.03.541.
1932. Slagboom PE, Droog S, Boomsma DI. Genetic determination of telomere size in humans: a twin study of three age groups. Am J Hum Genet. 1994;55(5):876–82.
1933. Bischoff C, Graakjaer J, Petersen HC, et al. The heritability of telomere length among the elderly and oldest-old. Twin Res Hum Genet. 2005;8(5):433–9. https://doi.org/10.1375/183242705774310141.
1934. Andrew T, Aviv A, Falchi M, et al. Mapping genetic loci that determine leukocyte telomere length in a large sample of unselected female sibling pairs. Am J Hum Genet. 2006;78(3):480–6. https://doi.org/10.1086/500052.
1935. Broer L, Codd V, Nyholt DR, et al. Meta-analysis of telomere length in 19,713 subjects reveals high heritability, stronger maternal inheritance and a paternal age effect. Eur J Hum Genet. 2013;21(10):1163–8. https://doi.org/10.1038/ejhg.2012.303.
1936. von Zglinicki T. Oxidative stress shortens telomeres. Trends Biochem Sci. 2002;27(7):339–44. https://doi.org/10.1016/S0968-0004(02)02110-2.
1937. Farzaneh-Far R, Lin J, Epel ES, et al. Association of marine omega-3 fatty acid levels with telomeric aging in patients with coronary heart disease. JAMA. 2010;303(3):250–7. https://doi.org/10.1001/jama.2009.2008.
1938. Werner C, Fürster T, Widmann T, et al. Physical exercise prevents cellular senescence in circulating leukocytes and in the vessel wall. Circulation. 2009;120(24):2438–47. https://doi.org/10.1161/CIRCULATIONAHA.109.861005.
1939. Song Z, von Figura G, Liu Y, et al. Lifestyle impacts on the aging-associated expression of biomarkers of DNA damage and telomere dysfunction in human blood. Aging Cell. 2010;9(4):607–15. https://doi.org/10.1111/j.1474-9726.2010.00583.x.
1940. Soares-Miranda L, Imamura F, Siscovick D, et al. Physical activity, physical fitness, and leukocyte telomere length: the Cardiovascular Health Study. Med Sci Sports Exerc. 2015;47(12):2525–34. https://doi.org/10.1249/MSS.0000000000000720.
1941. Polhemus DJ, Trivedi RK, Gao J, Li Z, Scarborough AL, Goodchild TT, Varner KJ, Xia H, Smart FW, Kapusta DR, Lefer DJ. Renal sympathetic denervation protects the failing heart via inhibition of neprilysin activity in the kidney. J Am Coll Cardiol. 2017;70(17):2139–53. https://doi.org/10.1016/j.jacc.2017.08.056.
1942. Fillingame RH, Angevine CM, Dmitriev OY. Coupling proton movements to c-ring rotation in F(1)F(o) ATP synthase: aqueous access channels and helix rotations at the a-c interface. Biochim Biophys Acta. 2002;1555(1–3):29–36.
1943. Kennedy DO. B vitamins and the brain: mechanisms, dose and efficacy – a review. Nutrients. 2016;8(2):68. https://doi.org/10.3390/nu8020068.
1944. Rodella LF, Favero G. Atherosclerosis and current anti-oxidant strategies for atheroprotection. Curr Trends Atherogenesis. 2012 (InTech, Open Access). https://doi.org/10.5772/53035.
1945. Ross R. Atherosclerosis – an inflammatory disease. N Engl J Med. 1999;340:115.
1946. Greenland P, Gidding SS, Tracy RP. Commentary: lifelong prevention of atherosclerosis: the critical importance of major risk factor exposures. Int J Epidemiol. 2002;31:1129–34. https://doi.org/10.1093/ije/31.6.1129.
1947. Caro P, Gomez J, Lopez-Torres M, Sanchez I, Naudiand A, et al. Effect of every other day feeding on mitochondrial free radical production and oxidative stress in mouse liver. Rejuvenation Res. 2008;11:621–9.
1948. Seals DR, Edward F. Adolph distinguished lecture: the remarkable anti-aging effects of aerobic exercise on systemic arteries. J Appl Physiol. 2014;117(5):425–39. https://doi.org/10.1152/japplphysiol.00362.2014.

1949. Betteridge DJ. The case for intensive lipid management: The opportunities and issues for cardiologists. PACE-CME Lecture. 2011. https://pace-cme.org/2011/06/16/the-case-for-intensive-lipid-management-the-opportunities-and-issues-for-cardiologists/
1950. Freire MO, Van Dyke TE. Natural resolution of inflammation. Periodontol 2000. 2013;63(1):149–64. https://doi.org/10.1111/prd.12034.
1951. Mozaffarian D, Wu JHY. Omega-3 fatty acids and cardiovascular disease: effects on risk factors, molecular pathways, and clinical events. J Am Coll Cardiol. 2011;58(20):2047–67. https://doi.org/10.1016/j.jacc.2011.06.063.
1952. Harris WS, Mozaffarian D, Lefevre M, et al. Towards establishing dietary reference intakes for eicosapentaenoic and docosahexaenoic acids. J Nutr. 2009;139(4):804S–19S. https://doi.org/10.3945/jn.108.101329.
1953. Giudetti AM, Cagnazzo R. Beneficial effects of n-3 PUFA on chronic airway inflammatory diseases. Prostaglandins Other Lipid Mediat. 2012;99(3–4):57–67. https://doi.org/10.1016/j.prostaglandins.2012.09.006.
1954. Calder PC. Fatty acids and inflammation: The cutting edge between food and pharma. Eur J Pharmacol. 2011;668(Supplement 1):S50–8.
1955. Quarles RH, Macklin WB, Morell P. Myelin formation, structure and biochemistry. In: Basic neurochemistry: molecular, cellular, and medical aspects. Siegel: Elsevier, Inc; 2006.
1956. Michael-Titus AT, et al. Omega-3 fatty acids and traumatic neurological injury: from neuroprotection to neuroplasticity? Trends Neurosci. 2014;37(1):30–8. https://doi.org/10.1016/j.tins.2013.10.005. Epub 2013 Nov 22.
1957. Ashraf MZ, Srivastava S. Oxidized phospholipids: introduction and biological significance. In: Kostner G, editor. Lipoproteins; 2012. https://doi.org/10.5772/50461.
1958. Predonzani A, Calì B, Agnellini AH, Molon B. Spotlights on immunological effects of reactive nitrogen species: when inflammation says nitric oxide. World J Exp Med. 2015;5(2):64–76. https://doi.org/10.5493/wjem.v5.i2.64. eCollection 2015 May 20.
1959. Rapozzi V, Della Pietra E, Bonavida B. Dual roles of nitric oxide in the regulation of tumor cell response and resistance to photodynamic therapy. Redox Biol. 2015;6:311–7. https://doi.org/10.1016/j.redox.2015.07.015. Epub 2015 Jul 31. Review.
1960. Emanuele MA, Wezeman F, Emanuele NV. Alcohol's effect on female reproductive function. Alcohol Res Health. 2002;26(4):274–81. National Institute on Alcohol Abuse and Alcoholism (NIAAA). June, 2003. https://pubs.niaaa.nih.gov/publications/arh26-4/274-281.htm
1961. Erez A. Arginosuccinate acidura: from monogenic to a complex disorder. Genet Med. 2013;15:251–7. https://doi.org/10.1038/gim.2012.166. Epub 2013 Jan 10.
1962. Kelm M. Nitric oxide metabolism and breakdown. BBA. 1999;1411:273–89. https://doi.org/10.1016/S0005-2728(99)00020-1.
1963. Tiso M, Schechter AN. Nitrate reduction to nitrite, nitric oxide and ammonia by gut bacteria under physiological conditions. PLoS One. 2015;10(3):e0119712. https://doi.org/10.1371/journal.one.0119712.
1964. Lai WK, Kan MY. Homocysteine-induced endothelial dysfunction. Ann Nutr Metab. 2015;67:1–12. https://doi.org/10.1159/000437098.
1965. Leiva E, Wehinger S, Guzmán L, Orrego R. Role of oxidized LDL in atherosclerosis. In: Kumar SA, editor. Hypercholesterolemia; 2015. https://doi.org/10.5772/59375.
1966. Frostegard J, Haegerstrand A, Gidlund M, Nilsson J. Biologically modified LDL increases the adhesive properties of endothelial cells. Atherosclerosis. 1991;90:119–26.
1967. Rajavashisth TB, Andalibi A, Territo MC, Berliner JA, Navab M, Fogelman AM, Lusis AJ. Induction of endothelial cell expression of granulocyte and macrophage colony-stimulating factors by modified low-density lipoproteins. Nature. 1990;344:254–7.
1968. Yla-Herttuala S, Lipton BA, Rosenfeld ME, Sarkioja T, Yoshimura T, Leonard EJ, Witztum JL, Steinberg D. Expression of monocyte chemoattractant protein 1 in macrophage-rich areas of human and rabbit atherosclerotic lesions. Proc Natl Acad Sci U S A. 1991;88:5252–6.
1969. Catapano AL, Maggi FM, Tragni E. Low density lipoprotein oxidation, antioxidants, and atherosclerosis. Curr Opin Cardiol. 2000;15:355–63.
1970. Quinn MT, Parthasarathy S, Fong LG, Steinberg D. Oxidatively modified low density lipoproteins: a potential role in recruitment and retention of monocyte/macrophages during atherogenesis. Proc Natl Acad Sci U S A. 1987;84:2995–8.
1971. Forstermann U, Sessa WC. Nitric oxide synthases: regulation and function. Eur Heart J. 2012;33:829–37, 837a–837d.
1972. Blair A, Shaul PW, Yuhanna IS, Conrad PA, Smart EJ. Oxidized low density lipoprotein displaces endothelial nitric-oxide synthase (eNOS) from plasmalemmal caveolae and impairs eNOS activation. J Biol Chem. 1999;274:32512–9.
1973. Cominacini L, Rigoni A, Pasini AF, Garbin U, Davoli A, Campagnola M, Pastorino AM, Lo Cascio V, Sawamura T. The binding of oxidized low density lipoprotein (ox-LDL) to ox-LDL receptor-1 reduces the intracellular concentration of nitric oxide in endothelial cells through an increased production of superoxide. J Biol Chem. 2001;276:13750–5.
1974. Chen M, Masaki T, Sawamura T. LOX-1, the receptor for oxidized low-density lipoprotein identified

from endothelial cells: implications in endothelial dysfunction and atherosclerosis. Pharmacol Ther. 2002;95:89–100.
1975. Kataoka H, Kume N, Miyamoto S, Minami M, Moriwaki H, Murase T, Sawamura T, Masaki T, Hashimoto N, Kita T. Expression of lectinlike oxidized lowdensity lipoprotein receptor-1 in human atherosclerotic lesions. Circulation. 1999;99:3110–7. Role of Oxidized LDL in Atherosclerosis. https://doi.org/10.5772/5937573.
1976. Li D, Mehta JL. Antisense to LOX-1 inhibits oxidized LDL-mediated upregulation of monocyte chemoattractant protein-1 and monocyte adhesion to human coronary artery endothelial cells. Circulation. 2000;101:2889–95.
1977. Li D, Chen H, Romeo F, Sawamura T, Saldeen T, Mehta JL. Statins modulate oxidized low-density lipoprotein-mediated adhesion molecule expression in human coronary artery endothelial cells: role of LOX-1. J Pharmacol Exp Ther. 2002;302:601–5.
1978. Cominacini L, Fratta Pasini A, Garbin U, Pastorino A, Rigoni A, Nava C, Davoli A, Lo Cascio V, Sawamura T. The platelet-endothelium interaction mediated by lectin-like oxidized low-density lipoprotein receptor-1 reduces the intracellular concentration of nitric oxide in endothelial cells. J Am Coll Cardiol. 2003;41:499–507.
1979. Valente AJ, Irimpen AM, Siebenlist U, Chandrasekar B. OxLDL induces endothelial dysfunction and death via TRAF3IP2: inhibition by HDL3 and AMPK activators. Free Radic Biol Med. 2014;70C:117–28.
1980. Rosen P, Nawroth PP, King G, Möller W, Tritschler H-J, Packer L. The role of oxidative stress in the onset and progression of diabetes and its complications: a summary of a Congress Series sponsored by UNESCO-MCBN, the American Diabetes Association and the German Diabetes Society. Diabetes Metab Res Rev. 2001;17(3):189–209. https://doi.org/10.1002/dmrr.196.
1981. Rocha VZ, Libby P. Obesity, inflammation, and atherosclerosis. Nat Rev Cardiol. 2009;6(6):399–409. https://doi.org/10.1038/nrcardio.2009.55. Epub 2009 Apr 28. Review.
1982. Zuo L, Chuang CC, Hemmelgarn BT, Best TM. Heart failure with preserved ejection fraction: defining the function of ROS and NO. J Appl Physiol. 2015;119(8):944–51. https://doi.org/10.1152/japplphysiol.01149.2014.
1983. Yuste JE, Tarragon E, Campuzano CM, Ros-Bernal F. Implications of glial nitric oxide in neurodegenerative diseases. Front Cell Neurosci. 2015;9:322. https://doi.org/10.3389/fncel.2015.00322. eCollection 2015. Review.
1984. Mion G, Villevieille T. Ketamine pharmacology: an update (pharmacodynamics and molecular aspects, recent findings). CNS Neurosci Ther. 2013;19(6):370–80. https://doi.org/10.1111/cns.12099. Epub 2013 Apr 10.
1985. Chen Y, Liu L. Modern methods for delivery of drugs across the blood-brain barrier. Adv Drug Deliv Rev. 2012;64(7):640–65. https://doi.org/10.1016/j.addr.2011.11.010. Epub 2011 Nov 28.
1986. Witcher KG, Eiferman DS, Godbout JP. Priming the inflammatory pump of the CNS after traumatic brain injury. Trends Neurosci. 2015;38(10):609–20. https://doi.org/10.1016/j.tins.2015.08.002. Review.
1987. Kroemer G, Galluzzi L, Brenner C. Mitochondrial membrane permeabilization in cell death. Physiol Rev. 2007;87(1):99–163. Review. https://doi.org/10.1152/physrev.00013.2006.
1988. Li R, Jia Z, Trush MA. Defining ROS in biology and medicine. Reactive oxygen species (Apex, NC). 2016;1(1):9–21. https://doi.org/10.20455/ros.2016.803.
1989. Kelly FJ. Oxidative stress: its role in air pollution and adverse health effects. Occup Environ Med. 2003;60:612–6. https://doi.org/10.1136/oem.60.8.612.
1990. Garrido N, Meseguer M, Simon C, Pellicer A, Remohi J. Pro-oxidative and anti-oxidative imbalance in human semen and its relation with male fertility. Asian J Androl. 2004;6(1):59–65.
1991. Kar SK, Choudhury I. An empirical review on oxidative stress markers and their relevance in obsessive-compulsive disorder. Int J Nutr Pharmacol Neurol Dis. 2016;6:139–45.
1992. Nisar A, Mamat AS, Hatim MI, Aslam MS, Muhammad MS. Identification of flavonoids (quercetin, gallic acid and rutin) from catharanthus roseus plant parts using deep eutectic solvent. Recent Adv Biol Med. 2017;3:1–6. https://doi.org/10.18639/RABM.2016.02.347628.
1993. Pillon NJ, Soulage CO. Chapter 19: lipid peroxidation by-products and the metabolic syndrome. In: Catala A, editor. Lipid peroxidation; 2012. https://doi.org/10.5772/46019
1994. Noble A, Johnson R, Thomas A, Bass P. Arterial blood pressure. In: The cardiovascular system, systems of the body series. 2nd ed. Edinburgh: Elsevier; 2010.
1995. Konturek SJ, Konturek PC, Brzozowski T, Bubenik GA. Role of melatonin in upper gastrointestinal tract. J Physiol Pharmacol. 2007;58(Suppl 6):23–52. Review.
1996. Varga ZV, Giricz Z, Liaudet L, Haskó G, Ferdinandy P, Pacher P. Interplay of oxidative, nitrosative/nitrative stress, inflammation, cell death and autophagy in diabetic cardiomyopathy. Biochim Biophys Acta Mol basis Dis. 2015;1852(2):232–42. https://doi.org/10.1016/j.bbadis.2014.06.030.
1997. Klabunde RE. Adrenergic and cholinergic receptors in the heart. http://www.cvphysiology.com/Blood%20Pressure/BP010
1998. Bhatia LS, Curzen NP. Non-alcoholic fatty liver disease: a new and important cardiovascular risk factor? Eur Heart J. 2012;33(10):1190–200. https://doi.org/10.1093/eurheartj/ehr453. Epub 2012 Mar 8.

1999. Maintz L, Novak N. Histamine and histamine intolerance. Am J Clin Nutr. 2007;85(5):1185–96. https://doi.org/10.1093/ajcn/85.5.1185.

2000. Calabriso N, Massaro M, Scoditti E, D'Amore S, Gnoni A, Pellegrino M, Storelli C, De Caterina R, Palasciano G, Carluccio MA. Extra virgin olive oil rich in polyphenols modulates VEGF-induced angiogenic responses by preventing NADPH oxidase activity and expression. J Nutr Biochem. 2016;28:19–29. https://doi.org/10.1016/j.jnutbio.2015.09.026.

2001. Kitada M, Koya D. Renal protective effects of resveratrol. Oxid Med Cell Longev. 2013;2013, Article ID 568093, 7 pages. https://doi.org/10.1155/2013/568093.

2002. Price NL, et al. SIRT1 is required for AMPK activation and the beneficial effects of resveratrol on mitochondrial function. Cell Metab. 2012;15(5):675–90. https://doi.org/10.1016/j.cmet.2012.04.003.

2003. Hong Y. Sympathovagal imbalance in type 2 diabetes – role of brainstem thyrotropin-releasing hormone. In: Masuo K, editor. Type 2 diabetes. IntechOpen. https://doi.org/10.5772/56541.

2004. Miller AH, Maletic V, Raison CL. Inflammation and its discontents: the role of cytokines in the pathophysiology of major depression. Biol Psychiatry. 2009;65:732–41. https://doi.org/10.1016/j.biopsych.2008.11.029. (p737).

2005. Even N, Devaud JM, Barron A. General stress responses in the honey bee. Insects. 2012;3:1271–98. https://doi.org/10.3390/insects3041271.

2006. Saladin K. Chapter 15: the autonomic nervous and visceral reflexes. In: Anatomy. New York: The McGraw-Hill; 2004.

2007. Sundman E, Olofsson PS. Neural control of the immune system. Adv Physiol Educ. 2014;38:135–9. https://doi.org/10.1152/advan.00094.2013.

2008. Cohen BH, Gold DR. Mitochondrial cytopathy in adults: what we know so far. Cleve Clin J Med. 2001;68(7):625–42.

2009. Finkelman BS, Putt M, Wang T, Wang L, Narayan H, Domchek S, DeMichele A, Fox K, Matro J, Shah P, Clark A, Bradbury A, Narayan V, Carver JR, Tang WHW, Ky B. Arginine-nitric oxide metabolites and cardiac dysfunction in patients with breast cancer. J Am Coll Cardiol. 2017;70(2):152–62. https://doi.org/10.1016/j.jacc.2017.05.019. Erratum in: J Am Coll Cardiol. 2017 Nov 28;70(21):2738.

2010. Chrysostomou A, Turnbull DM. Mitochondria, the synapse, and neurodegeneration. In: Reeve A, Simcox E, Duchen M, Turnbull D, editors. Mitochondrial dysfunction in neurodegenerative disorders. https://doi.org/10.1007/978-3-319-28637-2_9.

2011. Bhatt DL, Steg PG, Miller M, Brinton EA, Jacobson TA, Ketchum SB, Doyle RT Jr, Juliano RA, Jiao L, Granowitz C, Tardif JC, Ballantyne CM; REDUCE-IT Investigators. Cardiovascular risk reduction with icosapent ethyl for hypertriglyceridemia. N Engl J Med. 2018. https://doi.org/10.1056/NEJMoa1812792. [Epub ahead of print].

# Index




N. L. DePace, J. Colombo, *Clinical Autonomic and Mitochondrial Disorders*,
https://doi.org/10.1007/978-3-030-17016-5

Printed by Printforce, the Netherlands